This book is due for return on or before the last date shown below.

Caffey's Pediatric Diagnostic Imaging

EDITOR-IN-CHIEF

Brian D. Coley, MD

Professor
Departments of Radiology and Pediatrics
University of Cincinnati College of Medicine
Radiologist-in-Chief
Department of Radiology
Cincinnati Children's Hospital Medical Center
Cincinnati, Ohio

Caffey's Pediatric Diagnostic Imaging

Twelfth Edition

VOLUME II

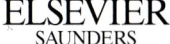

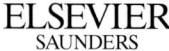

ELSEVIER
SAUNDERS

1600 John F. Kennedy Blvd.
Ste 1800
Philadelphia, PA 19103-2899

CAFFEY'S PEDIATRIC DIAGNOSTIC IMAGING   ISBN: 978-0-323-08176-4

Notices

Knowledge and best practice in this field are constantly changing. As new research and experience
broaden our understanding, changes in research methods, professional practices, or medical treatment
may become necessary.

Practitioners and researchers must always rely on their own experience and knowledge in evaluating
and using any information, methods, compounds, or experiments described herein. In using such
information or methods they should be mindful of their own safety and the safety of others, including
parties for whom they have a professional responsibility.

With respect to any drug or pharmaceutical products identified, readers are advised to check the most
current information provided (i) on procedures featured or (ii) by the manufacturer of each product to
be administered, to verify the recommended dose or formula, the method and duration of
administration, and contraindications. It is the responsibility of practitioners, relying on their own
experience and knowledge of their patients, to make diagnoses, to determine dosages and the best
treatment for each individual patient, and to take all appropriate safety precautions.

To the fullest extent of the law, neither the Publisher nor the authors, contributors, or editors, assume
any liability for any injury and/or damage to persons or property as a matter of products liability,
negligence or otherwise, or from any use or operation of any methods, products, instructions, or ideas
contained in the material herein.

Senior Content Strategist: Don Scholz
Content Development Manager: Maureen Iannuzzi
Publishing Services Manager: Patricia Tannian
Project Manager: Carrie Stetz
Design Direction: Ellen Zanolle

Printed in China

Last digit is the print number: 9   8   7   6   5   4   3   2   1

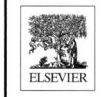

To my family:
Elizabeth, Ian, Connor, and Kate;

To my teachers:
Gordon, Rosengard, Halasz, Mattrey, Olson,
Talner, Leopold, Forrest, Shultz, Patterson, Johnson,
Babcock, Siegel, Slovis, and others;

To my students, residents, and fellows
whom I have been privileged to teach;

To my many brilliant colleagues
who have taught and guided me;

And to the children whom I hope
to have played some role in helping:

Thank you all.

Tribute to Drs. John P. Caffey, Frederic N. Silverman, and Thomas L. Slovis

Caffey's Pediatric Diagnostic Imaging (titled *Caffey's Pediatric X-Ray Diagnosis* for the first nine editions) is the oldest continuous comprehensive textbook in this subspecialty. First published in 1945, it was the first English language text on the subject since Thomas Morgan Rotch's 1910 *The Roentgen Ray in Pediatrics*.

This book began as a labor of love for John Caffey in an era without computers, digital images, or internet bibliographic searches. Each chapter was meticulously dictated, typed, corrected, and typed again. Each radiograph was carefully selected from Dr. Caffey's own teaching file at Babies Hospital in New York City. Dr. Caffey, initially trained as a pediatrician, was an astute clinician who stressed that the radiographic findings were only one part of the diagnostic evaluation; proper patient care required the integration of the history, physical examination, laboratory data, and imaging. Despite the great effort involved, he was the sole author of the first four editions.

With the 1967 fifth edition, former Caffey fellow Dr. Frederic N. Silverman of Children's Hospital Cincinnati participated in preparation of the text, and continued as a co-editor of the sixth and seventh editions. With the death of Dr. Caffey in 1978, Dr. Silverman became sole editor of the eighth edition in 1985. Also trained as a pediatrician, he, too, stressed the importance of the physical examination and the need for accurate clinical information to properly interpret imaging studies.

Over time, Dr. Silverman added authors and expanded sections. Due to the increasing amount of information, he edited a one-volume *Essentials of Caffey's Pediatric X-Ray Diagnosis* in 1989 aimed at trainees, which was my first exposure to this text. Dr. Jerald P. Kuhn joined Silverman as co-editor with the 1993 ninth edition, and then succeeded him as editor. For the 2003 tenth edition, Dr. Kuhn added Drs. Jack O. Haller and Thomas L. Slovis as co-editors, two important figures in pediatric radiology education. Dr. Slovis (also originally trained as a pediatrician) lead the production of the eleventh edition, which was a significant modernization of the text and figures. This addition had eight associate editors overseeing subsections of the text, reflecting the growing complexity and expertise required in delivering pediatric imaging care.

In an era when information is so readily obtainable, it is easy to forget the importance books such as Caffey's have played in education and training. For decades, this was the definitive source of pediatric imaging information, crafted by experts in the field who brought their understanding of the literature and practical experience to the interested reader. Caffey and Silverman devoted more than half of their lives to creating the best book possible in an era when the work was done with typewriters, carbon paper, film, and darkrooms. That this book has survived is testimony to the quality of their work. Dr. Slovis continued that care and attention to detail to reflect the modernization of pediatric imaging, while at the same time continuing to stress the importance of the physical examination and keeping the child at the center of our focus. The impact of Caffey, Silverman, and Slovis on the education of prior generations of pediatric imagers cannot be underestimated and is certain to continue far into the future.

Brian D. Coley
Editor, twelfth edition
2013

Contributors

Sami Abedin, MD Department of Radiology, University of Missouri–Kansas City, Kansas City, Missouri

Brent Adler, MD Associate Clinical Professor, Department of Radiology, The Ohio State University, Nationwide Children's Hospital, Columbus, Ohio

Prachi P. Agarwal, MD Clinical Associate Professor, Department of Radiology, Division of Cardiothoracic Radiology, University of Michigan, Ann Arbor, Michigan

Kimberly E. Applegate, MD Professor of Radiology and Pediatrics, Director of Practice Quality Improvement, Department of Radiology and Imaging Sciences, Emory University School of Medicine, Atlanta, Georgia

E. Michel Azouz, MD Pediatric Radiologist, Medical Imaging, Montreal Children's Hospital; Pediatric Radiologist, Shriners Hospital for Children, Montreal, QC, Canada

Paul Babyn, MDCM Radiologist-in-Chief, Hospital for Sick Children, Toronto, ON, Canada; Head of University of Saskatchewan and Saskatoon, Health Region, Royal University Hospital; Professor of Medical Imaging, University of Saskatchewan, Canada

D. Gregory Bates, MD Clinical Associate Professor of Radiology, Ohio State University College of Medicine and Public Health; Assistant Chief, Clinical Operations and Section Chief Fluoroscopy, Nationwide Children's Hospital, Columbus, Ohio

Mary P. Bedard, MD Associate Neonatologist, Neonatal-Perinatal Medicine, Children's Hospital of Michigan, Detroit, Michigan

Gerald G. Behr, MD Department of Radiology, Morgan Stanley Children's Hospital of New York-Presbyterian and Columbia University, New York, New York

Sadaf T. Bhutta, MBBS Associate Professor, Department of Radiology, University of Arkansas for Medical Sciences, Little Rock, Arkansas

Larry A. Binkovitz, MD Associate Professor, Department of Diagnostic Radiology, Mayo Clinic, Rochester, Minnesota

Susan Blaser, MD Department of Diagnostic Imaging, The Hospital for Sick Children, Toronto, ON, Canada

Stefan Bluml, MD Associate Professor of Research Radiology; Director, New Imaging Technologies; Departments of Radiology and Pediatrics, Children's Hospital, Keck School of Medicine, University of Southern California, Los Angeles, California

Danielle K.B. Boal, MD Professor of Radiology and Pediatrics, Department of Radiology, Pennsylvania State University College of Medicine; Professor of Radiology and Pediatrics, Department of Radiology, Milton S. Hershey Medical Center, Hershey, Pennsylvania

Phillip M. Boiselle, MD Department of Radiology, Beth Israel Deaconess Medical Center and Harvard Medical School, Boston, Massachusetts

Timothy N. Booth, MD Professor, Department of Radiology, Children's Medical Center, University of Texas Southwestern Medical Center, Dallas, Texas

Emma E. Boylan, BA Department of Medical Imaging, Ann and Robert H. Lurie Children's Hospital of Chicago, Chicago, Illinois

Dorothy Bulas, MD Professor of Pediatrics and Radiology, Department of Diagnostic Imaging and Radiology, Children's National Medical Center, Washington, DC

Angela Byrne, MD Department of Radiology, Children's Hospital of British Columbia, Vancouver, BC, Canada

Alicia M. Casey, MD Department of Medicine, Division of Respiratory Diseases, Boston Children's Hospital and Harvard Medical School, Boston, Massachusetts

Christopher I. Cassady, MD Clinical Associate Professor, Department of Radiology, Baylor College of Medicine; Chief of Fetal Imaging, Pediatric Radiology, Texas Children's Hospital, Houston, Texas

Kim M. Cecil, PhD Departments of Radiology, Pediatrics, Neuroscience and Environmental Health, Cincinnati Children's Hospital Medical Center, University of Cincinnati College of Medicine, Cincinnati, Ohio

Rafael C. Ceschin, MD Department of Radiology, Children's Hospital of Pittsburgh of UPMC; Department of Biomedical Informatics, University of Pittsburgh, Pittsburgh, Pennsylvania

Frandics P. Chan, MD, PhD Associate Professor, Department of Radiology, Stanford University Medical Center, Stanford, California

Teresa Chapman, MD Staff Radiologist, Seattle Children's Hospital; Assistant Professor, Department of Radiology, University of Washington, Seattle, Washington

Grace R. Choi, MD Assistant Professor, Department of Pediatrics, Northwestern University Feinberg School of Medicine; Attending Physician, Pediatrics, Division of Cardiology, Ann and Robert H. Lurie Children's Hospital of Chicago, Chicago, Illinois

Winnie C.W. Chu, MB ChB Department of Imaging and Interventional Radiology, Prince of Wales Hospital and The Chinese Univerisity of Hong Kong, Hong Kong SAR, China

Harris L. Cohen, MD Professor and Chairman, Department of Radiology; Professor, Pediatrics and Obstetrics & Gynecology, University of Tennessee Health Science Center; Medical Director, Radiology, LeBonheur Children's Hospital, Memphis, Tennessee

Brian D. Coley, MD Professor, Departments of Radiology and Pediatrics, University of Cincinnati College of Medicine; Radiologist-in-Chief, Department of Radiology, Cincinnati Children's Hospital Medical Center, Cincinnati, Ohio

Moira L. Cooper, MD Associate Clinical Professor, University of Victoria, Victoria, BC, Canada

Hannah Crowley, MD Department of Radiology, Children's Hospital of Pittsburgh of UPMC, Pittsburgh, Pennsylvania

J.A. Gordon Culham, MD Professor, Department of Radiology, University of British Columbia; Pediatric Radiologist, Department of Radiology, British Columbia's Children's Hospital, Vancouver, BC, Canada

Pedro Daltro, MD Clinica de DiagnOstico Por Imagem, Rio de Janeiro, Brazil

Amy R. Danehy, MD Division of Pediatric Neuroradiology, Boston Children's Hospital; Instructor in Radiology, Harvard Medical School, Boston, Massachusetts

Alan Daneman, MB BCh Radiologist, Department of Diagnostic Imaging; Division Head of General Radiology and Body Imaging, The Hospital for Sick Children; Professor, Medical Imaging, University of Toronto, Toronto, ON, Canada

Karunamoy Das, MD King Fahad Hospital, Dammam, Saudi Arabia

Andrew deFreitas, MD Assistant Professor of Pediatrics, Northwestern University Feinberg School of Medicine; Director, Adult Congenital Heart Disease, Ann and Robert H. Lurie Children's Hospital of Chicago, Chicago, Illinois

Katyucia de Macedo Rodrigues, MD Research Fellow, Radiology, Boston Children's Hospital; Research Fellow, Radiology, A.A. Martinos Center/Massachusetts General Hospital, Boston, Massachusetts

Jonathan R. Dillman, MD Assistant Professor, Department of Radiology, Section of Pediatric Radiology, University of Michigan Health System, Ann Arbor, Michigan

Lincoln O. Diniz, MD Department of Radiology, Cincinnati Children's Hospital Medical Center, Cincinnati, Ohio

Mary T. Donofrio, MD Associate Professor of Pediatrics, George Washington University; Director of the Fetal Heart Program, Children's National Heart Institute, Children's National Medical Center, Washington, DC

Andrea Schwarz Doria, MD, PhD, MSc Staff Radiologist/Clinician-Scientist, Department of Diagnostic Imaging; Scientist, Research Institute, The Hospital for Sick Children; Associate Professor, Faculty of Medicine, University of Toronto, Toronto, ON, Canada

Adam L. Dorfman, MD Clinical Associate Professor, Departments of Pediatrics and Radiology, University of Michigan, Ann Arbor, Michigan

Laura A. Drubach, MD Department of Radiology, Division of Nuclear Medicine, Boston Children's Hospital and Harvard Medical School, Boston, Massachusetts

Josée Dubois, MD, MSc Professor, Department of Radiology, Radio-Oncology, and Nuclear Medicine, University of Montreal; Chief, Department of Medical Imaging, CHU Sainte-Justine, Montreal, QC, Canada

Jerry Dwek, MD Clinical Adjunct Assistant Professor of Radiology, University of California at San Diego; Department of Radiology, Rady Children's Hospital and Health Center, San Diego Imaging, San Diego, California

Eric L. Effmann, MD Professor of Radiology, Department of Radiology, University of Washington; Division Chief, General Diagnosis, Department of Radiology, Seattle Children's Hospital, Seattle, Washington

Wendy D. Ellis, MD Assistant Professor, Department of Radiology, Vanderbilt University, Nashville, Tennessee

Monica Epelman, MD Department of Radiology, The Children's Hospital of Philadelphia, Philadelphia, Pennsylvania

Eric N. Faerber, MD Professor of Radiology and Pediatrics, Drexel University College of Medicine; Director, Department of Radiology, St. Christopher's Hospital for Children, Philadelphia, Pennsylvania

Nancy R. Fefferman, MD Assistant Professor of Radiology, Department of Radiology; Section Chief, Pediatric Radiology, NYU School of Medicine, New York, New York

Kate A. Feinstein, MD Professor of Radiology and Surgery; Section Chief, Pediatric Radiology, Comer Children's Hospital at University of Chicago, Chicago, Illinois

Celia M. Ferrari, MD Department of Radiology, Hospital de Ninos Sor Maria Ludovic, La Plata, Argentina

Tamara Feygin, MD Assistant Professor of Radiology, University of Pennsylvania School of Medicine, Neuroradiology, The Children's Hospital of Philadelphia, Philadelphia, Pennsylvania

Kristin Fickenscher, MD Assistant Professor and Fellowship Program Director, Radiology and Pediatrics, University of Missouri-Kansas City; Pediatric Radiologist, Children's Mercy Hospital and Clinics, Kansas City, Missouri

A. Michelle Fink, MD Department of Medical Imaging, The Royal Children's Hospital, Melbourne, Australia

Martha P. Fishman, MD Department of Medicine, Division of Respiratory Diseases, Boston Children's Hospital and Harvard Medical School, Boston, Massachusetts

Donald P. Frush, MD Chief of Pediatric Radiology, Duke University, Durham, North Carolina

Andre D. Furtado, MD Department of Pediatric Radiology, Department of Pediatrics, Division of Neurology, Children's Hospital of Pittsburgh of UPMC, Pittsburgh, Pennsylvania

Ana Maria Gaca, MD Assistant Professor, Department of Radiology, Duke University Medical Center, Durham, North Carolina

Asvin M. Ganapathi, MD Department of Surgery, Duke University Medical Center, Durham, North Carolina

Seth Gibson, DO Department of Radiology, University of Missouri-Kansas City; Radiology Fellow, Children's Mercy Hospitals and Clinics, Kansas City, Missouri

Hyun Woo Goo, MD Department of Radiology and Research Institute of Radiology, Asan Medical Center, University of Ulsan College of Medicine, Seoul, Korea

P. Ellen Grant, MD Associate Professor, Department of Radiology; Director, Fetal-Neonatal Neuroimaging and Developmental Science Center, Boston Children's Hospital, Boston, Massachusetts

J. Damien Grattan-Smith, MBBS Department of Radiology, Children's Healthcare of Atlanta, Atlanta, Georgia

S. Bruce Greenberg, MD Professor of Radiology and Pediatrics, Department of Radiology, University of Arkansas for Medical Sciences, Little Rock, Arkansas

John P. Grimm, MD Assistant Professor, Children's Hospital Los Angeles, Keck School of Medicine, University of Southern California, Los Angeles, California

R. Paul Guillerman, MD Associate Professor of Radiology, Baylor College of Medicine, Edward B. Singelton Department of Pediatric Radiology, Texas Children's Hospital, Baylor College of Medicine, Houston, Texas

Stephen M. Henesch, DO Director of Pediatric Radiology, Radiology Consulting of Long Island; Imaging Services Department, Good Samaritan Hospital Medical Center, West Islip, New York

James René Herlong, MD Associate Clinical Professor of Pediatrics, University of North Carolina School of Medicine; Division Chief, Pediatric Cardiology, Sanger Heart and Vascular Institute, Charlotte, North Carolina

Marta Hernanz-Schulman, MD Professor of Radiology and Pediatrics, Vanderbilt University Medical Center; Medical Director, Diagnostic Imaging, Monroe Carell, Jr. Children's Hospital at Vanderbilt, Nashville, Tennessee

Melissa A. Hilmes, MD Assistant Professor, Department of Radiology & Radiological Sciences, Vanderbilt University School of Medicine, Nashville, Tennessee

Hollie A. Jackson, MD Associate Professor, Department of Radiology, Children's Hospital Los Angeles, Keck School of Medicine, University of Southern California, Los Angeles, California

J. Herman Kan, MD Associate Professor, Baylor College of Medicine; Section Chief, Musculoskeletal Imaging, E.B. Singleton Pediatric Radiology, Texas Children's Hospital, Houston, Texas

Ronald J. Kanter, MD Professor, Departments of Pediatrics & Medicine; Director, Pediatric Electrophysiology, Duke University Medical Center, Durham, North Carolina

Sue Creviston Kaste, DO Professor of Radiology, University of Tennessee Health Science Center; Member, Radiological Sciences, St. Jude Children's Research Hospital, Memphis, Tennessee

Paritosh C. Khanna, MD Department of Radiology, Seattle Children's Hospital, Seattle, Washington

Stanley T. Kim, MD Assistant Professor, Department of Radiology, Northwestern University Feinberg School of Medicine, Chicago, Illinois

Sunhee Kim, MD Assistant Professor, Department of Diagnostic Radiology, University of Pittsburgh, Children's Hospital of Pittsburgh of UPMC, Pittsburgh, Pennsylvania

Joshua Q. Knowlton, MD, MPH Pediatric Radiologist, Department of Radiology, Children's Mercy Hospital, Kansas City, Missouri

Amy B. Kolbe, MD Pediatric Radiology Fellow, Department of Radiology, Mayo Clinic, Rochester, Minnesota

Korgün Koral, MD Associate Professor, Department of Radiology, University of Texas Southwestern Medical Center; Department of Radiology, Children's Medical Center, Dallas, Texas

Rajesh Krishnamurthy, MD Director of Cardiovascular Imaging, EB Singleton Department of Pediatric Radiology, Texas Children's Hospital; Associate Professor of Radiology and Pediatrics, Baylor College of Medicine, Houston, Texas

Anita Krishnan, MD Pediatric Cardiologist, Children's National Medical Center, Washington, DC

Ralph Lachman, MD Emeritus Professor, Radiology & Pediatrics, UCLA School of Medicine; International Skeletal Dysplasia Registry, Medical Genetics Institute, Cedars-Sinai Medical Center, Los Angeles, California; Consulting Clinical Professor, Stanford University, Stanford, California

Tal Laor, MD Professor of Radiology and Pediatrics, University of Cincinnati College of Medicine; Co-Section Chief, Musculoskeletal Imaging, Department of Radiology, Cincinnati Children's Hospital Medical Center, Cincinnati, Ohio

Bernard F. Laya, MD, DO Associate Professor of Radiology; Director, Institute of Radiology, St. Luke's Medical Center, Global City, Taguig City, The Philippines

James Leach, MD Associate Professor, Department of Radiology, Cincinnati Children's Hospital Medical Center; Associate Professor, Department of Radiology, University of Cincinnati College of Medicine, Cincinnati, Ohio

Henrique M. Lederman, MD Professor of Radiology, Department of Diagnostic Imaging, Federal University of Sao Paulo; Chief, Center of Diagnostic Imaging, Pediatric Oncology Institute, Sao Paulo, Brazil

Edward Y. Lee, MD, MPH Associate Professor of Radiology and Chief, Division of Thoracic Imaging; Director, Magnetic Resonance Imaging, Departments of Radiology and Medicine, Pulmonary Division, Boston Children's Hospital and Harvard Medical School, Boston, Massachusetts

Craig W. Lillehei, MD Department of Surgery, Boston Children's Hospital and Harvard Medical School, Boston, Massachusetts

Andrew J. Lodge, MD Assistant Professor, Department of Surgery; Assistant Professor, Department of Pediatrics, Duke University Medical Center, Durham, North Carolina

Lisa H. Lowe, MD Professor, Department of Pediatrics, Children's Mercy Hospitals and Clinics; Professor, Academic Chair and Residency Program Director, Department of Radiology, University of Missouri-Kansas City, Kansas City, Missouri

Jimmy C. Lu, MD Clinical Assistant Professor, Departments of Pediatrics and Radiology, University of Michigan, Ann Arbor, Michigan

Cathy MacDonald, MD Assistant Professor, Department of Medical Imaging, University of Toronto; Staff Radiologist, Department of Diagnostic Imaging, The Hospital for Sick Children, Toronto, ON, Canada

Maryam Ghadimi Mahani, MD Clinical Assistant Professor, Department of Radiology, University of Michigan, Ann Arbor, Michigan

Diana V. Marin, MD Pediatric Radiologist, Department of Radiology, Miami Children's Hospital, Miami, Florida

John B. Mawson, MB, CHB (NZ) Assistant Professor, Department of Radiology, University of British Columbia; Pediatric Radiologist, Department of Radiology, British Columbia's Children's Hospital, Vancouver, BC, Canada

Charles M. Maxfield, MD Associate Professor of Radiology and Pediatrics, Duke University Medical Center, Durham, North Carolina

William H. McAlister, MD Professor of Radiology and Pediatrics, Department of Pediatric Radiology, Washington University Medical School, St. Louis, Missouri

M. Beth McCarville, MD Associate Member, Department of Radiological Sciences, St. Jude Children's Research Hospital, Memphis, Tennessee

James S. Meyer, MD Associate Professor of Radiology, University of Pennsylvania School of Medicine; Associate Radiologist-in-Chief, Department of Radiology, Children's Hospital of Philadelphia, Philadelphia, Pennsylvania

Sarah S. Milla, MD Assistant Professor, Department of Radiology, New York University Langone Medical Center, New York, New York

Elka Miller, MD Chief/Medical Director and Research Director, Diagnostic Imaging Department, Children's Hospital of Eastern Ontario; Assistant Professor, Department of Radiology, University of Ottawa, ON, Canada

David M. Mirsky, MD Pediatric Neuroradiology Fellow, The Children's Hospital of Philadelphia, Philadelphia, Pennsylvania

David A. Mong, MD Department of Radiology, The Children's Hospital of Philadelphia, Philadelphia, Pennsylvania

Kevin R. Moore, MD Vice Chair of Radiology; Director of MR Imaging, Department of Medical Imaging, Primary Children's Medical Center; Adjunct Associate, Professor of Radiology, Department of Radiology, University of Utah, Salt Lake City, Utah

Oscar Navarro, MD Assistant Professor, Department of Medical Imaging, University of Toronto; Staff Radiologist, Department of Diagnostic Imaging, The Hospital for Sick Children, Toronto, ON, Canada

Marvin D. Nelson Jr, MD, MBA Chairman, Department of Radiology, Children's Hospital Los Angeles; Professor, Department of Radiology, Keck School of Medicine, University of Southern California, Los Angeles, California

Beverley Newman, BSc, MB BCh Associate Professor, Department of Radiology, Lucile Packard Children's Hospital at Stanford University, Stanford, California

Julie Currie O'Donovan, MD Pediatric Radiologist, Department of Radiology, Nationwide Children's Hospital; Clinical Assistant Professor of Radiology, The Ohio State University Medical Center, Columbus, Ohio

Robert C. Orth, MD, PhD Assistant Professor of Radiology, Baylor College of Medicine, Edward B. Singleton Department of Pediatric Radiology, Texas Children's Hospital, Houston, Texas

Deepa R. Pai, MHSA, MD Assistant Clinical Professor, Department of Radiology, Section of Pediatric Radiology, University of Michigan, Ann Arbor, Michigan

Michael J. Painter, MD Department of Pediatric Radiology, Department of Pediatrics, Division of Neurology, Children's Hospital of Pittsburgh of UPMC, Pittsburgh, Pennsylvania

Harriet J. Paltiel, MD Radiologist, Boston Children's Hospital; Associate Professor of Radiology, Harvard Medical School, Boston, Massachusetts

Ajaya R. Pande, MD Department of Radiology, Children's Hospital of Pittsburgh of UPMC, Pittsburgh, Pennsylvania

Ashok Panigrahy, MD Radiologist-in-Chief, Associate Professor of Radiology, Children's Hospital of Pittsburgh of UPMC, Pittsburgh, Pennsylvania

Angira Patel, MD, MPH Assistant Professor of Pediatrics, Department of Pediatric Cardiology, Northwestern University Feinberg School of Medicine; Attending Physician, Pediatric Cardiology, Ann and Robert H. Lurie Children's Hospital of Chicago, Chicago, Illinois

Grace S. Phillips, MD Assistant Professor, Department of Radiology, University of Washington School of Medicine; Division Chief, Computed Tomography, Department of Radiology, Seattle Children's Hospital, Seattle, Washington

Avrum N. Pollock, MD Associate Professor of Radiology, Department of Radiology, Division of Neuroradiology, The Children's Hospital of Philadelphia, Philadelphia, Pennsylvania

Andrada R. Popescu, MD Radiology Fellow, Ann and Robert H. Lurie Children's Hospital of Chicago, Chicago, Illinois

Tina Young Poussaint, MD Professor of Radiology, Harvard Medical School; Attending Neuroradiologist, Department of Radiology, Boston Children's Hospital, Boston, Massachusetts

Sanjay P. Prabhu, MBBS Instructor in Radiology, Harvard Medical School; Attending Neuroradiologist, Department of Radiology, Boston Children's Hospital, Boston, Massachusetts

Sumit Pruthi, MD Assistant Professor, Department of Radiology & Radiological Sciences, Vanderbilt University, Memphis, Tennessee

Anand Dorai Raju, MD Department of Radiology, LeBonheur Children's Hospital, Memphis, Tennessee

Brenton D. Reading, MD Assistant Professor of Radiology, Department of Pediatric Radiology, University of Missouri-Kansas City, Kansas City, Missouri

Brian Reilly, RT(R) 3D Imaging Specialist, Department of Medical Imaging, Ann and Robert H. Lurie Children's Hospital of Chicago, Chicago, Illinois

Ricardo Restrepo, MD Department of Radiology, Miami Children's Hospital, Miami, Florida

John F. Rhodes, MD Associate Professor, Departments of Pediatrics & Medicine; Chief, Duke Children's Heart Center; Director, Pediatric & Adult Congenital Cardiac Catheterization Laboratory, Duke University Medical Center, Durham, North Carolina

Michael Riccabona, MD University Professor, Department of Radiology, Division of Pediatric Radiology, Universitätsklinikum-LKH Graz, Auenbruggenplatz, Graz, Australia

Cynthia K. Rigsby, MD Professor of Radiology and Pediatrics, Northwestern University Feinberg School of Medicine; Division Head, Body Imaging and Vice Chair, Medical Imaging, Ann and Robert H. Lurie Children's Hospital of Chicago, Chicago, Illinois

Douglas C. Rivard, DO Assistant Professor, Department of Radiology, Children's Mercy Hospital and Clinics, Kansas City, Missouri

Richard L. Robertson, MD Radiologist-in-Chief, Division of Pediatric Neuroradiology, Boston Children's Hospital; Associate Professor of Radiology, Harvard Medical School, Boston, Massachusetts

Ashley J. Robinson, MD Department of Radiology, Children's Hospital of British Columbia, Vancouver, BC; Department of Diagnostic Imaging, The Hospital for Sick Children, Toronto, ON, Canada

Joshua D. Robinson, MD Division of Cardiology, Children's Memorial Hospital, Department of Pediatrics, Northwestern University Feinberg School of Medicine, Chicago, Illinois

Caroline D. Robson, MB ChB Operations Vice Chair and Division Chief of Neuroradiology, Department of Radiology, Boston Children's Hospital; Associate Professor, Department of Radiology, Harvard Medical School, Boston, Massachusetts

Diana P. Rodriguez, MD Radiologist, Boston Children's Hospital, Boston, Massachusetts

Nancy Rollins, MD Medical Director, Department of Radiology, Children's Medical Center; Professor, Department of Radiology, University Texas Southwestern Medical Center, Dallas, Texas

Lucy B. Rorke-Adams, MD Senior Neuropathologist, Division of Neuropathology; Clinical Professor, Pathology and Laboratory Medicine, Perelman School of Medicine at the University of Pennsylvania, Philadelphia, Pennsylvania

Arlene A. Rozzelle, MD Associate Professor, Department of Surgery, Wayne State University School of Medicine; Chief, Plastic & Reconstructive Surgery, Children's Hospital of Michigan; Director, CHM Cleft/Craniofacial Anomalies Program Director, CHM Vascular Anomalies Team, Children's Hospital of Michigan, Detroit, Michigan

Gauravi Sabharwal, MBBS Section Head, Pediatric Radiology, Henry Ford Hospital and Health Network; Clinical Assistant Professor of Radiology, Wayne State University School of Medicine, Detroit, Michigan

Vincent J. Schmithorst, PhD Department of Radiology, Children's Hospital of Pittsburgh of UPMC, Pittsburgh, Pennsylvania

Erin Simon Schwartz, MD Associate Professor of Radiology, Perelman School of Medicine at the University of Pennsylvania; Clinical Director, The Lurie Family Foundation's Magnetoencephalography Imaging Center, Department of Radiology, Division of Neuroradiology, The Children's Hospital of Philadelphia, Philadelphia, Pennsylvania

Jayne M. Seekins, DO Instructor, Department of Radiology and Radiological Sciences, Vanderbilt University, Nashville, Tennessee

Sabah Servaes, MD Assistant Professor, Department of Radiology, The Children's Hospital of Philadelphia, Philadelphia, Pennsylvania

Virendersingh K. Sheorain, MD Radiology Fellow, University of Tennessee Health Science Center, Memphis, Tennessee

Richard M. Shore, MD Divison Head, General Radiology and Nuclear Medicine, Medical Imaging, Ann & Robert H. Lurie Children's Hospital of Chicago; Professor, Radiology, Northwestern University Feinberg School of Medicine, Chicago, Illinois

Sudha P. Singh, MBBS, MD Assistant Professor, Department of Radiology and Radiological Sciences, Vanderbilt University, Nashville, Tennessee

Carlos J. Sivit, MD Professor of Radiology and Pediatrics, Case Western Reserve School of Medicine; Vice Chairman, Clinical Operations, University Hospitals Case Medical Center, Cleveland, Ohio

Thomas L. Slovis, MD Professor, Department of Pediatric Imaging, Wayne State University School of Medicine; Emeritus Chief, Pediatric Imaging, Children's Hospital of Michigan, Detroit, Michigan

Christopher J. Smith, MD University of Missouri-Kansas City School of Medicine, Kansas City, Missouri

Gloria Soto, MD Department of Radiology, Clinica Alemana de Santiago, Santiago, Chile

Vera R. Sperling, MD Assistant Clinical Professor, Department of Radiology, Children's Hospital of Pittsburgh of UPMC, Pittsburgh, Pennsylvania

Stephanie E. Spottswood, MD, MSPH Associate Professor of Radiology, Department of Diagnostic Imaging, Monroe Carell, Jr. Children's Hospital at Vanderbilt University, Nashville, Tennessee

Gayathri Sreedher, MD Department of Pediatric Radiology, Children's Hospital of Pittsburgh of UPMC, Pittsburgh, Pennsylvania

Jan Stauss, MD Medical X-Ray Consultants, Eau Claire, Wisconsin

Peter J. Strouse, MD Professor and Director, Section of Pediatric Radiology, Department of Radiology, University of Michigan Health System, Ann Arbor, Michigan

George A. Taylor, MD Radiologist-in-Chief Emeritus, Department of Radiology, Boston Children's Hospital; John A. Kirkpatrick Professor of Radiology (Pediatrics), Department of Radiology, Harvard Medical School, Boston, Massachusetts

Paul Thacker, MD Instructor, Pediatric Radiology, Children's Mercy Hospitals and Clinics, Kansas City, Missouri

Darshit Thakrar, MD Advanced Pediatric Radiology Fellow, Department of Medical Imaging, Children's Memorial Hospital, Northwestern University Feinberg School of Medicine, Chicago, Illinois

Mahesh M. Thapa, MD Program Director, Radiology Medical Education, Seattle Children's Hospital; Associate Professor, Department of Radiology, UW Medicine, Seattle, Washington

Jean A. Tkach, PhD Associate Professor, Department of Radiology, Imaging Research Center, Cincinnati Children's Hospital Medical Center, Cincinnati, Ohio

Alexander J. Towbin, MD Assistant Professor of Radiology, Department of Radiology, Cincinnati Children's Hospital Medical Center, Cincinnati, Ohio

Donald A. Tracy, MD Assistant Professor of Radiology, Tufts University School of Medicine; Chief of Pediatric Radiology, Tufts Medical Center and Floating Hospital for Children, Boston, Massachusetts

Jeffrey Traubici, MD Assistant Professor, Medical Imaging, University of Toronto; Radiologist, The Hospital for Sick Children, Toronto, ON, Canada

S. Ted Treves, MD Chief, Division of Nuclear Medicine and Molecular Imaging, Radiology, Boston Children's Hospital; Professor of Radiology and Director of the Joint Program in Nuclear Medicine Radiology, Harvard Medical School, Boston, Massachusetts

Shreyas S. Vasanawala, MD, PhD Assistant Professor, Department of Radiology, Stanford University, Stanford, California

Arastoo Vossough, PhD, MD Assistant Professor of Radiology, University of Pennsylvania; Department of Radiology, Children's Hospital of Philadelphia, Philadelphia, Pennsylvania

Robert G. Wells, MD Associate Professor of Radiology and Pediatrics, Medical College of Wisconsin; Pediatric Radiologist, Pediatric Diagnostic Imaging, Milwaukee, Wisconsin; Director, Pediatric Radiology, Northwestern Lake Forest Hospital, Lake Forest, Illinois

Sjirk J. Westra, MD Associate Professor of Radiology, Department of Radiology, Massachusetts General Hospital and Harvard Medical School, Boston, Massachusetts

Elysa Widjaja, MBBS, MRCP, MD, MPH Neuroradiologist, Department of Diagnostic Imaging, The Hospital for Sick Children; Associate Professor, Medical Imaging, University of Toronto, Toronto, ON, Canada

Sally Wildman, DO Pediatric Radiologist, Department of Radiology, Nationwide Children's Hospital; Assistant Professor, Department of Radiology, The Ohio State University Medical Center, Columbus, Ohio

Peter Winningham, MD Department of Radiology, University of Missouri–Kansas City, Kansas City, Missouri

Jessica L. Wisnowski, PhD Department of Pediatric Radiology, Department of Pediatrics, Division of Neurology, Children's Hospital of Pittsburgh of UPMC, Pittsburgh, Pennsylvania; Department of Radiology, Children's Hospital Los Angeles; Brain and Creativity Institute, University of Southern California, Los Angeles, California

Ali Yikilmaz, MD Associate Professor of Radiology, Department of Pediatric Radiology, Erciyes University Medical Center, Erciyes University; Department of Pediatric Radiology, Children's Hospital, Kayseri, Turkey

Adam Zarchan, MD Assistant Clinical Professor, Department of Diagnostic Radiology, University of Kansas-Wichita; Pediatric Radiologist, Wesley Medical Center, Wichita, Kansas

Giulio Zuccoli, MD Radiology Department, Children's Hospital of Pittsburgh of UPMC, Pittsburgh, Pennsylvania

Evan J. Zucker, MD Radiology Resident, Tufts Medical Center and Floating Hospital for Children; Clinical Associate in Radiology, Tufts University School of Medicine, Boston, Massachusetts

Foreword

The twelfth edition of *Caffey's Pediatric Diagnostic Imaging* reflects the evolution of a powerful educational tool. It is shorter as a book but infinitely longer when one includes the many online images, videos, and supplemental text.

Since the 1945 first edition, the organization of topics and their placement in "The Book" has varied from purely anatomic to organ system and disease. In 1972, the sixth edition, the neonatal section first appeared and continued through the most recent edition. Modality chapters were specifically noted in the table of contents when Dr. Frederic Silverman became the editor of the eighth edition in 1985. The incorporation in 2003, when Drs. Jerald Kuhn, Thomas Slovis, and Jack Haller shared the editorship, of an initial section on the "Effects of Radiation" followed by "Neonatal Imaging" emphasized the importance of these topics in our practice. Chapters on prenatal imaging first formally appear with this edition.

Through the years the authorship has grown from Dr. John Caffey alone to Drs. Caffey and Silverman to literally more than 100 hundred experts. This is important because the authors are not only pediatric radiologists, but also superb pediatric subspecialists and scientists in the technical aspects of multimodality imaging. This mix has brought us back to our clinical roots.

Caffey's Pediatric Diagnostic Imaging is more than an imaging text. The twelfth edition reflects the evolution of pediatric radiology and pediatric medicine. The initial section, "Radiation Effects and Safety," expresses our concern for the safety of our patients in the broad context of radiation, use of magnetic resonance imaging, and contrast effects.

Neonatal and perinatal imaging has been incorporated into organ system chapters to emphasize the continuum of an abnormality throughout the patient's life. The concept of "the best test" has allowed elimination of the modality approach, and each test is discussed when appropriate in the disease state. Interventional radiology has been incorporated into those chapters when it is useful.

Dr. Brian Coley and his team have a done a superb job of making our educational experience more efficient. The continual change we see with each edition not only reflects the need for us to "keep up" with the science, but also emphasizes what is best for our patients.

Congratulations, Brian.

Thomas L. Slovis, MD
Professor Emeritus
Department of Radiology
Wayne State School of Medicine
Emeritus Chairman
Department of Imaging
Children's Hospital of Michigan
Detroit, Michigan

Preface

How and where we seek information differ today from 1945, when the first edition of *Caffey's Pediatric X-Ray Diagnosis* was published. There was no Internet, Google, or PubMed; you could make a Photostat of an article, but no Xerox machines existed yet. Journals of the day contained the latest research, but the synthesis of that knowledge with practical experience came in the form of the textbook. Historically, the landmark textbooks were written by the most influential leaders in their fields and were usually solo efforts (one can speculate whether ego or difficulties of collaboration played the greater part). A small number of valuable and influential texts have outlived their creators, evolving over years through the efforts of new authors and editors. Sir William Osler's *The Principles and Practice of Medicine* was published from 1892 to 2001; Sir Vincent Zachary Cope's *Early Diagnosis of the Acute Abdomen,* currently in its twenty-second edition, first appeared in 1921. Other such venerable texts still being published include Harrison's *Principles of Internal Medicine* (1950), Nelson's *Textbook of Pediatrics* (1945), and Goodman & Gilman's *The Pharmacological Basis of Therapeutics* (1941). *Caffey's Pediatric Diagnostic Imaging* has also proven its lasting value and importance over almost six decades.

But how we collect, store, and access information has changed. Even the most technophobic among us obtains information regularly via electronic means. For those of us fond of our computers and mobile devices, we can indulge in a deluge of data at any time or location. The ability to find information and answers to specific questions is a tremendous benefit to medical care and education. The quality of the information retrieved online, however, is sometimes unclear. Further, freely available Internet content is often truncated and condensed to suit a culture of shortened attention span. How well are subtleties or syntheses conveyed by a single screen page summary or bullet point list? As we learn more about the science of education, what is the best method of presenting information to learners both young and old?

Are books such as this one still relevant? Clearly, I have a somewhat biased viewpoint. I believe that well-constructed prose from an author with expert knowledge and practical real-world experience, coupled with illustrative images and diagrams, is a powerful and efficient way to transmit information and facilitate learning. Lists of facts and bullet point paragraphs cannot convey more complex concepts and syntheses. No matter what the medium, content counts. And books such as this one have tremendously valuable content.

That said, there is ongoing debate as to the best medium in which to disseminate complex and comprehensive content. Books are simple to use. They are familiar. It is easy to flip from section to section, to go back a few pages without losing your place. You can take notes in the margins. Books can also be heavy and cumbersome. They are costly to manufacture. Electronic formats have their pros and cons as well. A light, portable laptop or tablet may contain thousands of books' worth of information. Images can be manipulated as in actual practice. Video and animations can augment the learning experience. Online texts can be accessed anywhere with an Internet connection. Content length need not be dictated by physical page limitations. However, the device screen size dictates and somewhat limits the amount and method of information display. Moving back and forth between content sections can be awkward.

The twelfth edition of this text reflects the conflict and state of flux in publishing. There is a physical book. There are more explanatory diagrams and illustrations with better use of color, and I have tried to continue the work of Dr. Slovis in updating and improving the images. This edition adds a significant online and electronic presence. Additional images, animations, and videos are available online to supplement the print volume and to allow those who prefer electronic media to take advantage of the material in an alternate way.

The authors and section editors have contributed significant updates regarding newer imaging modalities, the understanding of disease processes, imaging appropriateness, and the importance of minimizing radiation exposure. As with the last edition, there has been input from many clinical specialists, providing perspective on the important role of imaging in the care of children. The authors and section editors have my thanks.

I would like to thank the team at Elsevier. Rebecca Gaertner and Kristina Oberle helped to get this edition started. Maureen Iannuzzi and Don Scholz were my main partners in this project. I especially appreciate Maureen's hard work in keeping us on task and her sense of humor. Carrie Stetz oversaw the layout and proof part of the production, helping to give the book its updated look.

I hope that this twelfth edition of Caffey is helpful to you and to the patients you serve.

Brian D. Coley, MD

Preface to First Edition

Shadows are but dark holes in radiant streams, twisted rifts beyond the substance, meaningless in themselves.

He who would comprehend Röntgen's pallid shades need always to know well the solid matrix whence they spring. The physician needs to know intimately each living patient through whom the racing black light darts, and flashing the hidden depths reveals them in a glowing mirage of thin images, each cast delicately in its own halo, but all veiled and blended endlessly.

Man — warm, lively, fleshy man — and his story are both root and key to his shadows; shadows cold, silent and empty. —
JOHN CAFFEY

Within a few weeks after Röntgen announced his now renowned discovery to the world in December 1895, the x-ray method of examination was applied to infants and children. The Vienna letter of February 29 (M. Rec. 49:312, 1896) contained a roentgen print of the arm of an infant made of Kreidl in Vienna: this is the second reproduction of a roentgen image in the American literature. Credit for the first recorded roentgen examination of an infant in the United States undoubtedly belongs to Dr. E.P. Davis of New York City, who described the roentgen shadows cast by the trunk of a living infant and the skull of a dead fetus in March 1896. In his remarkable article (The study of the infant body and the pregnant womb by the roentgen ray, Am. J. M. Sc. 111:263, 1896), Dr. Davis also included three drawings of shadows visualized by means of a skiascope—shadows of the feet, elbows, and orbit of a living infant. Feilchenfeld's discussion of spina ventosa in May 1896 is probably the first roentgen description of morbid anatomy in children (Berlin. Klin. Wchnschr. 33:403, 1896). There were only two roentgen pediatric publications in 1896; the number increased to 14 in 1897.

In 1898, Escherich of Graz had had sufficient experience with pediatric roentgen examinations to write a general exposition on the merits and weaknesses of the method (La valeur diagnostique de la radiographie chez les enfants, Rev. d. mal. de l'enf. 16:233, May 1898). This is a highly interesting and illuminating discussion in which Escherich points out the roentgen examination was already not being used as commonly in young patients as in adults. He states that a roentgen laboratory was established especially for children at Graz in 1897, and it seems probable that this was the first of its kind. A single film is reproduced—a print of an infantile hand and forearm which shows rachitic changes. The uncertainties of the mediastinal shadows, which still bedevil us, were fully appreciated by Escherich, and he was quite unhappy about this baffling structure "in which so many important infantile lesions lie concealed." He was enthusiastic in regard to the possible estimation of the state of hydration of soft tissues in infantile diarrhea from their roentgen densities.

Reyher's German monograph in 1908 is the earliest review of the world literature of pediatric roentgenology which I have found (Reyher, P.: Die roentgenologische Diagnostik in der Kinderheilkunde, Ergebn. d. inn. Med. U. Kinderh. 2:613, 1908). In it there are 276 references to articles published during the first 12 years following Röntgen's discovery, and these furnish a good key for the study of the early writings in this field. The appendix contains 40 small but clear roentgen prints.

Rotch's *The Roentgen Ray in Pediatrics* appeared in 1910—the first book in any language devoted exclusively to pediatric x-ray diagnosis and still, I believe, the only one in English. Dr. Thomas Morgan Rotch was Professor of Pediatrics, Harvard University, and an outstanding podiatrist of his time.★ In this pioneer treatise he stresses the importance of mastering the shadows of normal structure before attempting the recognition and interpretation of the abnormal, and he carefully correlates the clinical findings with the roentgen findings in the cases illustrated; 42 of 264 figures depict the "normal living anatomy of infants and children." This material was taken largely from the files of the Boston Children's Hospital, and the author's statement that more than 2,300 cases were available for study demonstrates that roentgen examination had long been a commonplace in his clinic. Dr. Rotch's early fostering of roentgen examination of infants and children, his appreciation of the special problems in applying this method to the young, his careful anatomic roentgen studies and his text, monumental for this time, all mark him as the father of pediatric roentgenology in America.

Two years later—1912—the first German book, Reyher's *Das Roentgenverfahren in der Kinderheilkunde*, was published. Later and more familiar texts are Gralka's *Roentgendiagnostik im Kindesalter* (1927), Becker's *Roentgendiagnostik und Strahlentherapie in der Kinderheilkunde* (1931), and the *Handbuch der Roentgendiagnostik und Therapie im Kindesalter* by Engel and Schall (1933). As far as I have been able to determine, no book on pediatric roentgen diagnosis has been published in English during the 35 years which have passed since Rotch's unique publication in 1910. The absence of pediatric roentgenology in the flood of medical texts which has streamed from the American and English presses during the last three decades constitutes a dereliction unmatched in other equally important fields of medical diagnosis—a literary developmental hypoplasia which it is hoped *Pediatric X-Ray Diagnosis* will remedy.

This book stems from the roentgen conferences held semimonthly at the Babies Hospital during the last 20 years. The films reproduced herein were all selected from our own roentgen files save those for which credit to others is

---

★Jacobi, A.: In memoriam Thomas Morgan Rotch, Am. J. Dis. Child. 8:245, 1914.

indicated in the legends. The purpose of the author is two-fold: description of shadows cast by normal and morbid tissues, and clinical appraisal of roentgen findings in pediatric diagnosis. Roentgen physics, technique, and therapy have been omitted intentionally. As references and acknowledgments testify, the writer has borrowed freely from the literature and is indebted to many contributors for subject matter and illustrations. To all of them I am sincerely grateful. In the broad and deep field of pediatric diagnosis, selection of the most appropriate material has posed many dilemmas. In the main, data have been chosen which have proved the most useful and instructive in solving the common and important diagnostic problems which have arisen during two decades in a large and busy pediatric hospital and out-patient clinic.

The limitations of space do not permit adequate recognition here of all those to whom credit is due for the making of this book. The roentgen examinations which are its foundation could not have been made without the cooperation of thousands of patients—many weak and pain weary; to all of these I am profoundly thankful. Intimate clinical contacts have been maintained and essential collateral examinations have been made possible through the sustained collaboration of my colleagues—attending physicians and surgeons, resident physicians and nurses. I am under deep and solid obligation to Dr. Rustin McIntosh who read the entire manuscript; his discerning criticism and valuable suggestions are responsible for numerous corrections and improvements in the text. The sympathetic reception given to our early endeavors by Dr. Ross Golden will always be remembered gratefully, as well as his continuing wise and friendly counsel. We have benefited much and often from the discipline of the necropsy table—from the instructive dissections of Dr. Martha Wollstein, Dr. Beryl Paige, and Dr. Dorothy Anderson.

To none, however do I owe more than to my loyal coworkers in the roentgen department of the Babies Hospital—Edgar Watts, Cecelia Peck, Moira Shannon, Mary Fennell, and Mary Jean Cadman—for their gentle handling of patients, unfailing industry, and superlative technical skill. Mrs. Cadman typed the manuscript; I am grateful to her for the speedy completion of a thorny chore. The drawings are the work of Alfred Feinberg, and they reflect his rich experience in medical illustration.

The final phase in the preparation of the manuscript was saddened by the death of Mr. H.A. Simons, President of the Year Book Publishers. His stimulating enthusiasm and generosity were indispensable to the completion of the book during these unsettled war years. His passing was a grievous loss. The task of publication has fallen to the capable and patient hands of Mr. Paul Perles and Mrs. Anabel Ireland Janssen.

John Caffey
Babies Hospital
New York 32
June 10, 1945

Contents

SECTION 4

Respiratory System

VOLUME II

SECTION 8

Musculoskeletal System

Video Contents

Videos are available at the *Caffey's Pediatric Diagnostic Imaging* collection online at www.expertconsult.com.

SECTION 6

Gastrointestinal System

Chapter 84

Embryology, Anatomy, and Normal Findings

MARY P. BEDARD

This chapter provides an overview of the embryology of the abdominal wall and peritoneal cavity, as well as the solid and hollow viscera, within the context of the normal anatomic findings.

Abdominal Wall and Peritoneal Cavity

During the third week of gestation the intraembryonic mesoderm differentiates, forming the lateral plates.[1,2] Mesoderm from paravertebral myotomes invades the lateral plates during the sixth week. The leading edges of the lateral plates will differentiate into the right and left rectus abdominis muscles. The main portion of the mesoderm splits into three layers and forms the external oblique, internal oblique, and transverse abdominis muscles. Approximation of the right and left recti is complete by the twelfth week except for the umbilical ring.

The aponeurosis of the external oblique muscles forms the anterior and posterior rectus sheaths.[1] These sheaths join in the midline to form the linea alba. The lowest portion of the aponeurosis ends in the inguinal ligament. The external inguinal ring is an opening in the aponeurosis between the inguinal ligament inferiorly and the tendinous portion superiorly. The spermatic cord in males and the round ligament in females pass through the inguinal canal.

Closure of the cephalic, caudal, and lateral folds leads to the formation of the intraembryonic coelom.[3,4] The mesoderm surrounding the coelom splits into two layers, the somatic mesoderm and the splanchnic mesoderm. The somatic layer forms the parietal peritoneum, which lines the inner abdominal wall, and the splanchnic layer forms the visceral peritoneum, which covers the abdominal organs. The space between the parietal and visceral peritoneum is the peritoneal cavity.

Hepatic and Biliary System

The liver, gallbladder, and biliary duct system arise as a ventral outgrowth from the caudal end of the foregut early in the fourth week of development (Fig. 84-1).[5,6] This outgrowth, known as the hepatic diverticulum, extends into the septum transversum, which is the future diaphragm. The hepatic diverticulum grows rapidly and divides into cranial and caudal portions. The larger cranial portion forms the primordium of the liver parenchyma. Proliferating endodermal cells develop into cords of hepatocytes and into the epithelial lining of the biliary system. The connective tissue, hematopoietic cells, and Kupffer cells are derived from the mesoderm of the septum transversum. The caudal portion expands to form the gallbladder, and its stalk becomes the cystic duct. The two major intrahepatic ducts join to form the common hepatic duct. The stalk connecting the hepatic and cystic ducts to the duodenum becomes the common bile duct.

The liver grows rapidly, with the right lobe growing faster than the left lobe. Intrahepatic ducts appear in the region of the hilus and grow peripherally. This ductal system is complete by the tenth week of gestation, and bile formation is seen in the twelfth week. The extrahepatic biliary tree initially is formed as a solid cord that canalizes by the tenth to twelfth week of gestation. Bile is excreted into the duodenum via the common bile duct and is responsible for the characteristic dark green color of meconium.

The liver is the largest of the abdominal organs, with the right lobe being larger than the left lobe.[7] It occupies most of the right upper quadrant, extends across the midline, and is relatively larger in infants than in older children and adults. The superior portion of the liver is in direct contact with the diaphragm and is known as the *bare area* because it is not covered by peritoneum. The posterior margin abuts the inferior vena cava, the right adrenal gland, and the distal esophagus. Inferiorly, the liver is in contact with the colon, gallbladder, and right kidney. The left lobe is in contact with the stomach. The visceral surface of the liver contains the porta hepatis with its vessels and biliary ducts.

Traditional nomenclature in the United States divides the liver into five segments. However, hepatic segmental anatomy as described by Couinaud is more useful in defining surgically resectable segments (Fig. 84-2).[8] In Couinaud's system, the right and left lobes of the liver are divided by the middle hepatic vein and the Cantlie line, a line between the inferior vena cava and the gallbladder fossa. The caudate lobe is segment I. Segments II to IV are in the left lobe and segments

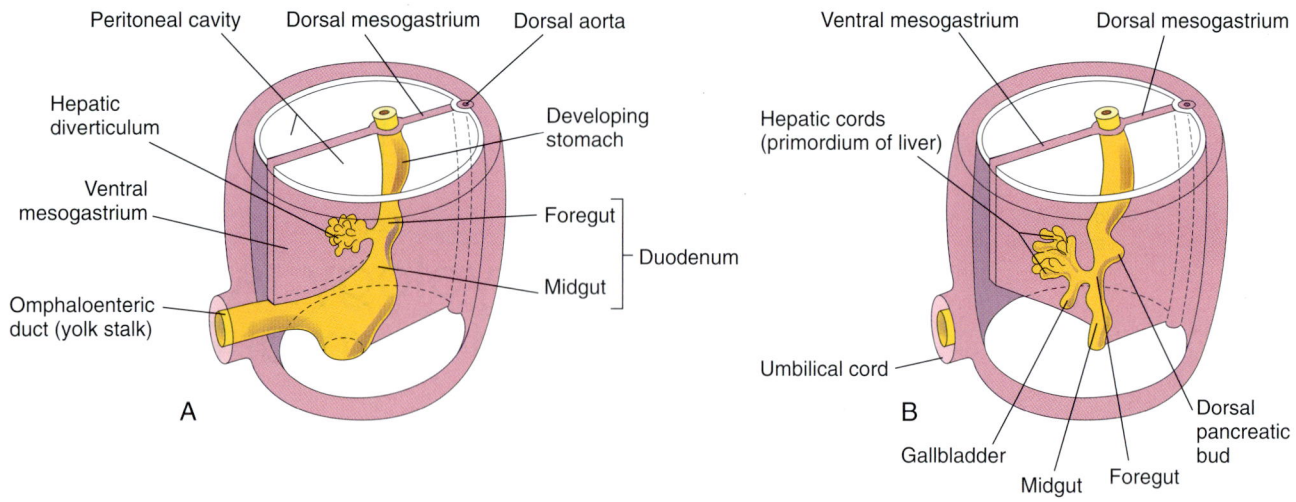

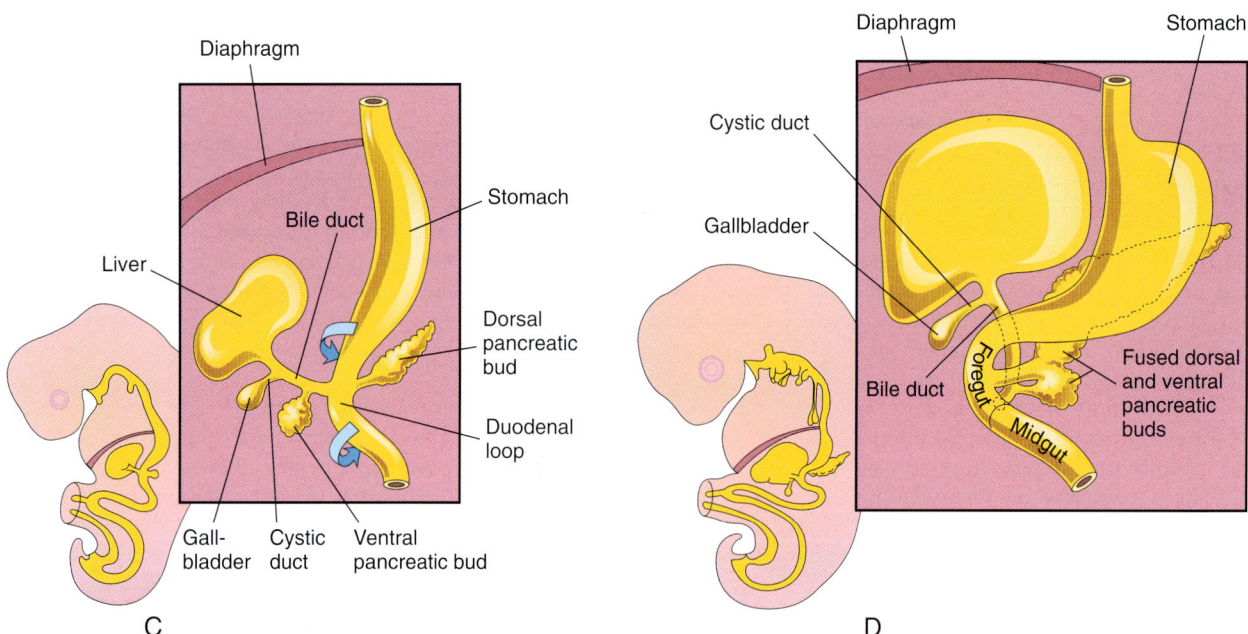

Figure 84-1 Schematic illustrations of hepatic embryology. **A,** Hepatic embryology at 4 weeks. **B** and **C,** Hepatic embryology at 5 weeks. **D,** Hepatic embryology at 6 weeks. Note hepatic diverticulum extending into the ventral mesentery and dividing into cranial (liver primordium) and caudal (gallbladder and common bile duct) buds. Also note that the entrance of the bile duct into the duodenum shifts gradually to a posterior position, which explains why the bile duct passes posterior to the duodenum. (From Moore KL, Persaud TVN. The digestive system. In: Moore KL, Persaud TVN, eds. *The developing human: clinically oriented embryology.* 8th ed. Philadelphia: WB Saunders; 2007.)

V to VIII are in the right lobe. The left hepatic vein divides the left lobe into posterior segment II and anterior segments III and IV; segments III and IV are separated by the umbilical fissure and falciform ligament. The right hepatic vein divides the right lobe into posterior segments VI and VII and anterior segments V and VIII. The superior segments (VII and VIII) are separated from the inferior segments (V and VI) by the right portal vein.

Spleen

The spleen begins to develop during the fifth week of gestation.[9,10] It is derived from a mass of mesenchymal cells in the dorsal mesogastrium that coalesce to form the spleen. Failure of these cells to fuse completely gives rise to accessory spleens, which are quite common. As the stomach's greater curvature rotates to the left, the spleen is carried with it into the left upper quadrant. It lies in a niche formed by the diaphragm, the stomach, the left kidney and adrenal gland, the phrenicocolic ligament, and the chest wall (Fig. 84-3). The splenic hilum is a depression along the medial surface through which the splenic artery, vein, and nerves pass. The two major ligaments that hold the spleen in place are the gastrosplenic and the splenorenal ligaments. Other ligaments that support the spleen are the splenophrenic, splenocolic, splenopancreatic, colophrenic, and pancreaticocolic ligaments.

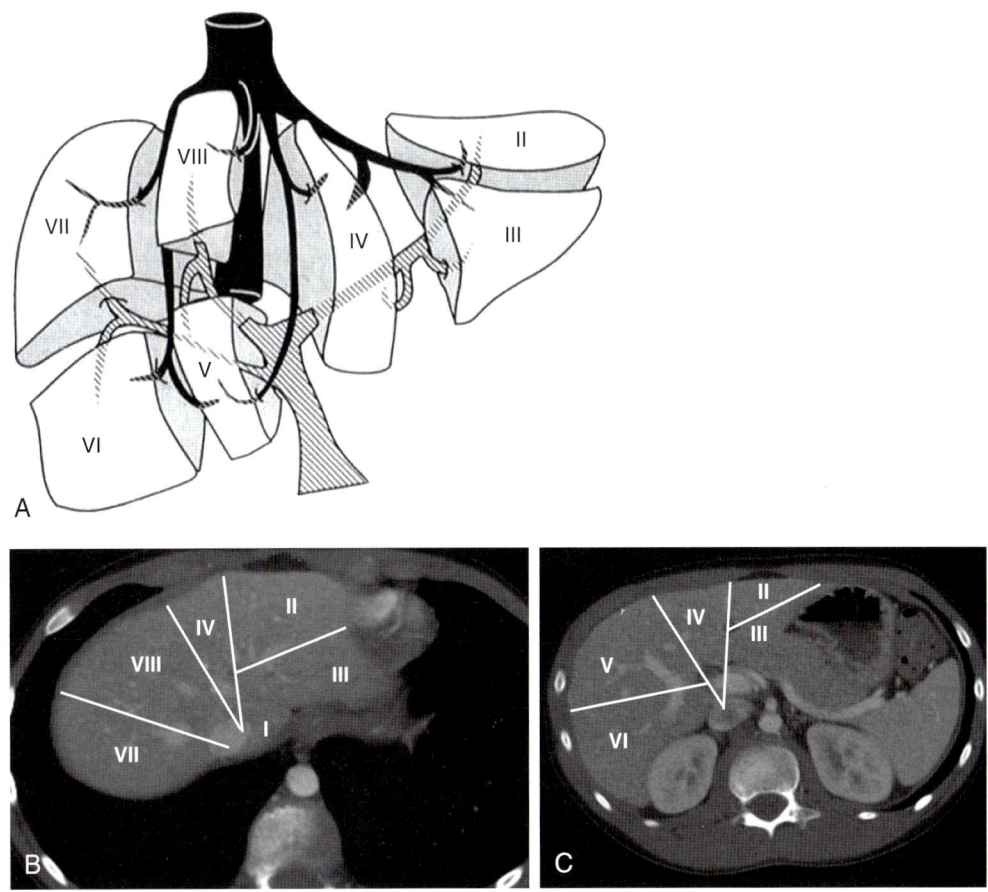

Figure 84-2 **A,** Schematic illustration of hepatic segmental anatomy according to Couinaud. Diagonally shaded vessels indicate the portal venous supply to each segment. Hepatic veins are solid black. Not shown are the bile ducts, which drain within the portal triads with the portal venous system and hepatic arteries. **B** and **C,** Segmental anatomy as seen on computed tomography. (**A,** From Gazelle GS, Lee MJ, Mueller PR. Cholangiographic segmental anatomy of the liver. *Radiographics.* 1994;14:1005. Reprinted with permission.)

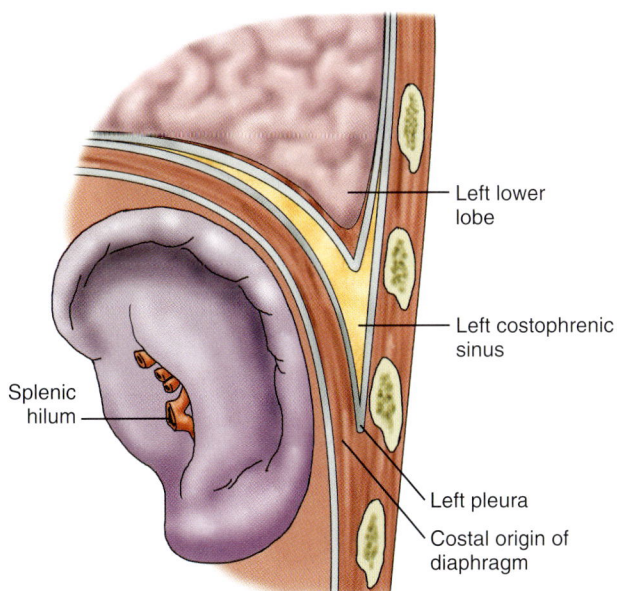

Figure 84-3 Location of the spleen. (From Skandalis JE, Gray SW, eds. *Embryology for surgeons.* 2nd ed. Baltimore: Williams & Wilkins; 1994.)

The embryonic spleen is a site of hematopoiesis in some mammalian species, such as rodents, but current evidence suggests that splenic hematopoiesis does not occur in the human fetus.[11] The spleen is an important lymphatic organ and plays a role in providing protection from infection caused by encapsulated organisms. Lymphocytes begin to appear in the spleen around 11 weeks of gestation. The spleen also filters damaged red blood cells and foreign particles and acts as a reservoir for platelets.

Pancreas

The development of the pancreas is closely related to duodenal development. The dorsal pancreatic bud arises from the dorsal side of the duodenum, and the ventral pancreatic bud arises from the liver diverticulum (Fig. 84-4).[12-14] The larger dorsal bud appears first and arises cranial to the smaller ventral bud. It will form the tail, body, and part of the head of the pancreas. The ventral bud develops at the site of entry of the common bile duct and forms part of the pancreatic head and the uncinate process. As the duodenal loop rotates, the ventral bud is carried dorsally to lie in a position posterior to the dorsal bud, with which it fuses. After fusion of the pancreatic buds, the duct systems anastomose. The main pancreatic duct is formed proximally from the ventral bud and the distal

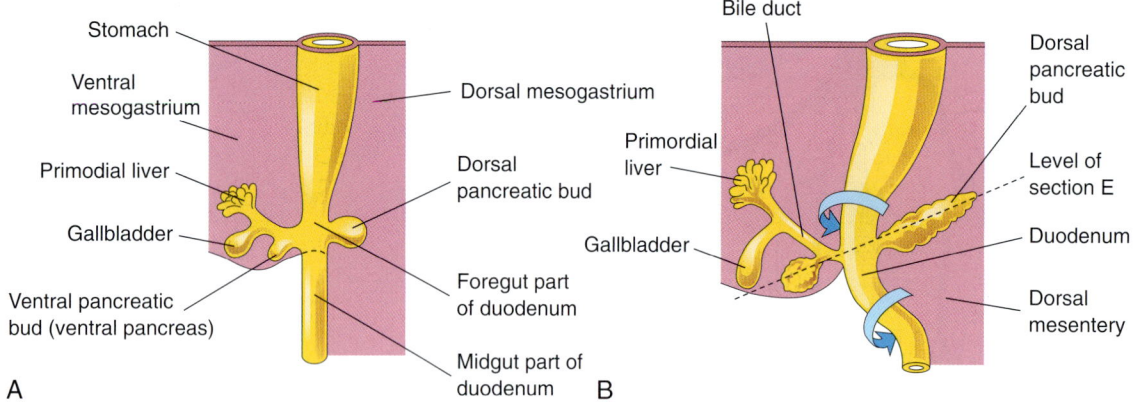

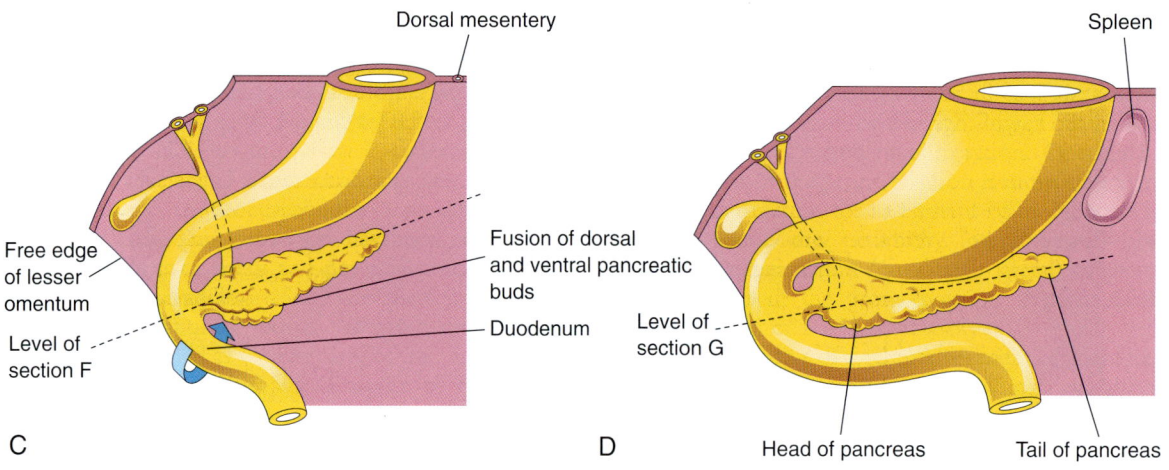

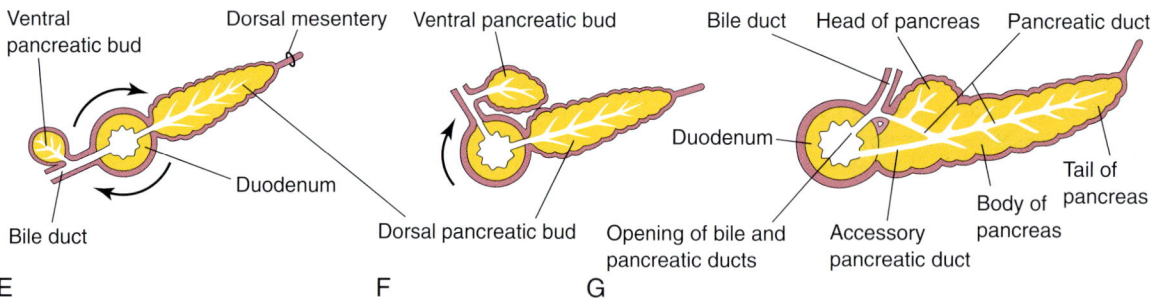

Figure 84-4 **A** to **D,** Illustrations of successive stages in the development of the pancreas from the fifth to the eighth weeks. **E** to **G,** Transverse sections through the duodenum and the developing pancreas. Growth and rotation (*arrows*) of the duodenum bring the ventral pancreatic bud toward the dorsal bud; these two structures subsequently fuse. Note that the bile duct initially attaches to the ventral aspect of the duodenum and is carried around to the dorsal aspect as the duodenum rotates. The pancreatic duct is formed by the union of the distal part of the dorsal pancreatic duct (duct of Santorini) and the entire ventral pancreatic duct (duct of Wirsung). The proximal part of the dorsal pancreatic duct usually is obliterated, but it may persist as an accessory pancreatic duct. (*From Moore KL, Persaud TVN. The alimentary or digestive system. In: Moore KL, Persaud TVN, eds. Before we are born: essentials of embryology and birth defects. 7th ed. Philadelphia: Saunders Elsevier; 2008.*)

portion is formed from the dorsal pancreatic bud. The proximal portion of the duct from the dorsal bud either disappears or persists as the accessory pancreatic duct. Islet cells appear at the end of the second month of gestation, and acinar cells develop during the third month. The islet cells secrete insulin, glucagon, somatostatin, and pancreatic polypeptide. Acinar cells produce digestive enzymes that are secreted into the second portion of the duodenum.

The pancreas lies horizontally in the retroperitoneum.[15] The head of the pancreas lies to the right of the midline in the curve of the duodenum. The uncinate process is an extension of gland substance at the junction of the inferior

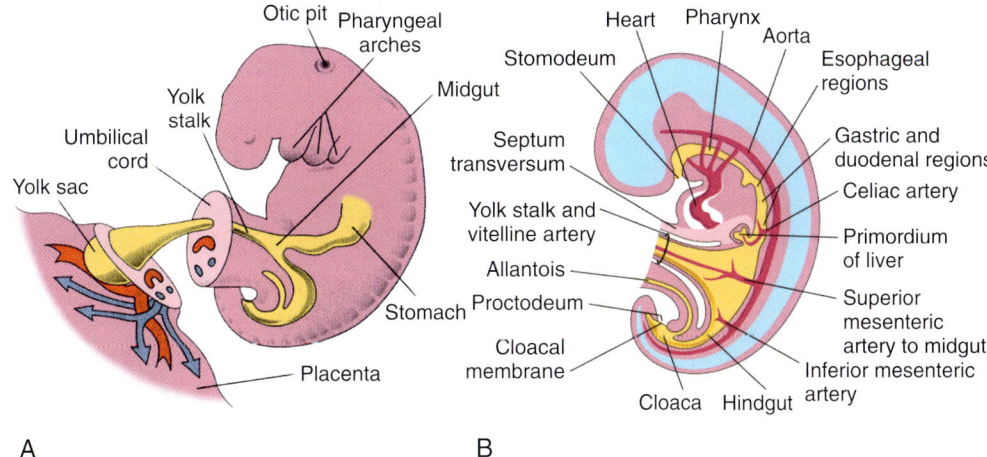

Figure 84-5 Early digestive tract. **A,** A lateral view of a 4-week embryo showing the relationship of the primordial gut to the yolk sac. **B,** A drawing of a median section of the embryo showing the early digestive system and its blood supply. The primordial gut is a long tube extending the length of the embryo. Its blood vessels are derived from the vessels that supplied the yolk sac. (**A,** Modified from Moore KL, Persaud TVN. The digestive system. In: Moore KL, Persaud TVN, eds. *Before we are born: essentials of embryology and birth defects.* 5th ed. Philadelphia: WB Saunders; 1998. **B,** From Moore KL, Persaud TVN, eds. *Before we are born: essentials of embryology and birth defects.* 7th ed. Philadelphia: Saunders Elsevier; 2007.)

and left margins of the pancreatic head. The anterior surface of the pancreatic head is in contact with the transverse colon, gastroduodenal artery, and several loops of small intestine. The posterior surface is adjacent to the inferior vena cava, common bile duct, renal veins, and abdominal aorta. The anterior surface of the uncinate process is in contact with the superior mesenteric artery and vein.

The pancreatic body is in contact with the stomach anteriorly and the posterior portion abuts the abdominal aorta, splenic vein, left kidney and adrenal gland, and the origin of the superior mesenteric artery. The small intestine lies inferior to the pancreatic body. The tail lies in contact with the gastric surface of the spleen and the splenic flexure of the colon. The tail may be more bulbous than the head or body in children and is narrower in adults.

Gastrointestinal Tract

The primitive gastrointestinal tract forms during the third to fourth week of gestation.[16-19] It is marked by the oropharyngeal membrane at the cranial end and the cloacal membrane caudally (Fig. 84-5). It is divided into three parts: the foregut, midgut, and hindgut. The foregut includes the esophagus, stomach, and proximal duodenum and receives most of its arterial supply from the celiac axis, with the exception of the esophagus, which is proximal to the lower esophageal sphincter. The midgut is supplied by the superior mesenteric artery and includes the distal duodenum, jejunum, ileum, cecum, appendix, ascending colon, and approximately two thirds of the transverse colon. The hindgut is supplied by the inferior mesenteric artery and comprises the remainder of the transverse colon, the descending and sigmoid colon, and the upper two thirds of the rectum.

Esophagus

The esophagus begins as a ventral diverticulum from the primitive foregut that will give rise to the trachea and the esophagus.[18-21] As this diverticulum elongates, a partition forms, the tracheoesophageal septum, which ultimately leads to separation of the esophagus from the trachea at 34 to 36 days of gestation. Elongation of the esophagus initially occurs cranially, and the relative final length of the esophagus is reached at 7 weeks. Epithelial proliferation with partial to complete obliteration of the esophageal lumen occurs, which normally recanalizes by the tenth week. The muscular coat of the esophagus is derived from the surrounding splanchnic mesenchyme. In the upper third of the esophagus, striated muscle is present that is innervated by the vagus nerve, whereas in the lower third, smooth muscle innervated by the splanchnic plexus is present.

The esophagus begins at the level of C7 and ends at the esophagogastric junction, which is usually at the T10–11 vertebral body level (Fig. 84-6). The caliber varies with peristaltic activity but is slightly narrower at both ends than along its intrathoracic course. Extrinsic impressions are caused by the aorta, the left mainstem bronchus, and the diaphragm (Fig. 84-7).

The esophageal mucosa normally has thin, smooth longitudinal folds that flatten when the esophagus is distended by gas or barium. When fully distended, the distal esophagus enlarges and forms a fusiform shape commonly termed the *esophageal vestibule* or *phrenic ampulla.* The upper margin of the vestibule is radiographically delineated by a transient contractile area that forms bilateral, semilunar indentations termed the *A ring, inferior esophageal sphincter,* or *Wolf ring.* The lower margin is also delineated by a transient contractile region termed the *B ring, transverse mucosal fold, lower esophageal ring, Schatzki ring,* or *lower esophageal diaphragm.* In young infants the vestibule spans the diaphragmatic hiatus so that the upper part lies within the thorax and the lower part lies within the abdomen.

Stomach

The stomach arises as a tubular dilatation at the distal end of the foregut at 4 to 5 weeks of gestation.[16,18,19,22] The dorsal

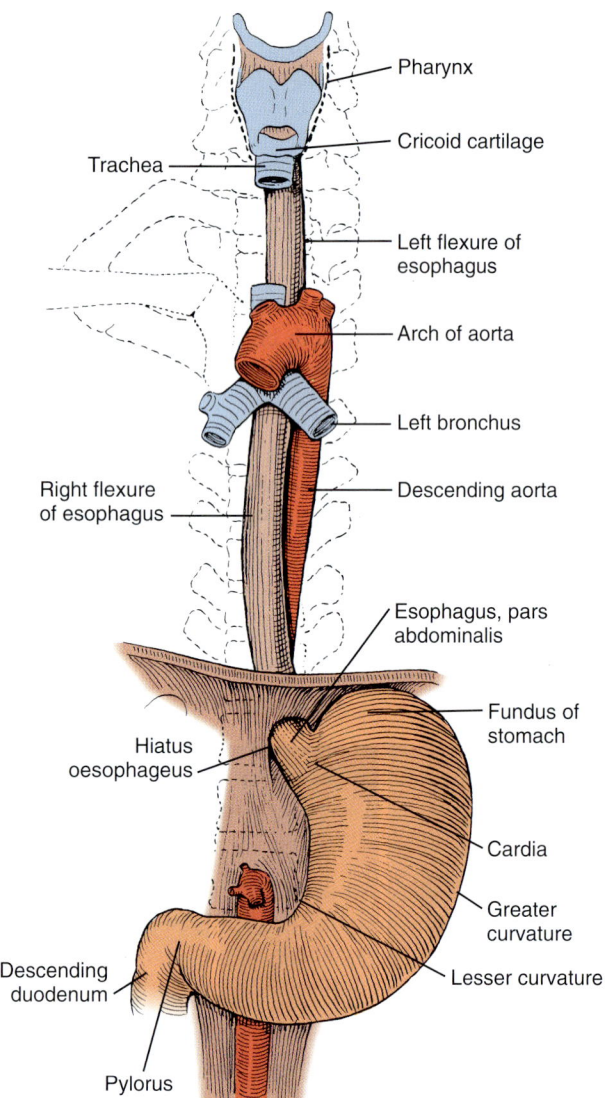

Figure 84-6 A semischematic drawing of the normal esophagus depicting its relation to the trachea, aorta, diaphragm, and stomach. (Modified from Schaegger JP. *Morris' human anatomy.* 10th ed. New York: McGraw-Hill; 1943. Reprinted with permission.)

border grows more rapidly than the ventral border, leading to a 90-degree clockwise rotation on its longitudinal axis. As a result, the dorsal border rotates to the left and becomes the greater curvature, whereas the ventral border rotates to the right and becomes the lesser curvature of the stomach. This process explains why the right vagus nerve innervates the posterior wall of the stomach and the left vagus nerve innervates the anterior surface.

The stomach lies below the left hemidiaphragm with its long axis transverse to the long axis of the body.[22] The stomach is relatively fixed proximally by the esophagogastric junction and distally by the fixed retroperitoneal position of the first portion of the duodenum. The stomach also is fixed to neighboring structures by four major peritoneal folds or ligaments: gastrophrenic, gastrohepatic, gastrosplenic, and gastrocolic ligaments.

The stomach is divided into four regions (Fig. 84-8). The cardia is a small, ill-defined area immediately adjacent to the

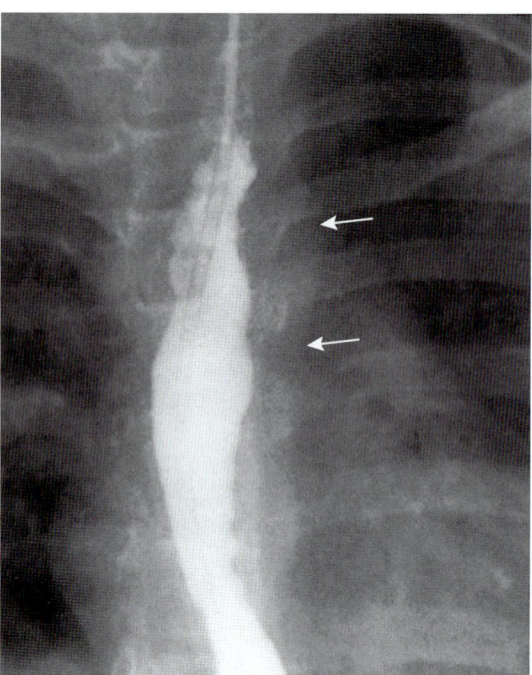

Figure 84-7 A barium swallow study demonstrates the impression of the aortic knob (*upper arrow*) and the left main stem bronchus (*lower arrow*) on the barium-filled esophagus. These impressions are normal and are not to be confused with mediastinal abnormalities.

esophagogastric junction and just to the left of the midline. The fundus is the most bulbous portion of the stomach. It projects upward, above the cardia and gastroesophageal junction, and is in contact with the left hemidiaphragm and the spleen. The body is the largest part of the stomach and is bounded by the greater and lesser curvatures. The incisura angularis, a sharp indentation two thirds of the distance down the lesser curvature, marks the beginning of the gastric antrum. The antrum extends to the junction of the pylorus with the duodenum. The normal size, shape, and position of the stomach vary with the volume of gastric content and the age of the individual. In infancy, the stomach is high and transverse, whereas in older children and adults it is more longitudinal and J-shaped.

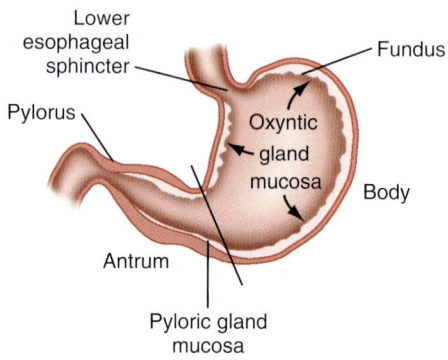

Figure 84-8 Anatomic regions of the stomach. (From Redel CA, Zwiener RJ. Anatomy and anomalies of the stomach and duodenum. In: Feldman L, Sleisenger MH, Scharschmidt BF, eds. *Gastrointestinal and liver disease.* 6th ed. Philadelphia: WB Saunders; 1998.)

Duodenum

The duodenum is derived from the caudal portion of the foregut and the cranial portion of the midgut.[16,18,19] The junction of these two parts is just distal to the common bile duct. The duodenal segment elongates rapidly, forming a C-shaped loop. As the stomach rotates, the duodenal loop rotates to the right, causing the duodenum to be pressed against the posterior abdominal wall, which leads to fusion and resorption of peritoneal layers such that the duodenum becomes a retroperitoneal structure. Because it is derived from both foregut and midgut, the duodenum receives its blood supply from both the celiac and superior mesenteric arteries. During the fifth and sixth weeks of development, the duodenal lumen is temporarily obliterated by proliferation of epithelial cells. Recanalization then occurs and usually is complete by the tenth week. Unlike the rest of the midgut, the duodenum does not herniate into the extraembryonic coelom.

The duodenum is the most proximal portion of the small intestine.[22] The first portion of the duodenum begins at the pylorus and ends at the neck of the gallbladder. It is loosely attached to the liver by the hepatoduodenal portion of the lesser omentum; the second, third, and fourth portions are retroperitoneal. The second or descending portion extends from the neck of the gallbladder and is in contact with the head of the pancreas. The common bile duct enters in its midportion. The third portion is horizontal and courses to the left across the midline, anterior to the spine, aorta, and inferior vena cava. Anteriorly, the third portion is covered by peritoneum and is crossed by the superior mesenteric artery and vein. The fourth portion ascends along the left side of the aorta and turns ventrally to become the jejunum at the level of the duodenojejunal flexure. The duodenojejunal flexure is retroperitoneal and is also fixed by the ligament of Treitz.

Midgut

The midgut is the portion of the gut that opens ventrally into the yolk sac.[16,19,23] It elongates rapidly so that, by the beginning of the sixth week, it forms a U-shaped ventral loop that projects into the extraembryonic coelom, creating a "physiologic" umbilical cord hernia. The stalk at the apex of the loop is the omphalomesenteric duct (Fig. 84-9). The midgut proximal to the apex of the loop is small bowel and the midgut distal to the apex is colon. During the sixth week of gestation, a diverticulum forms on the antimesenteric border of the distal portion of the midgut, which will give rise to the cecum and appendix. A Meckel's diverticulum is the result of persistence of the proximal portion of the omphalomesenteric duct. If this connection remains patent, it is known as an omphaloileal fistula.

While the bowel is in the extraembryonic coelom, it undergoes a 90-degree counterclockwise rotation around the superior mesenteric artery (see Fig. 84-9, B). During this rotation, the jejunum and ileum grow more rapidly than the colon; this rotation brings the proximal midgut (jejunum and ileum) to the right and the distal portion (large intestine) to the left. The bowel abruptly returns to the abdominal cavity at about 10 weeks of development (see Fig. 84-9, C and D).

The forces responsible for this sudden return are unknown. The small bowel enters first, passes posterior to the superior mesenteric artery, and ends up occupying the central part of the abdomen. As the large intestine returns to the abdominal cavity, it undergoes a 180-degree counterclockwise rotation, with the cecum ending up below the liver. Further growth of the ascending colon forces the cecum down into the right lower quadrant (see Fig. 84-9, E).

Fixation of the midgut begins during the twelfth week of gestation. The mesenteries of the ascending and descending colon fuse with the posterior abdominal wall and become retroperitoneal. As a result of the fusion of the mesenteries of the ascending and descending colon and of the duodenum to the posterior abdominal wall, the small bowel mesentery becomes fan shaped, with a broad-based attachment extending from the left upper quadrant to the right lower quadrant (Fig. 84-10). This broad attachment limits the mobility of the mesentery and prevents a midgut volvulus around the superior mesenteric artery. Failure of complete rotation (malrotation) leads to a narrow mesenteric pedicle, which, in conjunction with the lack of mesenteric attachments, may result in midgut volvulus.

Hindgut

The hindgut begins in the mid to distal transverse colon and terminates at the cloaca. The hindgut is supplied by the inferior mesenteric artery.[16,19,24] The watershed region between the superior and inferior mesenteric arteries is located in the mid to distal transverse colon.

Around day 13 of gestation, a ventral diverticulum of the hindgut, the allantois, forms. The hindgut distal to the allantois disappears around the sixth week of gestation (Fig. 84-11). The junction of the allantoic stalk and the hindgut is the site of the cloaca. The cloaca, which is lined with endoderm, is in direct contact with the ectodermally lined proctodeum (anal pit). The area of contact between these two surfaces is the cloacal membrane. A wedge of mesenchyme, the urorectal septum, develops in the angle between the allantois and the hindgut (see Fig. 84-11, C and D). As the urorectal septum grows toward the cloacal membrane, it produces infoldings of the lateral walls of the cloaca. These folds grow toward each other and fuse, forming a partition that divides the cloaca into two parts: the rectum and upper anal canal dorsally and the urogenital sinus ventrally. The area of fusion of the urorectal septum with the cloacal membrane forms the perineal body. The anal membrane ruptures at the end of the eighth week, allowing the intestinal tract to communicate with the amniotic cavity. Transient occlusion of the colon occurs between the fifth and eighth weeks of gestation. After return of the intestine to the abdominal cavity, the mesentery of the descending colon fuses with the left posterior abdominal wall.

Normal Anatomy of the Small Intestine

The small intestine is a tubular structure within the abdominal cavity that is located between the stomach and the colon[25]

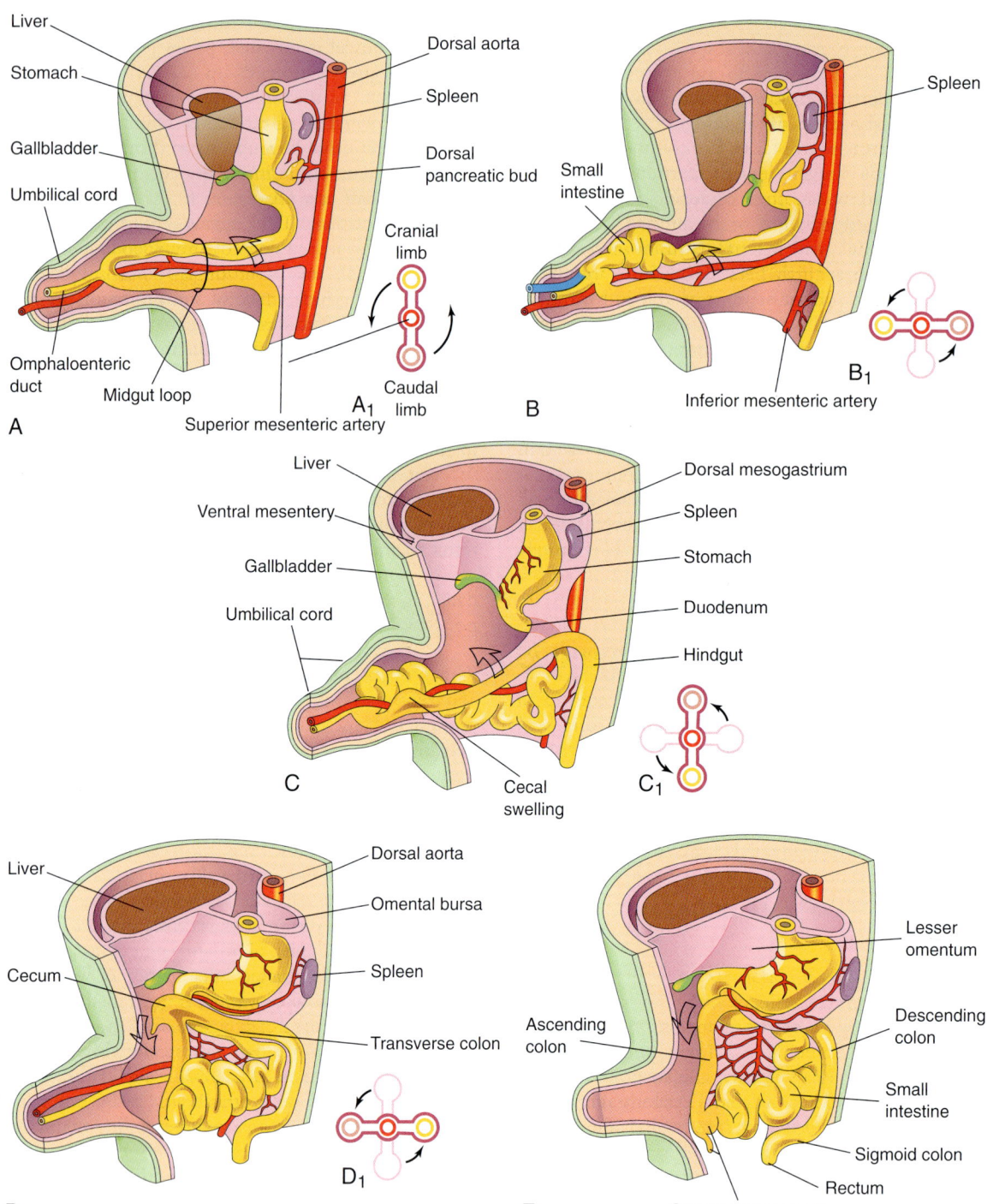

Figure 84-9   Illustrations of the rotation of the midgut, as seen from the left. **A,** During the sixth week, the midgut loop is situated in the proximal part of the umbilical cord. **A₁,** Transverse section through the midgut loop, showing the initial relationship of the limbs of the midgut loop to the superior mesenteric artery. **B,** A later stage, showing the beginning of midgut rotation. **B₁,** Illustration of the 90-degree counterclockwise rotation that carries the cranial limb of the midgut to the right. **C,** At approximately 10 weeks, the intestines return to the abdomen. **C₁,** Illustration of a further rotation of 90 degrees. **D,** By approximately 11 weeks, all of the intestines return to the abdomen. **D₁,** A further 90-degree rotation of the gut, for a total of 270 degrees. **E,** The later fetal period showing the cecum rotating to its normal position in the lower right quadrant of the abdomen. (From Moore KL, Persaud TVN. The alimentary or digestive system. In: Moore KL, Persaud TVN, eds. *Before we are born: essentials of embryology and birth defects.* 7th ed. Philadelphia: Saunders Elsevier; 2008.)

and consists of the duodenum, jejunum, and ileum. The length of the small intestine increases from approximately 200 cm at birth to 6 m in the adult.

The anatomy of the duodenum is discussed earlier in this chapter. Jejunum comprises the proximal two fifths of the small bowel; the remainder is ileum, although no morphologic demarcation exists between the two segments. The jejunum and ileum are suspended by a broad-based mesentery attached to the posterior peritoneal wall and thus are freely mobile within the abdominal cavity, although secured at both ends. The proximal third of the small bowel occupies the left upper quadrant, the middle third is in the midportion of the abdomen and right upper quadrant, and the distal third lies on the right side of the abdomen and pelvis. The caliber of the small intestine tapers as it progresses distally, with the diameter of the terminal ileum being about one third smaller than the first portion of the jejunum. The external surface is smooth while the internal surface has transverse and spiral folds that are covered by villi. The jejunum has more visible folds than the ileum (Fig. 84-12).

Normal Anatomy of the Colon

The colon extends from the ileocecal valve to the anus and is divided into the ascending, transverse, descending, and sigmoid portions and the anus (Fig. 84-13).[25] In the newborn it is 30 to 40 cm long, and it reaches 1.5 m in length in the adult. The cecum is the beginning of the ascending colon; it lies in the right lower quadrant, although it often is higher in infants, in whom it may be located above the iliac crest. The appendix is a blind outpouching of the cecum.

The ascending colon, which is retroperitoneal, extends upward along the right side of the peritoneal cavity to the underside of the liver. The colon turns medially at the hepatic flexure and emerges into the peritoneal cavity as the transverse colon. It courses right to left to reach its highest point in the left upper quadrant at the splenic flexure. The transverse colon is suspended by the mesocolon and is freely mobile. At the splenic flexure the colon again becomes retroperitoneal and turns caudally to become the descending colon, running along the left lateral abdominal wall to the pelvic brim. At this point it emerges into the peritoneal cavity as the sigmoid colon. The sigmoid colon is an S-shaped, redundant segment of variable length. The narrowest portion of the colon is in the sigmoid segment. In children the sigmoid colon tends to extend upward, and it is not unusual for the apex of the sigmoid to extend to the right upper quadrant. The rectum begins at the peritoneal reflection and follows the curve of the sacrum, ending at the anal canal. The distal one third of the rectum is retroperitoneal.

Key Points

The liver is the largest of the abdominal organs.

The embryonic spleen is not a site of hematopoiesis in the human fetus.

The gastrointestinal tract begins to form during the third week of gestation.

The foregut receives blood supply from the celiac axis, the midgut from the superior mesenteric artery, and the hindgut from the inferior mesenteric artery.

The midgut returns to the abdominal cavity from the extraembryonic coelom between the tenth and eleventh weeks of gestation.

Normal rotation of the bowel leads to a broad based mesentery with proximal and distal attachments; incomplete rotation (malrotation) leads to a narrow mesentery without attachments and therefore is conducive to midgut volvulus.

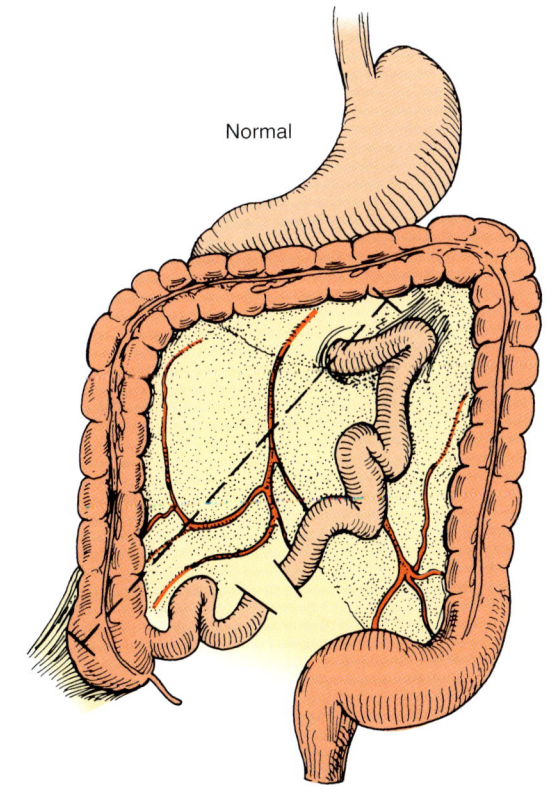

Normal

Figure 84-10 Normal rotation and fixation of the midgut. Note the broad-based fixation between the left upper and right lower quadrants, which fixes the superior mesenteric artery so it cannot be the "root" of a volvulus. (From Ross AJ III. Organogenesis, innervation, and histologic development of the gastrointestinal tract. In: Polin RA, Fox WW, eds. *Fetal and neonatal physiology.* 2nd ed. Philadelphia: WB Saunders; 1998.)

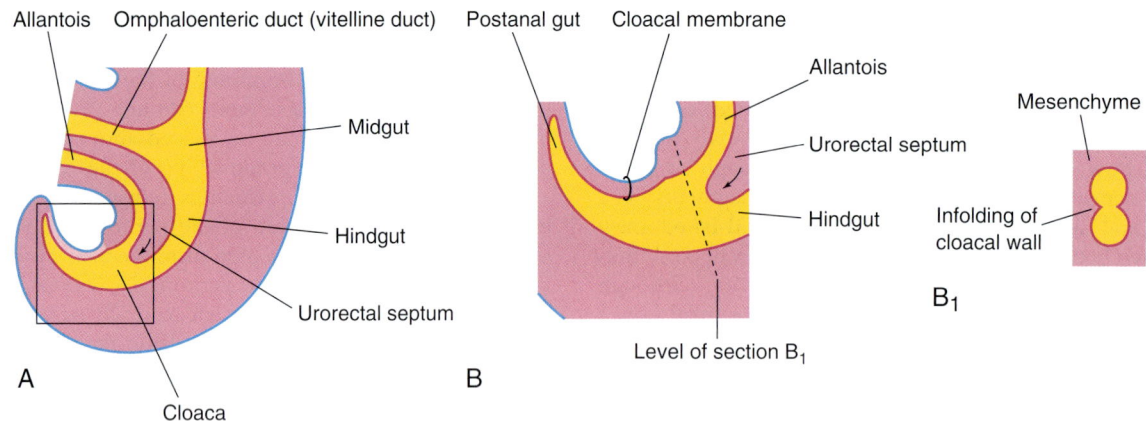

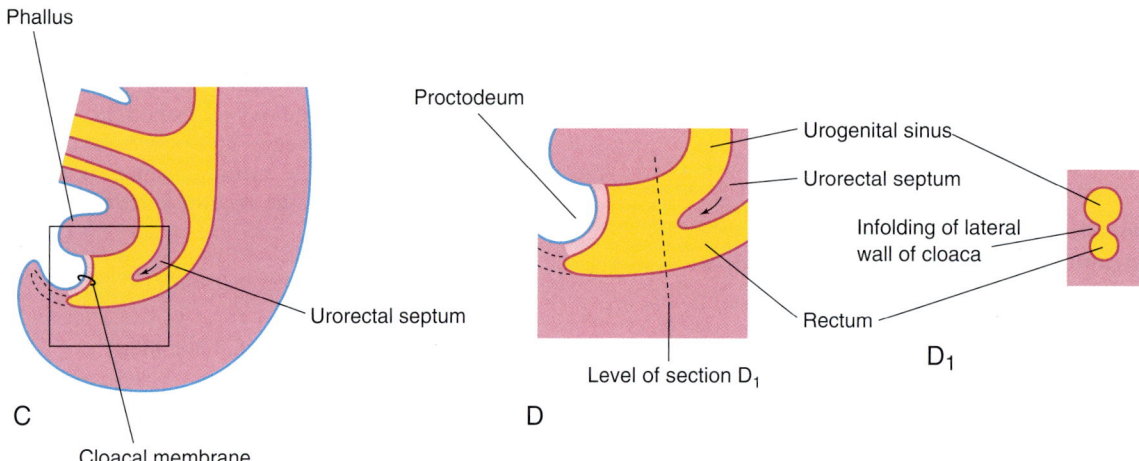

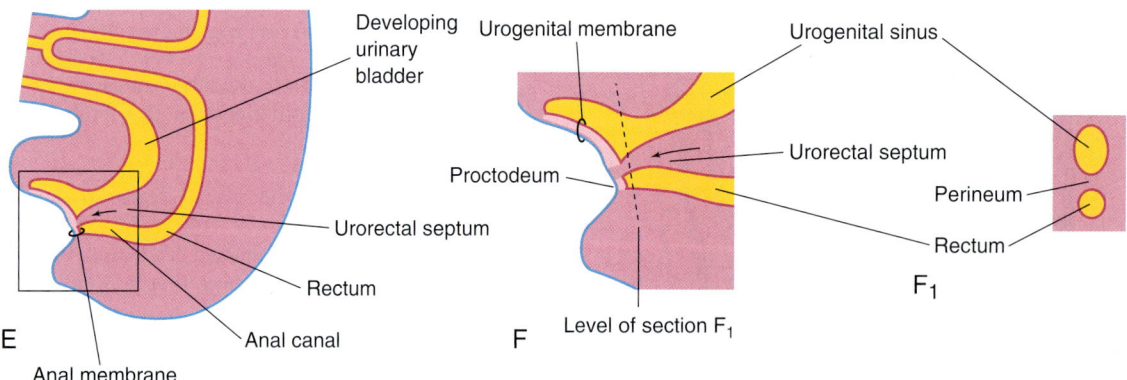

Figure 84-11 Illustrations of successive stages in the partitioning of the cloaca into the urogenital sinus and the rectum by the urorectal septum. **A, C,** and **E,** Views from the left side at 4, 6, and 7 weeks, respectively. **B, D,** and **F,** Enlargements of the cloacal region. **B₁, D₁,** and **F₁,** Transverse sections of the cloaca at the levels shown in **B, D,** and **F,** respectively. Note that the postanal gut, or tailgut (shown in **B**), degenerates and disappears as the rectum forms from the dorsal part of the cloaca (shown in **C**). The arrows indicate the growth of the urorectal septum. (From Moore KL, Persaud TVN. The alimentary or digestive system. In: Moore KL, Persaud TVN, eds. *Before we are born: essentials of embryology and birth defects.* 7th ed. Philadelphia: Saunders Elsevier; 2008.)

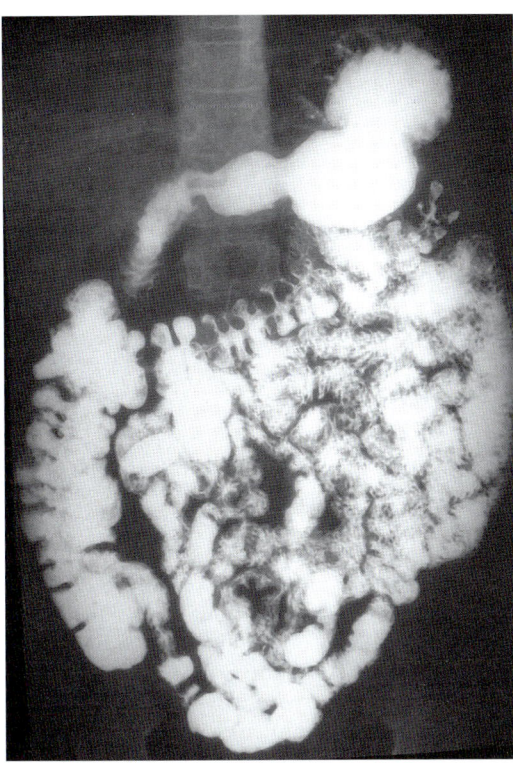

Figure 84-12 Normal small intestine. An overhead radiograph from an upper gastrointestinal series with small bowel follow-through shows contrast in the stomach, duodenum, jejunum, ileum, and ascending portion of the colon. The jejunal loops in the left upper quadrant have normal visible folds, and the ileum is relatively featureless.

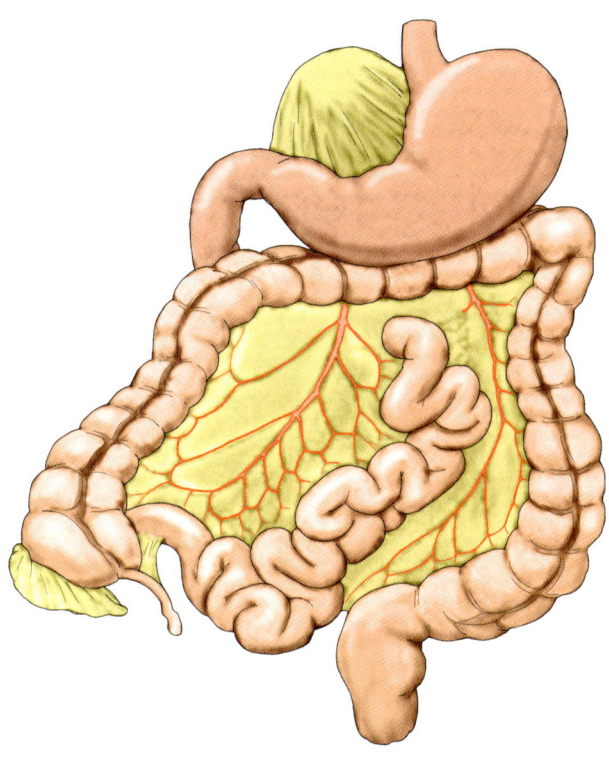

Figure 84-13 Schematic figure of a normal colon framing the peritoneal cavity and small bowel, from the cecum in the right lower quadrant, through hepatic and splenic flexures, to the sigmoid and rectum. (From Hernanz-Schulman M. Imaging of neonatal gastrointestinal obstruction. *Radiol Clin North Am.* 1999;37:1163-1186.)

Suggested Readings

Moore KL, Persaud TVN. *Before we are born: essentials of embryology and birth defects*. 7th ed. Philadelphia: Saunders; 2008.

O'Rahilly R, Müller F. *Human embryology & teratology*. 2nd ed. New York: Wiley-Liss; 1996.

Polin RA, Fox WW, Abman SG, eds. *Fetal and neonatal physiology*. 3rd ed. Philadelphia: Saunders; 2004.

Sadler TW. *Langman's medical embryology*. 8th ed. Philadelphia: Lippincott Williams & Wilkins; 2000.

Skandalis JE, Gray SW, eds. *Embryology for surgeons*. 2nd ed. Baltimore: Williams & Wilkins; 1994.

References

Full references for this chapter can be found on www.expertconsult.com.

Chapter 85

Imaging Techniques

MARTA HERNANZ-SCHULMAN, STEPHANIE E. SPOTTSWOOD, and
SHREYAS S. VASANAWALA

When the first edition of Caffey's classic textbook of pediatric radiology was published in 1945, its title was *Caffey's Pediatric X-ray Diagnosis*, denoting the single modality available at the time. In the intervening seven decades, 11 additional editions of the book have been published, and the title has changed to *Caffey's Pediatric Diagnostic Imaging* to reflect the diversity of tools now accessible to the pediatric radiologist. Indeed, technology has accelerated at an increasing rate, paralleling a continuing change in the capabilities and applications of existing modalities. This expansion has been coupled with increasing awareness of safety and potential stochastic effects of radiation, further adding to the complexity of choosing and implementing optimal pediatric imaging strategies. This short review is intended as an overview of the various modalities as applied to the diagnostic imaging of the pediatric gastrointestinal (GI) tract.

Plain Films and Fluoroscopy

OVERVIEW

Evaluation of the GI system includes the hollow viscera (from the esophagus to the rectum); solid viscera (the liver, spleen, and pancreas); and the peritoneal cavity and retroperitoneal spaces, in which all entities are contained. Although considerable overlap can exist among various modalities and newer applications continue to be defined, plain films usually are the initial imaging modality used in assessment of the GI system.

Chest radiographs can point out some abnormalities of the esophagus, such as achalasia and, notably, esophageal atresia, which requires no further imaging for diagnosis. Abdominal radiographs can assess calcifications, which would be expected in cases of meconium peritonitis or can be present in abdominal masses such as a hepatoblastoma or in persons with appendicitis. Intramural air, free intraperitoneal air, portal venous air, and the double bubble sign of duodenal atresia are identified on plain films and point to the correct diagnosis in the appropriate clinical setting. Inflammatory conditions such as Crohn disease may be suspected by assessing the gas pattern. Dilated bowel loops typically direct the radiologist toward consideration of an ileus pattern or obstruction. In such cases, decubitus views and prone cross-table lateral views of the rectum can help differentiate between these possibilities and direct further diagnostic imaging.

Air is the inherent contrast medium in plain film diagnosis, and the abdominal series is based on distribution and movement of gas. The basic plain film evaluation typically consists of supine and horizontal-beam images. Left-side-down decubitus and upright views are used for evaluation of free intraperitoneal air and air-fluid levels. The left-side-down decubitus view further directs air toward the right colon for evaluation of the right lower quadrant and into the rectum for evaluation of obstruction. Obtaining a film with the patient in the prone position is more effective in directing gas to the rectum for assessment of its caliber when concern exists about the possibility of a bowel obstruction; a horizontal-beam film (cross-table lateral) of the rectum with the patient in the prone position is particularly helpful in these cases.

The mainstay of further assessment of suspected pathology of the hollow viscera remains fluoroscopy, although sonography, computed tomography (CT), scintigraphy, and, increasingly, magnetic resonance imaging (MRI) also are applicable and will be discussed later in this chapter. To limit the radiation dose, fluoroscopy should be intermittent; pulsed fluoroscopic techniques can decrease the radiation dose substantially without loss of clinical information.[1,2] Capture and storage of the fluoroscopic images can be used liberally to document such findings as viscus distension, course of contrast, and peristaltic activity, with spot films reserved for areas in which greater anatomic detail is of diagnostic importance, such as mucosal abnormalities and potential perforation with contrast leaks.

Fluoroscopic studies typically require use of enteric contrast material for diagnosis.[3,4] Barium, an inert substance that is not absorbed, remains the primary contrast medium used in fluoroscopic procedures, whether it is administered orally to evaluate the esophagus and upper GI tract or rectally in a contrast enema. Several barium preparations are available; barium sulfate powder (96% wt/wt) can be diluted with sterile water for infant upper GI examinations to the desired concentration of 40% to 60% wt/vol. Premixed suspensions (60% wt/vol) can be used in older children, adolescents, and adults. Enema kits containing 97% barium wt/wt can be mixed with water to a final concentration of 15% to 33% barium wt/vol for infants, older children, and adolescents. Although adverse reactions to barium products are rare—reportedly 2 per million or less[5]—they do occur and may present as a rash, loss of consciousness, and anaphylaxis, typically related to any one of several additives, such as methylparaben and carboxymethylcellulose.[5-7] Aspiration of barium in small quantities is tolerated, but aspiration of a large volume of barium can be fatal.[8,9]

Table 85-1

Commonly Used Types of Contrast Media in Fluoroscopy of the Gastrointestinal Tract

Contrast Medium	Organically Bound Iodine (mg/mL)	Osmolality (mOsm/kg)	Viscosity (37°C)	Comments
High Osmolar, Ionic				
Gastrografin (meglumine diatrizoate and diatrizoate sodium)	367	1600		Potential for aspiration, dehydration, precarious electrolyte balance; may cause problems if patient has an underlying bowel injury
Conray 30 (iothalamate meglumine)	141	600	1.5	Lower gastrointestinal tract
Low Osmolar, Nonionic				
Omnipaque (iohexol)				
140	140	322	1.5	Young infants
180	180	408	2	Infants and young children
240	240	520	3.4	Young children or ostomy evaluations
300	300	672	6.3	Not used
350	350	844	10.4	Not used

Data from package inserts.

Barium is contraindicated in cases in which viscus perforation is suspected. In such cases, a low-osmolality, nonionic, water-soluble iodinated medium such as iohexol is used (Table 85-1). It is important that hypertonic media such as ionic or high-osmolality media (e.g., diatrizoate or iothalamate) not be used orally because of the risk of aspiration and consequent pulmonary edema.[10-12]

Gastrografin (diatrizoate meglumine and diatrizoate sodium) is an ionic, markedly hypertonic iodine solution with an osmolality (mOsm/kg) of approximately 1600; a 1:5 dilution approximates serum osmolality (285) but also dilutes the iodine concentration. Ionic hyperosmolar media can be absorbed from the GI tract and thus pose a risk in patients with a history of hypersensitivity, particularly to iodine, and potentially in patients with thyroid disease. Hyperosmolar media cause severe pulmonary complications of edema and pneumonitis if aspirated and can cause major fluid shifts into the bowel lumen, leading to a decrease in intravascular volume, an increase in serum osmolarity, and a decrease in cardiac output. In patients with underlying bowel disease, additional injury is possible.[13,14]

Omnipaque (iohexol) is a nonionic water-soluble iodinated contrast medium that is available in concentrations of 140, 180, 240, 300, and 350 mg of iodine. It is poorly absorbed from the intact GI tract, with renal excretion of 0.1% to 0.5% of the administered dose. Isovue (iopamidol) also has been used in the evaluation of the pediatric GI tract, but currently only Omnipaque is officially approved for this purpose. It must be emphasized that the osmolality of both of these media is greater than that of blood and that no agent is safe in the tracheobronchial tree, and thus great care and close fluoroscopic monitoring is necessary in all patients in whom aspiration is a potential complication.[15]

Barium is the standard agent used in the evaluation of the colon. However, in cases of potential perforation, water-soluble agents are used and can be diluted to approximate the tonicity of serum. Higher osmolality contrast media are used rectally for therapeutic purposes in cases of uncomplicated meconium ileus after diagnosis with a low-osmolarity agent. Gastrografin (diatrizoate meglumine and diatrizoate sodium)

was the original agent described for this purpose.[16] However, this agent can be associated with large fluid shifts and systemic complications in severely ill infants.[13] Full-strength iothalamate meglumine 30% also can be used successfully for this purpose. Close attention to water and electrolyte balance, along with surgical standby, are mandatory.

Air also can be used during fluoroscopic procedures. For example, air provides an excellent way to distend a viscus during fluoroscopic transpyloric tube placement without obscuring the tube or adjacent bowel loops, and it is the preferred agent in the reduction of intussusception.

Specific procedures are outlined in the following sections, and indications and imaging protocols are discussed.

INDICATIONS AND PROTOCOLS

Esophagram and Upper gastrointestinal Series

An esophagram and an upper GI series usually are performed in conjunction and include evaluation of swallowing, along with evaluation of the esophagus, stomach, and duodenum to the duodenojejunal junction. Common indications include evaluation of esophageal problems, such as complications of esophageal atresia repair, postoperative strictures or acute postoperative leaks, radiolucent foreign bodies such as impacted food, and the degree and efficacy of peristalsis. This examination is *not* indicated to diagnose esophageal atresia in most cases, because a chest radiograph with use of a coiled enteric tube typically is diagnostic, and the study may lead to unintended aspiration. Evaluation of the stomach in young infants includes assessment of gastric emptying as well as evaluation of the mucosa and focal lesions such as gastric duplication cysts. Evaluation of the duodenum is crucial in pediatric patients to document normal intestinal rotation. Small bowel follow-through has been largely supplanted by cross-sectional imaging in the diagnosis and monitoring of inflammatory bowel disease and therefore is undertaken much less frequently than in years past.

The examination is begun in the lateral projection, with the child lying on his or her left side to maintain the ingested contrast agent within the fundus of the stomach. Images of the esophagus are obtained from the nasopharynx to the esophagogastric junction, with special attention paid to nasopharyngeal aspiration, tracheal aspiration, masses, fistulas, and esophageal peristalsis and distensibility. The child is then laid supine, and the esophagus is examined in the anteroposterior projection. When the evaluation of the esophagus is completed, the barium in the fundus will be directed into the duodenum by turning the child into the prone right anterior oblique position. Gastric emptying is assessed, along with distensibility of the antrum, pylorus, duodenal bulb, and descending duodenum. Once the contrast material has reached the junction of second and third portions of the duodenum, the child is quickly placed in the supine position for assessment of the duodenojejunal junction, which is visible through the air-filled antrum. The duodenojejunal junction should lie to the left of the spine, at approximately the same level as the duodenal bulb. Once this assessment is accomplished, the child is quickly turned again, this time for a lateral projection to document the posterior course of the ascending and descending limbs of the normally rotated retroperitoneal duodenum. Evaluation for reflux can be performed after this portion of the study, if desired, or this can be done through other means such as scintigraphy or esophageal probe. A final image documents gastric emptying (Fig. 85-1).

A small bowel follow-through procedure usually requires ingestion of a larger amount of a contrast agent, typically barium, although in premature infants one can use a nonionic water-soluble contrast agent. Radiographs are obtained at regular intervals based on the course of the contrast medium through the bowel loops, with fluoroscopic evaluation as needed. Images of the terminal ileum with and without compression are obtained once the contrast has reached the cecum. In ill infants in the neonatal intensive care unit who do not require visualization of the ligament of Treitz, a "portable" small bowel follow-through procedure can be done, with the contrast material administered at the bedside and portable radiographs obtained at the appropriate intervals.

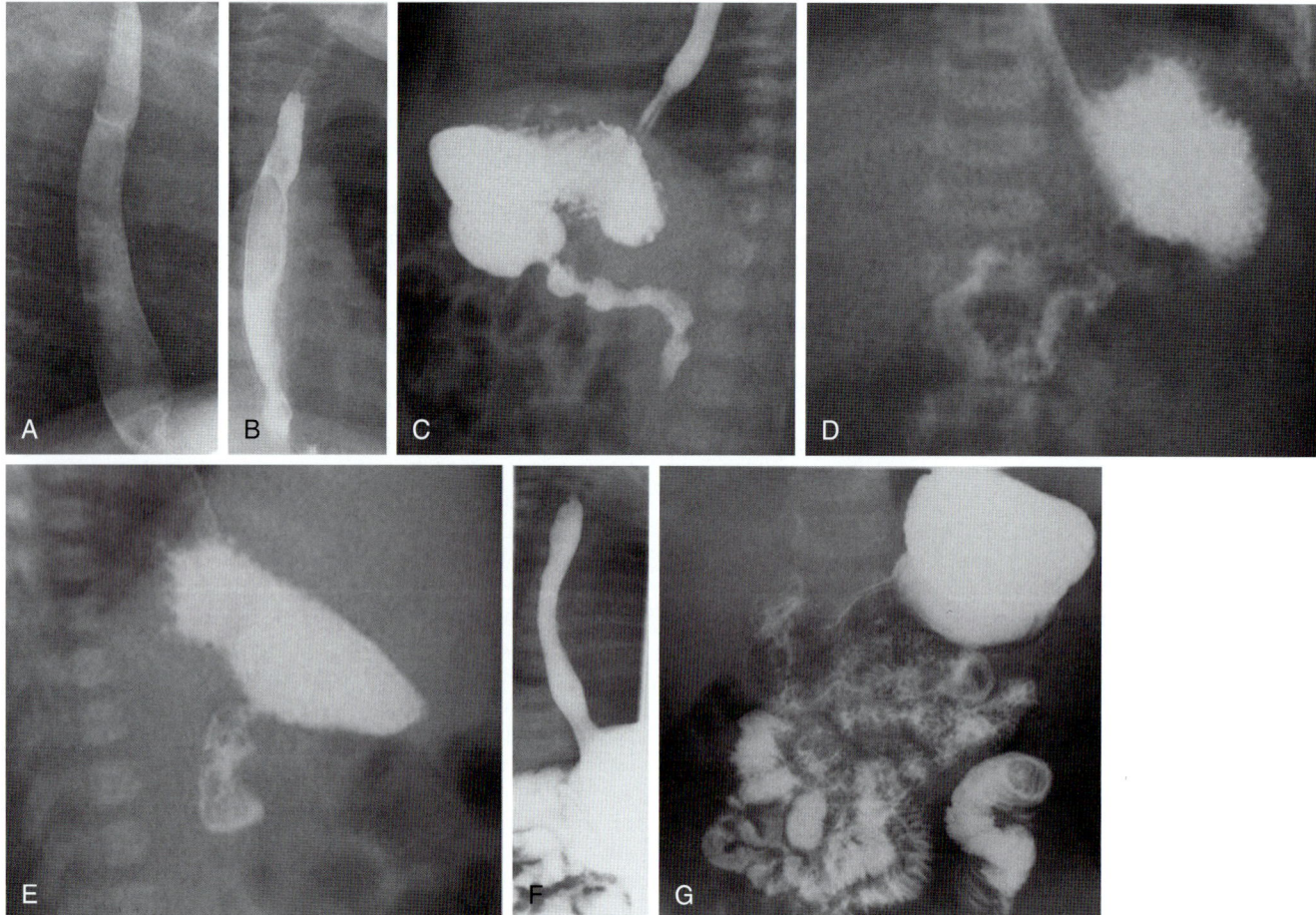

Figure 85-1   Typical upper gastrointestinal series showing reflux in otherwise healthy infant. **A** and **B,** Lateral and anteroposterior views of the esophagus during drinking show full distensibility without intrinsic or extrinsic mass lesions. **C,** Oblique imaging (right anterior oblique) directs ingested contrast material to the gastric outlet and shows prompt emptying and a normal pylorus and first and second portions of the duodenum. **D,** An anteroposterior image immediately following **C** shows progress of contrast material to the normally located gastroduodenal junction at the ligament of Treitz. **E,** A subsequent lateral view of the duodenum shows the posterior retroperitoneal location of parallel ascending and descending limbs. **F,** After further drinking and gastric filling, an episode of reflux to the cervical esophagus is documented. Note the wide open gastroesophageal junction, a typical appearance during reflux. **G,** An image recorded at the completion of the study shows good progress of contrast material through the small bowel.

Contrast Enema

Although contrast enema has been superseded by other procedures (such as endoscopy) for previous indications (such as polyp identification), this examination remains extremely useful in many pediatric clinical settings, such as evaluation of distal bowel obstruction in the neonate, evaluation of complications of surgery or of disease such as necrotizing enterocolitis, and reduction of ileocolic intussusception.

The choice of contrast medium and the technique used for the contrast enema vary with the indication for the procedure, as previously discussed. Barium typically is used unless a perforation is suspected, in which case an iso-osmolal water-soluble medium is used. In newborns suspected of having distal bowel obstruction, an iso-osmolal water-soluble medium is used, and changed to a hyperosmolal medium is used as a therapeutic option if meconium ileus is encountered. Air is the contrast of choice in patients with intussusception during fluoroscopic reduction.

A catheter with a small tip is placed in the rectum and secured with tape to both buttocks, which are then taped together using manual pressure. Use of a balloon-tipped catheter is usually unnecessary and, we believe, inadvisable in young infants because of the potential for rectal injury. Fluoro-grab images can be recorded liberally to document the progression of contrast material and to document findings; spot filming is needed in areas in which increased detail is important, such as mucosal abnormalities or if a subtle leak or perforation is encountered.

Sonography

OVERVIEW

Sonography has become an extraordinarily useful modality in the evaluation of patients with GI symptoms. In addition to the availability of spectral as well as frequency shift and amplitude color Doppler imaging, advances with newer equipment include recording of motion cine images, harmonic imaging, extended field-of-view imaging, and three-dimensional (3D) capability.

INDICATIONS AND PROTOCOLS

The utility and application of sonography in pediatric patients is extensive. The major advantage of sonography over CT is the obvious lack of ionizing radiation, but other very important advantages include the lack of need for sedation, and the multiplanar imaging capabilities. In general, scanning should be performed with the transducer that has the highest frequency necessary to penetrate the anatomy to be imaged and that will allow optimal spatial resolution; linear transducers are preferred if the access window will allow it. Curved array transducers allow a broader field of view; sector transducers may be necessary when the access window is limited or to image deeper structures in larger patients.

The primary role of sonography in the diagnosis of pyloric stenosis has become firmly established. Sonography is also extremely useful in the assessment of patients with clinically equivocal symptoms of appendicitis, although this setting punctuates its well-known operator dependence (e-Fig. 85-2), with published sensitivities ranging between 40% and 100%.[17-19] Sonography also is extremely useful in the evaluation of mesenteric adenopathy (e-Fig. 85-3), in highly detailed assessment of the bowel wall (Fig. 85-4),[20] in evaluation of small and large bowel intussusception (e-Fig. 85-5),[21] and coupled with Doppler, in the effective estimation of disease activity in patients with Crohn disease.[22]

The role of sonography in the diagnosis of solid organ pathology is likewise extensive and can be the final diagnostic tool for many abnormalities. Sonographic detail is particularly well visualized in young children, in whom high frequency and linear transducers can be used to access even the deeper abdominal structures. Indications include evaluation of biliary tract abnormalities, such as choledochal cysts, although additional imaging may be performed with MR depending on the specific clinical circumstances. Sonography may be performed as the initial modality to investigate suspected liver masses, and any subsequent CT or MRI protocols can be tailored on the basis of sonographic findings.

Although vascular structures are seen easily with contrast-enhanced CT, the direction and velocity of flow can be evaluated with Doppler sonography. Analysis of waveform pattern can identify hepatofugal flow in collateral vessels in patients with portal hypertension, along with vascular stenosis or thrombus. In patients with heterotaxy, abdominal sonography is helpful in assessing a splenic mass (located along the greater curvature of the stomach) and the associated vascular anomalies, such as interruption of the inferior vena cava, a preduodenal portal vein, and infradiaphragmatic total anomalous pulmonary venous connection[23,24] (e-Fig. 85-6).

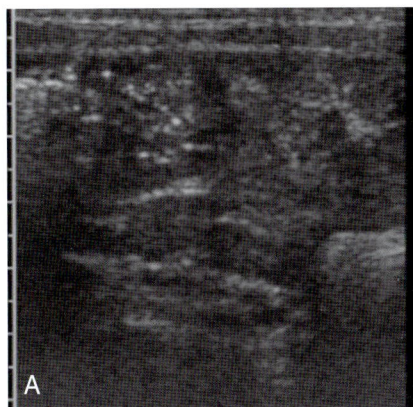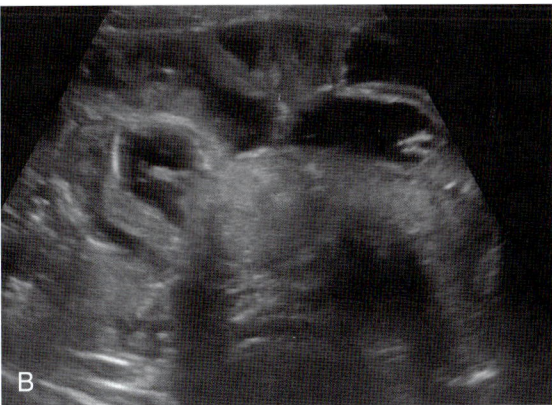

Figure 85-4 Ultrasound appearance of normal and abnormal loops of bowel. **A,** A transverse image through the right lower quadrant demonstrates normal, collapsed loops of small bowel. **B,** A transverse image through the mid abdomen in a 14-month-old boy with vomiting and diarrhea consistent with gastroenteritis reveals multiple distended, fluid-filled loops of bowel.

Computed Tomography

OVERVIEW

CT is a particularly useful modality in pediatric abdominal imaging. The introduction of scanners with multichannel technology and volumetric acquisition permits very rapid examinations with isotropic reconstructions in multiple planes, with decreasing need for sedation.[25,26] These new capabilities require development of newer protocols to accommodate more complex and sophisticated diagnostic demands. The timing and rate of contrast administration, with the ability to scan during a specific phase of intravascular contrast distribution, demand particular attention to technical details and new approaches to image interpretation.[27,28] The pediatric radiologist is further challenged by the need to balance image detail with radiation dose and implementation of the ALARA, or "as low as reasonably achievable" concept, with the increasing recognition of the potential risks of radiation exposure for pediatric patients.[29,30] Improvements in equipment aimed at reducing radiation exposure include innovations such as improved collimators and iterative reconstructive algorithms. Although significant challenges persist, much progress has been made through educational and awareness-raising social marketing campaigns such as the Image Gently Campaign of The Alliance for Radiation Safety in Pediatric Imaging (www.imagegently.org).[31]

INDICATIONS AND PROTOCOLS

Unlike sonography, CT images are sequential, standardized, and much less operator dependent, and therefore CT is particularly useful in patients with complex disease affecting multiple organ systems, because it provides reliable monitoring of change in the extent of the disease during therapy and follow-up. CT also helps solve problems in patients with unusual multi-organ abnormalities. Evaluation of both intraabdominal and extraabdominal multiorgan pathology can be accomplished with great anatomic detail (e-Figs. 85-7 and 85-8) because evaluation of solid organ, hollow viscera, and peritoneal cavity pathology is rapidly accomplished with great anatomic detail and physiologic information. The relative lack of operator dependence and high sensitivity and specificity of CT in the imaging diagnosis of appendicitis has led to its increasing use when this diagnosis is clinically equivocal, with a documented reduction in negative appendectomies.[32] However, this success has led to overuse in patients with abdominal pain; therefore physical examination, followed by ultrasound when the diagnosis is clinically uncertain, is recommended by most pediatric radiologists, with CT reserved for more difficult cases.[17,18] MRI is receiving increasing attention as a viable substitute for CT scanning in many indications, such as inflammatory bowel disease.[33]

CT protocols vary and undergo change with the ongoing introduction of new applications and advances in equipment capability; generalizable protocols applicable to pediatric patients can be downloaded at http://www.imagegently.org. However, some underlying principles underscore most successful pediatric examinations. Administration of intravenous contrast material is extremely important, particularly in pediatric patients in whom a paucity of intraabdominal fat decreases intrinsic intraabdominal contrast.[27,34] CT angiography requires a rapid contrast bolus injection, which in pediatrics can be challenging because of the caliber of IV access. Lowering kVp is important in patients in whom high-contrast structures are of interest, such as those undergoing angiography or bone examinations; in neonates, the kVp can be decreased to as low as 80, with some adjustment of the milliamperes-second (mAs) to produce acceptable image quality.[29] Precontrast images are seldom necessary and serve to increase the radiation exposure without adding diagnostic information. If necessary (e.g., to identify the presence of calcifications in an abdominal mass), the mAs of the precontrast scans can be decreased significantly and the scan should be limited to the appropriate specific area (e.g., scan only the mass, not the entire abdomen). The use of oral contrast material is usually important when outlining some types of intraperitoneal pathology, such as abscess or masses, but in other cases, its use is more controversial.[35] Positive oral contrast material will mask mucosal enhancement; use of water-density contrast material may be more appropriate in such cases.

Despite radiation concerns, CT remains an important lifesaving modality in pediatric diagnosis. As with any other tool, it needs to be used judiciously, according to the principles of appropriateness, justification, optimization, and training.[36]

Magnetic Resonance Imaging

OVERVIEW

MRI increasingly is being used for pediatric GI applications. The introduction and increasing use of imaging at 3 T and advances in parallel imaging and coil design expand the range of pediatric applications. In addition to congenital and acquired hepatobiliary abnormalities, indications for MRI increasingly include bowel abnormalities, such as inflammatory bowel disease and appendicitis.

PATIENT PREPARATION AND EQUIPMENT REQUIREMENTS

Adequate patient preparation is essential, because MRI often is time-consuming and requires extensive hospital resources. Considerations include the need for sedation, fasting requirements, and the need for oral contrast media.

Preparation begins with assessment of the need for sedation or anesthesia. Generally, children younger than 6 years who cannot hold their breath for 20 seconds will need sedation or anesthesia. Sedation is avoided in patients undergoing MR enterography examinations because of the need to use oral contrast media.

Patients should refrain from oral intake for 4 hours before the examination to ensure gallbladder distension in examinations of the biliary tree, as well as to minimize artifacts from bowel peristalsis. For all cases requiring vascular assessment, power injection of contrast material in appropriate-aged children is optimal and requires adequate peripheral venous access. Finally, once the patient is on the MR table, a respiratory monitoring pillow or belt should be placed with care.

Use of an oral contrast agent is essential for enterography examinations. A number of choices are acceptable, although most regimens consist of a biphasic agent, that is, one that gives the bowel lumen a long T2 and T1 relaxation time. Agents include VoLumen (E-Z-Em, New York, NY), mannitol, polyethylene glycol l, and locust bean gum (a type of galactomannan) solutions. Little difference is seen in efficacy of these choices, although patient tolerance may vary.[37] Most important is rapid consumption of a large volume of the contrast agent; 25 mL per kilogram of body weight over an hour is adequate. Placing the patient in the right decubitus position for the final 15 minutes before the start of imaging aids in emptying of the stomach.

Antiperistaltic agents also are required for enterography examinations. Glucagon, the more commonly used intravenous agent, can be used with either of two strategies: (1) half of the dose at the beginning of the examination and half just before administration of intravenous contrast material, or (2) the entire dose just before intravenous contrast material is administered. The dose, from 0.5 mg to 1 mg, varies between facilities. Although glucagon causes nausea and vomiting, it is well tolerated by most patients if it is given as a slow intravenous push over 1 minute and if, before it is administered, the patient is instructed to expect a brief period of nausea.

Equipment specifications are important because of children's smaller sizes, with the consequent need for improved signal to noise and faster acquisition times to decrease the need for and length of sedation. Although the literature to date is still sparse on pediatric abdominal imaging at 3 T,[38,39] increasing experience suggests that most children will benefit from the higher signal. Phased array surface coils are now standard, typically with eight to 32 channels. In the following situations, 1.5 T often provides improved image quality compared with 3 T: when the patient is very large, when ascites is present, when enterography examinations are being performed (1.5 T results in fewer banding artifacts in steady-state imaging), and during hepatic iron quantification.

INDICATIONS AND PROTOCOLS

Hepatic tumors are well evaluated by MRI relative to CT,[40] with the goal of imaging being tumor characterization, staging, and assessment of resectability. For lesion characterization, determination of the T2-weighted signal and enhancement characteristics is essential.[41] Staging and resectability of tumors (such as hepatoblastomas) require delineation of anatomic boundaries, lymph node involvement, vascular invasion, and delineation of the biliary tree, according to accepted staging systems such as PRETEXT (PRETreatment tumor EXTension) outlined by the International Childhood Liver Tumor Strategy Group.[42,43] Biliary and pancreatic diseases also are well assessed by MRI.[44,45] Common indications include cholelithiasis, pancreatitis, sclerosing cholangitis,[46,47] ductal plate malformations and choledochal cysts,[48-50] and biliary complications of liver transplantation. In the case of liver transplantation, assessment of vascular complications often is essential. Diffuse liver disease, such as fibrosis, steatosis,[51-53] and iron deposition, can be quantified by MRI. Fibrosis has been quantitatively assessed by elastography,[54] as well as qualitatively by T2-weighted imaging and delayed contrast enhancement.[55] Although steatosis can be assessed by spectroscopic methods,[56] more commonly steatosis, as well as iron deposition, are assessed by multi-echo gradient echo imaging.[53,57] MR enterography is most commonly performed for evaluation of inflammatory bowel disease.[58-60] The goals of MR include detection of bowel inflammation, distinction of active inflammation from chronic fibrosing disease, and fistula/abscess detection and characterization. Fistulography, particularly for fistula in ano, is performed well by MRI.[61] The goals of the examination include detection of fistulae, classification (i.e., intersphincteric, transsphincteric, suprasphincteric, or extrasphincteric), and abscess detection.

Suggested protocols are provided in Table 85-2, with examples in Figures 85-9 and 85-10 and e-Figures 85-11 and 85-12 and details provided in the following sections. In general, matrix, field of view, and slice thickness should be adjusted to the patient size and thus are not emphasized in the following sections.

Table 85-2

Common Pulse Sequences for Hepatobiliary and Bowel Magnetic Resonance Imaging

Pulse Sequence	Scan Time	Tumors	MRCP	Indication Transplant	Liver Iron/Fat	Enterography	Fistulography
Localizer (1.5 T: SSFSE, HASTE, SSH-TSE; 3 T: FIESTA, TrueFISP, Balanced FFE)	20 sec–3 min	x	x	x	x	x	x
Two-dimensional T2 (FSE, TSE, TSE)	3-4 min	x	x	x	Optional		Two planes
Volumetric T2 (CUBE, SPACE, VISTA)	4-5 min	Optional	x	x			x
Single shot (SSFSE, HASTE, SSH-TSE)	2-3 min		x	x		x	
Balanced steady state (FIESTA, True-FISP, balanced FFE)						x	
Diffusion	1-3 min	x		Optional		Optional	Optional
Dual echo (LAVA-Flex, VIBE-Dixon)	30 sec	x		x	x		
Multi-echo gradient echo	30 sec				x		
Noncontrast MRA	4-5 min			x			
SPGR (LAVA, VIBE, THRIVE)	30 sec	Full echo	Optional with gadoxetate	Partial echo		x	x

CUBE, three-dimensional turbo spin echo (TSE) with variable flip angle (GE Healthcare); FFE, fast field echo; FIESTA, fast imaging with steady-state acquisition; FSE, fast spin echo; HASTE, half-Fourier acquisition single shot TSE; LAVA, volume interpolated gradient refocused echo (GRE) (GE Healthcare); MRA, magnetic resonance angiography; MRCP, magnetic resonance cholangiopancreatography; SPACE, three-dimensional TSE with variable flip angle (Siemens); SPGR, spoiled gradient; SSFSE, single shot fast spin echo; SSH-TSE, single shot TSE; TrueFISP, true fast imaging with steady-state precession (Siemens); TSE, turbo spin echo; VIBE, volume interpolated GRE (Siemens).

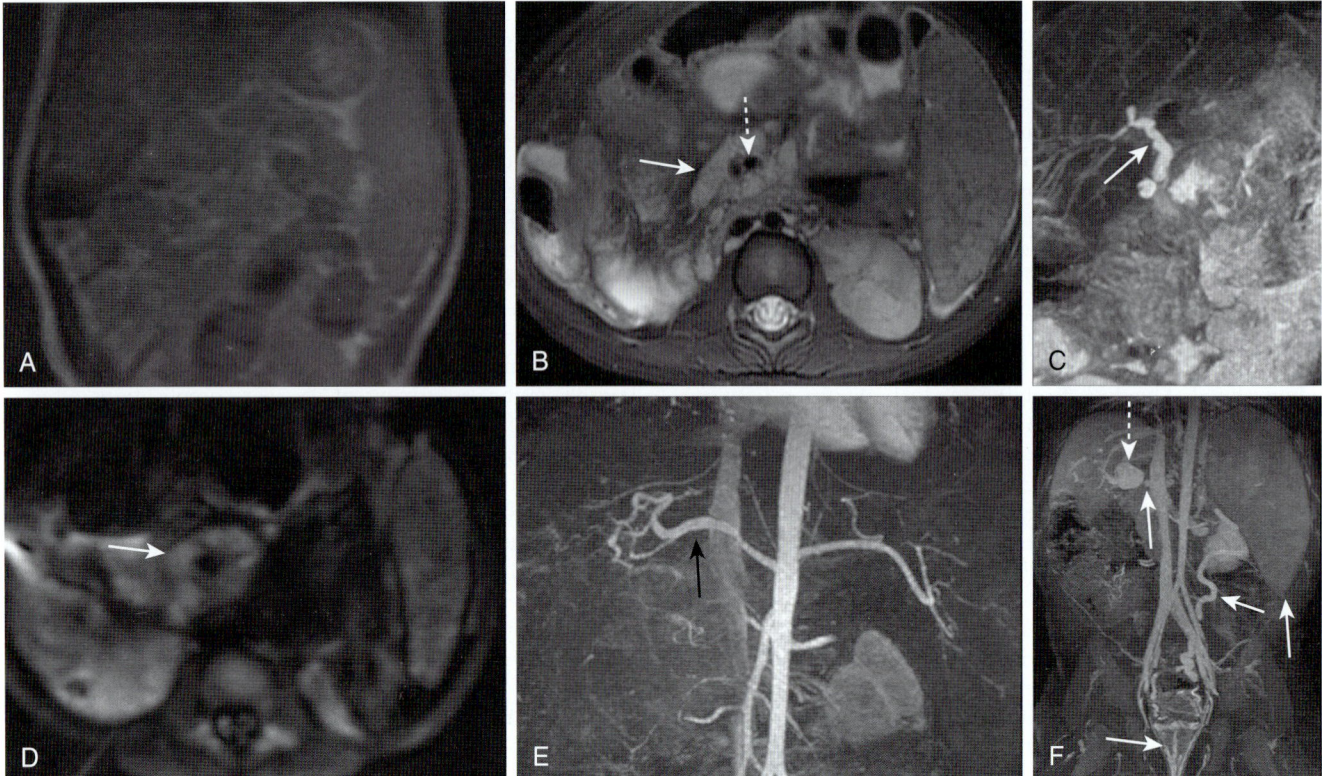

Figure 85-9 Volumetric, diffusion, and angiographic imaging of a 1-year-old girl with a left lobe lateral segment liver transplant. **A,** A localizer is performed quickly. **B,** Axial fat-suppressed T2-weighted imaging shows lymph nodes (*solid arrow*) and surrounding mesenteric vessels (*dashed arrow*), suggesting posttransplant lymphoproliferative disorder. **C,** Maximum intensity projection of a volumetric T2-weighted image showing patent bile ducts (*arrow*). **D,** Axial diffusion again showing lymph nodes (*arrow*). **E,** A contrast-enhanced angiogram (spoiled gradient with fat suppression) in the arterial phase showing a patent hepatic artery (*black arrow*). **F,** Venous phase imaging shows the proximal portal vein (*small arrow*), poststenotic dilation of the intrahepatic portal vein (*dashed arrow*), hemorrhoidal varices (*medium arrows*), and splenomegaly (*large arrow*).

Localizers

At 1.5 T, three-plane single shot fast spin echo with low bandwidth (20 kHz), matrix, and repetition time are performed as localizers. If diagnostic single shot images are required, adjustments can be made to the matrix (320 × 256), slice thickness (4 to 5 mm), and echo time (TE) (200 ms) and images acquired with respiratory triggering.[62] At 3 T, localizers may be more efficiently achieved with balanced steady-state imaging to decrease specific absorption rate, especially for small patients. All localizer sequences should employ parallel imaging.

Conventional T2-Weighted Imaging

Conventional T2-weighted imaging can be performed with fast spin echo. Here parallel imaging is not optimal, because the primary emphasis is on tissue characterization with high

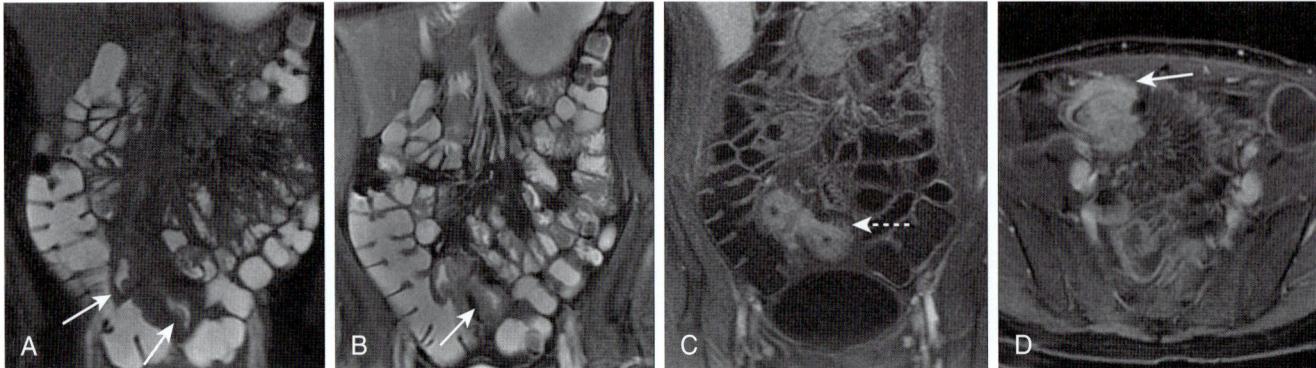

Figure 85-10 Magnetic resonance enterography. A 20-year-old girl with typical findings of Crohn disease. **A,** Single shot imaging shows a thickened terminal ileum with submucosal edema (*arrows*). **B,** Balanced steady state imaging shows wall thickening (*arrow*). **C,** Hyperemia and early transmural enhancement is seen after contrast administration, as well as a "comb sign" (*dashed arrow*). **D,** Delayed imaging shows persistent enhancement of the terminal ileum (*arrow*).

signal/noise ratio (SNR). Sequences should be performed at least in the axial plane, and respiratory triggering or navigation is significantly helpful in improving image quality.[63,64] Typical TEs are 80 to 90 ms at 1.5 T and 70 to 80 ms at 3 T. Fast recovery may be used to improve SNR. Current literature is mixed on the ability of T2-weighted single shot images to provide an equivalent alternative to longer conventional sequences,[65] and thus protocols almost always include conventional T2-weighted imaging.

Volumetric T2-Weighted Imaging

Volumetric T2-weighted sequences have been described mostly for musculoskeletal imaging and neuroimaging.[66-68] These pulse sequences are similar to fast spin echo in that a 90° excitation is required, which excites a slab rather than a slice. These sequences permit thin slices (1 to 2 mm) and reformatting in arbitrary planes. Parallel imaging is essential to maintain a reasonable scan time of 4 to 5 minutes. Navigation or respiratory triggering is important in optimizing image quality, along with a high bandwidth (e.g., 62 kHz). For dedicated MR with cholangiopancreatography examinations, a higher TE (>500 ms) can be used to permit excellent maximum intensity reformation of the biliary tree and pancreatic duct. For other examinations, a TE of 70 to 90 ms permits delineation of relevant anatomy.

Single Shot Imaging

Although volumetric imaging usually displays the bile ducts well,[69] image quality likely will be suboptimal in patients with voluntary or involuntary motion, such as irregular breathing and peristalsis. Thus single shot imaging is complementary[70] for biliary imaging and essential for bowel imaging. In patients with irregular breathing, the user can hand trigger acquisition of each slice by observing the respiratory belt tracing, enabling reasonable assessment of bile ducts in even the most challenging patients.

T1-Weighted Imaging

Dual echo imaging (spoiled gradient with both in-phase and opposed-phase echoes) offers volumetric images at high spatial resolution, as well as with fat-water separation. These sequences can be performed while the patient hold his or her breath, and data can be processed to yield four image sets from one acquisition: water, in-phase, opposed-phase, and fat. Typical parameters are high bandwidth (100 kHz), 4-mm slice thickness, and 12° to 15° flip angle.

Dynamic Gadolinium

Several contrast agents are now available. Consideration should be given to macrocyclic agents, such as gadobutrol (Gadavist), because they may provide enhanced safety in the setting of renal insufficiency. If the primary clinical concern is evaluation of the vascular structures, gadobenate dimeglumine (MultiHance) is a reasonable option, given its higher relaxivity and longer intravascular residence time. The agent has approximately 5% hepatobiliary elimination. Gadofoveset trisodium (Ablavar) recently has been approved by the Food and Drug Administration for assessment of aortoiliac disease

in adults, and it may be an option if vascular evaluation is the sole clinical question. Finally, gadoxetate disodium (Eovist) may be a good option if the primary clinical concern is biliary.[71-77] This agent has 50% hepatobiliary excretion in the setting of normal hepatic and renal function and thus provides a functional as well as an anatomic MR with cholangiopancreatography examination. This agent also is preferred in the setting of evaluation of suspected focal nodular hyperplasia. Although the literature is still limited, gadoxetate may prove useful for characterization of other liver tumors. Even though the gadoxetate dose of 0.025 mmol/kg contains only a quarter of the gadolinium of other agents, its higher T1 relaxivity still allows adequate first-pass hepatic imaging. For all agents, the rate of single dose administration at 1 mL/sec followed by a saline solution flush is acceptable.

For dynamic gadolinium studies, a 3D spoiled gradient sequence with intermittent fat suppression can be performed. Generally, if a patient can hold his or her breath, the matrix and number of slices are adjusted to make the scan time match the patient's ability. If the patient cannot hold his or her breath, quiet breathing with a scan time of approximately 30 seconds can be used. Three phases are acquired in rapid succession followed by delayed imaging at 3 minutes after administration of contrast material.

Scan delay and choice of echo time are significantly different depending on whether the goal of the examination is tumor characterization or vascular assessment. If tumor characterization or detection of bowel wall enhancement is the primary goal, a scan delay should be set to ensure that the center of k-space is acquired at 30 seconds after half the contrast agent is administered:

$$\text{Scan delay} = 30 \text{ seconds} - (\text{scan duration} + \text{bolus duration})/2$$

For tumor characterization, the minimum full echo time should be chosen to maximize SNR.

If vascular assessment is the primary goal, a timing run can be performed with fluoroscopic triggering and centric k-space acquisition or sequential k-space acquisition and calculation of the scan delay, substituting the time to abdominal aortic peak enhancement for 30 seconds in the aforementioned equation. For vascular or bowel enhancement, the minimum echo time (i.e., a fractional echo) should be used to minimize spin dephasing artifacts from flowing blood or field inhomogeneity near the bowel wall from enteric gas, as well as to minimize scan time.

Noncontrast Magnetic Resonance Angiography

Although contrast-enhanced MR angiography (MRA) has become the dominant MR method of vascular assessment, the administration of gadolinium contrast material may be contraindicated in some patients with renal insufficiency. Additionally, the technique has little room for error because intravenous contrast material can be given only once; an injection-scan timing mismatch or patient motion during the scan cannot be rectified, which is particularly problematic in patients who require sedation. Thus noncontrast-enhanced techniques improve the reliability of MRI as a modality for assessment of abdominal vasculature.

Although time-of-flight–based approaches have been used, these sequences produce limited image quality in the abdomen. Noncontrast-enhanced techniques based on balanced steady-state approaches have been gaining favor.[78] A variation of this method is based on a respiratory-triggered inversion pulse covering the imaged volume, as well as a region inferior to it,[79] followed by a balanced steady-state echo train. Thus blood flowing from superior to the inverted region is bright, producing MRA. These sequences have pitfalls similar to time-of-flight–based techniques, including flow-related dephasing, slow-flow–related signal dropout, and intrinsic high T1-weighted signal, but on the whole they provide a nice complement to contrast-enhanced MRA.

Iron/Fat Quantification

Although MRI methods of hepatic iron quantification based on a T2-weighted signal and a composite of signals (proton density, T2-weighted, T2★-weighted, and T1-weighted) have been used, the most common approach is based solely on T2★-weighted imaging. T2★-weighted measurement can be performed on any scanner, although a dedicated pulse sequence and image reconstruction facilitates completion of the examination. These examinations generally are performed on 1.5 T scanners, because the T2★-weighted value depends on field strength, and the vast majority of the calibration literature is based on 1.5 T data.

T2★ may be calculated by running a gradient echo sequence multiple times at different TE values but with a fixed repetition time of approximately 150 ms. Typically values should range from approximately 1 to 20 ms, and the user should avoid prescanning between sequences (or the transmit and receive gains may change). A region of interest then can be drawn in the same area of the liver on each of the resulting series of images. Thus mean signal at each TE is known and will demonstrate an exponential decay relationship (signal = $Ae^{-R2^{\star} \cdot TE} + B$, where $R2^{\star} = 1/T2^{\star}$). R2★ and hence T2★ can be determined by various software packages using logarithms and linear regression.

This process for determining T2★ is time-consuming for data acquisition, because the patient must hold his or her breath for each TE. An alternative is multi-echo gradient echo sequences, in which a series of gradient echoes are obtained at various TEs after each excitation. The multi-echo approach can be performed with two-dimensional (2D) acquisition of a single slice of the liver or a 3D volume acquisition. Whether 2D or 3D, the acquisition requires that the patient hold his or her breath just once, which has the advantage of avoiding slice misregistration issues; it also is easier on the patient and facilitates patient throughput. When coupled with an image reconstruction algorithm that performs a fit to determine R2★, image maps are obtained. Although the pulse sequences and reconstruction programs are not widely available, all major MRI vendors are actively addressing this issue.

One of the challenges of pediatric hepatic iron determination is the wide range of T2★-weighted values that are acquired in practice. Obtaining accurate T2★-weighted values over such a wide range can be challenging. A long series of echoes with long TEs in a patient with a short T2★ will have mean signal over a region of interest dominated by noise, giving an overestimation of T2★. Conversely, a series of echoes with short TEs to address this situation will yield minimal signal decay in a patient with a long T2★, again resulting in poor estimation of T2★. Thus the longest TE

used to determine T2★ should be based in part on the T2★. One approach is to acquire two datasets (one with a long TE and one with a short TE) and use the appropriate one.

For assessment of steatosis, qualitative evaluation may be performed by dual echo imaging (in/opposed phase gradient echo). For quantitative assessment, low flip angle multi-echo imaging may be used, or alternatively spectroscopy can be performed.[80-82] In general, the gradient echo methods are faster and easier, although considerable care must be taken for quantitative accuracy to be maintained.

Nuclear Medicine

OVERVIEW

Nuclear scintigraphy plays an important role in the evaluation of hepatobiliary dysfunction and disorders of the gastrointestinal tract in infants and children. Although some of the studies offer unique diagnostic information, others provide functional information complementary to that obtained with sonography, CT, MRI, and fluoroscopy. Radionuclide imaging of the GI system can be divided into two major categories: imaging of the hepatobiliary system and spleen (Table 85-3) and imaging of the GI tract (Table 85-4).

Table 85-3

Radionuclide Imaging of the Liver, Biliary System, and Spleen

Study	Radiopharmaceutical Agent	Indication

Hepatobiliary scan	Tc-99m IDA	Hepatitis
		Biliary atresia
		Choledochal cyst
		Acute cholecystitis
		Bile plug syndrome
		Caroli disease
		Trauma—bile leak
		Liver transplantation
		  Assess vascularity
		  Assess parenchymal
		    function
		  Evaluate bile drainage
		  Evaluate possible bile leak
		  Evaluate possible
		    obstruction

Liver-spleen scan	Tc-99m sulfur colloid	Hepatitis Hepatic mass (e.g., FNH) Diffuse hepatic disease Abnormal LFTs Hepatitis Congenital abnormalities Diaphragmatic hernia Splenogonadal fusion Wandering spleen Ectopic/accessory spleen Functional asplenia
Hemangioma scan	Tc-99m–labeled RBCs	Liver Hemangioma
Splenic sequestration scan	Tc-99m–labeled, heat-damaged RBCs	Hypersplenism

FNH, Focal nodular hyperplasia; *IDA,* iminodiacetic acid derivative; *LFT,* liver function test; *RBC,* red blood cell; *Tc,* technetium.

Table 85-4

Radionuclide Imaging of the Gastrointestinal Tract

Study	Radiopharmaceutical Agent	Indication
GE reflux	Tc-99m sulfur colloid	Gastric regurgitation Early satiety Recurrent pneumonia Pulmonary aspiration Preoperative: Nissen fundoplication, gastrostomy tube
Salivagram	Tc-99m sulfur colloid	Pulmonary aspiration
Meckel diverticulum	Tc-99m pertechnetate	GI bleeding
GI bleeding (labeled RBCs)	Tc-99m pertechnetate	GI bleeding Asplenia
Infection (labeled WBCs)	Tc-99m HMPAO	Inflammatory bowel disease Appendicitis Abscess

GE, Gastroesophageal; *GI*, gastrointestinal; *HMPAO*, hexamethylpropyleneamine oxime; *RBC*, red blood cell; *Tc*, technetium; *WBC*, white blood cell.

Hepatobiliary scintigraphy provides an anatomic and dynamic physiologic evaluation of biliary function. Splenic scintigraphy is useful in the evaluation of splenic sequestration, accessory spleens, posttraumatic splenosis, postsurgical residual splenic tissue, and a wandering spleen with torsion. GI scintigraphy allows the dynamic assessment of swallowing, gastric emptying, gastroesophageal reflux, esophageal transit, colonic transit, and tracheobronchial aspiration. Red blood cell labeling allows the anatomic localization of intestinal bleeding, and white blood cell labeling can be used for the localization of sites of abdominal infection inflammation. Finally, ectopic mucosa scintigraphy is used for evaluation of suspected Meckel diverticulum.

PATIENT PREPARATION AND EQUIPMENT REQUIREMENTS

Sedation usually is not required for GI radionuclide examinations. However, correct anatomic positioning beneath the camera is essential, and some type of restraint usually is required even with cooperative children. Rarely, patient sedation is necessary for lengthy examinations.

Some of the studies discussed in this section require a period of fasting before imaging. Hepatobiliary imaging typically is performed after premedication with phenobarbital, and Meckel diverticulum imaging can be enhanced with pentagastrin (not currently available in the United States), histamine H2 blockers, or glucagon.[83]

Standard imaging parameters vary, but imaging usually is performed with children in the supine position with either a single-head or dual-head gamma camera, using a low-energy, all-purpose collimator or, preferably, a low-energy, high-resolution collimator. The photopeak and window settings should be predetermined for technetium-99m (^{99m}Tc) (140 keV, 15% to 20%).

Radiopharmaceutical Agents

The radionuclide used in all but positron emission tomography (PET) and molecular imaging studies is ^{99m}Tc, which is administered either intravenously or orally, usually combined with a nonradioactive compound (pharmaceutical agent). The resulting radiopharmaceutical agent (e.g., ^{99m}Tc sulfur colloid) is directed to the target tissue (e.g., the reticuloendothelial system of the liver, spleen, and bone marrow). Ionizing radiation from the internalized radiopharmaceutical agent emanates in the form of gamma rays that deposit energy into the imaging detector. The information sought by the clinician dictates the specific radiopharmaceutical agent used.

The dose of a radiopharmaceutical agent used in a child should be determined by the minimal dose required to yield a high-quality diagnostic examination. Administered activity typically is calculated on the basis of either body surface area or weight. Recent work by Gelfand and colleagues[84] determined that weight-based formulas result in lower radiation exposures, especially in young infants. The group has worked with The Alliance for Radiation Safety in Pediatric Imaging (www.imagegently.org) and published weight-based consensus guidelines for recommended doses of radiopharmaceutical agents in children[84] and is supported by the Society for Pediatric Radiology, the Society of Nuclear Medicine, and the American College of Radiology.

INDICATIONS AND PROTOCOLS

Hepatobiliary Scintigraphy

Hepatobiliary scintigraphy is a useful adjunct to sonography in the evaluation of infants with jaundice and cholestasis, as well as in older children with hyperbilirubinemia. Its value in jaundiced neonates is the timely differentiation of neonatal hepatitis and biliary atresia, because surgical intervention in patients with biliary atresia is most successful when it is performed early in life. Postoperatively, hepatobiliary imaging may be requested to confirm patency of the bilioenteric anastomosis. Imaging with sonography, CT, and MRI frequently is diagnostic for choledochal cysts, but hepatobiliary imaging is a useful adjunct. Similarly, the evaluation of Caroli disease often is facilitated with hepatobiliary imaging. Cystic duct patency can be assessed in older children with suspected acute cholecystitis. Hepatobiliary imaging is highly sensitive and specific for the detection of spontaneous, postoperative, or posttraumatic biliary leaks.[85] Other clinical indications are listed in Table 85-3.

Currently, ^{99m}Tc mebrofenin is used widely for hepatobiliary imaging because it has a high hepatic extraction; it is transported into the hepatocytes and then excreted with bile into the bile ducts. The radiopharmaceutical agent is administered intravenously, and static anterior images of the abdomen are acquired in the supine position every 5 minutes for 30 minutes. A simultaneous dynamic acquisition is suggested during the first 30 minutes. Delayed images may be obtained at 45 minutes, 60 minutes, and up to 24 hours, as necessary, to visualize the gallbladder and biliary tree and excretion into the duodenum. A normal scan typically demonstrates radiopharmaceutical uptake in the liver by 5 minutes, in the biliary tree by 15 minutes, and in the small bowel by 15 to 45 minutes (Fig. 85-13). In patients with neonatal hepatitis, delayed and diminished uptake by the liver occurs, but the

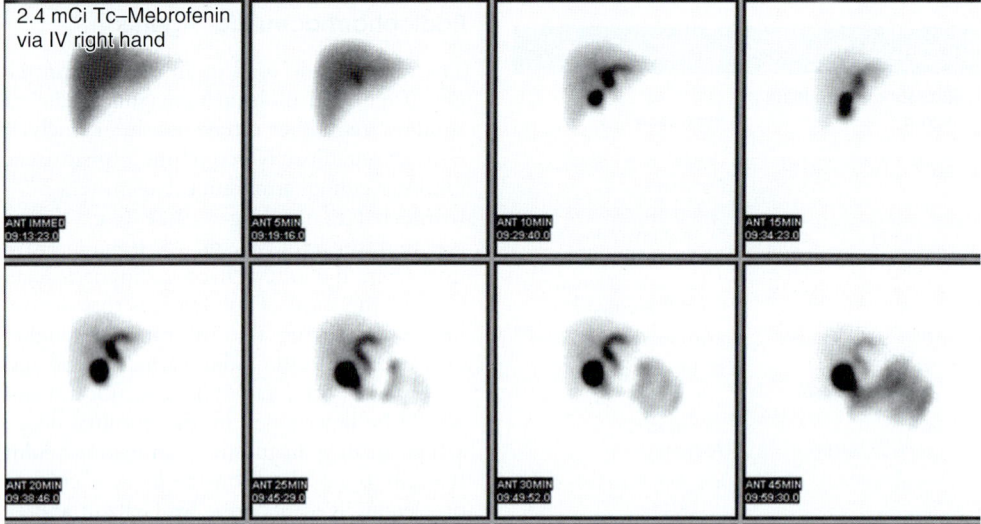

Figure 85-13 Normal results of a hepatobiliary study in a 5-year-old with right upper abdominal pain. Anterior static images of the abdomen were obtained every 5 minutes for 45 minutes after the intravenous (*IV*) administration of technetium (*Tc*)-99m mebrofenin. Homogeneous radiotracer accumulation is seen throughout the liver, with prompt visualization of the intrahepatic ducts by 5 minutes, the common bile duct and gallbladder by 10 minutes, and the small bowel by 25 minutes.

radiopharmaceutical agent eventually reaches the small bowel. In patients with biliary atresia, radiopharmaceutical uptake by the liver is usually adequate, but the radiotracer never reaches the bowel, even on delayed 24-hour images (e-Fig. 85-14).

When differentiation between biliary atresia and neonatal hepatis is required, premedication with phenobarbital (5 mg/kg per day for 5 days) improves hepatic extraction of tracer,[86] and 3 to 5 days of premedication is recommended in the setting of elevated conjugated hyperbilirubinemia. A child should fast for 2 to 4 hours; 2 hours is sufficient for infants. Prolonged fasting is not recommended.

When the possibility of cholecystitis is a concern, the same protocol is used without phenobarbital premedication but with continuous imaging for 1 hour. When the gallbladder is visualized, a right anterior oblique or right lateral view is acquired. Delayed images at 2, 4, and 24 hours may be necessary. If the gallbladder is not visualized at 45 to 60 minutes, in lieu of further delayed imaging, intravenous morphine sulfate (0.04 mg/kg) may be administered, followed by dynamic 1-minute imaging for 30 minutes. If cholecystokinin cholescintigraphy is requested, 0.02 µg/kg of cholecystokinin (Sincalide or Kinevac) is administered as a slow infusion over 30 minutes after the gallbladder is visualized. A normal gallbladder ejection fraction is >35%. When leakage of bile is a concern, the same protocol is used, without administration of phenobarbital.

Liver-Spleen Scintigraphy

The traditional liver-spleen scan is seldom used because of advances in sonography, CT, and MRI, which provide far greater spatial and contrast resolution and more precise anatomic details. However, several important indications for the liver-spleen scan still exist, including the evaluation of congenital anomalies, such as the location of accessory or ectopic spleens, the evaluation of functional asplenia, the functional evaluation of hepatitis and cirrhosis, and the diagnostic differentiation of certain hepatic masses, such as focal nodular hyperplasia. Some authors have reported its utility in the assessment of children with heterotaxy syndrome; however, differentiating a normal abdominal situs from asplenia with a midline, transverse liver can be difficult when the splenic fossa is occupied by liver tissue. CT or MRI makes this distinction more clearly.[24] The physiologic basis of the liver-spleen scan is the phagocytosis of radioactive colloid particles by the reticuloendothelial cells of the liver, spleen, and bone marrow. Normal images reveal homogeneous distribution of the radiopharmaceutical agent in the liver and spleen, which can be evaluated for size, position, configuration, and any focal areas of radiotracer deficit. Functional asplenia is better documented with ^{99m}Tc-labeled, heat-damaged red blood cell imaging.

No patient preparation is necessary for the liver-spleen scan. The child receives an intravenous injection of ^{99m}Tc sulfur colloid, and static images are obtained from multiple projections approximately 15 minutes after injection, with the child lying supine. Dynamic images also may be acquired, depending on the clinical indication.

Splenic Sequestration Scintigraphy

Splenic sequestration scintigraphy is used in children with hypersplenism, which results in acceleration of the normal sequestration and phagocytosis of abnormal erythrocytes, neutrophils, and platelets. Spleen scintigraphy also can be used to identify accessory spleens, posttraumatic "splenosis," and to evaluate splenic uptake in a "wandering" spleen (see Chapter 95).

No patient preparation is necessary. Red blood cells are withdrawn from the patient, labeled with ^{99m}Tc pertechnetate, and then denatured (in a warm temperature bath at 49.5°C for 12 to 15 minutes) to improve splenic localization. The child receives an intravenous injection of the ^{99m}Tc-labeled, heat-damaged red blood cells, and static images are obtained from multiple projections approximately 15 minutes after injection. Images diagnostic of hypersplenism reveal rapid clearance of the radiolabeled red blood cells from the blood pool and greater than normal splenic uptake.

Scintigraphy of the Gastrointestinal Tract

Radionuclide imaging of the GI tract is a sophisticated, systematic technique that allows anatomic and functional imaging of the esophagus and stomach, small bowel, and colon. Anatomic location of GI bleeding or GI infection can be accomplished with dynamic imaging of the entire GI tract.

These studies usually are more sensitive than conventional radiographic and fluoroscopic studies because dynamic, uninterrupted imaging can be performed for longer periods and with less radiation exposure. The physiologic information obtained with GI scintigraphy complements the anatomic information provided by radiography and fluoroscopy.

Gastroesophageal Reflux Scintigraphy

Gastroesophageal reflux in infants and young children manifests clinically with vomiting and failure to thrive in severe cases; it is associated with recurrent bronchitis and pneumonia, peripheral airway disease, esophagitis, and GI bleeding. Radionuclide imaging can detect and quantify gastroesophageal reflux, as well as pulmonary aspiration. The sensitivity is greater than with conventional barium fluoroscopy because the chest and abdomen can be monitored continuously; the only disadvantage is the lower anatomic resolution.

Patient preparation requires fasting for 2 to 4 hours. A ^{99m}Tc sulfur colloid–labeled liquid or solid meal is administered. Infants can be fed infant formula or saved breast milk, using a similar volume to that typically used for regular feedings, and the radiolabeled meal should replace the regularly scheduled feeding. Alternatively, an infant feeding volume can be calculated at 10 to 20 mL/kg. Older children should fast for 2 to 4 hours, and an age-appropriate volume of whole milk, whole chocolate milk, or PediaSure typically is administered. If the liquid meal is given via a nasogastric tube, the position of the tube should be verified with radiography and adjusted if the tip is in the esophagus, distal stomach, or small intestine. If the child is receiving continuous feedings, these should be stopped 2 to 4 hours before the examination. The meal should be introduced into the stomach quickly— preferably within 10 minutes. The radiolabeled meal should be followed with radiopharmaceutical-free liquid. The child is then placed supine, and a computer acquisition is immediately obtained dynamically at 60 seconds/image for 30 minutes. At our institution, we image 15 minutes in the supine position, followed by 15 minutes in the prone position. A 3- to 4-hour delayed image over the lungs may be obtained to evaluate for possible pulmonary aspiration.

A study with normal findings shows the radiopharmaceutical agent in the stomach but no activity in the esophagus or lungs. If reflux is detected, the number of episodes is counted over the entire imaging period, and the proximal extent is noted (Fig. 85-15).

Gastric Emptying Scintigraphy

Gastric emptying imaging is useful in the evaluation of early satiety, bloating, or abdominal pain, for evaluation of accelerated gastric emptying, and for the preoperative assessment of children with reflux who are undergoing Nissen fundoplication and gastrostomy tube placement. The gastric emptying study can be performed with a liquid or solid meal. Liquid gastric emptying studies can be performed in combination with a gastroesophageal reflux study. The advantages of the gastric emptying study compared with fluoroscopic studies are that they use real food, rather than barium, they can be performed with a liquid or solid meal, and they are quantitative. The disadvantages are that meal content, volume, and imaging techniques are not standardized; normal pediatric gastric emptying standards are not firmly established. Despite these limitations, gastric emptying imaging studies are considered the gold standard for the evaluation of gastric emptying.

Imaging techniques vary widely, and there is little standardization of technique, test meal content, and test meal volume. Patient preparation requires fasting for 2 to 4 hours. A ^{99m}Tc sulfur colloid–labeled liquid or solid meal is administered with techniques similar to that previously described for the gastroesophageal reflux examination.

Liquid gastric emptying studies can be performed in combination with a gastroesophageal reflux study. When performed separately, images are obtained in the left anterior oblique position for 90 to 120 minutes. When performed in combination with the gastroesophageal reflux study, images are obtained with a dual-head camera in the anterior and posterior projections in the supine position only. An ambulatory child can move between acquisition of images, but walking about is discouraged.

A study with normal findings reveals radiotracer in the stomach on the initial images, followed by progressive emptying of the stomach (see Fig. 85-15). Computer processing is performed by drawing a region of interest around the stomach at selected time points to calculate fractional emptying. A time-activity curve is then generated and plotted on a linear scale using the geometric mean of the anterior and posterior counts. A half-time for emptying ($T_{1/2}$) is calculated, that is, the length of time required for the initial number of counts to decrease by 50%. In normal studies the time-activity curve should exhibit a continuous decline in activity over time.

Reported normal values are variable. Seibert and colleagues[87] showed 60-minute gastric emptying values of 48% ± 16% in infants and 51% ± 7% in children who were fed a radiolabeled milk formula (roughly, a gastric emptying $T_{1/2}$ of 60 minutes in each age group). A different study performed with healthy infants who were fed radiolabeled milk demonstrated a $T_{1/2}$ of 87 ± 29 minutes.[88] Singh et al.[89] developed a standard solid meal (^{99m}Tc-labeled "Technecrispy cake"), determined a standard meal volume (30 g), and prospectively established normal gastric emptying values in healthy children, which typically are normalized by each individual nuclear medicine laboratory or imaging department.

Esophageal Transit Scintigraphy

Esophageal transit scintigraphy may be used to evaluate esophageal motility disorders such as achalasia, diffuse esophageal spasm, and impaired motility from esophagitis and esophageal atresia/tracheoesophageal fistula.

Patient preparation requires fasting for 2 to 4 hours. The child is positioned supine with the mouth at the very top of the field of view and the stomach at the lower field of view, A small radioactive marker may be placed over the cricoid cartilage for an anatomic reference. The child is instructed to swallow a ^{99m}Tc sulfur colloid radiolabeled bolus of liquid (water or milk) as computer acquisition begins. A practice swallow of 5 mL of unlabeled water is recommended. Posterior images are acquired over the mouth and stomach at 5 seconds/frame for 1 to 3 minutes. Regions of interest are drawn around the upper, middle, and lower thirds of the esophagus and stomach, and a time-activity curve is generated. The normal transit time through the esophagus is generally less than 10 seconds.

Colonic Transit Scintigraphy

Colonic transit scintigraphy is useful in patients with chronic constipation to establish whether the cause is slow colonic transit or functional fecal retention. Differentiation between these two patterns is important because the treatment strategy is different for each.

Patient preparation requires discontinuance of laxatives for 5 days before the transit study, and 4 hours of patient fasting is recommended. A ^{99m}Tc sulfur colloid radiolabeled liquid or solid meal is administered orally. Anterior and posterior images are obtained in the supine position at 0 to 2, 6, 24,

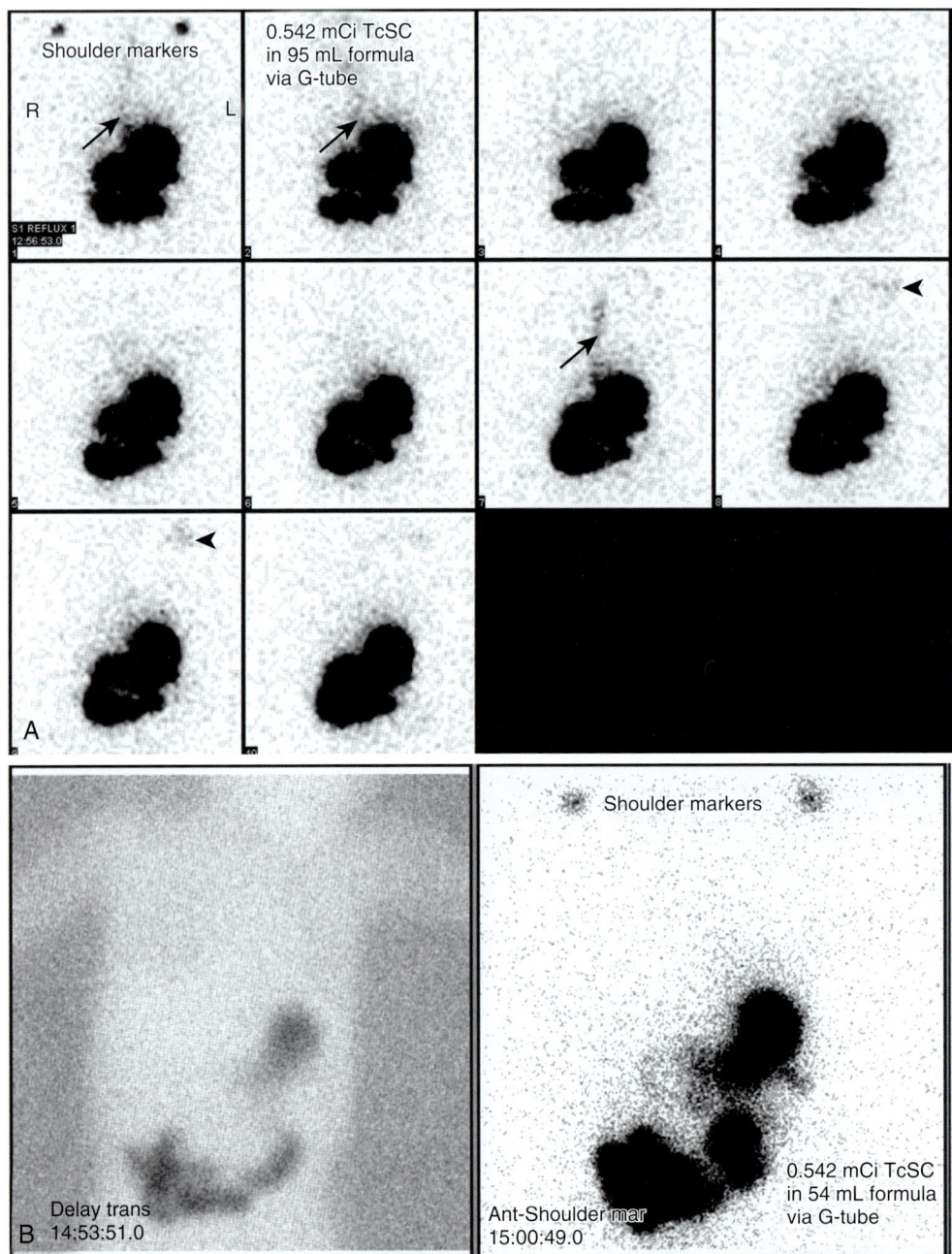

Figure 85-15   A combined gastroesophageal reflux and gastric emptying imaging study in a 1-year-old child with persistent emesis. **A,** Initial images of the chest and abdomen reveal three episodes of reflux (*arrows* in the first, second, and seventh images), with subsequent visualization of the radiopharmaceutical agent in the child's mouth (*arrowheads* in the eighth and ninth images). **B,** Three-hour delayed transmission and routine supine image of the chest and upper abdomen reveal no pulmonary aspiration.

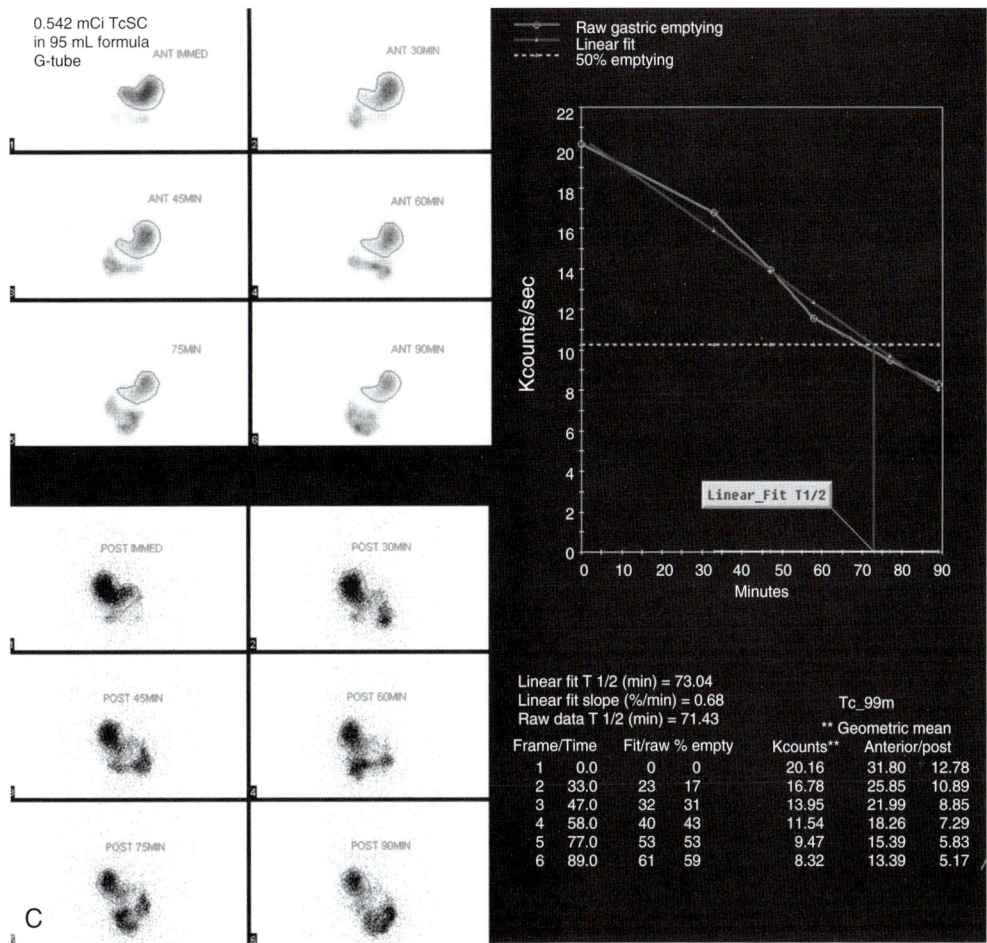

Figure 85-15, cont'd. **C,** Progressive gastric emptying is occurring. A time-activity curve constructed from regions of interest drawn around the stomach reveals a half time for emptying of 73 minutes, which is within normal limits. *TcSC,* Technetium-99m sulfur colloid.

30, and 48 hours. Radioactivity is measured in six regions (precolonic, ascending, transverse, descending, rectosigmoid colon, and evacuated feces). An examination with normal results shows radioactivity in the cecum by 6 hours and evacuation by 30 to 58 hours. Retention in the proximal colon at 48 hours indicates "slow colonic transit," whereas retention in the rectum at 48 hours indicates "functional fecal retention."[90,91] Quantitative assessment of transit also can be performed with geometric center analysis.[92]

Salivagram

The salivagram allows the dynamic assessment of swallowing in patients suspected of having primary aspiration with feeding.

Fasting is not required. The child is positioned supine, and a small dose of ^{99m}Tc sulfur colloid mixed in 0.1 to 0.5 mL of water or saline solution is placed on the anterior tongue and allowed to mix with oral secretions. Rapid dynamic images of the neck, chest, and upper abdomen are acquired from the posterior projection every 60 seconds for 1 hour. Static images are then obtained at 1 hour and 3 hours. Detection of any radiopharmaceutical agent in the tracheobronchial tree is abnormal (Fig. 85-16).

Meckel Scintigraphy

Meckel diverticulum is a congenital anomaly resulting from incomplete closure of the omphalomesenteric duct; it is present in approximately 2% of the population.[93] Most of these diverticula are asymptomatic and are lined by ileal mucosa. However, those that contain ectopic gastric mucosa are capable of producing hydrochloric acid and pepsin, thereby inducing mucosal ulceration. Peptic ulceration causes acute GI hemorrhage in children, usually in the first 2 years of life. A Meckel diverticulum can be quite small and difficult to differentiate from bowel loops by anatomic imaging. The Meckel scan is the study of choice for unexplained GI bleeding in children. Those diverticula with ectopic gastric mucosa can be detected with scintigraphy because the radiopharmaceutical agent accumulates within the ectopic gastric mucosa. Bleeding enteric duplication cysts containing ectopic gastric mucosa also can be detected.

Pharmacologic pretreatment is not considered necessary to produce a high-quality Meckel scan. However, if a false-negative study is suspected, a follow-up examination with pentagastrin or an H2 blocker can increase diagnostic sensitivity. Pentagastrin stimulates gastric secretions and increases gastric mucosa uptake of the pertechnetate. It also stimulates

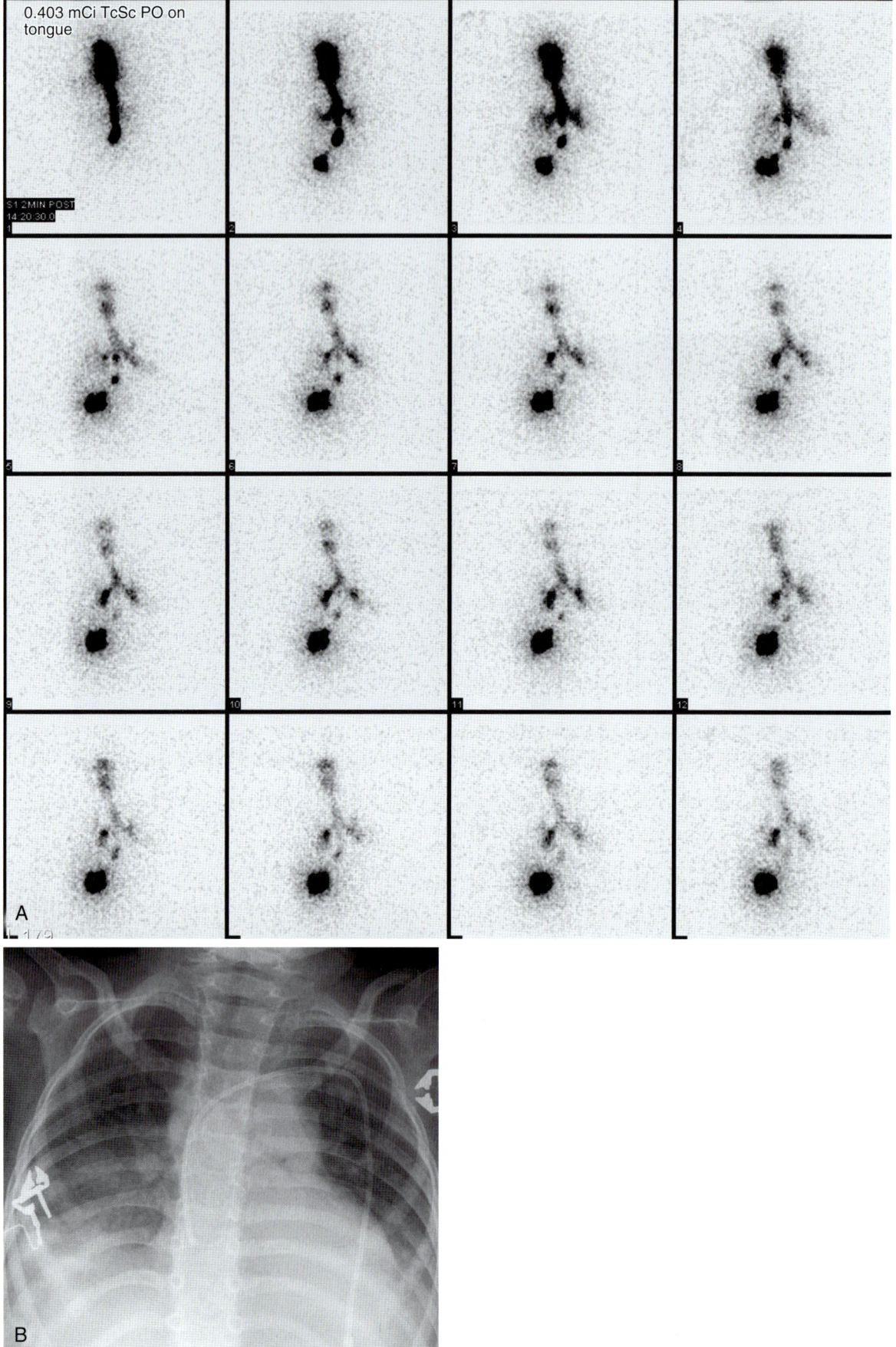

0.403 mCi TcSc PO on tongue

S1 2MIN POST
14 20 30.0

A

B

Figure 85-16 A salivagram. **A,** A radionuclide salivagram (posterior images) obtained in a child with recurrent pneumonia and neuromuscular inco-ordination demonstrates technetium-99m sulfur colloid (*TcSC*) outlining the tracheobronchial tree. Some of the swallowed radiopharmaceutical agent is seen in the stomach. **B,** A chest radiograph obtained the same day reveals bibasilar lung opacity, consistent with aspiration pneumonitis.

secretion of pertechnetate and GI motility. Histamine H2 blockers (e.g., cimetidine, ranitidine, and famotidine) block secretions from the cells and increase gastric mucosa uptake. Glucagon may be given to decrease intestinal peristalsis.[94]

The child is placed in the supine position under the gamma camera and receives an intravenous injection of [99mTc] pertechnetate. Multiple static anterior images of the abdomen are acquired for 30 minutes. Dynamic images also are obtained at 60 seconds per image. The images are processed to allow cinematic display of the dynamic images and summed 5-minute static images.

A study with normal findings reveals radiotracer accumulation in the stomach and the urinary bladder, sometimes with faint uptake by the kidneys. An abnormal study demonstrates accumulation of radiotracer in ectopic tissue simultaneously with the appearance of gastric mucosa, usually between 6 and 10 minutes after injection. The abnormality is usually a small, rounded focus of radiopharmaceutical agent uptake in the right lower abdomen (e-Fig. 85-17). Single photon emission tomography (SPECT) imaging co-registered with simultaneously acquired low-dose CT (SPECT/CT) on a hybrid scanner has proved useful in discriminating between a Meckel diverticulum and possible artifact from urinary or other visualized activity.[95,96]

Gastrointestinal Bleeding Scintigraphy

Lower GI bleeding in infants and children has many causes that are largely age-specific. When entities such as volvulus and intussusception are excluded, radionuclide imaging is useful for localizing a bleeding source. Radiolabeled red blood cells are useful in patients who are bleeding slowly or intermittently.

No patient preparation is necessary. A sample of the patient's blood is obtained (1 to 3 mL), anticoagulated, and labeled with [99mTc]. The tagged autologous cells subsequently are reinjected into the patient. The child is placed supine, with the imaging camera positioned anteriorly over the abdomen. After a bolus intravenous injection of [99mTc]-labeled red blood cells, a dynamic flow study is performed for 1 minute, followed by a static image obtained every 5 minutes for 30 minutes. If the images do not immediately reveal bleeding, delayed images are obtained at 45 minutes and 60 minutes; they can be obtained up to 24 hours after injection. A cinematic display also is processed when bleeding is detected. A positive study reveals activity in a location and configuration consistent with bowel, displays progressively increased intensity over time, and exhibits movement through the GI tract over time.

Gastrointestinal Inflammation and Infection Scintigraphy

The radionuclide labeling of white blood cells can be used for the localization of sites of abdominal infection, including appendicitis,[97] and for the localization and evaluation of the intensity and extent of inflammatory bowel disease (Crohn disease and ulcerative colitis).

Data suggest that [99mTc] hexamethylpropyleneamine oxime–labeled leukocyte imaging may be superior to CT[98] for assessing the extent and activity of inflammatory bowel disease, and a review of these techniques has been published more recently.[99] Labeled leukocyte imaging may be used as a screening study to determine if a child should undergo more invasive testing. The study also is useful for patients who refuse endoscopy or contrast radiography or for those who have luminal narrowing that precludes endoscopic evaluation.

The radiopharmaceutical agent used is [99mTc] hexamethyl-propyleneamine oxime. In children, the minimal amount of blood needed for labeling is 10 to 15 mL, depending on the child's size and circulating leukocyte count. Images are acquired at 30 minutes and 2 to 3 hours after the injection of the labeled white blood cells. The patient should void before each image acquisition. SPECT imaging may be performed after planar imaging for improved localization of the disease. A study with normal findings reveals uptake of the radiolabeled leukocytes by the liver, spleen, bone marrow, kidneys, and urinary bladder. Normal bowel activity due to hepatobiliary excretion is seen in 20% to 30% of children by 1 hour. Abnormal bowel activity may be seen in 15 to 30 minutes and usually increases in intensity during the next 2 to 3 hours.

Positron Emission Tomography

PET using fluorine-18 ([18F]) fluorodeoxyglucose has been reported as a noninvasive, sensitive alternative to conventional studies in the identification and localization of intestinal inflammatory and infectious processes in children. Specific inflammatory conditions investigated using [18F]-fluorodeoxyglucose PET imaging include inflammatory bowel disease,[100-102] chronic granulomatous disease,[31] appendicitis,[103] and fever of unknown origin.[104]

PET imaging using [18F]-dihydroxyphenylalanine has been used to distinguish focal from diffuse pancreatic disease in infants with hyperinsulism. Patients with focal disease may undergo resection of the offending adenoma, whereas those with diffuse disease may be treated with octreotide or subtotal pancreatectomy.[105,106] The imaging techniques for these PET studies are beyond the scope of this chapter.

Molecular Imaging

Molecular imaging techniques that use tiny concentrations of radiotracers have been used as probes in animal models and human tissue samples to characterize, measure, and treat disease processes at the cellular or molecular level. Such techniques show promise in preclinical studies of patients with inflammatory bowel disease, but translation into routine clinical use in children awaits further evaluation.[107]

References

Full references for this chapter can be found on www.expertconsult.com.

Chapter 86

Prenatal Gastrointestinal and Hepatobiliary Imaging

CHRISTOPHER I. CASSADY

Evaluation of the organs in the gastrointestinal tract and within the peritoneal cavity is a standard part of the full prenatal ultrasound scan for anatomy screening.[1] In circumstances when ultrasound cannot accurately determine the extent or nature of an abnormality, fetal magnetic resonance imaging (MRI) can be useful. Sequence selection includes standard single-shot fast spin echo (SSFSE) T2-weighted images at 3- to 5-mm slice thickness and steady-state free-precession imaging (SSFP) at overlapping intervals. Echo-time lengths range from 80 to 250 ms; longer lengths are advantageous for delineation of cystic abnormalities. T1-weighted fast gradient echo (GRE) sequences may be useful in the fetal abdomen, specifically for identification of the liver, which is mildly hyperintense, and very bright signal meconium.[2] Imaging modalities using ionizing radiation have no role in the evaluation of a fetus with a gastrointestinal (GI) tract abnormality, which can be categorized into one of several general categories: obstructions, ventral wall defects, masses and solid organ abnormalities, echogenic bowel, and peritoneal abnormalities.

Intestinal Obstructions

Etiology Interruption of the fetal GI tract can occur at any point from the esophagus to the anus, and the etiology for the loss of continuity is not the same at each site. The cause of esophageal atresia (EA) with or without a fistula (communicating between the trachea and the esophagus distal to the atretic level) is not known but is believed to be a result of failure of the tracheal bud to develop normally from the primitive foregut (see Chapter 97).[3,4] EA occurs in approximately 1 in 4000 live births and can be associated with a number of additional abnormalities in the fetus. Most commonly these abnormalities include those comprising the VACTERL complex (*v*ertebral, *a*nal, *c*ardiac, *t*racheo*e*sophageal, *r*enal, and *l*imb anomalies) and those seen in Down syndrome, such as common atrioventricular canal, absent or hypoplastic nasal bone, and nuchal thickening. EA occurs most commonly with a distal fistula (84%).[5]

Gastric atresia is the rarest atresia and is almost always pyloric with a distended proximal stomach. It likely results from vascular impairment during fetal development and is associated with epidermolysis bullosa.[6,7]

In contrast to pyloric atresia, duodenal atresia (DA) is relatively common, and along with EA is associated with Down syndrome. The etiology of DA may be exceptional in that it is believed to be due to dysfunction in embryonic recannulation of this segment of the proximal small bowel (see Chapter 103).[8]

Atresias distal to the duodenum are thought to be the result of ischemia or other focal insult to the bowel and may be multiple. Thus it is prudent not to assume that the most proximal obstruction is the only site. Small bowel atresias are the most common cause of fetal and neonatal bowel obstructions, with colonic segments affected much more rarely (in 10% of all atresias).[9,10] Although most atresias are sporadic, some populations are prone to multiple atresia syndromes.[11,12] Meconium ileus in persons with cystic fibrosis also can have small bowel atresia, and colonic atresia can be seen in persons with Hirschsprung disease.[13,14] Anorectal atresia/malformation deserves special consideration because it often is seen in combination with other malformations, such as VACTERL, caudal regression, cloacal malformation, or the Currarino association.

Imaging of the Esophagus Despite the likelihood of a distal fistula that might allow for flow of fluid into the gut, the most consistent clues to the diagnosis of EA on ultrasound are a persistently small-volume stomach and polyhydramnios. Distension of a proximal esophageal pouch typically is intermittent and therefore unreliably witnessed either on ultrasound or MRI, although in the rare cases where it is vital to make a prenatal diagnosis, serial midline sagittal MRI with cine SSFP sequences may prove useful (Fig. 86-1).[15]

Imaging of the Stomach A lack of visualization of the stomach is most likely EA with or without a distal fistula. Other considerations in the differential diagnosis of a small stomach at fetal imaging include congenital microgastria; oligohydramnios/anhydramnios, with a lack of fluid to swallow and distend the stomach; diminished swallowing function (e.g., in arthrogryposis, with little to no fetal movement); or obstruction to normal swallowing, including from increased intrathoracic pressure (Fig. 86-2). A markedly distended stomach, on the other hand, might raise concern for outlet obstruction, as with pyloric atresia. Gastric volvulus rarely has been reported in utero and is more of a risk when

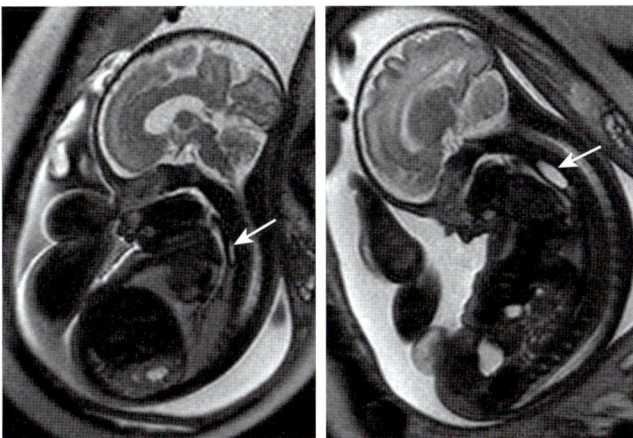

Figure 86-1 Esophageal atresia. Serial imaging may show intermittent phenomena: A sagittal single-shot fast spin echo image in the neck and chest shows a small amount of fluid in the proximal esophagus that distends to a pouch on a later sequence (*arrows*). Cine steady-state free-precession sequences are especially useful for serial imaging because of their fast acquisition times.

the stomach is not in its normal location.[16] A right-sided stomach in situs ambiguous or inversus should be evident as long as one is careful to establish the orientation of the fetus to the mother during the examination (Fig. 86-3).

Imaging of the Duodenum DA appears on imaging as the classic fluid-filled double bubble of dilated stomach and duodenal bulb (Fig. 86-4). Duodenal stenosis sometimes can be distinguished by hyperperistalsis of the dilated proximal duodenum, whereas in DA, no peristalsis may exist at all. DA is

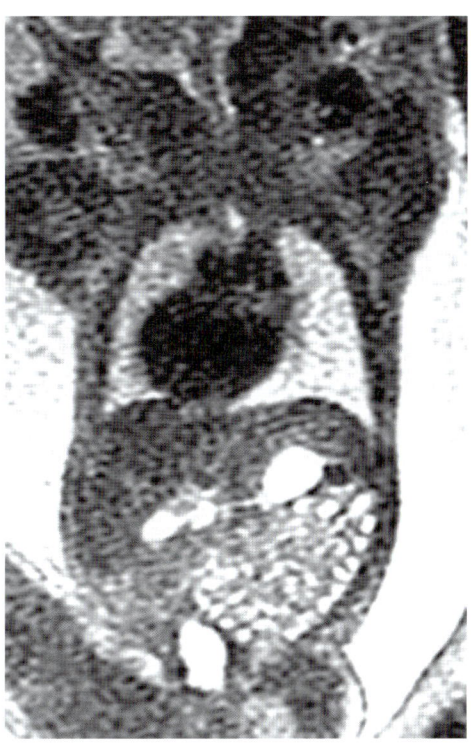

Figure 86-3 Heterotaxia. Coronal single-shot fast spin echo T2-weighted magnetic resonance image shows dextrocardia. The abdominal situs is normal, and a spleen is present.

associated with malrotation of the bowel in approximately 29% of cases.[8] Other causes for proximal obstruction include an adhesive Ladd band in a patient with primary midgut malrotation, or annular pancreas. As with other obstructions to the GI tract above the level of the distal jejunum, a fetus

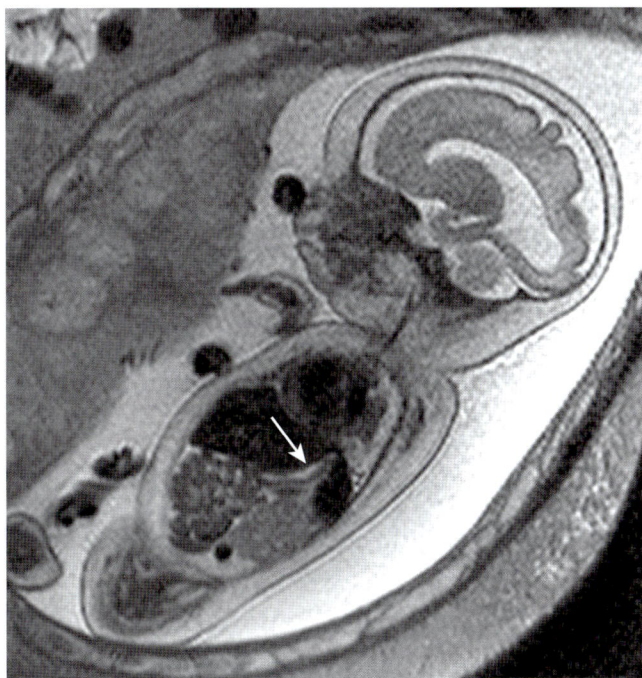

Figure 86-2 A small collapsed stomach (*arrow*) in a fetus with hydrops, hypotonia, and limited swallowing. Note the lack of any motion artifact in the amniotic fluid.

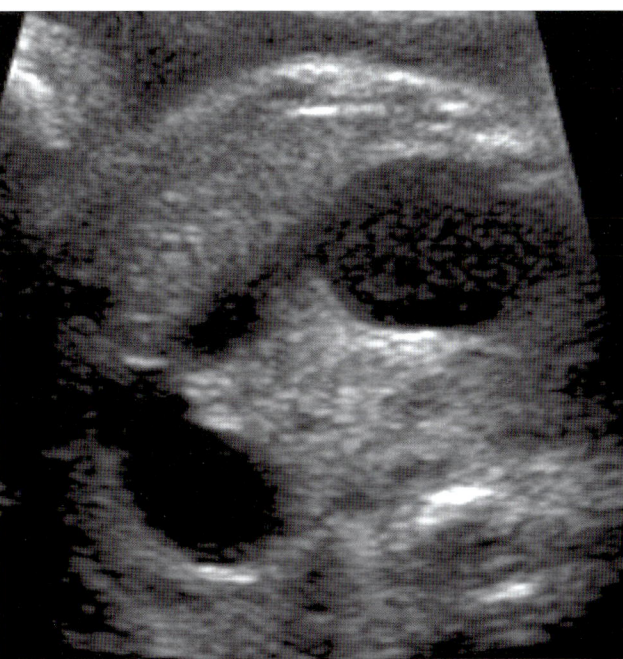

Figure 86-4 Duodenal atresia. Axial ultrasound of the stomach, pylorus, and dilated duodenum ("double bubble").

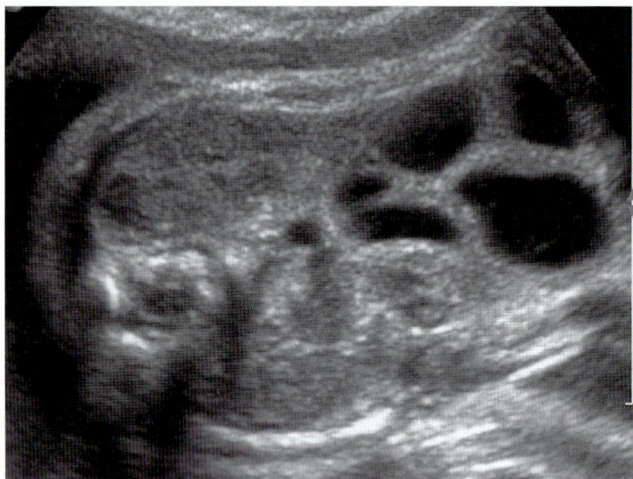

Figure 86-5 Ileal atresia. A coronal sonogram of the abdomen shows multiple dilated small bowel loops.

with duodenal obstruction typically has polyhydramnios; the more proximal the atresia, the earlier and the more frequently an abnormally large amniotic fluid volume tends to present.[17]

Imaging of the Small Bowel The small bowel is considered to be dilated if it is larger than 7 mm; the colon is usually up to 15 mm in the third trimester, while the normal rectum, which should be the largest segment, can be larger[18-20] (Fig. 86-5). In proximal jejunal atresia, more loops will be dilated than just the double bubble seen with DA ("triple bubble" in very proximal jejunal atresia) (Fig. 86-6); distal jejunal atresia and ileal atresia, on the other hand, may be more difficult to distinguish prospectively because multiple dilated, fluid-filled loops are seen in both conditions, and typically a normal amniotic fluid volume is present. Other considerations for a distal bowel obstruction parallel those in newborn imaging and include meconium ileus in a fetus with cystic

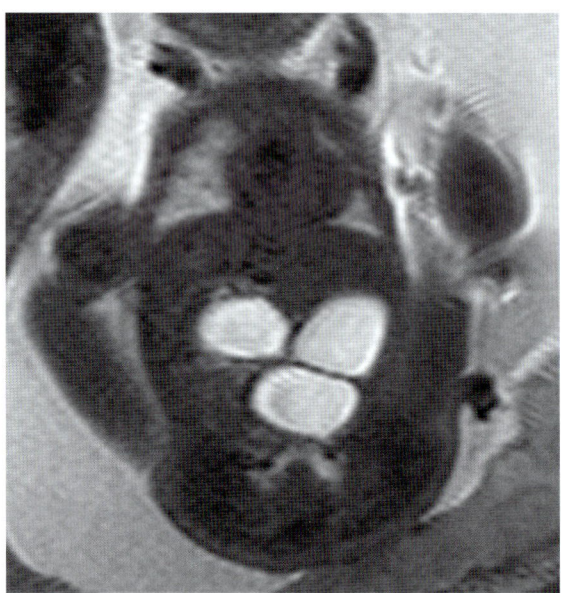

Figure 86-6 Proximal jejunal atresia. A single-shot fast spin echo coronal image with a dilated stomach, duodenal bulb, and proximal jejunum ("triple bubble").

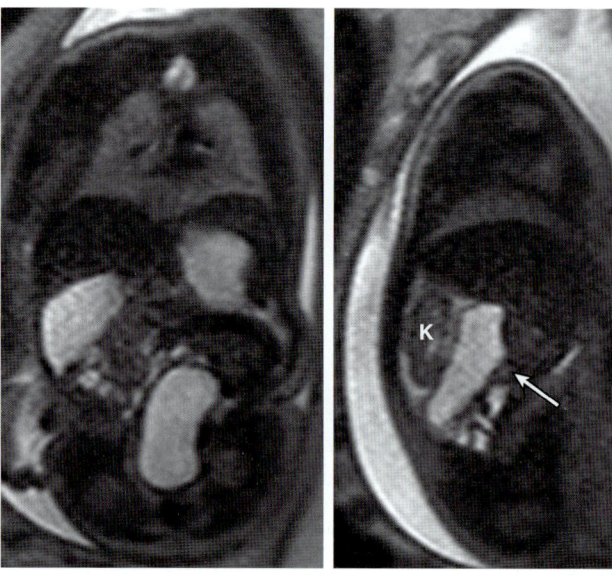

Figure 86-7 Duodenal obstruction due to Ladd's band in malrotation. Coronal (*left*) and sagittal (*right*) single-shot fast spin echo images show the stomach in the left upper quadrant and a dilated segment of bowel in the right upper quadrant (*arrow*) ventral to the right kidney (*K*). The ultrasound clip shown in Video 86-1 is remarkable for hyperperistalsis of this segment.

fibrosis; midgut volvulus; volvulus around a residual of the omphalomesenteric duct; and total colonic aganglionosis (Hirschsprung disease). One clue to the diagnosis of meconium ileus might be the presence of hyperechoic debris filling distended loops near the point of obstruction in the distal small bowel on ultrasound; MRI shows that the internal contents are hyperintense on T1-weighted images but intermediate on T2 imaging, consistent with meconium. One would expect low-signal T2 contents with the more simple intraluminal fluid in the fetus with ileal atresia.[21-23] Vigorous hyperperistalsis of the bowel is indicative of obstruction (Fig. 86-7 and Video 86-1). Cases of in utero volvulus, although uncommon, have been prospectively identified when the dilated ischemic segments are thick walled, nonperistaltic, and have internal echogenicity from hemorrhage.[24]

Imaging of the Colon Colonic atresias are difficult to diagnose specifically unless the obstructed segment can be identified with certainty in the expected location of the colon, or interhaustral notches can be separated from valvulae conniventes on ultrasound. Meconium typically is seen in the rectum by 20 weeks' gestation, in the left colon by 24 weeks' gestation, and in the right colon by 31 weeks' gestation, but this pattern may be altered by the pathology that is present.[25] On FSE T2-weighted sequences, meconium has a very low signal, whereas it shows a high signal on T1 weighting.

In general, when dilated loops are discovered, ultrasound is sufficient to diagnose the level of obstruction as proximal versus distal and to generate a focused differential diagnosis. Fetal MRI is reserved for complex cases or for those in which other abnormalities are suspected and might be confirmed by additional imaging.[26] The advantage of MRI is in its larger field of view and reproducible multiplanar capability, showing the anatomy relative to other landmarks.[27] This advantage usually is demonstrated well with single-shot T2-weighted sequences in multiple planes, whereas the addition of GRE

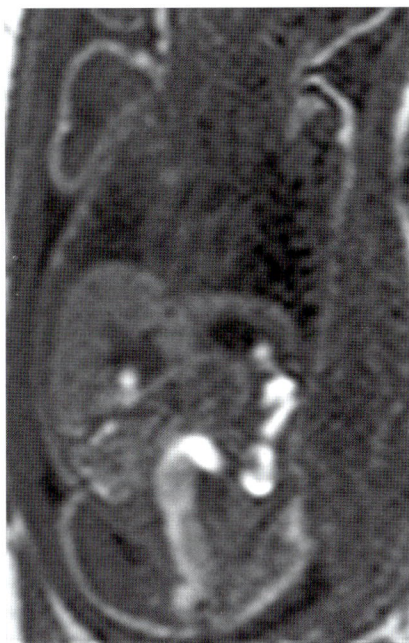

Figure 86-8 **Meconium.** A coronal T1-weighted gradient echo image showing T1 high-signal meconium in the colon.

Although one might anticipate that bowel loops would be dilated in cases of anorectal atresia, such dilation is uncommon, and the diagnosis often is made on the basis of a high level of suspicion because of associated features.[29] On ultrasound and MRI, the diagnosis may be suspected if the characteristic hypoechoic configuration of the anal musculature (Fig. 86-10) is absent. Also, a cord or ridge of abnormal fibrous tissue at the perineum may be imaged by ultrasound or MRI (Fig. 86-11). If a fistula between the colon and the urinary tract allows mixing of meconium and urine, intraluminal precipitant calcifications may be detected (Fig. 86-12).

Congenital diarrhea syndromes have been reported as showing dilation of the bowel to the rectum but without meconium signal on T1-weighted imaging, reflecting the loss of normal meconium.[30] Therefore lack of colonic meconium is not exclusive to mechanical small bowel obstructions. Differential considerations include secretory sodium or chloride diarrheas, megacystis-microcolon-hypoperistalsis syndrome, pseudoobstruction, and total colonic aganglionosis (Hirschsprung disease).[25,28,30,31]

Treatment and Follow-up At this time, no criteria have been established for intervention in the fetus based on bowel obstruction unrelated to ventral wall defects, aside from amnioreduction for polyhydramnios. Selected patients may have amniocentesis to evaluate for the possibility of chromosomal abnormalities or cystic fibrosis. Follow-up is performed with ultrasonography, with a plan to have the newborn evaluated at birth by the appropriate pediatric specialists.

T1-weighted sequences to show the distribution of high-signal meconium can provide useful additional information (Fig. 86-8). It is crucial to understand that meconium is not exclusively restricted to the colon, can normally be seen in the distal ileum, and may be in dilated loops proximal to distal obstructions (Fig. 86-9).[28] Box 86-1 lists causes of nonvisualization of meconium in the colon.

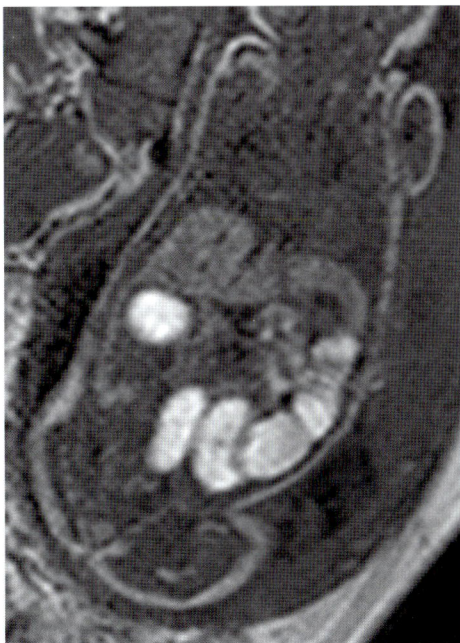

Figure 86-9 **Meconium ileus.** A gradient echo T1-weighted image at 32 weeks demonstrates dilated small bowel containing high-signal meconium.

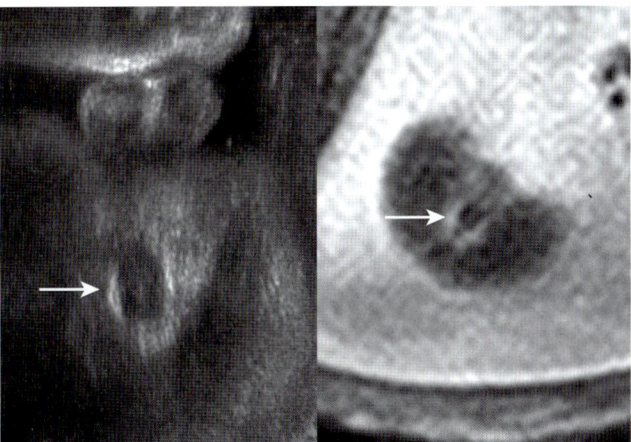

Figure 86-10 The normal hypoechoic configuration of the anal musculature at the perineum on ultrasound and axial single-shot fast spin echo T2-weighted magnetic resonance (*arrows*).

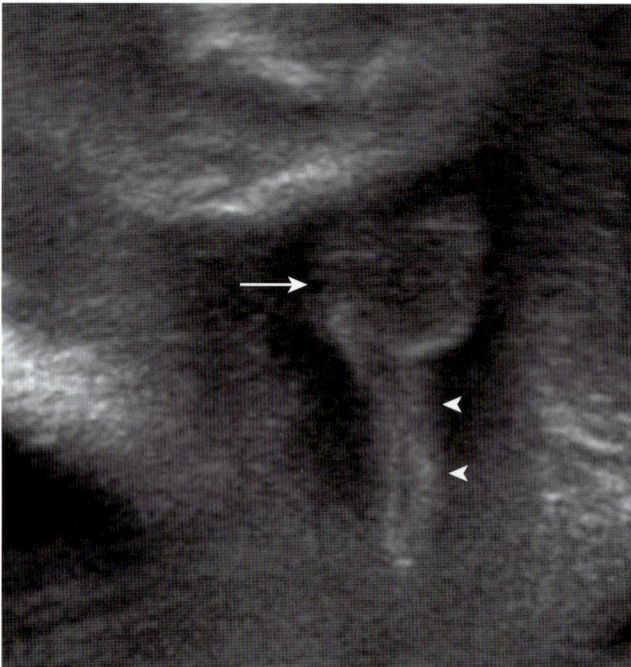

Figure 86-11 Typical configuration of the perineal cord (*arrowheads*) that may be seen from the genitalia toward the level of anal atresia. The arrow indicates the scrotum in this male fetus.

Ventral Wall Defects

Etiology Normal herniation of the midgut into the proximal umbilical cord occurs in the eighth gestational week, and after undergoing 270 degrees of rotation, the midgut returns to the abdominal cavity for fixation by the end of the twelfth week. Visualization of either the liver or bowel in the umbilical cord after 12 weeks is abnormal. Ventral wall defects include all abnormalities in which extrusion of internal anatomic structures to the outside of the fetal abdomen and/or pelvis occurs. In general, these abnormalities are thought to occur from a failure of the normal infolding and fusion of

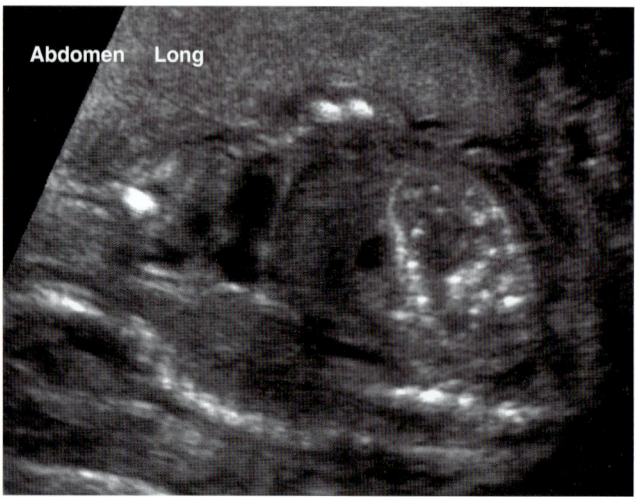

Figure 86-12 Cloacal malformation. An oblique coronal ultrasound shows multiple small echogenic calcifications within dilated colon in the left abdomen, resulting from mixing of meconium and urine.

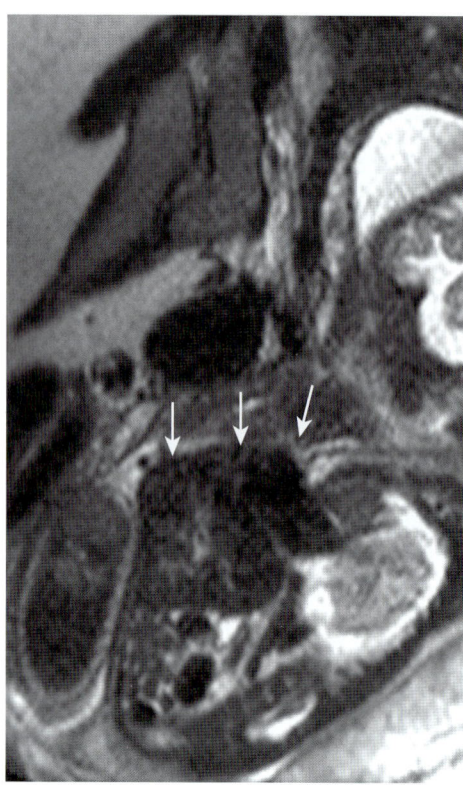

Figure 86-13 Pentalogy of Cantrell. A sagittal single-shot fast spin echo image through the chest shows herniation of low-signal liver and even lower-signal heart (*arrows*) through a ventral wall defect.

the embryonic disc.[32] If craniad infolding fails, the resulting defect would be to the abdominal wall and lower chest, resulting in findings in the spectrum of the pentalogy of Cantrell (omphalocele, sternal defect, ventral mediastinal diaphragmatic hernia, pericardial defect, and ectopia cordis) (Fig. 86-13). Lateral fold defects lead to an omphalocele, which is the most common isolated ventral wall defect and is contained by a membrane (parietal peritoneum and amnion) unless ruptured (Fig. 86-14).[33] Caudal fold failure results in bladder or cloacal exstrophy, which primarily affect the genitourinary tract. In bladder exstrophy, the ventral wall of the bladder, inferior rectus musculature, and skin are absent, and the residual dorsal wall of the bladder is continuous with the abdominal wall. Cloacal exstrophy is more complex; persistence of the infraumbilical cloacal membrane is thought to prevent normal anterior abdominal wall closure and separation of the urogenital system from the rectum, and as a result, two hemibladders are separated by bowel. Closed spinal defects, renal and genital malformations, and club feet may occur. Both bladder and cloacal exstrophy include diastasis of the pubic symphysis and may have more complex pelvic bone deformities (Fig. 86-15). OEIS complex describes the particular association of **o**mphalocele, bladder **e**xstrophy, **i**mperforate anus, and **s**pinal defect,[34] but this complex is believed by many persons to be a synonym for cloacal exstrophy.[35]

Body stalk anomaly is a severe form of ventral wall defect that results from failure of folding along multiple planes and is not compatible with extrauterine life (Fig. 86-16).[36]

Gastroschisis is a type of ventral wall defect that may be unrelated to embryonic disc folding. It is possible that a

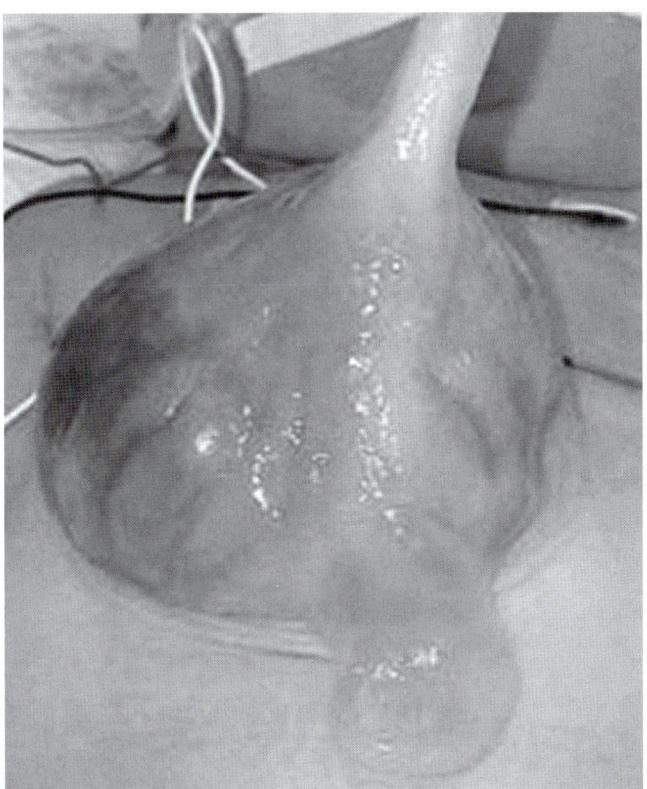

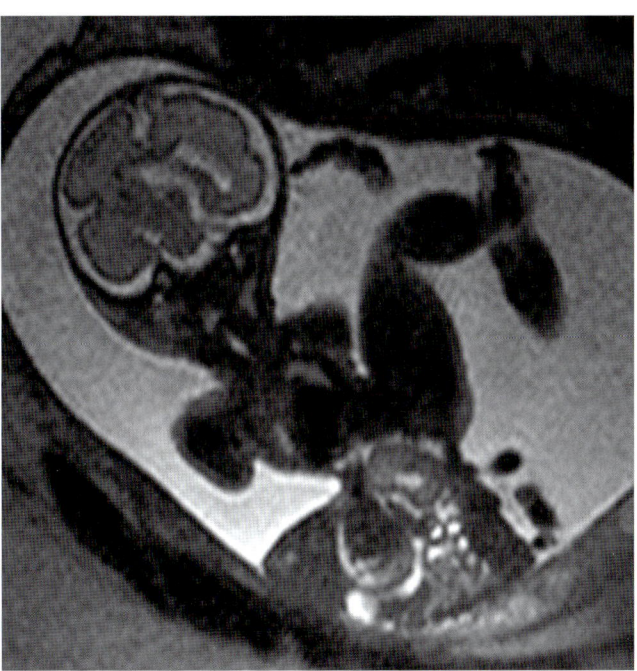

Figure 86-16 **Limb-body wall complex.** Extrusion of all abdominal contents in limb-body wall complex. Typically a very short umbilical cord and significant fetal contortion are present.

Figure 86-14 **Omphalocele.** This photograph of a newborn shows a large anterior wall defect with a surrounding membrane. The umbilical cord is inserting at the apex.

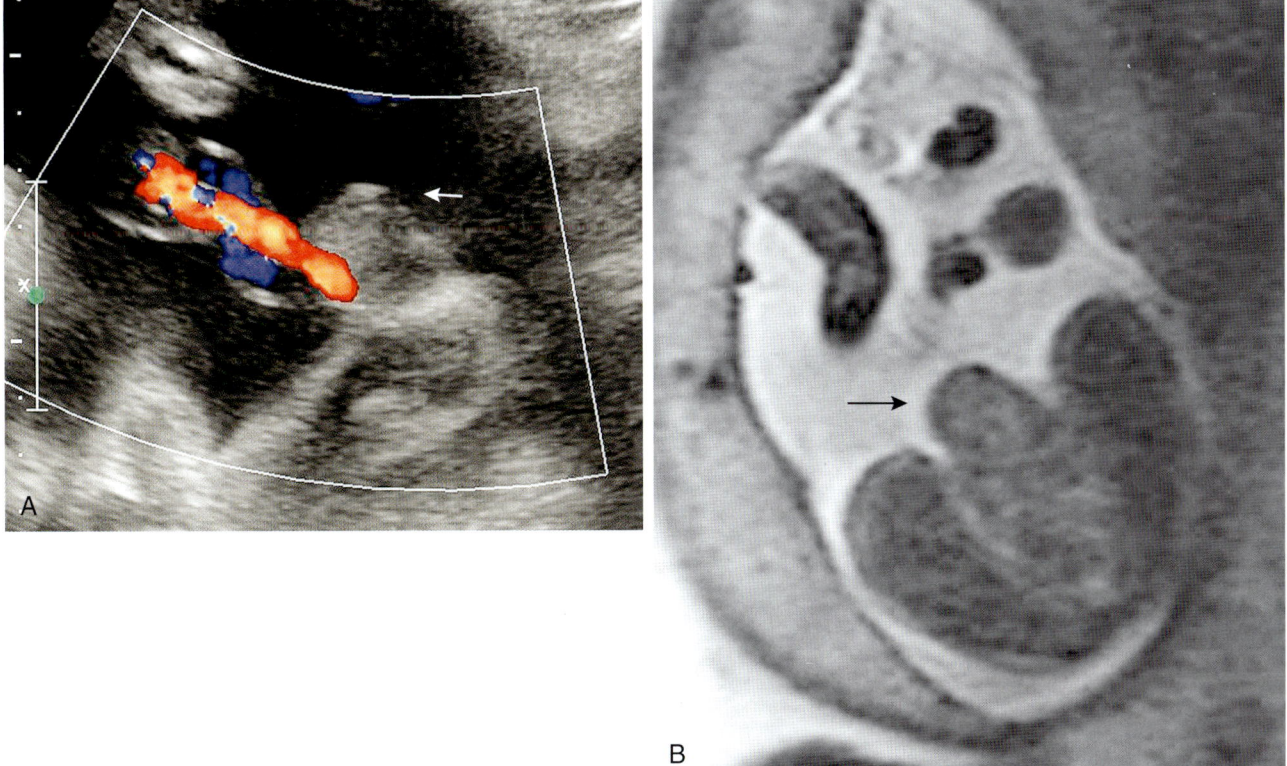

Figure 86-15 **A,** A longitudinal sonogram of the anterior pelvis shows a small outpouching just below the low-lying umbilical cord insertion (*arrow*). No bladder is noted. **B,** An axial single-shot fast spin echo T2-weighted magnetic resonance image of the pelvis confirms the presence of a soft tissue outpouching below the cord insertion (*arrow*). No bladder is present.

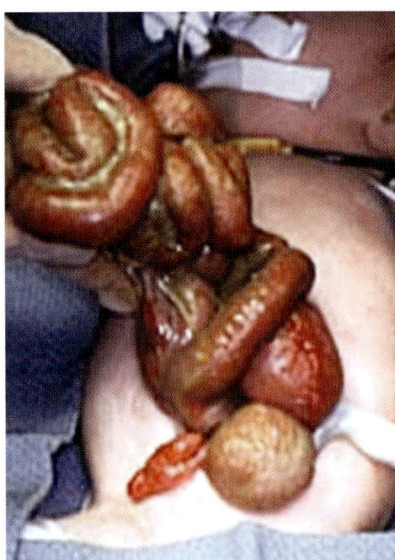

Figure 86-17 *Gastroschisis.* This newborn has a large amount of dilated bowel protruding outside the abdominal cavity at the level of the umbilicus. No covering membrane is present.

vascular insult results in a through-and-through defect in the layers of the abdominal wall adjacent to the umbilicus, almost universally on the right, through which the bowel herniates without a covering membrane; other hypotheses have been proposed, but the cause is not yet known (Fig. 86-17).[37,38] The risk of bearing a fetus with gastroschisis is reportedly increased in young primigravida women and also has been associated with the use of agents that may cause vasoconstriction, such as tobacco and salicylates.[39,40]

Because of the lack of skin covering in this constellation of defects, the maternal alpha-fetoprotein levels can be elevated, and further subsequent screening with ultrasound leads to the prenatal diagnosis.

Imaging Visualization of liver or bowel within the umbilical cord beyond the twelfth week of gestation is evidence of an omphalocele. A giant omphalocele is defined when more than 50% of the liver is extracorporeal or the defect is greater

than 5 cm wide.[41,42] Wharton's jelly pseudocysts may be found in association with the defect, located near the cord insertion site on the omphalocele.[43] When the defect is small, the differentiation of a small, skin-covered umbilical hernia from omphalocele is difficult. Ultrasound typically can diagnose these defects readily and accurately define the extruded anatomy (Fig. 86-18). When ultrasound fails to reveal the pertinent details, MRI can be useful and relies on standard single-shot FSE T2-weighted imaging; the liver tends to have a higher signal than other abdominal structures on T1-weighted sequences, which is useful for identification of the position of the liver in questionable cases. Characteristically, however, when fetal MRI is requested in cases of omphalocele, it is because of an interest in assessing for additional abnormalities or a need to calculate MR-derived lung volumes. Newborns with giant omphalocele have a tendency to need long-term ventilatory support and may have pulmonary hypoplasia.[42,44,45] Echocardiography is indicated, because 50% of fetuses with omphalocele have congenital heart disease. Ascites may be present but tends to decrease through gestation. Note that if a normal bladder is not seen over time or in repeated studies, exstrophy must be considered.

Gastroschisis is differentiated from omphalocele by the lack of a covering membrane of the herniated viscera and the normal insertion of the umbilical vessels at the abdominal wall (Fig. 86-19). MRI generally is not necessary for evaluation of this diagnosis because gastroschisis almost always is an isolated defect without additional fetal malformations or lung hypoplasia.[32] Closure of the abdominal wall defect in utero with subsequent severing of the extruded bowel, thus leading to extensive atresia/congenital short-gut syndrome, has been reported.[46] Additionally, on rare occasions the membrane covering an omphalocele may rupture, thus simulating gastroschisis on imaging because of the free-floating appearance of the bowel. Differentiation is made by examining the relationship of the umbilical vessels to the extruded bowel. If the liver is extruded, it is an omphalocele (Fig. 86-20).

Treatment and Follow-up Fetuses in whom omphalocele is diagnosed are tested for chromosomal abnormalities because the incidence of aneuploidy is 40% to 60%, especially if only bowel is herniated.[47] The outcome for patients with

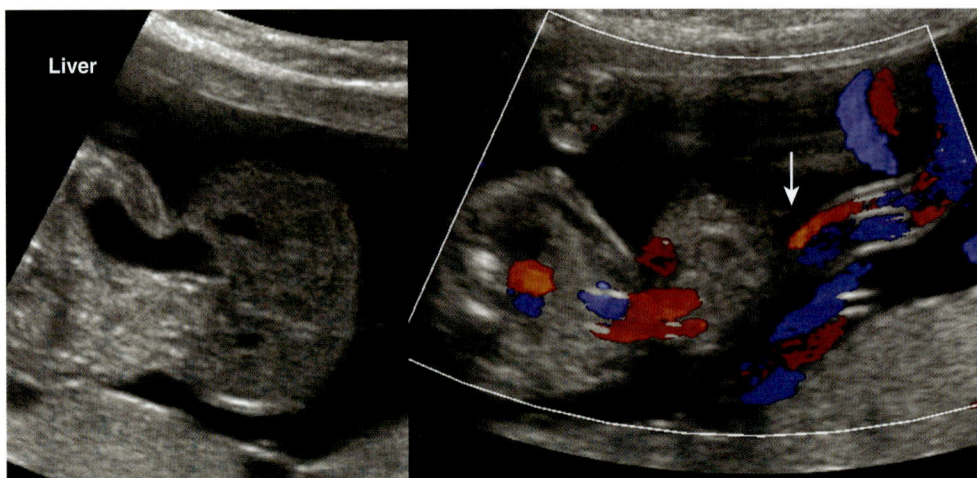

Figure 86-18 *Omphalocele containing liver and distal stomach.* The umbilical cord inserts into the omphalocele sac (*arrow*). The spine is on the left.

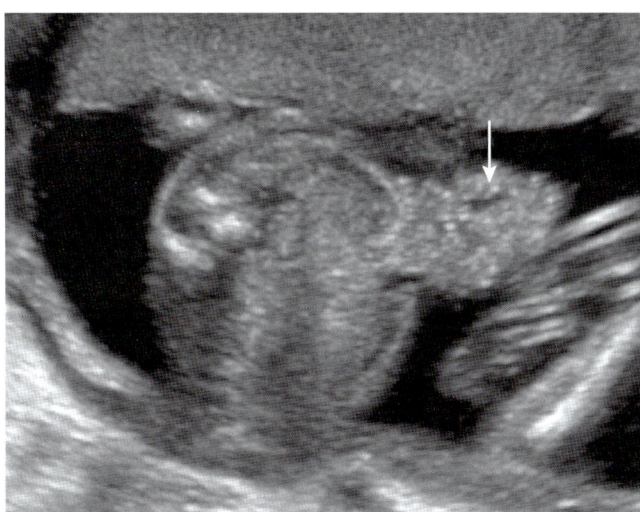

Figure 86-19 Gastroschisis. A transverse sonogram shows a right para-umbilical defect with herniation of small bowel loops (*arrow*) into the amniotic cavity with no surrounding membrane.

omphalocele is usually dependent on the severity of other anomalies, including cardiac defects.[48] Repair of omphaloceles in the newborn period has a high rate of success, especially with surgical techniques emphasizing gradual reduction for larger lesions.[33,49,50]

Gastroschisis, unlike omphalocele, is not associated with chromosomal abnormalities, although the occurrence of

extraintestinal abnormalities is approximately 6%.[51] Fetuses with gastroschisis experience complications that occur in the part of the bowel that is directly exposed to amniotic fluid during pregnancy; perforation or atresia occurs in up to 20% of cases.[51] Although dilation of the herniated loops is poorly correlated to worsened prognosis, sustained distension of intraabdominal bowel loops is of concern.[52] Postnatally, these patients may require resection of portions of their bowel, and short-gut syndrome may develop. These children are at risk for presentation with necrotizing enterocolitis and perforation even months after undergoing repair.[53,54]

In fetuses with either omphalocele or gastroschisis, bowel rotation does not occur, and these patients, by definition, have midgut malrotation.

Echogenic Bowel and Peritoneal Abnormalities

Etiology Echogenic bowel is a nonspecific ultrasound finding that should not be ignored, although in most cases no subsequent fetal or neonatal problem develops.[55] In cases in which this finding is a marker for an abnormality, the problem could be as varied in etiology as infection (e.g., cytomegalovirus or parvovirus), intrauterine growth retardation, or aneuploidy (e.g., trisomy 21), or the direct cause of the increased conspicuity of the bowel might remain unclear. In other cases, the etiology may be more obvious; for example, in persons with cystic fibrosis, the meconium is more viscous and may present as hyperechoic contents within the bowel lumen. If bleeding has occurred into either the amniotic fluid or GI tract, swallowed intraluminal fluid can appear bright on ultrasound.

Abnormalities of the peritoneum in the fetus include ascites and calcifications. The etiology of fetal ascites can be classified under five general categories, ranging from serous through chylous, hemorrhagic, bilious, and related to the urinary tract (Box 86-2).[56-65]

Imaging When the bowel is as echogenic as the fetal skeleton, it is considered abnormal (Fig. 86-21).[66] It has been

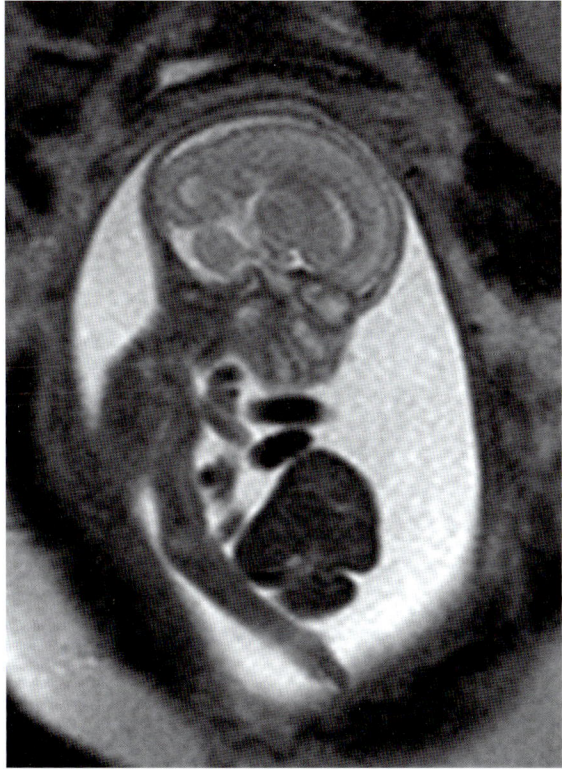

Figure 86-20 Ruptured omphalocele. A sagittal single-shot fast spin echo magnetic resonance image shows liver outside the fetal abdomen without a covering membrane.

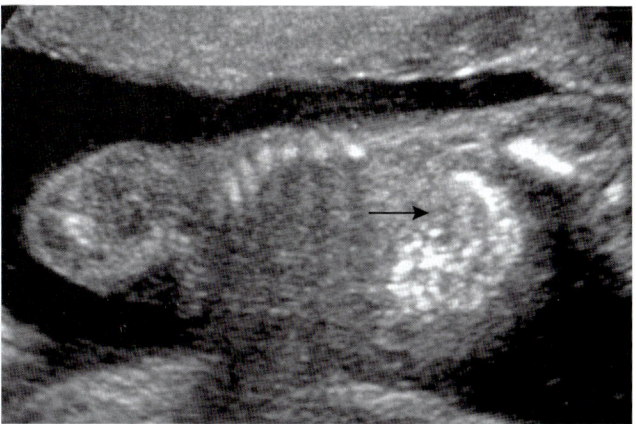

Figure 86-21 Echogenic bowel. A longitudinal sonogram of a 20-week fetus with echogenic bowel (*arrow*) that is as echogenic as the adjacent bone. Intrauterine growth retardation was present.

Box 86-2 Causes of Fetal Ascites

Serous
- Bowel perforation (fluid may be complex)
- Hydrops: immune and nonimmune (most common cause)
- Ruptured or torted ovarian cyst
- Cardiac decompensation
- Hypoproteinemia
- Hepatic dysfunction (storage disorders, mass, infection)

Bilious
- Perforation of a choledochal cyst

Chylous
- Thoracic duct obstruction, increased intrathoracic pressure
- Lymphatic malformation (e.g., Klippel-Trenaunay syndrome)
- Mesenteric lymphangiomatosis

Hemorrhagic
- Rupture of a vascular tumor
- Trauma

Uriniferous
- Perforation of the collecting system or bladder
- Cloacal malformation, urogenital sinus

---

recommended that transducer frequencies of 5 MHz or less be used for confirmation, because higher frequencies may make the bowel appear unnecessarily bright.[67] Although most of these patients are healthy, the finding of abnormally bright bowel in the fetus should prompt a careful ultrasound search for additional abnormalities, with consideration of further imaging by MRI for evaluation of the neural axis if infection is suspected.

Imaging of fetal ascites should be directed toward determining whether the fluid can be related to a particular organ system. Anatomy should be examined carefully, whether on ultrasound or MRI, for abnormalities of the urinary or reproductive tracts, biliary system, chest, and bowel. The presence of septations or loculation might suggest protein contamination from blood products, bowel pathology, or abdominal lymphangiomatosis. In some case, ascites may be a physiological consequence of a condition (e.g., hypoproteinemia, hydrops, or infection) not directly related to an anatomic abnormality. It is important to look for any evidence of calcifications in the peritoneum, especially along the liver capsule, that would indicate meconium peritonitis and the implied disruption of bowel integrity, as from perforations secondary to obstruction or ischemia. Calcifications in the parenchyma of the liver or spleen would be a clue to the presence of aneuploidy or infection, or rarely may be related to portal emboli.[68,69] Calcification inside the bowel lumen is an indication of GI-genitourinary fistula (see Fig. 86-12).[70]

Treatment and Follow-up Treatment and follow-up are directed toward the cause of the finding and could include in utero intervention (e.g., intrauterine transfusion) and post-natal surgery, depending on the etiology. Fetuses who have isolated fetal ascites with a normal karyotype and a negative infection screen have a good prognosis.[71,72]

Masses and Other Organ Abnormalities

Etiology The etiology of masses in the fetal abdomen may be related to abnormally enlarged or infiltrated viscera or to the presence or development of an abnormal structure.

Visceromegaly includes hepatosplenomegaly, which may be the result of viral infection, fetal hydrops, glycogen or lysosomal storage disorders, Beckwith-Wiedemann syndrome, or the presentation in utero of anemia or hematologic malignancy (particularly for trisomy 21), and amniotic fluid testing may be necessary.[57,65,73-75] Considerations for isolated hepatomegaly include increased right heart pressure; the liver also might appear enlarged if it lies transversely across the abdomen, as in heterotaxy. Neoplasia also may present with visceromegaly, with the organ being either a repository for metastatic disease, such as neuroblastoma diffusely metastatic to the liver,[76,77] or the site of a primary intraperitoneal tumor, most frequently in the fetal liver (Fig. 86-22).[78-80] Intrauterine torsion also can present with visceromegaly from edema.[78-80] A special note should be made of megacystis-microcolon-hypoperistalsis syndrome, which can be considered in patients, more commonly female, with gross bladder enlargement and no colonic meconium on T1-weighted MRI (Fig. 86-23).[25,81]

The category of abnormal structures presenting as mass lesions includes intraperitoneal cysts or fluid collections, such as meconium peritonitis as a result of perforation of the bowel, or, as recently reported, as a result of reflux of meconium into the peritoneum through the uterus in a fetus with

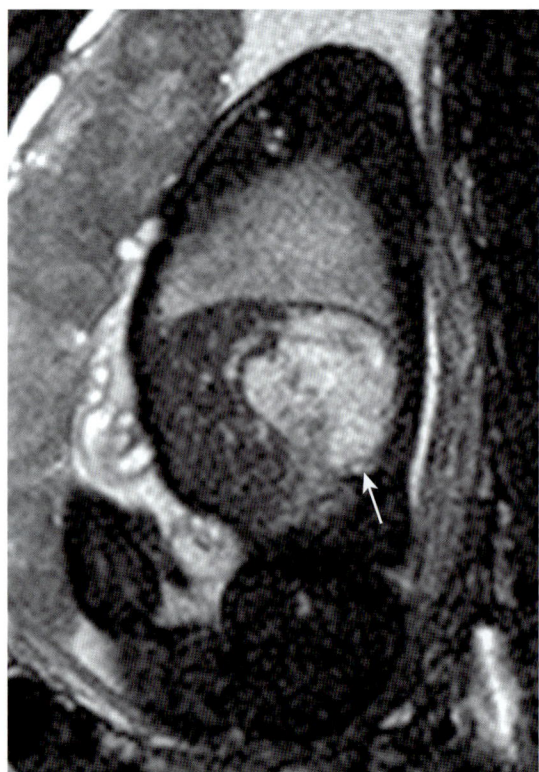

Figure 86-22 Rapidly involuting congenital hemangioma. A sagittal T2-weighted image of a high-signal mass lesion (*arrow*) in the posterior right lobe of the liver.

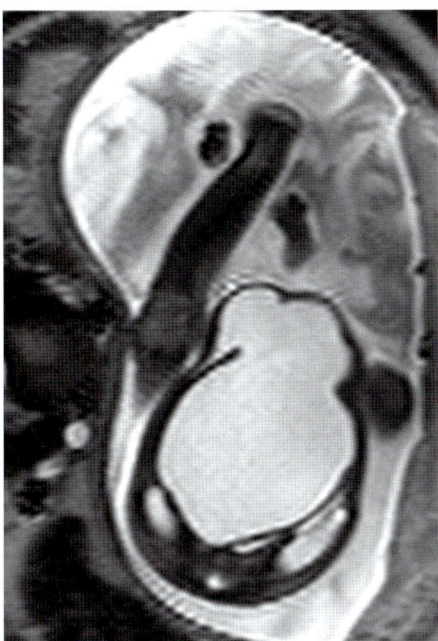

Figure 86-23 Megacystis-microcolon-hypoperistalsis syndrome. An axial single-shot fast spin echo image in a female fetus with hydronephrosis and marked bladder distension. Normal amniotic fluid volume was present. No meconium could be identified in the bowel on T1-weighted imaging.

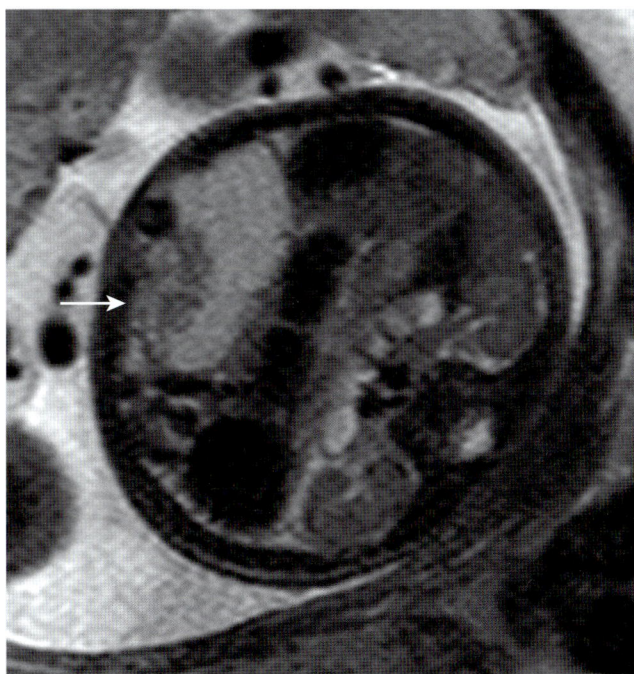

Figure 86-25 Meconium pseudocyst. Magnetic resonance shows a medium to moderately high signal collection containing debris (*arrow*) on T2-weighted imaging, consistent with meconium mixing.

cloacal malformation (Figs. 86–24 and 86–25).[82] Box 86-3 lists the origins of cystic masses in the abdomen and pelvis, and Box 86-4 describes solid masses that have been reported. Occasionally a "pseudomass" is described inside of a bowel lumen, such as the stomach; in this particular case, it is thought to represent debris such as blood products and may be seen after a history of intervention (e.g., amniocentesis).[83] Note that most commonly, masses in the fetal abdomen are related to the genitourinary tract; these masses are discussed in greater detail in Chapter 113.

Box 86-3 Intraperitoneal Cystic Masses in the Fetus*

Gastrointestinal tract: duplication, meconium pseudocyst, segmental dilatation of the ileum (ileal dysgenesis)

Biliary: choledochal cyst

Hepatic: epithelial cyst, mesenchymal hamartoma, vascular malformation

Splenic: congenital epithelial cyst, epidermoid

Lymphatic: mesenteric cyst, mesenteric lymphangiomatosis

Ovarian†: follicular cyst, torsion (late), teratoma

*Most cystic masses in the fetal abdomen are related to the genitourinary tract.
†Technically retroperitoneal, but may seem to present as an intraperitoneal mass. Note that other retroperitoneal masses, such as cystic neuroblastoma in the adrenal, may seem to be intraperitoneal depending on size.

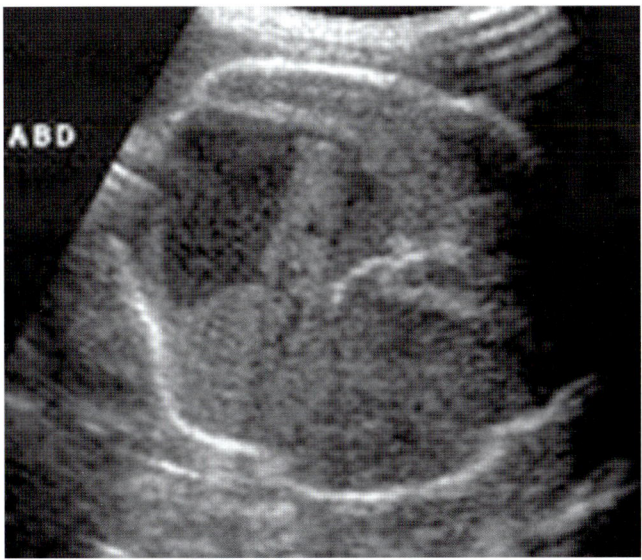

Figure 86-24 Meconium pseudocyst. A transverse sonogram shows a large loculated heterogeneous collection with a calcified rim within the abdomen. A sigmoid perforation was identified after delivery.

Box 86-4 Intraperitoneal Solid Masses in the Fetus

Hepatic: hepatoblastoma, hemangioendothelioma, rapidly involuting congenital hemangioma, torsion of accessory lobe, mesenchymal hamartoma, teratoma, infarction

Splenic: torsion

Ovarian*: torsion (early), teratoma

Pulmonary*: infradiaphragmatic sequestration

*Technically retroperitoneal, but may seem to present as an intraperitoneal mass.

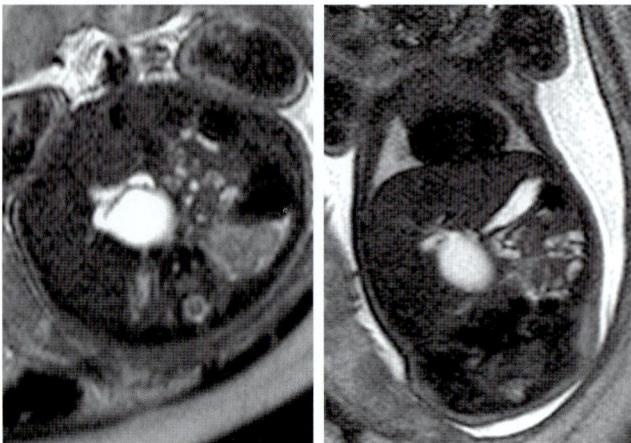

Figure 86-26 Choledochal cyst. Axial and coronal T2-weighted single-shot fast spin echo images of a cystic mass at the margin of the liver demonstrate a connection to the biliary system.

Some abnormalities are related to the absence of expected structures. For example, the spleen may be absent, and the gallbladder may be in abnormal position or absent; these findings suggest heterotaxy, which would mandate careful evaluation of the cardiac axis and configuration and other viscerovascular structures. The gallbladder usually can be detected on serial ultrasound[84] and is identified consistently on MRI.[85] Its absence would suggest biliary atresia and polysplenia if found within the heterotaxy complex. A gallbladder also may be indistinguishable in a fetus with cystic fibrosis.

Calcifications and/or debris in the gallbladder can be a sign of fetal hemolysis, but most are incidental and do not cause complications.[86] Small stones typically resolve without intervention. Finally, organs may be displaced from their normal position in persons with splenogonadal fusion, the so-called *wandering spleen,* and of course with diaphragmatic hernias.

Imaging Careful delineation of the organ of involvement and of the pertinent anatomy can suggest the correct diagnosis (Fig. 86-26). When calcifications are identified, infection should be considered.[87] The use of a high-resolution linear transducer in the appropriate patient can be extremely advantageous in delineating fine detail, such as subtle calcifications, the presence within a large cyst of a daughter cyst indicative of ovarian origin, or the characteristic bowel signature of a duplication cyst. For all abnormalities, in addition to identifying the organ of origin, Doppler evaluation will help to understand whether a primary vascular lesion (increased flow) or torsion/ischemia (decreased flow) should be advanced in the differential diagnosis (Fig. 86-27).

Ultrasound generally delineates well the origin of fetal abdominal masses from solid organs. Masses are investigated by MRI when the organ of origin or the extent of involvement is imprecisely detailed by ultrasonography. In addition to the use of GRE, T1-weighted and FSE T2-weighted sequences, SSFP T2-weighted sequences are useful because of their ability to delineate adjacent structures and high–signal blood flow. This effect can be very helpful in identifying primary vascular lesions (Fig. 86-28) or enlarged vessels supplying tumors. In addition, fetal MRI may be indicated in the evaluation of the liver in conditions of potential iron overload, in which the signal from the liver is abnormally low.[88,89]

Umbilical venous varix is a vascular lesion that is variably associated with in utero complications.[90] Other vascular anomalies of the venous system, including absence of the ductus venosus or agenesis of the portal veins, have been described and require meticulous delineation of the associated portosystemic shunt pathway by ultrasound Doppler or bright-blood (SSFP) MRI for accurate diagnosis.[91,92.]

Treatment and Follow-up Depending on the diagnosis, alterations in planning and timing of delivery may be indicated; amniocentesis and in utero therapies may be considered (e.g., intrauterine transfusion for fetal anemia). In general, therapy is targeted at providing the safest environment in which appropriate treatment can be directed for the fetus or neonate. To date, there are no clear indications for fetal surgery for gastrointestinal anomalies, although imaging evaluation can alter both the timing and mode of delivery. Open fetal surgery has been reserved for conditions determined to be terminal without intervention in a previable fetus, and has been limited to excisions of malformations and tumors of the chest, head and neck, and coccyx (e.g., sacrococcygeal teratoma).[93-95]

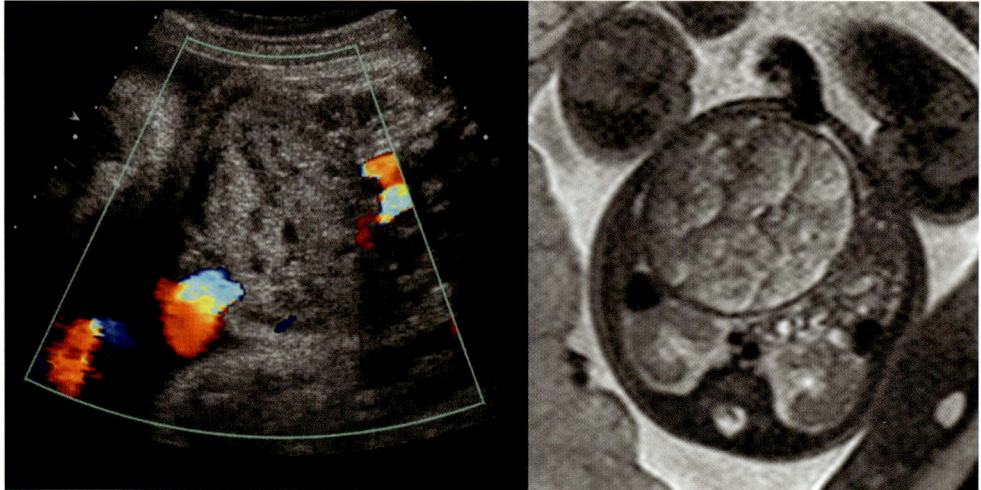

Figure 86-27 Ovarian torsion. A solid-appearing but avascular mass is delineated in this female fetus with both ultrasound and magnetic resonance imaging.

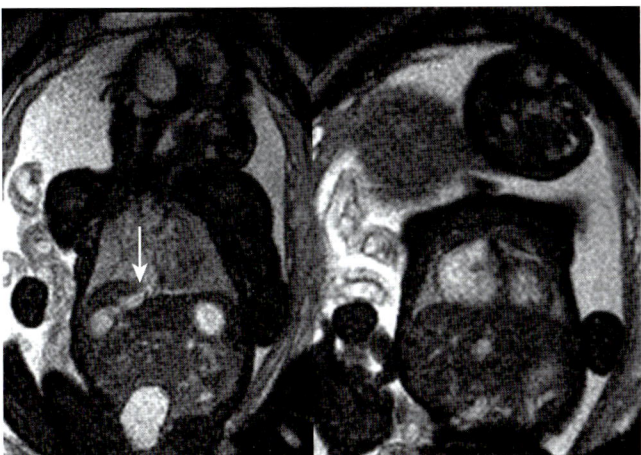

Figure 86-28 **Hepatic vascular malformation.** Balanced steady-state free-precession coronal imaging shows an enlarged draining vein (*arrow, left*) and enlarged right atrium (*right*) as a result of congenital vascular malformation in the liver.

WHAT THE CLINICIAN NEEDS TO KNOW

- Dilated or echogenic bowel loops
- Expected level of obstruction
- Presence of mass, calcification, or ascites
- Assessment of vascularity
- Associated and/or additional abnormalities

Key Points

Ultrasound is for screening of fetal bowel abnormalities and will answer almost all questions. MRI can be useful for targeted questions unanswered by ultrasonography, including evaluation of microcolon and abnormal meconium signal distribution.

Ventral wall defects are distinguished by what is herniated from the fetal abdomen, the presence of a covering membrane, and the relationship of the umbilical vessels to the herniated viscera.

When fetal ascites is encountered, a careful search for an anatomic abnormality to the cardiac, pulmonary, biliary, genitourinary, and gastrointestinal systems is indicated.

Precise identification of the organ(s) of origin will determine an appropriate differential diagnosis for fetal abdominal masses.

Suggested Readings

Brugger PC. MRI of the fetal abdomen. In: Prayer D, ed. *Fetal MRI.* Berlin: Springer-Verlag; 2011.

Dubois J, Grignon A. Abdomen (digestive tract, wall and peritoneum). In: Avni FE, ed. *Perinatal imaging: from ultrasound to MR imaging.* Berlin: Springer-Verlag; 2002.

Hertberg BS, Nyberg DA, Neilsen IR. Ventral wall defects. In: Nyberg D, McGahan JP, Pretorius DH, et al, eds. *Diagnostic imaging of fetal anomalies.* Philadelphia: Lippincott, Williams and Wilkins; 2003.

Nyberg DA, Neilsen IR. Abdomen and gastrointestinal tract. In: Nyberg D, McGahan JP, Pretorius DH, et al, eds. *Diagnostic imaging of fetal anomalies.* Philadelphia: Lippincott, Williams and Wilkins; 2003.

Samuel N, Dicker D, Feldberg D, et al. Ultrasound diagnosis and management of fetal intestinal obstruction and volvulus in utero. *J Perinat Med.* 1984;12(6):333-337.

References

Full references for this chapter can be found on www.expertconsult.com.

Chapter 87

The Abdominal Wall and Peritoneal Cavity

SUMIT PRUTHI, SUDHA P. SINGH, and MELISSA A. HILMES

Peritoneal Cavity

Overview The peritoneum is a thin serosal membrane of mesodermal origin that comprises a single layer of mesothelial cells resting on a basement membrane.[1] It is divided into visceral and parietal components, and the space between the two components constitutes the peritoneal cavity. The layer covering the abdominal viscera, omentum, and the mesenteries is designated *visceral,* whereas the layer covering the abdominal walls, undersurface of the diaphragm, anterior surface of the retroperitoneal viscera, and the pelvis is designated as *parietal.* The peritoneum is continuous in males, whereas in females it is discontinuous at the ostia of the oviducts to allow communication between the peritoneal cavity and extraperitoneal pelvis.

The layers of peritoneum that invest blood vessels, lymphatics, nerves, adipose tissue, and connective tissue within the abdomen and the pelvis form the various peritoneal ligaments, omentum, and mesenteries. A ligament usually supports a structure within the cavity, whereas a mesentery usually suspends the structure to the retroperitoneum. Omentum is a specialized ligament that connects the stomach to another structure. These ligaments and mesenteries not only serve to suspend and support the visceral organs but also divide the peritoneal cavity into multiple compartments that dictate the location and routes of spread of malignancies and infection.

The mesothelial cells produce a small amount of sterile fluid within the peritoneal cavity that is continuously circulated by the movement of the diaphragm and peristalsis of bowel, and the fluid provides a frictionless surface over which the viscera can move, a site for fluid transport, and local bacterial defense.[1] Peritoneal fluid predominantly flows up the right paracolic gutter into the right supramesocolic compartment, and 90% of the fluid is cleared by the subphrenic lymphatics to the supradiaphragmatic nodes.[2] Areas of relative stasis include 1) the rectouterine pouch or cul-de-sac (pouch of Douglas) in females, 2) the rectovesical region in males, 3) the right lower abdomen at the end of the small bowel mesentery, 4) the left lower abdomen along the sigmoid mesocolon, 5) the right paracolic gutter, and 6) the right subhepatic/subdiaphragmatic space (Morison pouch).[2]

Entities Affecting the Peritoneum

PNEUMOPERITONEUM

Overview The term *pneumoperitoneum* refers to the presence of air within the peritoneal cavity. Benign postoperative pneumoperitoneum is a separate entity that results from accumulation of free air following abdominal surgery. Usually, free peritoneal air clears more rapidly in children than in adults, but the timing can be variable. The timing of clearance usually depends upon the amount of air initially trapped after surgery, which in most cases is related to the patient's body habitus; obese patients trap less air than thin patients.[3] Several studies have demonstrated clearing of free air in 68% to 90% of children postoperatively by 24 hours, but free air can be seen for as long as 6 to 7 days postoperatively in 2% to 3% of cases.[3]

Etiology Free intraperitoneal air is most commonly a consequence of gastrointestinal (GI) tract perforation.[4] In the neonate, this usually results from intestinal obstruction, necrotizing enterocolitis, or spontaneous gastric or bowel perforation, usually at the ileocecal region (Box 87-1).[5] Necrotizing enterocolitis is the most common cause of pneumoperitoneum in the neonatal intensive care unit.[6]

Free intraperitoneal gas sometimes results from mediastinal extension in newborns supported by mechanical ventilation. Rarely, nasogastric or nasoduodenal tubes may perforate the bowel. The position of the tube is often a clue to the perforation (e-Fig. 87-1).

In children beyond the neonatal period, perforated peptic ulcers and inflammatory bowel disease (IBD) are other causes of pneumoperitoneum; it should be noted that pneumoperitoneum is rarely found with appendiceal perforation, because the omentum usually seals off the perforation very quickly.[7] Trauma, both accidental and nonaccidental, may also result in pneumoperitoneum.

Clinical Presentation Pneumoperitoneum may be suspected clinically because of the history of an underlying disease that predisposes to bowel perforation, detection of acute abdominal distension with increased tympany on physical examination, clinical deterioration of the patient, and

Box 87-1 Causes of Pneumoperitoneum in Newborns

With Perforation of the Gastrointestinal Tract

- Gastric perforation, spontaneous or iatrogenic (nasogastric tubes)
- Duodenal ulcer with perforation
- Isolated perforation of the small bowel or colon in the absence of associated abnormality
- Perforation of Meckel diverticulum (ectopic gastric mucosa with ulceration)
- Necrotizing enterocolitis
- Colonic perforation (secondary to instrumentation, enema tip, thermometer)
- Perforation secondary to intestinal obstruction (atresia, meconium ileus, Hirschsprung disease, neonatal small left colon)
- Secondary to postsurgical anastomotic leak

Without Perforation of the Gastrointestinal Tract

- Pulmonary air leaks (pneumomediastinum) with or without other manifestations of alveolar leaks
- Idiopathic (extremely rare)

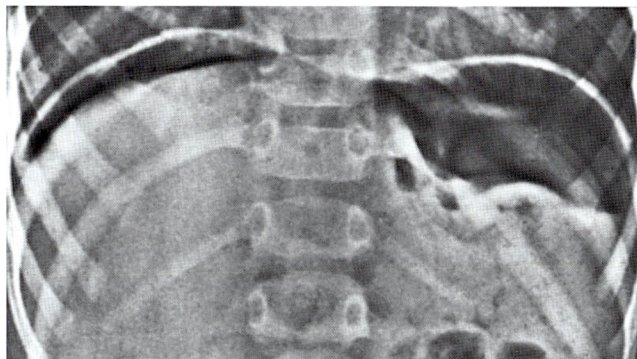

Figure 87-2 Free intraperitoneal air. An upright examination of the abdomen in a 2-year-old boy with perforated gastric ulcer. Air is easily demonstrated between the diaphragm and the liver on the right side and between the diaphragm and the spleen and stomach on the left.

occasional fortuitous discovery on imaging examinations of the chest or abdomen.

Imaging   A single, supine abdominal radiograph is usually the most common imaging study requested for patients with suspected abdominal pathology. The cited overall detection rate of free intraperitoneal air on supine imaging ranges from 56% to 59%; detection rates as high as 80.4% have been quoted on supine abdominal radiographs; and the rate is 78.7% on supine chest radiograph.[4] It is important to be familiar with the various signs of intraperitoneal free air on supine radiographs, because this may be the only initial study requested by the patient's primary care giver.

Once suspected, the diagnosis can be confirmed on horizontal–beam plain radiographs. Upright radiographs will show air collecting between the diaphragm and the liver on the right and between the diaphragm and the liver, spleen, stomach, or colon on the left (Figs. 87-2 and 87-3). Young children and those too ill to sit or stand can be examined in the decubitus position. The decubitus view should be obtained with the right side up to allow the liver to fall away from the wall of the peritoneal cavity; this allows visualization of free peritoneal air between the liver and the abdominal wall. Both techniques are considered equally effective, and the choice usually depends upon the patient's age and clinical status and the preference of the radiologist.[4]

If decubitus or upright imaging is difficult to obtain, a supine view using a horizontal-beam technique can be utilized. On the horizontal-beam supine radiograph, free peritoneal air may collect between the anterior surface of the liver and the anterior abdominal wall (Fig. 87-4), but small amounts of free air may be more difficult to detect, particularly if located over loops of bowel.

Tension pneumomediastinum can dissect along the retroperitoneum and the subadventitial layer of the mesenteric vessels and can rupture freely into the peritoneal cavity. The latter is usually suspected because of the history of assisted ventilation and the presence of pneumomediastinum on the

chest radiograph. A ruptured viscus permits both air and fluid to escape into the peritoneal cavity, causing abnormal extraluminal air-fluid levels (compares Figs. 87-3 and 87-4). Dissecting pneumomediastinum results in only air within the peritoneal space, thus a significant air-fluid level is not identified in the peritoneal space on horizontal-beam examination. The differentiation may remain difficult in patients with preexistent ascites, therefore correlation with chest radiographs, clinical history, and physical findings may be required to make the distinction.

Multiple signs related to pneumoperitoneum are described on plain radiographs (Table 87-1) based on the location and volume of air and its relationship to adjacent structures. The lucency caused by the free air rising to an anterior position in the abdomen is most easily detected when it projects over the liver, thus many right upper quadrant signs of free air are described.[8] The normal liver is uniform in radiodensity and is typically denser than the heart. Air overlying the liver on a supine radiograph decreases the radiodensity of that portion of the liver over which it lies.

Small amounts of free air may appear only as subtle, localized collections in the right upper quadrant on supine radiographs. Linear collections represent air in the right subhepatic space, known as the *hepatic edge sign*, whereas triangular collections are seen with air in the Morison pouch (e-Fig. 87-5); this is known as the *Doge cap sign*, because it

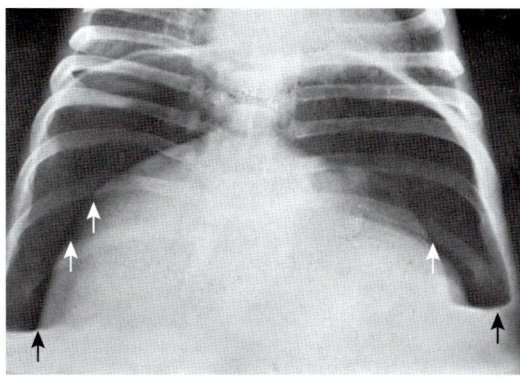

Figure 87-3 Pyopneumoperitoneum. Massive amount of free air in the abdomen below the diaphragm (*white arrows*) with air-fluid levels (*black arrows*) on an upright film.

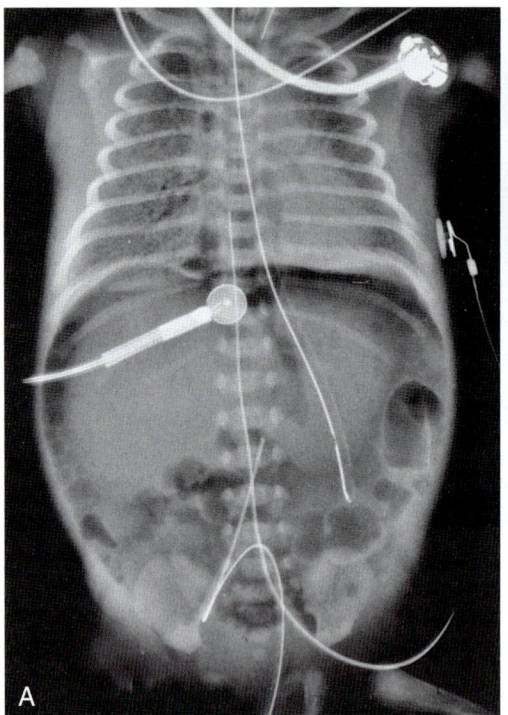
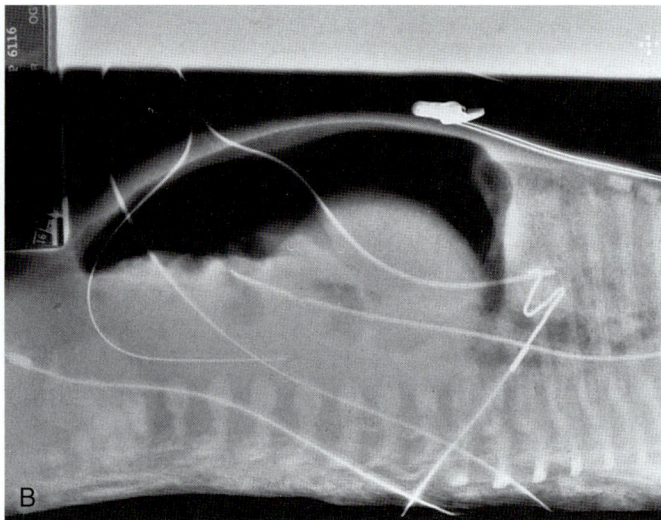

Figure 87-4   Pneumoperitoneum. **A,** Anteroposterior view of the chest and abdomen in a newborn with pulmonary interstitial emphysema, pneumo-mediastinum, and pneumoperitoneum. A large amount of gas is in the peritoneal cavity, the Rigler sign is positive, and density of the liver is decreased compared with the extraperitoneal soft tissues. The falciform ligament per se is not visualized because of the obscuring umbilical venous catheter. **B,** Cross-table lateral view of the same patient demonstrates large pneumoperitoneum without air-fluid levels, suggesting that the air has dissected into the peritoneum from the chest.

resembles the cap worn by the Venetian Doge.[9,10] A linear collection of air may also be located in the fissure of the liga-mentum teres.[11]

The *Rigler sign* refers to visualization of the outer edge of the bowel wall caused by the presence of air on both sides of the wall (e-Fig. 87-6). The telltale *triangle sign* is a trian-gular focus of extraluminal air seen on the cross-table lateral view of the abdomen, created by the external surface walls of adjacent bowel loops and the anterior abdominal wall, as the air collects at the highest point in the peritoneal space.[12]

Radiographic Signs of Pneumoperitoneum

Bowel-Related Signs	Right Upper Quadrant Signs	Peritoneal Ligament-Related Signs	Miscellaneous Signs
Rigler sign	Hyperlucent liver sign	Falciform ligament sign	Football sign
Triangle sign	Anterior-superior oval sign	Inverted V sign	Cupola sign
	Fissure for ligamentum teres sign	Urachus sign	Left-sided anterior-superior oval sign
	Doge cap sign		Subphrenic radiolucency
	Hepatic edge sign		Focal radiolucency
	Dolphin sign		

A sufficiently large amount of free air can be seen as a large, ovoid lucency overlying the abdominal contents (Fig. 87-7). As the liver falls away from the anterior peritoneal surface in the supine position, free peritoneal air can dissect along both sides of the falciform ligament, which attaches the liver to the anterior abdominal wall. The ligament, when outlined by free peritoneal air, appears as a very thin, vertical, opaque line (e-Fig. 87-8). The distension of the flanks caused by the free intraperitoneal air and the outline of the falciform ligament centrally are the elements of the well-known *football sign,* so termed because of its similarity to a football; the falciform ligament represents the central thread in the ball (see Fig. 87-7). A less commonly encountered sign of pneu-moperitoneum is the *inverted V sign,* caused by air outlining the medial umbilical folds in the pelvis.[13]

Apart from plain radiographs, ultrasound (US) can also be used in the detection of pneumoperitoneum by detecting gas over the liver, with a reported sensitivity of 93%, specific-ity of 64%, and accuracy of 90%.[14] However, we do not believe that US should be considered definitive in diagnosing or excluding a pneumoperitoneum without associated exten-sive expertise and experience, and US findings should be confirmed by appropriate radiographic evaluation.

Although not typically performed for assessment of pneu-moperitoneum, computed tomography (CT) is an extremely sensitive method to identify small amounts of intraperitoneal or extraperitoneal air and intraperitoneal air-fluid levels. CT is superior to upright radiography in demonstrating free intra-peritoneal air,[15] and it can be optimized by reviewing abdom-inal images using lung-window parameters (e-Fig. 87-9 and Fig. 87-10).

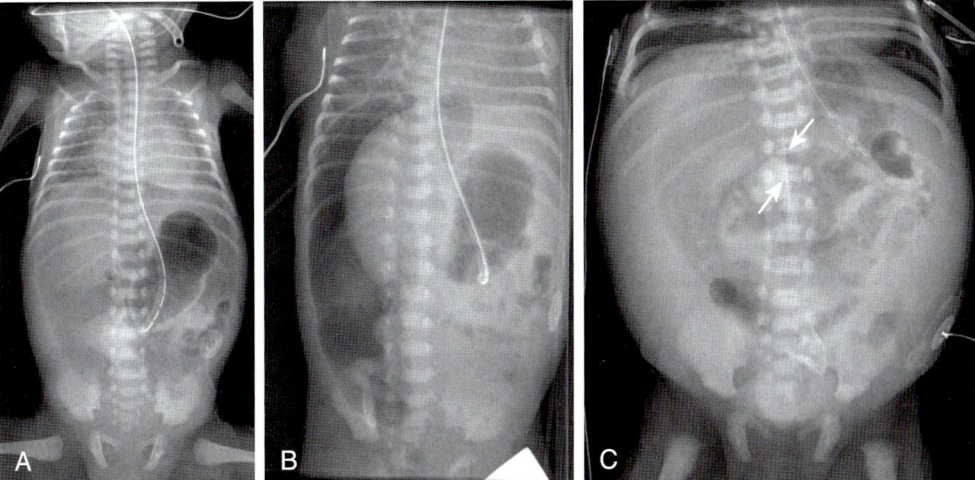

Figure 87-7 Pneumoperitoneum with "football sign." **A,** Supine radiograph in a 5-day-old 30-week-gestation premature infant shows a large lucency over the entire abdomen. **B,** Decubitus view in the same infant confirms the large pneumoperitoneum. Multiple intestinal perforations were found at surgery. **C,** Another patient with pneumoperitoneum demonstrates the classic football sign on abdominal imaging. Gas outlines the falciform ligament (*arrows*), and a large lucency overlies the upper abdomen centrally as the gas accumulates anteriorly. At surgery, this patient was found to have a colonic perforation.

Mimics and Potential Pitfalls

A *pseudo-Rigler sign* occurs when two loops of dilated air-filled bowel lie adjacent to one another. The line seen in the pseudo-Rigler sign is thicker than with free peritoneal air, because it represents a double thickness of bowel wall (from the two adjacent bowel loops), whereas the line in patients with free peritoneal air—a true Rigler sign—represents a single bowel wall. However, this is not always a reliable differentiation, because the underlying disease-causing perforation may lead to a thickened bowel wall. In equivocal cases, a horizontal-film radiograph should be obtained for clarification.[16]

ASCITES

Overview It is normal for a small amount of fluid to be present in the peritoneal cavity. This is more common in females, and it may be seen incidentally on cross-sectional imaging. *Ascites* refers to abnormal or pathologic accumulation of fluid within the peritoneal cavity.

Etiology Pathologic intraperitoneal fluid collections stem from a variety of causes and most commonly result from sequestration of fluid from the splanchnic vascular bed. Other causes of pathologic intraperitoneal fluid include hemoperitoneum, urinary ascites, bile, pancreatic juices, chylous fluid,

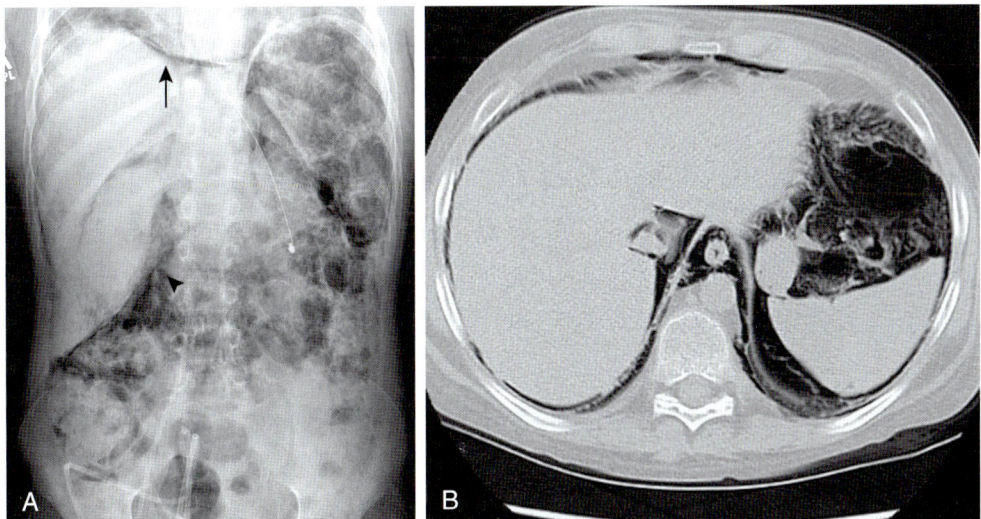

Figure 87-10 Pneumatosis intestinalis. **A,** Radiograph of the abdomen and pelvis in a patient who underwent bone marrow transplantation for refractory recurrent neuroblastoma. Abundant pneumatosis intestinalis has resulted in pneumoperitoneum (*arrow*) and pneumoretroperitoneum (*arrowhead*). **B,** Computed tomographic image through the upper abdomen viewed with lung windows confirms the pneumoperitoneum, pneumoretroperitoneum, and pneumomediastinum. Note absence of air-fluid levels.

and cerebrospinal fluid (CSF). *Transudative ascites* is most commonly found in patients with hepatobiliary disease, especially cirrhosis; heart failure; hyponatremia; renal failure; peritonitis; and Budd-Chiari syndrome. *Exudative ascites* can occur secondary to peritoneal infections and peritoneal metastases. Perforation of the GI tract results in the escape of both air and fluid into the peritoneal cavity. In children, the most common causes for ascites are hepatic, renal, and cardiac disease.[17]

The lesser sac, Morison pouch, paracolic gutters, pelvis, and recesses formed by many of the peritoneal ligaments are all sites where fluid can collect (Fig. 87-11). Typically, small amounts of ascites collect in the pelvis when the patient is supine. As the amount of fluid increases, it moves cephalad along the paracolic gutters into the subhepatic spaces and Morison pouch, and it can sometimes be identified in the fossa of the ligamentum teres (e-Fig. 87-12). Ascites eventually spreads through the peritoneal cavity and into the mesenteric recesses (Fig. 87-13); in cases of inflammation, loculations may occur. Encysted collections of CSF may be seen adjacent to the tip of a ventriculoperitoneal shunt tube ("CSF pseudocyst"), usually as a result of an inflammatory response around the shunt tube tip (Fig. 87-14).

Clinical Presentation   The clinical hallmark of ascites is abdominal distension, which in itself is a nonspecific sign. The clinical findings are in part governed by the underlying etiology. Early satiety and dyspnea can be seen with increasing accumulation of fluid within the abdominal cavity.[17]

Abdominal compartment syndrome is an uncommon sequela of acute accumulation of large-volume ascites and may arise secondary to collection of any material that leads to intraabdominal hypertension. The increased pressure in the confined space leads to progressive organ failure with significant

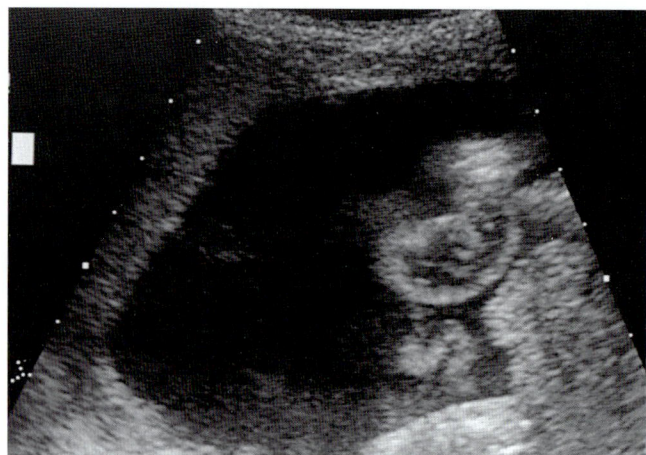

Figure 87-13   **Ascites.** Transverse sonogram through the left lower quadrant demonstrates a massive ascitic fluid collection that outlines thick-walled loops of intestine in a patient with graft-versus-host disease following bone marrow transplantation.

associated mortality. It is most commonly described after trauma but can also be seen in the setting of surgery and other entities, such as pancreatitis. The diagnosis is usually made at the bedside with measurement of intravesical pressure.[18] The criteria for diagnosis of abdominal compartment syndrome include elevation of intraabdominal pressure to 20 mm Hg or higher, coupled with impaired function of at least one organ; typically, it affects respiratory or renal function.[19] On CT this syndrome can be suggested by a ratio of anteroposterior to transverse diameters of the abdomen exceeding 0.81 (Fig. 87-15).[19] However, abdominal measurements on a single CT scan may be nonspecific, because an increased anteroposterior abdominal dimension may be seen with chronic ascites. Other findings on imaging include an elevated diaphragm, the presence of hemoperitoneum and increasing girth on serial examinations, attenuated inferior vena cava or renal veins, and shock bowel. Although not specific, a combination of these findings in the appropriate clinical setting or worsening of these findings on sequential imaging studies should raise the possibility of abdominal compartment syndrome.[18]

Imaging   Diagnosis of ascites is usually made based on clinical history, physical examination, and aspirated fluid analysis. Imaging is usually performed to confirm the clinical ascites, estimate its volume, and identify loculations, septations, or internal echoes or to assist in sampling or draining of ascitic fluid.

Abdominal radiographs are only sensitive to large amounts of intraperitoneal fluid. In such cases, the gas-filled bowel loops will appear centrally located within the abdomen (e-Fig. 87-16). Separation of bowel loops may also occur as a result of ascites, but this appearance can be simulated by large amounts of intraluminal fluid or by thick-walled bowel loops (e-Fig. 87-17).[20]

US is an extremely sensitive imaging modality for ascites.[21] Simple ascites usually appears as anechoic fluid and can be seen in the various peritoneal recesses.[22] Septations, loculations, and internal echoes usually suggest complex fluid, which can be seen in the setting of blood, chyle, inflammatory cells, or peritoneal metastases (e-Fig. 87-18). Ascites

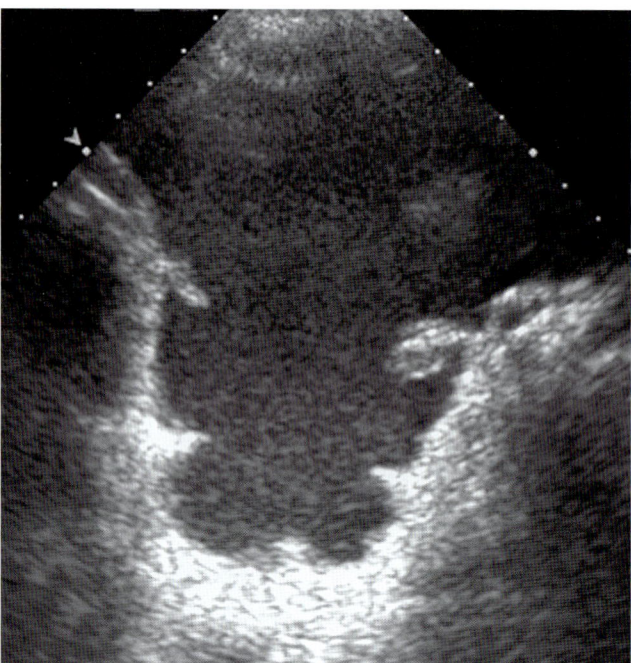

Figure 87-11   **Complex ascites.** Transverse ultrasound image through the deep pelvis in a 6-year-old patient with epithelioid sarcoma demonstrates abundant complex ascites. The thickening of the lateral peritoneal surface indicates peritoneal disease.

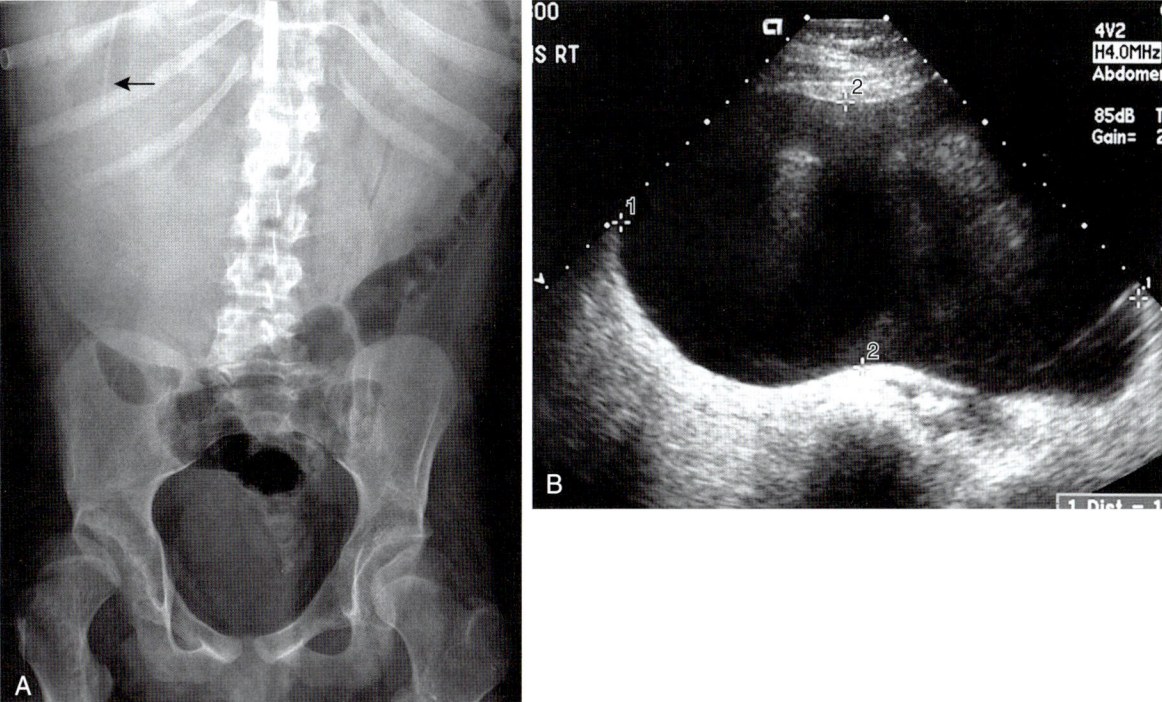

Figure 87-14 Cerebrospinal fluid pseudocyst. **A,** Abdominal radiograph demonstrates a large soft tissue mass that occupies the entire upper abdomen, especially the right abdomen. The tip of a ventriculoperitoneal shunt is seen in the right upper quadrant (*arrow*). **B,** Transverse image through the entire upper abdomen confirms a large cystic mass surrounding the tip of the shunt.

occasionally will pass through the esophageal hiatus or through patent pleuroperitoneal canals to present as intrathoracic fluid.[23]

CT is equally sensitive to detect ascites, although it does not visualize internal septations, which are easily seen on US. Because of radiation exposure, CT is not the first-line modality in the evaluation of ascites. Additional information related to the cause of ascites may be discernible, depending on the underlying condition.[24]

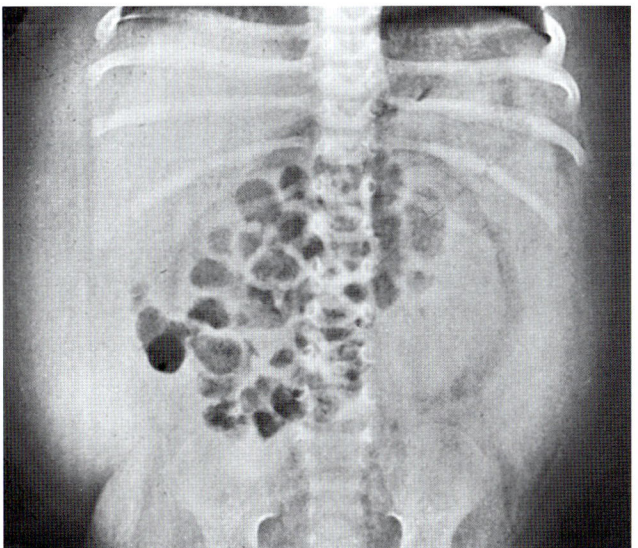

Figure 87-15 Ascites. Anteroposterior views of the abdomen in a 16-month-old infant with severe nephrotic syndrome. Abdominal distension is noted, and numerous loops of gas-containing intestine are seen floating in the center of the abdomen.

Treatment The course, prognosis, and treatment of ascites depend entirely on the cause. Drainage of the ascitic fluid can usually provide symptomatic relief, however, in most cases treatment is aimed at the underlying disorder. The treatment for abdominal compartment syndrome includes emergent drainage or decompressive laparotomy. The mortality rate in abdominal compartment syndrome remains high, at approximately 60% to 70%.[18]

PERITONITIS

Overview Peritonitis is a generalized or loacalized inflammatory process that affects the peritoneum. Acute generalized peritonitis is usually of infectious etiology and can be further subclassified as primary and secondary. *Primary peritonitis,* also called *spontaneous bacterial peritonitis,* is a primary infection of the peritoneal cavity that does not result from intraabdominal pathology. *Secondary peritonitis* results from secondary infection of the peritoneum, usually from urogenital or GI sources, particularly perforation.[25] Abscesses may develop locally and at sites where fluid is likely to accumulate, which are at times distant from the perforation site. The subhepatic and subphrenic spaces are common distant sites for abscess formation.

Etiology *Primary peritonitis* may occur spontaneously in patients without underlying pathology, and it is usually seen in association with postnecrotic cirrhosis and nephrotic syndrome.[25] Access of organisms to the peritoneal cavity through the fallopian tubes is another putative cause of this condition, supported by the increased occurrence in patients with intrauterine contraceptive devices.[25]

Secondary peritonitis in children is most commonly caused by a perforated appendix. Other causes of bowel perforation

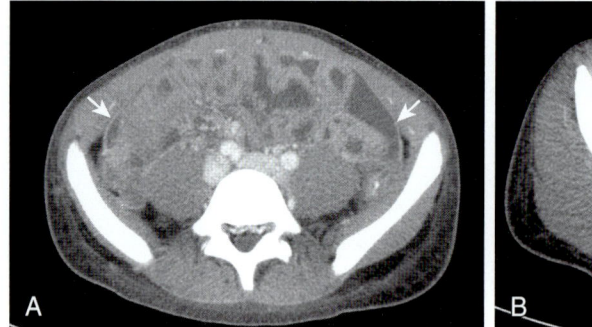
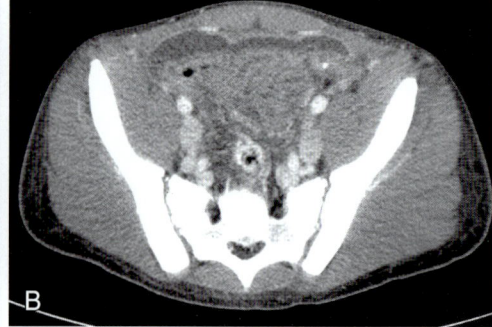

Figure 87-20 Peritonitis. **A,** Postcontrast computed tomographic image in a 14-year-old boy with perforation occurring after severe retching following a Heller myotomy shows low-attenuation fluid within the pelvis and between bowel loops. The peritoneal lining is enhancing (*arrows*) consistent with a clinical diagnosis of peritonitis. **B,** Image caudal to *A* shows similar findings.

that could potentially result in secondary peritonitis include inflammatory bowel disease, incarcerated hernias, complications of Meckel diverticulum, midgut volvulus, intussusception, hemolytic uremic syndrome, necrotizing enterocolitis, typhlitis, and traumatic perforation.[17] Peritoneal dialysis is another cause of peritonitis in children and is the most common cause of dialysis failure.[26]

Granulomatous peritonitis is usually associated with infectious etiologies such as tuberculosis, histoplasmosis, or pneumocystosis, most often in immunocompromised hosts. Tuberculosis that involves the peritoneum occurs in approximately 4% of patients with tuberculosis[27] but is reported to occur in 10% of children aged less than 10 years.[28] Noninfectious causes for granulomatous peritonitis include foreign material, such as talc and barium, meconium, bowel contents, bile, or gallstones.[2] *Meconium peritonitis* is a sterile peritonitis that results from prenatal perforation of the bowel; this is discussed in Chapter 103.

Clinical Presentation Patients usually come to medical attention with fever (≥39.5°C), diffuse abdominal pain, nausea, and vomiting. Signs of peritoneal inflammation can be elicited on physical examination; these signs include rebound tenderness,

abdominal wall rigidity, and decreased or absent bowel sounds from a paralytic ileus.[17] Patients with infectious granulomatous peritonitis secondary to histoplasmosis or pneumocystosis are nearly always immunocompromised.[2]

Imaging Abdominal radiographs in patients with peritonitis often show a nonspecific, adynamic ileus pattern with dilated bowel, multiple intraluminal air-fluid levels, and evidence of ascites; in addition, the properitoneal fat plane may be obliterated (e-Fig. 87-19). US may demonstrate intraperitoneal fluid with internal echoes and septations, and abscesses are identified as focal collections of mixed echogenicity.

CT demonstrates enhancement of the peritoneal lining with associated dense ascites (Fig. 87-20). Abscesses appear as focal fluid collections with relatively high attenuation values and densely enhancing walls (Fig. 87-21). On magnetic resonance imaging (MRI), abscesses in the peritoneum show similar findings as elsewhere, with high T2 signal and dense peripheral enhancement. Both gallium citrate– and indium-labeled white blood cells have been used as scintigraphic agents in the diagnosis of abscesses, although these are often unnecessary.

Granulomatous peritonitis is secondary to a spectrum of lesions, as discussed above. *Peritoneal tuberculosis* has been

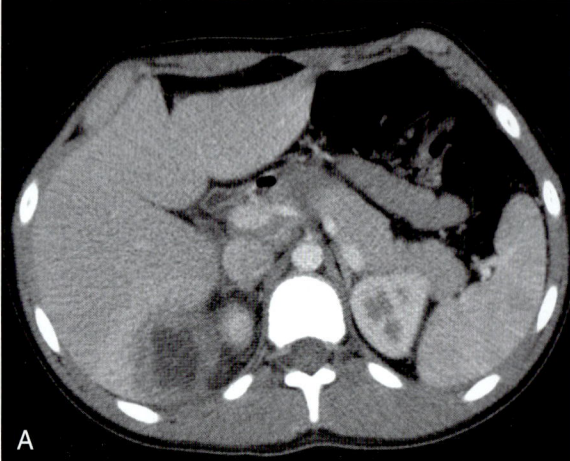
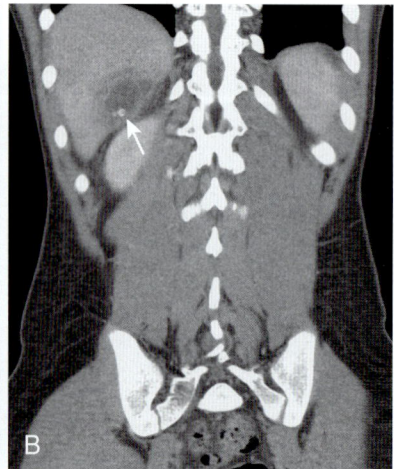

Figure 87-21 Ruptured appendicitis with intraabdominal abscess. **A,** Postcontrast computed tomographic scan in a patient with perforated appendicitis shows an irregular, thick-walled, peripherally enhancing abscess adjacent to the right lobe of the liver. **B,** Coronal reformat reveals the location of the mass in the subhepatic/parahepatic region. In addition, two hyperdense foci are seen (*arrow*) within the mass, most consistent with appendicoliths.

subdivided into three overlapping subtypes—a wet type, a fibrotic variety, and a dry, plastic type—with decreasing ascites and increasing soft tissue components along the spectrum.[2,29] The wet type is the most common and is characterized by ascites, which on CT is often (but not always) of high density[2,28,29] with free or localized fluid collections. Dry plastic or fibrotic fixed patterns are characterized by a relative lack of ascites and a variable amount of peritoneal and omental nodules and masses, peritoneal adhesions, and fibrotic fixation of the small bowel and mesentery as the predominant features.[2] Omental involvement is usually seen as diffuse, infiltrating, ill-defined enhancing lesions that produce a "smudged" appearance of the omentum (Fig. 87-22). The findings in tuberculosis are indistinguishable from those in histoplasmosis.[2] Although no single CT feature is diagnostic of peritoneal tuberculosis, additional imaging features that help in diagnosis include concomitant central, low-attenuation lymph node enlargement, miliary microabscesses in the liver or spleen, splenic or lymph node calcification, and inflammation that involves the terminal ileum and cecum.[29,30]

Treatment The treatment of peritonitis includes correction of the underlying etiology and supportive therapy. General supportive measures include vigorous intravenous rehydration and correction of electrolyte disturbances and infection control. Early control of the infection can be achieved medically, operatively, and through image-guided percutaneous interventions.

ABDOMINAL WALL AND PERITONEAL CALCIFICATION

Overview Abdominal wall calcification is uncommon in infants and children. The etiology depends upon the location of the calcification—whether it is skin, muscles, soft tissue, or peritoneum—and on the age of the patient. Most causes of intraabdominal calcification are related to specific organs, and these are discussed in the appropriate chapters.

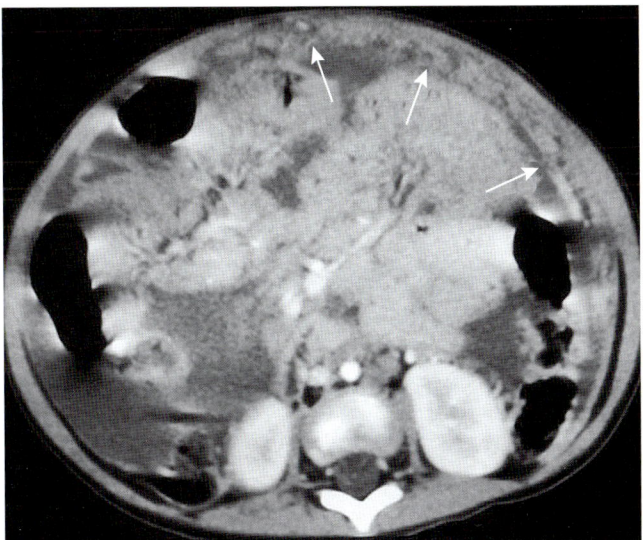

Figure 87-22 Tuberculous peritonitis in a 14-month-old girl. Contrast-enhanced computed tomographic image shows a large amount of ascites displacing bowel loops centrally, with studding of the peritoneal surface (*arrows*).

Etiology Fat necrosis is of one of the causes of abdominal wall calcification in neonates and infants.[31] Although there are many causes of fat necrosis, the majority are associated with neonatal asphyxia, sepsis, gestational diabetes, and hypothermia.[32] Older children with hypothermia, hepatic failure, and renal failure may also experience subcutaneous fat necrosis.[31]

Abdominal wall calcification may be seen in fibrodysplasia ossificans progressiva and in myositis ossificans, but these lesions are more common in the thoracic wall than in the abdominal wall. Calcifications secondary to dermatomyositis are more likely to be in the extremities than in the trunk, but calcifications can be found in the abdominal wall. Subcutaneous hemangiomas may contain phleboliths. Abdominal wall calcification in infants has also been described following subcutaneous emphysema and in prune-belly syndrome.[33]

The most common cause of peritoneal calcification in the neonate is meconium peritonitis,[34] discussed in Chapter 103. Peritoneal calcification in older children is rare. Intestinal perforation with subsequent peritonitis may cause calcification, as can granulomatous tuberculous peritonitis. Other causes include peritoneal dialysis, calcification along surgical scars, hyperparathyroidism, and peritoneal malignancies such as ovarian adenocarcinoma.[34]

Clinical Presentation Subcutaneous fat necrosis appears clinically as firm, erythematous plaques. In addition to the underlying condition, patients may develop hypercalcemia, particularly when involvement is extensive.[35]

Imaging Most abdominal wall and peritoneal calcifications are detected fortuitously on plain radiographs and/or CT scans obtained for other clinical indications. Correlation with any underlying predisposing disease, location, and shape of the calcification may help identify the underlying etiology. Peritoneal calcification associated with calcified lymph nodes is significantly more likely to be associated with malignancy, and a sheetlike appearance of peritoneal calcification was associated significantly more frequently with benign disease.[34]

Anterior Abdominal Wall Abnormalities

Overview Anterior abdominal wall defects encompass a variety of conditions, most commonly omphalocele and gastroschisis. *Omphalocele* refers to a defect larger than 4 cm that occurs in the midline and typically contains both gut and the liver and may or may not include other abdominal organs covered by a bilayer consisting of the peritoneum as the inner layer and the amnion as the outer layer, with Wharton's jelly in between. It is differentiated from the less common *umbilical cord hernia* in that the latter is less than 4 cm, does not contain liver, has a normal abdominal wall, and has few associated anomalies. *Gastroschisis* has no covering membrane and contains only gut, although a gonad may occasionally protrude through the defect, located adjacent to the umbilical cord insertion, typically on the right. Umbilical hernia, unlike the above defects, is covered by skin, tends to become apparent several weeks after birth, and is not associated with malrotation.[36]

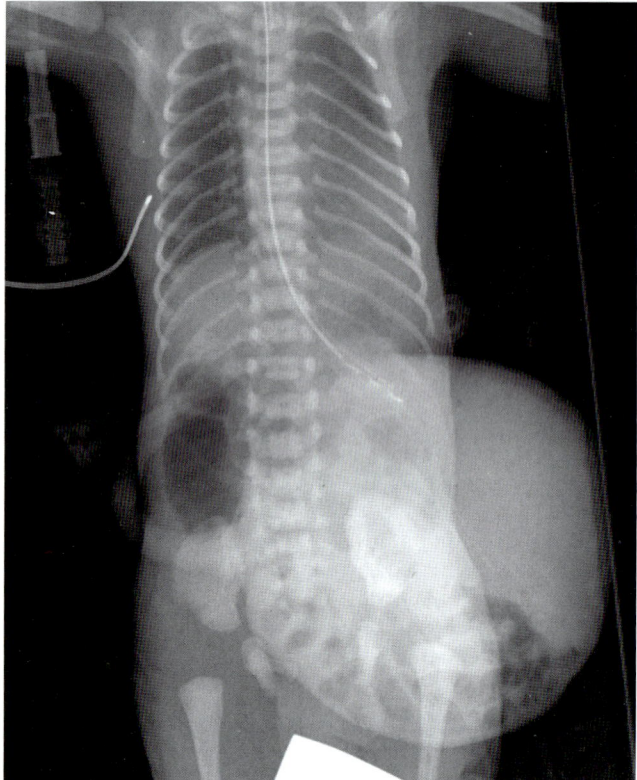

Figure 87-23 **Omphalocele.** Frontal view of the chest and abdomen in a neonate shows a large anterior wall defect covered by a membrane and containing the liver, which is well visualized adjacent to air-filled and mildly distended bowel loops. The umbilical cord inserts on the omphalocele.

OMPHALOCELE

Overview   Omphaloceles constitute the second most common anterior abdominal wall defect, with a prevalence of approximately 1 to 5 in 10,000 live births; it is more common in boys.[36,37]

Etiology   An omphalocele forms when fusion fails in the lateral folds of the body wall, the rectus muscles fail to meet in the midline, and the herniated bowel fails to return into the peritoneal cavity, with the umbilical cord inserting into the covering membrane (Fig. 87-23 and e-Fig. 87-24).[36,37] The herniated viscera are covered by an outer layer of amnion and Wharton jelly and an inner membrane of parietal

peritoneum.[37] Involvement of the cephalic folds results in the spectrum of pentalogy of Cantrell/ectopia cordis: midline supraumbilical abdominal wall defect, pericardial and diaphragmatic defects, cardiac or ventricular diverticulum herniation through the defect, congenital heart disease, and sternal clefts (Fig. 87-25).[37,38] Failure of caudal fold development results in cloacal exstrophy.[36,37]

Clinical Presentation   Associated anomalies are present in 50% to 70% of cases. Chromosomal anomalies, especially trisomies, occur in 40% to 60%.[39] Absence of liver in the sac, smaller defects, and abnormal amounts of amniotic fluid are associated with an increased incidence of other anomalies, and 50% of these patients have congenital heart disease. Omphaloceles also are associated with Beckwith-Wiedemann syndrome and omphalocele–bladder exstrophy–imperforate anus–spinal defect complex.[39] Intrauterine growth retardation and prematurity commonly coexist.[37]

Imaging   The diagnosis is usually made on antenatal US. Antenatal evaluation includes assessment of the umbilical cord insertion, presence or absence of a covering membrane, contents of the omphalocele, and coexisting anomalies.[40] Multiple associated anomalies indicate a poorer prognosis, as do oligohydramnios and polyhydramnios.

Treatment   Definitive treatment is surgical and may consist of primary closure or a staged procedure. If primary closure is not possible, the sac may be covered with nonadherent dressings to prevent trauma to the sac and exposure of the underlying bowel until delayed closure is possible.[36,37]

GASTROSCHISIS

Overview   The prevalence of gastroschisis has been rising over the past three decades, particularly in infants born to young mothers, for reasons that remain unclear,[36,37,41] with a prevalence of approximately 2 to 5 per 10,000 live births.[42] Gastroschisis is not usually associated with chromosomal abnormalities or congenital anomalies outside of the GI tract. Complex gastroschisis results when associated GI complications are present.[43]

Etiology   The etiology of gastroschisis remains uncertain, but it is postulated to result from ischemia to the paraumbilical abdominal wall and results in its involution. The defect occurs much more commonly on the right and may be

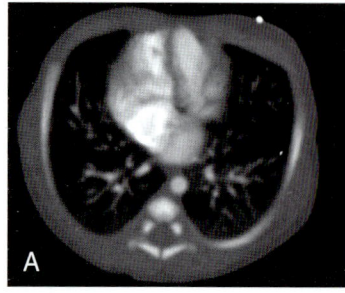 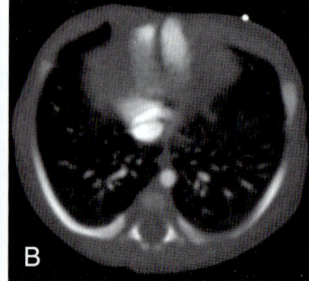 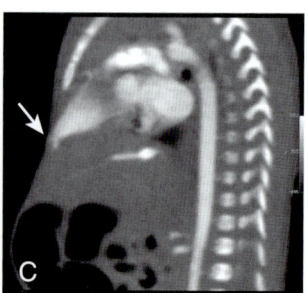

Figure 87-25 **Pentalogy of Cantrell.** Neonate with an inferior sternal defect and protrusion of anterior abdominal wall with deficient epigastric abdominal wall musculature. **A** and **B,** Axial images from a contrast-enhanced computed tomographic scan show a midline heart with a left ventricular diverticulum. **C,** Sagittal reformat demonstrates the herniating left ventricular diverticulum to better advantage (*arrow*). (Courtesy Marta Hernanz-Schulman, MD, Nashville, TN.)

related to mistiming of the involution of the right omphalo-mesenteric artery and right umbilical vein, with herniation of the bowel through the defect.[37] A vascular genesis of the defect is supported by reported incidence in cases of maternal use of vasoactive compounds, such as cocaine and cigarettes.[44]

Clinical Presentation Infants with gastroschisis are typically born prematurely. At birth the bowel may appear normal, but soon after, it may be covered with fibrinous exudates.[36] The maternal α-fetoprotein level is elevated, because the lack of covering membrane allows the bowel loops to be exposed to the amniotic fluid. The incidence of associated anomalies is approximately 10% to 20%, most involve the GI tract,[45] and include antenatal perforation, necrosis, atresia, and volvulus, sometimes resulting in congenitally short bowel.[36,46]

Imaging On prenatal US, gastroschisis is characterized by a normal umbilical insertion; a defect located adjacent to the umbilicus, most commonly on the right; and absence of a covering sac (e-Fig. 87-26 and Fig. 87-27). Dilatation of the bowel loops on prenatal imaging has been found to correlate with complex gastroschisis, with poorer survival and increased morbidity.

Treatment In the immediate postnatal period, close attention to heat preservation and fluid balance is important, because the large surface area of the exposed bowel leads to heat and fluid loss. Rapid coverage of the exposed bowel is a priority and may be accomplished with a Silastic silo bag. The defect itself may need to be surgically enlarged, if the bowel is at risk of vascular compromise.[37] Whenever possible, surgery as soon as possible after delivery is advocated.[36]

OMPHALOMESENTERIC DUCT AND URACHAL REMNANTS

Omphalomesenteric Duct Remanant

Overview *Omphalomesenteric duct remnant* refers to a variety of conditions that range from a Meckel diverticulum to ligamentous and umbilical abnormalities (Fig. 87-28).

Etiology The *omphalomesenteric duct,* also called the *vitelline duct,* connects the primitive midgut, the future ileum, to the yolk sac remnant; normally, it obliterates during the fifth to seventh week of embryonic development. However, if this process does not proceed normally, a spectrum of abnormalities may ensue. Closure of the duct with failure of complete involution results in a ligamentous remnant. The spectrum of abnormalities has been subdivided into three general categories.[47] In a *type 1 abnormality,* the entire duct is open (Fig. 87-29). A *type 2 abnormality* refers to a duct that is open at one end but ends blindly at the other; when open at the ileal end, it represents a *Meckel diverticulum* (see Chapter 103). A *type 3 abnormality* refers to focal patency along the course of the duct.

Clinical Presentation Patients with a type 1 abnormality will come to medical attention with fecal material draining from the umbilicus. Patients in whom the duct is open only along the umbilical end are seen with discharge from the umbilicus that consists of secretions produced by the lining of the tract. A type 3 abnormality, or *vitelline duct cyst,* is often asymptomatic but may become infected, in which case it can manifest with acute symptoms. Omphalomesenteric duct remnants or attachments may also lead to mechanical bowel obstruction.

Imaging In a type 1 abnormality, contrast injected through the umbilicus passes directly into the ileum. In a type 2 defect, contrast injection reveals a blind-ending sinus tract of varying length. Imaging over the palpable abnormality in a type 3 defect may demonstrate a simple or complex cystic mass. These may also occur as incidental findings in asymptomatic patients.

Treatment Management depends on the clinical presentation. Definitive treatment is surgical with resection of the omphalomesenteric duct remnant.[48]

Urachal Remnant

Overview The urachus connects the bladder and the allantois; when normally obliterated, it becomes the median umbilical ligament. In a manner analogous to the omphalomesenteric duct, the urachus can be open throughout its course from the bladder to the skin surface at the umbilicus. Alternatively, a portion of the urachus can be open as a

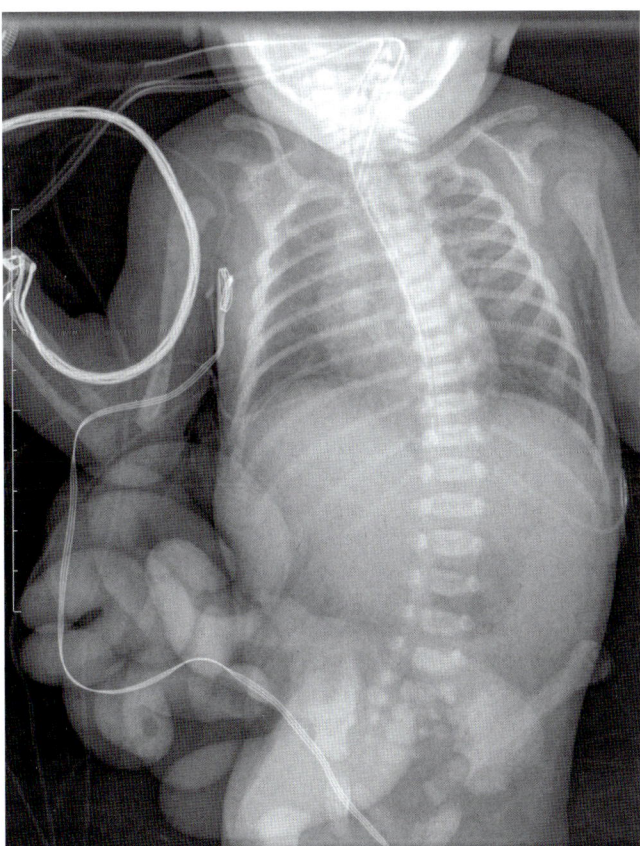

Figure 87-27 **Gastroschisis.** Frontal view of the chest and abdomen of a newborn shows bowel loops outside the abdominal cavity. The bowel loops are not covered by a membrane, and the umbilical cord inserts into the anterior abdominal wall to the left of the defect.

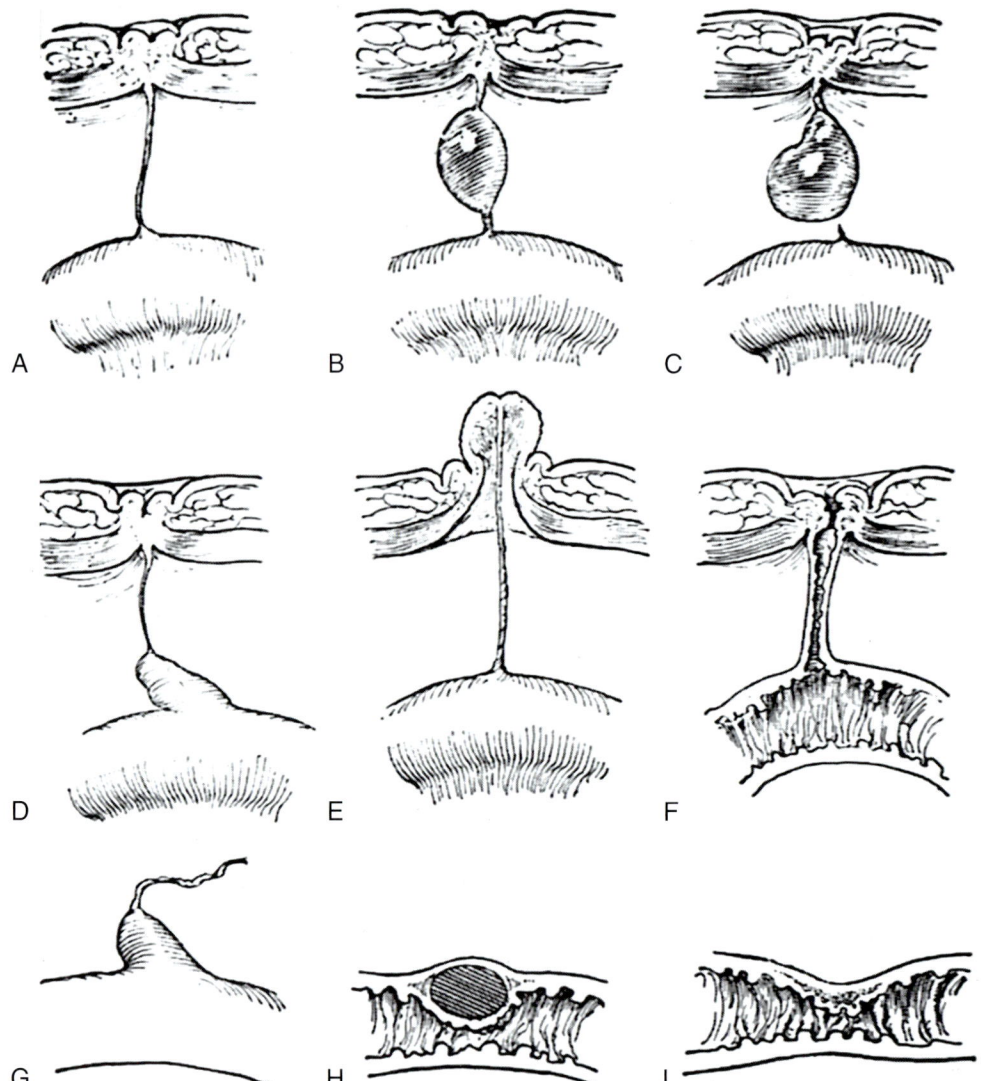

Figure 87-28   Variants of omphalomesenteric duct remnants. **A,** Persistent cord between the ileal wall and the closed umbilicus. **B,** Cyst in the same cord. **C,** Cyst anchored at the umbilical end of the cord but free at the ileal end. **D,** Meckel diverticulum attached to the closed umbilicus by a closed cord. **E,** Everted mucocele of the umbilicus with the cord attached to the ileal wall. **F,** Fecal fistula open at both the umbilical and ileal ends. **G,** Meckel diverticulum open at the ileal end but blind at the umbilical end, which is unattached. **H,** Intramural cystic diverticulum. **I,** Local stenosis of the ileum at the site of the mouth of the omphalomesenteric duct. (From Cullen TS. *Embryology, anatomy and diseases of the umbilicus.* Philadelphia: Saunders; 1916)

blind-ending sinus, from either the dome of the bladder, as a vesicourachal diverticulum, or from the umbilicus, as an umbilicourachal sinus; this is seen in approximately 15% of cases. If only the midportion remains patent, it is known as a *urachal cyst,* seen in approximately 30% of cases.[49]

Etiology   Urachal remnants result from failure of obliteration of a portion or of the entire embryonic urachus.

Clinical Presentation   In an infant with a fully patent urachus, leaking of urine is typically noticed in the neonatal period. Other urologic abnormalities—such as hypospadias, posterior urethral valves, or renal ectopia—may be present in a few cases.[49] Umbilicourachal sinuses may have intermittent discharge. Vesicourachal diverticula, although typically asymptomatic, may serve as a reservoir for stone formation or for development of malignancy in adulthood.[49,50]

Imaging   The patent urachus may be seen as a fluid-filled tubular structure that extends from the anterior-superior aspect of the bladder to the umbilicus on US or CT. Voiding cystourethrograms may demonstrate the patent connection to the umbilicus, or injection of the umbilical sinus tract may demonstrate the lesion. The vesicourachal diverticulum appears as an extension of the bladder at its anterosuperior portion and is often found in patients being imaged for prune-belly syndrome.[49] An urachal cyst is seen as a well-circumscribed cyst in the anterior abdominal wall on US or CT, with mural thickening and increased enhancement if complicated by infection (Fig. 87-30).[51]

Treatment   Definitive treatment is surgical, using either an open or laparoscopic technique with complete resection of the urachal remnants. If infection has supervened, this is treated before surgical resection.

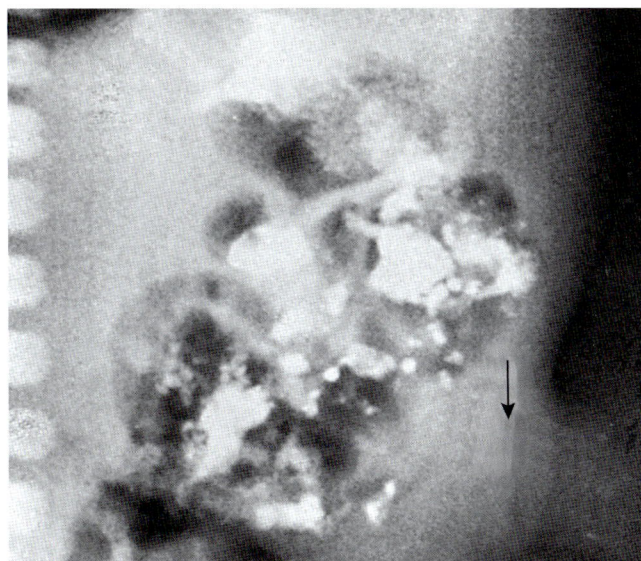

Figure 87-29 Type I patent omphalomesenteric duct remnant. Lateral view of the abdomen from an upper gastrointestinal series demonstrates barium flowing from the ileum through a patent omphalomesenteric duct (*arrow*) to the umbilicus and the anterior abdominal wall.

GROIN AND PELVIC HERNIAS

Overview Inguinal hernias may be direct or indirect, depending on their relationship to the inferior epigastric vessels. Direct inguinal hernias, with the hernia sac medial to the epigastric vessels, are acquired, rather than congenital, and are uncommon in children. Indirect inguinal hernias, with the hernia sac lateral to the epigastric vessels, are the most common form of inferior abdominal wall herniation. The true incidence of inguinal hernias is difficult to determine, but it ranges from 0.8% to 4.4% in children and is more common in boys.[52] Premature infants are at increased risk of developing inguinal hernia, with an approximate 30% incidence.[53] Patients with bladder exstrophy, Ehlers-Danlos syndrome, or prune-belly syndrome also have an increased incidence of inguinal hernia.[52]

Etiology The processus vaginalis normally closes between the thirty-sixth and fortieth weeks of gestation. However, if it remains open, as in indirect inguinal hernia, abdominal contents can herniate through the inguinal ring into the scrotum in boys (Fig. 87-31). In girls, abdominal contents or ovaries can herniate through the canal of Nuck into the labia majora (Fig. 87-32; see also Fig. 87-31).

Although femoral hernias, hernias through the obturator foramen, sciatic hernias, and perineal hernias are rare in children, these need to be included in the differential diagnosis of pelvic masses that extend into the buttock or perineum.

Clinical Presentation Most inguinal hernias in children are asymptomatic, but incarceration or strangulation can occur (e-Fig. 87-33) and can lead to intestinal obstruction. Asymptomatic patients usually come to medical attention with an intermittent painless bulge in the inguinal region, scrota, or labia that is noticed when the abdominal pressure rises, such as during crying, straining, or coughing.[52,53] If the bowel loop becomes entrapped or incarcerated in the hernia, the patient may exhibit signs and symptoms of bowel obstruction, such as abdominal distension or vomiting. If the hernia is not reduced, the blood supply to the trapped bowel loops may be compromised, leading to bowel necrosis and perforation. Incarceration occurs most frequently in the first 6 months of life.[53]

Imaging Inguinal hernias may be seen on radiographs as a loop of bowel in the scrotum (see Fig. 87-31, *A*), but they are often obscured by gonadal shielding. Herniating bowel loops may be an incidental finding on small bowel series, and contrast enema with reflux into the small intestine in infants with intestinal obstruction may show a pinched-off loop at the entrance to the inguinal canal.

In patients with equivocal clinical findings, US is highly accurate (95%) in demonstrating an inguinal hernia (Fig. 87-34; also see Fig. 87-31, *B*).[54] If the bowel loops are filled with fluid, US can identify the intestinal wall surrounding the intraluminal fluid and may show bubbles of air or peristalsis, and color Doppler US may show blood flow in the wall of the herniated bowel loop. These findings help differentiate a hernia from a hydrocele.

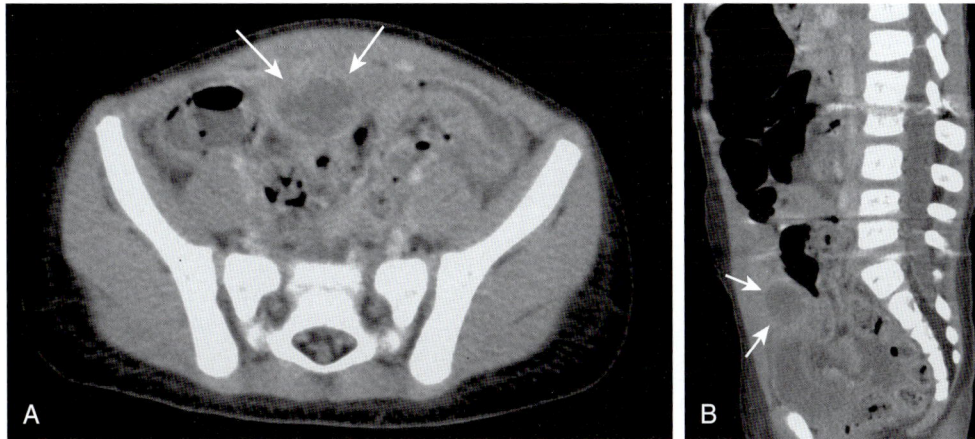

Figure 87-30 Infected urachal cyst. **A,** Contrast-enhanced computed tomographic scan of the abdomen and pelvis shows a thick-walled cyst (*arrows*) with surrounding inflammation just superior to the urinary bladder. This infected urachal cyst was later removed intraoperatively. **B,** Midline sagittal reformat shows its location with respect to the bladder and umbilicus to better advantage.

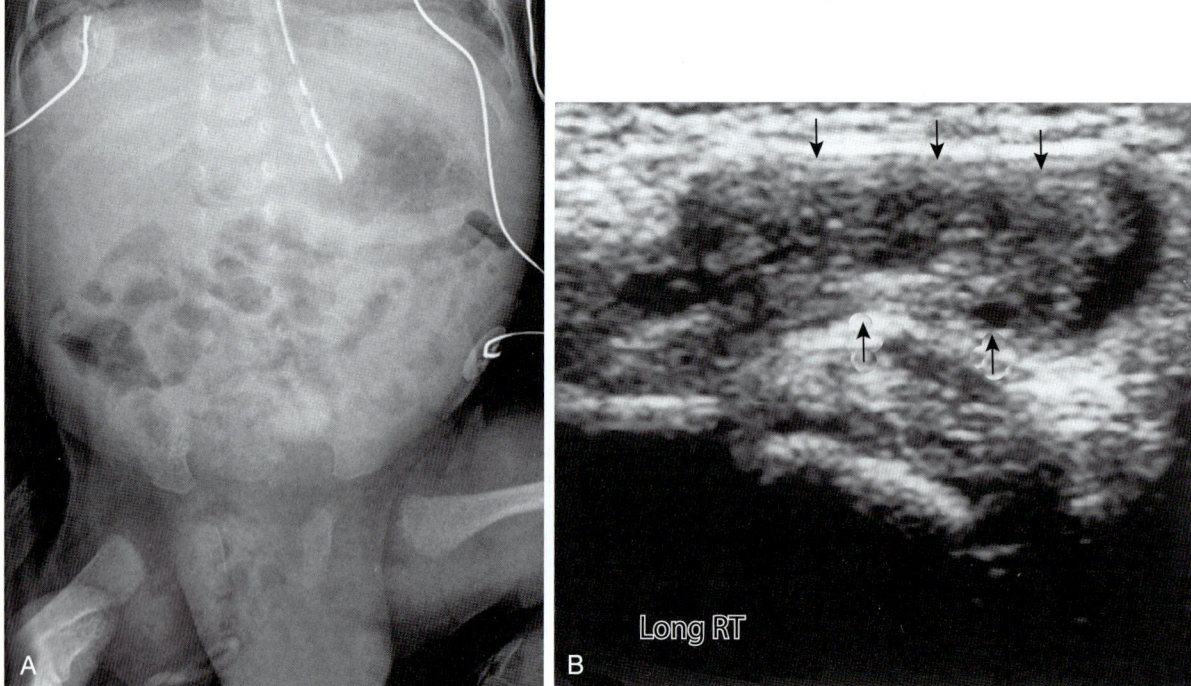

Figure 87-31 Inguinal hernia. **A,** Anteroposterior view of the abdomen and pelvis in a newborn boy shows an enlarged scrotum, with multiple air-filled loops of intestine within it, secondary to indirect right inguinal hernia. **B,** Ultrasound in the inguinal region of an infant girl with a labial mass confirms a herniated ovary (*arrows*) in the canal of Nuck.

Although hernias may be seen with CT (see Fig. 87-30) and MRI,[55,56] these studies are rarely indicated as first-line modalities for diagnosing hernias; usually, they are incidental findings when these examinations are performed for other reasons.

Treatment The treatment of inguinal hernia is surgery. It may be performed using an open or laparoscopic technique.[57]

Benign and Malignant Neoplasms

CYSTIC NEOPLASMS

Overview Abdominal cystic lesions include lymphatic malformations; lesions related to the bowel, such as duplication cysts; and cysts related to the urogenital system, such as urachal cysts. The term *mesenteric cyst* has been previously applied to cysts of variable histopathologic origin.[58,59] More recent literature classifies such "mesenteric cysts" based on histopathologic features, such as lymphatic, mesothelial, enteric, urogenital, or dermoid cysts or mature cystic teratomas and pseudocysts.[60,61] This section will discuss lymphatic and mesothelial cystic peritoneal lesions.

LYMPHATIC MALFORMATIONS

Overview *Lymphatic malformations,* formerly known as *lymphangiomas,* are the most common type of vasculolymphatic malformation to affect the peritoneal cavity and mesentery.[62] Lymphatic malformations have an endothelial lining with walls that contain smooth muscle and lymphatic spaces.[60,63]

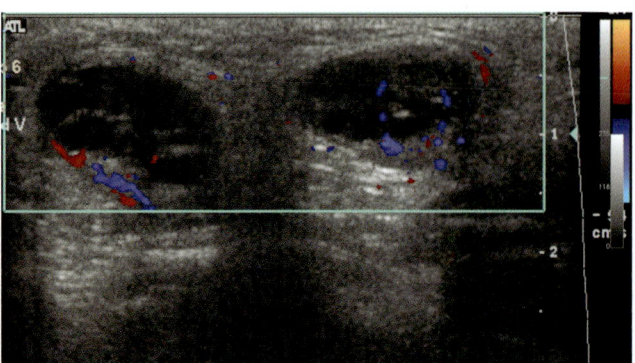

Figure 87-32 Canal of Nuck hernia. Transverse ultrasound image through labia majora in a newborn with bilateral palpable labial masses demonstrates ovaries herniated through the canal of Nuck into the labia.

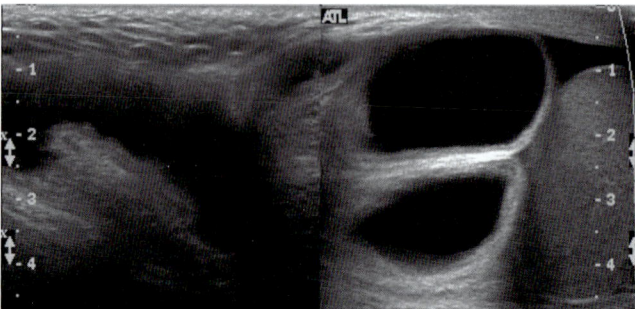

Figure 87-34 Inguinal hernia. Composite oblique ultrasound image along the inguinal canal from a scrotal sonogram demonstrates an inguinal hernia that contains moderately distended fluid-filled bowel loops. During real time imaging, the herniated bowel loops demonstrated peristalsis. The normal right testis is seen lower in the scrotal sac.

Etiology Lymphatic malformations do not have a clear origin and have been variously postulated to be developmental, congenital, or neoplastic.[64-66] A prevalent hypotheses suggests that they result from the proliferation of abnormal lymphatic channels that do not communicate with the systemic lymphatics.[67]

Clinical Presentation Lymphatic malformations may be encountered incidentally, either as a palpable abdominal mass—which, if sufficiently large, could be mistaken for ascites—or during imaging for another reason. When symptomatic, lymphatic malformations may manifest with small bowel obstruction secondary to acute enlargement of the cyst or to segmental volvulus of adjacent bowel loops, with symptoms that include abdominal distension, pain, vomiting, and peritonitis or septic shock.[59,62,67,68]

Imaging On US, lymphatic malformations are typically seen as thin-walled, fluid-filled, single or multiple cysts, often with thin septations.[11] In the presence of hemorrhage or infection, internal echoes may be detected. Ascites, often chylous, can also be present.[62] Despite the internal echoes, Doppler interrogation will reveal no internal flow within the echogenic but cystic component, differentiating it from a solid mass. On real time visualization, movement of the internal echoes can be seen and documented on video clip.

CT shows cystic or multicystic lesions with thin or imperceptible walls, and internal septations may enhance as a result of the presence of vascular structures. The CT attenuation of the cyst contents may be lower than water because of their chylous nature, but usually they are homogenous.[62,64]

On MRI, lymphatic malformations are typically of low signal on T1- and high signal on T2-weighted sequences.[69] Internal hemorrhage may be manifested as increased signal intensity on both T1- and T2-weighted sequences,[69] and internal septations are seen as linear structures that may enhance; the peripheral rim and septations may enhance, but the majority of the lesion does not enhance and should not enhance centrally.[69] MRI may aid in distinguishing large lymphangiomatous masses that have hemorrhaged from complex intraperitoneal fluid (Fig. 87-35). Cross-sectional imaging is useful to assess the entire extent of the lesion and to define the relationship with adjacent structures.

Treatment Lymphatic malformations may be treated with sclerotherapy or surgical resection. The decision largely depends on the location and size of the lesion. Staged sclerotherapy and/or surgical resection may be required, particularly with multicentric lesions or lesions that extend into the retroperitoneum. The prognosis is generally good, with a low recurrence rate.[67]

CYSTS OF MESOTHELIAL ORIGIN

Overview Cysts of mesothelial origin include simple mesothelial cysts, benign cystic mesotheliomas, and malignant cystic mesothelioma. Simple cysts are unilocular and are usually 1 to 5 cm in size, whereas benign cystic mesotheliomas are large and multilocular.[60] Mesothelial cysts are lined by flat cuboidal or columnar cells without lymphatic structures; this distinguishes these lesions from lymphatic malformations.[60,63]

Benign cystic mesothelioma is a rare, usually multilocular peritoneal lesion that most commonly arises from the peritoneal surface of the pelvis. This lesion has many alternative names that include *peritoneal inclusion cyst, multilocular inclusion cyst,* and *benign multicystic mesothelioma.*[1] Although most commonly found in middle-aged women, it can also occur in children.[1,70-72]

Etiology The cause of mesothelial cysts remains unclear, although theories postulate developmental, neoplastic, and reactive etiologies. The reactive hypothesis suggests that a stimulus produces chronic irritation that can lead to reactive and loculated proliferation of mesothelial cells, resulting in a cystic fluid collection with mesothelial lining.[72]

Clinical Presentation Similar to lymphatic malformations, mesothelial cysts can be detected incidentally as asymptomatic masses,[63,68] or they may present with acute abdominal symptoms that can mimic appendicitis.[58,59,73]

Imaging Because differentiation from cystic lymphatic malformations is based on histologic elements, imaging findings in these lesions are very similar to those in lymphatic malformations.[70]

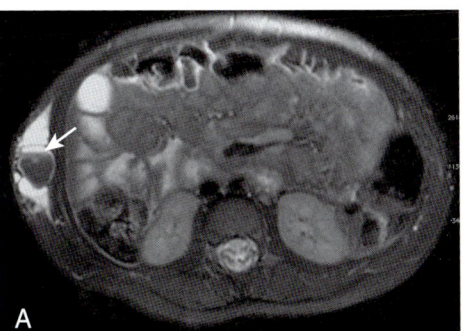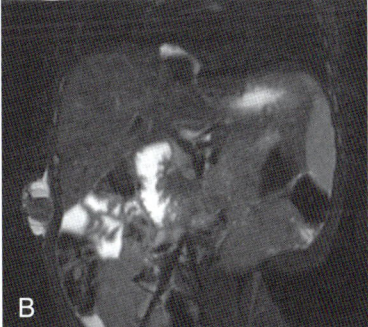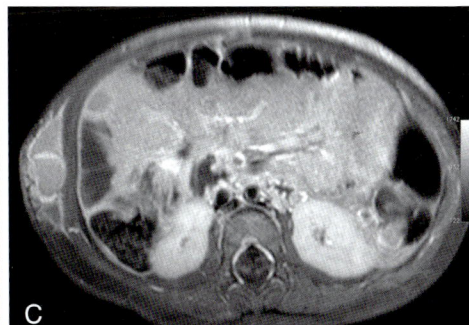

Figure 87-35 Abdominal wall lymphatic malformation. A 16-month-old girl with 2 weeks of localized swelling in the right flank. **A** and **B,** Axial and coronal T2-weighted magnetic resonance images with fat saturation show a multiloculated cystic lesion within the subcutaneous tissues of the abdominal wall with some mass effect upon the underlying musculature. Most of the locules are hyperintense on T2, with a large T2 hypointensity within and a fluid level (*arrow*) consistent with a hematocrit level. **C,** After the administration of contrast, T1-weighted, fat-suppressed image shows that the septations enhance, but the internal contents do not, which is typical of a lymphatic malformation. No solid components were detected.

Treatment The goal is complete surgical resection,[67] because these tumors recur in as many as 75% of cases; in addition, malignant degeneration has been reported in adult patients.[70]

OTHER BENIGN LESIONS

Lipoblastoma

Overview Lipoblastoma is a rare, benign, mesenchymal fat-containing tumor seen almost exclusively in infants and children. Multiple series support that these tumors affect children under 8 years of age, with 70% to 90% affecting children under 3 years of age, with a slight male predilection.[74-79] The most common sites involved are the subcutaneous and superficial soft tissue of the neck and extremities.[74,76,77] Approximately 7% of lipoblastomas occur in the abdomen.[80] Lipoblastoma differs from lipoblastomatosis in that it is a well-circumscribed, encapsulated lesion, whereas lipoblastomatosis is a diffuse, infiltrating process.[74,80]

Etiology Lipoblastomas arise from embryonal white fat, in contradistinction to hibernomas, which arise from brown fat.[79] The etiology of the lesions is not known, but lipoblastomas demonstrate chromosomal abnormalities with deletions or abnormal sequencing. The vast majority of cases have characteristic cytogenetic abnormality containing 8q11-13 clonal chromosomal rearrangement that affects *PLAG1*.[81-83] Distinction from liposarcoma, particularly the myxoid variety, may be difficult: histologic criteria are based on a uniform growth pattern, absence of nuclear atypia, and cytogenetics; clinical criteria include patient age, because liposarcomas in children younger than 10 years are very rare.[78,83]

Clinical Presentation Clinical manifestations depend upon mass size and location and its effect on adjacent structures. Lipoblastomas frequently manifest as rapidly growing painless masses. Abdominal lipoblastomas may result in symptoms of vomiting, anorexia, abdominal pain, and diarrhea secondary to mass effect upon adjacent structures.[80]

Imaging Imaging features of lipoblastoma reflect the underlying pathology, and they vary depending upon the extent of underlying myxoid stroma versus adipose tissue.[83] Abdominal radiographs may demonstrate radiolucency,[84] although US may be the first imaging to confirm the presence of a mass and to assess its characteristics and location. A lipoblastoma is seen as a homogenously hyperechoic solid lesion, but mixed echogenicity and fluid-filled spaces can be present.[83,85] On CT and MRI, lipoblastoma appears as a lobular, fat-containing, well-circumscribed mass, often with internal septations (Fig. 87-36), but the amount of fat will depend on the maturity of the cells that make up the tumor, with the proportion of mature adipocytes positively correlating with fat attenuation and signal characteristics respectively on CT and MRI.[83] If fat is the predominant component, the lipoblastoma is usually indistinguishable from a lipoma, with the diagnosis suggested based on patient age. If myxoid stroma is the predominant component, as seen in very young children, imaging will reflect decreased fat[85] and a variable amount of contrast enhancement.[83]

Differential diagnosis includes liposarcoma, which may be difficult to distinguish based solely on imaging findings.[78,83] Benign cystic teratomas also contain fat, but these may be distinguished from lipoblastoma by calcification or ossification.[83]

Treatment and Follow-up Treatment for lipoblastoma is complete surgical resection, but the lesions may locally recur in up to 9% to 25% of cases. Recurrences are more often seen with lipoblastomatosis, likely related to incomplete resection. Current management suggests that extensive surgery is not justified to achieve complete resection, because the lesions have no malignant potential, and spontaneous regression and maturation into lipoma may occur.[83,86,87]

Desmoid Tumors

Overview Desmoid tumors are histologically benign but locally aggressive, nonmetastasizing tumors that belong to a group of disorders known as *fibromatoses*.[88,89] Approximately 37% to 50% of desmoids arise in the abdominal region.[90] In the abdominal wall, desmoid tumors arise from the aponeuroses of fascia and near surgical scars.[89]

These tumors can occur sporadically or in association with familial adenomatous polyposis (FAP) and Gardner syndrome, and they occur in as many as 20% of affected patients.[89,91] They can also occur in FAP patients after prophylactic colectomy and are one of the leading causes of death after colectomy in these patients.[92,93]

Etiology The etiology of desmoid tumors is unknown but is thought to be multifactorial.[90] Their development within the setting of the polyposis syndromes suggests a genetic correlation. Desmoid tumors tend to develop after trauma and often arise 6 to 30 months after colectomy in FAP patients[91] or after chemotherapy or radiation treatment.[88] There is also evidence of hormonal influence, and some tumors express estrogen receptors.[88] These lesions are more common in women, with a ratio as high as 4:1.[90]

Clinical Presentation Abdominal desmoids may be asymptomatic. However, as they enlarge, they may infiltrate adjacent structures and lead to symptoms related to compression of bowel, vascular, or other retroperitoneal structures.[90]

Imaging Desmoid tumors vary in imaging characteristics, depending upon the amounts of collagen, proliferating fibroblasts, fibrosis, and vascularity. The fibrous and cellular composition of desmoid tumors varies with the stage of their evaluation.

On US, the margins may be ill defined or irregular, and the echogenicity is variable. CT density and margins likewise vary. On MR, desmoid tumors typically demonstrate decreased signal intensity on T1- and variable signal intensity on T2-weighted sequences compared with muscle. An association has been found between increased tumor cellularity, as shown on T2-weighted images, and a tendency to rapid tumor growth.[89] Enhancement patterns are variable (Fig. 87-37). MRI is a useful method for staging desmoid tumors, assessing stage of activity, and detecting recurrence.

Treatment Surgical resection has been the mainstay of treatment; however, many abdominal desmoids are discovered when they are no longer easily resectable, particularly with sufficiently wide margins to prevent recurrence, thus

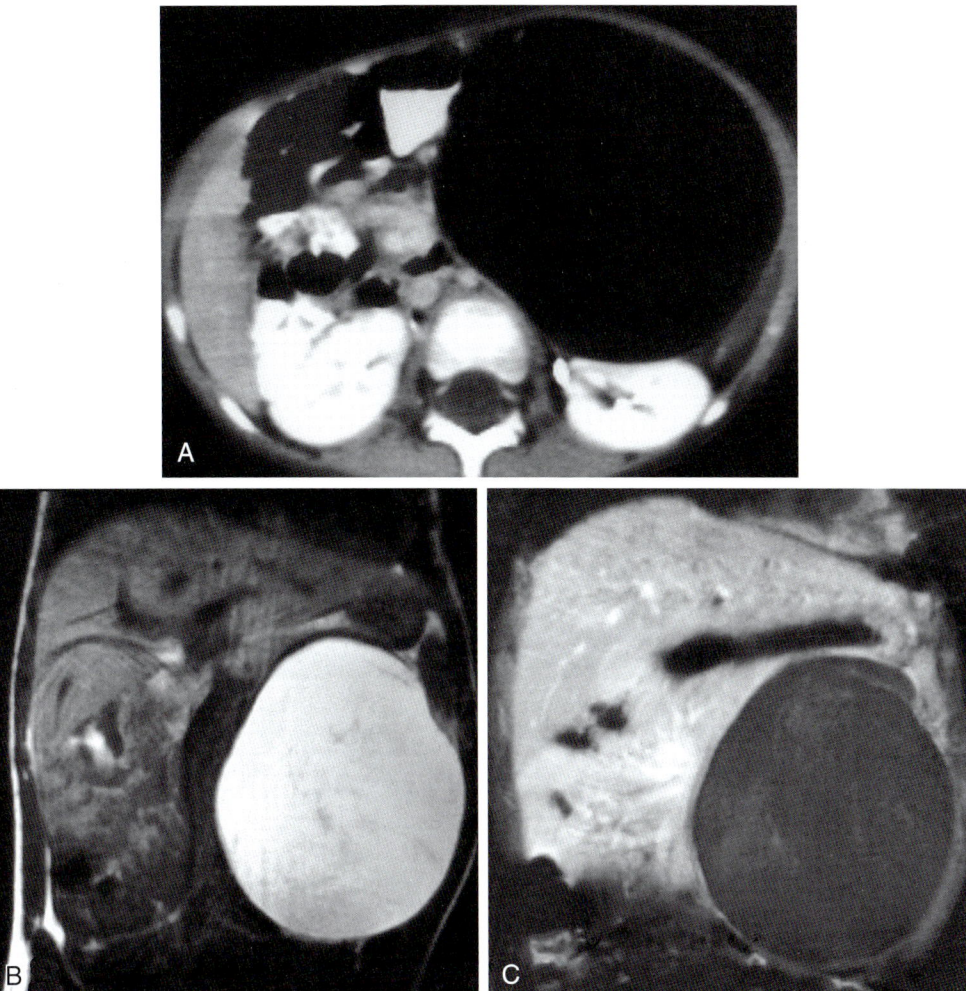

Figure 87-36 Lipoblastoma. Encapsulated left upper quadrant lipoblastoma attached to the pancreatic tail of a 2-year-old girl. **A,** Contrast-enhanced computed tomographic image through the midabdomen shows a large fatty mass. Coronal magnetic resonance T1-weighted sequences without (**B**) and with (**C**) fat saturation depict the fatty nature of the entire mass as well as some internal septations.

risking significant morbidity and mortality.[93] The goal of resection is negative margins; positive margins or incomplete resection are treated with adjuvant radiotherapy.[73,91,94] Other systemic therapies have been tried, including steroids, antiestrogen agents such as tamoxifen, nonsteroidal antiinflammatory agents such as sulindac, and chemotherapeutic agents such as vinblastine and methotrexate.[91,94]

Pseudomyxoma Peritonei

Overview Pseudomyxoma peritonei occurs when the omental and peritoneal surfaces are caked with copious amounts of mucinous or gelatinous material.[2]

Etiology Pseudomyxoma peritonei arises from an appendiceal lesion in most patients, through rupture of an appendiceal mucinous adenoma into the peritoneal cavity. Abundant amounts of mucus, which may or may not contain epithelial cells, spreads through peritoneal pathways and accumulates in spaces such as the cul-de-sac, Morison pouch, and paracolic gutters.[2,95] Pseudomyxoma peritonei may also originate in, or may secondarily involve, the ovary.[95]

Clinical Presentation Pseudomyxoma peritonei is more common in adults and affects women more than men.[95] Patients typically present with abdominal pain and weight loss, despite increasing abdominal size.[2]

Imaging Imaging findings are generally similar to those seen in massive ascites. US reveals ascitic fluid that demonstrates nonmobile internal echoes.[2] Septations and occasionally solid-appearing masses can be seen. On CT the mucinous material is typically low density and accumulates in dependent areas as discussed above. Scalloping of visceral surfaces, particularly the liver, is an important imaging sign to differentiate pseudomyxoma peritonei from ascites.[2] On imaging it is difficult to differentiate the benign form of pseudomyxoma peritonei from peritoneal mucinous carcinomatosis. Adenopathy, pleural involvement, enhancing masses, and invasion of visceral organs favors a malignant process.[2]

Treatment The treatment for the benign forms of pseudomyxoma peritonei consists mainly of surgical evacuation and appendectomy, with the potential need for resection of other involved structures. Malignant causes need additional

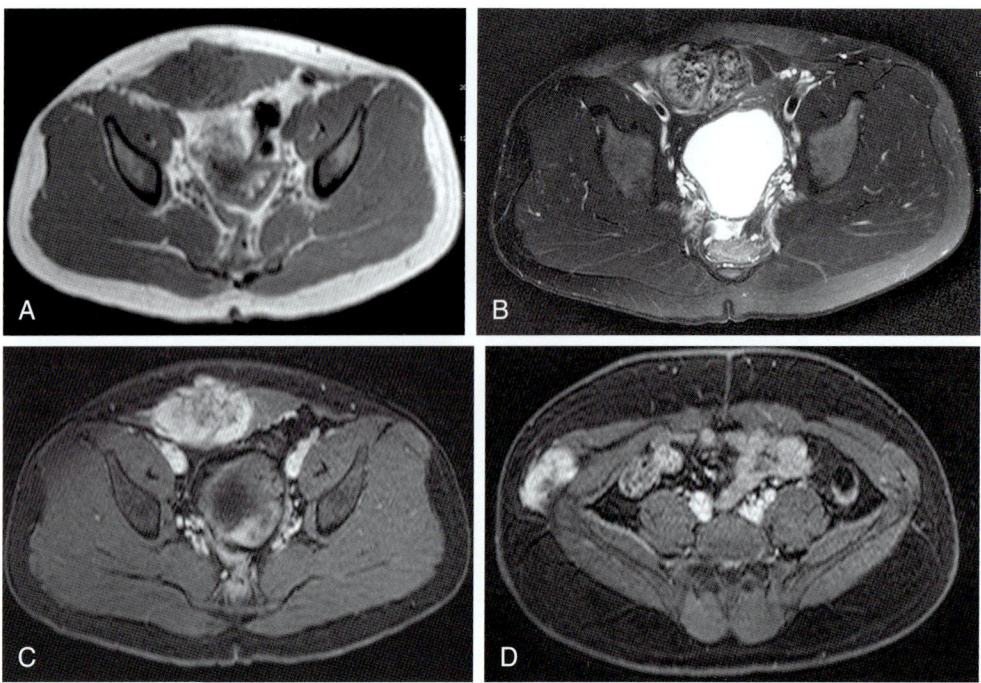

Figure 87-37 Desmoid tumor. A 16-year-old girl had an abdominal wall mass for 1 year. **A,** Axial T1-weighted magnetic resonance image shows a relatively well-defined rounded mass within the right rectus muscle. **B,** Axial T2-weighted image with fat saturation shows a heterogenous appearance to the mass. **C,** T1-weighted fat saturation after administration of contrast shows avid enhancement, especially when compared with adjacent muscle. **D,** An additional lesion with similar imaging characteristics is also identified more laterally in the abdominal wall.

treatment, such as intraperitoneal instillation of chemotherapeutic agents and radiotherapy.[96,97]

Malignant Lesions

PERITONEAL METASTASES AND CARCINOMATOSIS

Overview Peritoneal metastatic spread is rare in pediatric patients. Germ cell tumors or carcinoma of the colon account for up to 47% of cases of peritoneal carcinomatosis in pediatric patients.[98] Other tumors that can be seen with diffuse peritoneal dissemination include Wilms tumors, neuroblastoma, teratoma, desmoplastic small round cell tumor (DSRCT), and non-Hodgkin lymphoma.[98,99]

Etiology Malignancy disseminates throughout the peritoneum by intraperitoneal seeding, direct invasion, hematogenous spread, or lymphatic dissemination.[2] Peritoneal metastases frequently occur in the presence of other sites of metastatic disease. Seeding may occur at the time of operative intervention through tumor rupture and intraperitoneal spillage, with rare instances of intraabdominal spread of intracranial disease via a ventriculoperitoneal shunt.

Malignant cells migrate through the normal circulation of the peritoneal fluid. The adhesion of tumor cells to mesothelial cells is believed to be mediated through the expression of intercellular adhesion molecules.[2,100] Ascites results when disseminated disease interferes with the absorptive capacity of the mesothelial lining of the peritoneum.[100]

Clinical Presentation Peritoneal metastases may initially be asymptomatic; with progression of disease, patients come to medical attention with abdominal enlargement, ascites, nausea, and abdominal pain.[98,99] Approximately 20% are seen with bowel obstruction and 50% with ascites.[100,101] CT may demonstrate solitary or multiple masses, diffuse peritoneal thickening, peritoneal enhancement, and tumor studding of the peritoneal surfaces.[98] Diffuse caking is a feature of peritoneal metastases from rhabdomyosarcoma, non-Hodgkin lymphoma, and germ cell tumors (e-Figs. 87-38 and 87-39).[98]

MRI detection of peritoneal implants may be improved over CT because of the inherent tissue contrast and multiplanar capabilities.[2] Peritoneal implants tend to be hypointense on T1- and hyperintense on T2-weighted sequences, with variable enhancement.[100] Delayed images obtained 10 to 15 minutes after gadolinium administration may show lesions better, because they are slow to enhance.[2,100] However, respiratory and bowel motion may degrade identification of peritoneal and serosal lesions. Positron emission tomography (PET) or CT scan may also help to identify peritoneal carcinomatosis with greater confidence, depending on the size of the lesions.[2]

Treatment Surgical cytoreductive procedures aimed at removal of gross or bulky disease has been reported, followed by hyperthermic intraperitoneal chemotherapy. However, tumor recurrence rates as high as 70% are reported.[100]

DESMOPLASTIC SMALL ROUND CELL TUMOR

Overview DSRCT is a rare and aggressive abdominal malignancy that belongs to the small, round, blue cell tumor family.[101-103] Intraperitoneal involvement is most common, and less common sites include paratesticular, pleural, lung, ovary, sinus, central nervous system, kidney, and stomach.[102,104,105]

Etiology   The etiology of DSRCT is unknown; it has been hypothesized that the tumor originates from the mesothelial, submesothelial, or subserosal mesenchyma.[100] Pathologically DSRCTs are part of the small, blue, round cell family that includes Ewing sarcoma, neuroblastoma, Wilms tumor, rhabdomyosarcoma, and primitive neuroectodermal tumors. Immunocytochemical staining is usually required to distinguish DSRCTs from other small round cell tumors.[106]

Clinical Presentation   DSCRTs typically affect adolescents and young adults aged 15 to 25 years, and there is a strong male predilection with ratios that range from 3:1 to 9:1. Patients generally come to medical attention with vague abdominal pain and/or distension, and palpable abdominal masses may be present on physical exam.[101,104]

Imaging   On CT imaging, DSRCT is usually seen as multiple, scattered peritoneal masses without an apparent primary parenchymal source. The masses are generally of low attenuation and have a variable degree of central necrosis or hemorrhage with mild to moderate contrast enhancement.[102,107] US and MRI findings for DSRCT are variable and nonspecific (e-Fig. 87-40). The utility of fluorodeoxyglucose PET/CT is still evolving and is currently used to evaluate metastatic progression and response to systemic therapy.[108,109]

Tumor spread by direct peritoneal seeding results in multiple omental and mesenteric masses. Liver metastases, both intrahepatic (hematogenous) and serosal, are seen in up to 50% of patients (Fig. 87-41, *B*).[104,107] Other hematogenous metastatic lesions are less common. In addition, hydronephrosis and small-bowel obstruction may result from mass effect. Multiple studies have found a correlation between retroperitoneal lymphadenopathy and ascites with a dominant or large pelvic mass (see Fig. 87-41).[1,104,110] Although imaging features are usually nonspecific, the combination of a dominant pelvic mass, scattered small peritoneal masses, retroperitoneal lymphadenopathy, and ascites is somewhat characteristic for this entity. Primary differential diagnostic considerations include peritoneal carcinomatosis, rhabdomyosarcoma, neuroblastoma, lymphoma, and germ cell tumors.[104,110,111]

Treatment   Treatment generally includes a combination of chemotherapy and surgical resection. Chemotherapy may be useful for presurgical treatment, to reduce tumor bulk prior to resection, because improved outcomes have been reported in patients with complete resection.[102,103,112] However, DSRCT is an aggressive malignancy that has a poor prognosis despite treatment, with a reported 29% survival at 3 years.[112]

MISCELLANEOUS TUMORS

Rhabdomyosarcoma comprises about half of pediatric soft tissue sarcomas but is less common in the trunk (Fig. 87-42).[113] Abdominal wall and other truncal rhabdomyosarcomas have

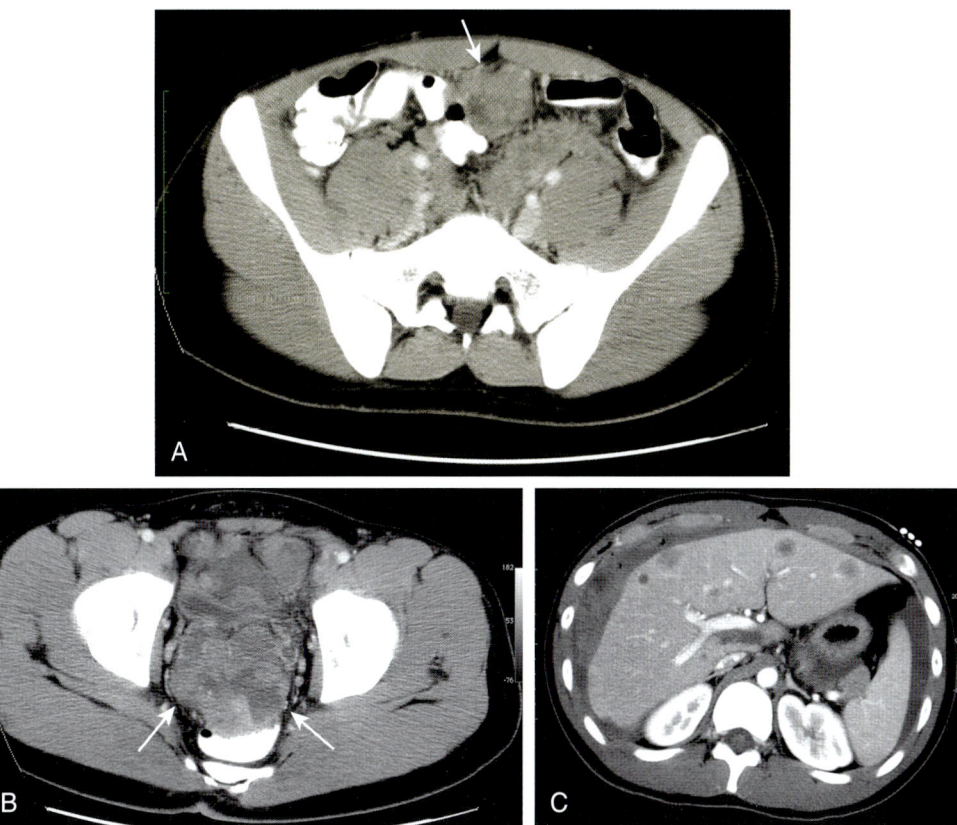

Figure 87-41   Desmoplastic small round cell tumor. **A** and **B,** Contrast-enhanced computed tomographic images in a 17-year-old boy show multiple heterogenously enhancing pelvic masses (*arrows*) with a dominant mass seen within the rectovesical pouch. **C,** Metastatic spread and peritoneal seeding are evident as multiple enhancing nodules within the liver with a large, heterogenous, peritoneal subcapsular mass indenting the hepatic surface.

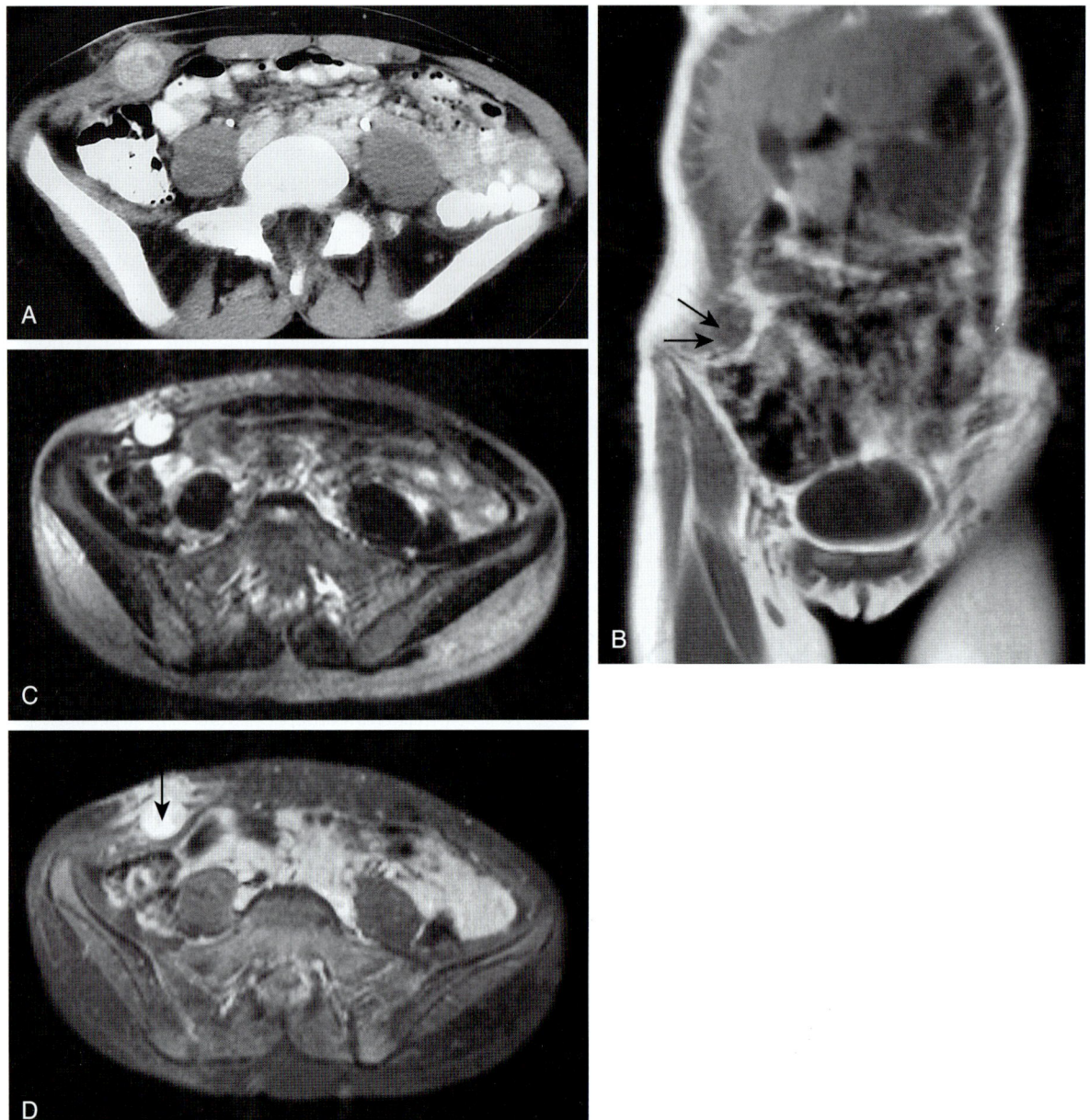

Figure 87-42 Embryonal rhabdomyosarcoma. A 13-year-old girl with a firm subcutaneous mass in the right lower abdominal wall. **A,** Contrast-enhanced computed tomographic image of the lower abdomen shows a heterogenously enhancing mass that causes focal enlargement of the right lateral oblique muscles. Edema is evident within the subcutaneous fat overlying the mass. Local infiltration by tumor cannot be excluded on this image. **B,** Oblique, coronal, noncontrast T1-weighted MR image shows the 3-cm round tissue mass within the right lateral oblique muscles (*arrows*). **C,** On an axial T2-weighted magnetic resonance image, the mass exhibits intense signal (as it did on short-tau inversion recovery sequence, not shown). **D,** Intense enhancement is seen with intravneous contrast administration in the soft tissue mass and in the overlying subcutaneous fat (*arrow*). This finding warrants concern about tumor infiltration.

a poorer prognosis when compared with other sites.[113] The truncal lesions are more likely to be of the embryonal than the alveolar type, tend to present with advanced disease, and are more likely to be greater than 5 cm at presentation. The ability to undergo gross total resection influences the prognosis, and gross total resection should be the goal of therapy.

Synovial sarcoma is a rare malignancy constituting 5% to 6% of pediatric soft tissue sarcomas, It most often originates in the extremities and near large joints, but it may rarely affect the anterior abdominal wall.[114]

Leiomyosarcoma often originates in the retroperitoneum, genitourinary, or GI tract and lower extremity.[115] Rarely,

such a lesion may arise in the omentum (Figs. 87-43 and 87-44).

Liposarcoma has been briefly discussed; the presence of fat may help to distinguish this tumor from other sarcomas. Although more commonly seen in the retroperitoneum, it is the least frequent soft tissue sarcoma to occur in childhood.[116]

Fibrosarcoma has two forms in children: the *congenital* or *infantile form* occurs in children up to 2 years of age, and the *childhood form* affects the 10- to 15-year-old age group (Fig. 87-45). The histology of the two forms is similar, but the infantile form has a distinct chromosomal translocation.

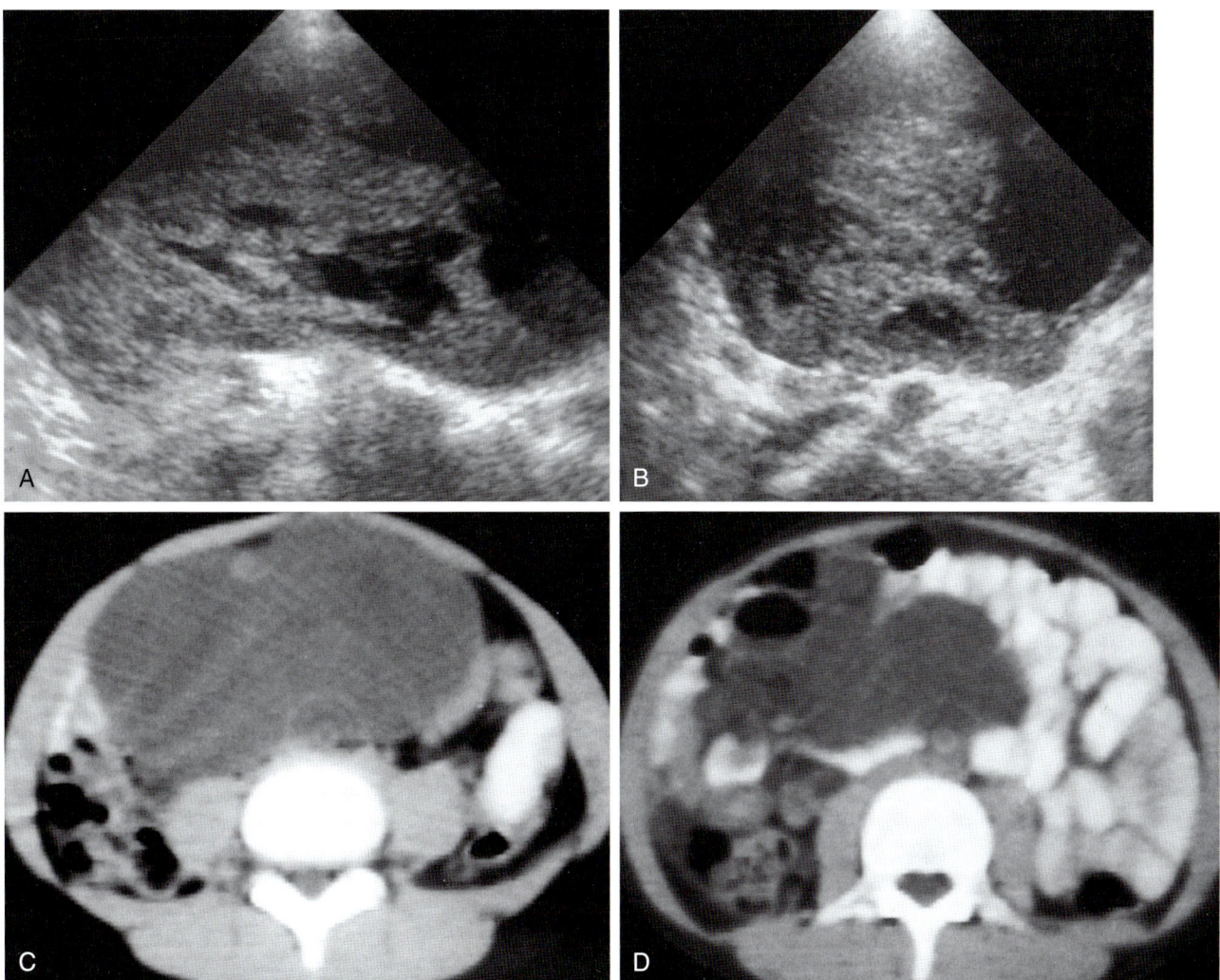

Figure 87-43   Leiomyosarcoma. Longitudinal (**A**) and transverse (**B**) ultrasound images through the midabdomen in a 10-year-old boy show a large, heterogenous, solid and cystic mass. **C** and **D,** Computed tomographic images without intravenous contrast show a large, homogenous, low-density, midline soft tissue mass displacing bowel.

Infantile fibrosarcoma has been reported to involve the trunk and retroperitoneum in children.[115,117] After complete surgical resection, the prognosis is better for the congenital or infantile form than for the childhood/adult form.[117]

Malignant mesenchymomas are very rare soft tissue tumors seen predominantly in adults. These tumors contain at least two distinct histologic sarcoma subtypes and are considered to be high-grade tumors with an overall poor prognosis. The most common sites of primary malignant mesenchymoma are the retroperitoneum or the thigh, but these have been reported in various locations.[118] CT findings are of a soft tissue mass with mixed attenuation that often contains areas of necrosis and calcification, with heterogenous enhancement and moderate vascularity (Fig. 87-46). Using MR imaging, these lesions are typically heterogenous on T2-weighted images.[119] Treatment includes a combination of surgical incision, radiation therapy, and chemotherapy.

Malignant mesothelioma of the peritoneum is rare in children and does not seem to be related to radiation or asbestos exposure.[1,120] Children with peritoneal malignant mesothelioma come to medical attention with ascites and multiple tumor nodules along the peritoneal surface (see e-Fig. 87-38).[120]

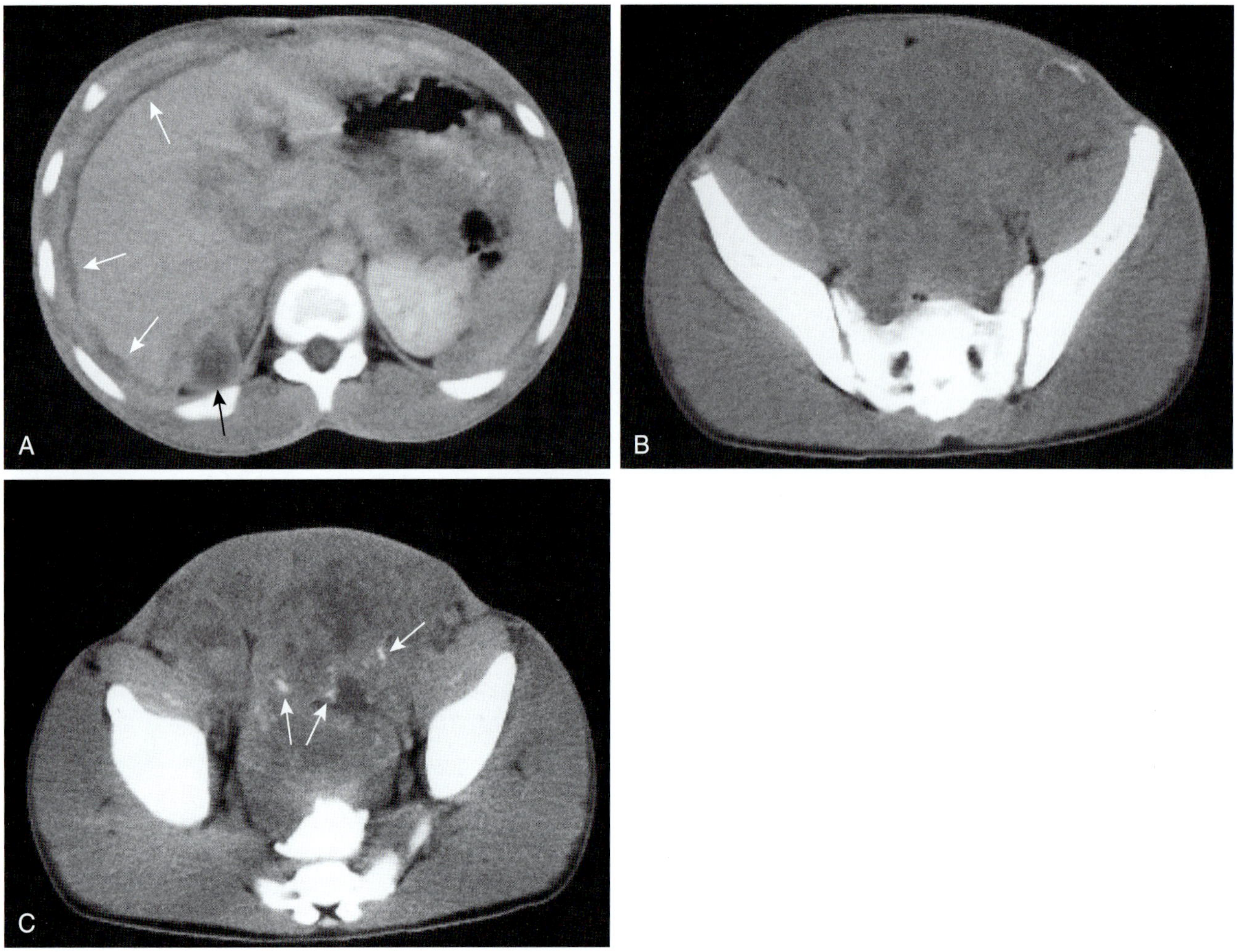

Figure 87-44   Leiomyosarcoma. **A,** Contrast-enhanced computed tomographic image in a 16-year-old boy shows extensive peritoneal metastases around the liver (*white arrows*) and surrounding the pancreas in addition to a cystic peritoneal metastasis (*black arrow*). **B,** Lower image in the upper pelvis shows that the mass occupies most of the lower abdomen and pelvis. **C,** Another image lower in the pelvis shows scattered calcifications (*arrows*). Bowel contrast is present in the rectum.

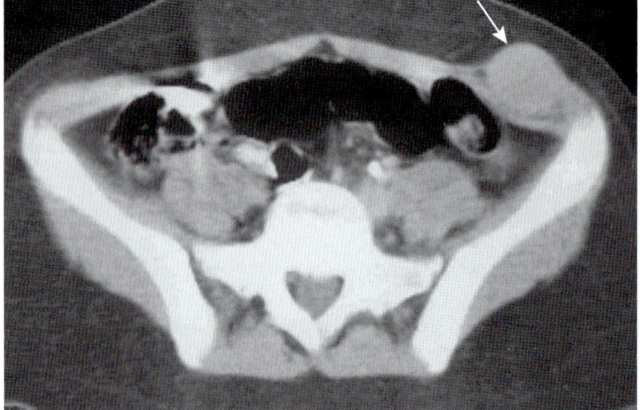

Figure 87-45   Fibrosarcoma. Contrast-enhanced computed tomographic image through the upper pelvis in a 14-year-old girl shows a well-defined, round 3-cm mass in the left anterior abdominal wall. The mass expands and is isointense with the left lateral oblique muscles (*arrow*).

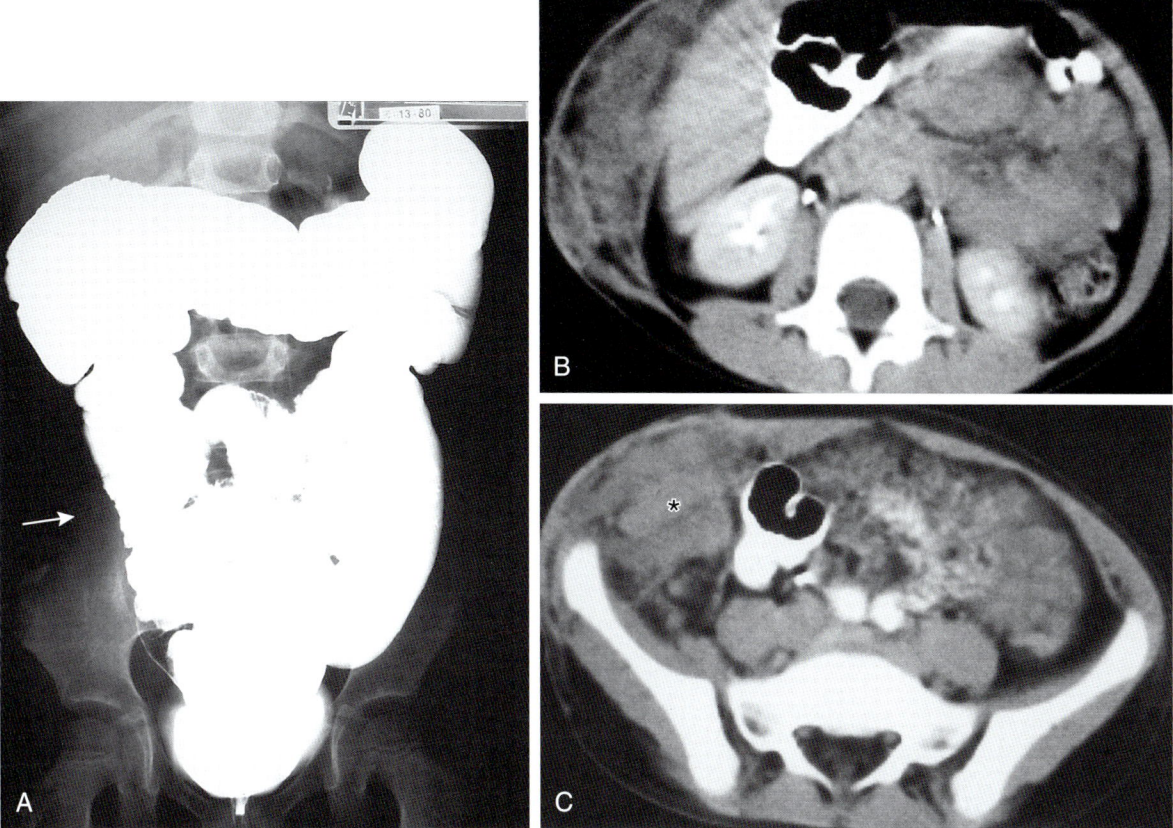

Figure 87-46 Recurrent mesenchymoma in a 5-year-old girl originally diagnosed at age 3 years. **A,** Abdominal radiograph from a barium enema demonstrates a normal colon with displacement of the right colon (*arrow*) from the adjacent abdominal wall mesenchymoma. **B** and **C,** Axial computed tomographic images after intravenous and oral contrast administration show expansion of the anterolateral abdominal wall by heterogenous infiltrative soft tissue (*asterisk*). Extension from the subcutaneous location (**B** and **C**) infiltrates the abdomen, with mass effect on adjacent structures, most notably the right colon, as depicted in **A.**

Key Points

Upright radiographs and decubitus abdominal radiographs for detection of free air have similar sensitivity.

Abdominal compartment syndrome is a clinical diagnosis that includes elevation of intraabdominal pressure to 20 mm Hg or greater, coupled with impaired function of at least one organ.

Fat necrosis is of one of the causes of abdominal wall calcification in neonates and infants. The majority of such calcifications are associated with neonatal asphyxia, sepsis, gestational diabetes, and hypothermia.

Peritoneal calcification associated with calcified intraabdominal lymph nodes is more likely to be associated with a malignant process.

Lipoblastomas can have a variable amount of macroscopic fat and may not appear completely fatty on imaging.

MR imaging is preferred for detection of peritoneal implants given the inherent tissue contrast and multiplanar capabilities.

Scalloping of visceral surfaces, particularly the liver, is one of the most important imaging signs to differentiate pseudomyxoma peritonei from ascites.

DSRCTs usually are seen as multiple, scattered peritoneal masses without an apparent primary parenchymal source.

Suggested Readings

Agarwal A, et al. Peritoneal calcification: causes and distinguishing features on CT. *AJR Am J Roentgenol.* 2004;182(2):441-445.

Bellah R, et al. Desmoplastic small round cell tumor in the abdomen and pelvis: report of CT findings in 11 affected children and young adults. *AJR Am J Roentgenol.* 2005;184(6):1910-1914.

Chiu YH, et al. Reappraisal of radiographic signs of pneumoperitoneum at emergency department. *Am J Emerg Med.* 2009;27(3):320-327.

Ledbetter DJ. Gastroschisis and omphalocele. *Surg Clin North Am.* 2006;86(2):249-260, vii.

Patel A, et al. Abdominal compartment syndrome. *AJR Am J Roentgenol.* 2007;189(5):1037-1043.

References

Full references for this chapter can be found on www.expertconsult.com.

Chapter 88

Congenital Hepatobiliary Anomalies

JOSHUA Q. KNOWLTON and LISA H. LOWE

Fibropolycystic liver disorders are a group of associated congenital anomalies of the liver caused by malformation of the embryonic ductal plates (Fig. 88-1). They include choledochal cysts, Caroli disease, hepatic fibrosis, biliary hamartomas, and cystic liver disease. The specific type of fibropolycystic disorder depends on the size of the embryonic duct with faulty development (Table 88-1).

Choledochal Cyst

Overview Choledochal cysts, which are among the most frequent of congenital hepatobiliary anomalies, are a fusiform or saccular dilation of the bile ducts. The Todani classification system is commonly used to categorize these anomalies into five general types (with several subtypes) that differ based on etiology, pathogenesis, appearance, and presentation (Fig. 88-2).[1]

The most common choledochal cyst is the Todani type I, found in 80% to 90% of cases.[2] It involves variable lengths and degrees of common bile duct dilatation and is further classified into subtypes.[2] Todani type IA, IB, and IC describe cystic dilation of the common bile duct, segmental dilation below the cystic duct, and fusiform dilation, respectively. Todani type II choledochal cysts are found in only 2% of cases and consist of one or more diverticula of the common bile duct.[3] Todani type III occurs in 1.5% to 5% of cases and involves dilation of the intraduodenal portion of the duct, forming a cystlike mass, termed a "choledochocele," with both the common bile and pancreatic ducts emptying into it. Todani type IVA consists of multiple intrahepatic and extrahepatic biliary dilatations and occurs in 10% of patients with choledochal cysts.[1,3] Type IVB, which involves multiple extrahepatic biliary cysts without intrahepatic involvement, is rare. Todani type V is synonymous with Caroli disease.[1] Todani type IVA also has been described as a type I cyst with intrahepatic involvement, and controversy exists about whether it is actually a type V (Caroli disease) cyst with common duct enlargement.

Etiology Several theories for the pathogenesis of the type I choledochal cysts exist. In addition to the ductal plate malformation described previously, other theories have suggested cyst formation as a result of obstruction of the distal biliary duct and/or reflux of pancreatic enzymes into the biliary tree because of anomalous proximal insertion of the pancreatic duct into the common bile duct (ductal malunion).[4,5] This ductal malunion could permit reflux of pancreatic enzymes into the common bile duct, with subsequent inflammation and weakening of the wall, a pathologic mechanism that occurs in about 60% of patients.[5] This anomalous ductal connection has been demonstrated on endoscopic retrograde cholangiopancreatography (ERCP) (Fig. 88-3). Type I choledochal cysts are more common in girls than in boys in Western countries, but the sex ratio is equal in Asia.[2,3] About 65% of all reported cases are from Japan.[2]

It has been theorized that type II choledochal cysts result from prenatal rupture of the common bile duct with subsequent healing.[3] Type III choledochal cysts may be the sequelae of ampullary obstruction or congenital duplication of the duodenum at the ampulla. The intrahepatic cysts seen in types IV and V are thought to be due to primary ductal ectasia resulting from ductal plate malformation.

Clinical Presentation Choledochal cysts may present in infancy with cholestatic jaundice, which clinically is inseparable from neonatal hepatitis or biliary atresia.[2] In older children and young adults, the clinical presentation is variable. A characteristic triad of abdominal pain, obstructive jaundice, and fever has been reported, but few patients present with all three components. Abdominal pain is the most characteristic presentation, followed by obstructive jaundice, fever, pale stools, splenomegaly, hepatomegaly, and a palpable mass.[6] The most common complication of a choledochal cyst is ascending cholangitis.[7] Long-term complications, such as hepatic cirrhosis with subsequent portal hypertension, can occur.[6] Carcinoma of the biliary tree has a twentyfold increased incidence in patients with choledochal cysts. This risk is low in the first decade but increases with advancing age.[8] Spontaneous cyst rupture also has been reported.[6]

Imaging When the clinical presentation points to a hepatobiliary problem, sonography usually is the initial imaging study requested. The markedly dilated common bile duct is readily discernible in types I and IV choledochal cysts. The gallbladder usually can be identified adjacent to the dilated common duct (Fig. 88-4). Most frequently, the intrahepatic ducts are normal, but varying degrees of dilation may be present as a result of obstruction. Sludge or stones may be

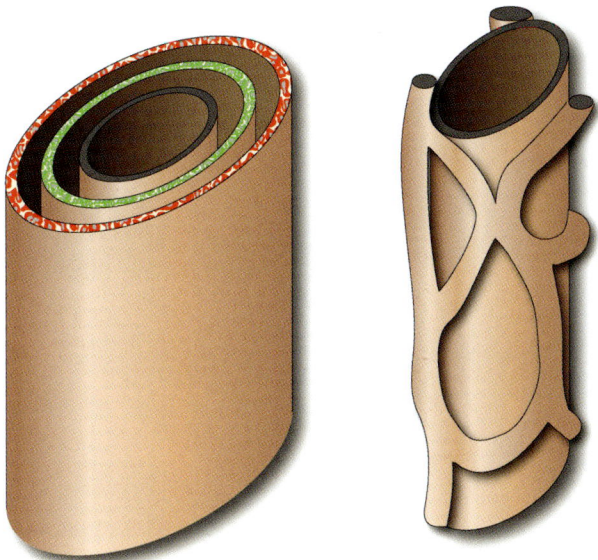

Figure 88-1 *Schema of ductal plate.* A bilayer of hepatocytes (green and red layers) surrounds the portal venous structures (central black), forming the lumina of primitive bile ducts (*left*). A process of organized resorption leads to the normal organization of biliary ducts within the portal triads. Failure of this process leads to ductal plate malformations.

identified within the dilated ducts.[9] Type III cysts may cause mass effect at the ampulla of Vater (Fig. 88-5, *A* and *B*).

Abdominal magnetic resonance imaging (MRI) with cholangiopancreatography (MRCP) often is performed to delineate anatomy (Fig. 88-6).[10-12] Hepatobiliary scintigraphy can prove useful in difficult cases by demonstrating communication between the choledochal cyst and the hepatobiliary ducts (Fig. 88-7).[9] Computed tomography (CT) does not demonstrate the biliary ductal anatomy as well as ultrasound and MRI, although it can be useful along with sonography to guide abscess drainage and to evaluate hepatic anatomy.[10,11]

Percutaneous transhepatic cholangiography (PTC) and ERCP are useful when placement of a percutaneous biliary drain may be helpful (Fig. 88-8). Some investigators prefer PTC to ERCP because it carries a lower risk of iatrogenic cholangitis.[7]

Treatment Because of the potential long-term sequelae, surgical excision and hepatojejunostomy are performed as definitive treatments. Patients with intrahepatic cysts are closely monitored for cholangitis, cholestasis, and stone formation. Antibiotics are administered in the setting of acute cholangitis. Medical therapy can be instituted to reduce the risk of

Table 88-1

Fibropolycystic Liver Disorder and Size of Ducts with Faulty Embryogenesis	
Disorder	**Duct Size**
Congenital hepatic fibrosis	Small
Biliary hamartoma	Small
Polycystic liver disease	Medium
Choledochal cyst	Large extrahepatic
Caroli disease	Large intrahepatic

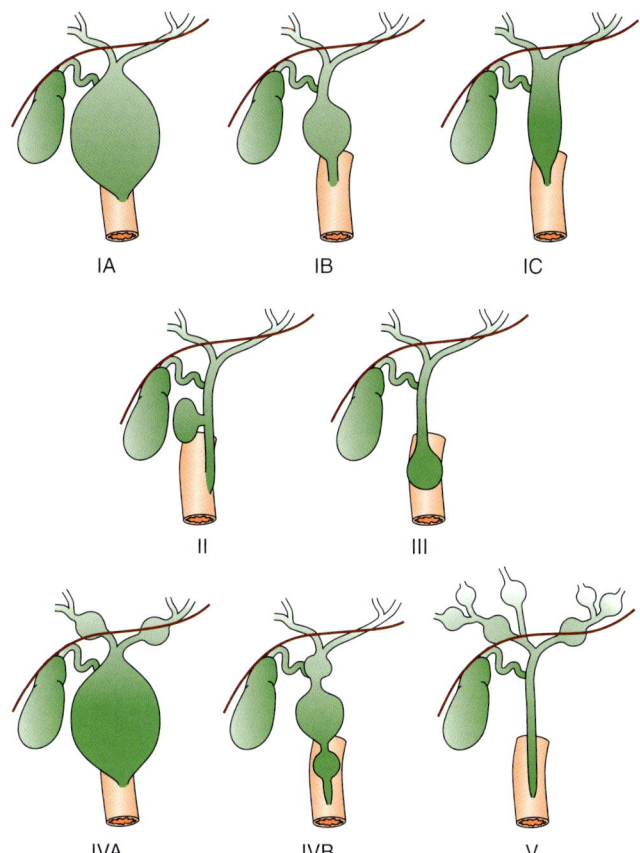

Figure 88-2 *Schematic of Todani classification of choledochal cysts based on cholangiographic morphology.* Type IA and IB involve cystic dilatation of the common duct, with IB limited to the area below the insertion of the cystic duct; IC is fusiform dilatation of the duct. Type II is a saccular diverticulum from the common bile duct, and type III is a choledochocele at the ampulla of Vater. Types IVA and IVB are multiple cystic dilations of the intrahepatic and extrahepatic biliary tree, and type V is equivalent to Caroli disease with numerous intrahepatic bile lakes throughout the biliary tree and liver. (From Kim OH, Chung HJ, Choi BG. Imaging of the choledochal cyst. *Radiographics.* 1995;15:69-88.)

cholestasis and promote bile flow; however, when extensive liver damage and cirrhosis occurs, a liver transplant may be necessary.

Caroli Disease and Caroli Syndrome

Overview Caroli disease, also classified as Todani type V choledochal cyst, is a segmental nonobstructive dilation of the intrahepatic bile ducts. It is characterized by multiple hepatic cysts in continuity with the biliary system, representing ectatic intrahepatic ducts,[7] and can be associated with stone formation, cholangitis, and hepatic abscesses.[13] In Caroli syndrome, which is discussed further below, hepatic fibrosis is also present.

Etiology Leading theories on the etiology of Caroli disease include maldevelopment of the large intrahepatic ductal plates. Other postulated mechanisms include occlusion of the hepatic artery in the neonatal period with associated ischemia of the bile ducts versus abnormal growth rate of the biliary epithelium and supporting connective tissues with lack of the normal involution of ductal plates. This process leads to

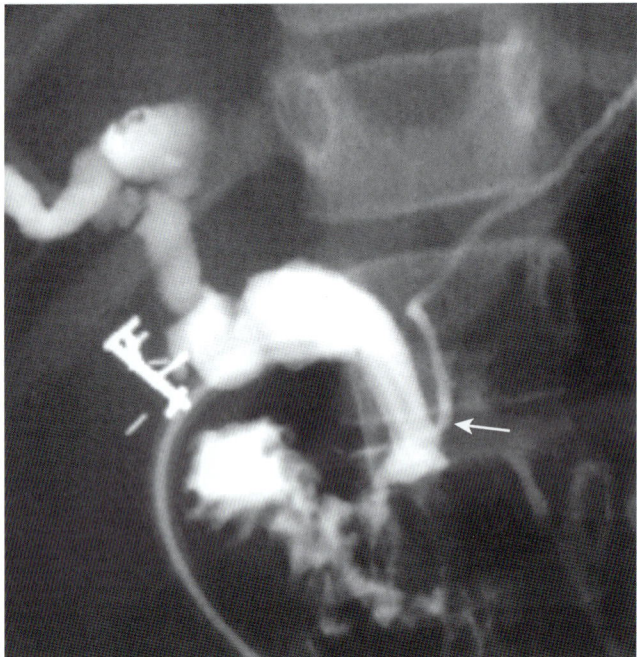

Figure 88-3 Endoscopic retrograde cholangiopancreatography in a child with a choledochal cyst reveals dilation of the common bile duct and a relatively proximal insertion of the pancreatic duct (*arrow*).

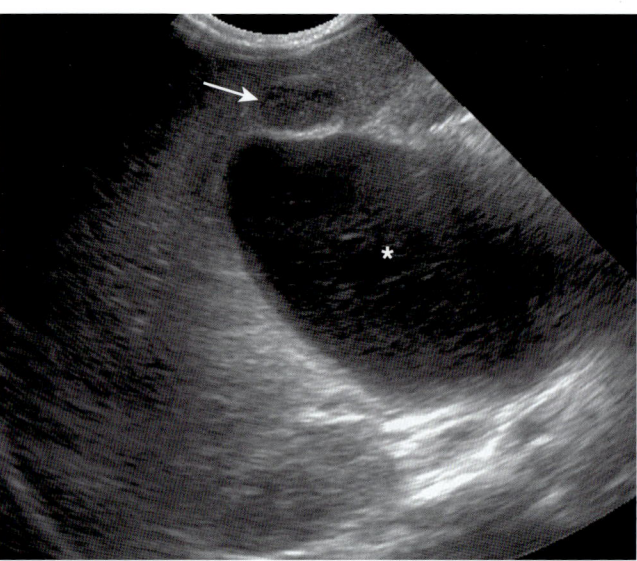

Figure 88-4 Choledochal cyst (Todani type I) in an 8-day-old girl with jaundice. Transverse sonogram shows a large fusiform cyst in the porta hepatis (*asterisk*) just beneath a small, contracted sludge filled gallbladder (*arrow*).

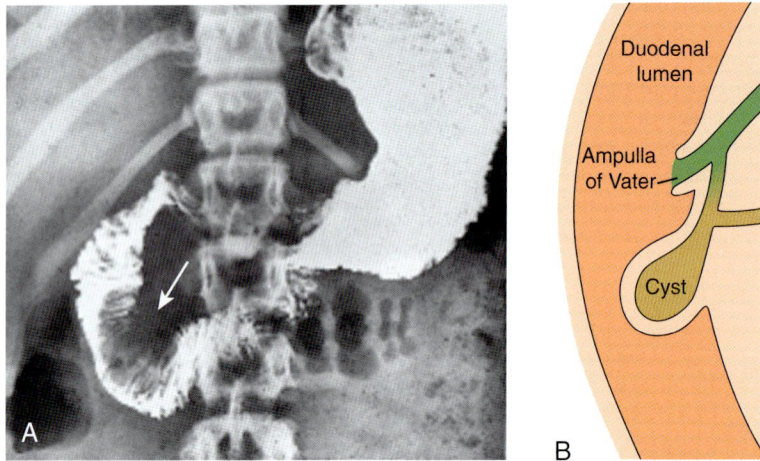
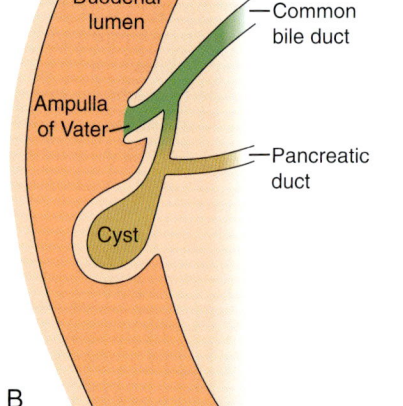

Figure 88-5 Choledochocele (Todani type III) in a 12-year-old girl with abdominal pain. **A,** Upper gastrointestinal tract image shows a large filling defect (*arrow*) coincident with the site of the Ampulla of Vater. **B,** Drawing of findings of choledochocele confirmed at surgery.

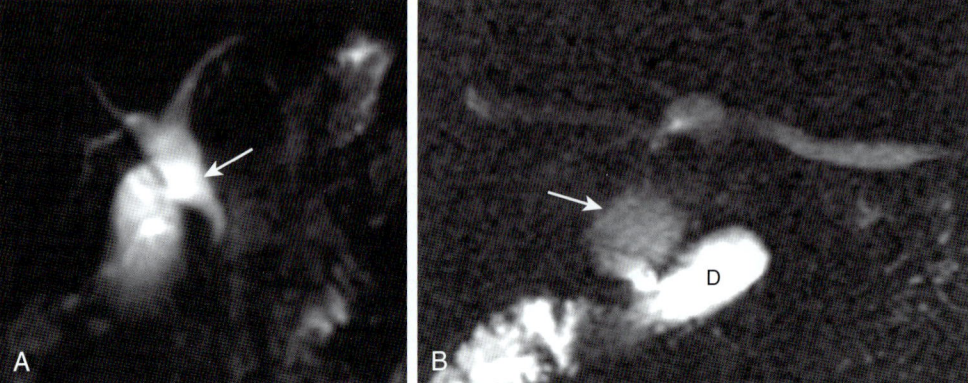

Figure 88-6 A choledochal cyst (Todani type I). **A,** Magnetic resonance imaging with cholangiopancreatography (MRCP) in a 10-day-old boy with jaundice demonstrates dilatation of the common bile duct (*arrow*). **B,** A choledochal cyst (Todani type I) in a 6-year-old boy with abdominal pain. MRCP reveals dilation of the common bile duct (*arrow*) draining into the normal duodenum (*D*).

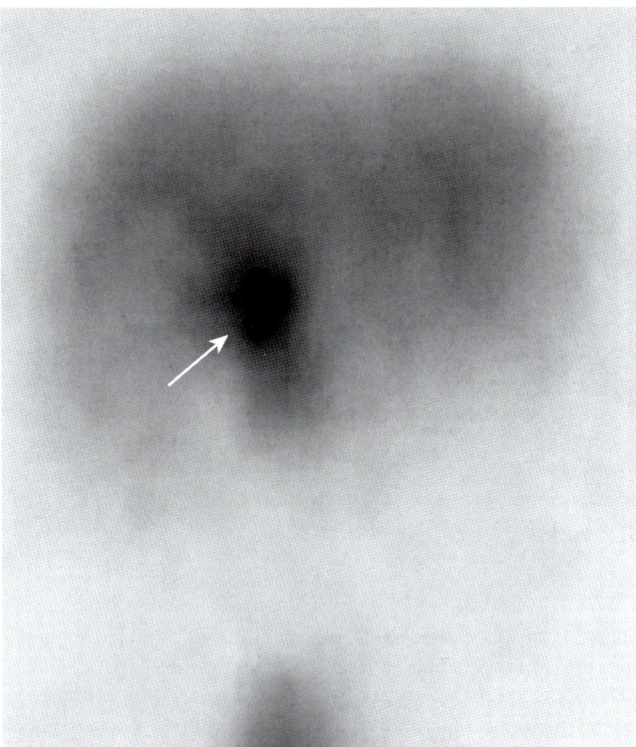

Figure 88-7 Delayed image from a technetium-99m–labeled hepatoiminodiacetic acid confirms communication with the biliary tree, as radiotracer accumulates in the cyst (*arrow*). This area was photopenic on early scans (not shown).

ectatic biliary cysts surrounding the portal triads. In Caroli syndrome, which involves large and small ductal plate abnormalities, associated hepatic fibrosis is present. Caroli hepatic ductal ectasia also may be associated with extrahepatic ductal plate abnormalities and choledochal cysts (Todani IVA choledochal cyst), as discussed previously. An association also exists with renal disorders, including autosomal recessive polycystic kidney disease, medullary sponge kidney, and nephronopthisis.[7] Although it typically is a diffuse process,

monolobar Caroli disease has been reported, with 88% of cases involving the left lobe.[14]

Clinical Presentation Although the disease is present from birth, most patients do not present until later in life when abdominal pain resulting from cholangitis and cholestasis leads them to seek medical attention. The abdominal pain also may be related to hepatic abscesses (a consequence of cholangitis) or biliary stones (a consequence of cholestasis). Patients with associated hepatic fibrosis may present with symptoms and signs of portal hypertension as a result of the disease process.[13]

Imaging In most patients, sonography reveals very large and irregular ectatic ducts.[7,15] To distinguish Caroli disease from hepatic cysts, one must recognize that the ectatic ducts connect with one another and with the ductal system (Fig. 88-9). The ectatic ducts surround portal vein radicles that produce the central dot sign, which has been considered pathognomonic for Caroli disease.[16] Doppler interrogation can be used to confirm blood flow within these portal venous branches.[16] Biliary sludge and calculi are common findings within the dilated bile ducts.[7] If an abscess develops, one or more cysts will show mixed echogenicity rather than the anechoic appearance of uncomplicated cysts.

The kidneys should be examined in all patients with confirmed Caroli disease. Kidneys may be normal or polycystic, or they may show increased medullary echogenicity with loss of corticomedullary differentiation (Fig. 88-10). MRI and CT are excellent modalities to show the extent of disease. An enhancing "central dot" may be present that corresponds to the portal vein radicles seen sonographically.[17] If an abscess is present, the affected cyst may show higher attenuation or peripheral enhancement compared with adjacent uninfected cysts.[7] Biliary patency HIDA (hepato-iminodiacetic acid) scans have been used to demonstrate a connection to the biliary tree. Occasionally, PTC is used during abscess drainage.

Treatment Ursodeoxycholic acid can decrease complications that occur as a result of cholelithiasis. Broad-spectrum antibiotic coverage can be used to prevent and treat cholangitis.

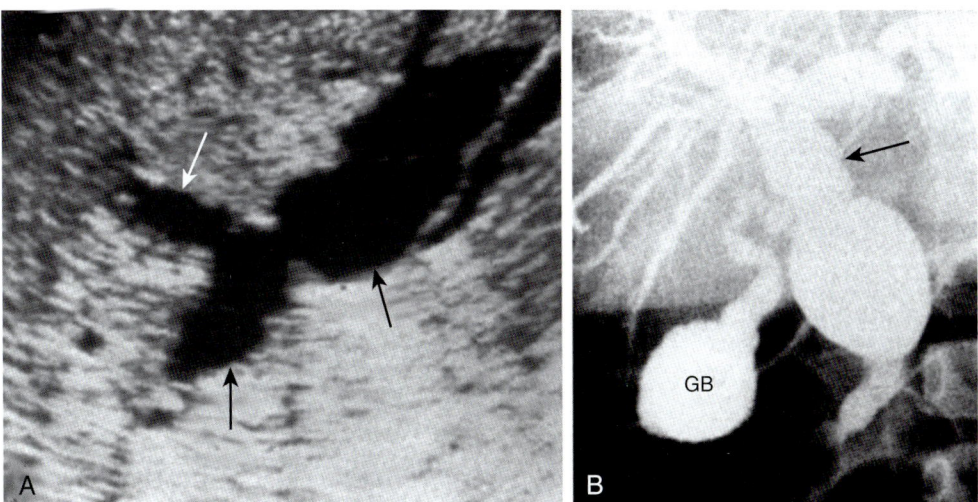

Figure 88-8 Choledochal cyst (Todani type IV) in a 1-year-old boy. **A,** A longitudinal sonogram shows marked saccular dilation of the intrahepatic and extrahepatic bile ducts (*arrows*). **B,** An operative cholangiogram confirms dilation of the intrahepatic biliary tree and common bile duct (*arrow*). The gallbladder (*GB*) is noted.

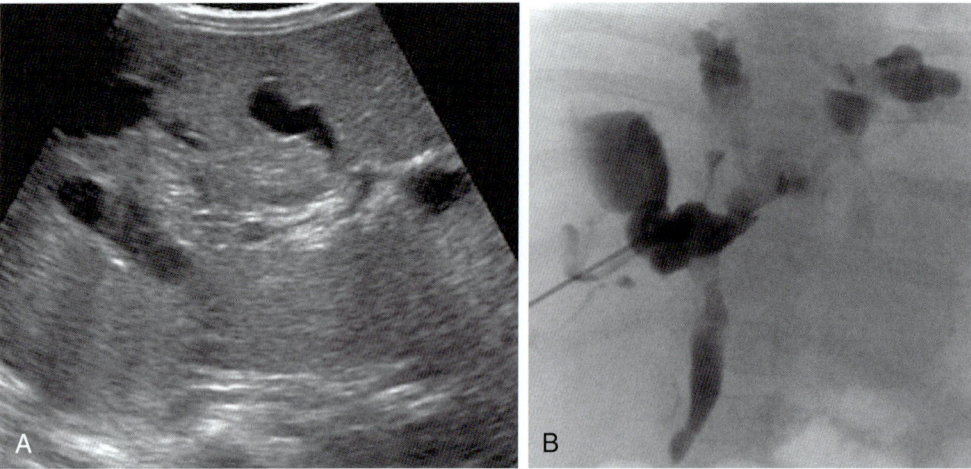

Figure 88-9   Caroli disease (type V choledochal cyst) in a 6-month-old girl with failure to thrive. **A,** A transverse hepatic sonogram shows multiple, large, hypoechoic, well-defined, variably shaped bile lakes scattered throughout the liver. **B,** A percutaneous transhepatic cholangiogram confirms variably shaped patulous bile lakes connected to the biliary tree.

Supplementation of fat-soluble vitamins may help alleviate symptoms of cholestasis. In addition, serologic screening for carcinogenic antigen (CA) 19-9 and carcinoembryogenic antigen (CEA) are helpful. Surgical resection has been used carcinogenic antigen successfully in patients with monolobar disease. For patients with diffuse involvement and progression beyond medical management, orthotopic liver transplant is the definitive treatment.[18]

Congenital Hepatic Fibrosis

Overview   Congenital hepatic fibrosis is a progressive condition that leads to portal hypertension. Autosomal recessive polycystic kidney disease is invariably associated with this condition.[19,20] The hepatic abnormality is expressed later in life and therefore depends on less severe renal involvement that affords sufficient longevity for the hepatic abnormalities to become manifest clinically.

Etiology   Congenital hepatic fibrosis is a ductal plate malformation involving the small interlobular ducts.[19] Periportal fibrosis occurs from scarring between adjacent biliary tracts and ductal plate remnants, resembling bile ducts. Hepatic fibrosis (due to malformation of small intrahepatic ductal plates) can be associated with Caroli disease, which is a large ductal plate anomaly; this association has been termed *Caroli syndrome.*[21]

Clinical Presentation   The onset of congenital hepatic fibrosis is variable, with less severe disease presenting later in childhood or in adulthood, frequently with splenomegaly and portal hypertension.[7,19,22] Major complications of congenital hepatic fibrosis include ascending cholangitis, hepatic failure, and an increased risk of hepatocellular carcinoma. An increased incidence of hepatocellular carcinoma is found in patients with congenital hepatic fibrosis as well.[7,23,24]

Imaging   Ultrasound is the initial imaging modality typically requested (Fig. 88-11, *A*). Increased hepatic echogenicity and poorly defined portal vessels are seen, with increased echogenicity of the portal triads. If associated with Caroli syndrome, large ectatic biliary cysts are seen encircling irregular portal vein radicals. Associated renal lesions also should be investigated with ultrasound.[7] Portal hypertension, supervening splenomegaly, and multiple collaterals bypassing the

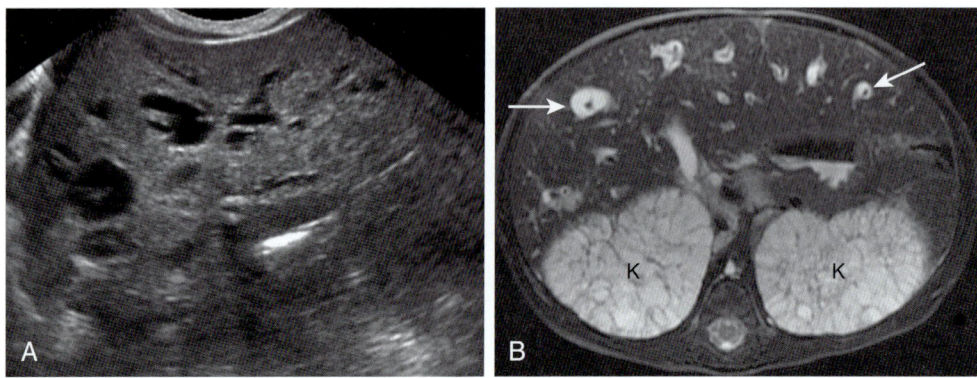

Figure 88-10   Caroli (type V choledochal cyst) disease in a 3-day-old girl with organomegaly and associated autosomal recessive polycystic kidney disease. **A,** Longitudinal sonograms through the liver show focal dilatation of the biliary ducts throughout the liver. **B,** Magnetic resonance imaging with cholangiopancreatography shows the central dot sign, seen as numerous T2 bright distended bile ducts each surrounding a portal vessel or "dot" (*arrows*). Associated enlarged, polycystic T2 bright kidneys (*K*) also are seen.

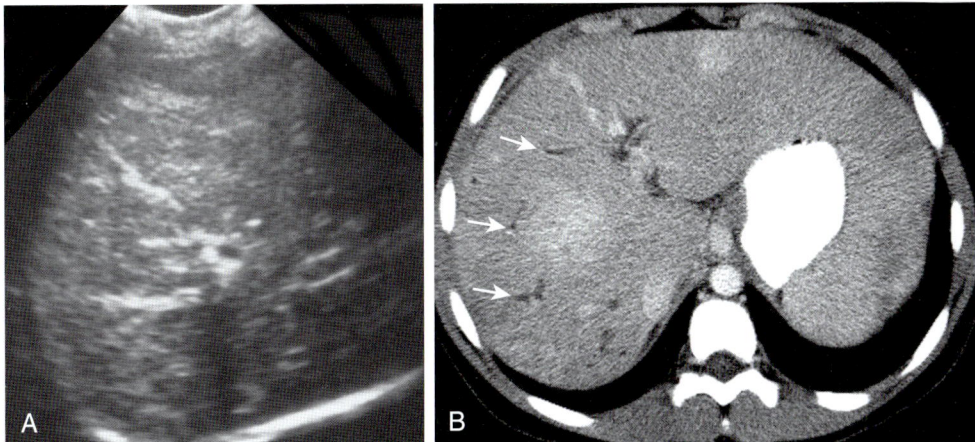

Figure 88-11   Congenital hepatic fibrosis complicated by portal hypertension in a 12-year-old girl. **A,** A transverse sonogram shows heterogeneous echogenicity of the liver with linear bands of hyperechogenicity due to advanced fibrosis. **B,** Axial contrast-enhanced computed tomography images show heterogeneous hepatic enhancement and linear branching hypoattenuating tubular structures indicating mild ductal dilation (*arrows*). Extensive collateral vessels caused by portal hypertension were present (not shown).

hepatic sinusoids can be seen with ultrasound, but they are more easily and completely revealed with contrast CT or MRI. CT and MRI reveal areas of hepatic parenchymal heterogeneity with variable CT attenuation (Fig. 88-11, *B*) and T1 and T2 MRI parenchymal signal.[7] Magnetic resonance angiography can demonstrate the vascular sequelae of portal hypertension, and MRCP is useful to ascertain the anatomy of the biliary tree.[19,21]

Treatment   Medical management of hepatic fibrosis and portal hypertension consists of diuretics as first-line pharmacotherapy used to reduce ascites and increase glomerular filtration. When hepatic cirrhosis and portal hypertension become severe, orthotopic hepatic transplant is a more definitive treatment.

Biliary Hamartomas

Overview   Biliary hamartomas, also known as microhamartomas and Von Meyenburg complex, are rare.[25] Patients usually have many well-defined, similar-sized lesions measuring less than 15 mm; their uniform size helps distinguish these lesions from metastatic disease, although a biopsy ultimately is required.[7,26] Because microhamartomas are small, they usually are asymptomatic and are identified at pathologic examination. A small increased risk of hepatobiliary carcinomas exists.[7]

Etiology   Biliary hamartomas result from ductal plate malformations of the small bile ducts. They usually are multiple and typically do not have associated abnormalities, although at times they can coexist with simple hepatic cysts or polycystic kidney and liver disease.[24,27]

Imaging   Biliary hamartomas are seen with ultrasound; they are predominantly hypoechoic with comet tail echoes and can have mild cyst wall irregularity. Increased heterogeneity of the hepatic architecture often is seen.[26] The lesions have low attenuation on CT, and on MRI they have a decreased signal with T1 weighting and an increased signal with T2 weighting (Fig. 88-12).[7]

Treatment   Most biliary hamartomas are asymptomatic, and thus no treatment is required. However, follow-up may be useful because of the rare possibility of malignancy.

Biliary Atresias

Overview   Biliary atresia (BA) is the most common cause of neonatal cholestasis and is the primary indication for pediatric liver transplantation. It is more common in Japan than in the United States.[28]

Etiology   The etiology of BA remains unknown; viral, genetic, and autoimmune origins have been suggested as possibilities. Recent theories suggest that BA and hepatitis are inflammatory cholangiopathies on two ends of a spectrum.[2]

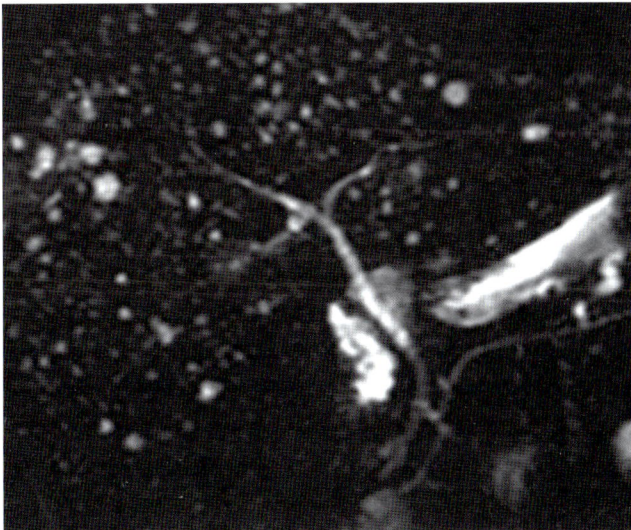

Figure 88-12   Biliary hamartomas. Magnetic resonance imaging with cholangiopancreatography demonstrates innumerable small, well-defined, bright foci throughout the liver. Note the normal size ductal system. (From Kim OH, Chung HJ, Choi BG. Imaging of the choledochal cyst. *Radiographics.* 1995;15(1):69-88. Reprinted with permission.)

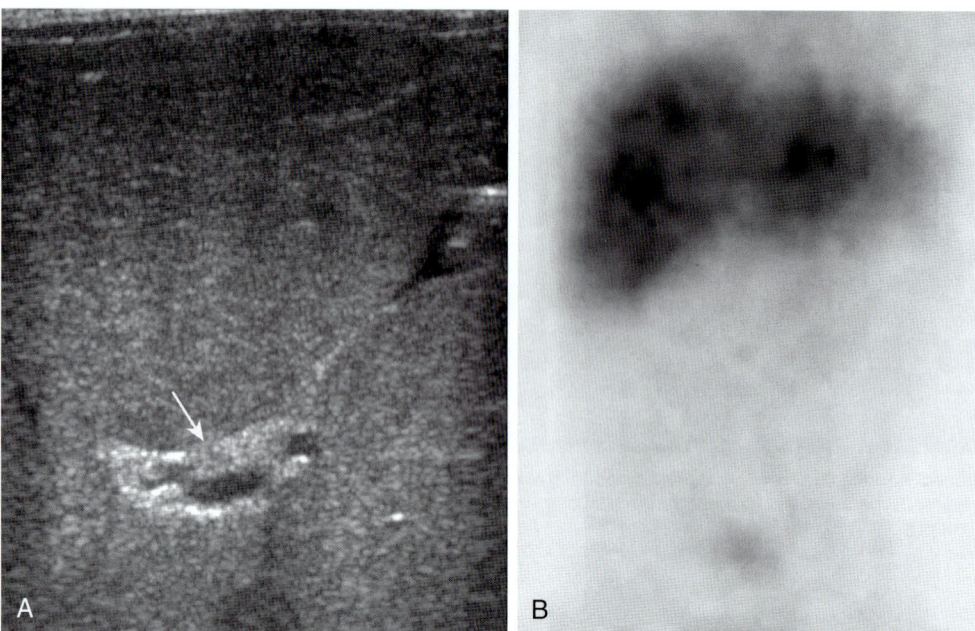

Figure 88-13 Biliary atresia in a 2-month-old boy with persistent jaundice. **A,** A transverse image at the porta hepatis shows increased echogenicity along the expected course of the common bile duct and common hepatic ducts (*arrow*). A small (9 mm) gallbladder was present (not shown). **B,** A delayed image from a technetium-99m–labeled hepatoiminodiacetic acid shows normal radiotracer uptake in the liver but lack of excretion into the biliary tree. This finding persisted on all images.

With severe inflammation, bile ducts are obliterated and BA develops. Less severe inflammatory cholangiopathy does not cause duct obliteration, and thus hepatitis ensues. Distinguishing between BA and hepatitis is important to determine therapy.[29]

Clinical Presentation BA usually presents in the first month of life with jaundice, light-colored stools, and direct hyperbilirubinemia.[2] If untreated, BA progresses to end-stage liver disease and death within the first 3 years of life.[28]

Imaging Ultrasound is the initial study for neonatal jaundice; it is used to exclude surgical lesions such as choledochal cysts. Key findings in children with BA include an absent or small gallbladder (<15 mm) and the presence of a triangular cord sign (>4 mm echogenic tissue at the porta hepatitis following the portal veins) (Fig. 88-13, *A*).[30] Identification of a triangular cord sign has been cited as 96% accurate for a diagnosis of BA. A small (measuring <15 mm) or absent gallbladder has been cited as 73% accurate for a diagnosis of BA compared with neonatal hepatitis; 90% of infants with neonatal hepatitis have a normal gallbladder.[31] Accuracy can be improved to 98% when ultrasound findings are combined.[32,33]

Biliary scintigraphy with technetium-99m iminodiacetic acid and phenobarbital pretreatment has been used to distinguish BA and neonatal hepatitis (Fig. 88-13, *B*). A study without excretion is difficult to interpret, but if excretion of a radiopharmaceutical agent into the bowel occurs, BA is excluded.[34,35] Postoperative use of nuclear scintigraphy has been advocated to assess restoration of biliary drainage after the portoenterostomy (Kasai) procedure.[36] MRCP may be useful in infants to further delineate biliary tree anatomy before surgery and after ultrasound.[3] ERCP typically is performed only when percutaneous intervention is needed.

Despite all of the aforementioned imaging techniques, making a definitive diagnosis of BA can be challenging. In some cases, even a biopsy is nondiagnostic, and diagnosis is confirmed via an intraoperative cholangiogram.[37,38]

Treatment BA is managed surgically with the Kasai procedure (hepatic portoenterostomy),[39] and neonatal hepatitis is managed medically. It is important to diagnose BA early because infants younger than 3 months who are treated with the Kasai procedure tend to have a good long-term prognosis compared with infants older than 3 months, who often require liver transplantation.[33]

Key Points

Fibropolycystic liver diseases, including biliary hamartomas, hepatic fibrosis, cystic liver disease, choledochal cysts, and Caroli disease (or Caroli intrahepatic ductal ectasia), are disorders that occur as a result of faulty development of the embryonic ductal plates.

Caroli disease (intrahepatic ductal ectasia) may be associated with choledochal cysts, hepatic fibrosis (Caroli syndrome), and renal disorders, including autosomal recessive polycystic kidney disease, medullary sponge kidney, and nephronophthisis.

The central dot sign seen on cross-sectional imaging, which occurs as a result of patulous bile ducts surrounding the portal veins, is diagnostic of Caroli intrahepatic ductal ectasia.

In utero biliary ductal inflammation causes a spectrum of cholangiopathy injury ranging from mild, self-limited hepatitis up to complete ductal obliteration and BA.

Ultrasound diagnosis of BA is 98% accurate when using a combination of the triangular cord sign and gallbladder size of less than 15 mm, which individually are 96% and 73% accurate, respectively.

Suggested Readings

Lowe LH. Imaging hepatobiliary disease in children. *Semin Roentgenol.* 2008;43:39-49.

Veigel MC, Prescott-Focht J, Rodriguez MG, et al. Fibropolycystic liver disease in children. *Pediatr Radiol.* 2009;39:317-327.

References

Full references for this chapter can be found on www.expertconsult.com.

Chapter 89

Acquired Biliary Tract Disease

BRENTON D. READING and LISA H. LOWE

Cholelithiasis and Choledocholithiasis

Overview Although in the past cholelithiasis was believed to be rare in children without hemolytic anemia, it is being diagnosed more frequently as a result of increased utilization of sonography. In fact, the sonographic finding of gallstones has been reported in fetuses, although most of these gallstones resolve spontaneously.[1]

Etiology Development of gallstones in infants may be related to immature physiologic regulation of bile salt secretion. Chronic cholestasis likely plays a role in the pathophysiology of cholelithiasis. Although gallstones in infants often are discovered incidentally, many predisposing conditions have been described (Box 89-1). Gallstones in infants resolve spontaneously less often than in fetuses. Further, stones in infants are rarely complicated by biliary tract perforation and peritonitis.[2]

Although most of the stones seen in older children are idiopathic, a number of underlying states have been associated with gallstones (Box 89-2). Prominent among these states are sickle cell disease and intestinal problems that interfere with normal enterohepatic circulation.[3] Patients with sickle cell disease and other hemolytic anemias have an increased incidence of gallstones with advancing age. Gallstones also have been reported after surgery and antibiotic therapy.[4]

Clinical Presentation Cholelithiasis usually is asymptomatic in infants and young children, with an increased incidence of symptoms in older children. When symptoms occur in older children and adolescents, they are similar to those seen in adults and include bloating, nausea, vomiting, and postprandial right upper quadrant colicky pain radiating to the shoulder. In younger children the presentation may be nonspecific (such as irritability), because young children may not be able to verbalize or relate their discomfort to the right upper quadrant or to a recent meal.[5]

Choledocholithiasis results from migration of stones from the gallbladder into the common duct. Stones are more likely to be symptomatic when they pass into the cystic duct or the common bile duct. The most common complication of gallstones in children is pancreatitis,[5] although the most common cause of pancreatitis is idiopathic or posttraumatic.[6]

Imaging Although radiolucent cholesterol stones are the most common type overall, they are rare in children, and thus the majority of pediatric gallstones are visible radiographically. Even so, sonography remains the primary imaging modality for the evaluation of cholelithiasis (Fig. 89-1). Three main sonographic criteria are used to diagnose gallstones: (1) echogenic focus, (2) acoustic shadowing, and (3) gravitational dependence. Most stones move with change in patient position, which should be a routine maneuver during hepatobiliary sonography (Fig. 89-2). Four general sonographic patterns of cholelithiasis are described. The first pattern includes the simple echogenic, shadowing, mobile stone, which may be single or multiple. The second pattern of cholelithiasis describes collections of very tiny, sandlike stones, termed *milk of calcium,* which may mimic gallbladder sludge; acoustic shadowing may be seen only in the aggregate (see Fig. 89-2).[7] Occasionally, if bile within the gallbladder is of high density, the stones may seem to float on the surface, giving an apparent fluid-fluid level. The last sonographic pattern of cholelithiasis relates to stones within a contracted gallbladder, in which case the stones produce an echogenic double arc known as the wall echo shadow (WES) complex. This pattern may be seen in patients with a chronically contracted gallbladder or those who have not fasted sufficiently (Fig. 89-3). Careful scrutiny must be used so as not to confuse the WES complex with emphysematous cholecystitis (air in the gallbladder wall), which is far more common in adults than in children.[8]

Sonography is less successful at revealing choledocholithiasis than it is at detecting cholelithiasis because of interference from gas in adjacent bowel. Therefore dilated extrahepatic bile ducts (Fig. 89-4) may be the only sonographic sign of a more distal obstructing stone. Computed tomography (CT) scans[9] might be obtained in children with biliary stones if other abdominal processes initially are clinically suspected. CT is inferior to sonography with regard to revealing the actual stone, but it readily demonstrates biliary dilation.[6] If no stone is seen on sonography yet evidence exists of biliary ductal dilation, magnetic resonance cholangiopancreatography (MRCP) may be helpful. With MRCP, stones are seen as low signal intensity filling defects within the gallbladder and the biliary tree (Figs. 89-5 and 89-6).[10]

Treatment and Follow-up Treatment of infantile gallstones generally is conservative and includes addressing the underlying cause of disease. Surgery, often laparoscopic, is the usual treatment of choice for symptomatic patients and patients with choledocholithiasis.[11]

Biliary Sludge

Overview The clinical significance of biliary sludge, which is particulate matter within the bile produced by cholestasis, is debated. Although most biliary sludge is a transient finding, particularly if it is associated with a transient predisposing condition, it may evolve into gallstones.[12]

Etiology Sludge is formed predominantly of calcium bilirubinate particles and, depending on the underlying process,

cholesterol crystals. Predisposing conditions that share the common pathway of biliary stasis include biliary outflow obstruction, intravenous hyperalimentation, hemolysis, and prolonged fasting.[13]

Clinical Presentation Biliary sludge usually is asymptomatic; however, it may cause symptoms, particularly if it is associated with microlithiasis or if "bile balls" migrate into the biliary ducts. When this migration happens, symptoms occur that are similar to those seen in patients with cholelithiasis.[12]

Imaging On sonography, sludge is echogenic without acoustic shadowing; it typically layers in the dependent portion of the gallbladder or other part of the biliary tree (such as a choledochal cyst) and demonstrates a fluid-sludge level (Fig. 89-7). Occasionally sludge coalesces within the gallbladder lumen, forming a tumefactive "sludge ball" that, when fixed, may mimic a polyp or mass.[8] Differential considerations include uncommon conditions such as hemobilia, biliary mucus, and parasitic infection.

Treatment and Follow-up Because biliary sludge generally is asymptomatic and resolves spontaneously with resolution of the underlying condition, it does not require separate treatment. However, follow-up in patients in whom the underlying condition does not remit is important to assess for resolution or evolution, particularly if the patient becomes symptomatic.[12]

Acute Cholecystitis

Overview Acute cholecystitis is uncommon in infants and children compared with adults. However, the mortality rate is at least 30% because of concomitant disease and the potential for rapid progression, with gallbladder gangrene occurring in more than 50% of cases and perforation in more than 10% of cases.[14]

Etiology Cholecystitis develops in a small percentage of children with cholelithiasis, and acute acalculous cholecystitis represents 50% to 70% of all cases of cholecystitis in children.[15] In most cases, the pathophysiology of acute cholecystitis involves obstruction of the cystic duct, which leads to gallbladder distention, followed successively by edema, ischemia, mural necrosis, and, in severe cases, perforation. The pathophysiology of acalculous cholecystitis is thought to

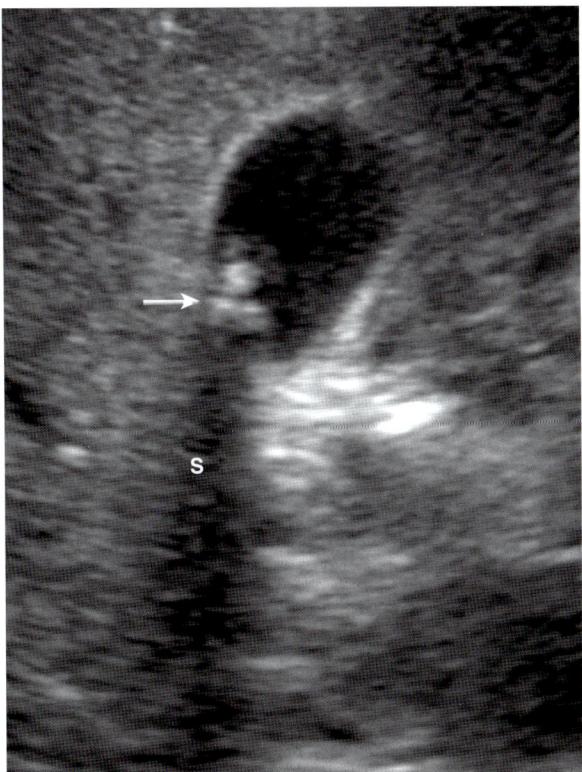

Figure 89-1 Cholelithiasis in a 17-year-old girl with abdominal pain. A transverse sonogram of the gallbladder shows cholelithiasis (*arrow*) with associated posterior acoustic shadowing (*S*).

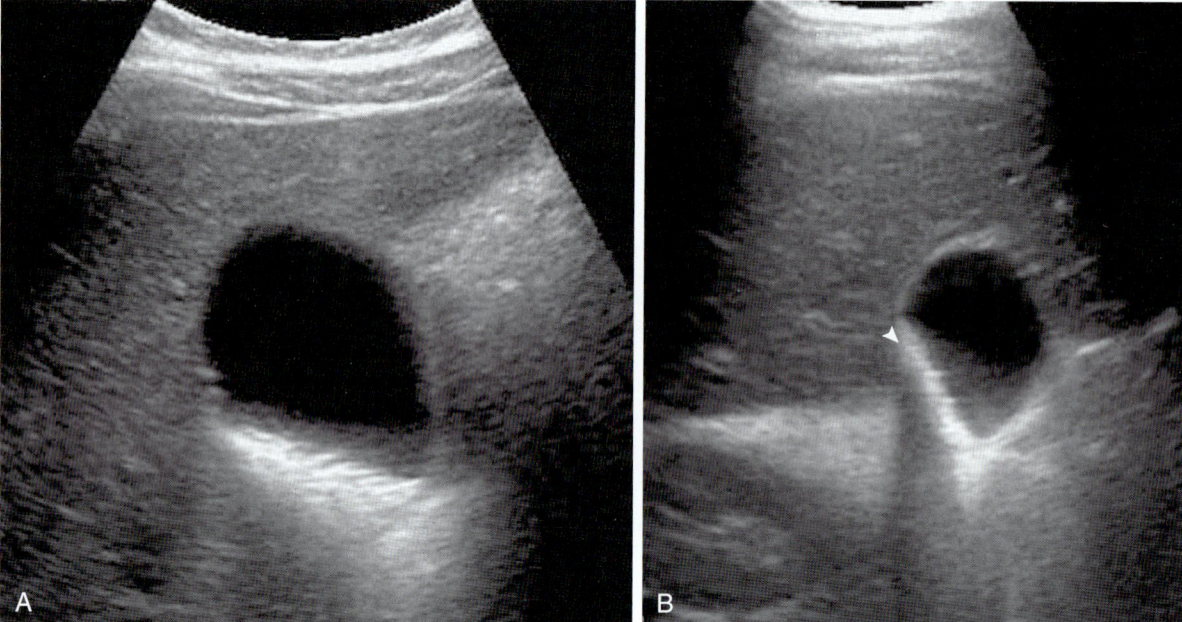

Figure 89-2   Cholelithiasis in a 16-year-old girl with right upper quadrant pain. Transverse sonograms in the supine (**A**) and decubitus (**B**) positions reveal echogenic layering of tiny stones. Note the change in stones with change in patient position, as well as diffuse shadowing of the stone aggregate (*arrowhead* in **B**).

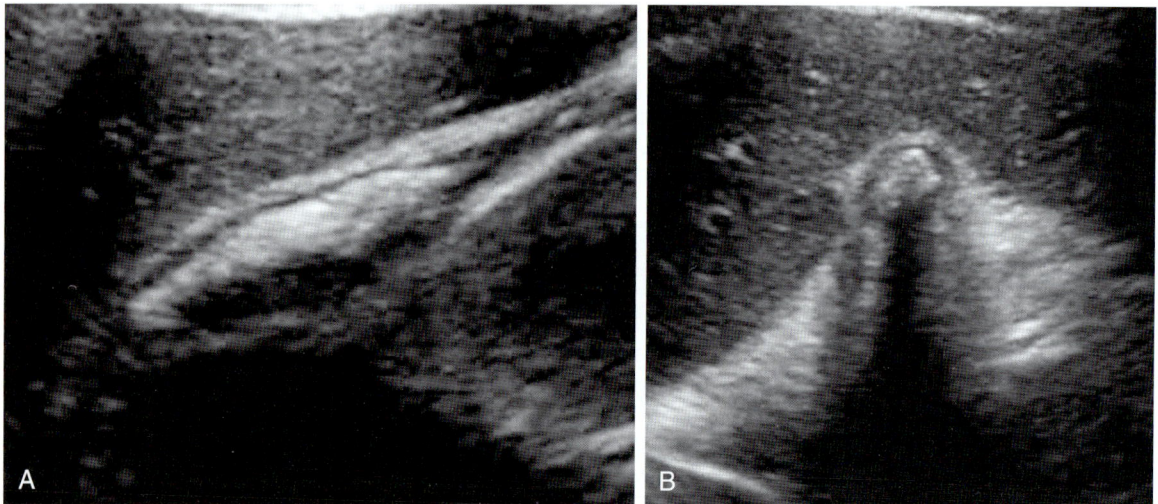

Figure 89-3   Cholelithiasis in a 16-year-old girl with abdominal pain. Longitudinal (**A**) and transverse (**B**) sonograms performed without fasting show the anterior gallbladder wall and multiple echogenic stones with posterior acoustic shadowing (wall-echo-shadow triad).

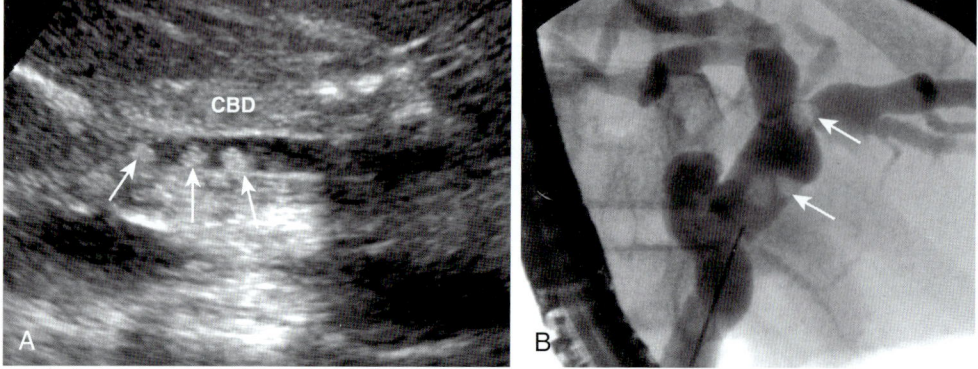

Figure 89-4   Choledocholithiasis in a 15-year-old girl with sickle cell disease and abdominal pain. **A,** Sonogram of the common bile duct (*CBD*) reveals three stones (*arrows*). **B,** Subsequent endoscopic retrograde cholangiopancreatography shows dilated bile ducts and intraluminal filling defects (*arrows*).

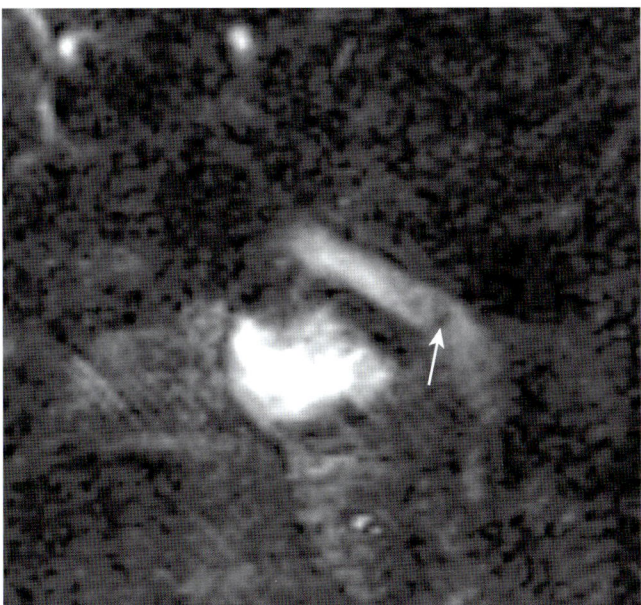

Figure 89-5 Choledocholithiasis in a 17-year-old boy with Duchenne muscular dystrophy and jaundice. Three-dimensional reformatted T2-weighted sequences from a magnetic resonance cholangiopancreatogram show a filling defect consistent with a stone (*arrow*) in the distal common bile duct. A small stone was removed at subsequent endoscopic retrograde cholangiopancreatography.

involve biliary stasis, dehydration, gallbladder ischemia, and elevated ampullary pressures as contributing factors.[14] In neonates with acute cholecystitis, the diagnosis may not be suspected, leading to a high mortality rate.

Clinical Presentation Making a diagnosis in cases of acalculous cholecystitis can be difficult. The condition is most dangerous when it occurs during a serious illness, and the development of symptoms and laboratory abnormalities (such as fever and leukocytosis) initially may be masked by the underlying condition. Patients who may experience acalculous cholecystitis include those with septicemia, postoperative patients, and patients who have sustained severe trauma or burns. Systemic infection may be more common in pediatric patients. Symptoms include jaundice, nausea, vomiting, and tenderness to palpation.[12,14-16]

Imaging Urgent imaging of possible acute cholecystitis is useful for rendering a diagnosis, determining the severity of disease, and discovering other potential causes of abdominal pain. Sonography is the initial imaging modality of choice, particularly to evaluate for gallstones and biliary obstruction.

The sonographic findings of calculous and acalculous cholecystitis are identical except for the lack of gallstones in the latter condition. Sonographic findings of cholecystitis when viewed individually are nonspecific, but when combined they may indicate a specific diagnosis. The best indicators of acute cholecystitis include cholelithiasis, a sonographic Murphy sign (tenderness when the gallbladder is compressed), and gallbladder wall edema with wall thickening greater than 3.5 mm (Fig. 89-8).[14,17] Intramural edema related to acute cholecystitis is usually striated, with multiple interrupted bands of hypoechogenicity. This appearance also has been associated with gangrenous cholecystitis. The interrupted layers of intramural edema seen with acute cholecystitis should not be confused with homogeneous gallbladder wall thickening, a common nonspecific finding seen in a variety of disorders such as ascites, hypoalbuminemia, congestive heart failure, hepatitis, portal hypertension, and gallbladder wall varices. Other sonographic findings of acute cholecystitis include gallbladder distention, pericholecystic fluid (especially with perforation), adjacent rim of hypoechogenicity or hypervascularity in the liver, biliary sludge, and, rarely, dirty shadowing as a result of air-producing infection (found most often in adults with diabetes). CT is not the modality of choice in most pediatric patients with cholecystitis, but if it is performed for other reasons, it shows similar findings (Fig. 89-9).

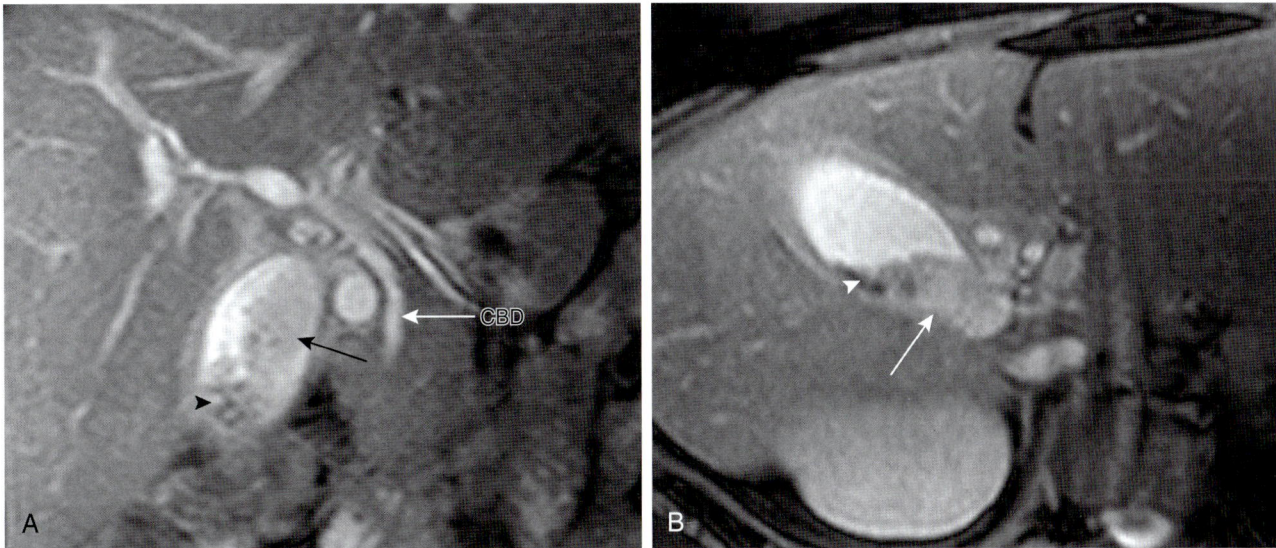

Figure 89-6 Cholelithiasis in a 12-year-old girl with abdominal pain. Coronal (**A**) and axial T2-weighted (**B**) magnetic resonance images reveal low signal intensity gallstones (*arrowheads*) and isointense sludge (*arrows*) within the gallbladder lumen. Note the normal common bile duct (*CBD*) (*long white arrow* in **A**).

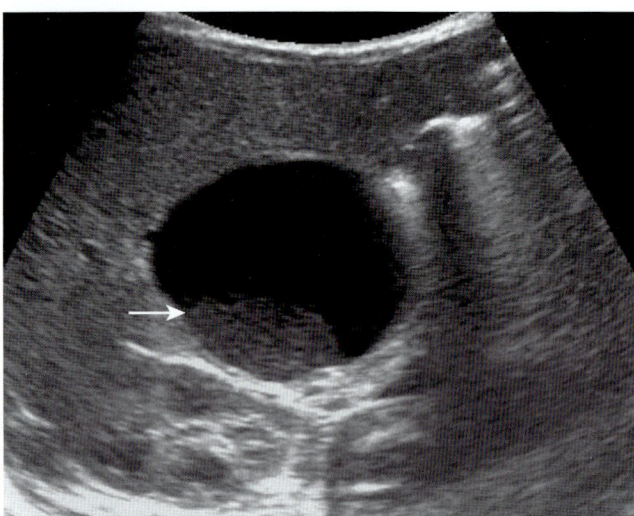

Figure 89-7 Biliary sludge in a 1-year-old boy with a choledochal cyst. A transverse sonogram shows layering echogenic material within the cyst; its echogenicity, which is less than that of a stone, and lack of shadowing distinguish it from a calculus.

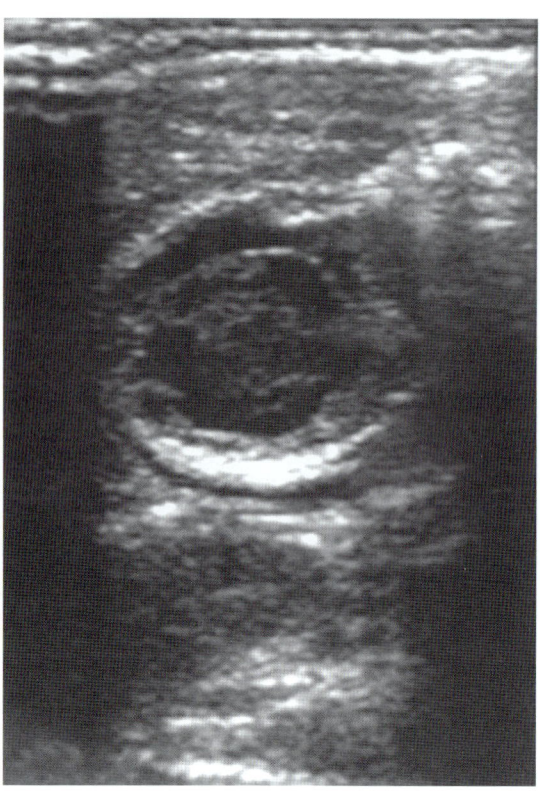

Figure 89-8 Acute cholecystitis in a 15-year-old girl with a history of cholelithiasis. A transverse sonogram through the gallbladder reveals a markedly thickened and edematous gallbladder wall with echogenic material in the lumen. The patient had a history of chronic, recurrent abdominal pain.

Hepatobiliary scintigraphy with technetium-99m–labeled iminodiacetic acid derivative is highly sensitive for the diagnosis of acute cholecystitis in adults and children. Normally, the gallbladder is opacified with a radiopharmaceutical agent in the first 30 minutes of the study or in the first hour with slow injection of intravenous morphine (which increases pressure in the sphincter of Oddi). However, with acute cholecystitis, gallbladder opacification does not occur. Occasionally a rim of increased activity is seen in the liver surrounding the gallbladder (the rim sign), and peritoneal activity may be seen with perforation (Fig. 89-10).[18]

Treatment and Follow-up Treatment for acute acalculous cholecystitis may differ depending on the patient's clinical status and underlying conditions. Children may be treated medically and observed prior to surgery.[16,19] Percutaneous cholecystostomy is increasingly a lifesaving, minimally invasive alternative. Gallbladder perforation is a surgical emergency that occurs in 3% to 15% of patients with acute cholecystitis.[20]

Cholangitis

Overview Cholangitis, or ascending cholangitis, refers to biliary duct obstruction with associated biliary infection. Primary sclerosing cholangitis (PSC) is a noninfectious idiopathic obliterative inflammatory fibrosis of the biliary tree.

Etiology Causes of ascending cholangitis are numerous and range from neoplasms (benign and malignant) to infection (suppurative, nonsuppurative, and human immunodeficiency virus) to autoimmune or chemotherapy-induced disorders.

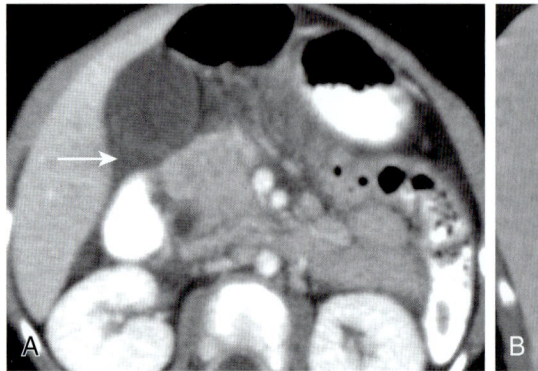
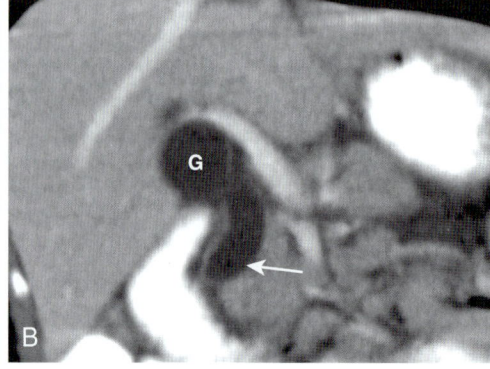

Figure 89-9 Cholecystitis and ascending cholangitis in a 25-month-old boy with subsequent confirmed passage of a gallstone. **A,** Axial image from a contrast-enhanced computed tomography scan of the abdomen demonstrates pericholecystic edema (*arrow*) on the axial image. **B,** A coronal reformatted image demonstrates a distended gallbladder (*G*) and dilation of the common bile duct (*arrow*).

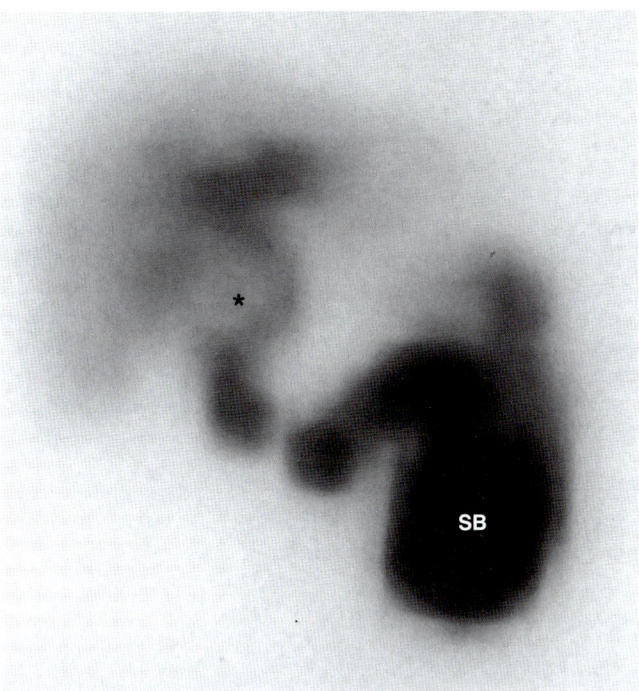

Figure 89-10 Acute cholecystitis in a 15-year-old girl with a history of cholelithiasis (same patient as in Fig. 89-8). A 4-hour image from a biliary patency scan shows hepatic uptake and excretion of technetium-99m–labeled iminodiacetic acid into the biliary tree and small bowel (*SB*) without gallbladder (*asterisk*) opacification. A halo of increased activity known as the rim sign surrounds the gallbladder fossa indicating hyperemia.

Appropriate therapy is directed toward relief of the underlying cause of obstruction, whether congenital or acquired.

The features of PSC suggest an autoimmune mechanism, but the pathophysiology of tissue damage has not been definitively determined. Associated disorders include inflammatory bowel disease, in particular ulcerative colitis (47%), idiopathic causes (24%), Langerhans cell histiocytosis (15%), and other immune system disorders (10%).[21] PSC also has been associated with cystic fibrosis.

The differential diagnosis of cholangitis includes sclerosing biliary cholangiocarcinoma, which is rare in children.

Clinical Presentation Boys are affected more often than girls and typically present in the second decade of life. Presentation is with jaundice, abdominal pain, and hepatomegaly. Alkaline phosphatase levels may be within normal limits. As many as 81% of patients may have underlying irritable bowel disease, possibly subclinical.[22]

Imaging With use of sonography, nonspecific dilation of the biliary system, hyperechoic portal triads, portal casts, thickened gallbladder wall, and cholelithiasis may be identified in persons with PSC. CT findings include focal dilation of the biliary tree and contrast enhancement of the bile duct walls caused by inflammatory changes. Magnetic resonance imaging may reveal peripheral wedge–shaped areas of high T2 signal in association with dilated bile ducts. T1 and T2 shortening along the periportal triads as a result of inflammation also may be detected. Key findings on cholangiopancreatography include multifocal stricture of the biliary tree with alternating areas of dilation, forming a classic "string of beads" appearance. Additional findings include the pruned-tree pattern (dilation limited to central ducts), cobblestone appearance (coarse mural irregularities), and pseudodiverticula (Fig. 89-11). MRCP has been found to be 84% sensitive and accurate in the diagnosis of PSC.[23]

Although cholangitis occasionally is segmental, the entire biliary tract usually is involved and intrahepatic biliary duct involvement is seen in 100% of cases, whereas the extrahepatic ducts are involved in 60% of cases.[24] The gallbladder is rarely involved.

Treatment and Follow-up Complications of sclerosing cholangitis include portal hypertension, biliary cirrhosis, secondary cholangitis, and cholangiocarcinoma. Treatment is aimed at palliation and may include medical therapy (such as ursodeoxycholic acid to promote bile flow), interventional dilation of strictures, and drainage of infected obstructed ducts. The median reported time for liver transplantation is approximately 12.7 years from initial diagnosis.[22,25]

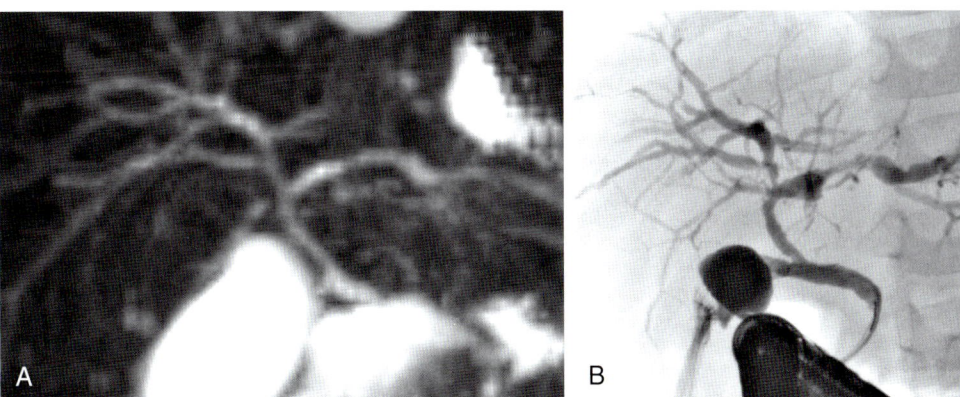

Figure 89-11 Sclerosing cholangitis in an adolescent boy with ulcerative colitis. **A,** Magnetic resonance cholangiopancreatography demonstrates irregularity, narrowing, and ductal beading throughout the biliary system. **B,** Endoscopic retrograde cholangiopancreatography in another patient demonstrates areas of abnormal biliary ductal dilation and strictures throughout the biliary duct system consistent with sclerosing cholangitis. (**A,** Courtesy Dr. Marta Hernanz-Schulman, MD, Nashville, TN.)

Box 89-3 Causes of Hydrops of the Gallbladder

Mucocutaneous lymph node syndrome (Kawasaki disease)
Obstruction
Familial Mediterranean fever
Scarlet fever
Leptospirosis
Ascariasis
Typhoid fever
Sepsis
Total parenteral nutrition

Hydrops of the Gallbladder

Overview Gallbladder hydrops is a rare cause of a right upper quadrant mass in children.

Etiology Gallbladder hydrops is thought to be related to transient cholestasis and obstruction of the biliary tree and usually is associated with preceding infectious disorders elsewhere in the body (Box 89-3), most notably mucocutaneous lymph node syndrome (Kawasaki disease) and parenteral hyperalimentation.

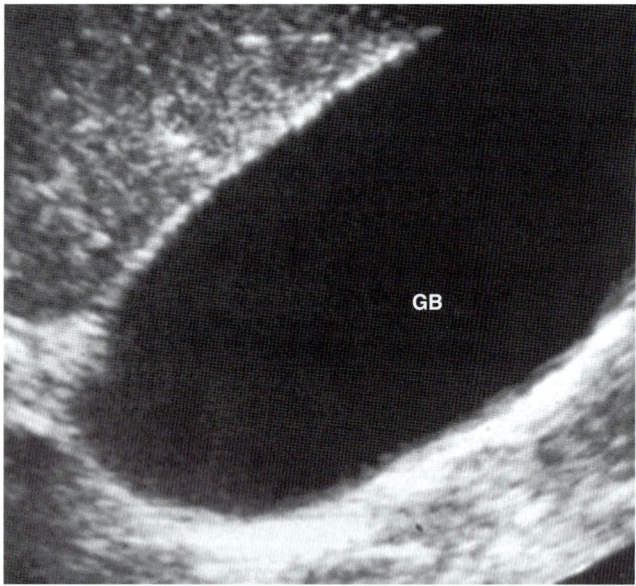

Figure 89-12 Hydrops of the gallbladder in a child with Kawasaki disease. A longitudinal sonogram shows a markedly enlarged, balloon-shaped gallbladder (*GB*). Hydrops resolved spontaneously as the patient's condition improved.

Clinical Presentation Hydrops of the gallbladder is more frequent in boys and usually presents in children ages 17 months to 7 years. Presentation may include jaundice, abdominal pain, right upper quadrant tenderness, vomiting, or a palpable mass.[26]

Imaging Sonography is the modality of choice in patients suspected of gallbladder hydrops. The findings consist of gallbladder dilation without gallbladder wall thickening. The gallbladder may resemble a balloon in which normal contours are lost (Fig. 89-12). A normal gallbladder length is 1.5 to 3 cm in infants (<1 year old) and 3 to 7 cm in older children.[27] Sludge is seen in some cases, and the biliary tree is otherwise normal. Serial sonographic studies may demonstrate resolution.[28]

Treatment and Follow-up Hydrops generally responds to conservative therapy, although gallbladder perforation has been reported in persons with Kawasaki disease.[29]

Key Points

Sonographic criteria for the diagnosis of cholelithiasis include an intraluminal echogenic focus in the gallbladder with acoustic shadowing and gravitational dependence.

Although acute calculous and acalculous cholecystitis cases are rare in children compared with adults, the mortality rate in children is higher because of frequent and rapid progression to gangrene and perforation.

Findings of sclerosing cholangitis on MRCP include multifocal biliary tree strictures alternating with ductal distension, forming a string-of-beads appearance; prominent opacification of central ducts, causing a pruned-tree appearance; cobblestone mucosal irregularity; and pseudodiverticula.

Suggested Readings

Albuquerque PA, Morales Ramos DA, Faingold R. Magnetic resonance imaging of the liver and biliary tree in children. *Curr Probl Diagn Radiol.* 2009;38(3):126-134.
Anupindi SA. Pancreatic and biliary anomalies: imaging in 2008. *Pediatr Radiol.* 2008;38(suppl 2):S267-S271.
Lowe LH. Hepatobiliary disease in children. *Semin Roentgenol.* 2008; 43(1):39-49.

References

Full references for this chapter can be found on www.expertconsult.com.

Chapter 90

Parenchymal Liver Disease

ADAM ZARCHAN, KRISTIN FICKENSCHER, and LISA H. LOWE

Hepatic Steatosis

Overview Hepatic steatosis (fatty liver) is the most common cause of chronic liver disease in pediatric patients. It can range from simple steatosis to nonalcoholic steatohepatitis, which can progress to cirrhosis. Obesity and insulin resistance are the most common risk factors for hepatic steatosis, but it also may be associated with a number of metabolic processes and toxins (Box 90-1). The incidence is 2.6% in the general population, with a higher percentage in obese children.[1] Adolescents are affected more often than younger children, with a higher prevalence in boys than girls. Fatty replacement of the liver may be diffuse or localized with areas of fatty sparing.

Clinical Presentation Hepatic steatosis often is asymptomatic and is found incidentally on imaging performed for other reasons, such as nonspecific abdominal pain. Laboratory studies may show elevated liver enzymes (i.e., alanine aminotransferase and aspartate aminotransferase).[1] Histologically, hepatocytes contain large cytoplasmic fat vacuoles filled with triglycerides. Pathologic diagnosis of hepatic steatosis is made when more than 5% of the total liver weight is replaced by fat.[2]

Imaging Ultrasound evidence of hepatic steatosis includes variable hepatomegaly, increased echogenicity of the liver parenchyma when compared with the adjacent kidney, and poor visualization of the intrahepatic vascular structures (Fig. 90-1).[2] Areas of fatty sparing are seen as hypoechoic foci within the fatty liver without mass effect and should not be mistaken for a mass. Ultrasound sensitivity for steatosis decreases with lower degrees of fatty infiltration. Increased obesity of the patient limits ultrasound quality because the increased extrahepatic fat further attenuates the ultrasound beam and decreases ultrasound sensitivity for liver abnormalities, including steatosis.

On computed tomography (CT), liver minus spleen attenuation of less than 1 Hounsfield unit (HU) can be used to screen for mild hepatic steatosis.[3,4] Moderate to severe cases are indicated by liver minus spleen attenuation of less than -10 HU or absolute hepatic parenchymal attenuation less than 40 HU on noncontrast CT.[4]

Conventional spin-echo magnetic resonance imaging (MRI) is less sensitive than CT and ultrasound for detection of steatosis. Imaging findings include increased signal intensity on T1-weighted images and decreased signal intensity on fat-saturated and short tau inversion recovery sequences. However, chemical shift imaging with in-phase and out-of-phase sequences that demonstrates loss of signal on out-of-phase images is highly specific for diagnosing hepatic steatosis.[2] This modality can be particularly helpful in differentiating this condition from neoplastic disease in equivocal cases, particularly in cases with focal fatty infiltration or sparing.

MR spectroscopy is a more recently described technique that may prove to be the most accurate method to quantitatively assess hepatic steatosis noninvasively. The area under the water and lipid peaks can be measured, allowing estimation of the hepatic fat fraction with a diagnostic accuracy of 80% to 85% in adult studies.[2,5,6]

The gold standard for diagnosis is biopsy and histologic evaluation. However, this approach is not without risk and is impractical in most pediatric patients with suspected hepatic steatosis.

Treatment Treatment focuses on reduction of obesity and insulin resistance with diet and exercise. The use of medications targeted at insulin resistance, such as metformin, is being investigated in the treatment of children with hepatic steatosis.[2,5]

Iron Deposition in the Liver

Overview Approximately 80% of the normal iron stores of 2 to 6 g are in the form of hemoglobin, myoglobin, and enzymes that contain iron, and 20% are in the storage form of ferritin and hemosiderin. In normal situations, trace levels of iron are found in the liver, spleen, and bone marrow. When excess iron is present in the body, deposition may occur in the liver, spleen, lymph nodes, pancreas, kidneys, pituitary, and gastrointestinal (GI) tract. The body can compensate for some excess iron (10 to 20 g) without the occurrence of tissue damage, in which case the term *hemosiderosis* is applied. However, if functional and structural impairment of organs occurs as a result of excess iron (50 to 60 g), the term *hemochromatosis* is applied.

Two forms of hemochromatosis exist: primary and secondary. The primary form is the result of a genetic disorder that causes excess iron absorption through the gastrointestinal tract. This iron becomes bound to transferrin and eventually is stored as crystalline iron oxide within the cytoplasm of periportal hepatocytes. With progressive disease, the pancreas,

Box 90-1 Causes of Hepatic Steatosis

Metabolic and Genetic Disorders
- Obesity
- Extreme malnutrition
- Total parenteral nutrition
- Cystic fibrosis

Steroids (Exogenous and Endogenous; e.g., Cushing Syndrome)
- Familial hyperlipoproteinemia
- Glycogen storage disease
- Wilson disease
- Galactosemia
- Reye syndrome
- Severe hepatitis
- Poorly controlled diabetes mellitus
- Chronic tuberculosis
- Chronic congestive heart failure

Hepatotoxins (Mostly Adults)
- Alcohol
- Chemotherapy
- Carbon toxins
- Phosphorus
- Amiodarone

synovium, heart, pituitary, and thyroid may be involved, but the Kupffer cells and reticuloendothelial cells of the bone marrow and spleen are spared.

The secondary, nongenetic form of hemochromatosis is more common than primary disease and may be the result of a myelodysplastic syndrome, anemia as a result of ineffective erythropoiesis, or exogenous sources from multiple transfusions, parenteral iron infusion, or ingestion. With secondary hemochromatosis, phagocytosis of intact red blood cells

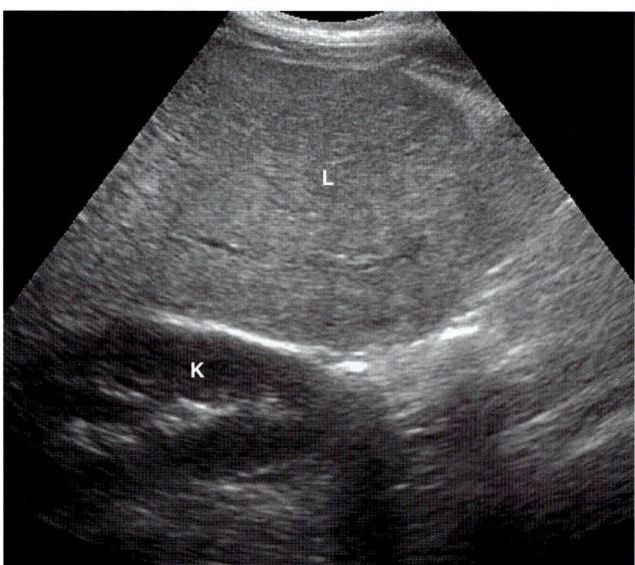

Figure 90-1 Glycogen storage disease in a 17-year-old girl. Longitudinal ultrasound image of the right hepatic lobe demonstrates diffuse increased echogenicity of the liver (*L*) parenchyma compared with the adjacent kidney (*K*). Also notice poorly defined portal triads.

causes initial iron deposition within the reticuloendothelial system (i.e., the liver, spleen, and bone marrow). Once the storage capacity of the reticuloendothelial system is saturated, iron may accumulate within parenchymal cells of the organs, including the liver hepatocytes, pancreas, and myocardium, in a pattern similar to that of primary hemochromatosis.

Clinical Presentation Patients with primary hemochromatosis usually become symptomatic in the second decade of life. Symptoms are related to organ injury from excess iron deposition and may include hyperpigmentation, hepatomegaly, arthralgia, diabetes as a result of pancreatic beta cell damage, congestive heart failure, and arrhythmia. Various other complications due to chronic hemochromatosis include periportal fibrosis, cirrhosis, and hepatocellular carcinoma. However, with early diagnosis and treatment, patients may have a normal life expectancy.[7] A neonatal form of primary hemochromatosis exists in which newborns (often younger than 12 hours old) present with fulminant hepatic failure, along with pancreatic and cardiac involvement.

Imaging Ultrasound findings are nonspecific and noncontributory to the diagnosis of hemochromatosis. CT has a low sensitivity (63%) but high specificity (96%) for the diagnosis of iron overload.[8] Noncontrast CT shows homogeneous increased density of the liver greater than 72 HU.[8] However, coincident steatosis can lower the HU number, causing false-negative examinations. False-positive results may be seen with Wilson disease, gold therapy, or long-standing amiodarone treatment.

MR is the imaging modality of choice for confirming the diagnosis, determining severity, and monitoring therapy in persons with hemochromatosis. Excess iron deposition causes a proportional decrease in signal intensity on T1- and T2-weighted sequences and is most pronounced on gradient echo sequences. Skeletal muscle is unaffected by hemochromatosis and serves as a good internal reference to compare the signal intensity of affected abdominal organs and bone marrow, which will be hypointense to skeletal muscle. On in-phase and out-of-phase imaging, decreased signal intensity is seen in the affected organs on the in-phase sequence (an opposite finding from steatosis). The key findings in primary hemochromatosis are low signal intensity within the liver and pancreas on T2-weighted images (Fig. 90-2). In contradistinction, secondary hemochromatosis demonstrates a low signal in the liver, spleen, and bone marrow (Fig. 90-3) with sparing of the pancreas.[9]

MR quantification of liver iron concentration (LIC) is possible, eliminating the need for multiple biopsies to monitor hemochromatosis. One proposed method uses multiple gradient echo sequences (T1, PD, T2, and T2★). Three regions of interest are placed on the right lobe of the liver and two on skeletal muscle; these values then can be placed in an online algorithm that estimates LIC.[10] A more recently described technique utilizes breath-hold multiecho T2★-weighted sequences and generation of a line plotting the natural log of hepatic signal intensity versus time to echo (TE). The slope of the line is R2★ where $1/R2★ = T2★$. The T2★ values then can be used to stratify different grades of LIC.[11]

Treatment Treatment of hemochromatosis consists of scheduled phlebotomy or chelation therapy to reduce iron levels.[7]

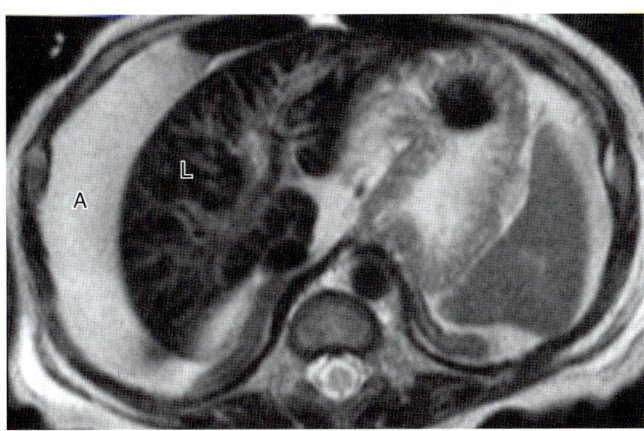

Figure 90-2 Primary hemochromatosis in an infant with multiorgan system failure. Axial T2-weighted magnetic resonance image reveals extensive ascites (A) surrounding a liver (L) of low signal intensity. (Courtesy Lynn Fordham, MD, University of North Carolina–Chapel Hill.)

As mentioned earlier, MR quantification of LIC may be used to follow treatment regimes, obviating the need for liver biopsies.

Glycogen Storage Diseases

Overview Glycogen storage diseases are autosomal recessive disorders that involve the abnormal storage and synthesis of glycogen and the catabolism of glucose. Six major types have been described, including von Gierke (type I), Pompe (type II), Cori (type III), Anderson (type IV), McArdle (type V), and Hers (type VI).[12]

Clinical Presentation von Gierke disease (VGD), which is attributed to glucose-6-phosphatase deficiency, is the most common glycogen storage disease that involves the liver. In

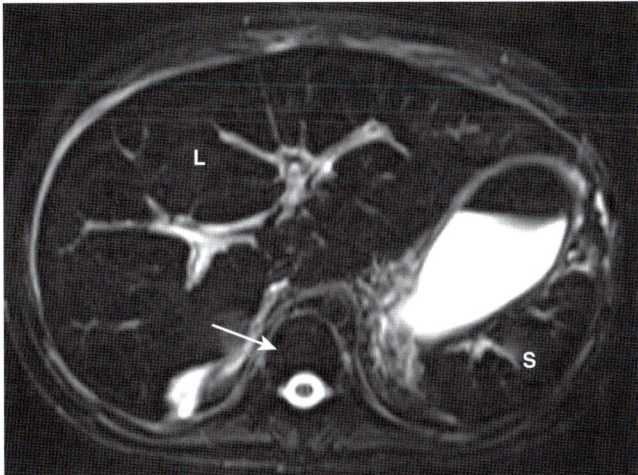

Figure 90-3 Secondary hemosiderosis due to multiple transfusions in a 10-year-old boy with a history of acute myelogenous leukemia. A T2-weighted axial magnetic resonance image shows low signal within the liver (L) and spleen (S) because of iron deposition. Also note low signal intensity of bone marrow (arrow).

VGD, histopathology shows excess intracytoplasmic accumulations of glycogen and small amounts of lipid within hepatocytes and proximal renal tubules. The clinical presentation of VGD includes failure to thrive, hepatomegaly, hypoglycemia, nephromegaly, jaundice, hyperlipidemia, and hyperuricemia.[12] Complications of VGD include hepatocellular carcinoma and hepatic adenomas (in up to 40% of patients), which may be multiple and generally increase in number and size with age.[12,13] Serial screening is required to monitor for neoplasia.

Imaging Sonography shows hepatomegaly with diffuse hepatic hyperechogenicity because of the combination of fatty replacement and glycogen deposition (e-Fig. 90-4).[14,15] Superimposed hepatic adenomas are common. They are seen as well-defined masses with variable echogenicity (depending on the relative change in liver echotexture) and often demonstrate increased sound transmission and refractory shadowing at the margins. Because hepatic attenuation is increased by glycogen but decreased by fat, the CT findings are variable depending on which factor predominates. When fatty replacement predominates, the result is diffusely low attenuation of the liver.[16] Hepatic adenomas likewise vary in appearance depending on the status of the liver; they appear hypodense when found in livers of normal attenuation (e-Fig. 90-5) but are variably hyperdense in the setting of a hepatic steatosis.

Treatment Hepatic adenomas should be followed up with serial imaging to monitor their typical pattern of slow growth. Malignant neoplasia should be suspected in cases of hyperattenuating or rapidly growing liver masses.[13]

Gaucher Disease

Overview Gaucher disease is a rare autosomal-recessive lysosomal storage disorder resulting from a deficiency of β-glucocerebrosidase enzyme. The abnormalities are the result of the accumulation of glucocerebroside in cells of the brain and reticuloendothelial system. The disease occurs worldwide, most commonly in Ashkenazi Jews.[17]

Clinical Presentation Three forms of Gaucher disease exist. Type 1 is the chronic nonneuropathic form and may present in childhood but commonly is recognized in the third to fourth decade. Type 2, the acute neuropathic or infantile form, rapidly leads to death and presents with severe hepatosplenomegaly, progressive seizures, mental retardation, spasticity, strabismus, and, rarely, skeletal manifestations. Type 3, the subacute neuropathic or juvenile form, is the rarest and presents between 2 and 6 years of age with hepatosplenomegaly, mild neurological symptoms, and late-onset skeletal disease.

Bone marrow histopathology reveals Gaucher cells (kerasin-laden histiocytes). Significant replacement of liver parenchyma by Gaucher cells leads to hepatomegaly. The course of the disease includes regenerating nodules and hepatic fibrosis, leading to cirrhosis and portal hypertension.[18] Splenic manifestations include infarcts and focal clusters of glucosylceramide-laden cells. Bone complications as a result of marrow replacement are common, including pathologic fractures, avascular necrosis, and osteomyelitis.

Imaging Ultrasound, CT, and MRI demonstrate findings of hepatomegaly and possible cirrhosis (e-Fig. 90-6, *A*).[16] On sonography, splenic lesions have variable echogenicity. They usually are hypodense on CT before administration of contrast, isointense on T1-weighted MRI, and hyperintense on T2-weighted MRI (e-Fig. 90-6, *B*).[19]

Treatment Treatment of Gaucher disease with enzyme replacement therapy is possible.[18] In general, the degree of liver and spleen enlargement correlates with disease severity. Thus quantification of hepatosplenomegaly (i.e., measurement of liver and spleen volume) has been used to determine treatment response.[20] Liver volume can be measured with sonography, CT, or MRI. The prognosis varies with the type, extent, and severity of disease.

α_1-Antitrypsin Deficiency

Overview α_1-antitrypsin deficiency is a rare autosomal recessive disorder and is the second most common cause of chronic severe pediatric liver disease. The α_1-antitrypsin enzyme normally is produced by the liver, but in this disease the protein is not secreted properly. This situation leads to deficient serum levels of α_1-antitrypsin, as well as buildup of abnormal protein in the hepatocytes, leading to inflammation, fibrosis, and cirrhosis.[21] Associated damage to lung parenchyma is thought to be due to unhindered neutrophil elastase digestion of collagen as a result of the deficiency of this protease inhibitor.

Clinical Presentation Although α_1-antitrypsin presents most commonly in the second decade as a result of lung disease (e.g., panacinar emphysema, bullae, and bronchiectasis), it also can present in the neonatal period with jaundice that mimics biliary atresia.[22] Other symptoms related to the liver include feeding difficulties, failure to thrive, ascites, and elevated liver enzymes. Rarely, children may present with symptoms of cirrhosis.

The diagnosis can be made by measuring the serum α_1-antitrypsin level and is confirmed with a liver biopsy.[21]

Imaging Infants presenting in the first months of life with elevated direct bilirubin levels may undergo scintigraphy with the intention of excluding biliary atresia. In these cases, scintigraphy cannot distinguish biliary atresia from α_1-antitrypsin deficiency because both conditions may show good hepatocyte uptake without biliary excretion as a result of a paucity of intralobular bile ducts in some cases of α_1-antitrypsin deficiency (e-Fig. 90-7).[22] Sonographic correlation may be helpful because infants with α_1-antitrypsin deficiency generally have normal sonographic findings of the liver and gallbladder. Abdominal cross-sectional imaging in older children typically reveals nonspecific findings of cirrhosis.[23]

Treatment No cure exists for α_1-antitrypsin deficiency, and the prognosis is extremely variable depending on disease severity, age at diagnosis, and therapeutic interventions. α_1-antitrypsin deficiency is second only to biliary atresia as an indication for liver transplantation in pediatric patients.[21,22]

Wilson Disease

Overview Wilson disease (hepatolenticular degeneration) is a rare autosomal-recessive disorder of copper metabolism localized to chromosome 13, and in which hepatic excretion of copper into the biliary system does not occur. Normally 95% of copper in the body is bound to the serum protein ceruloplasmin.[24] With copper toxicosis, accumulation begins in the liver, and when its copper binding capacity is reached, the basal ganglia, renal tubules, corneas, bones, joints, and parathyroid glands may be affected.

Clinical Presentation Wilson disease presents most often in children older than 7 years and in young adolescents with hepatic manifestations such as jaundice and hepatomegaly, or acute fulminant hepatitis. Older adolescents and adults with unrecognized, subclinical liver involvement present with a parkinsonian movement disorder (i.e., tremor, rigidity, dysarthria, and dysphagia) or psychosis. Elevated urine copper levels and low ceruloplasmin are the best screening tests for Wilson disease but are not always diagnostic in patients who present with hepatic disease. Serum ceruloplasmin levels are in the low to normal range in 45% of patients with Wilson hepatic disease.[25] A biopsy can be performed as well, in which case hepatic copper content is elevated (>250 µg/g dry weight).[25]

Imaging Hepatic changes are poorly seen with cross-sectional imaging because multiple processes are occurring in the liver simultaneously: copper accumulation, fatty replacement, hepatitis, cirrhosis, and liver necrosis. The liver is hyperechoic on sonography. Copper has a high atomic number, which increases attenuation on CT. However, hepatic attenuation usually remains normal because of concurrent steatosis, which lowers attenuation and thus may negate the hyperattenuation of copper (e-Fig. 90-8).[16] Hepatic MRI early in the course of the disease demonstrates hyperintensity on T1-weighted images and hypointensity on T2-weighted images, but these changes may be overshadowed once cirrhosis supervenes.[16,26,27]

Treatment Early treatment, optimally before the patient is symptomatic, is important, because chelation with penicillamine and zinc is effective in preventing toxic copper deposition in the liver and brain. Treatment of symptomatic patients should result in rapid improvement. Lifelong chelation therapy is required, and severe cases may require liver transplantation.[25]

Cirrhosis

Overview Cirrhosis is the end-stage of chronic liver disease in which parenchymal necrosis, nodular regeneration, and active parenchymal fibrosis distort normal lobular and vascular architecture.

Clinical Presentation In children, cirrhosis is the result of many different disease processes, including biliary, postnecrotic, and metabolic causes (Box 90-2). Cirrhosis

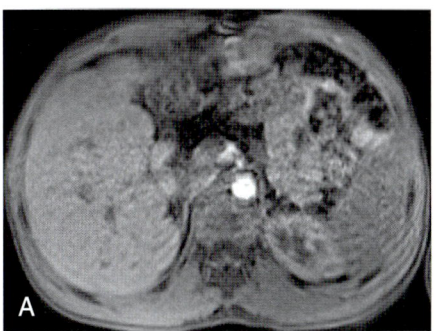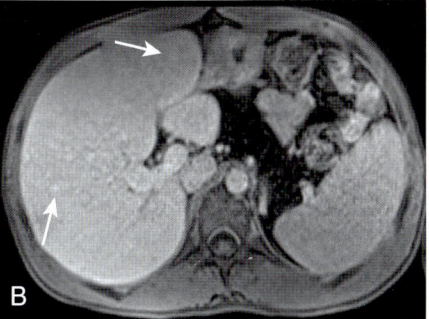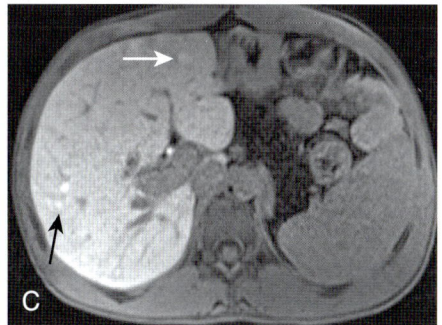

Figure 90-10   Cirrhosis with regenerative or well-differentiated dysplastic nodules in a 17-year-old boy with cystic fibrosis. Postcontrast magnetic resonance images after administration of Eovist (gadoxetate disodium), a hepatobiliary specific contrast agent. **A,** The arterial phase shows nodular contour of the liver with no abnormal enhancement. **B,** The venous phase demonstrates subtle areas of nodular enhancement (*arrows*). **C,** The delayed phase reveals more pronounced areas of nodular enhancement (*arrows*).

traditionally has been classified into three main categories: micronodular (Laënnec), with equal-sized nodules up to 3 mm; macronodular (postnecrotic), with variable-sized nodules ranging from 3 mm to 3 cm; and mixed cirrhosis.[28,29] Micronodular cirrhosis in children is caused by disorders such as biliary obstruction, hemochromatosis, and venous outflow obstruction; macronodular cirrhosis results from disorders such as viral hepatitis, Wilson disease, and α_1-antitrypsin deficiency.

Imaging   The sonographic features of cirrhosis include heterogeneous echogenicity of the liver and hepatic surface irregularity (e-Fig. 90-9, A). Other findings include regenerative nodules that may have relatively decreased echogenicity, a smaller right hepatic lobe, and compensatory enlargement of the caudate lobe and left lateral segment. Findings of portal hypertension often are seen, with collateral vessels and hepatofugal flow in the portal vein on Doppler interrogation.[28,30]

CT shows a small or normal-sized liver with surface nodularity and heterogeneous attenuation that is exaggerated after the administration of contrast material. Decreased attenuation in areas of fatty replacement and normal attenuation in areas of fibrosis and regenerating nodules are common. CT also may demonstrate findings of portal hypertension with development of collateral pathways including coronary to gastroesophageal, paraumbilical, splenorenal, gastrorenal, and hemorrhoidal varices (Fig. 90-9, *B*).[28,30]

Typical findings on MRI include morphologic changes already described on ultrasound and CT. Regenerating nodules typically are hypointense to liver on T2-weighted sequences and variable on T1-weighted sequences. No enhancement occurs on postcontrast arterial phase imaging, although enhancement may occur on delayed images when hepatobiliary-specific agents are used (Fig. 90-10). Dysplastic nodules have variable signal intensity on T1-weighted images. Hypointense signal on T2-weighted images is seen in low-grade dysplastic nodules, and hyperintense signal is present in high-grade dysplastic nodules. On postcontrast imaging, low-grade dysplastic nodules are indistinguishable from regenerating nodules, and high-grade dysplastic nodules are indistinguishable from well-differentiated hepatocellular carcinoma (HCC).[29] HCC complicating cirrhosis is characterized by variable signal on T1-weighted images and a hyperintense signal on T2-weighted images, in addition to arterial enhancement after administration of contrast material and rapid washout during the portal venous phase.[29,30]

Treatment   Complications of cirrhosis include ascites, portal hypertension, and HCC. Mortality most often is related to bleeding esophageal varices, hepatorenal syndrome, spontaneous bacterial peritonitis, and treatment related to ascites. Imaging follow-up and surveillance is performed with ultrasound. Further workup with contrast-enhanced MRI is performed when enlarging or suspicious nodules and/or increasing α-fetoprotein levels are present.[29,31]

Box 90-2   Causes of Cirrhosis in Children

Viral hepatitis
Hepatic fibrosis
Biliary atresia
Primary biliary cirrhosis
Cystic fibrosis
Budd-Chiari syndrome
Iron overload
Chronic biliary obstruction
α_1-antitrypsin deficiency
Glycogen storage disease
Tyrosinemia
Wilson disease
Galactosemia
Autosomal recessive polycystic kidney disease (hepatic fibrosis)
Osler-Weber-Rendu syndrome

Key Points

Hepatic steatosis is the most common chronic liver disease in pediatric patients because of the prevalence of childhood obesity.

In primary hemochromatosis, excess iron is stored in the hepatocytes of the liver, pancreas, heart, and pituitary. The spleen is spared except in severe cases complicated by cirrhosis.

In secondary hemochromatosis, excess iron is stored in the spleen, bone marrow, and Kupffer cells of the liver (the reticuloendothelial system). The pancreas and heart are notably spared, except in cases of severe disease.

Regenerating and low-grade dysplastic nodules are hypointense on T2-weighted images and do not enhance on postcontrast arterial phase imaging. Enhancement may be seen on delayed imaging when hepatobiliary specific contrast agents are used, such as Eovist (gadoxetate disodium).

High-grade dysplastic nodules and HCC are hyperintense on T2-weighted images with notable enhancement on postcontrast arterial phase imaging.

Suggested Readings

Boll DT, Merkle EM. Diffuse liver disease: strategies for hepatic CT and MR imaging. *Radiographics*. 2009;29:1591-1614.

Hanna RF, Aguirre DA, Kased N, et al. Cirrhosis-associated hepatocellular nodules: correlation of histopathologic and MR imaging features. *Radiographics*. 2008;28;747-769.

Lindback SM, Gabert C, Johnson BL, et al. Pediatric nonalcoholic fatty liver disease: a comprehensive review. *Adv Pediatr*. 2010;57:85-140.

Pariente D, Franchi-Abella S. Paediatric chronic liver diseases: how to investigate and follow up? Role of imaging in the diagnosis of fibrosis. *Pediatr Radiol*. 2010;40;906-919.

Queiroz-Andrade M, Blasbalg R, Ortego CD, et al. MR imaging findings of iron overload. *Radiographics*. 2009;29:1575-1589.

References

Full references for this chapter can be found on www.expertconsult.com.

Chapter 91

Infectious Causes of Liver Disease

BRENTON D. READING and LISA H. LOWE

Viral hepatitis is the most common diffuse infection of the liver in otherwise healthy children.[1] Although parasites are more common worldwide, they typically involve the biliary tree, as in ascariasis, or produce focal infections of the liver, as in echinococcosis or amebiasis. In immunocompromised patients, other infections, particularly fungal infections, become more common.

Viral Hepatitis

Overview Viral hepatitis presents a spectrum of clinical severity, which can range from subclinical infections to fulminant hepatitis or progression into cirrhosis.

Etiology Beyond the neonatal period, viral hepatitis is most commonly caused by the hepatitis A, hepatitis B, and hepatitis C viruses.[1] A number of other viruses have been implicated in childhood hepatitis, including mumps, measles, varicella-zoster, herpes simplex, cytomegalovirus, adenovirus, Coxsackie virus, and Epstein-Barr virus. Most affected patients have a short-lived acute disease with complete recovery. Complications include subacute and chronic active hepatitis, evolution into cirrhosis, and development of hepatocellular carcinoma.[2]

Imaging Diagnosis is made clinically and on the basis of laboratory data. If imaging is performed during the acute phase of the illness, the liver may be enlarged or normal in size. Sonography of the affected liver may demonstrate increased parenchymal echogenicity and heterogeneity.[3] Increased thickness of the portal triads related to periportal edema may be seen (Fig. 91-1), which leads to the "starry sky" pattern, and the gallbladder wall can appear thickened.[1,4-6] Lymphadenopathy may be present at the porta hepatis. Computed tomography (CT) scans sometimes show heterogeneous changes in attenuation, but more commonly they show hepatomegaly, gallbladder wall thickening, and periportal low attenuation (Fig. 91-2). In patients with fulminant hepatitis and subsequent hepatic regeneration, imaging differences have been described between necrotic areas and regenerating nodules. Regions of necrosis have central low attenuation on noncontrast CT relative to regions of regeneration. After intravenous (IV) administration of contrast material, areas of necrosis and regeneration may enhance similarly such that they become indistinguishable, or the regenerating nodules may show diminished enhancement,

which can simulate a neoplastic lesion. Similarly, magnetic resonance imaging (MRI) may show nonspecific periportal high intensity on T2-weighted images and hepatomegaly.[3] On MRI, areas of nodular regeneration show high signal on T1-weighted images and low signal on T2-weighted images relative to adjacent parenchyma.[4]

Although it is used less frequently today than in the past, nuclear scintigraphy may be performed in infants suspected of having biliary atresia or hepatitis. Because liver function is decreased, there is poor uptake of the radiopharmaceutical agent with delayed excretion through the biliary tree into the small bowel and vicarious excretion through the kidneys (Fig. 91-3).

Treatment and Follow-up Treatment of viral hepatitis varies from treatment of symptoms to antiviral medication to a liver transplant, depending on the type and severity of the disease. Fulminant hepatitis may be fatal without hepatic transplant.[4]

Pyogenic Abscess

Overview Pyogenic infection with hepatic abscess formation is caused by microbial liver infection with subsequent inflammatory cell response and pus accumulation. The mortality rate is 6% to 14%.[5] Immunocompromised patients with chronic granulomatous disease of childhood or those who have undergone bone marrow transplantation are at particularly high risk for liver abscesses. Other susceptible states include chemotherapy, congenital or acquired immunodeficiency, and intraabdominal infection, such as appendicitis and inflammatory bowel disease.[7] Hepatic abscesses are most common in the right hepatic lobe, and most are solitary.[6]

Etiology Staphylococci, streptococci, and *Escherichia coli* are the most common pathogens involved in a pyogenic abscess. However, *Klebsiella pneumonia,* which typically is more common in Asian countries, is increasing in incidence in North America.[6,7]

Imaging Hepatic abscesses often have an insidious presentation, leading to a delay in diagnosis. They range from single, well-defined, homogeneous, circular foci to heterogeneous, poorly defined, multiloculated, septated, debris- or gas-containing lesions (Fig. 91-4). Air-fluid levels may be related to gas-forming organisms. Enhanced through-transmission in a hypoechoic mass on ultrasound and lack of central flow

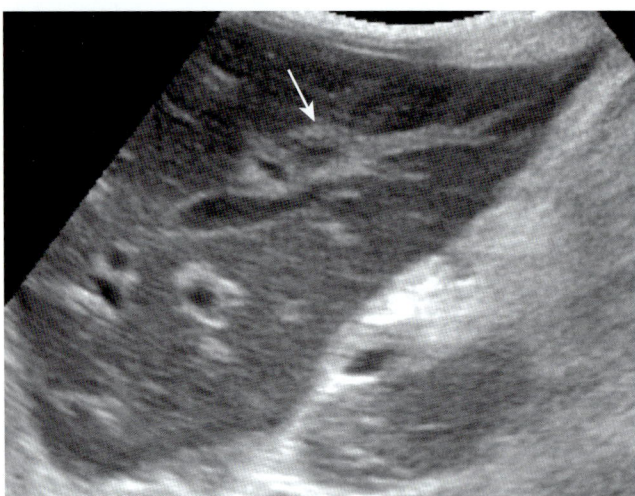

Figure 91-1 Periportal edema in a 12-year-old boy with viral hepatitis. A longitudinal sonogram demonstrates increased perivascular echogenicity along the portal triads (*arrow*).

with Doppler are useful in confirming a cystic, rather than a solid, lesion.[2] Other sonographic findings in persons with a pyogenic liver abscess include a hypoechoic or anechoic mass, a hypoechoic surrounding ring of edema, internal fluid–debris levels, and septations. Common CT findings include lack of central enhancement after contrast administration, an enhancing abscess wall, and a surrounding rim of low–attenuation hepatic edema.[2,8] Abscesses in patients with chronic granulomatous disease may heal with formation of granulomas, which frequently calcify. MRI of hepatic abscesses typically show decreased or nearly isointense signal on T1-weighted images, increased signal on T2-weighted images, and peripheral ringlike contrast enhancement.[8] Multiple abscesses are most commonly the result of biliary disease, biliary obstruction, or hepatic trauma. Hematogenous spread of pyogenic organisms may result in multiple abscesses (Fig. 91-5). A tuberculous abscess cannot be differentiated on imaging

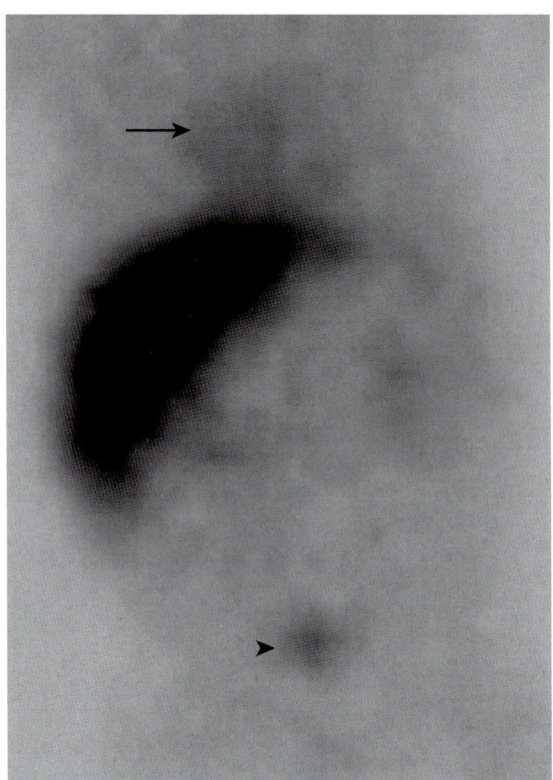

Figure 91-3 Hepatitis in a 7-week-old boy with persistent jaundice. A technetium 99m-labeled hepatoiminodiacetic scan (HIDA) shows poor uptake within the liver with a large amount of background activity in the heart (*arrow*) and vicarious excretion through the genitourinary tract (*arrowhead*).

studies from other pyogenic infections.[9] Resolved tuberculosis may result in hepatic calcifications.

Treatment and Follow-up Treatment of pyogenic abscesses ranges from antibiotics alone for small lesions (usually <5 cm) to percutaneous aspiration and catheter drainage for larger

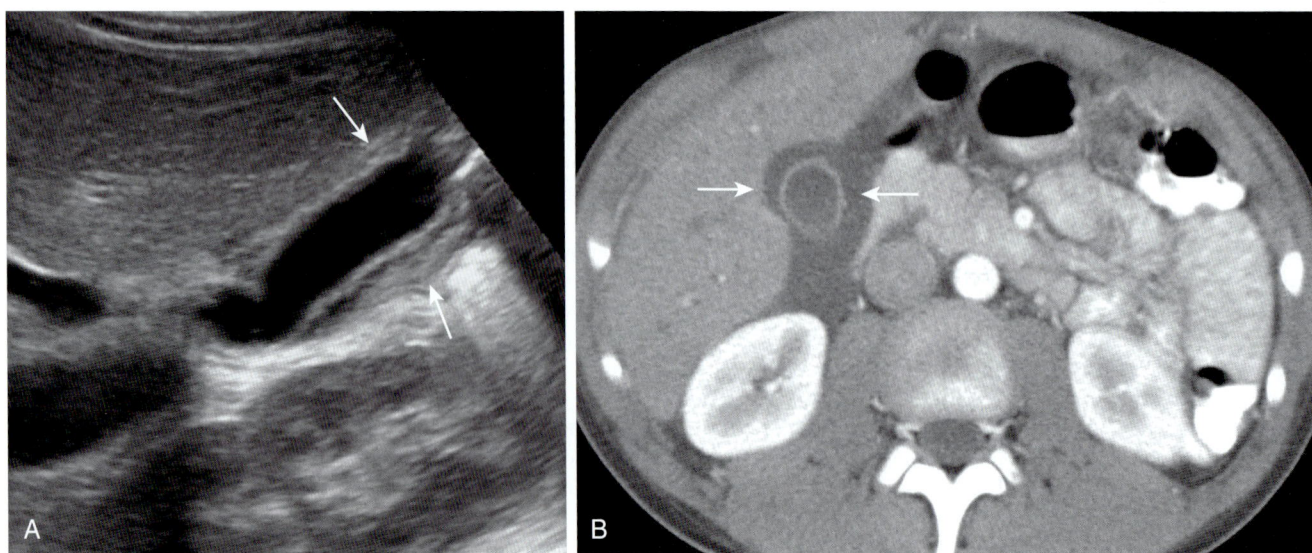

Figure 91-2 Gallbladder wall thickening in a 10-year-old boy with viral hepatitis. **A,** A longitudinal sonogram shows a thick, hyperechoic gallbladder wall (*arrows*). **B,** Computed tomography with intravenous contrast confirms gallbladder wall thickening (*arrows*) and periportal edema.

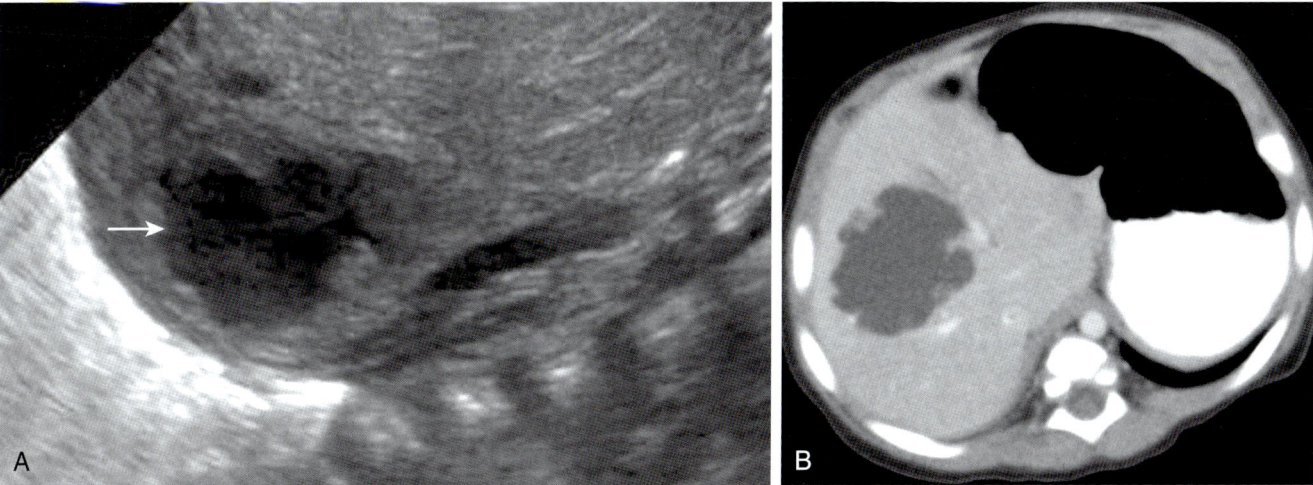

Figure 91-4 Pyogenic abscess in a 2-month-old boy with fever. **A,** A longitudinal sonogram of the right hepatic lobe reveals a hypoechoic region with irregular margins (*arrow*) and a halo of decreased parenchymal echogenicity. **B,** Axial contrast-enhanced computed tomography image confirms the low attenuation region. Staphylococcus was found upon subsequent percutaneous needle aspiration.

lesions. Percutaneous abscess drainage has markedly reduced case mortality from 40% to 2%.[2,5,10] Because amebic abscesses are readily treated medically, serology or aspiration diagnosis of this entity can help avoid drain placement.[11,12] The techniques used for percutaneous drainage in children are similar to those used for adults, although IV sedation or general anesthesia may be necessary.[13] The rare complications that occur after percutaneous drainage include bleeding, peritonitis, and less often, septicemia, pneumothorax, and empyema.[2] Surgical drainage is used only if catheter drainage fails or treatment of an underlying cause of abscess is required.[11]

Fungal Infections

Overview Fungal infection occurs frequently in the setting of immune compromise, such as leukemia and chronic granulomatous disease; a reported increase in systemic fungal

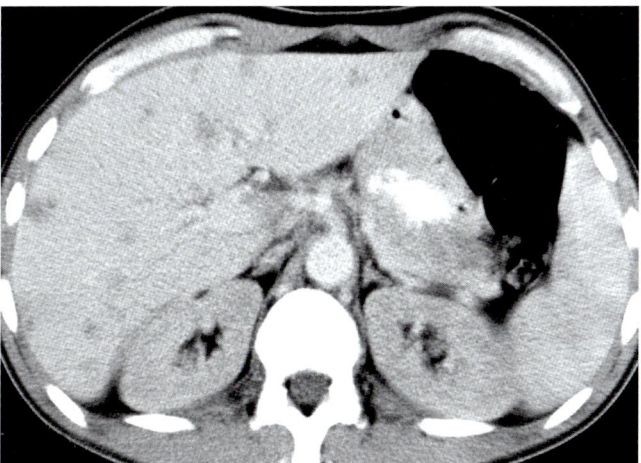

Figure 91-5 Multiple hepatic abscesses in a 17-year-old boy undergoing steroid therapy for inflammatory bowel disease. Axial computed tomography with intravenous contrast material identifies multiple low attenuation, poorly defined foci of variable size scattered throughout the liver.

infection may be the result of longer survival of immunocompromised hosts.[14,15]

Etiology The most common causative organism is *Candida albicans*, which may affect any organ system. However, other ubiquitous fungi such as *Aspergillus*, *Histoplasma*, *Coccidioides immitis* (in endemic areas), and opportnistic bacteria such as *Nocardia* have been identified in persons with immune compromise.[14]

Imaging The imaging appearance depends on the host's immune response. In neutropenic patients, disease is microscopic and lesions may be occult on imaging. Formation of microabscesses is possible when the patient recovers from neutropenia and mounts an immune response. On sonography, four imaging patterns of candidiasis within the liver are reported. All four patterns have multiple, small (<3 mm to 4 mm) lesions scattered diffusely throughout the liver parenchyma.[16] Early in the disease process, the "wheel-within-a-wheel" appearance is seen, representing a hyperechoic nidus of necrotic fungus, surrounded by echogenic inflammatory cells, in turn surrounded by a peripheral zone of fibrosis. The bull's-eye or target appearance, consisting of an echogenic center with a hypoechoic rim, is seen when the host mounts an immune response.[2] The most common appearance is seen later and consists of diffuse uniform hypoechoic foci throughout the liver resulting from formation of tiny microabscesses (<4 mm) and fibrosis (Fig. 91-6). Last is the pattern of calcified, hyperechoic tiny foci in persons with a healed or healing fungal infection (1 to 4 mm) (Fig. 91-7).[16,17] Findings on CT include multiple foci of low attenuation of variable size (2 to 20 mm), with or without enhancement and calcification.[2,16] Arterial phase scans have been shown to be more sensitive for detection.[18] MRI may reveal tiny lesions of low signal intensity on T1-weighted imaging and high signal intensity on T2-weighted imaging; T1-weighted gradient echo sequences have been reported to show greater sensitivity than the spin-echo sequence.[19] However, the appearance remains relatively nonspecific compared with the more distinct patterns described on sonography.[16]

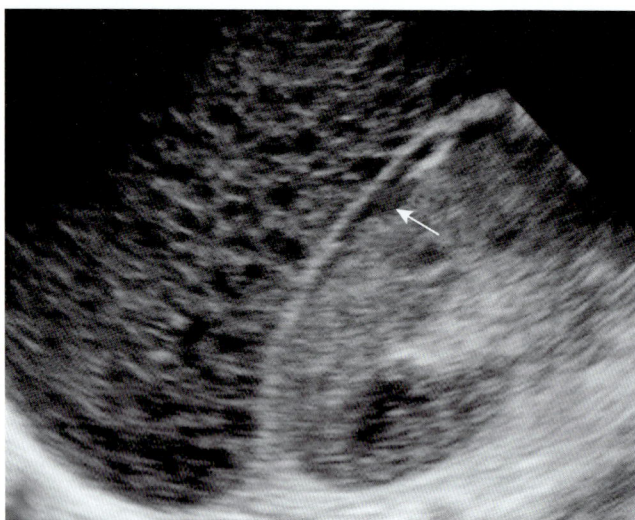

Figure 91-6 Hepatic candidiasis in a 7-month-old boy with immune deficiency. A longitudinal sonogram shows diffuse, homogeneous, hypoechoic foci consistent with microabscesses throughout the liver. A tiny amount of fluid in the Morrison pouch is noted (*arrow*) adjacent to the right kidney.

Treatment and Follow-up Systemic treatment with antifungal medications is the treatment of choice.[14]

Cat Scratch Disease

Overview Cat scratch disease usually is a self-limited infection that most often involves the lymph nodes. In 5% to 10% of cases it spreads systemically to variably involve the liver, spleen, bone, and, rarely, the central nervous system with meningoencephalitis or neuroretinitis. Patients with acquired immunodeficiency syndrome may present with bacillary

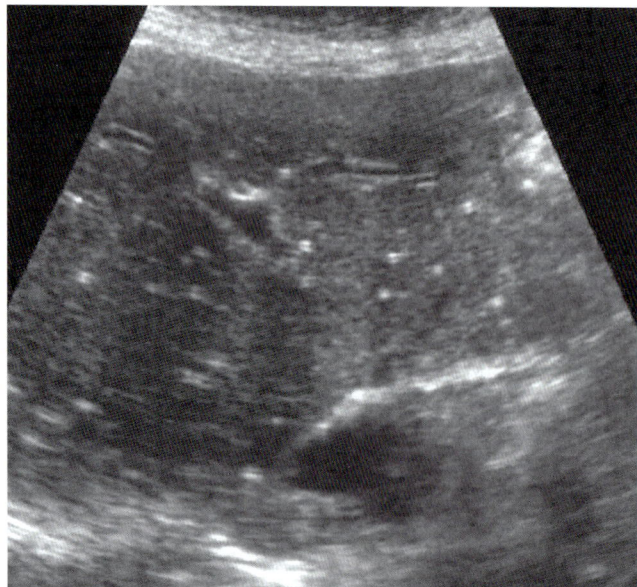

Figure 91-7 Candidiasis in a 17-year-old girl undergoing chemotherapy. A transverse sonogram of the liver shows tiny punctate foci of increased echogenicity resulting from diffuse calcified microabscesses.

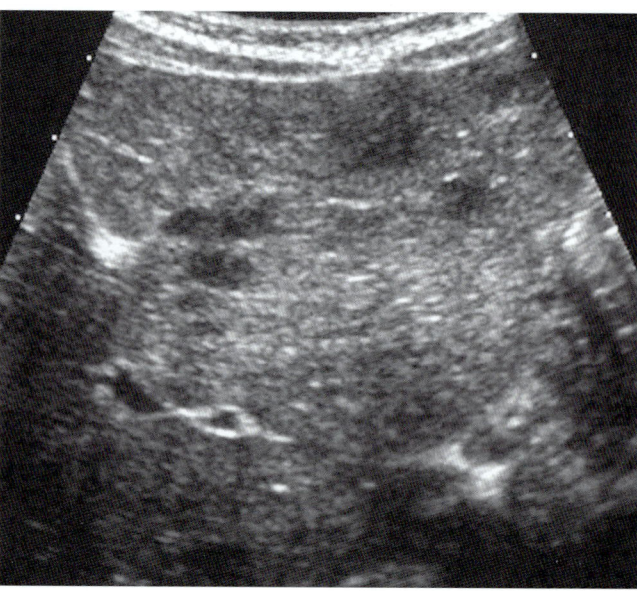

Figure 91-8 Cat-scratch disease in a 2-year-old boy with abdominal pain. A transverse sonogram of the left hepatic lobe demonstrates multiple hypoechoic lesions of variable size.

angiomatosis.[20,21] Children usually present with painful lymphadenopathy; however, systemic spread may cause low-grade fever and various complaints related to involvement of virtually any organ system.[20] The typical course of cat-scratch disease involves formation of granulomas, which heal spontaneously and may calcify.

Etiology Cat scratch disease is caused by *Bartonella henselae*. The disease is transmitted to the patient's lymphatic system, often by a cat scratch; occasionally the disease may be transmitted to humans via a flea or tick.[20] It is helpful to elicit a history of recent contact or exposure to a cat or kitten in making the diagnosis. The organism is difficult to culture, and diagnosis hinges on enzyme assay for identification of anti-*B. henselae* immunoglobulins.[22] A definitive diagnosis requires biopsy to detect deoxyribonucleic acid from the organism; however, a biopsy is rarely performed.

Imaging Sonography of a patient with cat scratch disease reveals numerous small hypoechoic, well-marginated, circular, homogeneous foci within the liver or spleen, in many cases associated with lymphadenopathy (Fig. 91-8). On CT, small low-attenuation lesions are found before administration of contrast material. Variable attenuation is seen after administration of contrast material, and marginal enhancement often is present.[23]

Treatment and Follow-up Most cases of cat scratch disease are self-limited and do not require antibiotic treatment. However, if antibiotic treatment is required, azithromycin has demonstrated effectiveness.[20]

Parasitic Infestations

ASCARIASIS

Overview Although rare in North America, ascariasis is estimated to affect 1 billion people worldwide; it is most prevalent in tropical and subtropical regions, particularly in areas with poor sanitation.[24]

Etiology   Ascariasis is an intestinal infection caused by *Ascaris lumbricoides*. It occurs when eggs are ingested and grow into larvae and subsequently into pencil-shaped round worms within the intestine. Larvae that penetrate through the intestinal wall enter the bloodstream and travel to the liver and may continue on to the lungs. Symptoms depend on the organ involved. The helminthic mass within the lumen of the bowel may lead to intestinal obstruction and segmental volvulus.[24] Worms may obstruct the biliary system, causing dilation and pain, as well as increasing the risk for bacterial superinfection.[25]

Imaging   On imaging studies, characteristic vermiform defects are seen inside the small intestine (Fig. 91-9), and if a small bowel follow-through is performed, the worms may ingest the contrast material, thus outlining their own gastrointestinal tracts.[26] The worms can be visible on sonography, within the bowel lumen, or within the biliary tree.[24,25]

Treatment and Follow-up   Treatment with antiparasitic medications is usually effective, with rapid resolution of symptoms.[24]

ECHINOCOCCOSIS

Overview   Echinococcosis or hydatid disease is a parasitic infection endemic in many parts of the world, with the major endemic regions encompassing sheep-grazing countries of the

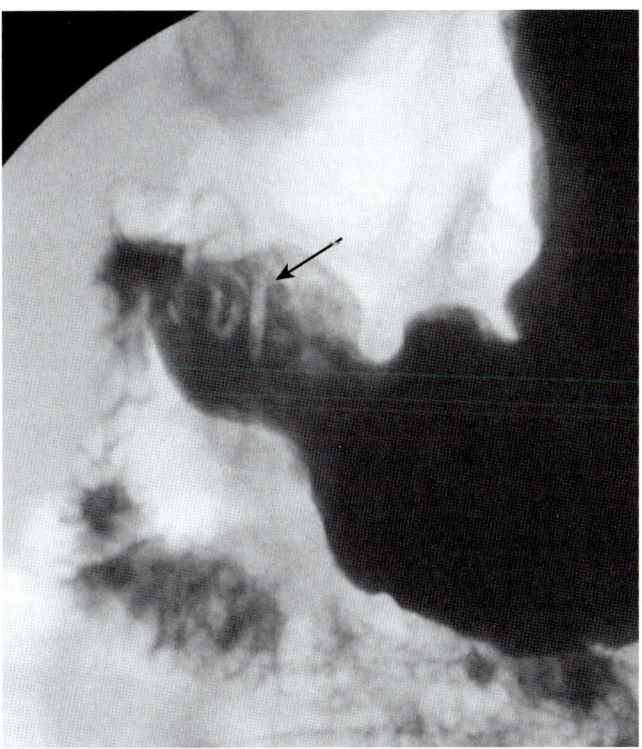

Figure 91-9   Ascariasis in an 8-year-old boy with vomiting since a recent Mexico vacation. Fluoroscopic image from an upper gastrointestinal study demonstrates a well-defined, vermiform-shaped structure coiled in the gastric antrum (*arrow*).

Mediterranean, Middle East, South America, and Australia. Although human disease most often affects the liver, multiple other organs may be affected, including the lung, peritoneum, genitourinary system, heart, and central nervous system.

Etiology   Hydatid disease refers to an infestation by the larval form of two main varieties of Echinococcus: *E. granulosus* and *E. multilocularis*. *E. granulosus* is more common, whereas *E. multilocularis* is more invasive.[27] The definitive hosts are specific carnivores, such as the dog or wolf; ruminants, particularly sheep, are intermediate hosts, and humans are accidental intermediate hosts.[28] Humans become infected by ingesting the parasite eggs in food or water contaminated with fecal material from the definitive host. After ingestion, the protective covering of the eggs is digested, releasing the larvae or oncosphere, which pass through the mucosa into the portal venous radicles, becoming lodged in the liver, where they may die or slowly grow to produce hydatid cysts.[16,27] *E. granulosus* forms a cyst with three histologic layers. The outermost layer, the pericyst, is a tough, collagenous membrane formed by the host response to the parasite; the middle layer is an acellular membrane that allows the passage of nutrients; and the inner layer is the germinal layer, which secretes both the middle layer and cyst fluid. The germinal layer and the middle layer together are known as the endocyst, although the middle layer is sometimes termed the ectocyst. The germinal layer is the layer from which brood capsules and scolices are secreted into cyst fluid, forming "hydatid sand." Daughter cysts may arise from brood capsules along the periphery of the endocyst.[29] Formation of multiple daughter cysts may result in starvation and death of the cyst. When contained cyst rupture occurs, separation of the endocyst from the pericyst occurs, resulting in a floating membrane (water lily sign); communicating rupture, on the other hand, results in spillage of cyst material into the biliary tree, whereas direct rupture into the peritoneal cavity will lead to spillage of both infectious scolices and antigenic cyst fluid, causing seeding of the peritoneum and possibly anaphylaxis.[2,27,28] Superinfection occurs only after cyst rupture, because the intact ectocyst is resistant to bacterial invasion.[30]

Imaging   The imaging appearance of *E. granulosus* and *E. multilocularis* is distinct. Hydatid cysts may be single or multiple; the right lobe is most commonly involved.[2]

Echinococcal cysts have been classified into three types, reflecting cyst contents and findings during various stages of development.[28] Type I cysts are simple fluid-filled cysts that may contain hydatid sand and septa but exhibit no other internal architecture. On ultrasound they are anechoic, but upon rolling the patient, hydatid sand is dispersed, resembling "falling snowflakes."[27] On CT, type I cysts are well-defined hypodense lesions with enhancement of the cyst wall and any internal septa. At MRI, the signal intensity follows water, although on T2 weighting, the cyst may manifest a rim of low signal intensity.[27] Type II cysts contain daughter cysts or internal matrix (Fig. 91-10). Ultrasound may demonstrate floating membranes or vesicles, and a "wheel spoke" appearance may arise from contact of multiple daughter cysts. On CT, the fluid within the mother cyst is of higher attenuation than that within the daughter cysts and may appear as a "rosette." They may have scattered calcifications (Fig. 91-11).

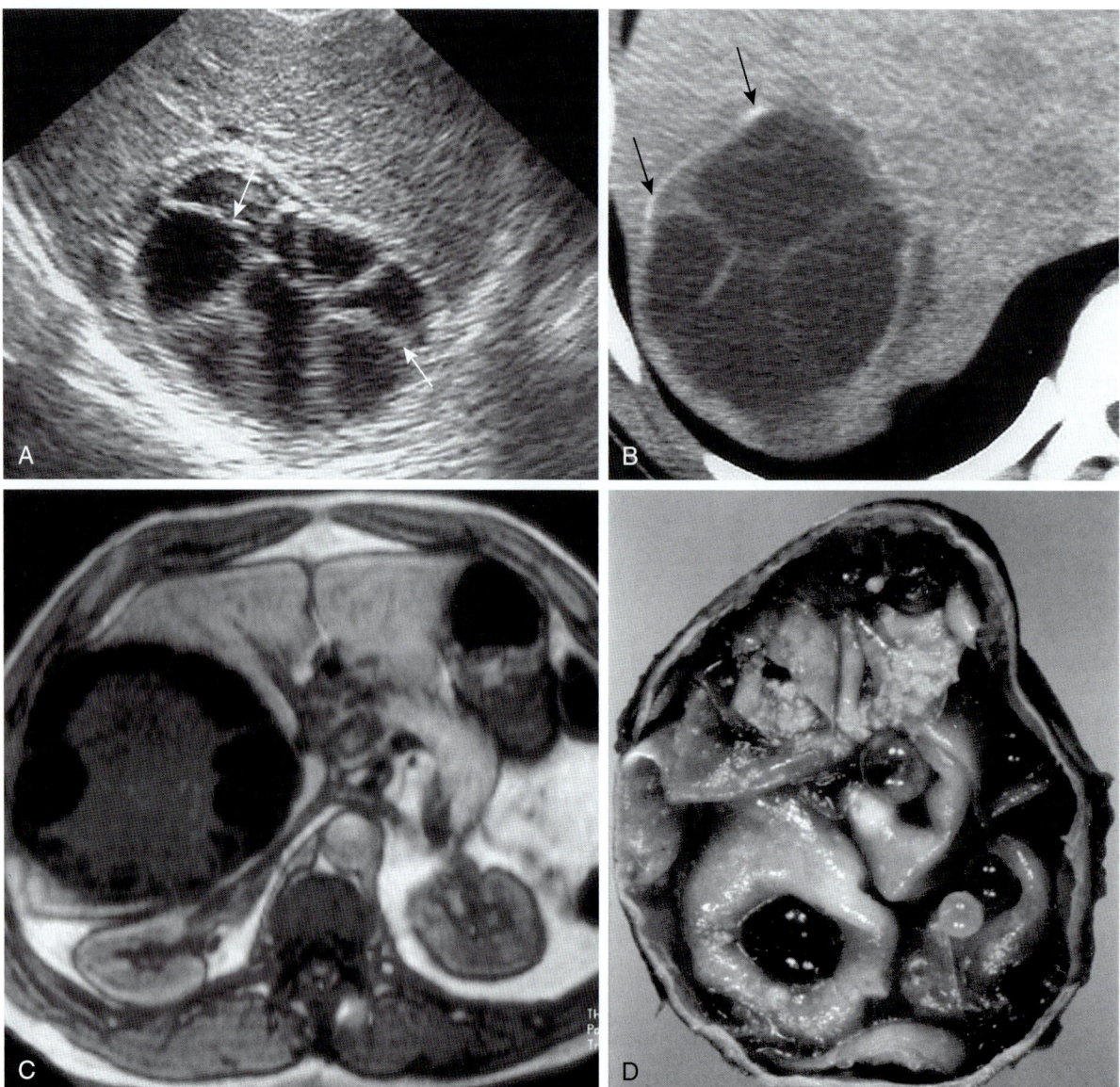

Figure 91-10 Echinococcal (hydatid) cyst. **A,** A longitudinal hepatic sonogram shows a type II, well-defined (*arrows*), multilocular lesion with a "spoke wheel" appearance. **B,** An axial unenhanced computed tomography image confirms a mass with multiple septations, daughter cysts, and peripheral calcifications (*arrows*). **C,** An axial T1-weighted gradient echo magnetic resonance image shows a hepatic hydatid cyst with a hypointense fibrous pericyst and extensive peripheral low-signal-intensity daughter cysts surrounding central intermediate-signal-intensity matrix that was bright on T2-weighted images (not shown). **D,** A gross specimen of a resected hydatid cyst reveals numerous daughter cysts. (From Mortele KJ, Segatto E, Ros PR. The infected liver: radiologic-pathologic correlation. *Radiographics*. 2004;24:937-955.)

On MRI the membranes have low signal intensity on both T1- and T2-weighted sequences.[27] Type III cysts are completely calcified and indicate cyst death.[27,28]

E. multilocularis (alveolaris), which is less common than *E. granulosus,* is distributed in North America and central and northern Eurasia, with foxes and rodents serving as the definitive and intermediate hosts.[31] The lesion grows by extension along its periphery, causing multilocular cysts as it invades the host tissues; central necrosis and calcification may be present. Its growth has been likened to that of a slow-growing tumor, with infiltration of biliary and venous structures within the liver.[32] Imaging features of *E. multilocularis* include hepatomegaly, multiple irregular lesions with increased echogenicity on sonography, decreased attenuation on CT, microcalcifications and dilation of intrahepatic bile ducts, vascular involvement, and involvement of parahepatic structures by direct of hematogenous extension.[31]

Treatment and Follow-up   In general, treatment of echinococcal cysts requires removal of the entire cyst and its contents. Partial capsectomy may be done but has the drawback of increased risk of recurrence. Percutaneous drainage, injection, and reaspiration often is successful and is applied in conjunction with antiechinococcal drugs, particularly albendazole. However, the diagnosis of echinococcal cysts should be made serologically before percutaneous drainage because the

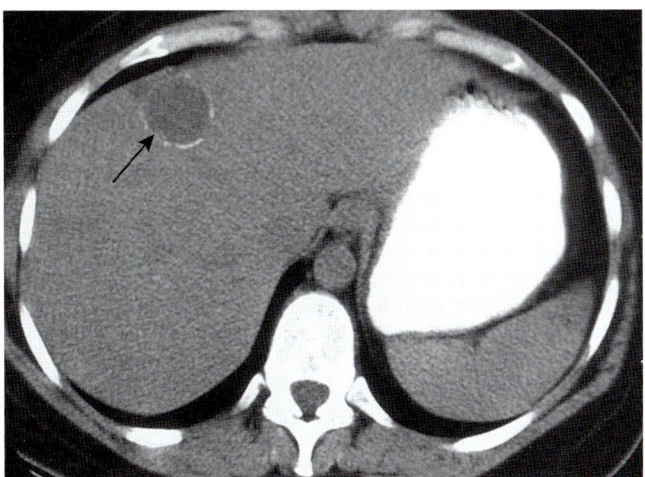

Figure 91-11 An echinococcal (hydatid) cyst. Axial unenhanced computed tomography images show peripheral calcification in hepatic echinococcal cyst (*arrow*).

differential diagnosis includes uncomplicated amebic and small pyogenic abscesses, which are treated with medical therapy alone.[33] Inoperable cases or cases with disseminated disease may benefit from administration of albendazole.[33,34]

AMEBIC ABSCESS

Overview Amebic infection is considered a leading parasitic cause of human mortality, affecting approximately 50 million people and resulting in 100,000 deaths annually.[12,35] Endemic areas include Africa, India, the Far East, and South America.[36] In the United States, about 1200 cases occur per year. With the availability of effective treatment, mortality from hepatic amebic abscess has gradually diminished from 2.0% to 0.2%.[12]

Amebic abscesses usually are solitary and often are found within the right lobe of the liver. The primary infection is often intestinal, with diarrhea and dysentery at presentation. The liver may become involved as a result of spread via the portal vein; however, some studies report that in 59% of cases there is no preceding history of diarrhea.[37,38] Extension across the diaphragm to involve the pleura may occur. Other extraintestinal sites include pericardium, brain, skin, and genital disease, but involvement at these sites is rare.[12,38] Perforation into the peritoneum will lead to peritoneal spread.[38]

Amebic abscesses can occur at any age but are most common in children younger than 3 years.[36] The presentation is usually acute right upper quadrant pain. Diagnosis can be made from fresh stool specimens collected from at least three separate bowel movements. Circulating antibodies can be identified with serologic tests at least 7 days after invasive disease has presented.[12]

Etiology Amebic abscesses are caused by the protozoan *Entamoeba histolytica*.

Imaging The cross-sectional imaging appearance of amebic abscesses is variable and shares imaging features with pyogenic abscess. Sonography, the initial modality of choice, reveals a homogeneous round or oval mass with internal debris.[11,36] Lesions are more common in the right lobe of the liver,

are often peripheral in location near the hepatic capsule, and have enhanced through-transmission. CT shows a low attenuation area with peripheral enhancement and a rim, or halo, of surrounding edema and may show internal septations (Fig. 91-12).[2] MRI of amebic abscesses shows heterogeneous low signal intensity on T1-weighted sequences and high signal intensity on T2-weighted sequences with a double-layered wall and peripheral enhancement after gadolinium administration.[2]

Treatment and Follow-up Treatment of amebic abscesses is medical, in distinction to pyogenic abscesses, which generally require percutaneous or surgical drainage. More than 90% of patients do well with prolonged antibiotic therapy (usually metronidazole). The initial response to antibiotics is generally rapid, and failure to respond in 24 to 72 hours may indicate superimposed bacterial infection, in which case percutaneous aspiration may be useful.[2] Percutaneous aspiration also may be useful if impending rupture is an immediate clinical concern.

SCHISTOSOMIASIS

Overview Schistosomiasis affects more than 250 million people worldwide, and approximately 600 million people are believed to be at risk for infection. The disease is endemic in South America, Africa, the Middle East, and the Far East and is rare in North America.[39,40]

Etiology Schistosomiasis is an infection with parasitic blood flukes. Three forms affect humans: *Schistosoma japonicum*, *Schistosoma mansoni*, and *Schistosoma hematobium*.[41] The latter affects the urinary system and will not be detailed in this chapter. The parasites penetrate the skin of humans (the definitive host) through contact with contaminated water, in which the intermediate host (a snail) releases the infective cercaria. The larvae mature and migrate to the venules of the urinary bladder (*S. hematobium*) or gastrointestinal tract

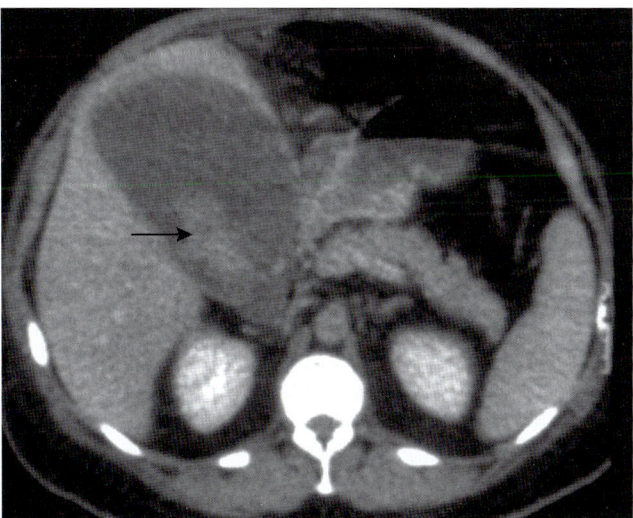

Figure 91-12 An amebic abscess. An axial computed tomography image shows a large, exophytic low-attenuation cyst with hyperdense central debris (*arrow*).

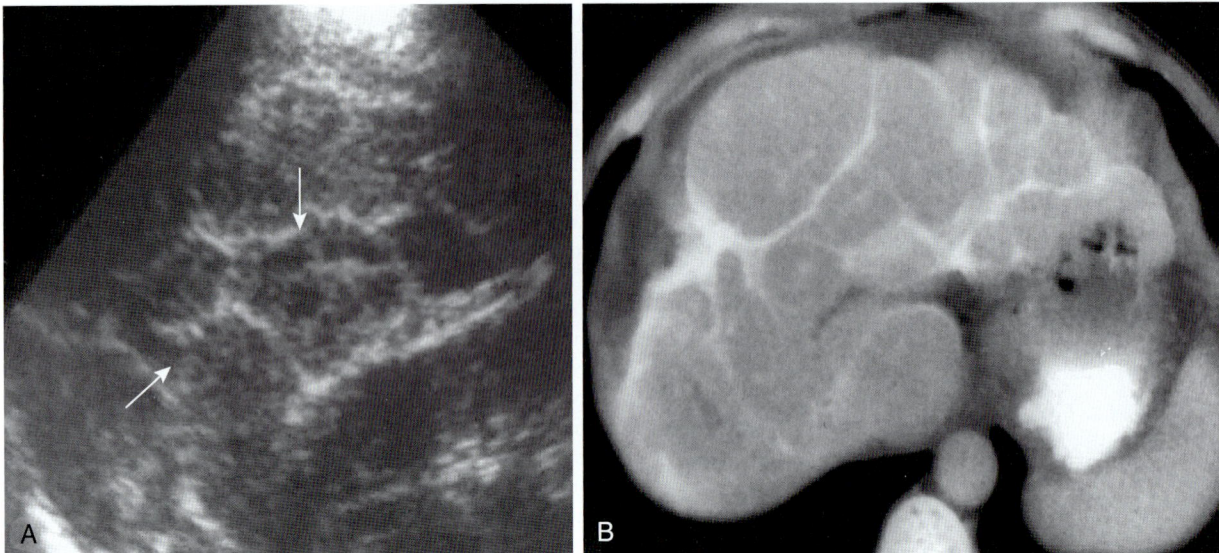

Figure 91-13 Schistosomiasis, *Schistosoma japonicum*. **A,** A longitudinal sonogram of the right lobe of the liver reveals hyperechoic septations (*arrows*) between polygonal areas of hepatic parenchyma. **B,** An axial computed tomography image of the liver confirms the characteristic "turtle back" or "tortoise shell" appearance of the liver resulting from septal fibrosis with calcification. (From Mortele KJ, Segatto E, Ros PR. The infected liver: radiologic-pathologic correlation. *Radiographics*. 2004;24:937-955.)

(*S. mansoni* and *S. japonicum*) to deposit eggs. Eggs deposited in the gastrointestinal tract spread via the mesenteric venules to the portal vein, where they incite an inflammatory granulomatous response, resulting in fibrosis and presinusoidal portal obstruction.[2]

Imaging The acute syndrome, also known as Katayama fever, can be suspected in persons who travel to endemic areas. Acutely, hepatosplenomegaly and hypoechoic lesions have been described in the liver, along with portal adenopathy.[42] Chronic schistosomiasis demonstrates the changes of hepatic fibrosis and portal hypertension. The smaller eggs of *S. japonicum* are deposited along the small portal radicles at the periphery of the liver, whereas the larger *S. mansoni* eggs are deposited along the large portal branches from the liver hilum. Periportal fibrosis in persons with *S. japonicum* therefore is distributed along the peripheral part of the liver and centrally in patients infected with *S. mansoni*. Fibrotic tracts in patients with *S. japonicum* form a "polygonal network" with a honeycomb or tortoise shell appearance and are likely to calcify. Fibrotic tracts in patients with *S. mansoni* do not tend to calcify and form a "Symmers' pipe-stem" fibrosis (Fig. 91-13).[39,42] Sonography reveals hyperechoic septa outlining polygonal areas that may resemble a fish scale network. On CT, dense fibrous and calcific septa distributed at right angles to the hepatic surface produce the classic CT appearance of "turtle back calcification" in persons with *S. japonicum* infection. MRI may show isointense periportal bands on T1-weighted images, which are bright on T2-weighted images and enhance after gadolinium contrast administration.[2,41]

Treatment and Follow-up Schistosomiasis infection is treatable with praziquantel.[41] However, hepatic fibrosis related to egg antigens trapped in the liver occurs in approximately 20% of infected patients despite effective treatment, and work continues to identify the patients at greatest risk of the development of hepatic fibrosis.[43]

Key Points

Treatment of hepatic infection depends on the causative pathogen, which must be determined to avoid morbidity and mortality related to incorrect therapy.

Small pyogenic (<5 cm) and amebic abscesses undergo medical therapy only. However, larger pyogenic (>5 cm) and amenable (totally intrahepatic) echinococcal abscesses are drained percutaneously.

Surgical removal is required for echinococcal cysts at risk for rupture (partially extrahepatic or crossing the diaphragm) to avoid life-threatening anaphylaxis.

Fungal hepatic infections typically occur in immunosuppressed children and are treated by removing the cause of immune suppression if possible, in addition to antifungal medications.

Cat scratch disease, a generally self-limiting disorder that rarely requires antibiotic therapy, may involve the skin, lymph nodes, liver, spleen, bones, and central nervous systems.

Suggested Readings

Balci NC, Sirvanci M. MR imaging of infective liver lesions. *Magn Reson Imaging Clin North Am.* 2002;10:121-135.

Doyle DJ, Hanbidge AE, O'Malley ME. Imaging of hepatic infections. *Clin Radiol.* 2006;61(9):737-748.

Oleszczuk-Raszke K, Cremin FJ, Fisher RM, et al. Ultrasonic features of pyogenic and amoebic hepatic abscesses. *Pediatr Radiol.* 1989;19:23.

Pedrosa I, Saiz A, Arrazola J, et al. Hydatid disease: radiologic and pathologic features and complications. *Radiographics.* 2000;20(3):795-817.

Restrepo RS, Raut AA, Riascos R, et al. Imaging manifestations of tropical parasitic infections. *Semin Roentgenol.* 2007;42:37-48.

References

Full references for this chapter can be found on www.expertconsult.com.

Chapter 92

Neoplasia

JOSÉE DUBOIS and LISA H. LOWE

Overview

Hepatic neoplasms constitute approximately 2% of all childhood tumors and approximately 6% of pediatric abdominal neoplasms. Two thirds of liver tumors in children are malignant, and they represent the third most common intraabdominal malignancy in the pediatric age group after Wilms tumor and neuroblastoma. The most common hepatic malignant tumors in order of frequency are hepatoblastomas, hepatocellular carcinomas (HCC), undifferentiated embryonal sarcomas, angiosarcomas, and embryonal rhabdomyosarcomas.[1] Benign hepatic tumors in pediatrics include tumors specific to children such as vascular tumors and mesenchymal hamartomas, as well as entities that also are seen in adults, such as focal nodular hyperplasia (FNH), hepatocellular adenoma, and nodular regenerative hyperplasia (NRH).

A differential diagnosis of liver tumors can be obtained based on the age of the patient, laboratory findings such as serum alpha fetoprotein (AFP) levels, and imaging characteristics (Table 92-1). However, the serum AFP level is normally elevated at birth (25,000-50,000 ng/mL) and does not reach adult levels (<25 ng/mL) until 6 months of age.[2,3]

Several imaging modalities are available to evaluate liver masses, including plain radiographs, ultrasonography, computed tomography (CT), magnetic resonance imaging (MRI), and radionuclide scintigraphy. Plain radiographs have a limited role but may reveal the liver as the organ of origin and show calcifications or mass effect on neighboring structures. Sonography is the study of choice in the initial investigation of hepatomegaly and pediatric abdominal masses to confirm the organ of origin and characterize the lesion. Sonographic information helps identify a preliminary differential diagnosis and decide on the appropriate subsequent imaging modality and optimal protocol. Additional cross-sectional imaging with CT, MRI, nuclear scintigraphy, and, rarely, angiography may be required to fully characterize a hepatic lesion before a biopsy is performed and treatment is undertaken.

Malignant Hepatobiliary Tumors

HEPATOBLASTOMA

Overview Hepatoblastoma is the most common primary malignant liver tumor in infants and children. Sixty-eight percent of cases are seen in the first year of life, and 90% occur in patients younger than 5 years, with a male predominance of 2 : 1.[3] Four percent of cases are congenital.[1,3-6]

Etiology Predisposing conditions include Beckwith-Wiedemann syndrome, familial adenomatous polyposis, type 1A glycogen storage disease, Gardner syndrome, fetal alcohol syndrome, Wilms tumor, and trisomy 18. It also is reported in premature infants, low-birth-weight infants, and in infants born of mothers taking oral contraceptives. A strong association exists between low birth weight and hepatoblastoma, raising the issue of potential contribution by a variety of iatrogenic exposures in the neonatal intensive care unit.[7]

Clinical Presentation Hepatoblastoma usually presents as a palpable mass in the right upper quadrant and may be confused with hepatomegaly. Nonspecific clinical symptoms include pain, weight loss, irritability, vomiting, and infrequently, jaundice and precocious puberty (related to the secretion of chorionic gonadotropins). Distant metastases are present in fewer than 10% of cases at diagnosis, with the lungs being the most common site, followed by the lymph nodes, bone, brain, eye, and ovary. Compression or invasion of the hepatic vasculature and inferior vena cava may occur. Serum AFP, which is markedly elevated in approximately 90% of patients with hepatoblastoma, can be used to monitor therapy and detect recurrence.

Hepatoblastoma is classified into two histologic types: the epithelial type, which represents the majority of these tumors, and the mixed epithelial mesenchymal type.[1-3] Hepatoblastoma is usually solitary, but these tumors may be multifocal or, less commonly, diffusely infiltrating. Multifocal disease may consist of a dominant mass with satellite nodules or multiple small masses. When it is solitary, hepatoblastoma is most commonly located in the right hepatic lobe (60% of cases).[8]

Imaging Plain radiographs may show hepatomegaly or a mass with or without calcifications. On sonography, hepatoblastomas are most often well-defined and hyperechoic relative to adjacent liver (Fig. 92-1 and e-Fig. 92-2). Epithelial-type hepatoblastomas are more homogeneous, whereas mixed tumors are more heterogeneous and often contain hyperechoic foci with acoustic shadowing indicating calcifications and hypoechoic or anechoic foci representing necrosis or hemorrhage.[9-11] Intravascular tumor thrombus may be seen within the hepatic or portal veins. Flow within the thrombus on color Doppler imaging is useful to differentiate neoplastic from nonneoplastic thrombus. Infiltrative hepatoblastomas

Table 92-1

Summary for Differential Diagnosis of Liver Tumor			
Tumor	**Age Group**	**Clinical Features**	**Imaging Features**
Hepatoblastoma	<5 y	AFP levels: elevated	Calcifications: coarse, chunky
			Solid mass
			Invasion veins
			Enhancement: less than adjacent liver
Hepatocellular carcinoma	10-14 y	AFP levels: elevated	Solid, focal, multifocal
		Underlying liver disease	Heterogeneous, hemorrhage, necrosis
			Invasion veins
			Local spread
Fibrolamellar carcinoma	Adolescent	AFP levels: normal	Fibrous scar: hypointense T2-weighted imaging, no enhancement
		No liver disease	Homogeneous
			Solitary mass
Undifferentiated embryonal sarcoma	6-10 y	AFP levels: normal	Cystic on CT and MRI
			Solid on ultrasound
			Enhancement: solid portion and septa
Embryonal rhabdomyosarcoma	<5 y	AFP levels: normal	Often located near porta hepatis with intraductal growth pattern
Liver hemangioma	<1 y	AFP levels: normal	Calcification (50%): fine, granular
		Cardiac heart failure	Enhancement: more than adjacent liver
		Coagulopathy	
		Hypothyroidism	
Mesenchymal hamartoma	<5 y	AFP levels: normal	Cystic lesion
			Enhancement: septa and solid portion enhancement
			No calcification
Focal nodular hyperplasia	Young children Adolescents	AFP levels: normal	Vascular, myxoid scar: hyperintense T2-weighted imaging, delayed enhancement
		Strong predilection girls	Homogeneous lesion enhancement
Adenoma	>10 y	AFP levels: normal	No central scar
		Oral contraceptive or androgenic steroid use	Heterogeneous: fat/hemorrhage
		Glycogen storage disease	Opposed-phase T1-weighted gradient echo or fat suppressed: evidence of fat and glycogen
Metastases			Multifocal
Hydatid cyst		History travel	Cystic lesion
Simple cyst			No enhancement
Choledochal cyst			Location in porta hepatis with communication with biliary tree

AFP, Alpha fetoprotein; *CT,* computed tomography; *MRI,* magnetic resonance imaging.

show diffuse heterogeneous echogenicity, with loss of normal parenchymal architecture.[9-11]

Unenhanced CT typically shows a well-circumscribed mass with decreased attenuation relative to the surrounding liver. Speckled or amorphous calcifications are seen in more than 50% of cases.[9] On contrast-enhanced computed CT, the tumor enhances in a heterogeneous fashion and may be hyperdense compared with liver parenchyma in the early arterial postcontrast phase; it usually is isodense or hypodense on delayed images. Peripheral enhancement can be seen. CT angiography can help define vascular invasion when present and assess its potential to be resected.

On MRI, epithelial-type hepatoblastomas are homogeneously hypointense on T1-weighted images and hyperintense on T2-weighted images relative to adjacent liver, and they enhance after intravenous (IV) administration of gadolinium contrast material.[9] Mixed-type tumors show more heterogeneous signal intensity. However, areas of calcification, necrosis, hemorrhage, and septation may influence the signal intensity.[9-11] Hemorrhage is most often hyperintense on T1-weighted images and bands of fibrosis or septation are hypointense on T1- and T2-weighted sequences.[9] Vascular invasion is demonstrated with gradient-echo sequences; tumor thrombus appears as a high signal on T1-weighted images and as a signal void on gradient-echo images. On postgadolinium arterial and venous phase images, the tumor thrombus enhances and shows a filling defect, respectively. MR angiography is useful for preoperative evaluation of the relationship of the tumor to the hepatic vasculature.

Hepatic scintigraphy currently is not performed in persons with a hepatoblastoma but may demonstrate increased activity on the initial angiographic phase as a result of tumor vascularity and photopenia on the delayed images. Rarely, increased uptake of the radiopharmaceutical agent may be seen on delayed images, which is a finding more typical of focal nodular hyperplasia. Currently, catheter angiography is rarely performed and usually shows tumor hypervascularity except in avascular areas of necrosis.[9-11]

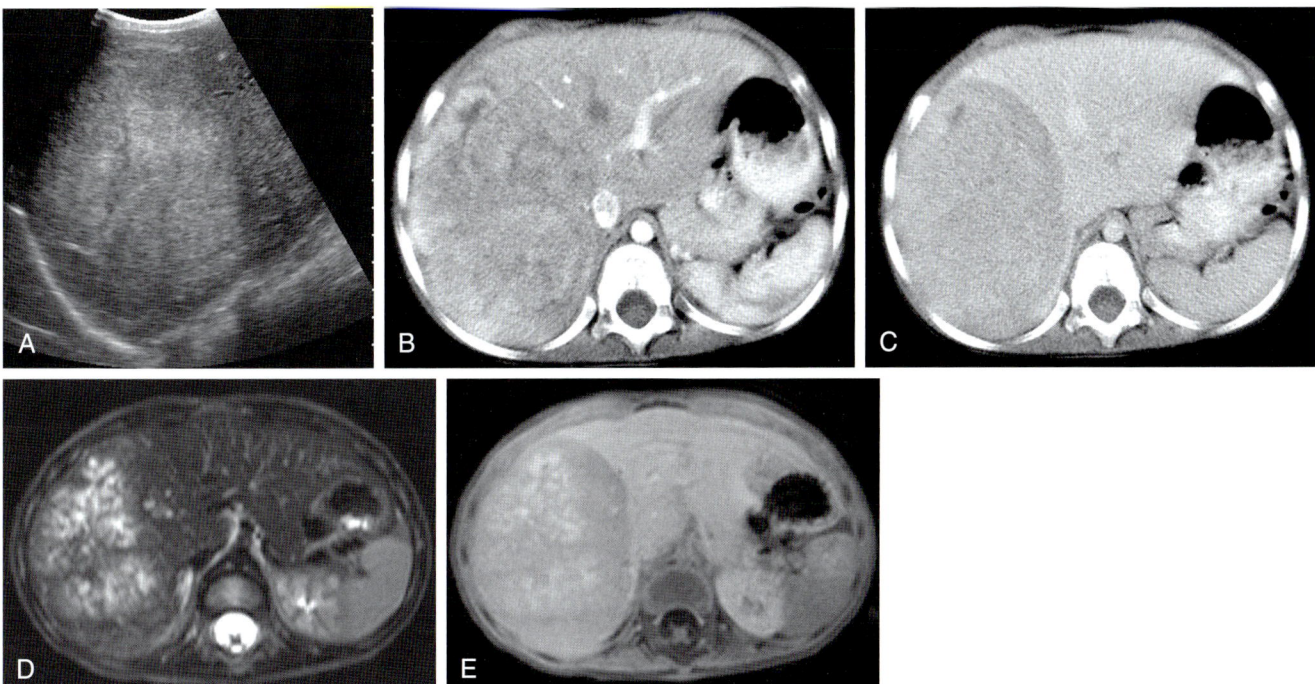

Figure 92-1 Hepatoblastoma. **A,** A longitudinal abdominal sonogram in a 3-year-old boy shows a well-defined lesion that is hyperechoic relative to the liver. **B,** A computed tomography (CT) scan in the early arterial postcontrast phase demonstrates a heterogeneous mass that is hyperdense compared with the liver. **C,** A CT scan in the delayed contrast phase shows a hypodense lesion. **D,** An axial T2-weighted magnetic resonance (MR) image shows hyperintense nodules with intervening hypointense septa. **E,** An axial T1-weighted MR image after intravenous administration of gadolinium demonstrates enhancement of the septa and capsule.

Treatment The treatment for hepatoblastoma is surgical resection. However, in about 40% to 60% of cases, the tumor cannot be resected at diagnosis.[12] Initial treatment with chemotherapy permits up to 85% of these tumors to become resectable.[3] The overall survival rate is reported to be 65% to 70%.[1,9-11] Imaging is crucial for assessment of the surgical resectability of hepatoblastomas at presentation and after the patient undergoes chemotherapy. Disseminated tumors have been treated successfully with chemotherapy and multiple resections of metastases. Radiofrequency ablation may be a promising treatment for recurrence.[13] Liver transplantation can be useful in lesions that are considered unresectable; the presence of pulmonary metastases is not considered an absolute contraindication to liver transplantation because of their sensitivity to chemotherapy.[9] Poor prognostic factors include AFP levels less than 100 ng/mL or more than 1,000,000 ng/mL, vascular invasion, and aneuploid nuclear content. Factors associated with favorable prognosis include single lobe involvement, pure fetal histologic composition, and AFP levels between 100 and 1,000,000 ng/mL.[9]

HEPATOCELLULAR CARCINOMA

Overview HCC, the second most common liver tumor in children after hepatoblastoma, accounts for 35% of primary pediatric hepatic malignancies.[14] It affects two age peaks in childhood: 4 to 5 years and (more commonly) 12 to 14 years. HCCs, like hepatoblastoma, occur more often in the right than in the left lobe of the liver and demonstrate a high propensity for vascular invasion, which is seen in approximately 75% of cases. Neoplastic cells vary from very

well-differentiated to poorly differentiated. The most helpful histologic feature in distinguishing HCC from metastases is the presence of bile canaliculi or bile pigment.[1] Kupffer cells also may be present.[9]

Etiology In nonendemic areas of the world, approximately half of HCCs arise in patients with underlying liver disease. Predisposing conditions include entities leading to cirrhosis, such as biliary atresia, infantile cholestasis, Alagille syndrome, hemochromatosis, hereditary tyrosinemia, glycogen storage disorder, α_1-antitrypsin deficiency, Wilson disease, galactosemia, and viral hepatitis (hepatitis B and C).

Clinical Presentation The clinical symptoms and presentation are similar to those of hepatoblastoma, in that patients often present with an abdominal mass, abdominal pain, fever, and cachexia. The serum AFP level is markedly elevated in 70% of patients.[14,15]

Imaging HCCs have three main growth patterns: solitary, multifocal, and diffuse/infiltrative.[9] The ultrasound findings of HCC are variable. With respect to liver parenchyma, smaller lesions may be isoechoic or hyperechoic, although most tend to be hypoechoic[9,10]; larger lesions are heterogeneous. Internal areas of increased echogenicity may represent acute hemorrhage, fat, or calcifications (which is less common than in hepatoblastoma), whereas areas of decreased echogenicity may represent necrosis. If a capsule is present, it may be detected as a thin halo of decreased echogenicity. Doppler demonstrates high-velocity arterial flow and is useful for identifying vascular invasion by showing blood flow within the substance of tumoral thrombus.[9]

On unenhanced CT, an HCC appears as a solitary mass or as multiple well-defined or poorly defined, hypointense to isodense masses.[10] The tumor shows variable enhancement after IV administration of contrast material and may contain low-attenuation regions of necrosis. The tumor capsule may also show a rim of low attenuation on unenhanced images that enhances on the delayed phase after injection of contrast material (Fig. 92-3).[9] Vascular tumor thrombi may be seen as intraluminal filling defects with a surrounding meniscus of contrast and can be better evaluated with angiographic sequences. When the tumor arises in a cirrhotic liver, differentiation from regenerating nodules may be difficult.

With MRI, the tumor typically is slightly hyperintense on T2-weighted images and hypointense on T1-weighted images, although the latter presentation tends to be more variable; hyperintense areas of fat or hemorrhage may be seen on T1-weighted images. If a fibrous pseudocapsule is present, MRI shows low signal intensity on T1- and T2-weighted pulse sequences.[16] After administration of gadolinium, in the early arterial phase, the lesion demonstrates enhancement and washes out with relatively low signal intensity during the portal venous phase. Vascular invasion appears as lack of a signal on spin-echo images and as an intravascular arterial enhancing mass with a delayed filling defect on dynamic gadolinium-enhanced images.[17]

Nuclear scintigraphy is rarely performed in patients with HCC and usually shows decreased uptake. Gallium scans, however, are characteristic and may help distinguish HCC, which is gallium-avid, from regenerating nodules, which are not gallium-avid. Fluorodeoxyglucose (FDG) positron emission tomography (PET) is useful in evaluating the degree of tumor differentiation. FDG uptake is variable in HCCs; uptake may be normal in well-differentiated tumors, with markedly elevated uptake usually seen in poorly differentiated tumors. FDG-PET may be useful in the staging of HCC or in distinguishing regenerating nodules in cirrhotic livers from HCC. Combining FDG-PET and gallium scintigraphy can be worthwhile when grading tumors.[18] For example, low-grade tumors typically show normal uptake on PET and increased uptake on gallium scans. However, gallium uptake also is seen in other processes, such as metastatic disease (lymphoma) and hepatic adenoma.

Treatment The treatment for HCC is complete surgical resection when possible, but approximately two thirds of children present with unresectable tumors as a result of multifocal or massive involvement of the liver, major vascular involvement, or metastases. HCC is relatively insensitive to systemic chemotherapy.[19] The impact of chemotherapy is unclear, with no evidence that it offers additional benefit in children with resectable localized HCC. Liver transplantation has been reported for an unresectable tumor but remains controversial.[14] Radiofrequency ablation and intraarterial chemotherapy have been reported, but the benefits require further investigation.[20,21] The prognosis is variable and is directly related to the resectability and histology of the lesion.

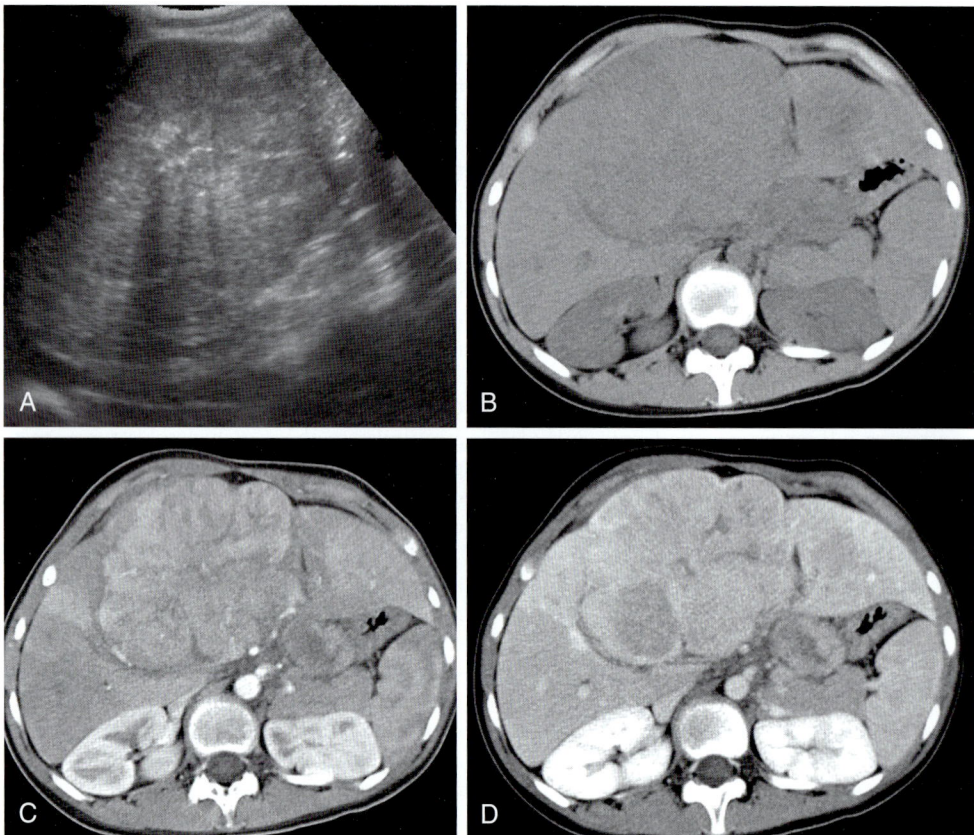

Figure 92-3 Hepatocellular carcinoma in a 14-year-old girl without underlying liver disease. **A,** An abdominal sonogram shows a heterogeneous hepatic lesion. **B,** An unenhanced computed tomography scan demonstrates the liver mass, with slightly decreased attenuation compared with adjacent normal liver parenchyma. Postcontrast arterial (**C**) and venous phase (**D**) images show enhancement during the arterial phase, which decreases during the venous phase. After administration of contrast material, the tumor margins are more conspicuous.

In tumors with favorable histology and complete resection, the 2-year survival rate may exceed 97%. However, without complete resection and with unfavorable histology, the 2-year survival rate may be less than 20%.[14] In places where the prevalence of tyrosinemia is especially high, routine neonatal screening and immediate treatment of positive cases by 2-(2-nitro-4-3 trifluoromethylbenzoyl)-1,3-cyclohexanedione (NTBC) have resulted in marked decrease in the prevalence of HCC in this population.[22] In Quebec, where the prevalence of tyrosinemia is especially high, routine neonatal screening and immediate treatment of positive cases with NTBC have resulted in 100% prevention of subsequent HCC to date in patients treated at birth. However, patients with delayed diagnosis who are treated with NTBC are at risk of having HCC develop.

FIBROLAMELLAR CARCINOMA

Overview Fibrolamellar carcinoma (FLC) is a variant of HCC that occurs in patients without underlying hepatic disease. It has distinctive clinical and pathologic features and represents approximately 5% to 8% of all cases of HCC. FLC tends to occur in younger patients, with a peak in the late teens; approximately 85% of patients with FLC are younger than 35 years, and it may be diagnosed in children as young as 10 years. The incidence is similar in males and females.[23]

Etiology The etiology of FLC is unknown. It has been reported in association with syndromes, including Wilms, Carney, Fanconi anemia, and familial adenomatous polyposis; these associations have been implicated in shared molecular pathways. FLC also has been associated with FNH, but currently evidence does not support such an association.[23]

Clinical Presentation Clinically, patients present with abdominal symptoms or pain and sometimes a palpable mass. Uncommon presentations are gynecomastia, jaundice, and venous compression or thrombosis.[9] Metastatic lymphadenopathy is seen in 70% of cases.[24] AFP levels generally are normal.[16] In 80% to 90% of patients, the gross pathological appearance is one of a large, circumscribed, and nonencapsulated mass.[16] Other patterns can be seen, including satellite lesions, multiple diffuse masses, or a bilobed mass. Fibrous tissue within a central scar is common (appearing in 30% of cases) and typically does not enhance after administration of contrast material. Calcifications are seen in 35% to 55% of tumors and are localized in the central scar.[16]

Imaging Plain radiographs may demonstrate hepatomegaly or calcifications. Ultrasound shows a well-defined mass with heterogeneous echo texture and isoechoic or hyperechoic areas.[25] If it is present, the central scar appears hyperechoic and may contain shadowing hyperechoic calcifications.

CT shows a hypoattenuating, well-defined, lobulated mass with calcifications in 30% to 55% of cases and a central scar in 45% to 60% of cases (Fig. 92-4). Adjacent lymphadenopathy often is present in the hepatic hilum at diagnosis. After IV injection of contrast material, in the early arterial phase, the tumor is hyperattenuating relative to the adjacent liver with variable attenuation during the portal venous phase. The central scar is hypoattenuating with little or no enhancement on CT.

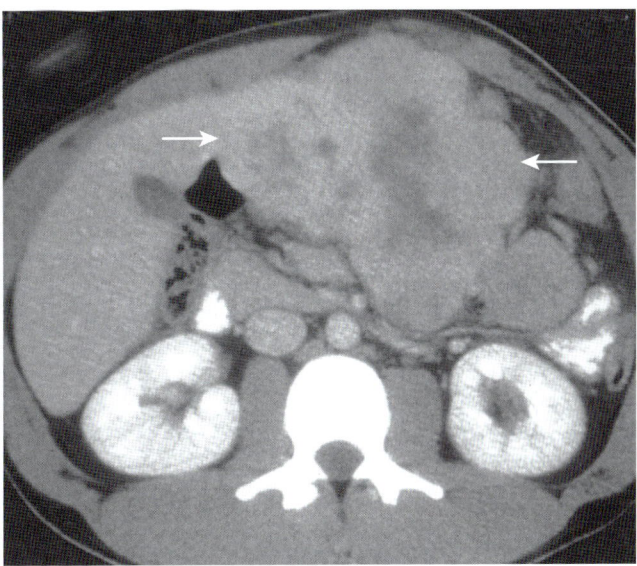

Figure 92-4 Fibrolamellar carcinoma in an 18-year-old girl. Axial contrast-enhanced computed tomography shows a lobulated mass (*arrows*) in the left lobe of the liver with a hypoattenuating central scar.

On T1-weighted MRI, the tumor is hypointense (86%) to isointense (14%), and it is slightly hyperintense (85%) to isointense (15%) on T2-weighted images. The fibrous scar is hypointense on T1-weighted images and hypointense on T2-weighted images, and it does usually not enhance after IV administration of contrast material.[9,11,15,25,26] These features are useful in distinguishing FLC from FNH, in which the central scar has increased signal on T2-weighted sequences and enhances with IV administration of contrast material.

Treatment The primary treatment of FLC is surgical resection, with surgical resectability considered to be the most important prognostic factor.[25] However, when the tumor is not resectable, orthotopic liver transplantation, systemic chemotherapy, or hepatic intraarterial chemoembolization is considered. Recent literature reports no significant difference in the prognosis of FLC compared with HCC in patients without underlying hepatic disease.[23,24] Normal hepatic function, younger age, absence of vascular invasion or thrombosis, lack of lymphadenopathy, and negative surgical margins are favorable prognostic indicators. The 5-year survival rate ranges from 30% to 67%.[20,21,23,24]

UNDIFFERENTIATED EMBRYONAL SARCOMA

Overview Undifferentiated embryonal sarcoma, previously called malignant mesenchymoma, embryonal sarcoma, or fibromyxosarcoma, is a rare, aggressive tumor of mesenchymal origin. Most commonly, the tumor affects children around 6 to 10 years of age with a slight male predominance.[27] In one review, this was the third most common malignant pediatric liver tumor, following hepatoblastoma and HCC.[28]

Etiology The etiology of undifferentiated embryonal sarcoma is uncertain. It has been linked to mesenchymal hamartoma as its malignant counterpart,[3,15] and some tumors have been reported to arise in a background of mesenchymal hamartoma.[29] On histology, an undifferentiated embryonal sarcoma shows primitive spindle-shaped, sarcomatous satellite cells closely packed in sheets or whorls and scattered throughout a background of loose myxoid tissue, which contains foci of hematopoiesis in 50% of cases.[27]

Clinical Presentation   The most common presenting symptoms include an abdominal mass, pain, and discomfort. An undifferentiated embryonal sarcoma usually is large at presentation, is solitary, involves the right lobe of the liver (in 75% of cases), and is predominantly solid with occasional cystic, necrotic, or hemorrhagic areas.[27] AFP levels are normal.[15]

Imaging   Plain radiographs show a large, typically noncalcified mass. On sonography, the tumor is solid and isoechoic to hyperechoic relative to normal liver with small anechoic spaces that correspond to necrosis, hemorrhage, or cystic degeneration.[27,30]

On CT, the tumor reveals predominantly water attenuation correlating with myxoid stroma (88% of tumor volume) (e-Fig. 92-5).[9,27] After administration of IV contrast material, a dense enhancing peripheral rim can be seen in relation to the pseudocapsule. Uncommon hyperattenuation regions may indicate hemorrhage and calcifications.

With MRI, the tumor shows low signal intensity on T1-weighted sequences and increased signal intensity on T2-weighted sequences (Fig. 92-6). A hypointense rim on T1- and T2-weighted images indicates a pseudocapsule. Bright areas on T1-weighted images correspond to regions of hemorrhage. Fluid levels, internal debris, and septa may be seen on T2-weighted images.[27,30] Heterogeneous enhancement of the tumor is seen after IV administration of gadolinium contrast material.[31] MRI permits excellent evaluation of tumor resectability, vascular invasion, and involvement of adjacent lymph nodes. Metastases usually are to the lungs and bone.

Treatment   Treatment consists of complete tumor resection. As late as three decades ago, the prognosis was poor, with death occurring within 12 months in many cases.[28] However, more recent reports of multimodal treatment show markedly improved survival rates. Patients with unresectable tumors that are not responsive to chemotherapy can be treated with liver transplantation.[9]

RHABDOMYOSARCOMA OF THE BILIARY TREE

Overview   Although rhabdomyosarcoma can be found throughout the body, involvement of the biliary ducts is one of the rarest forms of this mesenchymal tumor. It occurs almost exclusively in the pediatric age group and often in children younger than 5 years (in 75% of cases).[9]

Etiology   The tumor arises from the biliary tree beneath the biliary epithelium, with which the tumor is invested,[32] and grows as a polypoid mass within the biliary tree. Only the embryonal subtype of rhabdomyosarcoma arises in the biliary tree.[9] The tumor most commonly involves major extrahepatic bile ducts but can arise within the intrahepatic bile ducts, gallbladder, and cystic duct. Histologically, rhabdomyosarcoma demonstrates undifferentiated blue cells with scant cytoplasm and primitive nuclei that form a firm, lobulated mass with infiltrative margins and a well-defined pseudocapsule.[6,9,12,33]

Clinical Presentation   Jaundice, the most frequent manifestation, can be associated with abdominal distention, pain, nausea, vomiting, or fever. Elevated levels of conjugated bilirubin and alkaline phosphatase with normal levels of AFP are typical of the laboratory workup. At diagnosis, metastases are present in 30% of cases[9] and typically appear in the lung, appendicular skeleton, skull, and pericardium, although the tumor has a greater propensity to invade contiguous structures.[32] The clinical presentation may resemble that of hepatitis, which may lead to delay in obtaining diagnostic tests.[34]

Imaging   Multiplanar imaging demonstrates a mass within the biliary ducts. The tumor most frequently involves the common bile duct, in or near the porta hepatis. In large lesions, necrosis can be seen. Ultrasound may reveal a solitary, heterogeneous, relatively hypoechoic mass or multiple hypoechoic nodules associated with biliary duct dilation and intraductal extension.[9,35] Portal vein displacement without thrombosis is common.[35] CT shows a homogeneous or heterogeneous hypoattenuating or hyperattenuating intraductal mass with variable contrast enhancement associated with biliary dilatation (Fig. 92-7).[35,36] MRI usually shows low signal intensity on T1-weighted sequences and high signal intensity on T2-weighted sequences, with intense, heterogeneous enhancement after IV administration of contrast material.[9,35] Magnetic resonance cholangiopancreatography often demonstrates a partially cystic lesion in the common bile duct and a mass adjacent to the duct causing mural irregularity. Percutaneous cholangiography displays an intraluminal polypoid mass.[35-37] Gallium uptake can help localize metastatic disease.[35]

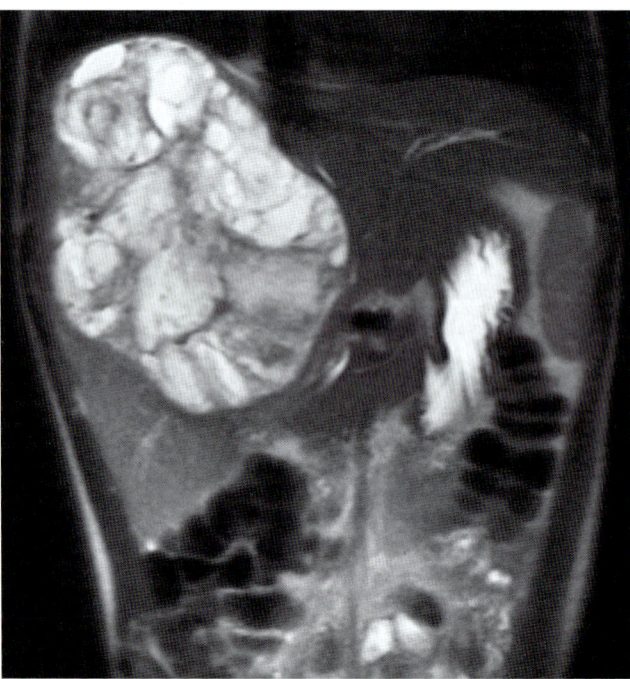

Figure 92-6   Undifferentiated embryonal sarcoma in a 13-year-old girl. A coronal T2-weighted magnetic resonance image shows a multiloculated mass of heterogeneous but predominantly high signal intensity in the right lobe of the liver. (Courtesy Lynn Fordham, MD.)

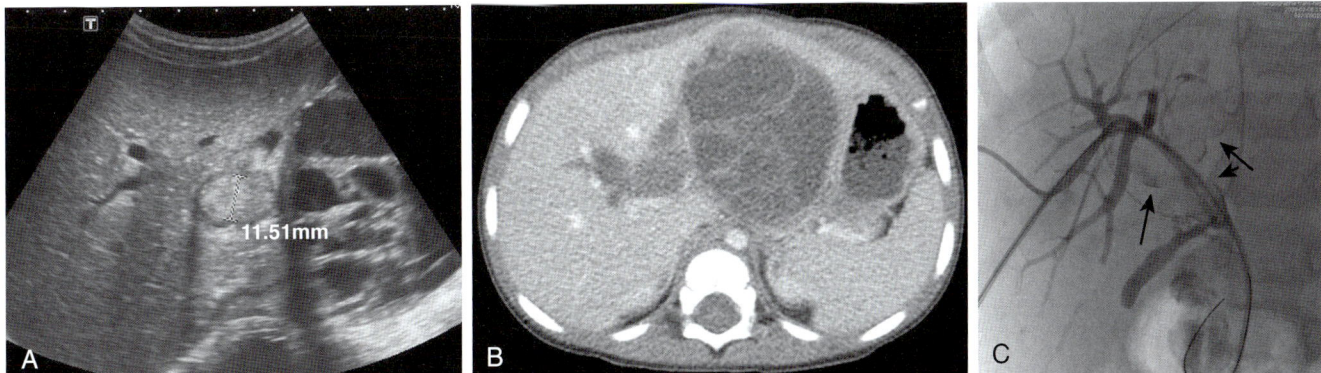

Figure 92-7 Embryonal rhabdomyosarcoma in a 20-month-old boy. **A,** A transverse sonogram shows a multicystic lesion with a mass in the biliary tree (measured). **B,** A computed tomography scan shows the hypoattenuating tumor in the common bile duct extending into the intrahepatic and extrahepatic bile ducts. **C,** Percutaneous cholangiography reveals multiple filling defect of the common bile duct (*short arrow*) with extension in the intrahepatic bile ducts (*long arrows*).

Treatment Multimodal therapy, including surgical resection, radiation, and chemotherapy, has improved outcome, with 78% survival in cases of local disease.[38] Concurrent internal or external biliary drainage is essential because some chemotherapeutic agents depend on hepatobiliary excretion, and the inability to excrete the agent may result in significant systemic toxicity.[38]

ANGIOSARCOMA

Overview Angiosarcoma is a rare, aggressive, malignant vascular tumor that generally develops after the first year of life. Histologically, the spindle cell form is especially common in children.[33,39] Immunohistochemical studies demonstrate reactivity of tumor cells to factor VIII–related antigen, CD31, and CD34, confirming the vascular nature of the tumor.[40]

Etiology Angiosarcoma typically presents in adults who have a history of exposure to thorium dioxide (Thorotrast), arsenic, and vinyl chloride[9,39]; however, as exposure to these toxins becomes rarer, some of these tumors arise de novo in adults with cirrhosis or are associated with hemochromatosis or the use of anabolic steroids. As a result, this tumor is considered the "quintessential example of malignant transformation secondary to environmental exposures."[41,42] In children, the tumors are very rare and typically arise without a history of exposure. Cases of the tumor arising in children with previously diagnosed infantile hemangioendotheliomas have been reported (e-Fig. 92-8).[39,43]

Clinical Presentation Clinical symptoms include hepatomegaly associated with pain, anorexia, and weight loss, as well as thrombocytopenia and consumptive coagulopathy.[42] At the time of diagnosis, 60% of cases have metastatic disease, most commonly to the lungs and spleen.[41,42]

Imaging Imaging findings are variable and depend on the patterns at presentation such as a localized mass versus a multifocal or diffuse lesion (see e-Fig. 92-8).

On ultrasound, the lesion is heterogeneous and the echogenicity varies depending on the amount of hemorrhage or necrosis. With CT, nodules hypoattenuate compared with normal liver. In the presence of hemorrhage, hyperattenuating foci can occur. Contrast enhancement is variable, often showing a centripetal enhancement pattern similar to hepatic venous malformations (formerly and inappropriately called "cavernous hemangiomas").[41,44] At MRI, the masses show low signal intensity relative to the liver on T1-weighted images with hyperintense foci (related to hemorrhage) and heterogeneous signal intensity on T2-weighted images. Dynamic MRI with contrast reveals a heterogenous pattern of enhancement.[42] FDG-PET/CT displays marked uptake in the tumors and is helpful for detection of metastases.

Prognosis The prognosis is dismal, with a rapid deterioration of the patients within 6 months from the diagnosis, regardless of treatment.[9,40,41]

CHOLANGIOCARCINOMA

Cholangiocarcinoma is a rare hepatic neoplasm accounting for fewer than 1% of all carcinomas. This neoplasm may complicate disorders that affect children, such as choledochal cysts and sclerosing cholangitis, but it usually occurs late in the disease process and thus presents mainly in adults.

HEPATIC METASTASES

Hepatic metastases in children usually are the result of neuroblastoma, lymphoma, leukemia, and Wilms tumor. The appearance of hepatic metastatic disease is highly variable, ranging from one or more focal lesions to a diffuse infiltrative pattern with loss of normal hepatic architecture, which most often is seen in children with neuroblastoma. Most discrete hepatic metastases are multiple, are hypoechoic on sonography, have low attenuation on CT with a tendency toward peripheral enhancement, and are hypointense on T1-weighted MRI and hyperintense on T2-weighted MRI.

Wilms tumor metastases most commonly are found in the lungs and adjacent lymph nodes. Hematogenous spread of Wilms tumor to the liver occurs in 15% of cases; however, the primary renal lesion often is very large at presentation, and if it arises from the right kidney, it may abut the liver, rendering direct hepatic invasion by the primary mass difficult to exclude with certainty. Most hepatic metastatic lesions

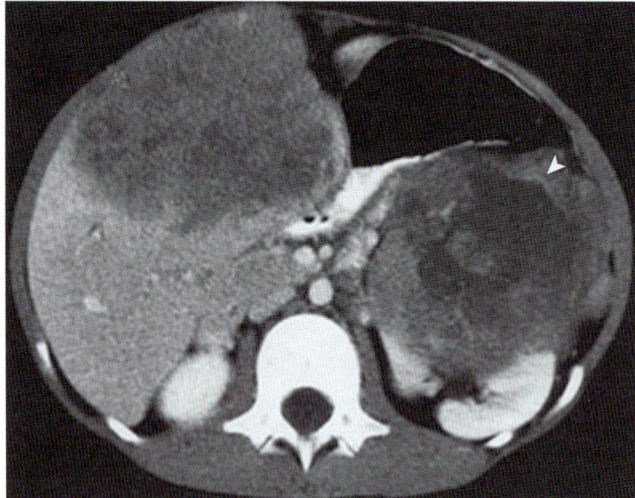

Figure 92-9 Metastatic Wilms tumor in a 4-year-old boy with clinical evidence of hepatomegaly. A postcontrast computed tomography image demonstrates heterogeneous enhancement within a hepatic metastasis from a Wilms tumor arising in the left kidney (*arrowhead*).

attributed to Wilms tumor are hematogenous and tend to be multifocal and heterogeneously enhancing; central necrosis, calcifications, or vascular invasion may be identified (Fig. 92-9).[44,45]

Neuroblastoma may present with metastatic spread to bone, regional lymph nodes, liver, brain, and lungs. Metastatic neuroblastoma to the liver has two typical patterns: (1) numerous discrete lesions of variable echogenicity, attenuation, and enhancement; and (2) diffuse infiltration with distortion of the normal hepatic architecture, leading to hepatomegaly (Fig. 92-10). The latter pattern is especially common with stage IV-S disease (a primary lesion limited to the organ of origin or a primary lesion with regional spread but without extension across the midline, along with involvement of the liver, skin, or bone marrow).

Leukemia often involves the liver at autopsy but typically is not visible with imaging. Lymphoma may present with

multiple discrete lesions or an infiltrative pattern similar to that of neuroblastoma. In addition, lymphoma often is associated with lymphadenopathy and splenic lesions.

Benign Hepatic Neoplasms

LIVER HEMANGIOMA

Overview   The International Society for the Study of Vascular Anomalies (ISSVA) has adopted terminology to address the classification of vascular anomalies, based on the classification by Mulliken and Glowacki proposed in 1982.[46] In this classification, vascular anomalies are divided into vascular tumors (exhibiting cellular proliferation and hyperplasia) and vascular malformations (lesions that arise by dysmorphogenesis and exhibit normal endothelial turnover).[47]

Despite these changes and recent literature,[47-49] improper terminology still in use leads to inappropriate description of findings in imaging studies and at times to misdiagnosis of vascular anomalies. For instance, in adults the term "liver hemangioma" continues to be erroneously applied instead of "venous malformation." According to the ISSVA classification, the proper name for liver vascular tumors in children is "liver hemangioma."

Liver hemangiomas are classified as infantile and congenital. Infantile hemangiomas usually begin growing after birth, although some are present at birth; they typically grow during the first year of life, enter an involuting phase between 1 and 7 years, and have an involuted phase between 8 and 12 years. Infantile hemangiomas are positive for glucose transporter-1 protein (Glut-1), a protein that facilitates the transport of glucose across erythrocyte cell membranes. Congenital hemangiomas are fully developed at birth and are characterized by Glut-1 negativity. Congenital hemangiomas in turn are subdivided into a rapidly involuting group, which involute more rapidly than infantile hemangiomas (usually within 12-14 months of age),[50] and a noninvoluting group, with some overlap between these groups.[47,50] The vascular tumors that appear most frequently in infancy are infantile hemangiomas. The differentiation among these tumors may be impossible at initial diagnosis because (1) there is no biopsy in most instances to identify the Glut-1 marker, and (2) contrary to skin lesions, it usually is not known whether the hepatic lesion is present and fully developed at birth. Infantile hemangioma is the most frequently occurring pediatric tumor, affecting 4% to 5% of infants.[47] Other vascular tumors seen in the pediatric age group include hemangioendotheliomas, tufted angiomas, and sarcomas.

A discussion of hemangiomas is not complete without a reference to vascular malformations. Vascular malformations are classified as slow-flow and high-flow lesions. Slow-flow lesions include capillary malformations, venous malformations, lymphatic malformations, capillary-venous malformations, and capillary-lymphatic-venous malformations. High-flow lesions include arteriovenous fistula and arteriovenous malformations. Complex-combined malformations are found in several syndromes: Klippel-Trenaunay, Parkes-Weber, blue rubber bleb, Proteus, and Maffucci.

Etiology   Hemangioma is a model of the angiogenesis concept proposed by Folkman et al.,[51] and its development is related to a combination of upregulation of factors that promote

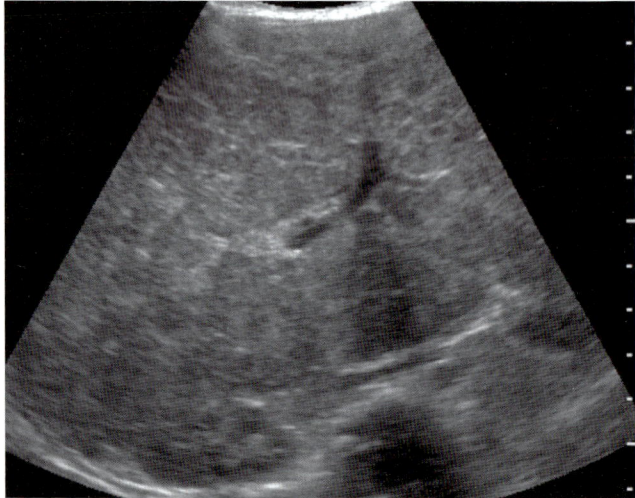

Figure 92-10 Metastatic infiltrative neuroblastoma in an 8-month-old boy with hepatomegaly. A transverse sonogram reveals loss of normal hepatic architecture with numerous discrete lesions of variable echogenicity.

angiogenesis and downregulation of its inhibitors. The trigger for this abnormal angiogenesis is unknown, although a viral cause and a somatic mutation have been postulated.[47]

Clinical Presentation Infantile hemangiomas occur more commonly in girls, with a female to male ratio of 3-5:1, and they are more common in fair-skinned individuals. Most liver hemangiomas are clinically silent and remain undetected. Others are discovered on prenatal ultrasound or postnatal imaging that is performed for various reasons. Even though most liver hemangiomas are asymptomatic, life-threatening complications may occur, especially in the setting of multifocal lesions or congestive heart failure related to an intralesional shunt, hypothyroidism resulting from overproduction of type III iodothyronine deiodinase, fulminant hepatic failure, and/or abdominal compartment syndrome. In some patients with liver hemangioma, consumptive coagulopathy may develop as a result of intralesional thrombosis, hemorrhage, and hemolysis.[52,53]

Liver hemangiomas may present as focal (Fig. 92-11), multifocal (e-Fig. 92-12), or diffuse lesions.[52] Focal lesions, which often are found at birth in asymptomatic children, can be associated with mild thrombocytopenia and anemia. They often occur in the absence of skin hemangioma. The Glut-1 marker is negative. This focal liver hemangioma likely corresponds to the cutaneous rapidly involuting congenital hemangioma, which characteristically regresses in an accelerated fashion by 12 to 14 months.[54-56]

Imaging On ultrasound, a well-defined hypoechoic or hyperechoic lesion is seen. The echotexture is sometimes heterogeneous, related to the central hemorrhage or necrosis.

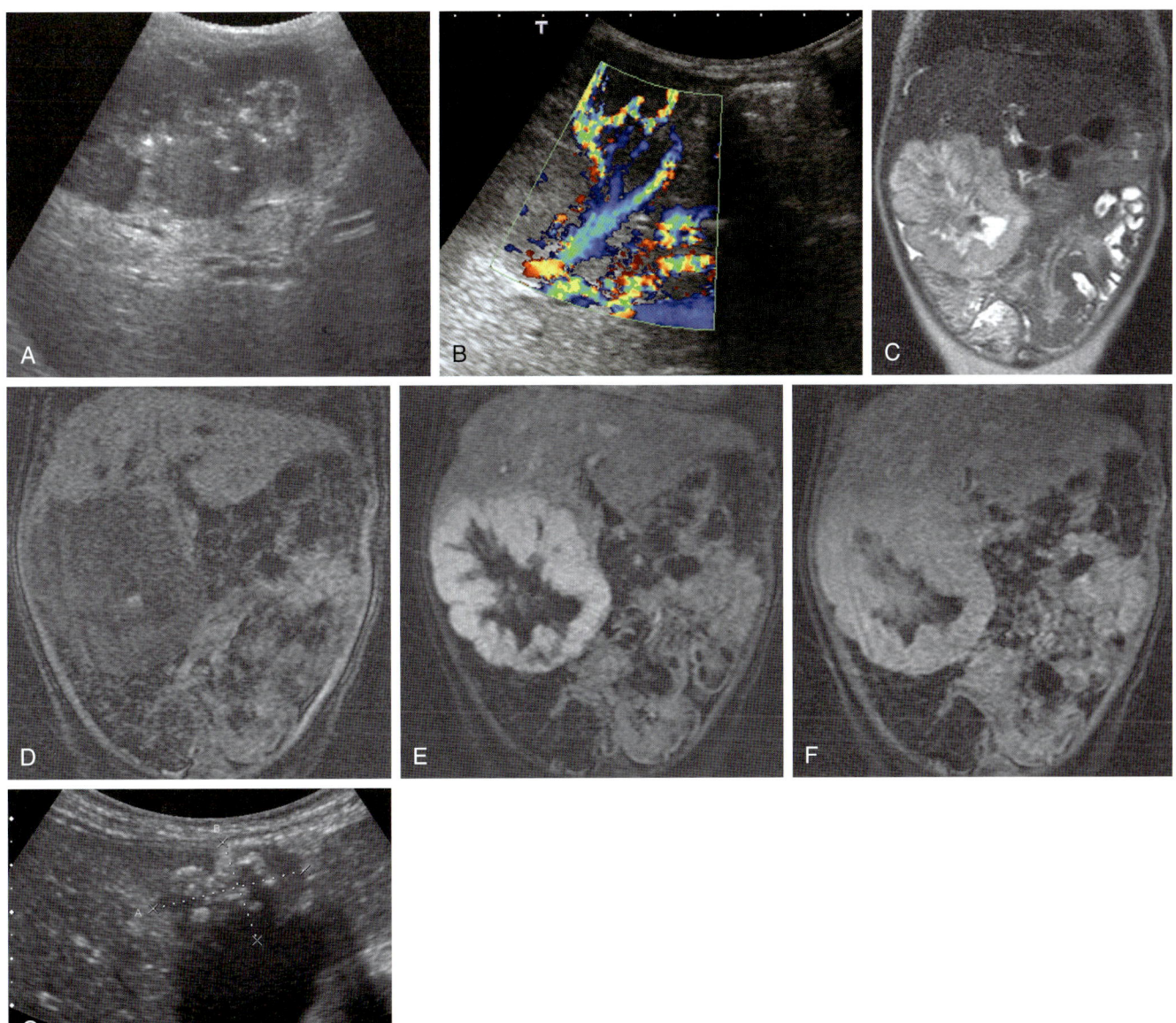

Figure 92-11 Liver hemangioma. **A,** A 2-month-old girl with an abdominal mass. Ultrasound imaging shows a well-defined hypoechoic lesion with hyperechoic calcifications. **B,** Color Doppler ultrasound demonstrates a hypervascular lesion. **C,** A coronal T2-weighted magnetic resonance (MR) image reveals a well-defined hyperintense and heterogeneous lesion without peripheral edema. Dynamic gadolinium MR imaging before administration of contrast material (**D**) and at 1 minute (**E**) and 10 minutes (**F**) shows centripetal enhancement with central necrosis and calcifications. **G,** Eighteen months later, ultrasound imaging reveals calcifications with significant regression of the lesion.

Color Doppler ultrasound demonstrates a variety of flow patterns depending on the presence of microshunts, portosystemic, or arteriovenous shunts, and on the stage of the lesion. These shunts are clinically significant when they are associated with cardiac failure.

On MRI, the lesion is well defined, solitary, hypointense on T1-weighted images, and hyperintense on T2-weighted images, without peripheral edema. After administration of gadolinium contrast material, the tumor shows centripetal enhancement and may contain internal vascular flow voids.[46] Heterogeneous signal is seen on all sequences if hemorrhage, thrombosis, and/or necrosis are present. Calcifications may occur in about 16% of cases.

Multifocal lesions frequently are associated with multiple cutaneous infantile hemangiomas with a Glut-1 positive marker.[54-56] Many of these lesions are asymptomatic; however, depending on the presence of arteriovenous or portosystemic shunts, cardiac failure may supervene and require treatment.

On ultrasound, small multifocal lesions are homogeneous and most are hypoechoic, although hyperechoic nodules may occur. The hepatic arteries and veins generally appear to be enlarged. Large feeding arteries and draining veins are seen in and around the vascular tumors. Direct arteriovenous or portosystemic venous shunts may occur.

On MRI, multiple nodular tumors present with T1 hypointense and T2 hyperintense signal, as well as homogeneous enhancement after injection of gadolinium contrast material. Flow voids are seen within and/or adjacent to the lesions as a result of large hepatic arteries or veins. Aortic tapering distal to the celiac trunk is a good indicator of increased hepatic flow and accordingly is a predictor of cardiac overload risk.[52]

Diffuse lesions present with extensive hepatic involvement, with the numerous small lesions in the liver leading to severe hepatomegaly and abdominal compartment syndrome, hypothyroidism due to overproduction of type III iodothyronine deiodinase that deactivates thyroid hormone, cardiac failure, and mental retardation.[53] Despite the size of the lesion, most diffuse liver hemangiomas show no cardiac failure in relation to the shunt. The enlarged infiltrated liver reveals numerous hypoechoic lesions. MRI findings are similar to those of the focal and multifocal lesions.

Treatment Symptomatic liver hemangiomas have been treated with corticosteroids followed by interferon-α-2a or vincristine. Recently, propranolol has demonstrated excellent efficacy as a first-line treatment for life-threatening soft tissue infantile hemangioma. More time is needed to determine the efficacy of this drug in liver hemangiomas. Catheter embolization in association with medical treatment is recommended for patients with cardiac failure related to arteriovenous or portosystemic shunts.[57] In patients with diffuse lesions, medical treatment is recommended, including the treatment of hypothyroidism. In selected instances, a liver transplant may be contemplated.

MESENCHYMAL HAMARTOMA

Overview Mesenchymal hamartoma is the second most common benign liver mass in children after vascular tumors. Most of them are discovered by 5 years of age.[3,58,59] Mesenchymal hamartomas affect boys slightly more often than girls

and have been diagnosed on prenatal ultrasound. Histologically, they are composed of disordered, primitive, fluid-filled mesenchyma, hepatic parenchyma, and bile ducts, in addition to stromal cysts of variable size without a capsule. Sampling of the hepatocyte component can generate confusion with hepatoblastoma.[60]

Etiology It is postulated that a mesenchymal hamartoma arises from primitive mesenchymal tissues through a developmental aberration of excessive and uncoordinated proliferation during embryogenesis.[59] Mesenchymal hamartoma generally is considered a congenital lesion related to a developmental anomaly. However, recent reports demonstrate balanced translocations at 19q13.4 and aneuploidy in some cases, suggesting that a mesenchymal hamartoma may represent a true neoplasm.[29,58,61]

Clinical Presentation The most common clinical presentation is painless abdominal distention. AFP levels are normal. The mass may be pedunculated and attached to the inferior surface of the liver.

Imaging On ultrasound and CT, mesenchymal hamartomas typically are multicystic, heterogeneous masses with septa of variable thickness (Fig. 92-13). When the cysts are tiny, the lesion is hyperechoic and simulates a solid lesion. Low-level echoes may be seen within the fluid related to gelatinous contents or hemorrhage. On CT, mesenchymal hamartomas are complex cystic masses. Their septations and solid components enhance after IV administration of contrast material. On MRI, the cystic regions are hypointense on T1-weighted images and hyperintense on T2-weighted images. The signal intensity varies, depending on the stromal content, the amount of protein within the cyst fluid, and the presence or absence of hemorrhage within the cyst. Septa and solid portions of the lesion usually are of decreased signal on T1- and T2-weighted images, with enhancement of septa and solid components.[10,11,62-64]

Treatment The treatment for mesenchymal hamartoma is surgical resection. Observation of mesenchymal hamartoma is not recommended because of rare reports of malignant transformation to undifferentiated embryonal sarcoma.[65,66] Long-term survival is reported at 90% even with incomplete resection.[3,59]

FOCAL NODULAR HYPERPLASIA

Overview FNH is a rare benign epithelial liver tumor that occurs more often in adults; approximately 7% of reported cases of FNH are in pediatric patients,[67] in whom the peak age at presentation is 2 to 5 years. FNH accounts for 2% of all primary pediatric hepatic tumors in children from birth to age 20 years with marked female predominance.[60] Histologically, FNH is composed of hepatocytes, Kupffer cells, radial fibrous septa with biliary epithelium unconnected to the biliary tree, and a central vascular scar. Foci of necrosis and hemorrhage are rare compared with hepatocellular adenoma.[6,60,67,68]

Etiology The etiology of FNH is not certain, but some investigators believe that FNH may represent a hyperplastic

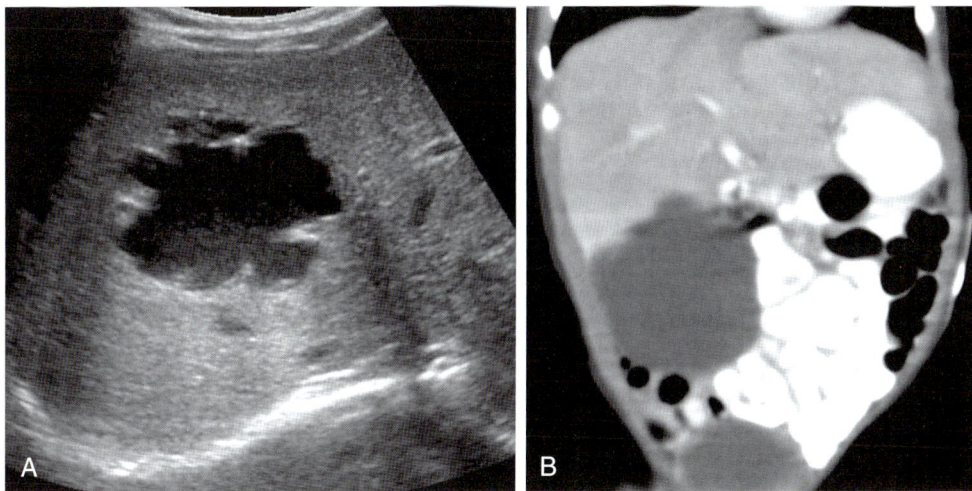

Figure 92-13   Mesenchymal hamartoma in a 1-week-old girl with a palpable abdominal mass. **A,** An axial sonogram demonstrates a well-defined, lobulated, hypoechoic mass with layering internal debris. **B,** A coronal reformat from a contrast-enhanced computed tomography image confirms the well-defined fluid attenuation lesion.

response to an underlying vascular malformation, as represented by the central scar, possibly related to vascular thrombosis, recanalization, and reperfusion.[60] Recent reports have noted the occurrence of FNH in oncologic patients, which is believed to be a manifestation of injury sustained to the vascular endothelium as a result of chemotherapy and/or radiotherapy.[69] Oral contraceptives and pregnancy are no longer considered risk factors for development of FNH.[67] FNH is most common in the right hepatic lobe and is multiple in 20% of cases.

Clinical Presentation   FNH is usually an incidental finding. Large lesions can present with an abdominal mass, as cited in approximately 20% of patients. Patients also may present with abdominal pain, rarely with tumor rupture or hemorrhage, because the lesion has a low tendency for hemorrhagic complications. No AFP elevation occurs.[6,9]

Imaging   On imaging, FNH is composed of a single, well-defined, often subcapsular mass with a characteristic vascular myxomatous central scar. However, atypical imaging features are common and necessitate multiple studies to obtain the diagnosis (Fig. 92-14).

On ultrasound, FNH is a well-defined homogeneous mass of variable echogenicity.[70] The central scar, which is seen in approximately 33% of cases on ultrasound, appears hyperechoic relative to the remaining mass.[67,70] On color Doppler ultrasound, increased blood flow is seen in the central scar extending to the periphery in a spoke-wheel pattern.[71,72] The flow has been reported as arterial, in contradistinction to intratumoral venous flow, as was seen in hepatic adenomas.[71]

On unenhanced CT, the mass and central scar are hypodense to isodense in comparison with the liver. A central scar is found in up to 60% of cases. After the administration of contrast material, the mass enhances brightly, with delayed enhancement and washes out of the central scar.[73]

On MRI, FNH is isointense to slightly hypointense to the liver on T1-weighted images and isointense to slightly hyperintense on T2-weighted images. The scar is hypointense on T1-weighted images and hyperintense on T2-weighted images. Dynamic IV gadolinium contrast imaging shows uniform enhancement, which is hyperintense during the arterial phase and isointense to slightly hyperintense on the delayed images, with either parallel or divergent enhancement of the central scar over time.[68,70,74] In contrast, the central scar in FLC does not enhance.[15] Hepatobiliary specific contrast agents, such as Eovist, also show arterial phase enhancement which persists for an extended period due to intralesional hepatocyte uptake and malformed bile ducts.

Only FNH contains sufficient Kupffer cells to cause normal to increased uptake on technetium-99m sulfur colloid scintigraphy, a finding that is nearly pathognomonic. Sulfur colloid scans may be used to distinguish between FNH and hepatic adenoma.[6,70-72]

Treatment   FNH has no malignant potential, and hemorrhage or rupture are rare. Conservative management with serial hepatic ultrasound examination is recommended for asymptomatic patients. Recommendations for symptomatic patients include discontinuation of oral contraceptives, surgical resection, ablative therapy, or embolization.[6]

HEPATIC ADENOMA

Overview   Hepatic adenoma is a relatively rare, benign tumor that is termed "adenomatosis" when more than four tumors are present, which occurs more often in adults than in pediatric patients. On histology, a hepatic adenoma consists of a solitary, spherical growth of hepatocytes within a pseudocapsule. The hepatocytes contain an increased amount of fat and glycogen and are organized in sheets along with thin-walled vessels, and dysfunctional Kupffer cells. Unlike FNH, this lesion does not exhibit a central scar or radiating septa.[15,60]

Etiology   The lesion is associated with use of steroids, and adolescents who use oral contraceptives are the most frequent pediatric patients with liver adenomas.[15,59] Hepatic adenomas also are associated with use of anabolic steroids, such as in the treatment of patients with Fanconi anemia, glycogen storage disease types I and III, galactosemia, and familial diabetes mellitus.[75,76]

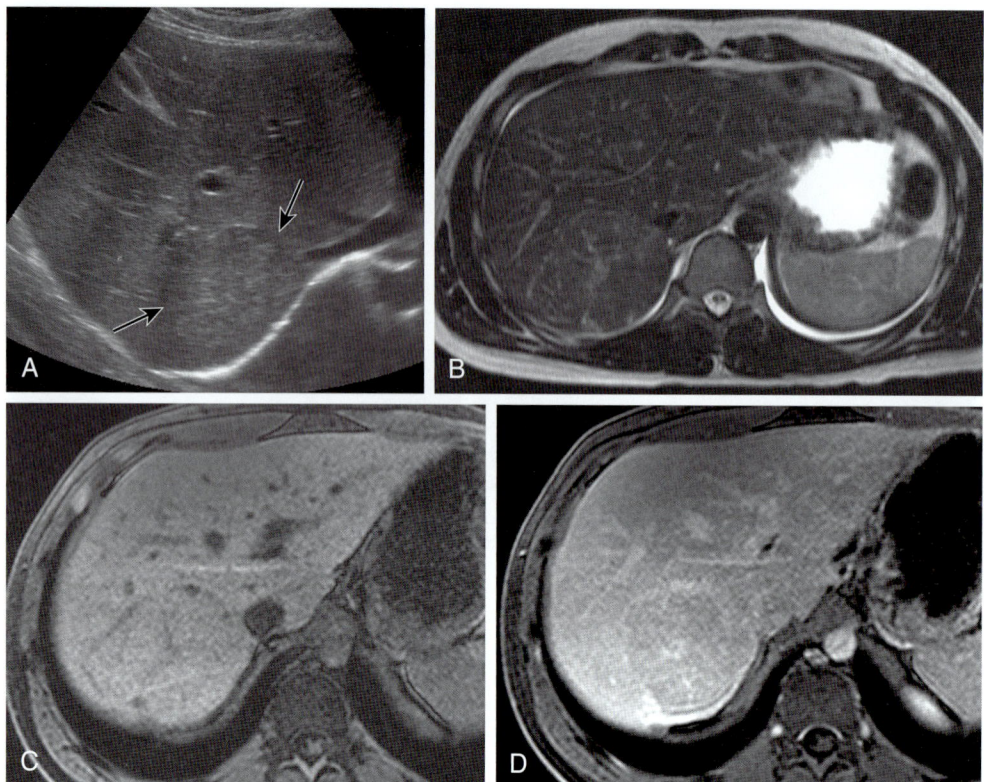

Figure 92-14 A 16-year-old boy with focal nodular hyperplasia. **A,** Transverse ultrasound imaging shows a homogeneous minimally hyperechoic lesion (*arrows*). **B,** Axial T2-weighted magnetic resonance (MR) imaging demonstrates a slightly hyperintense lesion with a hyperintense central scar. Dynamic gadolinium MR imaging was performed. **C,** A pregadolinium image shows an isodense lesion with a very subtle central scar. **D,** Five minutes after injection of gadolinium, the lesion is nearly isointense with enhancement of the central scar.

Clinical Presentation Patients often are asymptomatic. An association between hypervascular liver neoplasms, such as hepatic adenoma and FNH, and patients with congenital or acquired abnormal hepatic vasculature (e.g., portal vein absence or occlusion and congenital portosystemic shunts) has been reported. Intratumoral hemorrhage occurs in approximately 10% of patients and may result in abdominal pain; it rarely may result in intraperitoneal hemorrhage and hypovolemic shock.[76] Liver function is normal with no elevation of AFP levels.[77,78]

Imaging Imaging reveals that hepatic adenomas are solitary in approximately 80% of cases and multiple in 20% of cases. The ultrasound appearance of hepatic adenoma depends on the tumor content, such as lipid or hemorrhage. Hyperechoic masses related to the lipid content or hemorrhage may have a surrounding hypoechoic rim, and some may lack a well-defined wall (Fig. 92-15). Hypoechoic lesions to liver are more often seen in the setting of diffuse fatty infiltration and/or glycogen storage.[79] Color Doppler ultrasound imaging shows central venous flow, which differs from the arterial flow seen in persons with FNH.[71,80]

On unenhanced CT, hepatic adenomas usually are hypodense with a low-attenuation capsule (25%) and a well-defined border; the presence of hemorrhage or fat can result in heterogeneous attenuation (7%). Homogeneous enhancement is seen during the arterial phase of contrast injection, and the mass typically becomes isodense on delayed CT images.[78,79,81]

On MRI, most hepatic adenomas are mildly hyperintense to liver on T1- and on T2-weighted images.[78,82-84] On fat-suppressed or opposed-phase images, the signal drops out relative to the fat content.[78] This finding is not specific to adenomas and also can be seen in persons with HCC. The pseudocapsule is hypointense on T1-weighted images, has a variable signal on T2-weighted images, and may enhance.

Gallium uptake in hepatic adenomas is decreased, and they usually do not take up sulfur colloid, appearing as photopenic defects on both studies. Rarely a hepatic adenoma contains enough Kupffer cells to show uptake of sulfur colloid on scintigraphy, a finding typically associated with FNH.[80] With hepatobiliary agents, hepatic adenomas usually have early uptake, which persists on delayed images.[85]

Treatment Treatment options include discontinuation of oral contraceptives, dietary therapy in patients with glycogen storage disorder, or surgery. Some authors recommend surgery because of the risks of hemorrhage and the fact that HCC has been reported in solitary or multiple adenomas larger than 4 cm.[86] Radiofrequency ablation is an alternative to surgical resection.[87]

Inflammatory Pseudotumor of the Liver

Overview Inflammatory pseudotumor refers to an inflammatory mass that typically consists of fibrous tissue with plasma

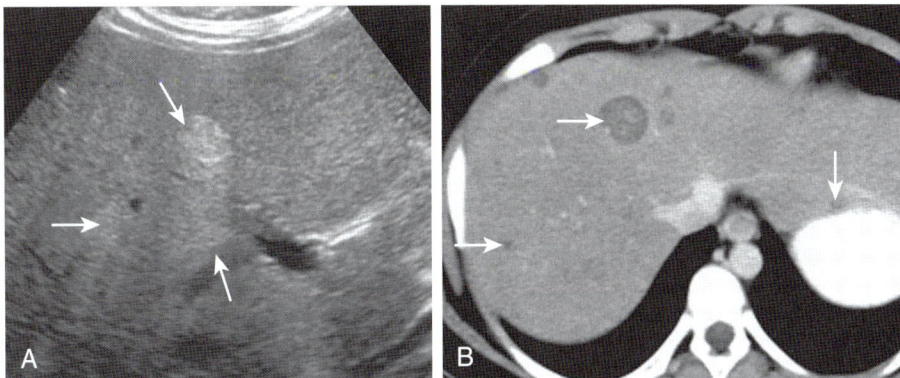

Figure 92-15 A hepatic adenomas in a 9-year-old girl with glycogen storage disease. **A,** An axial sonogram reveals hyperechoic foci within the liver (*arrows*). **B,** Axial contrast-enhanced computed tomography confirms multiple well-defined, hypoattenuating masses of varied size throughout the liver (*arrows*).

cells and mononuclear leukocytes; it lacks signs of anaplasia, and, prior to histologic analysis, it is difficult to distinguish from malignancy. It occurs most commonly in the lungs. Inflammatory pseudotumor of the liver is uncommon in children. Single or multiple well-defined hepatic masses occur. Single lesions, which have been termed type I, tend to occur centrally in the liver and may lead to biliary obstruction, portal pyelophlebitis, and portal hypertension. Multiple nodules have been termed type II lesions, involve both lobes, have an appearance indistinguishable from metastatic disease, and do not tend to be associated with biliary obstruction or the development of portal hypertension.[88]

Etiology The etiology of pseudotumor is unknown; inflammatory autoimmune and infectious causes have been postulated, including previous infection by the Epstein-Barr virus.[89,90]

Clinical Presentation The lesion tends to be more common in males.[90] Patients may present with fever, anorexia, and abdominal pain. Laboratory values may show liver enzyme elevations denoting biliary obstruction, as well as leukocytosis and elevation of the erythrocyte sedimentation rate and C-reactive protein. AFP values are normal.[88,91,92]

Imaging On ultrasound the lesions are solid and tend to be hypoechoic or heterogeneous (e-Fig. 92-16). On CT they are of low density; large single lesions tend to have a lower density core related to coagulation necrosis. Findings of biliary obstruction or pyelophlebitis may be seen. On delayed phase CT, they may show greater postenhancement attenuation than surrounding liver parenchyma.[93] On MRI, the lesion may be isointense to surrounding liver at both T1 and T2 weighting, necessitating IV contrast for evaluation.[94] The lesion is hypoechoic on sonography and of low attenuation on CT. It is not possible to reliably distinguish inflammatory pseudotumor from hepatic malignancy with imaging.

Treatment In some cases, the lesion may be resected based on a high preoperative probability of neoplasm, although a percutaneous biopsy may be diagnostic. Multiple lesions tend to be quiescent and involute.[88] Despite its relative rarity, it is important for clinicians, surgeons, and radiologists to be familiar with this diagnosis and consider it in the appropriate clinical setting.

Nodular Regenerative Hyperplasia

Overview NRH of the liver is a lesion characterized by regenerative nodules surrounded by atrophic liver in the absence of fibrosis, which is rarely seen in children.[67] Histologically, regenerative nodules are composed of focal proliferation of cells resembling hepatocytes within a supporting stroma.[67]

Etiology The etiology of this lesion is uncertain. This entity has been associated with small vessel vasculitis, with subsequent atrophy leading to compensatory hyperplasia of adjacent units. The entity has been linked to several other disorders such as collagen vascular diseases, hematologic disorders, cardiovascular diseases, neoplasms, metabolic disorders, and immunosuppressive or chemotherapeutic drugs.[60]

Clinical Presentation The lesion may be detected incidentally in asymptomatic patients, or it may be found in patients with portal hypertension but without cirrhosis. Malignant transformation to HCC has been reported.[60]

Imaging On imaging, NRH may be confused with FNH, adenomas, or metastases. Imaging findings are variable and depend on the size of the nodules.

The nodules are difficult to detect with ultrasound imaging because they are made of hepatocyte-like cells. Regenerative nodules may show heterogeneous echotexture with distortion of normal architecture. When detected, most nodules are hypoechoic, but they can be hyperechoic.[95,96] The nodules may bleed or lead to portal hypertension from pressure on portal radicles, and the liver may or may not be enlarged. On CT, lesions are of decreased attenuation compared with normal liver and do not enhance significantly after administration of IV contrast material.[95,96] On MRI, regenerative nodules are slightly hyperintense to adjacent liver on T1-weighted images and variable on T2-weighted images. A rim may be seen, which is hypointense or hyperintense on T1-weighted images and hyperintense on T2-weighting.[97]

Because of the presence of fat in the lesion, decreased signal intensity on fat-suppressed T1-weighted images may be seen. After injection of gadolinium, enhancement occurs during the portal phase such that the lesion is similar to the signal intensity of normal liver.[95]

Treatment   No specific treatment is recommended other than discontinuation of drugs associated with the NRH. If portal hypertension is present, a portocaval shunt may be needed.[60]

Key Points

Risk factors for development of hepatoblastoma, the most common pediatric primary hepatic tumor, include Beckwith-Wiedemann syndrome, familial adenomatous polyposis, glycogen storage disease, Gardner syndrome, fetal alcohol syndrome, Wilms tumor, trisomy 18, and prematurity.

Risk factors for HCC, the second most common liver tumor in children, include biliary atresia, infantile cholestasis, Alagille syndrome, hemochromatosis, hereditary tyrosinemia, glycogen storage disorders, α_1-antitrypsin deficiency, Wilson disease, galactosemia, and viral hepatitis.

The central fibrous scar in FLC is hypointense on T1-weighted images, hypointense on T2-weighted images, and does not enhance after IV contrast, which is distinct from the central scar in FNH, which has an increased signal on T2-weighted images and enhances after administration of contrast material.

Hepatic metastases in children are most often due to neuroblastoma, lymphoma, leukemia, and Wilms tumor.

Pediatric vascular masses have been reclassified according to the ISSVA, which divides lesions into vascular tumors (cellular mitosis) or vascular malformations (congenital dysmorphic vessels).

Mesenchymal hamartomas are cystic masses with variable solid components that enhance after administration of contrast. Most lesions present before 5 years of age.

FNH has a central scar in up to 60% of cases, which shows delayed enhancement and washout on CT and is hyperintense on T2-weighted images with postcontrast enhancement.

Hepatic adenomas are seen in persons who take birth control pills or anabolic steroids and in patients with glycogen storage disease.

Inflammatory pseudotumor is usually seen in the lungs. In the liver it can be associated with biliary obstruction and portophlebitis.

Suggested Readings

Christison-Lagay ER, Burrows PE, Alomari A, et al. Hepatic hemangiomas: subtype classification and development of a clinical practice algorithm and registry. *J Pediatr Surg*. 2007;42:62-68.

Chung EM, Cube R, Lewis RB, et al. From the Archives of the AFIP. Pediatric liver masses: radiologic-pathologic correlation. Part 1. Benign tumors. *Radiographics*. 2010;30:801-826.

Chung EM, Lattin Jr GE, Cube R, et al. From the Archives of the AFIP. Pediatric liver masses: radiologic-pathologic correlation. Part 2. Malignant tumors. *Radiographics*. 2011;31:483-507.

References

Full references for this chapter can be found on www.expertconsult.com.

Chapter 93

Vascular Abnormalities of the Liver

DOUGLAS C. RIVARD and LISA H. LOWE

Vascular abnormalities of the liver discussed in this chapter are divided into the following broad categories: portal hypertension, hepatopulmonary syndrome and pulmonary hypertension, Budd-Chiari syndrome, hepatovenous occlusive disease, and congenital vascular anomalies of the liver.

Portal Hypertension

Overview Portal hypertension is defined as a rise in pressure within the splanchnic venous system above 10 mm Hg. This increase in pressure may result from either increased resistance to hepatic venous drainage (presinusoidal and postsinusoidal) or increase in inflow pressure, such as is seen in persons with an arterioportal fistula.[1] The pathophysiology and clinical presentation of portal hypertension depend on the underlying hepatic disorder.

Etiology Cirrhosis, the most common cause of portal hypertension, is due to hepatic scarring resulting from chronic liver injury and is associated with deterioration of liver function. In pediatric patients, cirrhosis can result from a variety of conditions, including biliary atresia, cystic fibrosis, hemochromatosis, and Wilson disease (Box 93-1).[2] The Child-Turcotte-Pugh classification system provides a severity score that plays a part in treatment decisions.[3] Patients are stratified into grades A through C based on bilirubin elevation, albumin level, prothrombin time, ascites, and severity of encephalopathy.[3,4]

Patients with presinusoidal portal hypertension, such as extrahepatic portal vein occlusion, do not have intrinsic hepatic dysfunction. Extrahepatic portal vein occlusion is a relatively frequent cause of portal hypertension in children. It is increased in incidence in cases of complicated umbilical vein catheterization, sepsis, dehydration, hyperviscosity, shock, coagulopathy, and portal vein thrombosis, in persons with hypercoagulable syndromes (such as antithrombin III deficiency), and in persons with congenital portal venous webs, but it may occur without an identifiable cause.[2,5] Cavernous transformation of the portal vein is a result of porto-portal collaterals that develop along the thrombosed portal vein and that have been observed to occur in as little as 1 to 3 weeks after acute thrombus.[6]

Postsinusoidal obstruction includes primary liver disease with cirrhosis or hepatic vein obstruction, such as Budd-Chiari syndrome or hepatic venoocclusive disease, as seen in patients who have had bone marrow transplantation.[2]

Clinical Presentation Children may present with the consequences of portal hypertension, such as gastrointestinal bleeding, unexplained splenomegaly, and hypersplenism without jaundice, ascites, or cholestasis.[7,8]

Imaging Splenic enlargement may be the earliest imaging finding of portal hypertension. As resistance to portal flow increases, portal venous flow slows down, portal vein diameter decreases, and, with high resistance, portal venous flow may become reversed or even arterialized. In persons with a normal liver, the portal vein has a larger cross-sectional area than the splenic vein.[8,9] If instead the portal vein is smaller than the splenic vein, the presence of collaterals diverting portal flow away from the liver must be assumed (Fig. 93-1). Reversal of venous flow in the superior mesenteric and splenic veins also is suggestive of collaterals and spontaneous portosystemic shunting. Hepatopetal flow in the main portal vein does not exclude severe portal hypertension when collaterals are present or when lobe-to-lobe shunting occurs; hepatofugal flow is a late finding in persons with portal hypertension.[8,9]

The presence of a patent paraumbilical vein allows decompression of portal venous flow via the left portal vein, thus allowing hepatopetal flow in the main portal vein even in the presence of extreme portal hypertension, potentially creating a misleadingly normal main portal venous flow pattern. Because the paraumbilical veins are supplied by the left portal vein, intrahepatic portal flow may be directed toward them, causing reversal of flow in the right portal vein despite hepatopetal flow in the main portal vein. The paraumbilical veins are well visualized in the falciform fossa by color and power Doppler imaging, as well as by computed tomography angiography (CTA) and magnetic resonance angiography (MRA). Hepatic decompression by those veins may serve as relative protection against esophageal varices and variceal hemorrhage.

When portal venous pressure increases in the setting of portal hypertension, splanchnic venous return finds alternative drainage pathways connecting the portal circulation to the systemic circulation. Left gastric and splenic vein branches drain into the azygos system through esophageal and gastric varices, which in turn drain into the inferior vena cava (IVC) via the left renal vein. Paraumbilical veins (Fig. 93-2) communicate with inferior epigastric and internal mammary

Box 93-1 Causes of Portal Hypertension in Children

Increased Inflow Pressure or Volume
- Hepatic artery to portal vein fistula
- Total anomalous pulmonary venous return below the diaphragm
- Pulmonary sequestration with portal venous drainage

Presinusoidal Venous Obstruction
- Splenic vein occlusion (sinistral portal hypertension)
- Extrahepatic portal vein thrombosis/cavernous transformation of portal vein
- Posttransplantation portal vein stenosis, thrombosis, and occlusion
- Congenital hepatic fibrosis
- Schistosomiasis

Increased Sinusoidal Resistance
- Biliary atresia
- Cirrhosis
- Hepatitis: C, non-A non-B, autoimmune, neonatal
- Sclerosing cholangitis

Postsinusoidal Obstruction
- Budd-Chiari syndrome
- Glenn, Fontan systemic to pulmonary venous shunts
- Medications: 6-thioguanine

Idiopathic Portal Hypertension

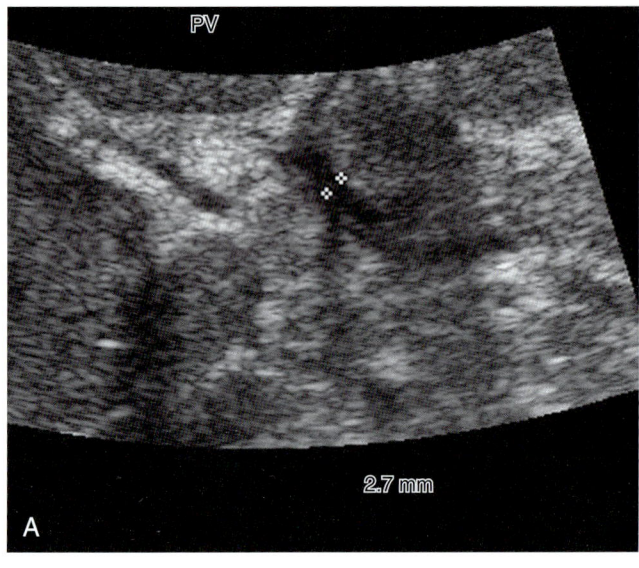

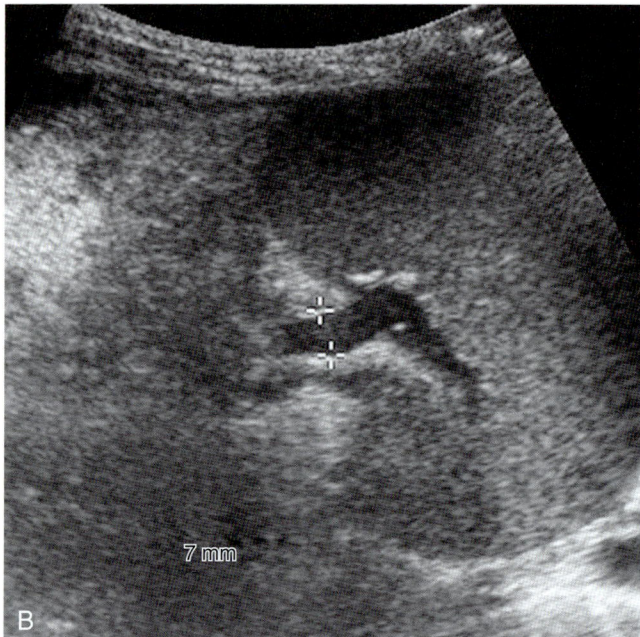

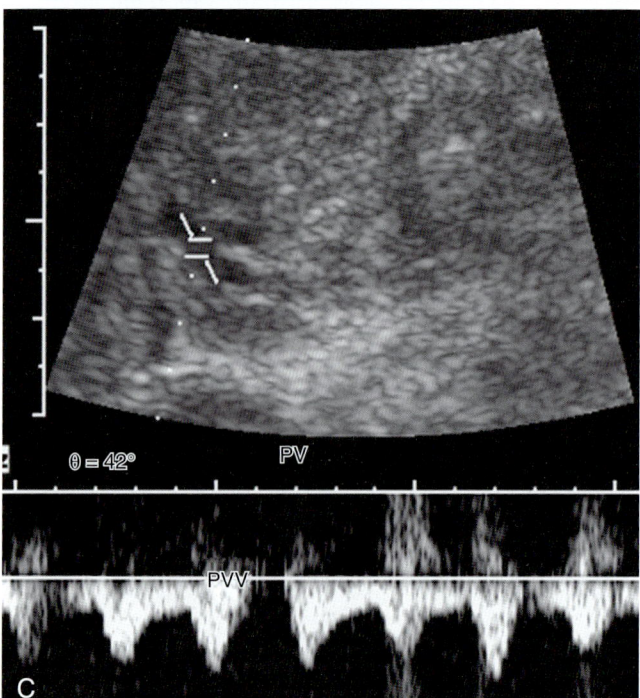

Figure 93-1 Severe portal hypertension following a Kasai portoenterostomy in a 2-year-old girl with biliary atresia. Ultrasound imaging was performed in preparation for liver transplantation. **A,** The main portal vein is very small, measuring 2.7 mm in diameter (calipers). Note the heterogeneous echotexture of the liver. **B,** The splenic vein is much larger, measuring 7 mm in diameter (calipers). This combination alerts one to the presence of collateral veins and varices. **C,** Spectral Doppler imaging of the main portal vein (*PV*), which is reversed and arterialized, reflects severe liver disease with high resistance to flow, causing the portal vein to become a draining vein to the hepatic artery through arterioportal communications.

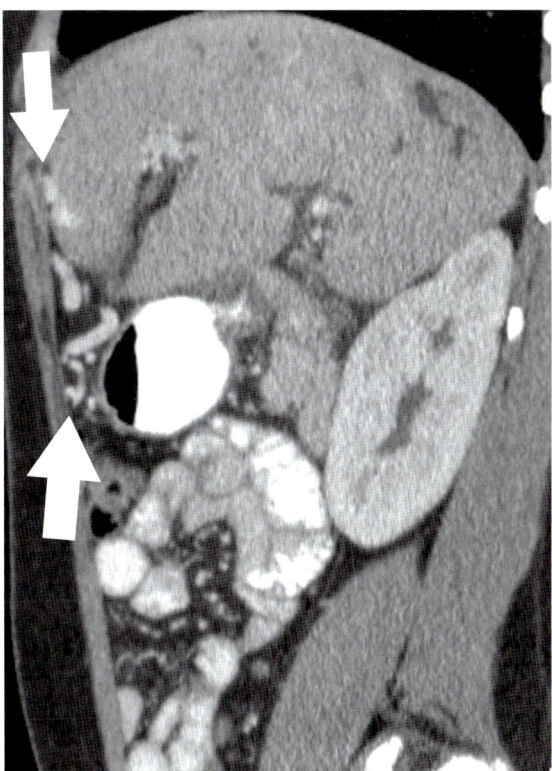

Figure 93-2 Paraumbilical collaterals in a 12-year-old girl with hepatic fibrosis, cirrhosis, and portal hypertension. A sagittal contrast-enhanced computed tomography image shows enhancing paraumbilical venous collaterals and enhancing internal mammary collateral vessels anterior to the liver (*arrows*).

abdominal wall venous networks to drain into the inferior and superior vena cava, respectively. These collateral pathways can be visualized with cross-sectional imaging.[6]

Additional collateral pathways develop with portal hypertension. Retroperitoneal and peripancreatic collaterals drain through renal and gonadal veins into the IVC and into paraspinal veins, which drain into the azygos system (Fig. 93-3). Inferior mesenteric branches drain into superior, middle, and inferior hemorrhoidal veins that lead to the iliac veins. Portosystemic collaterals also may form at enterocutaneous junctions in fistulas and enterostomies. Surgical anastomoses, such as a Roux-en-Y biliary-enteric anastomosis, may serve as sites of portoportal collaterals (Fig. 93-4). Finally, intercostal and phrenic veins also may serve as a means of portosystemic communication across the diaphragm.[6]

In patients with cavernous transformation of the portal vein, key cross-sectional imaging features include a tangle of venous channels in the liver hilum with no identifiable normal portal vein (Fig. 93-5). In most patients (76%), portoportal collaterals extend over a variable distance along the course of the intrahepatic portal branches. In extreme cases, no portal vein branches are demonstrated (Fig. 93-6). Preserved intrahepatic portal vein branches may be identified, some of which may demonstrate hepatofugal flow toward the cavernous vessels. Collateral veins may traverse the liver parenchyma to enter hepatic and capsular veins (Fig. 93-7). Doppler ultrasound imaging can be used to interrogate flow characteristics within the cavernous collaterals, revealing abnormal flow.[10]

Treatment and Prognosis A wide range of therapeutic options exist for children with portal hypertension, depending on the underlying cause and severity of liver disease. Treatments range from percutaneous transjugular intrahepatic portosystemic shunts to sclerotherapy and variceal ligation to

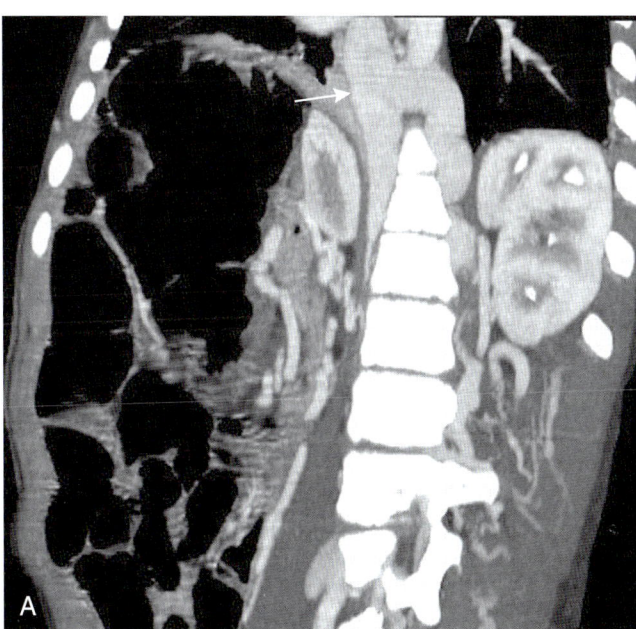
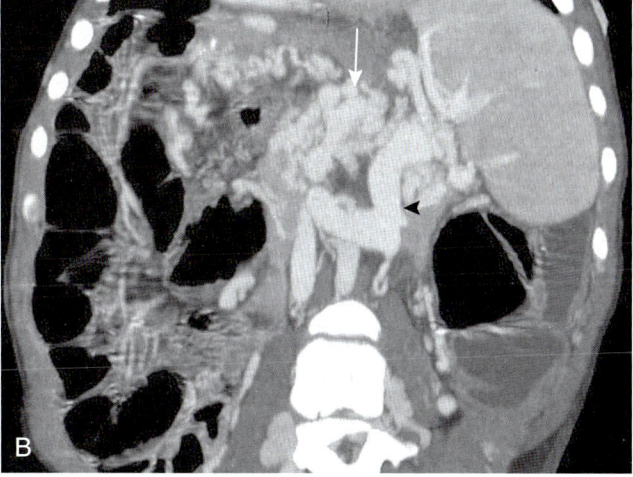

Figure 93-3 A liver transplant patient with an occluded portal vein and inferior vena cava. **A,** Retroperitoneal, paraspinal, and intraspinal venous collaterals are present. The azygos and hemiazygos veins are massively enlarged (*arrow*). **B,** Extensive pancreatic (*arrow*) and perisplenic collaterals are present, along with a splenorenal shunt (*arrowhead*).

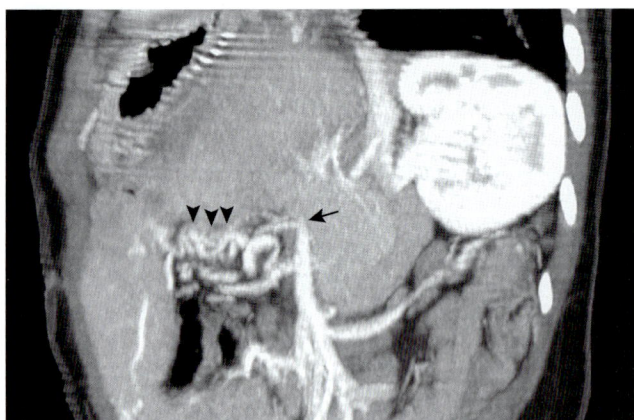

Figure 93-4 Nonacute portal vein thrombosis in an 11-year-old boy with a left lateral segment liver transplant. An oblique sagittal reformat of contrast-enhanced computed tomography shows that the extrahepatic portal vein is occluded (*arrow*), and multiple corkscrew collaterals from jejunal branches of the superior mesenteric vein are seen at the Roux-en-Y loop (*arrowheads*) used for the biliary anastomosis. The reconstituted central portal vein was identified on other images. Capsular collaterals are seen at the inferior edge of the liver.

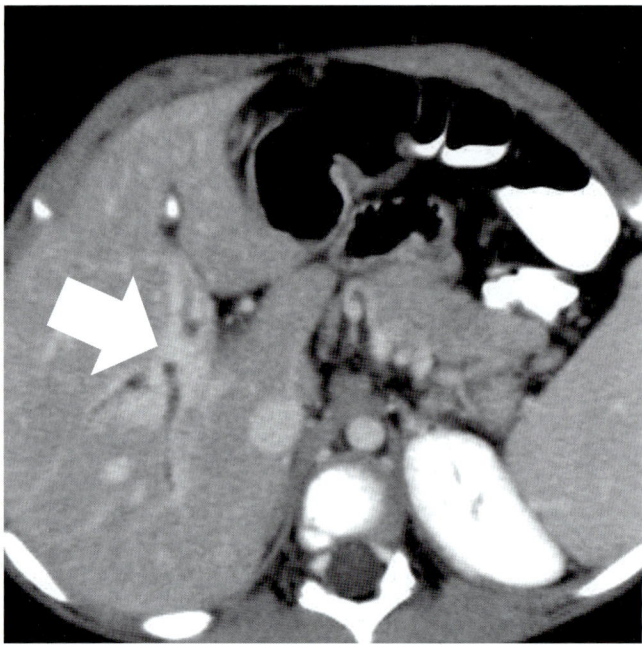

Figure 93-6 Cavernous transformation of the portal vein in a 3-year-old girl with biliary atresia and cirrhosis. No intrahepatic portal vein branches are seen anywhere in the liver. Tangles of intrahepatic collaterals (*arrow*) follow the expected course of the entire intrahepatic portal system.

surgical portosystemic shunts.[2,11] Endovascular therapies have become more refined and are used with increasing frequency.[12,13]

Surgical portosystemic shunts include splenorenal shunts, mesocaval shunts, and the mesoportal (Rex) bypass. In the splenorenal shunt, the distal splenic vein is connected end-to-side to the left renal vein (Fig. 93-8), leaving the superior mesenteric vein connected to the liver. The Rex bypass was first described in 1992 by de Ville de Goyet and coworkers[14] and is used in patients with extrahepatic portal vein obstruction.[15] In this bypass procedure, a venous graft is interposed between the superior mesenteric vein (inferior to the pancreas) and the left portal vein, restoring portal venous flow into the liver (Fig. 93-9). The Rex shunt may be definitive therapy for children with extrahepatic portal vein obstruction.[16] The collapsed intrahepatic portal system, which may be difficult to image before surgery because of exuberant intrahepatic collaterals that dominate portal flow, has been

shown to distend rapidly and accommodate the large volume of flow from the shunt. The shunt can be seen by all vascular imaging modalities and should demonstrate hepatopetal flow.[17]

Because the Rex shunt is a bypass graft, portal flow is hepatopetal. Portal vein flow is hepatofugal in patent mesocaval and proximal splenorenal shunts; it may be hepatopetal in the more selective distal splenorenal shunts, which are designed to decompress esophageal varices and preserve some portal venous flow. These shunts provide short- and long-term palliation in children with portal hypertension to prevent gastrointestinal hemorrhages and improve hypersplenism. In children with severe underlying liver disease, these shunts are temporizing procedures before liver transplantation.[18]

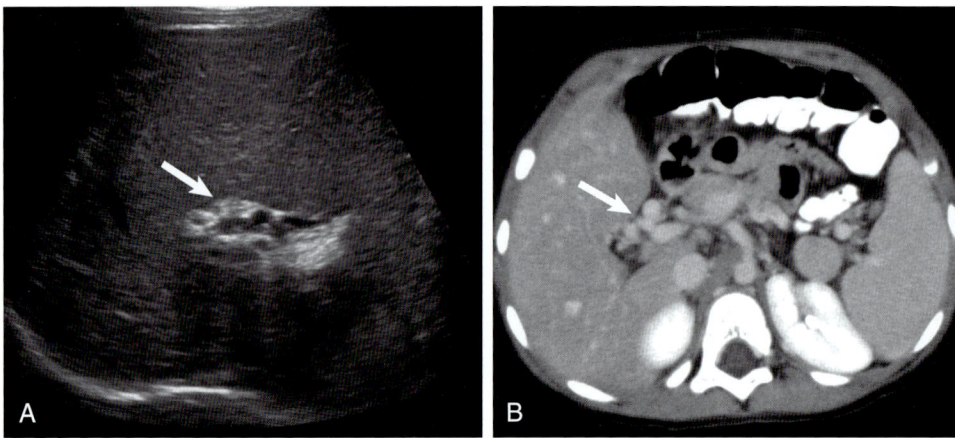

Figure 93-5 Cavernous transformation of the portal vein in a 3- year-old boy with cirrhosis. **A,** A transverse sonogram shows a tangle of periportal vessels without an identifiable normal portal vein (*arrow*). **B,** Axial contrast-enhanced computed tomography confirms multiple collateral vessels in the porta hepatis (*arrow*).

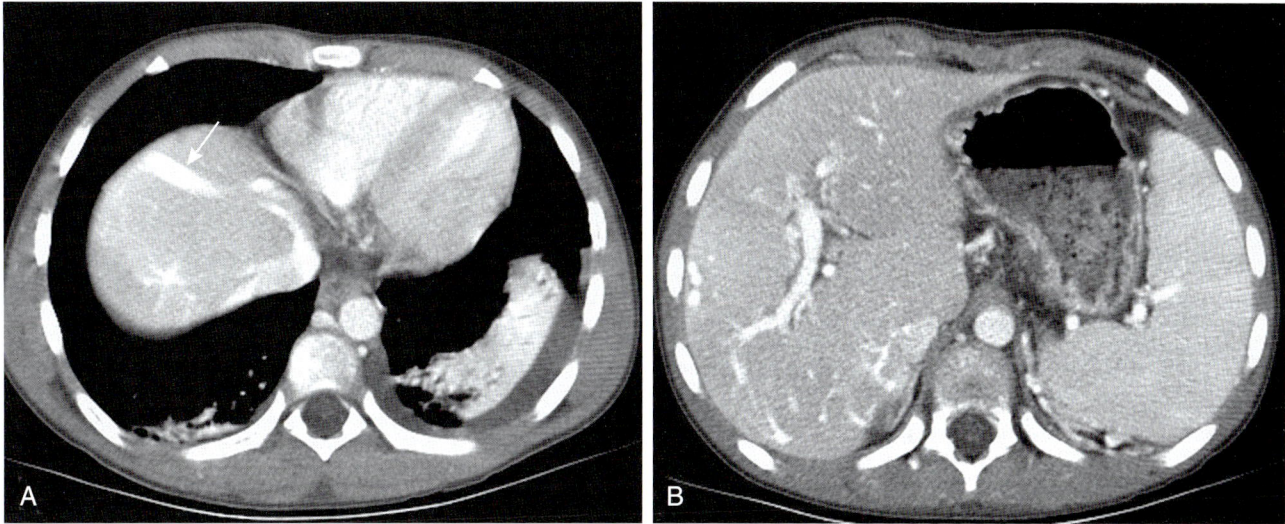

Figure 93-7 Portovenous and transcapsular collaterals in a patient with extrahepatic portal vein obstruction. Portovenous and transcapsular connections are present across the liver parenchyma. **A,** A high axial slice at the liver dome shows a peripheral large collateral vein (*arrow*) communicating with the left hepatic vein. **B,** A lower axial computed tomography slice shows numerous transcapsular venous collaterals that communicate with the intrahepatic portal vein branches.

Hepatopulmonary Syndrome

Overview Hepatopulmonary syndrome is defined as an elevated age-adjusted alveolar-arterial oxygen gradient that often leads to hypoxemia and pulmonary vascular dilation in patients with chronic liver disease.[19]

Etiology Hepatopulmonary syndrome is associated with hepatic vascular abnormalities (such as portal hypertension) that alter the normal portosystemic circulation and normal delivery of hepatic venous blood to the lungs, leading to right to left intrapulmonary shunting and pulmonary hypertension. The pathophysiology of hepatopulmonary syndrome has not

been fully elucidated, but most hypotheses agree on the role of increased pulmonary expression of endothelin B receptor, leading to nitric oxide overproduction mediated by endothelin-1 and nitric oxide synthetase. Endothelial and arterial wall changes produce either (1) ventilation-perfusion mismatch through vasodilatation and arteriovenous shunting or (2) pulmonary hypertension.[20]

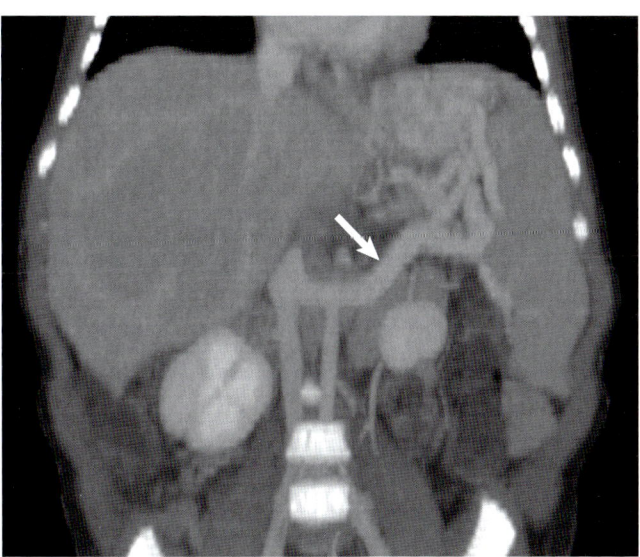

Figure 93-8 A distal splenorenal shunt in an 8-year-old boy. Coronal reconstruction from a computed tomography angiogram shows the splenic vein connected end to side (*arrow*) to the left renal vein draining into the inferior vena cava.

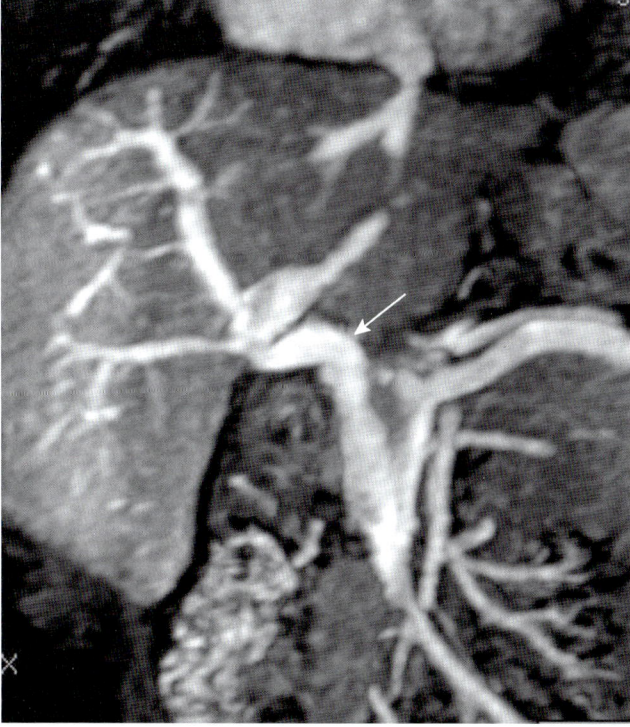

Figure 93-9 Rex (superior mesenteric to left portal vein) bypass. Angled coronal magnetic resonance angiography shows the harvested jugular vein (*arrow*) connecting the superior mesenteric vein below the pancreas to the left portal vein.

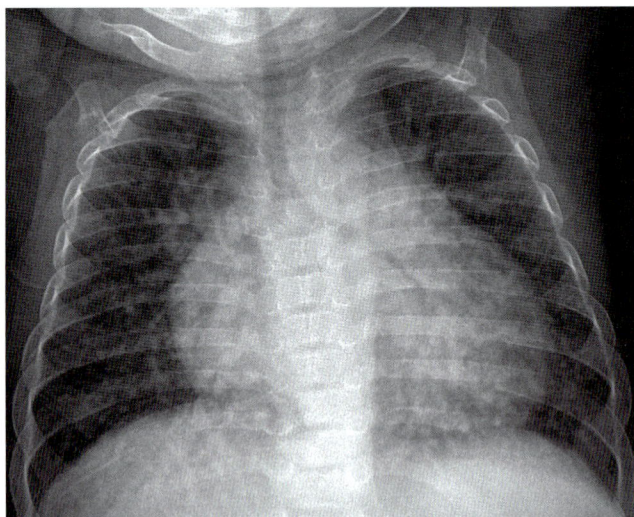

Figure 93-10 Hepatopulmonary syndrome in an 8-month-old boy with portal vein occlusion and cyanosis. A chest radiograph shows cardiomegaly and extensively increased pulmonary vascularity, representing diffuse pulmonary arteriovenous shunts.

Clinical Presentation The clinical presentation can range from relatively asymptomatic to the presence of cyanosis and clubbing.[19] Pulmonary manifestations may precede the clinical presentation of the liver disease and may progress rapidly within months of the initial presentation.

Imaging Plain radiographs may demonstrate increased vascular markings and cardiomegaly (Fig. 93-10). Computed tomography (CT) may outline enlarged vessels, predominantly in the lung bases. Echocardiography with contrast material injected into the antecubital vein will demonstrate echogenic bubbles in the pulmonary veins and in the left atrium as a result of intrapulmonary arteriovenous shunting.

Treatment and Prognosis The treatment of hepatopulmonary syndrome is aimed at the underlying disease, which affects prognosis. In patients in whom the syndrome is a consequence of a portovenous shunt, occlusion of the shunt can lead to regression of the intrapulmonary shunts and resolution of symptoms.[13,19,21]

Budd-Chiari Syndrome

Overview In persons with Budd-Chiari syndrome, obstruction of the hepatic veins and IVC at their confluence results in severe liver congestion, ascites, and portal hypertension.[22] As sinusoidal pressure increases, the pressure gradient between the portal venous system and the sinusoidal system is reversed, causing the portal vein to become a draining system for the hepatic artery. In complete Budd-Chiari syndrome, blood supply to the liver is solely from the hepatic artery. Because the caudate lobe has separate venous drainage, it is spared in most patients with Budd-Chiari syndrome.

Etiology The causes of Budd-Chiari syndrome include a caval web, thrombosis in hypercoagulable states such as nephrotic syndrome, tumor extension into the IVC as in

patients with hepatoblastoma or Wilms tumor, external compression, or liver transplantation; the syndrome also may be idiopathic.[22-24]

Clinical Presentation Clinically, collateral venous drainage develops in some patients, and they may be relatively asymptomatic. Other patients present with intractable ascites, liver failure, or gastrointestinal hemorrhage. Children who experience hepatic vein or IVC obstruction after liver transplantation may experience recurrence of portal hypertension.[25]

Imaging On cross-sectional imaging, hepatomegaly with ascites and poorly or nonvisualized hepatic veins are characteristic.[24,26] Portal venous flow usually is reversed in complete cases; however, in patients with partial hepatic vein occlusion, the flow may shunt from higher resistance segments into lower resistance segments, such as the caudate lobe. Intrahepatic portal-to-systemic collaterals may occur via transcapsular and paraumbilical veins, and extrahepatic collaterals occur via esophageal and gastric varices. These hemodynamic changes can be well demonstrated by Doppler ultrasound, CT angiography, and magnetic resonance (MR) imaging.[9,24,26]

On CT and CTA (Fig. 93-11), the liver parenchyma may demonstrate patchy, abnormal, wedge-shaped areas of attenuation with the apex pointing to the IVC. A heterogeneous, reticular, or mosaic pattern in the hepatic arterial phase that persists during the portal phase also may be observed. The caudate lobe retains a normal appearance, and the normal hepatic veins are not visualized. The portal vein may fill before its tributaries as a result of intrahepatic flow reversal. Similar findings are found on MRI and MR arteriography.

Treatment and Prognosis Treatment consists of medical control of ascites, percutaneous angioplasty when feasible, surgical creation of a diverting shunt, and liver transplantation in severe cases.[23,27] Prognosis of Budd-Chiari syndrome is highly variable depending on the timeliness of diagnosis and the ability to treat the underlying causes.[22]

Hepatic Venoocclusive Disease

Overview Hepatic venoocclusive disease (VOD) refers to severe endothelial and perivascular hepatocyte damage that may be followed by fibrosis and obliteration of the terminal hepatic venules.

Etiology Hepatic VOD develops most frequently in patients undergoing myeloablative therapy for bone marrow or stem cell transplantation. The reported frequency of VOD in patients who undergo bone marrow transplantation varies from 11% to 31% and is higher in patients who undergo bone marrow transplantation for malignant rather than nonmalignant indications. Risk factors include the presence of previous liver disease or other preexistent conditions such as osteopetrosis, repeat myeloablative procedure beyond second relapse, and specific chemotherapeutic regimens, such as the use of busulfan.[28] In patients who have not undergone bone marrow transplantation, the entity can occur when the patient has received hepatic radiation or actinomycin D, and it can also occur after liver transplantation. Because the damage occurs in the hepatic sinusoidal endothelial cells of the hepatic

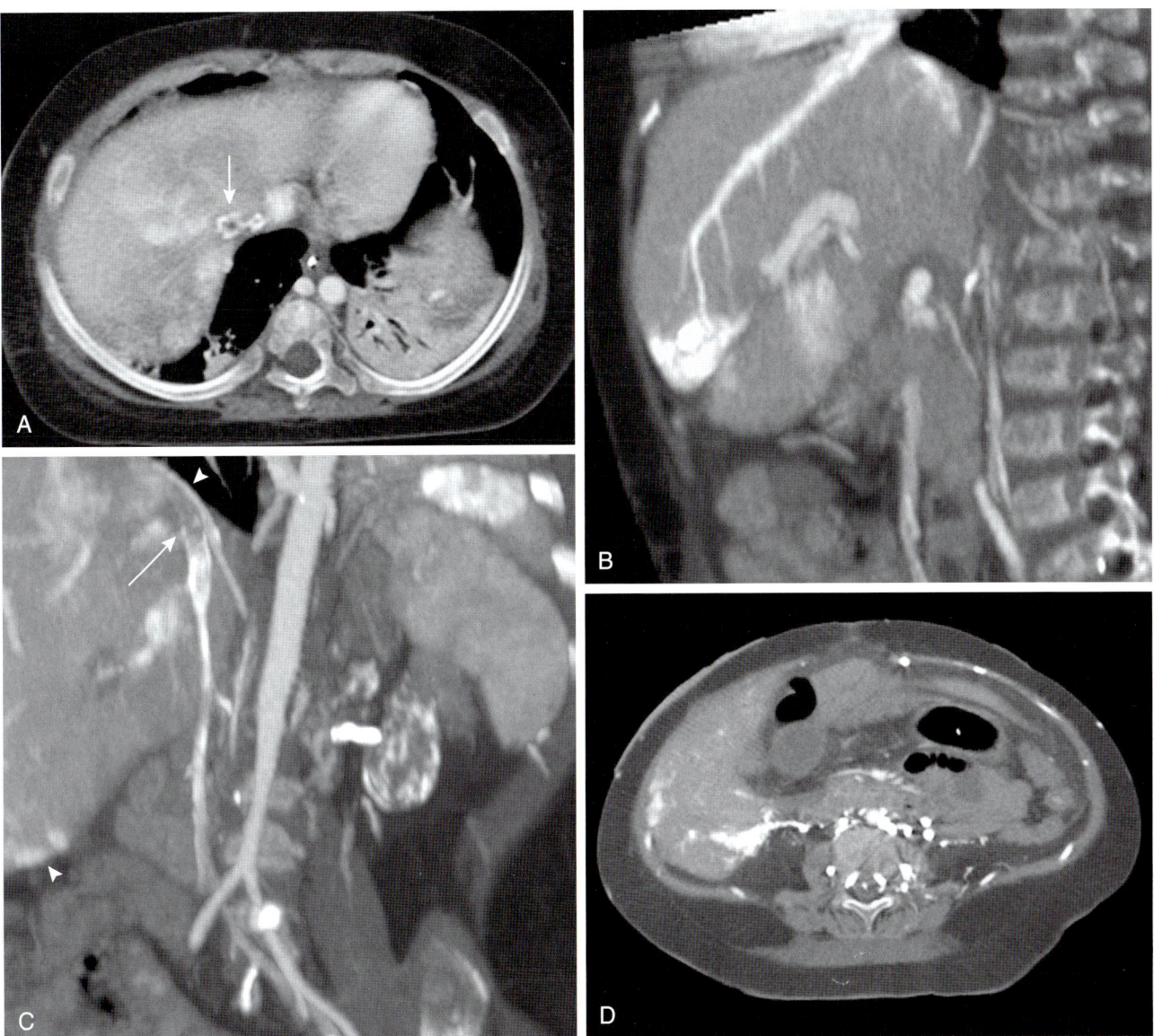

Figure 93-11 Budd-Chiari syndrome due to inferior vena cava (IVC) thrombosis. **A,** An axial image from computed tomographic angiography (CTA) shows a filling defect within the intrahepatic IVC (*arrow*). Note the patchy, inhomogeneous enhancement of the liver. **B,** Sagittal reformatting from CTA shows intense contrast retention peripherally in the territory of the obstructed hepatic vein and transcapsular collateral. **C,** Thrombus is seen in the IVC (*arrow*) in this coronal reconstruction. Transcapsular collaterals are seen at the liver dome and lower lateral edge (*arrowheads*). **D,** An axial lower CT slice shows extensive retroperitoneal, paraspinal, and transcapsular collaterals enhancing brightly.

venules, the term "sinusoidal obstructive disease" has been suggested.[29]

Clinical Presentation Patients present with fluid retention, abdominal pain, and hepatomegaly. The clinical diagnosis of hepatic VOD requires the presence of two of the following clinical criteria: jaundice, ascites or fluid retention, and painful hepatomegaly within the first 20 days after bone marrow transplantation.[30]

Imaging A constellation of findings may be identified on ultrasound imaging, including hepatomegaly, ascites, and thickening of the gallbladder wall. On Doppler imaging, decreased or reversed flow in the portal vein, increased resistive index of the hepatic artery, and the appearance of hepatofugal flow in the paraumbilical veins have been described

in patients with VOD[31] (Fig. 93-12). In some early cases, partial hemodynamic involvement may be present, resulting in flow reversal in only one segmental or lobar portal vein branch.[32] The entire constellation of findings is seldom present, and in many patients, no specific ultrasound findings may be observed.[31]

MRI findings include hepatomegaly, abnormal periportal cuffing, gallbladder wall thickening with intense wall signal on T2-weighted sequences, ascites, and pleural effusion.[33]

Treatment Treatment consists of supportive care and controlling the inflammation and the deposition of fibrin. Agents that have been used include antithrombotic agents such as prostaglandin E1 and heparin, which are of limited value. More promising is defibrotide, which is derived from porcine tissue and has antithrombotic and antiischemic properties,

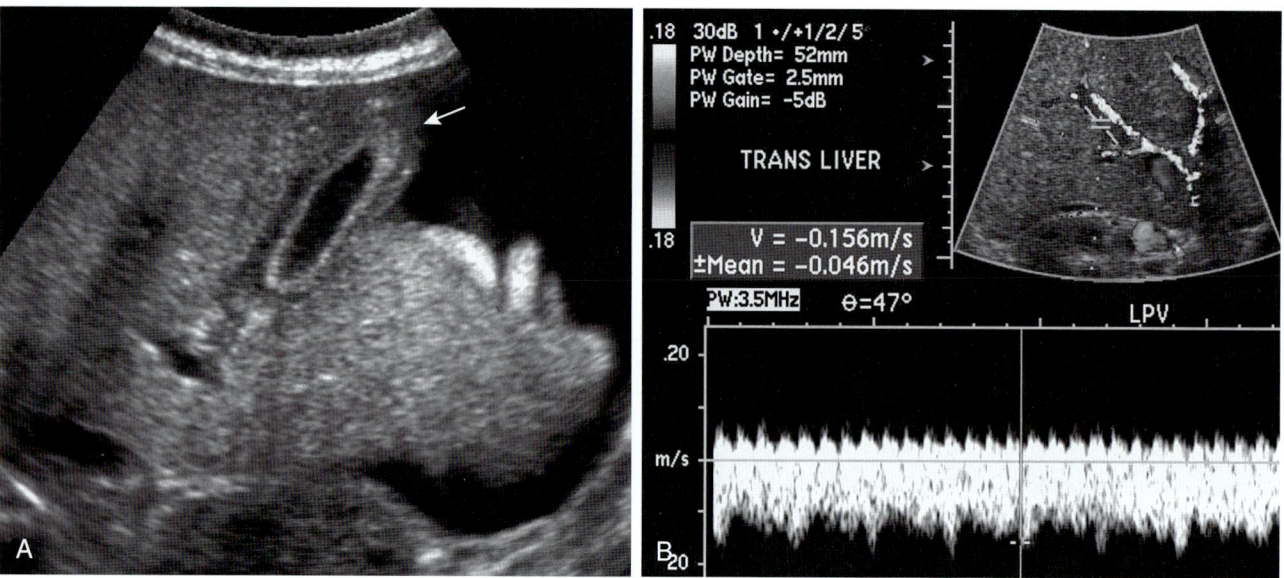

Figure 93-12 Hepatic venoocclusive disease. **A,** A longitudinal ultrasound image shows thickening of the gallbladder wall (*arrow*) and ascites. **B,** Doppler imaging shows reversal of portal venous flow.

with complete resolution seen in 35% to 55% of patients in reported uncontrolled clinical trials.[28,29,34]

Congenital Anomalies of Liver Vasculature

ANOMALIES OF THE PORTAL VEIN

Preduodenal Portal Vein

Overview Preduodenal portal vein is a rare anomaly in which the portal vein courses ventral to the duodenum and pancreatic head.

Etiology The proposed embryology is nonregression of the caudal anastomotic vein that connects the two vitelline veins ventral to the duodenum, where it then contributes to the formation of the portal vein.[35,36]

Clinical Presentation The anomaly is closely associated with the heterotaxy syndromes, particularly polysplenia[37] and malrotation, as well as splenic, pancreatic, cardiac, and duodenal anomalies. In approximately 50% of patients, an associated duodenal obstruction is present, such as intrinsic duodenal stenosis/membrane or malrotation with Ladd bands; however, the anomaly may be asymptomatic and discovered incidentally, particularly during workup of patients with heterotaxy or biliary atresia, because approximately 10% of patients with biliary atresia have associated heterotaxy/polysplenia.[36-39]

Imaging The preduodenal portal vein is seen as a vein anterior to the duodenum and pancreas, which can be visualized on cross-section imaging including ultrasound, CT, and MRI; it is particularly well visualized on sagittal images (Fig. 93-13).[36,37]

Treatment Treatment addresses correction of the underlying duodenal obstruction, if present. Awareness of this anatomic

abnormality is necessary because it can pose a surgical hazard during other hepatobiliary or proximal intestinal surgical procedures, particularly in patients with heterotaxy/polysplenia who have biliary atresia.[35,39]

Extrahepatic Congenital Portosystemic Shunts

Overview Abernethy[40] first described an extrahepatic portosystemic connection in 1793, and this malformation is now known as the Abernethy malformation. According to Morgan and Superina,[41] these malformations can be classified as type 1 or 2. Type 1 involves a complete shunt; no portal blood reaches the liver, as in congenital absence of the portal vein. In type 1a, the superior mesenteric and splenic veins do not join, and in type 1b, the superior mesenteric and splenic veins join before draining into the systemic circulation. Type 2 involves a partial shunt to the hepatic vein or IVC.[41,42]

Etiology Extrahepatic portosystemic shunts result from maldevelopment of the coordinated preservation and atresia of the left and right vitelline veins in the abdomen. Such maldevelopment could arise de novo, such as in patients with heterotaxy in whom orderly right-left processes are affected, with secondary hypoplasia of the portal venous system, or they may be a result of hypoplasia of the portal venous system with redirection of portal venous flow through extrahepatic channels.[43]

Clinical Presentation Extrahepatic portosystemic shunts are associated with other anomalies, such as polysplenia, biliary atresia, and cardiac and renal anomalies. They also are associated with the development of liver lesions, including focal nodular hyperplasia. Malignancies, including hepatoblastoma, hepatocellular carcinoma, and sarcoma, also have been reported in these patients. With the bypass of the hepatic circulation, systemic hyperammonemia also can be present, although hyperammonemic encephalopathy is more typically seen in older and adult patients, dependent in part on the

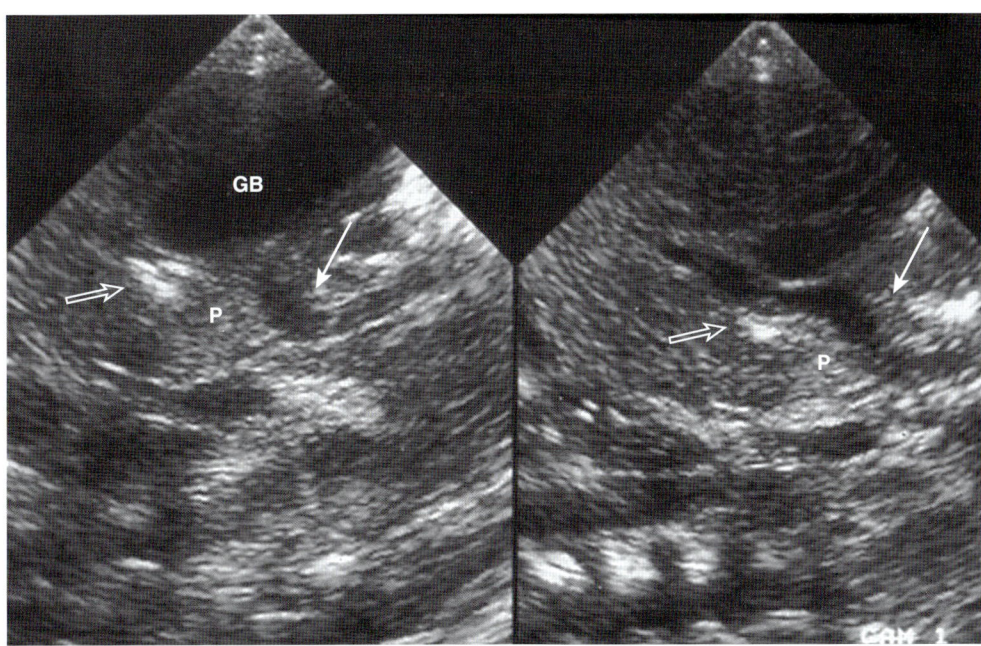

Figure 93-13 Preduodenal portal vein. Midline sagittal ultrasound imaging in an infant with polysplenia. The superior mesenteric vein (*solid arrow*) courses anterior to pancreas (*P*) and duodenum (*open arrow*) to enter the liver. *GB,* Midline gallbladder. (Courtesy Marta Hernanz-Schulman, MD, Nashville, TN.)

volume of the shunt; increased circulation of galactose and bile acids also occurs.[43-46]

Imaging   Absence of the portal vein may be noted prenatally, with congenital agenesis of the ductus venosus and umbilical vein drainage into the IVC or directly into the heart.[47]

When the portal vein is absent, the hepatic artery is larger than expected relative to the size of the liver and the patient's age.[44] When the portal vein is present, it is small (Fig. 93-14, *A*). The shunt's vascular connection may be demonstrated by ultrasound imaging, particularly with the aid of color Doppler imaging (Fig 93-14, *B*), but CTA and MRA are more likely to demonstrate its complete course and anatomy (Fig. 93-15). Associated hepatic parenchymal nodules may be demonstrated by all cross-sectional imaging modalities (Fig. 93-16).

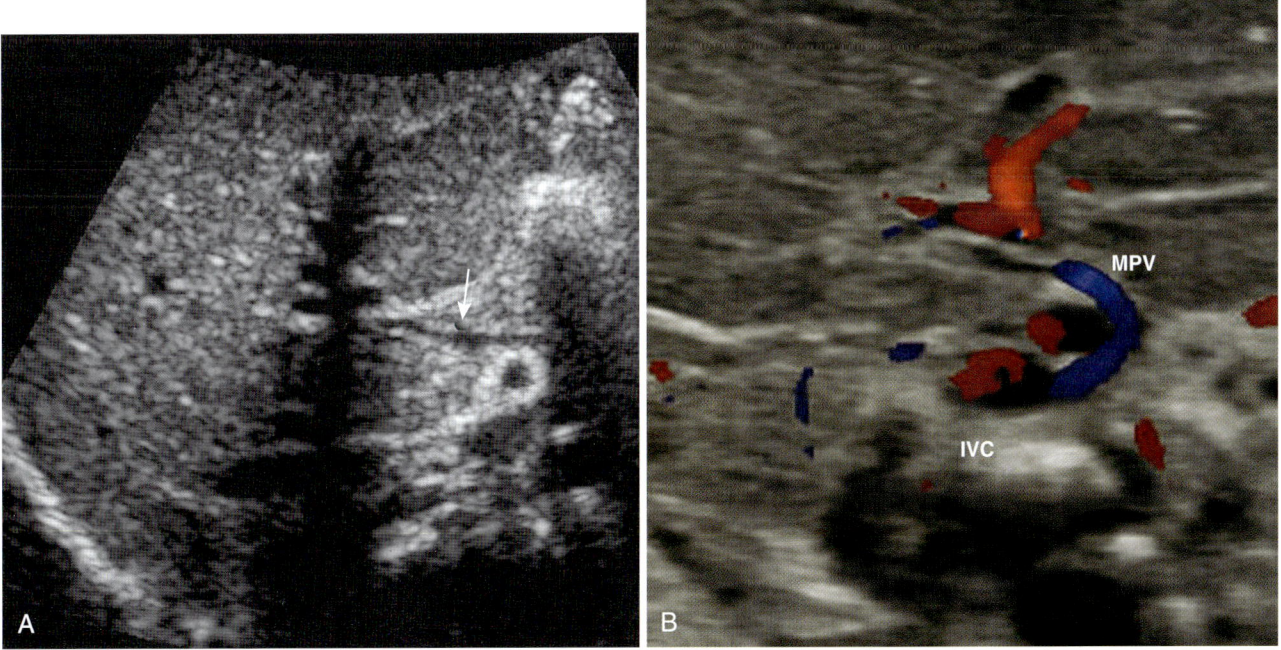

Figure 93-14   A congenital extrahepatic portosystemic shunt. **A,** A diminutive main portal vein is present (*arrow*). **B,** Transverse ultrasound Doppler imaging in another infant shows main portal vein (*MPV*) draining into the inferior vena cava (*IVC*).

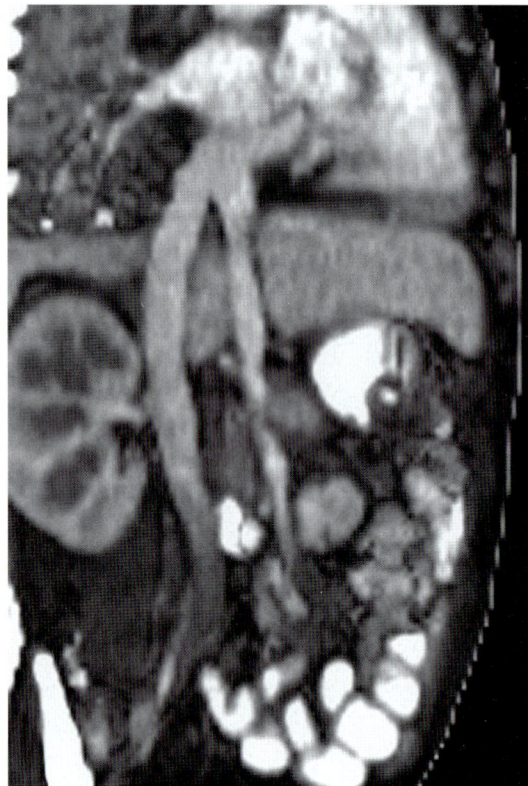

Figure 93-15 An extrahepatic portosystemic shunt. Computed tomographic angiography coronal oblique reformatting shows the superior mesenteric vein connecting to the suprahepatic inferior vena cava, bypassing the liver.

Treatment and Prognosis Treatment, particularly in symptomatic patients, is aimed at surgical or endovascular occlusion of the abnormal connection if evidence exists that intrahepatic flow can be restored; otherwise, extrahepatic portal hypertension will ensue. Surgical or endovascular

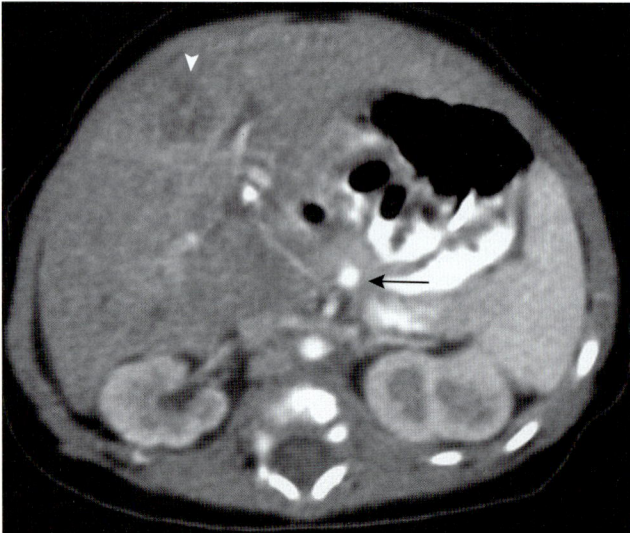

Figure 93-16 An extrahepatic portosystemic shunt and liver nodule. An axial computed tomography image shows the portosystemic shunt (*arrow*) in cross section, coursing cephalad toward the inferior vena cava. A liver nodule also is seen (*arrowhead*).

occlusion may be accomplished with a staged procedure, with narrowing of the shunt before complete occlusion is undertaken. Liver transplantation may be needed in persons with symptomatic extrahepatic shunts with agenesis of the portal vein and its branches.[44,46,48]

Intrahepatic Congenital Portosystemic Shunts

Overview Intrahepatic congenital portosystemic shunts also are relatively rare anomalies, in which one or more intrahepatic portosystemic venous shunts may be present. Park et al.[49] have classified intrahepatic portosystemic shunts into four types. Type I is a single large vein connecting the right portal and hepatic veins. Type II features peripheral single or multiple communications in one segment. Type III consists of an aneurysm connecting a peripheral portal vein and a hepatic vein branch. Type IV represents diffuse communications in multiple lobes. Type I is the most common.

Etiology Intrahepatic congenital portosystemic shunts represent persistent communications between the portal and hepatic venous derivatives of the embryologic vitelline veins, or between the vitelline and subcardinal veins.[44,50] A patent ductus venous represents a form of portosystemic shunt from the left portal vein into the IVC.

Clinical Presentation These shunts may be asymptomatic and diagnosed incidentally. When encountered in neonates, some of these shunts may resolve spontaneously within the first 12 to 24 months of life; however, the proportion of patients in whom this occurs is not known.[44]

When these shunts are clinically apparent, presentation can include jaundice, hyperammonemia, hypergalactosemia, encephalopathy, and pulmonary hypertension.[44,46] Type IV shunts may be associated with massive shunting and heart failure. Cutaneous hemangiomas have been described in neonates with intrahepatic portosystemic shunts.

Imaging Intrahepatic congenital portosystemic shunts often are demonstrated by ultrasound imaging, sometimes when evaluating a child with a cutaneous hemangioma. The nonuniform size of the portal vein and hepatic vein branches may locate additional communications. The flow pattern in the portal veins, and at times also in the splenic vein, may demonstrate a biphasic or triphasic pattern, reflecting bypass of the hepatic parenchyma. Intrahepatic shunts are well demonstrated by CTA and MRA (Fig. 93-17).

Treatment Asymptomatic children with mild metabolic abnormalities can be treated conservatively by dietary means and Doppler imaging follow-up, because some of these shunts may close spontaneously.[51] Contemporary literature has described endovascular treatment with increasing frequency using a variety of surgical techniques and devices.[48,50]

Subdiaphragmatic Anomalous Pulmonary Venous Connections

Overview Although anomalous pulmonary venous connections usually occur above the diaphragms, multiple subdiaphragmatic embryonal connections may persist, with

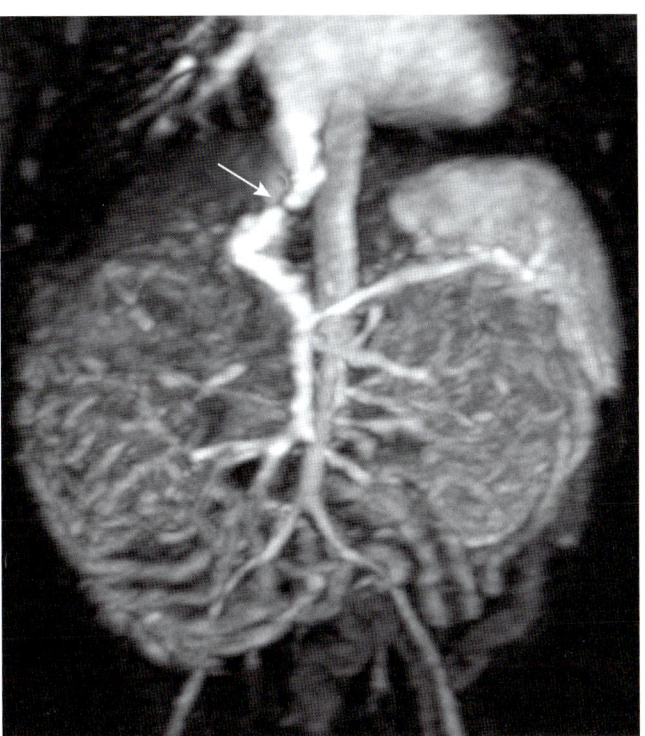

Figure 93-17 An intrahepatic portosystemic shunt in an infant with hyperammonemia. Magnetic resonance venography shows the anomalous connection (*arrow*) between the intrahepatic portal vein and the inferior vena cava. The portal vein was larger than normal on ultrasound.

subdiaphragmatic partial or total pulmonary venous drainage.

Etiology Pulmonary veins develop in the fourth week of gestation as a plexus that initially drains into both the cardinal veins and the umbilicovitelline venous system. As lung development proceeds, the common pulmonary vein is formed by the confluence of the four pulmonary veins and fuses with the posterior wall of the left atrium. If this normal fusion and drainage into the left atrium does not occur, embryonic connections to the splanchnic and umbilicovitelline systems persist.[38,52] Total anomalous pulmonary venous return below the diaphragm drains most frequently into the portal vein or ductus venosus.

Clinical Presentation Patients with infradiaphragmatic venous return are invariably obstructed and present with severe pulmonary edema. The obstruction may be at the level of the diaphragm, through intrinsic stenosis of the anomalous vessel, through closure of the ductus venosus, or through passage across the hepatic vascular bed in cases of drainage into the portal vein.[52,53]

Imaging On sonography, the anomalous common pulmonary vein is seen as a large vascular channel that enters the diaphragmatic hiatus anterior to the esophagus and inserts into the left portal vein or ductus venosus. CT and MRI show the same findings (Fig. 93-18).

Treatment and Prognosis Treatment of this anomaly is surgical (see Chapter 72).[54]

Hepatic Arteriovenous Malformations

Overview Arteriovenous malformations refer to a tangled collection of nonneoplastic vessels; they are much less common than infantile hemangiomas, although occasionally the two may be difficult to differentiate. Unlike hemangiomas, they do not regress and do not respond to medical therapy.[38,55]

Arterioportal fistulas refer to direct connections between the hepatic arterial and portal venous system, which can be intrahepatic or extrahepatic. Norton et al.[56] have classified these lesions according to their afferent supply: Type 1 is supplied by either the right or left hepatic artery; type 2 is supplied by both right and left hepatic arteries or their braches; and type 3 refers to a complex lesion, with vascular supply including extrahepatic arteries. Fistulas between the arterial and the systemic hepatic venous system are exceedingly rare, and when congenital, they are seen most often in the setting of other anomalies, such as hemorrhagic telangiectasia, hepatic carcinoma, and hemangioma.[10]

Etiology Congenital arteriovenous fistulas may be single or multiple and may be isolated lesions or part of the spectrum of Rendu-Osler-Weber syndrome (hereditary hemorrhagic telangiectasia) and Ehlers-Danlos syndrome. Most lesions are not congenital but are acquired in patients with biliary cirrhosis (such as children with biliary atresia) and after blunt or penetrating trauma (including after a liver biopsy).[55,57]

Clinical Presentation Arteriovenous malformations may present with congestive heart failure, hepatic ischemia, or portal hypertension.[55] Clinical manifestations of arterioportal fistulas are presinusoidal portal hypertension, with consequent ascites, splenomegaly, and gastrointestinal bleeding, as well as malabsorption and failure to thrive.[55,56] A murmur and thrill may be detectable over the right upper quadrant in approximately 50% of cases.[56] High-output heart failure may be seen in infants, mainly when the ductus venosus is patent; acute closure of the ductus venosus can result in fatal gastrointestinal bleeding.[55] If left untreated, further liver damage with hepatoportal sclerosis may aggravate the portal hypertension.[10] Acquired postbiopsy fistulas that are small and peripheral and produce no symptoms usually are self-limited.

Imaging Hepatic congenital arteriovenous malformations and arteriovenous fistulas can be diagnosed with ultrasound, CT, and MRI. In congenital arteriovenous malformations, ultrasound demonstrates a tangle of vessels of variable size.[55] The size of the hepatic artery is proportional to the size of the shunt; the draining hepatic veins are distended, and the aorta may taper after the takeoff of the hepatic artery. The hepatic artery demonstrates very high systolic Doppler shifts and high diastolic flow, whereas the hepatic veins demonstrate pulsatile or arterialized high-velocity flow.

In patients with arteriovenous fistulas, ultrasound demonstrates enlargement of the hepatic artery as well as dilatation of the portal vein at the site of the fistulous connection.[38] Portal venous flow is reversed on Doppler sonography in the draining vein of an arterioportal fistula and may be reversed in the main portal vein, depending on shunt size, as well as

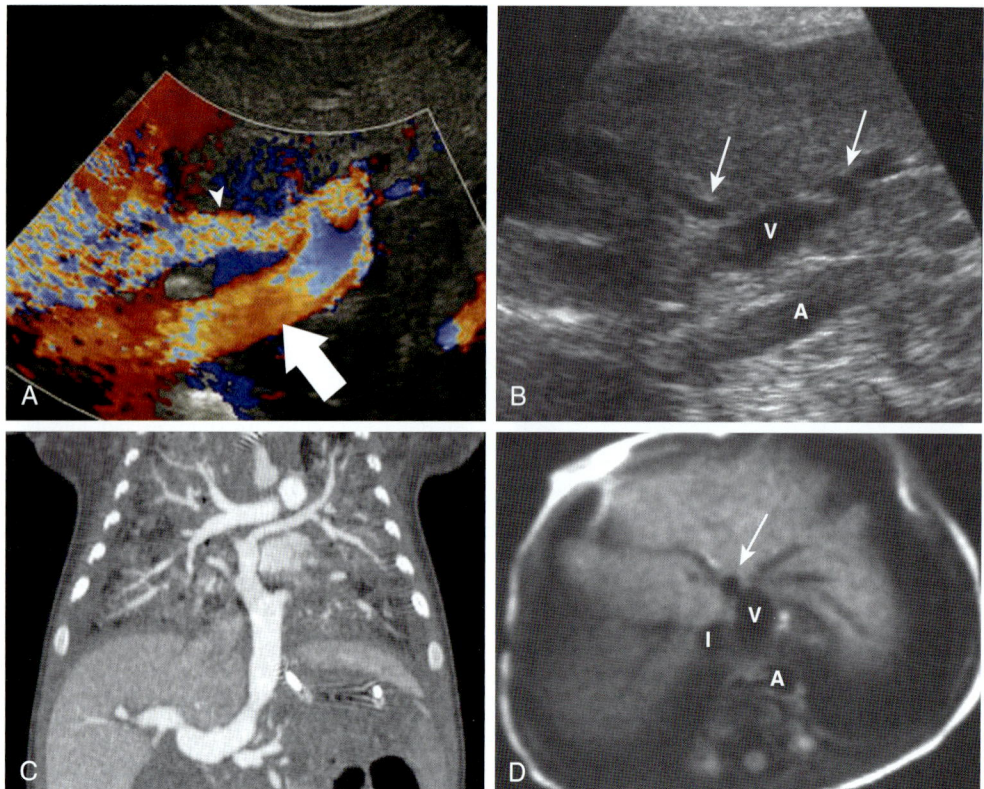

Figure 93-18 Total anomalous pulmonary venous return. **A,** A 2-week-old boy with pulmonary edema since birth. A transverse color Doppler ultrasound image shows a large common pulmonary vein (*arrow*) coursing caudally toward the portal vein (*arrowhead*). **B,** A sagittal gray-scale ultrasound image in a different child with asplenia shows the anomalous vein (*V*) entering the abdomen and joining the patent ductus venosus (*arrows*), partially outside the field of view. Note the stenosis at the junction between the anomalous vein and the ductus. **C,** Coronal reformatting from a computed tomography angiogram in another patient shows convergence of individual pulmonary veins into the common pulmonary vein, which in this case drains into the portal vein. Note the severe pulmonary edema. **D,** T1-weighted axial magnetic resonance in the same infant depicted in **B.** The anomalous vein (*V*) is seen transversely, with the dilated ductus venosus into which it drains (*arrow*) anteriorly. *A,* Aorta; *I,* IVC. (**B** and **D,** Courtesy Marta Hernanz-Schulman, MD, Nashville, TN.)

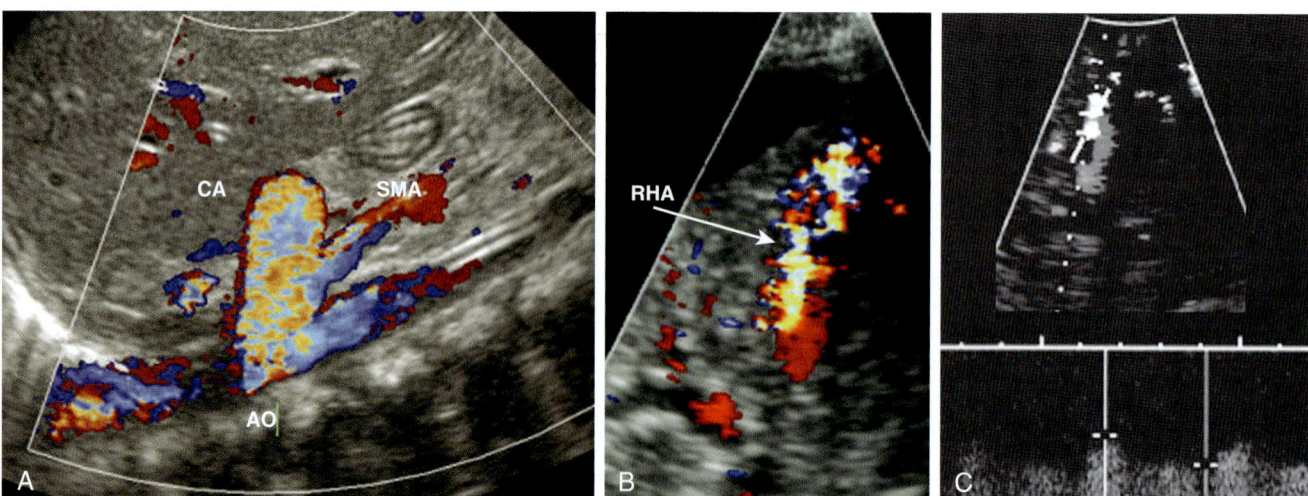

Figure 93-19 Congenital arterioportal shunts in two patients. **A,** A color Doppler image in a 4-month-girl with heart failure shows an enlarged celiac artery (*CA*) relative to the adjacent aorta (*AO*) and superior mesenteric artery (*SMA*), with color aliasing indicative of high flow velocity. **B,** Postbiopsy arterioportal fistula in an 8-year-old boy with a liver transplant. A color Doppler ultrasound image shows an intense high-velocity aliasing Doppler shift in a peripheral, small arteriovenous fistula arising from a right hepatic artery (*RHA*) branch (*arrow*) at the site of a previous liver biopsy. Ascites also is seen outlining the liver. **C,** Color (depicted in gray scale) and spectral Doppler images show a very high diastolic flow and a low resistive index in the hepatic artery branch leading into the fistula.

in the splenic and superior mesenteric veins.[1] The reversed portal venous flow usually is arterialized on spectral Doppler evaluation, with high flow velocity. The hepatic artery, or the branch that leads into the fistula, demonstrates high velocity and a decreased resistive index (Fig. 93-19). Ascites and bowel wall thickening may be present. The fistula is intensely visible by color and power Doppler imaging, with vibration artifact in the hepatic vein. CT and CTA demonstrate intense enhancement and rapid washout in malformations and fistulas; rapid appearance of the portal vein occurs during the arterial phase, with enhancement intensity similar to that of the aorta.[38] The enlarged arterial supply and venous drainage are well demonstrated by CTA, with early appearance of the draining veins.[38] The excellent temporal resolution of fast-sequence MRA allows visualization of the vascular nidus and identification of fast clearance in arteriovenous malformations and fistulas. Angiography shows similar findings (Fig. 93-20) and is reserved for imaging prior to therapeutic embolization.[55]

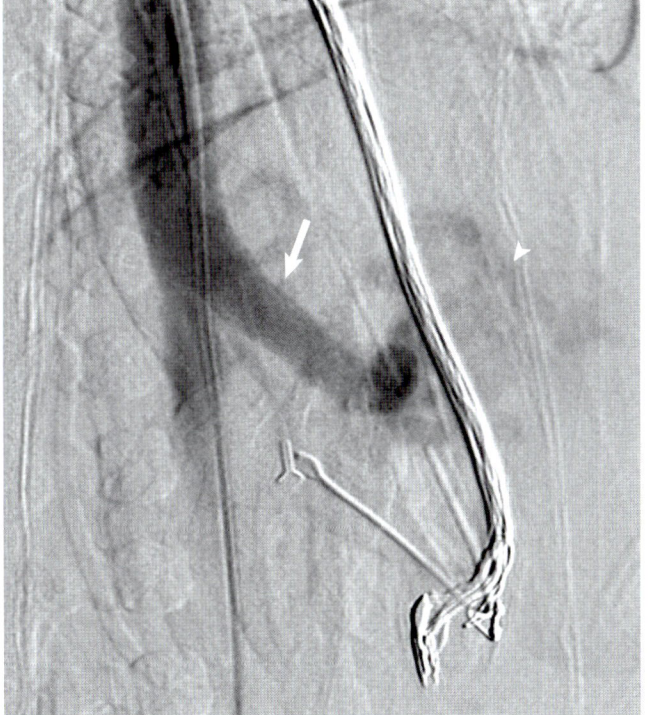

Figure 93-20 A lateral aortogram in same patient as depicted in Figure 93-19, *A*, confirms an enlarged celiac trunk (*arrow*) and decreased caliber of the more distal aorta. Early filling of the shunt vessels (*arrowhead*) is seen over the liver.

Treatment and Prognosis Congenital hepatic arteriovenous malformations and fistulas do not respond to medical management. Treatment is aimed at obliteration of the abnormal arteriovenous connection and consists of embolization, surgical ligation, hepatic lobectomy, or liver transplantation. Embolization of feeding vessels may lead to dilatation of subclinical channels and recurrence of the abnormal connection and may require further embolization of escalation of therapy.[1,38] Heparinization may be needed after embolization to prevent postembolization portal vein thrombosis.[55] As noted earlier, infants with biliary atresia and arterioportal shunt present a special problem; they are unlikely to tolerate interruption in hepatic arterial flow, and early liver transplantation may be the treatment of choice.[38,58,59] Prognosis depends on the severity of the underlying disease and the success of various treatments.

Suggested Readings

Alonso-Gamarra E, Parron M, Perez A, et al. Clinical and radiologic manifestations of congenital extrahepatic portosystemic shunts: a comprehensive review. *Radiographics*. 2011;31:707-731.

Altuntas B, Erden A, Karakurt C, et al. Severe portal hypertension due to congenital hepatoportal arteriovenous fistula associated with intrahepatic portal vein aneurysm. *J Clin Ultrasound*. 1998;26(7):357-360.

Biyyam DR, Chapman T, Ferguson MR, et al. Congenital lung abnormalities: embryologic features, prenatal diagnosis, and postnatal radiologic-pathologic correlation. *Radiographics*. 2010;30(6):1721-1738.

Cool CD, Deutsch G. Pulmonary arterial hypertension from a pediatric perspective. *Pediatr Dev Pathol*. 2008;11(3):169-177.

Dehghani SM, Haghighat M, Imanieh MH, et al. Tacrolimus related hypertrophic cardiomyopathy in liver transplant recipients. *Arch Iran Med*. 2010;13(2):116-119.

Fink MA, Berry SR, Gow PJ, et al. Risk factors for liver transplantation waiting list mortality. *J Gastroenterol Hepatol*. 2007;22(1):119-124.

Glassman MS, Klein SA, Spivak W. Evaluation of cavernous transformation of the portal vein by magnetic resonance imaging. *Clin Pediatr (Phila)*. 1993;32(2):77-80.

Hammon Jr JW, Bender Jr HW, Graham Jr TP, et al. Total anomalous pulmonary venous connection in infancy. Ten years' experience including studies of postoperative ventricular function. *J Thorac Cardiovasc Surg*. 1980;80(4):544-551.

Hammon Jr JW. Total anomalous pulmonary connection: then and now. *Ann Thorac Surg*. 1993;55(4):1030-1032.

Lassau N, Leclère J, Auperin A, et al. Hepatic veno-occlusive disease after myeloablative treatment and bone marrow transplantation: value of grayscale and Doppler US in 100 patients. *Radiology*. 1997;204(2):545-552.

Lee W, Chang S, Duddalwar VA, et al. Imaging assessment of congenital and acquired abnormalities of the portal venous system. *Radiographics*. 2011;31:905-926.

Mathieu D, Vasile N, Dibie C, et al. Portal cavernoma: dynamic CT features and transient differences in hepatic attenuation. *Radiology*. 1985;154(3):743-748.

Park JH, Cha SH, Han JK, et al. Intrahepatic portosystemic venous shunt. *AJR Am J Roentgenol*. 1990;155(3):527-528.

References

Full references for this chapter can be found on www.expertconsult.com.

Chapter 94

Liver Transplantation in Children

DOUGLAS C. RIVARD and LISA H. LOWE

Overview

The first liver transplantation was performed in 1963, with posttransplant survival reaching 1 year in 1968.[1] Subsequent use of immunosuppressants such as cyclosporine and tacrolimus, coupled with improved surgical techniques, has resulted in 1-year survival rates exceeding 90%.[2,3] The organ pool for children has been increased by reduced-size liver transplants, the sharing of organs between two recipients, and living related-donor transplantation.[4-6]

Liver transplantation is indicated in children with irreversible liver disease, liver failure, nonresectable liver tumors, vascular abnormalities, and some metabolic abnormalities (Box 94-1).[7] Biliary atresia with development of cirrhosis and portal hypertension after a Kasai portoenterostomy is performed accounts for more than 60% of liver transplants in children younger than 5 years. More than two thirds of patients with biliary atresia eventually require liver transplantation, with about one third of these procedures performed in the first year of life.[8]

Other cholestatic causes of cirrhosis include bile duct hypoplasia syndromes (e.g., Alagille), cystic fibrosis, and primary sclerosing cholangitis.[9-11] Children with cholestasis related to total parenteral nutrition may have underlying short-bowel syndrome and may require combined liver and small bowel transplantation.

Diffuse nonbiliary liver diseases necessitating transplantation include infectious and autoimmune hepatitis, neonatal hemochromatosis, graft-versus-host disease, and fulminant liver failure.[12-14] Congenital hepatic fibrosis is associated with autosomal recessive polycystic kidney disease; patients with these diseases may require combined liver and kidney transplantation.[15] Liver transplantation in persons with metabolic disorders is a well-established therapeutic option for glycogen storage disease, which involves a risk of liver adenomas and hepatocellular carcinoma; persons with tyrosinemia and Wilson disease have a risk of neurologic damage and cirrhosis.[16-18]

Most liver transplants performed in older children involve the use of a whole cadaveric liver (Fig. 94-1), whereas most young children receive reduced transplants. Liver segments are defined according to the segmental and vascular anatomy.[19] Most living donor transplants use the donor's left lateral segment or left lobe, although the right lobe also may be used. A cadaveric liver may be split between two recipients; however, both result in challenging vascular and biliary connections because of limited pedicle lengths.[5]

Left lobe and left lateral segment hila and their cut surfaces face to the right; however, they can be differentiated by the presence of the falciform ligament separating lateral segments two and three from medial segment four in the left lobe transplant, which is absent in left lateral segment grafts (Fig. 94-2). The small bowel, duodenum, colon, and right kidney often migrate into the vacated liver bed; a migrated cecum and right colon may imitate malrotation.

The portal vein usually is connected end-to-end to the recipient portal vein, with as much of the native portal vein preserved during hepatectomy as possible.[20] Children with older transplants may have had extension grafts, which may still be used in patients with unsuitable native portal veins.

The donor hepatic artery usually is anastomosed to the recipient's hepatic artery or celiac axis. The hepatic artery may be connected to the infrarenal aorta if technically required. In such cases the native hepatic artery is ligated and should not be confused with arterial occlusion on imaging. The bile duct typically is attached to a Roux-en-Y jejunal loop (Fig. 94-3).

In reduced-size transplants, the donor hepatic vein is connected to the recipient's modified hepatic vein orifice. In full-size liver grafts, the donor liver is removed with the intrahepatic inferior vena cava (IVC), which is then interposed between the infraatrial and distal native IVC. The donor IVC may be sutured distally and connected proximally, piggyback fashion, to the preserved native IVC. In patients with polysplenia and biliary atresia, vascular connections may be modified as a result of the frequent absence of the hepatic segment of the IVC, azygous continuation, malrotation, a preduodenal portal vein, and other anomalies.[5,20,21]

Vascular, biliary, infectious, and immunosuppression-related complications may befall liver recipients postoperatively, including posttransplant lymphoproliferative disease (PTLD). The most common complication of liver transplant is infection, but vascular thrombosis and primary graft nonfunction account for most cases of graft loss leading to retransplantation. Death in most pediatric liver recipients is caused by infection, neurologic complications, or multisystem organ failure. Enteric complications include bowel perforation and obstruction, gastrointestinal hemorrhage, and infectious enteritis. Neurologic complications include cerebral hemorrhage and infarction, infection, and drug toxicity.[22-24] Immunosuppressive drug-induced nephrotoxicity is common, but imaging features generally are nonspecific.

Other complications include hepatic parenchymal defects, pleural effusions, and splenic infarcts, which may occur after splenic artery ligation.[25,26] Right adrenal hemorrhage and

Box 94-1 Indications for Pediatric Liver Transplantation

- Cholestatic liver diseases
- Biliary atresia
- A₁-Antitrypsin deficiency
- Bile duct hypoplasia syndromes (e.g., Alagille syndrome and Byler syndrome)
- Cirrhosis as a result of chronic total parenteral nutrition
- Cirrhosis as a result of cystic fibrosis
- Sclerosing cholangitis associated with Langerhans cell histiocytosis
- Cystic fibrosis
- Tyrosinemia
- Urea cycle disorders
- Glycogen storage diseases
- Wilson disease
- Maple syrup urine disease
- Primary hyperoxaluria
- Crigler-Najjar syndrome
- Mitochondrial disease
- Hyperammonemia
- Viral hepatitis
- Congenital hepatic fibrosis
- Neonatal hepatitis
- Neonatal hemochromatosis
- Autoimmune hepatitis
- Medication-induced liver failure
- Graft-versus-host disease
- Acute liver failure
- Idiopathic portal hypertension
- Neoplastic diseases (hepatoblastoma, hepatocellular carcinoma, extensive infantile hemangiomas, metastatic neuroendocrine tumor)
- Hilar inflammatory pseudotumor

right phrenic nerve injury are potential complications seen after the standard transplant operation, but they rarely occur after a cava-sparing operation.

Imaging

Postoperative imaging is centered on evaluation of vascular and enteric complications. Therefore an understanding of specific surgical practice is essential.

Portable sonography may be used during surgery, mainly when vascular anastomoses are difficult or revised and their patency is uncertain. Vascular patency is evaluated daily with Doppler ultrasound for the first few posttransplant days because the fate of the transplant is much improved if vascular occlusions are diagnosed and managed early. The frequency of required ultrasound examinations then decreases, based on individual needs and clinical concerns.[27,28]

Early postoperative ultrasound may be challenging because of poor acoustic windows caused by dressings, open incisions, free intraabdominal air, and body wall edema. The flow patterns in all vessels vary in the early postoperative period because of edema of the anastomosis and surrounding tissues, as well as hemodynamic changes in the graft's vascular bed. Vascular patency, flow direction, pulsatility pattern, and velocity can be evaluated using gray-scale, spectral, and color Doppler ultrasound techniques. The color velocity scale may need to be adjusted for each vessel separately to avoid aliasing in the faster flowing vessels, which can lead to ambiguity of flow direction. Efforts must be made to interrogate at the anastomoses, where stenosis, thrombosis, and occlusion are most likely.[27]

Early findings seen in otherwise normal liver grafts include increased periportal echogenicity (low attenuation on computed tomography [CT] and increased signal on water-sensitive magnetic resonance [MR] sequences) related to transient lymphatic engorgement (Fig. 94-4), right pleural effusion, subhepatic fluid collections, and biliary air in recipients with choledochojejunostomies.[25,26]

Periodic long-term ultrasound screening of liver recipients is mandatory because vascular complications may be clinically silent. CT, CT angiography (CTA), magnetic resonance cholangiopancreatography (MRCP), and magnetic resonance angiography (MRA) are used to determine the need for biliary and vascular interventions in selected patients. CT remains the primary modality for evaluating many intraabdominal complications, such as infection and PTLD. New magnetic resonance imaging (MRI) sequences have increased the utility of MRI in these patients, with the obvious advantage of avoiding ionizing radiation.[29]

Pretransplant Imaging

Preoperative imaging is tailored to the patient's underlying disease and coexistent conditions. The goals are to document vascular patency, define visceral and vascular anatomy, exclude contraindications, and evaluate the extent of liver disease and portal hypertension.

Pertinent anatomic features for surgical planning include a small, absent, or occluded portal vein; IVC thrombosis; biliary atresia associated with polysplenia syndrome and absent

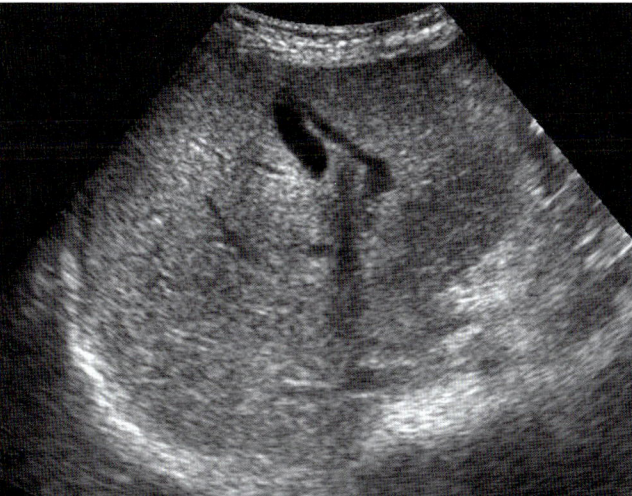

Figure 94-1 Transverse ultrasound image of a whole liver transplant. Fluid along the falciform ligament demarcates the left lateral and medial segments. A right lobe is also present.

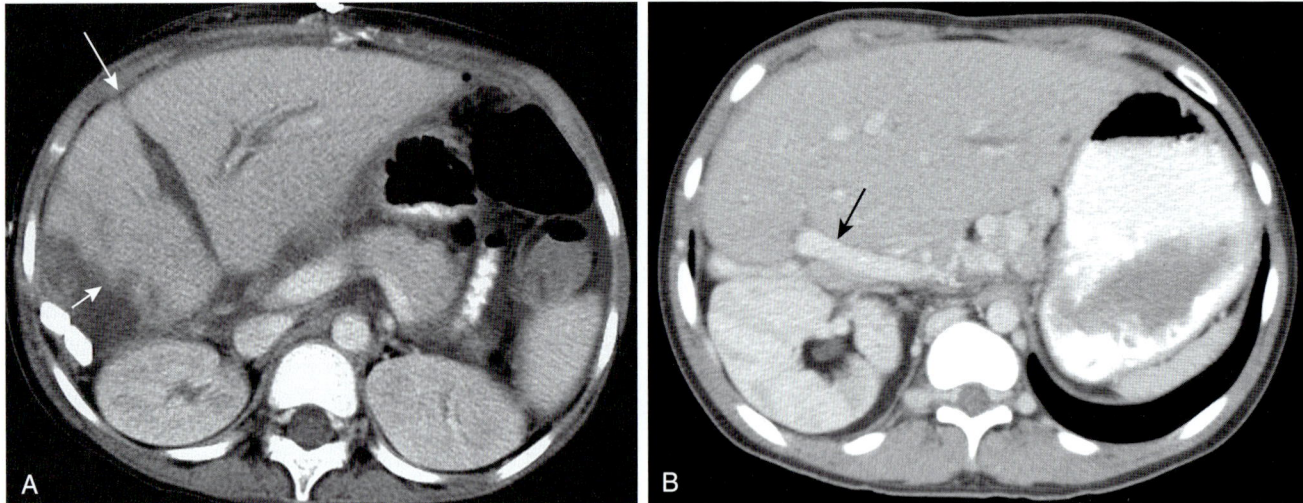

Figure 94-2 **Segmental liver grafts. A,** Computed tomography (CT) of a left lobe liver graft. Note the ill-defined, irregular cut edge with adjacent fluid (*short arrow*). Fluid along the falciform ligament (*long arrow*) separates the left lateral segment (segments two and three) from the medial segment (segment four). **B,** CT of a left lateral segment graft. Note the course of the portal vein entering from the right (*arrow*) and the absence of the falciform ligament. Also note the position of the right kidney in the upper abdomen.

intrahepatic IVC, with hepatic veins draining into the right atrium; systemic drainage of the splenic veins; congenital portosystemic shunts; and malrotation. Transplantation may be impossible when both the portal and superior mesenteric veins are occluded or in cases of nonresponsive metastatic hepatoblastoma. Detection of hepatocellular carcinoma in a patient with cirrhosis changes the transplant urgency and requires tumor staging and decisions about pretransplant therapy, which affect the timing and feasibility of transplantation.[27]

Ultrasound is the method used most often in the preoperative evaluation of pediatric transplant candidates. Doppler ultrasound assesses vascular patency and hemodynamics. CT with intravenous contrast is excellent for showing vascular and visceral anatomy, unimpeded by overlying bowel gas. MRI may supply hemodynamic information and is superior to ultrasound in depicting varices, collaterals, and spontaneous splenorenal shunts. Bone radiographs may detect rickets, osteopenia, and fractures, and chest radiographs may show cardiomegaly and vascular prominence in patients with hepatopulmonary disease (see Chapter 93).[29,30] Angiography is seldom needed but is reserved for patients for whom additional information might be required.

Vascular Complications

HEPATIC ARTERY

Overview Hepatic arterial complications include thrombosis, occlusion, stenosis, peripheral arteriovenous fistula, and aneurysm. Acute arterial thrombosis may be catastrophic and result

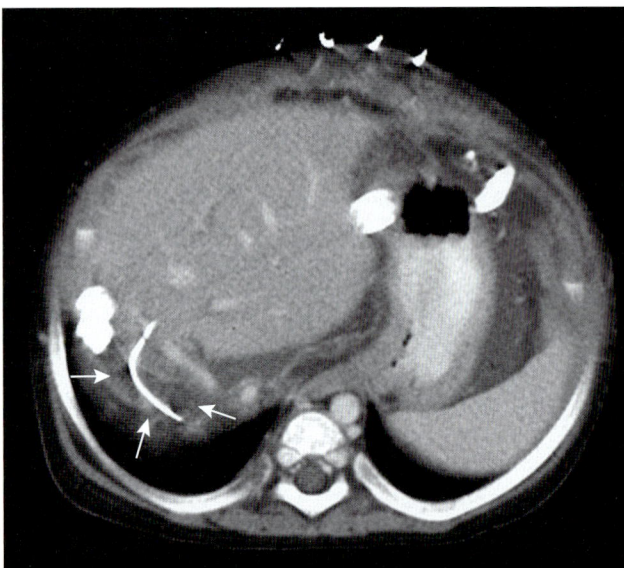

Figure 94-3 The Roux-en-Y biliary anastomosis and loop are marked early after transplantation by a small biliary stent (*arrows*). Being an efferent loop from the liver, it frequently does not fill with intestinal contrast, making it difficult to differentiate from a pathologic fluid collection. Diffuse mesenteric edema and skin staples are noted.

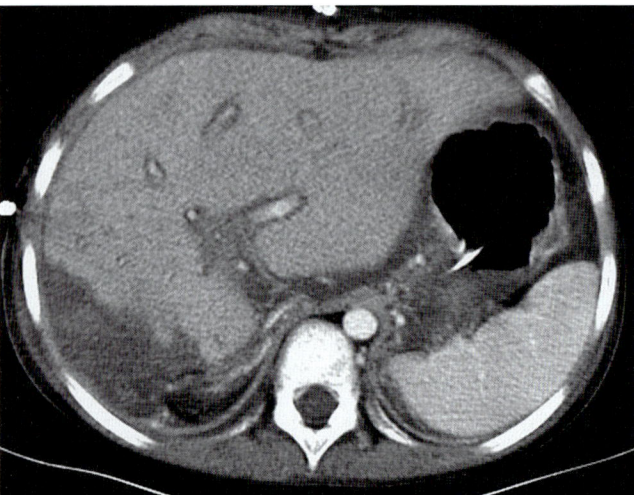

Figure 94-4 Early computed tomography findings in liver transplantation. Diffuse periportal hypoattenuation, irregularity of the liver cut surface edge, and adjacent fluid are present.

in acidosis, sepsis, and organ necrosis. Early hepatic artery thrombosis is associated with a high incidence of transplant loss.[31] If the problem is diagnosed within the first 2 to 3 days and the patient is still asymptomatic, most transplanted livers with hepatic artery thrombosis may be salvaged. However, if elevated liver function tests, bile leak, liver abscess, or sepsis have supervened, graft loss may reach 75%.[32]

Imaging   The hepatic artery is much more difficult to visualize by gray-scale ultrasound than the portal vein because of its small size. It is best evaluated by color and power Doppler ultrasound.[25] It is easier to follow the artery to its anastomosis when it is attached to the native hepatic artery or celiac axis rather than to the infrarenal aorta, where much of its course might be obscured by bowel gas. Both CTA and MRA are useful in showing hepatic artery anatomy, course, and complications (Fig. 94-5).[26]

The hepatic artery flow pattern may vary considerably in the early postoperative days, demonstrating both high and low resistive indices, without consistent prognostic implications.

The diagnosis of hepatic artery thrombosis is made by the inability to detect hepatic artery signal on color and spectral Doppler ultrasound.[25] Acute arterial thrombosis is treated by thrombectomy, revision, and occasionally retransplantation.[33] High-grade narrowing is manifested by turbulence and severely attenuated velocity distally with a parvus-tardus pattern in intrahepatic branches, with narrow systolic peaks and absent diastolic flow beyond the anastomosis.[31]

Later onset hepatic artery occlusion may manifest with biliary leaks, strictures, and infection, including peribiliary abscess and sepsis because the biliary tree depends on hepatic arterial supply. In long-standing hepatic artery occlusion, hilar or transcapsular collaterals may result in a detectable arterial Doppler signal.[31]

Stenosis of the hepatic artery may be silent or may manifest with biliary complications and infection. High velocity and turbulence may be seen at the stenotic site. The flow pattern is abnormal, with a low-amplitude, parvus tardus representing a systolic acceleration time longer than 0.08 second and a resistive index lower than 0.5.[31] Very high-grade stenosis manifests with narrow and low-amplitude systolic peaks and absence of diastolic flow. The stenosis itself is usually extrahepatic and difficult to demonstrate directly by Doppler ultrasound (Fig. 94-6).[26,31] The hemodynamic changes of hepatic artery stenosis may be more dramatic than its appearance on CTA or MRA.

Hepatic artery pseudoaneurysm may occur at the anastomosis or within the liver at a biopsy site.[26,31] Liver biopsy also is a cause of intrahepatic arteriovenous fistulas.[33]

VENOUS SYSTEM

Overview   Obstructive lesions of the portal vein, hepatic vein, and IVC may manifest with progressive ascites, deterioration of liver function, gastrointestinal bleeding, decreased platelet count, and increased spleen size. Pulmonary hypertension and intrapulmonary shunting may develop. Doppler signal in the intrahepatic portions of the portal vein do not exclude stenosis or obstruction, which may be present in the extrahepatic segment, with intrahepatic flow reconstituted by collateral vessels.[29] Portal vein, hepatic vein, and IVC stenosis result in flow acceleration at the stenosis and a jet of increased flow at the poststenotic segment, which appears as a contrasting color as a result of aliasing when the scale is adjusted to the velocity below the stenosis. The jet velocity is proportional to the pressure gradient across the stenosis.[25,26]

Imaging

Portal Vein   Ultrasound of the transplant portal vein requires visualization of its entire course. One must measure the diameter at any site of narrowing and interrogate the portal vein by spectral and color Doppler along its extrahepatic and hilar course, as well as its major intrahepatic branches. The curved course of the portal vein in left lobe and left lateral segment transplants and the size discrepancy between donor and recipient veins frequently cause dilation at the neohilum because of altered flow dynamics (Fig. 94-7) with a "yin-and-yang" swirling pattern on color Doppler. This pattern has not been proved clinically important. Anastomotic and periportal edema causing relative narrowing with jet formation is very common in the early postoperative period; these instances of edema are most often transient but may progress or persist and should be monitored. Complications include early thrombosis, stenosis, and late occlusion (Fig. 94-8).[25,26]

A hypoechoic thrombus may not be recognized by gray-scale ultrasound but shows absence of signal on color Doppler imaging. Reversal of superior mesenteric or splenic vein flow also is seen. Early thrombosis usually is treated by surgical thrombectomy and revision. Early posttransplant reversal of entire portal vein flow may reflect extensive hepatic necrosis and arterioportal shunting—an ominous sign associated with frequent organ loss.[26]

Later onset of portal vein thrombosis or occlusion may be clinically silent, manifesting with increasing plasma levels of

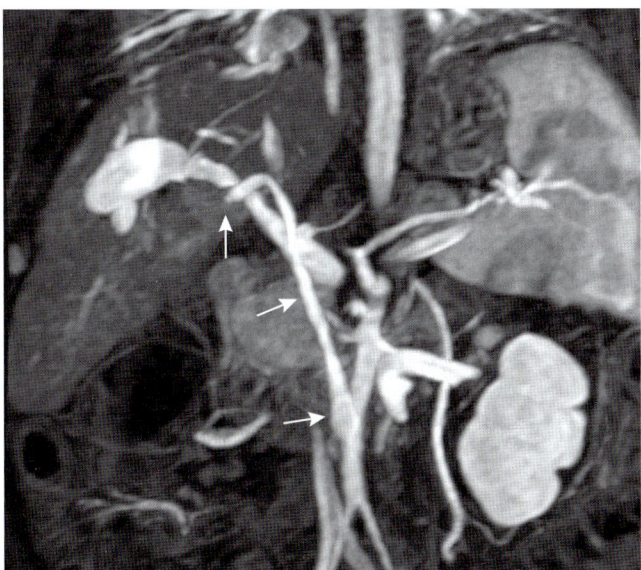

Figure 94-5   Hepatic artery occlusion. Magnetic resonance angiography shows the origin of the transplant hepatic artery from the infrarenal aorta (*arrows*). It is occluded near the liver.

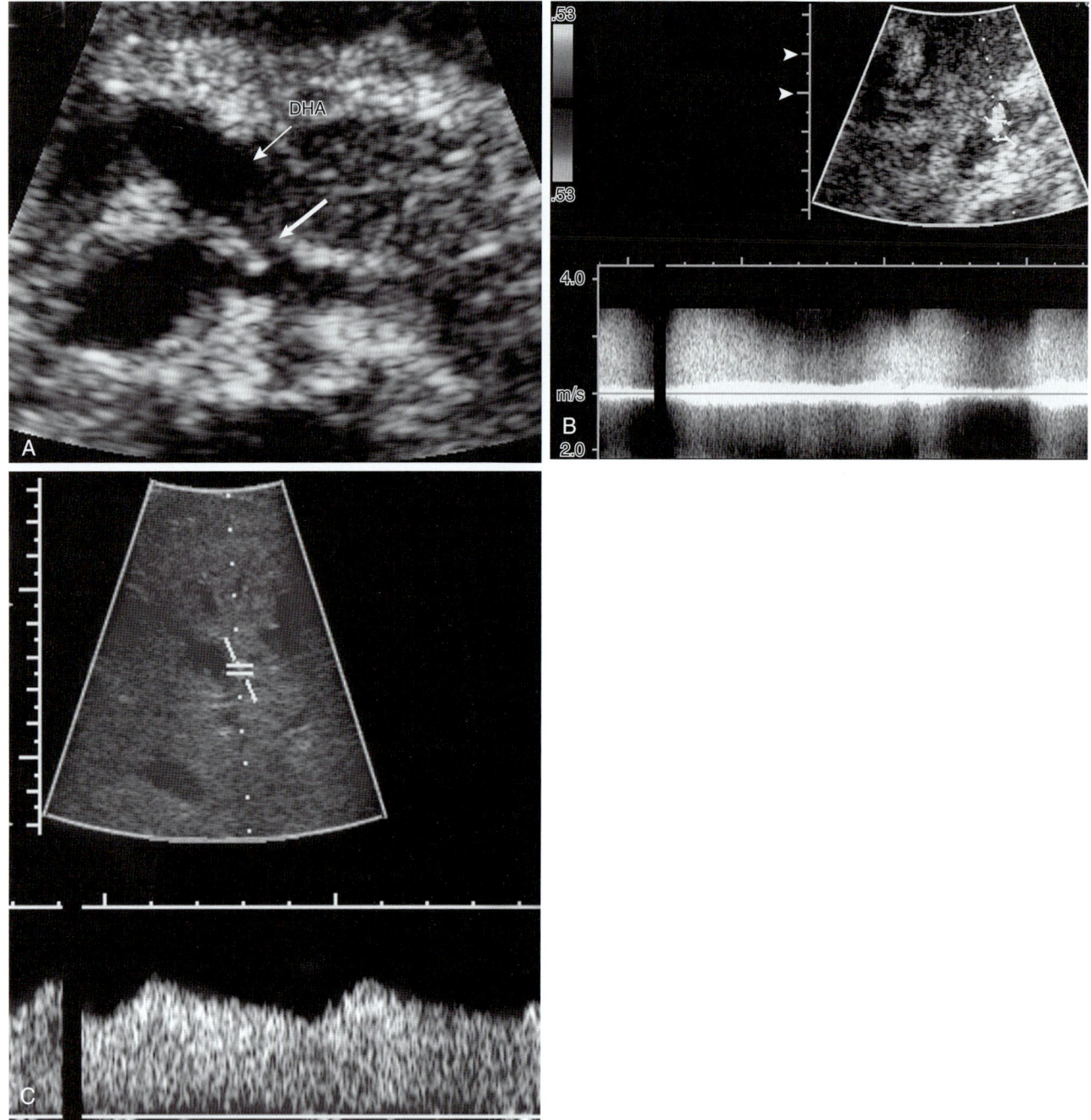

Figure 94-6   Ultrasound and Doppler characteristics of hepatic artery stenosis. **A,** Transverse ultrasound shows stenosis immediately distal to the celiac axis (*thick arrow*). The donor hepatic artery (*DHA*) distal to the anastomotic stenosis is marked by a thin arrow. **B,** Spectral and color Doppler at the stenosis show extreme turbulence and high velocity. The normal arterial signal is difficult to recognize because of aliasing. **C,** Spectral and color Doppler in an intrahepatic hepatic artery branch show a slow systolic upstroke (tardus phenomenon), and relatively high diastolic flow. Resistive index was also abnormally low.

hepatic enzymes, an enlarging spleen, and gastrointestinal bleeding. Intrahepatic portal venous flow frequently is reconstructed from collaterals recruited from superior mesenteric vein branches via varices in the Roux-en-Y loop and from transcapsular collaterals. In the latter event, flow in the receiving portal vein branches may be reversed with segment-to-segment shunting.

Stenosis usually occurs at anastomoses and in extension grafts (Fig. 94-9).[34] Because of the curved extrahepatic course of the portal vein, it may be difficult to demonstrate stenosis by ultrasound. The jet created at the stenotic site dissipates, such that flow velocity measured at the hilum is frequently normal despite a hemodynamically significant portal vein stenosis more proximally.[26] The jet also may exaggerate the dilation of the portal vein at the hilum. Following successful angioplasty, the jet velocity decreases and the diameter at the stenotic site increases (Fig. 94-10). Less operator-dependent CT and MRI are highly useful and more consistent than ultrasound in the evaluation of portal vein occlusion and stenosis.[29,31,35]

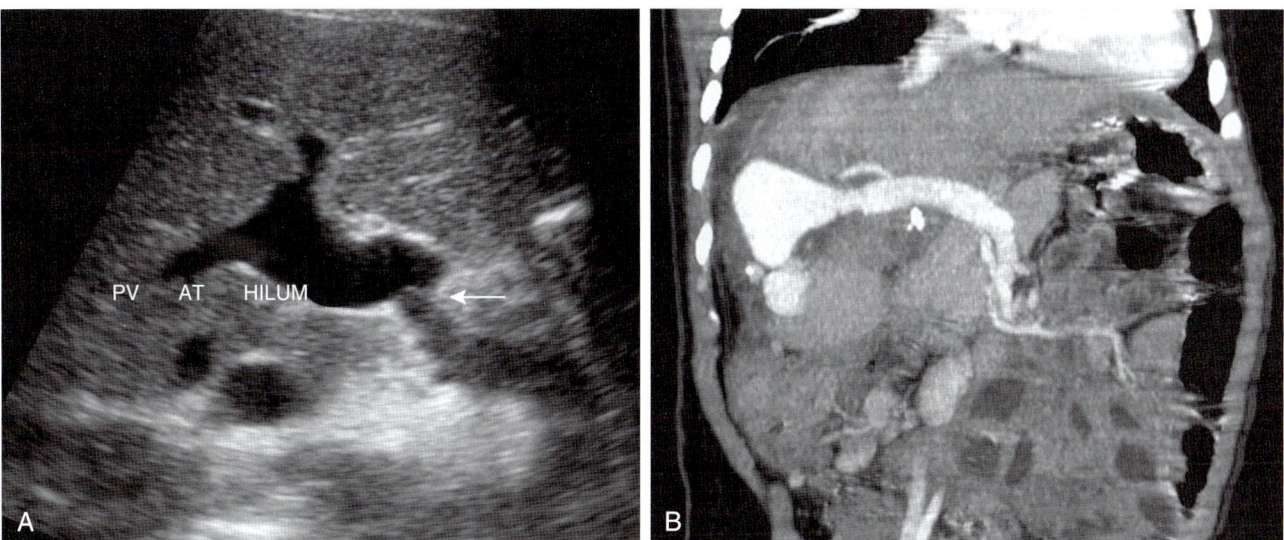

Figure 94-7   Portal vein in segmental transplantation. **A,** An ultrasound image shows a size discrepancy (*arrow*) between the native and donor portal veins and dilation of the donor portal vein (*PV AT HILUM*). **B,** Coronal reconstruction from computed tomography angiography demonstrates the extrahepatic portal vein coursing from the left to the right edge of the transplant, near the right abdominal wall. The portal vein is dilated at the neohilum. Note slight narrowing at the anastomosis in this early transplant.

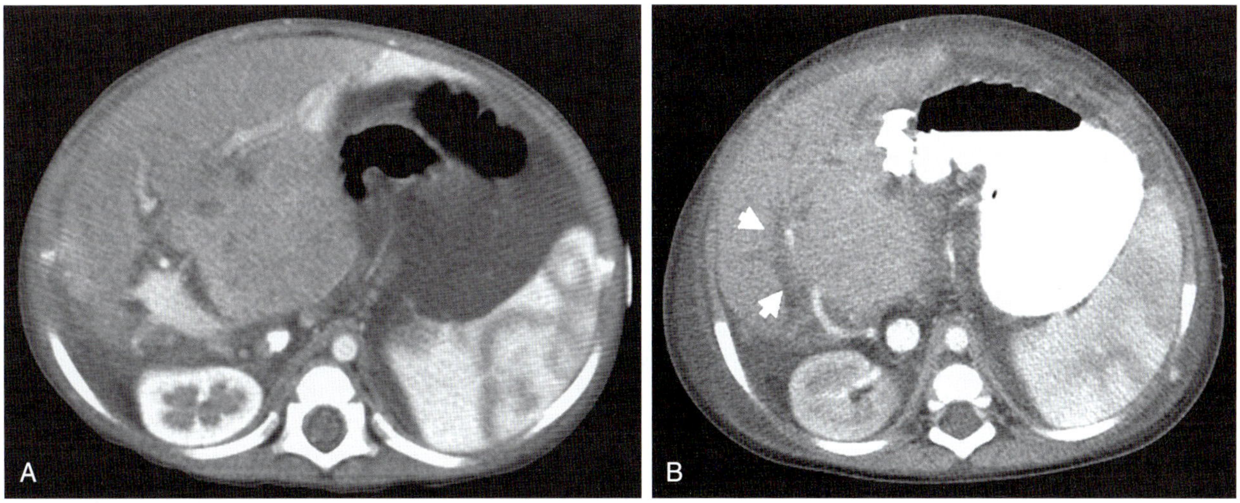

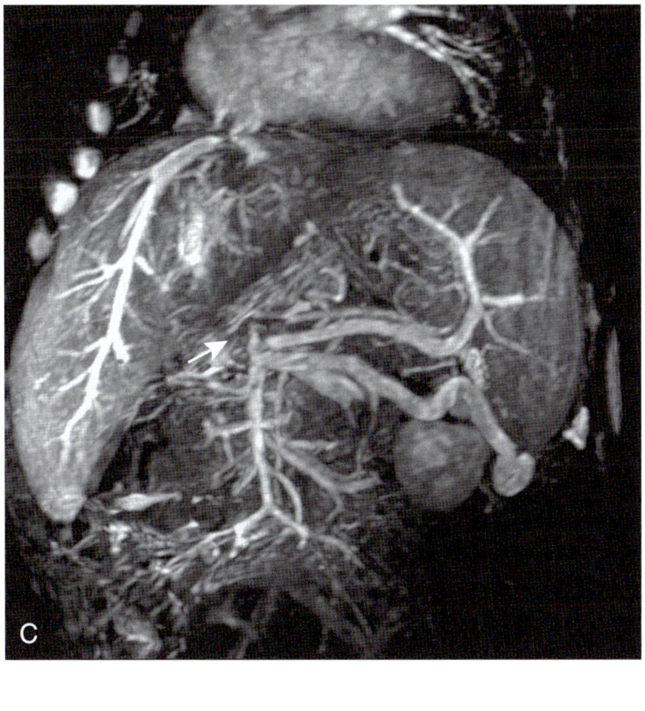

Figure 94-8   Portal vein occlusion. **A,** Contrast-enhanced computed tomography (CT) in an infant after left lateral segment graft shows that the portal vein and the hepatic artery are well seen in the neohilum. **B,** At 4-month follow-up, contrast-enhanced CT shows a lucent band where the portal vein previously had been seen (*arrows*). The patient underwent successful thrombolysis. **C,** Long-standing portal vein occlusion. Magnetic resonance venography shows occlusion of the entire portal vein from the splenomesenteric confluence (*arrow*). A large venous collateral is seen from the confluence to the left flank.

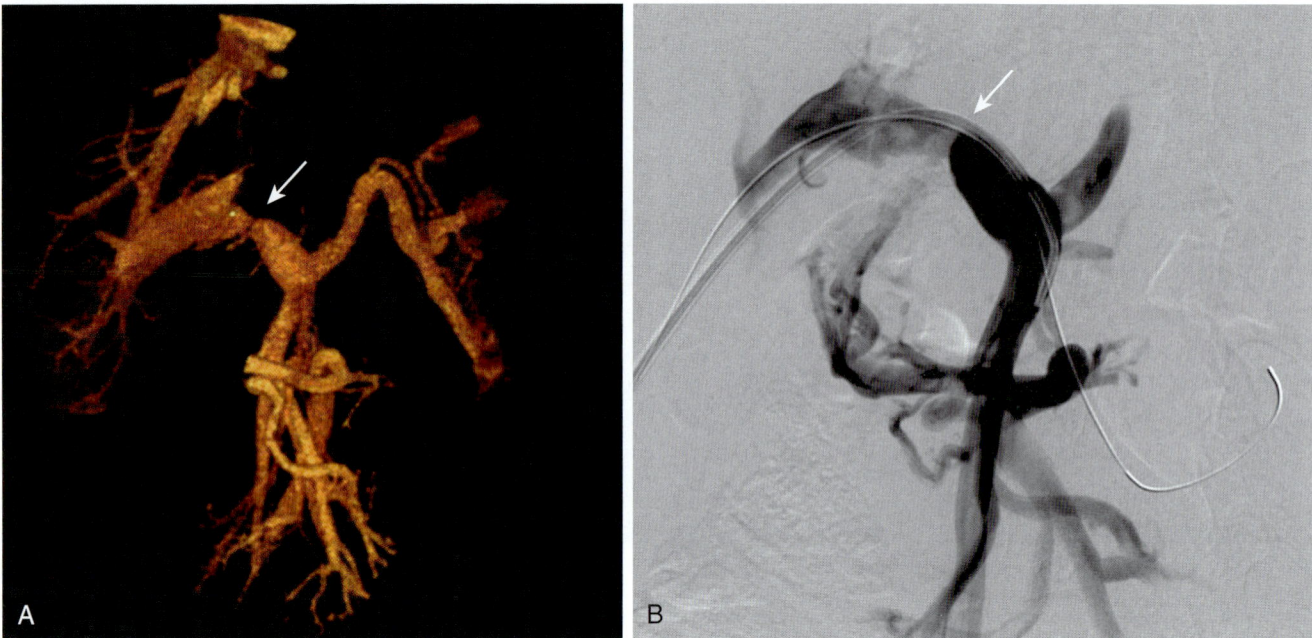

Figure 94-9 Portal vein stenosis. **A,** Reconstructed images from contrast-enhanced computed tomography shows anastomotic stenosis (*arrow*) in a patient with a whole liver transplant. **B,** A portal venogram in the same patient confirms the portal vein stenosis (*arrow*).

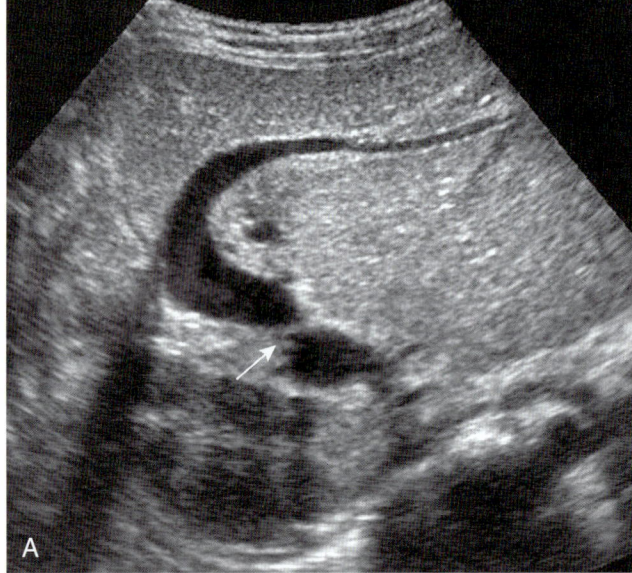

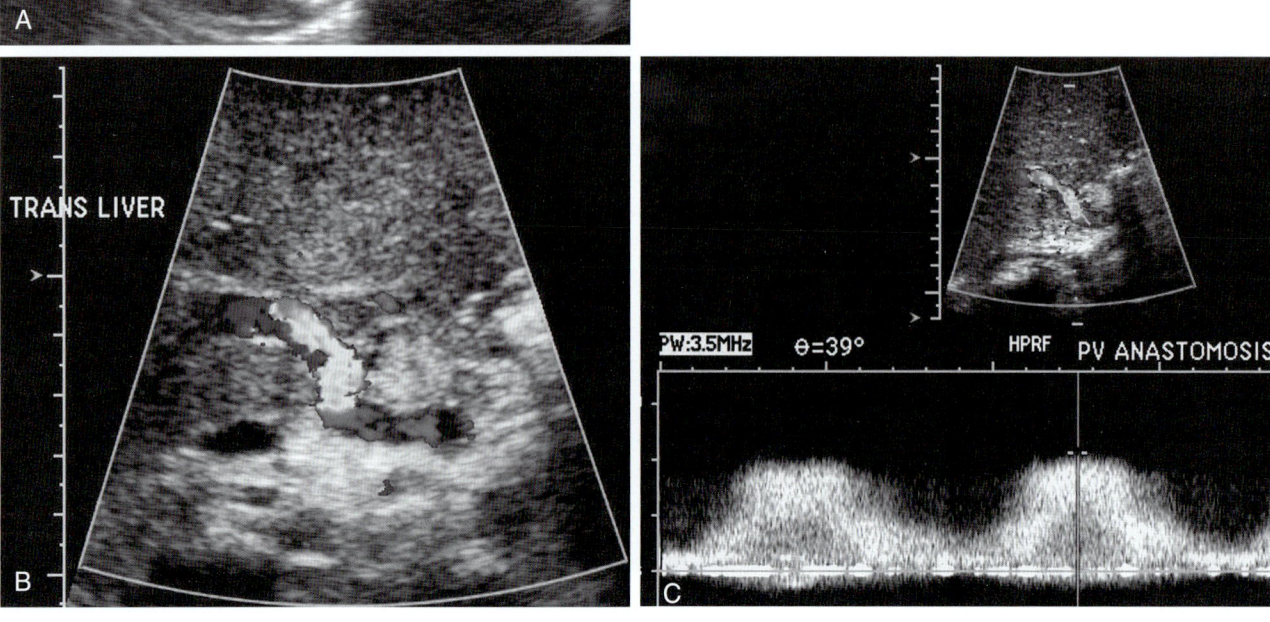

Figure 94-10 Ultrasound and Doppler characteristics of portal vein stenosis. **A,** Ultrasound of a child with a left lateral segment graft. The stenosis (*arrow*) is outside the liver hilum, beyond the portal vein curvature. **B,** On color Doppler, the velocity scale is adjusted such that aliasing demonstrates the higher velocity jet outlining the stenotic site. **C,** On spectral and color Doppler with sampling at the jet, maximal flow velocity is obtained to assess the hemodynamic impact of the stenosis. The maximal jet velocity exceeds 2 m/sec.

Hepatic Vein   Hepatic vein stenosis occurs mainly in reduced-size transplants at the anastomosis to the recipient IVC. In a posttransplant patient with the onset of portal hypertension, special efforts must be made to evaluate the hepatic veins and IVC if a portal vein complication is not seen. Stenosis is near the diaphragm, making it difficult to demonstrate by ultrasound (Fig. 94-11). Doppler ultrasound demonstrates increased flow velocity and a jet with loss of triphasic flow.[31,36] A caveat is that triphasic flow may be absent without obstruction. CTA and MRA are excellent to demonstrate or confirm the diagnosis.[26]

Inferior Vena Cava   IVC stenosis and obstruction may occur at the anastomosis. Anastomotic stenosis and obstruction may be short or long segment and may result from compression or graft torsion (Fig. 94-12). The clinical manifestations of IVC stenosis or obstruction depend on the location. If the problem is at or above the hepatic veins, it manifests with ascites and portal hypertension. If it is at a lower level, it may be clinically silent.[26]

IVC obstruction can be diagnosed by all cross-sectional modalities; however, several pitfalls may be encountered with Doppler ultrasound. Flow in the hepatic veins may be normal and triphasic if the IVC obstruction is distal to their insertion (Fig. 94-13). On the other hand, when the obstruction is proximal to the hepatic vein insertion, hepatic venous blood may enter the IVC and flow retrograde to decompress into systemic collaterals. In patients with a surgical portosystemic shunt, IVC obstruction prevents adequate decompression, sometimes reversing flow in the shunt and increasing preexistent varices.[31,34]

BILIARY COMPLICATIONS

Bile leaks and strictures occurring early after transplantation are related to technical surgical problems, such as anastomotic leak and narrowing or kinking. Biliary complications with a later onset commonly are associated with ischemia and infection as a result of arterial occlusion or stenosis.[31] Biliary strictures are more common in reduced-size liver transplants than in full-sized ones.[37] Inspissated bile and biliary compression by a mucocele or cystic duct remnant have been described.[29] Chronic rejection may be associated with loss of bile ducts and mild chronic dilation.

Ultrasound identifies biliary dilation and is the primary screening modality. When bile duct dilation is found, further imaging is indicated.[25] MRCP increasingly is used to assess biliary obstruction and the need for intervention.[38-40] Direct transhepatic cholangiogram usually is performed as part of the therapeutic approach (Fig. 94-14).

FLUID COLLECTIONS

Early postoperative bleeding from leaking anastomoses or inadequate hemostasis leading to visible fluid collections occurs in as many as 15% of recipients. Up to half of these patients undergo operative exploration. Most fluid collections occur at the cut edge, contain serous fluid, blood, or bile, and are transient and clinically insignificant. Other collections may result from an anastomotic bile leak, abscess, or bowel perforation. The imaging appearance of perihepatic fluid collections is nonspecific; most contain some debris.[25]

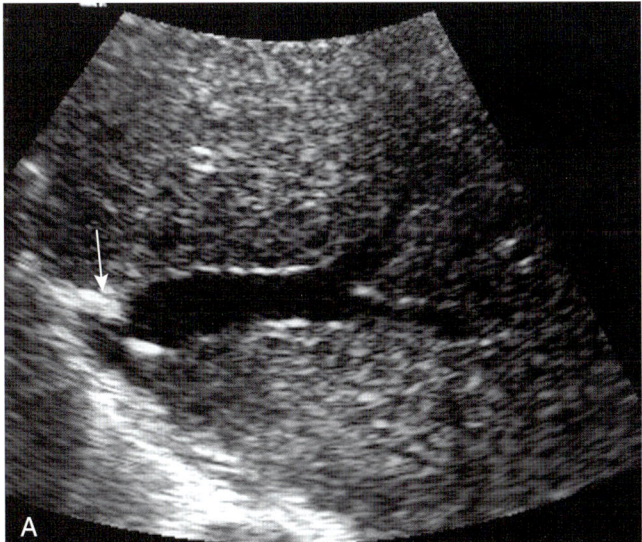

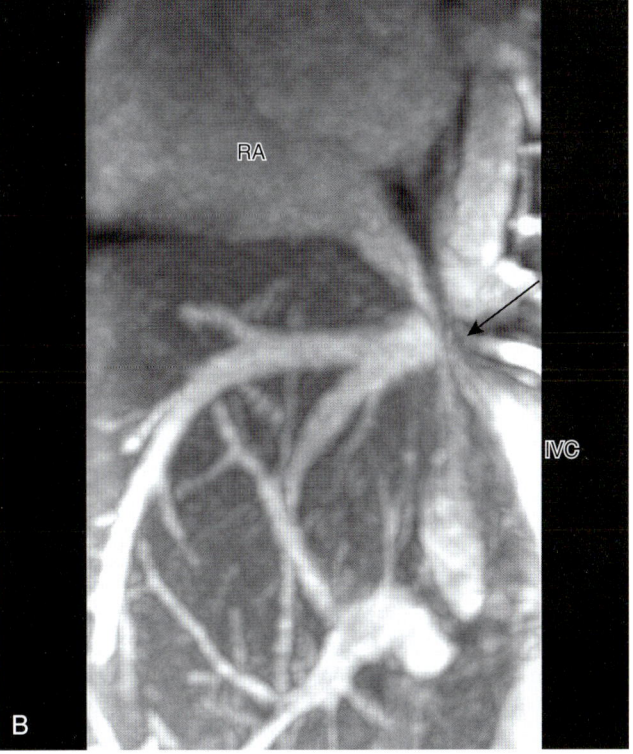

Figure 94-11   Hepatic vein stenosis. **A,** Ultrasound imaging demonstrates stenosis (*arrow*) at the typical high location near the diaphragm, where it may be very difficult to identify. **B,** Sagittal plane magnetic resonance venography confirms tight stenosis (*arrow*) and retraction of both the hepatic veins and the inferior vena cava (*IVC*). *RA,* Right atrium.

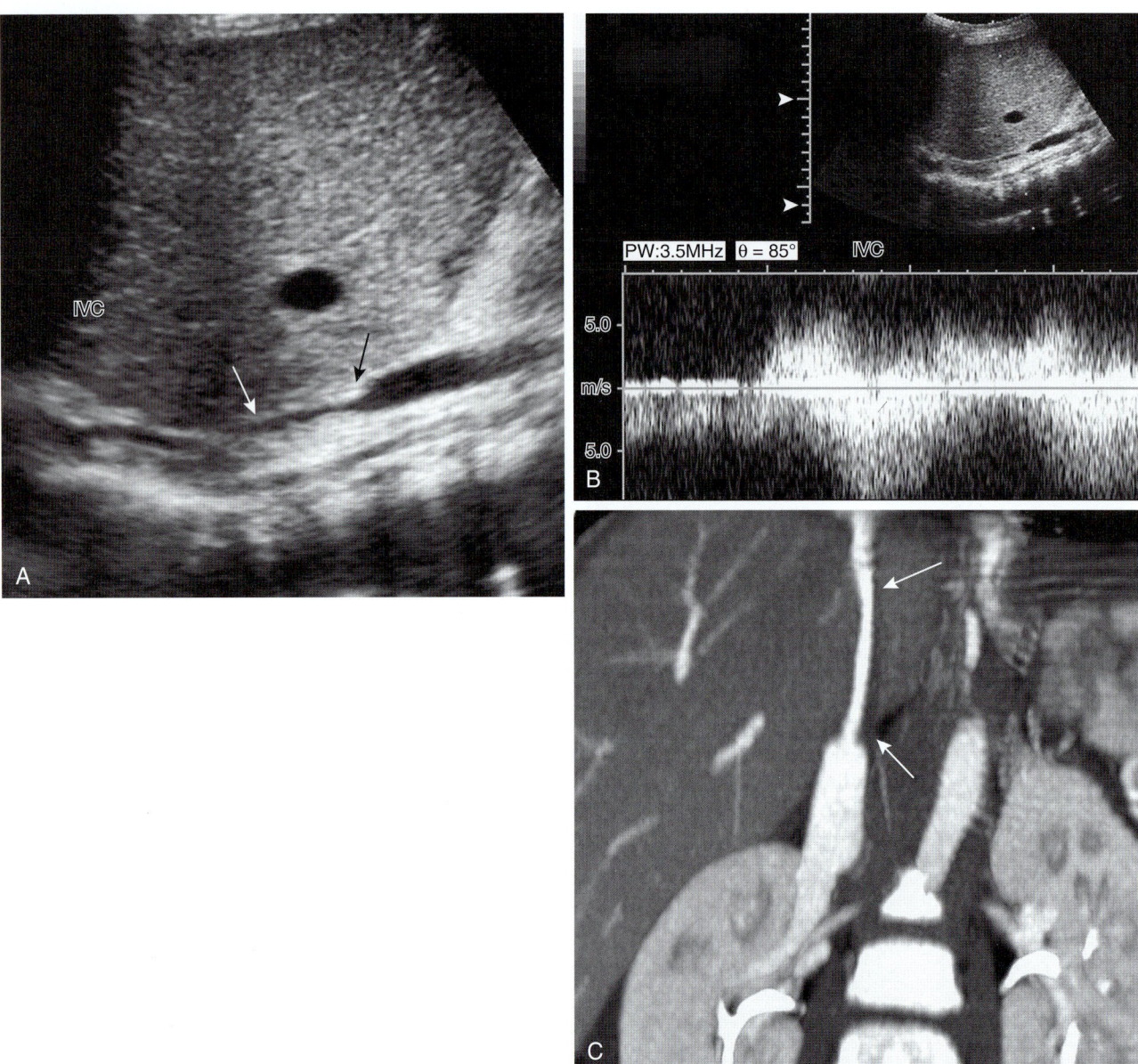

Figure 94-12 Long-segment inferior vena cava (IVC) stenosis. **A,** A longitudinal ultrasound image shows a long-segment IVC narrowing (*arrows*) along the posterior aspect of the transplanted liver graft. **B,** Spectral Doppler identifies extremely high-velocity and turbulence at the stenotic site. **C,** Sagittal reconstruction of computed tomographic angiography shows the long-segment IVC narrowing (*arrows*).

Specific diagnosis may require fluid aspiration or surgery (Fig. 94-15).

When a fluid collection is suspected, it is important to realize that although the blind end of the Roux-en-Y loop may dilate, the normal loop at the hilum of the transplanted liver may mimic a fluid collection on ultrasound and may not fill with oral contrast during CT scanning.[28,34]

Mycotic arterial pseudoaneurysms at anastomoses may rupture, producing abrupt exsanguinations.[25] Thus fluid collections near an artery should be interrogated carefully.

Ascites is also common in the days after transplantation and usually is self-limited. If large in amount or prolonged in duration, an evaluation for the cause may be required.

INFECTION

Postoperative infection develops in most liver recipients at some time, although consequent mortality is less than 10%. Bacterial and fungal infections are most common during the first postoperative month. Risk factors include hepatic artery occlusion, immunosuppression, central venous catheters, and nosocomial exposure. Viral and opportunistic infections usually occur between 30 and 180 days after transplantation.[41] Ultrasound and CT are the mainstay for assessing intraabdominal infections, particularly abscesses.[42] Cholangitis may prompt evaluation with MRCP or percutaneous transhepatic cholangiography.[38]

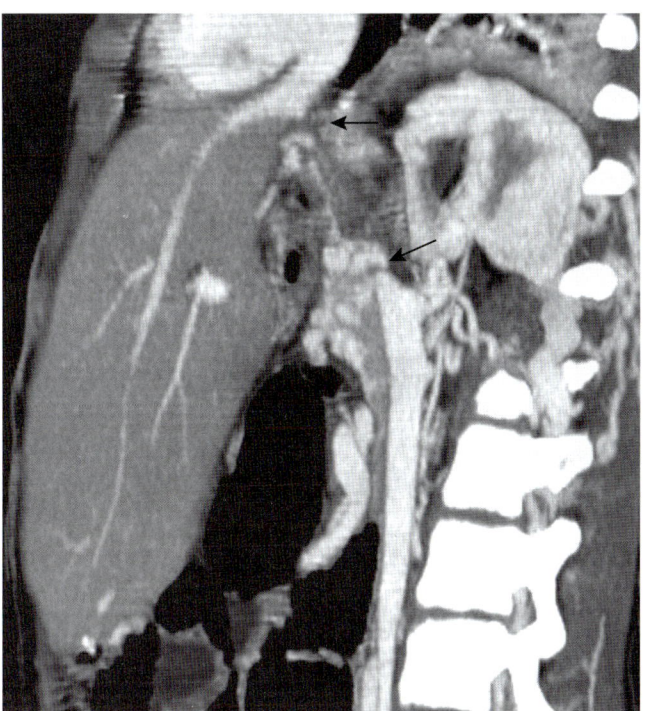

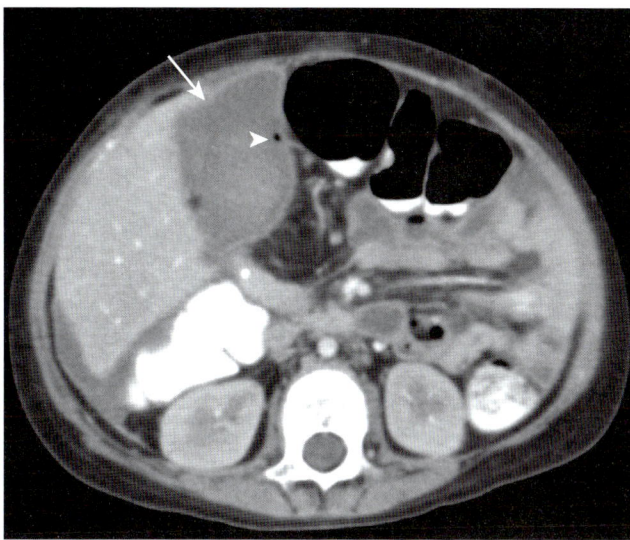

Figure 94-15 Infected bile collection. Computed tomography shows a fluid collection (*arrow*) containing a small gas bubble (*arrowhead*). Image-guided aspiration confirmed an infectious etiology.

Figure 94-13 Complete occlusion of the inferior vena cava along the posterior aspect of the liver segment (*arrows*). Note that the obstruction is caudal to the hepatic veins, which drain into the proximal inferior vena cava and right atrium undisturbed.

REJECTION

Imaging plays a relatively minor role in the diagnosis of rejection, which is established mainly by liver biopsy. Rejection may be associated with mild degrees of nonobstructive bile duct dilation and an increase in hepatic arterial resistive indices. However, neither hepatic arterial waveforms nor flow pattern in the hepatic veins have proved to be predictive of rejection.[35]

POSTTRANSPLANTATION LYMPHOPROLIFERATIVE DISEASE

PTLD represents a spectrum of abnormalities of lymphoid proliferation linked with Epstein-Barr virus (in 98% of pediatric patients) and immune cell proliferation that ranges from polyclonal reversible B cell proliferation to aggressive monoclonal B cell lymphoma. T cell, Burkitt lymphoma, and Hodgkin disease are less common.[43] Risk factors for the development of PTLD are seronegativity for Epstein-Barr virus at transplantation, young age, intensity and type of immunosuppression (especially antilymphocyte antibody), cytomegalovirus infection, and type of transplant.[39] PTLD develops in children about three times as often as in adults, reported at 9.7% versus 2.9%, respectively.[44] The time from transplantation to the development of PTLD averages about 8 months in children, although it may be shorter in patients treated with tacrolimus, occurring as early as within a few weeks.[45] Survival is better in patients with polyclonal PTLD and those with limited disease. In persons with polyclonal disease, PTLD may reverse completely with modifications of immune suppression.[46]

Sites of involvement in children include lymphoid tissue (particularly Waldeyer ring, pericardial, and mesenteric nodes), the gastrointestinal tract, the spleen, and the transplanted liver (Fig. 94-16). Newly enlarged tonsils and adenoids in a child with a transplanted liver should raise suspicion of PTLD. Unusually large mesenteric nodes are common in children with PTLD, although lack of normal standards makes it difficult to set a threshold size for diagnosis. Central nervous system involvement is uncommon.[40] The appearance of PTLD in the transplanted liver consists of multiple nonspecific focal lesions.[47]

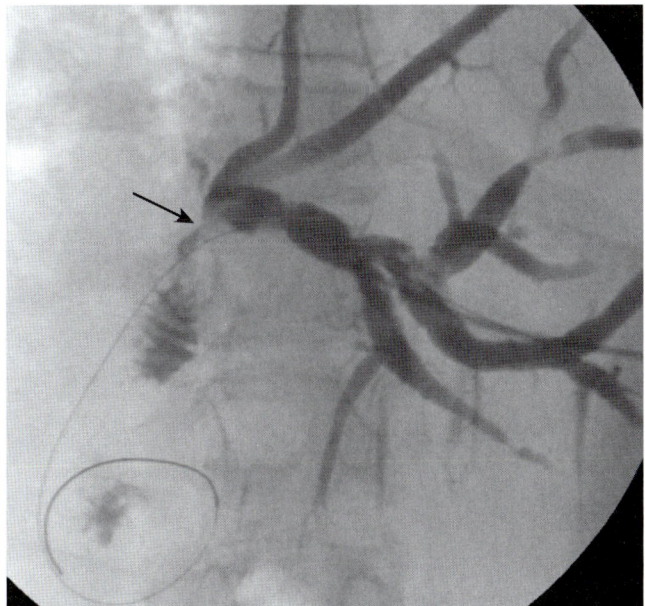

Figure 94-14 A percutaneous cholangiogram shows a tight stricture at the anastomosis between the donor left bile duct and the recipient Roux-en-Y loop (*arrow*).

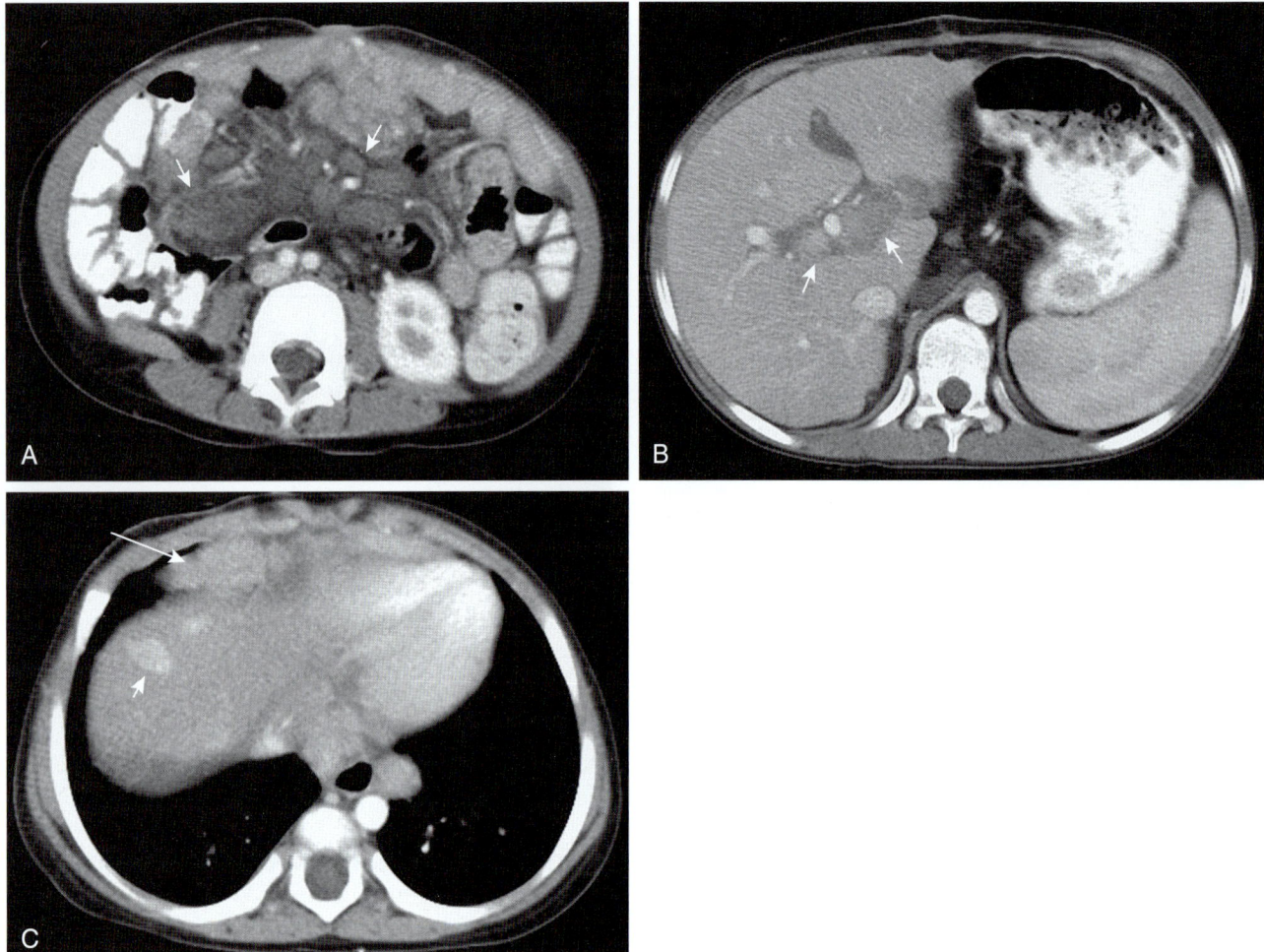

Figure 94-16 Posttransplantation lymphoproliferative disease. **A,** A computed tomography (CT) scan of the abdomen shows multiple enlarged mesenteric lymph nodes (*arrows*). **B,** A high CT slice reveals lymphadenopathy in the hilum of the transplanted liver (*arrows*). **C,** CT slice at the level of the diaphragm demonstrates an enhancing liver nodule (*short arrow*) as well as pericardial (*long arrow*) and posterior mediastinal lymphadenopathy.

Key Points

Pretransplant imaging should include information on the patency and size of the portal vein and IVC, abdominal anatomic anomalies, coexisting conditions, and the absence of hepatic neoplasm.

Early posttransplantation flow patterns may suggest vascular stenosis as a result of edema of the anastomosis and surrounding tissues. These findings are usually reversible but should be monitored.

Doppler signal in the intrahepatic portions of the hepatic artery and portal vein may be present in spite of stenosis or obstruction in the extrahepatic segment as a result of collateral vessels. When evaluating transplant vessels, screening ultrasound must be performed at the anastomosis, the narrowest portion, and at the site of maximal jet seen by color Doppler ultrasound.

Reversal of portal venous flow in a lobar or segmental branch is a strong indication of main portal vein occlusion.

Suggested Readings

Bhargava P, Vaidya S, Dick AAS, et al. Imaging of orthotopic liver transplantation: review. *AJR Am J Roentgenol*. 2011;196(3 suppl): WS15-WS25.

Spada G, Riva S, Maggiore G, et al. Pediatric liver transplantation. *World J Gastroenterol*. 2009;15(6):648-674.

References

Full references for this chapter can be found on www.expertconsult.com.

Chapter 95

The Spleen

STEPHANIE E. SPOTTSWOOD and MARTA HERNANZ-SCHULMAN

The spleen is maintained in its normal position by ligaments formed by peritoneal folds. The two major ligaments are the gastrosplenic ligament and the splenorenal ligament (Fig. 95-1). Other ligaments that help support the spleen are the phrenicosplenic, splenocolic, pancreaticosplenic, phrenocolic, and pancreaticocolic ligaments.

The spleen is the largest of the body's lymphatic structures and the second largest organ of the reticuloendothelial system. A combination of red pulp (75%) and white pulp (25%) constitute the splenic parenchyma,[1] which is surrounded by a relatively tough capsule. The red pulp is composed of the splenic cords and vascular sinuses and contains a large number of erythrocytes, whereas the white pulp is composed largely of lymphocytes and macrophages. The unique anatomy of the spleen is closely linked to its function and lends itself to some normal variations seen on computed tomography (CT) and magnetic resonance imaging (MRI). The primary function of the embryonic spleen is erythropoiesis, which is maximal in the middle of the second trimester and subsequently diminishes. The spleen is later responsible for filtering red blood cells that are aged or lack contractility, as well as antigen-coated cells, bacteria, and foreign particles. The spleen also acts as a platelet reservoir, releasing platelets in response to epinephrine or consuming platelets in case of splenomegaly.[1] These functional aspects of the pediatric spleen can be evaluated scintigraphically.

Imaging

Plain radiographs of the abdomen may reveal the spleen in the left upper quadrant, displacing the stomach medially and the colon inferiorly. The spleen may be obscured when large amounts of gas or stool are present in the gastrointestinal tract.

The spleen is easily identified on abdominal ultrasonography. It has a homogeneous sonographic texture, is slightly more echogenic than are the kidneys, and is isoechoic to slightly hyperechoic to the liver. The splenic hilar vessels usually are well visualized (Fig. 95-2), but intrasplenic vessels typically require color Doppler imaging for identification.

On CT, the normal spleen has a higher attenuation than the liver. Transient heterogeneous splenic enhancement patterns often are encountered during the first minute of contrast-enhanced CT, particularly with the rapid bolus

technique (e-Fig. 95-3). This normal phenomenon is thought to be a result of variations in blood flow through the red and white pulp of the spleen; it is more pronounced with contrast injection rates of 1 mL/sec or greater and in children older than 1 year. Common patterns of heterogeneity have been described as: (1) archiform, consisting of ring-like or zebra-stripe bands of alternating density; (2) focal areas of low density; and (3) diffuse, mottled areas of inhomogeneity.[2] More uniform enhancement is seen approximately 70 seconds after initiation of the contrast injection.

On MRI, the spleen signal intensity varies with age (Table 95-1; Fig. 95-4). In the neonate, the spleen is T1 and T2 isointense to hypointense with respect to the liver. The T2 hypointensity is because of immaturity of the white pulp. After age 8 months, the spleen is T2 hyperintense relative to the liver because of white pulp maturation, and it maintains this appearance through adulthood.[3]

Scintigraphic splenic imaging with technetium-99m (^{99m}Tc)–labeled sulfur colloid, which is removed from the blood by the reticuloendothelial system, is useful for the identification of splenic ectopia, as well as several entities discussed later in this chapter. It is not useful in cases of heterotaxy because splenic and hepatic tissue cannot be distinguished when neither location nor shape is an identifying criterion. Similarly, selective spleen scans can be misleading when the spleen is absent (e-Fig. 95-5).

Angiography is rarely used for intrasplenic disease; CT angiography and MR angiography offer excellent visualization of the spleen and its vessels.

Accessory Spleens

Overview The most common congenital anomaly of the spleen is the presence of one or more accessory spleens, or splenuli. These accessory spleens are present in 20% to 35% of postmortem examinations of the normal population[4] and usually are found incidentally at autopsy or on imaging studies. They number six or fewer and are located most commonly in the splenic hilum, in association with the splenic vessels, or in the gastrosplenic ligament. However, accessory spleens can be found virtually anywhere in the abdomen. They rarely exceed 2 cm in diameter and can be confused with splenic hilar or parapancreatic lymph nodes.

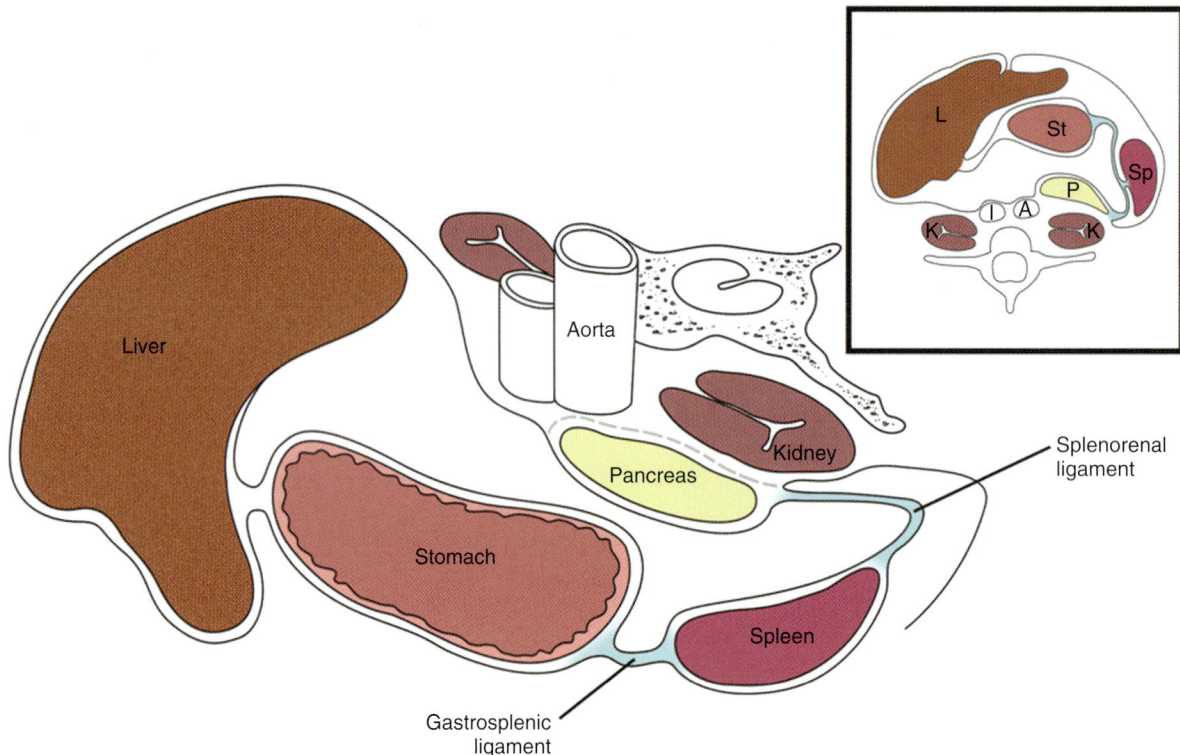

Figure 95-1   An oblique axial two-dimensional rendering of the fetal abdomen reveals the position of the gastrosplenic and splenorenal ligaments, which arise from the dorsal mesogastrium.

Etiology   Normally, the spleen forms from the coalescence of multiple small splenic masses. Accessory spleens therefore are not uncommon.

Clinical Presentation   The presentation is incidental, when accessory spleens are found during imaging for unrelated reasons.

Imaging   Accessory spleens can be identified on ultrasound, CT, or MRI, but when in question, the definitive imaging study is a ^{99m}Tc sulfur colloid liver-spleen scan.

Treatment   Accessory spleens are considered a normal variant of development and require no treatment.

Wandering Spleen

Overview   A wandering spleen is a congenital anomaly that results from maldevelopment of the splenic suspensory ligaments, including the gastrosplenic, splenorenal, and phrenicocolic ligaments. Acquired cases also have been described and may be a consequence of splenomegaly, traumatic injury, or ligamentous laxity.

Etiology   Normally, during embryonic life, the residuum of the dorsal mesogastrium fuses with the posterior peritoneum, helping to support the spleen in its normal position. When this fusion does not take place, the dorsal mesogastrium may

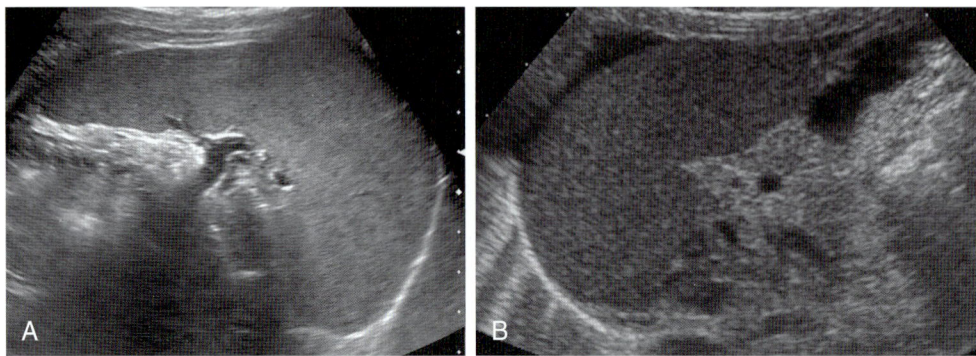

Figure 95-2   Normal spleen. **A,** A normal spleen in a 15-year-old girl. A transverse ultrasound image shows normal homogeneous parenchymal echotexture and hilar vessels. **B,** A normal spleen in a 3-month-old infant with ascites.

Table 95-1

Magnetic Resonance Signal Intensity of Spleen Relative to Liver by Age		
Age	**T1**	**T2**
Neonate	Isointense/hypointense	Isointense/hypointense
Postneonate infant	Hypointense	Minimally hyperintense
>8 mo	Hypointense	Hyperintense
>1 yr	Hypointense	Hyperintense

persist as a long mesentery, allowing the spleen to migrate, yielding the so-called "wandering spleen." The most common location for the ectopic spleen is the left lower quadrant.

Clinical Presentation The clinical presentation is variable; patients may be asymptomatic or present with a mobile mass on physical examination. More typically the presentation is an acute abdomen because of torsion of the vascular pedicle, with subsequent ischemia, impaired venous return, acute enlargement, and painful capsular tension.[5]

Imaging The abnormal position and orientation of the spleen can be identified by ultrasound, CT, or radionuclide imaging. It is important to pay close attention to the abnormal orientation and location of the spleen. Typically, no splenic tissue can be identified in the left upper quadrant, although a small accessory spleen may remain in the normal anatomic location. If the spleen undergoes torsion, a "whorled" appearance of the splenic artery in the splenic pedicle has been described as a characteristic CT sign of torsion[6] (Fig. 95-6, *A* and *B*). The twisted spleen has little uptake on radionuclide scintigraphy[7] and no contrast enhancement on CT (Fig 95-6, *C* and *D*). Color Doppler sonography shows lack of flow in the splenic hilar vessels (Fig. 95-6, *E*) and also may demonstrate the whorled appearance at the splenic hilum. Because of the defective ligamentous support, gastric volvulus has been associated with a wandering spleen[8] (Fig. 95-6, *F*).

Treatment Treatment is operative, consisting of a splenopexy if the spleen is viable or a splenectomy if it is nonviable.[9]

Splenogonadal Syndrome

Overview Splenogonadal syndrome is a rare anomaly in which a portion of the spleen is conjoined with left gonadal tissue. Although this congenital anomaly is uncommon, identifying it is important because 30% to 50% of cases result in unnecessary orchiectomy because of concern that a extratesticular neoplasm may be present.[10]

Etiology Splenogonadal fusion results when a portion of the splenic anlage fuses with primitive left gonadal tissue between the fifth and eighth weeks of gestation. Despite the fused splenic tissue, a normal spleen is present in the left upper quadrant. The splenogonadal fusion shows a splenic cord continuous with the ectopic, fused splenic tissue in approximately 55% of cases; it is discontinuous in approximately 45% of cases.[10] Splenogonadal fusion has been reported in association with transverse testicular ectopia.[11]

Clinical Presentation Splenogonadal fusion is much more common in males, with a male to female ratio of 16:1. The condition may be asymptomatic and discovered incidentally or at autopsy. It may be associated with left cryptorchidism, inguinal hernia, or testicular torsion, particularly when it is continuous. Multiple other anomalies may be present, particularly in the continuous type. In females, fusion of splenic tissue with the left ovary or mesovarium occurs; this connection does not result in ovarian ectopia.

Imaging Sonography can reliably demonstrate the extratesticular location of a palpable scrotal mass in these cases. The mass is typically oval or round and of similar echotexture to the adjacent normal testis, but often it has a slightly different size or configuration (e-Fig. 95-7, *A*). Color Doppler sonography shows abundant vascularity in the splenic tissue (e-Fig. 95-7, *B*). Radionuclide imaging with ^{99m}Tc sulfur colloid adds specificity to the diagnosis by revealing radiopharmaceutical uptake in the ectopic splenic tissue either in the left hemiscrotum or in the left inguinal canal when associated with cryptorchidism. A linear pattern extending from the left upper quadrant of the abdomen to the pelvis or scrotum may be detected in the continuous type (e-Fig. 95-7, *C*).

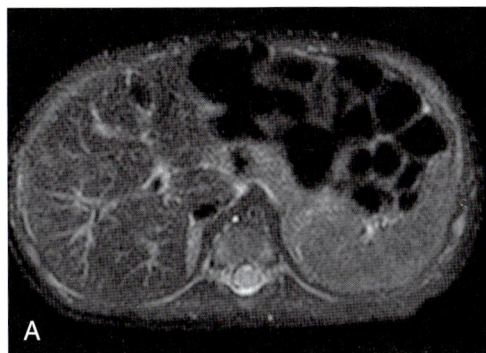
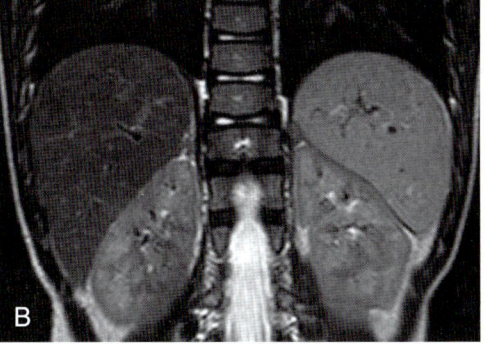

Figure 95-4 Change in spleen T2 signal with age. **A,** An axial T2-weighted fat-suppressed image of the upper abdomen in a 2-month-old child shows that the spleen is nearly isointense to liver. **B,** An axial T2-weighted fat-suppressed image of the upper abdomen in a 4-year-old child shows hyperintensity of the spleen compared with the liver.

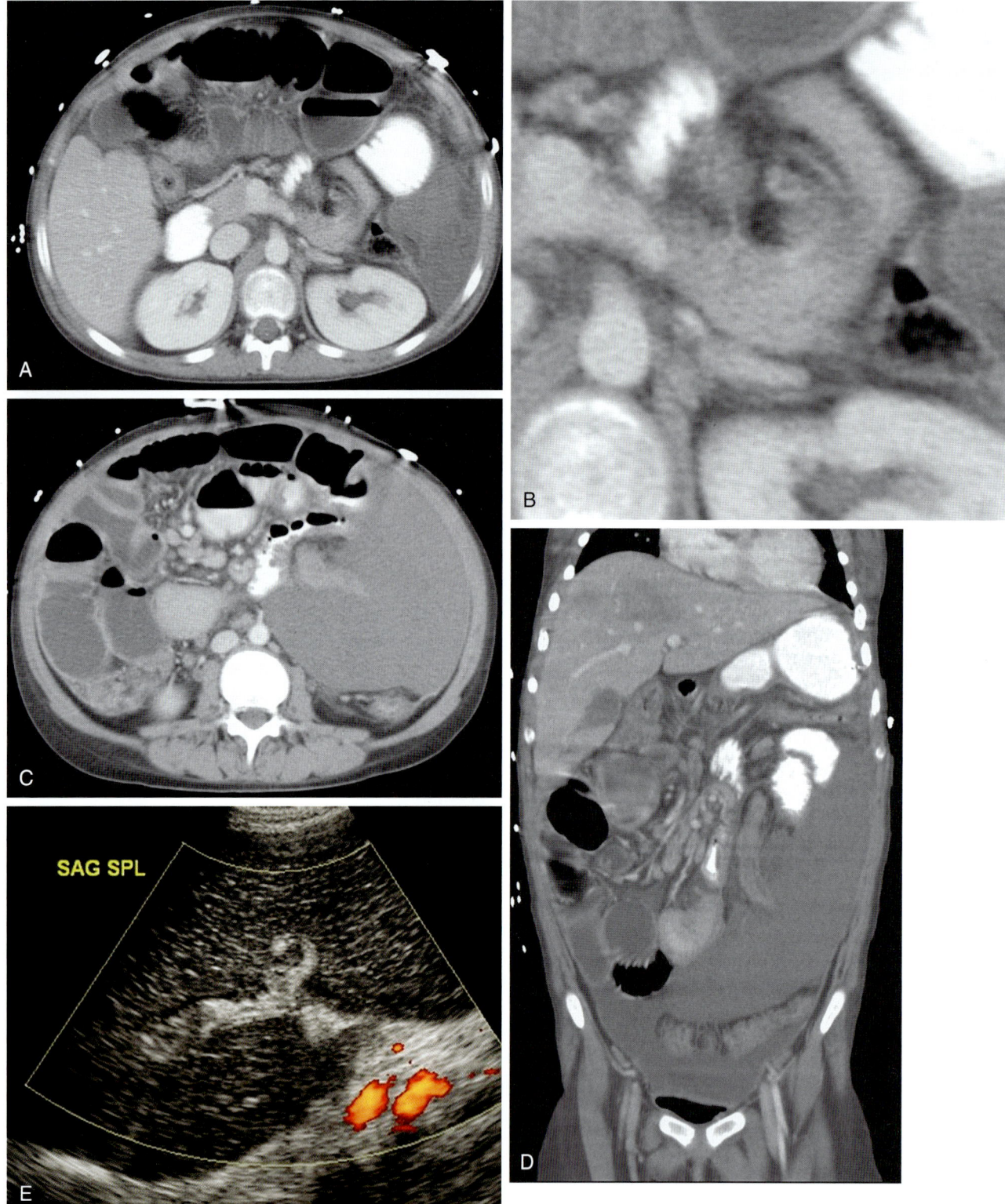

Figure 95-6 A wandering spleen in a 14-year-old girl with Niemann-Pick disease and the acute onset of abdominal pain. **A,** A contrast-enhanced computed tomography (CT) image of the abdomen shows a "whorled" appearance of the splenic vessels and pancreatic tail at the expected location of the splenic hilum. The spleen shows low attenuation without contrast enhancement as a result of absent perfusion. **B,** A close-up view of "whorled" hilar vessels and the pancreatic tail from **A**. **C,** Below the level of **A**, the caudal location of the splenic mass is shown. **D,** Coronal reformatting underscores the displacement and abnormal orientation of the spleen and again shows lack of contrast enhancement. **E,** A color Doppler ultrasound image shows no vascular flow into the spleen. Also note the abnormal echotexture of the spleen. *SAG SPL,* Sagittal spleen.

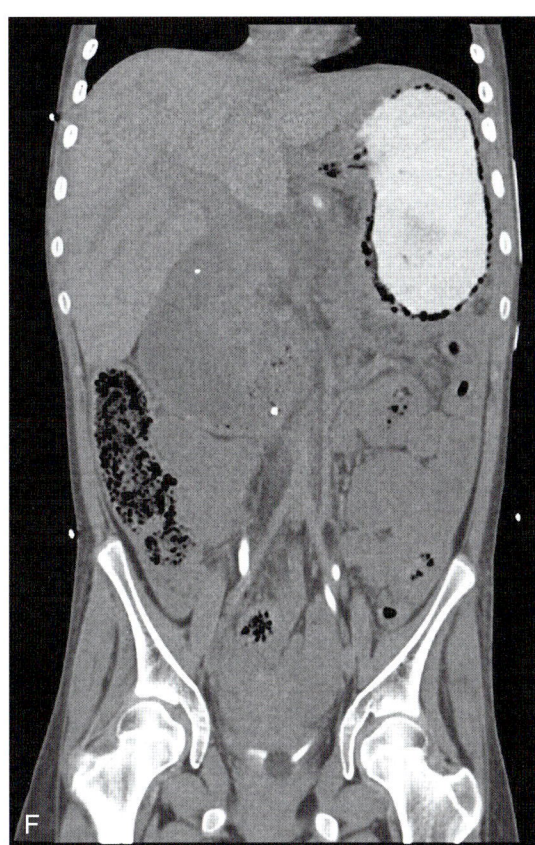

Figure 95-6, cont'd.   **F,** One year after undergoing a splenectomy, the child presented with hypotension and abdominal distention. Coronal reconstruction of abdominal CT scan performed with oral contrast reveals reversal of the usual relationship of the gastric fundus and gastric outlet, consistent with gastric volvulus. Note the gastric pneumatosis. (Courtesy Jeanne G. Hill, MD, MUSC.)

Although it is not the imaging modality of choice, contrast-enhanced CT may reveal a rounded, enhancing, well-circumscribed soft tissue mass in the left hemiscrotum or left hemipelvis that may or may not continue cephalad toward the spleen.[12] MRI is useful to obtain further detail.[11]

Treatment   When the diagnosis is confirmed by means of imaging and the child is asymptomatic, no treatment is necessary. However, if surgical exploration is performed, the splenic tissue can be dissected safely off the tunica albuginea and the testis can be preserved.

Splenorenal Fusion

Overview   Splenorenal fusion is a rare developmental anomaly in which congenital fusion of splenic and renal tissue is present. Fusion usually involves the left kidney and rarely the right kidney.[13,14] Unlike posttraumatic splenosis, patients with congenital splenorenal fusion demonstrate an intact spleen with a separate blood supply. Recognition of this anomaly is important to prevent an unnecessary nephrectomy for a presumed malignancy.

Etiology   One theory to explain the origin of this anomaly is that fusion of the mesogastrium and left posterior peritoneum brings the splenic anlage and the left mesonephric ridge in close proximity during the eighth week of gestation, allowing the two organs to fuse as they migrate toward the pelvis.[15] Alternatively, it is postulated that splenic cells could migrate caudally to reach the metanephros and retroperitoneum, where there is no barrier to crossing the midline; this theory would explain reported right-sided fusion anomalies.[13] Splenorenal fusion also may be acquired from posttraumatic or postsplenectomy splenosis, where splenic tissue implants on the kidney and regrowth occurs.[14,15]

Clinical Presentation   The condition may present incidentally on imaging, or it may cause symptoms as a result of the effect of the mass or hypersplenism, manifesting as anemia and thrombocytopenia.

Imaging   Conventional imaging with ultrasound, CT, or MR typically will not reliably distinguish this entity from a renal or retroperitoneal malignancy. When suspected, the diagnosis can be made reliably with ^{99m}Tc sulfur colloid imaging, or, in the case of hypersplenism, with ^{99m}Tc-labeled, heat-damaged red blood cell imaging.

Treatment   When the diagnosis is confirmed by means of imaging and the child is asymptomatic, no treatment is necessary.

Abnormal Visceroatrial Situs

Overview   Abnormal visceroatrial situs is a spectrum of abnormalities related to isomerisms of the atrial appendages, which typically involve abnormalities of the spleen. The normal visceroatrial anatomy is known as "situs solitus," which means "usual position." "Situs inversus" refers to mirror-image visceroatrial anatomy. Patients with situs inversus frequently are asymptomatic, although they have a slightly higher incidence of congenital heart disease than do patients with situs solitus. "Situs ambiguous," also called "visceroatrial heterotaxia," refers to deranged visceroatrial asymmetry. Patients with this abnormality are divided into two major groups: those with a tendency toward right-sided symmetry and those with a tendency toward left-sided symmetry. Therefore each patient, within broad categories, has a unique constellation of anatomic findings that must be evaluated and described individually.[16,17] Recognition of the spectrum of situs anomalies and the altered anatomy is important because of the increased risk in these children for anomalies such as congenital heart disease, malrotation with potential for development of midgut volvulus, and immunodeficiency in patients with asplenia.[16,18-20]

Etiology   Although the external human features are largely symmetric, asymmetry is characteristic of viscerovascular anatomy. In patients with heterotaxy, although it is not yet not fully understood, derangement of embryonic left-right recognition at the molecular level is present, which relates to abnormalities in ciliary movement, planar cell polarity, asymmetric gene cascades, and genes that generate a barrier for specific gene products to cross the embryonic midline. Underlying causative mechanisms include teratogenic exposures and genetic factors.[21-27]

Clinical Presentation Patients with right-sided atrial isomerism typically have asplenia, which is associated with immune deficiency and overwhelming sepsis, particularly as a result of *Streptococcus pneumoniae*.[28] The ambiguous atrium resembles the right atrium, and severe congenital cardiac lesions typically are present, usually with diminished pulmonary blood flow and often with associated total anomalous pulmonary venous return with or without obstruction. Patients thus will present with cyanosis and/or pulmonary edema.[16,17] Despite modern palliative procedures, mortality remains high, with 5-year survival reported at 20%, regardless of whether the diagnosis is made before or after birth.[27,29] Intestinal malrotation is common.

Patients with left-sided atrial isomerism typically have multiple splenules, known as polysplenia. Congenital heart disease often is present, although some patients with polysplenia are asymptomatic, and the diagnosis may be made incidentally.[30] In a study of a large series of people with left atrial isomerism, approximately 14% of patients had a normal heart and presented with extracardiac abnormalities. This condition is associated with biliary atresia in as many as 10% of patients.[31] Intestinal malrotation is common.

Imaging In patients with situs ambiguus, plain radiographs may denote abnormal situs, with discordance of heart, stomach, and liver position. On chest radiographs, patients with right-sided atrial isomerism may demonstrate bilateral right lungs with identification of the minor fissure and eparterial bronchi. Patients with left-sided isomerism, on the other hand, may demonstrate bilateral left-sided hila with hyparterial bronchi. However, hilar anatomy often is not clear because of overlying thymus. The plain film appearance may be indistinguishable from normal and falsely suggest situs solitus in some patients.[32]

Ultrasound, CT, and MRI confirm absence of the spleen in the vast majority of patients with right-atrial isomerism and may identify other anomalies such as horseshoe adrenals fused in the midline (e-Fig. 95-8).[33,34] Subdiaphragmatic total anomalous venous connections are easily identified, because the anomalous vessel courses anterior to the esophagus into the abdomen.[16] The inferior vena cava (IVC) is nearly invariably present and may lie to the right or left of the aorta, crossing the midline anterior to the aorta to enter the atrium, if necessary.[16,32]

In patients with left-sided atrial isomerism, because splenic tissue develops in the dorsal mesogastrium,[25] ultrasound, CT, and MRI will identify the splenules dorsal to the stomach along the greater curvature, whether the stomach lies on the left or the right.[16] The appearance of the splenules is variable and ranges from a conglomerate of multiple splenules to a sometimes septated, largely single splenic mass (Fig. 95-9 and e-Fig. 95-10). Interruption of the intrahepatic IVC is seen at least 50% of patients, with either right- or left-sided azygous continuation.[16] When the IVC is present, it may lie to the right or left of the aorta. A preduodenal portal vein may be seen. In patients presenting with biliary atresia, it is important to evaluate the continuity of the IVC and the course of the portal vein, because these vascular derangements are important in patients who are later referred for liver transplantation.

Treatment Treatment is individualized on the basis of the associated anomalies. Patients with asplenia are at risk for sepsis and need to be treated for immunodeficiency. Patients with congenital heart disease or gastrointestinal anomalies of midgut malrotation and biliary atresia typically require surgical correction.

Splenomegaly

Overview Splenomegaly refers to enlargement of the spleen, usually as a result of excessive destruction of abnormal blood cells, excessive antigenic stimulation, storage or infiltrative disorders, or portal venous congestion. Hypersplenism, in contrast, refers to the syndrome of sequestration by the enlarged spleen of blood cell lines, particularly platelets.

Etiology The spleen may become enlarged in several inherited conditions (Box 95-1). The hemolytic anemias frequently cause splenomegaly, with hereditary spherocytosis, hereditary elliptocytosis, and thalassemia being the most common. Sickle cell anemia initially leads to splenomegaly, followed by splenic atrophy as a result of multiple infarcts; the

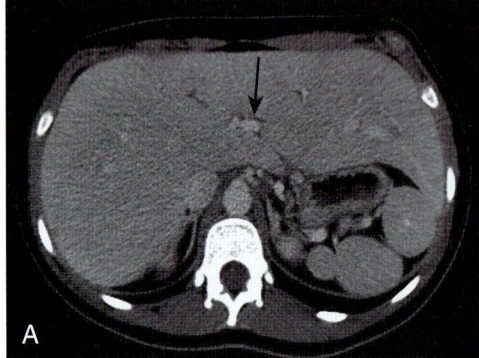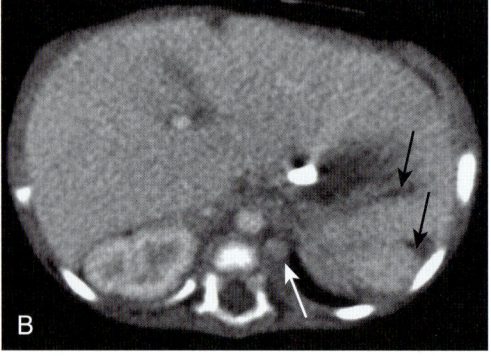

Figure 95-9 Polysplenia. **A,** Multiple splenules are present in the left upper quadrant, behind the stomach. Note the midline liver. The inferior vena cava (IVC) is intact, located to the right of the aorta. Note the midline liver, centrally located portal vein (*arrow*), which was noted to be preduodenal on lower sections. **B,** A 2-month-old infant with complex congenital heart disease and single ventricle anatomy. Note two splenules (*arrows*) in the left upper quadrant behind the stomach, and the left-sided azygous continuation of the interrupted IVC. The left azygous vein drained into the left-sided superior vena cava. (**A,** Courtesy Marta Hernanz-Schulman, MD, Nashville, TN.)

Box 95-1 Causes of Splenomegaly in Children

Infection

- Bacterial, viral (e.g., Epstein-Barr), fungal protozoan

Congestive States Related to Portal Hypertension

- Liver cirrhosis
- Portal or splenic vein thrombosis
- Right heart cardiac failure

Lymphohematogenous Disorders

- Hodgkin lymphoma
- Non-Hodgkin lymphoma
- Lymphoproliferative disease
- Hemolytic anemias (e.g., acute splenic sequestration in sickle cell anemia)
- Thalassemia
- Extramedullary hematopoiesis

Storage Diseases

- Gaucer, Niemann-Pick, mucopolysaccharidoses

Immunologic—Inflammatory

- Idiopathic thrombocytopenic purpura
- Systemic lupus erythematosus
- Juvenile rheumatoid arthritis

Cysts

- Congenital
- Acquired

Benign Neoplasms/Masses

- Hemangioma
- Lymphangioma
- Hamartoma

Miscellaneous

- Sarcoidosis
- Langerhans cell histiocytosis
- Collagen vascular diseases

pathophysiology is sequestration of impaired red blood cells by the spleen, leading to splenomegaly, anemia, and thrombocytopenia.

Splenomegaly is observed in neonates who have undergone extracorporeal membrane oxygenation cannulation. The proposed mechanism is sequestration of damaged blood cells in the extracorporeal membrane oxygenation circuit.[35]

Splenomegaly also can occur in a variety of acquired disorders, including infection and neoplasm (discussed in the following sections). Acquired causes of portal hypertension, such as cavernous transformation of the portal vein or cirrhosis of the liver in patients with cystic fibrosis, may present with splenomegaly.

Clinical Presentation Patients with splenomegaly present with the signs and symptoms of the underlying condition. Acute splenic sequestration crisis is manifested clinically by sudden enlargement of the spleen and a rapid decrease in the hematocrit level. This condition typically occurs in young children, with 76% of episodes occurring before 2 years of age. Clinically the episode can manifest emergently, with hypovolemic shock potentially progressing to death within a few hours.[36] The condition is rare beyond age 8 years as a result of the development of splenic fibrosis. Once a child has a sequestration crisis, a higher risk of recurrence exists.

Imaging Plain radiographs of the abdomen may reveal an enlarged spleen in the left upper quadrant, displacing the stomach medially and the colon inferiorly.

Ultrasound allows ready detection of splenomegaly. Splenic measurements are readily determined using the coronal imaging plane with the splenic hilum in view. The upper limit of normal at age 15 years and older is 12.0 cm for girls and 13.0 cm for boys.[37] More recently, several other authors have investigated normal spleen size with sonography in larger cohorts of pediatric patients, with similar results.[38-41] These authors all found a strong correlation between spleen length and body height (Tables 95-2 and 95-3). In a study of 712 children aged 7 to 15 years, investigators correlated splenic measurements with age, sex, body weight, height, body surface area, and body mass index.[42] The authors found the strongest correlation with body weight and determined a predicted spleen length according to the following formula: $69.875 + BODY\ WEIGHT\ [kg] \times 0.371$. Another group determined that a normal splenic measurement should not exceed 1.25 times the length of the left kidney.[41] As a general rule, the tip of the spleen should not extend below the inferior pole of the left kidney (e-Fig. 95-11).

CT and MRI also readily reveal an enlarged spleen and may allow for more standardized and reproducible measurement. Spleen volume can be readily measured with CT or MRI. CT measurements of normal pediatric spleen volume correlate with body weight in a linear relationship.[43]

The imaging findings are nonspecific as to cause unless evidence exists of extramedullary hematopoiesis or infarcts or ancillary findings are identified, such as varices in patients with congestive splenomegaly (Fig. 95-12). Extramedullary

Table 95-2

Spleen Length in Children and Adolescents*

Group	No.	10th Percentile	Median	90th Percentile	Upper Limit
0-3 mo	28	3.3	4.5	5.8	6.0
3-6 mo	13	4.9	5.3	6.4	6.5
6-12 mo	17	5.2	6.2	6.8	7.0
1-2 yr	12	5.4	6.9	7.5	8.0
2-4 yr	24	6.4	7.4	8.6	9.0
4-6 yr	39	6.9	7.8	8.8	9.5
6-8 yr	21	7.0	8.2	9.6	10.0
8-10 yr	16	7.9	9.2	10.5	11.0
10-12 yr	17	8.6	9.9	10.9	11.5
12-15 yr	26	8.7	10.1	11.4	12.0
15-20 yr (male)	5	9.0	10.0	11.7	12.0
15-20 yr (female)	12	10.1	11.2	12.6	13.0

* All measurements are in centimeters. Upper limits are the next highest whole integer over the 90th percentile.

From Rosenberg HK, Markowitz RI, Kolberg H, et al. Normal splenic size in infants and children: sonographic measurements. *AJR Am J Roentgenol.* 1991;157:119-121.

Table 95-3

Length of Spleen in Children vs. Body Height and Age*					
Body Height (cm)	No.	Age Range (mo)	Mean ± SD	Range	Normal Limits
48-64	52	1-3	53 ± 7.8	33-71	30-70
54-73	39	4-6	59 ± 6.3	45-71	40-75
65-78	18	7-8	63 ± 7.6	50-77	45-80
71-92	18	12-30	70 ± 9.6	54-86	54-85
85-109	27	36-59	75 ± 8.4	60-91	55-95
100-130	30	60-83	84 ± 9.0	61-100	60-105
110-131	36	84-107	85 ± 10.5	65-102	65-105
125-149	29	108-131	86 ± 10.7	64-114	65-110
137-153	17	132-155	97 ± 9.7	72-100	75-115
143-168	21	156-179	101 ± 11.7	84-120	80-120
152-175	12	180-200	101 ± 10.3	88-120	85-120

* All measurements are in centimeters.
From Konus OL, Ozdemir A, Akkaya A, et al. Normal splenic size in infants and children: sonographic measurements. *AJR Am J Roentgenol.* 1998;171:1693-1698.

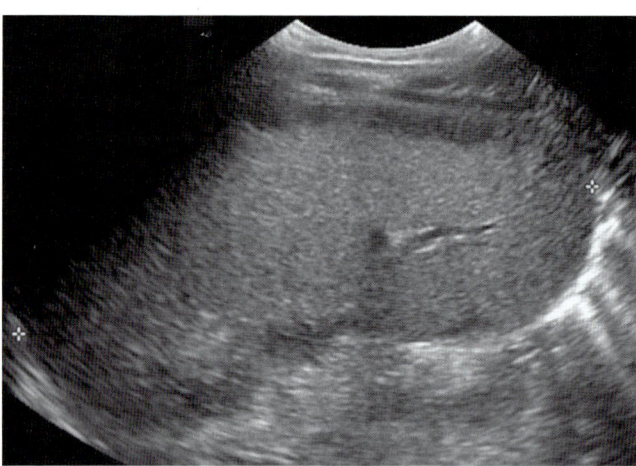

Figure 95-13 Splenic sequestration crisis. An ultrasound image of the spleen of a young child with an acute splenic sequestration crisis demonstrates numerous peripheral hypoechoic lesions. (Courtesy Sarah Fitch, MD, MCV, Richmond, VA.)

hematopoiesis may demonstrate focal areas of increased echogenicity on sonography, whereas infarcts may appear as hypoechoic areas. The storage diseases generally cause nonspecific splenomegaly,[44] but Gaucher disease may lead to focal hypoechoic foci, reflecting collections of Gaucher cells.[45] The

focal collections occasionally may be hyperechoic as a result of fibrosis.

In patients with sickle cell anemia who are experiencing an acute sequestration crisis, hypoechoic splenic lesions can be seen peripherally on sonography (Fig. 95-13) as a result of hemorrhage or infarction. Low attenuation lesions are demonstrated on contrast-enhanced CT; they typically are peripheral in location, with intervening areas of hemorrhage. T2-weighted MR sequences reveal that these lesions are markedly hyperintense.[46]

Treatment Treatment of splenomegaly is directed at the underlying cause. Splenectomy is used sparingly in children. A partial splenectomy can be performed laparoscopically or via interventional radiology selective transarterial embolization.

The long-term management of sequestration syndrome in patients consists of increased awareness of symptoms (primarily worsening anemia) and signs (an enlarging spleen) and, in some cases, short-term chronic transfusion; a splenectomy may be required.[36] In most patients with sickle cell disease, splenic function is diminished because of splenic infarcts, and autosplenectomy is frequent by age 5 to 6 years. Transfusion has been shown to transiently reverse hyposplenia, and hypertransfusion programs have documented splenic regrowth and reversal of functional hyposplenia.[47-49] Bone marrow transplantation has demonstrated recovery of splenic function in children with sickle cell disease.[50]

Infectious Diseases

Overview Splenic abscesses are uncommon lesions that are rare in the pediatric population.[51] Involvement of the spleen in systemic infectious disease is most common in immunocompromised patients, with increasing incidence as a result of the increased use of steroids and chemotherapeutic agents.[52] Bacterial, fungal, and granulomatous agents frequently are involved. Splenic involvement also can occur in immunecompetent hosts with cat scratch disease, granulomatous

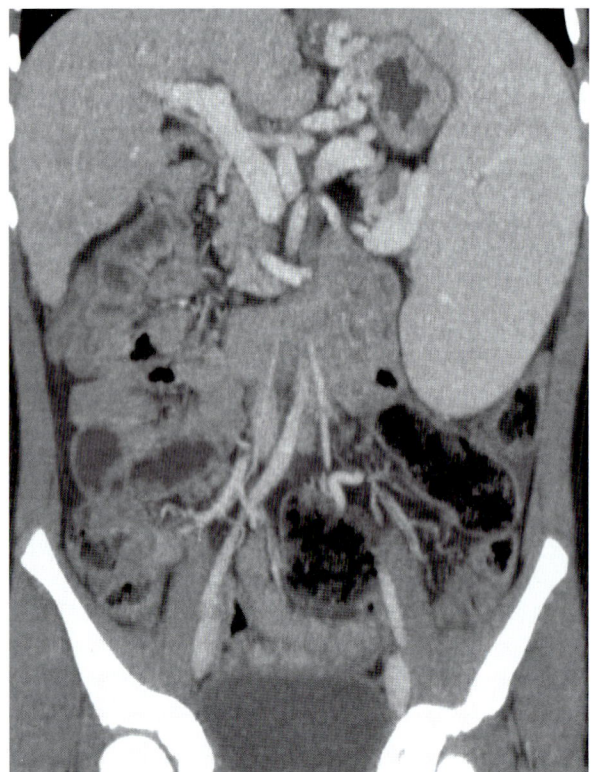

Figure 95-12 Splenomegaly as a result of portal hypertension in an 11-year-old girl with liver disease. Coronal reconstruction of a contrast-enhanced computed tomography scan of the abdomen shows splenic extension to the left lower quadrant. Multiple variceal collaterals are depicted clearly.

diseases such as histoplasmosis, parasitic diseases such as echinococcus, and viral infections. Viral infections, including infectious mononucleosis, are more likely to cause nonspecific splenomegaly as a result of reactive hyperplasia of the spleen's reticuloendothelial tissue.

Etiology Bacterial splenic abscesses can develop via several routes, which include hematogenous spread, such as in subacute bacterial endocarditis or cat scratch disease; spread from a contiguous infection, such as pancreatitis or perinephric abscess; and seeding in a spleen compromised by infarction or trauma.

Clinical Presentation Symptoms can be nonspecific and may be related to the systemic illness or splenomegaly. Patients may present with fever, lethargy, and weight loss. Abdominal distension, tenderness, and leucocytosis often are found.[51] Cat scratch disease, a relatively common infection in children, is caused by *Bartonella henselae* and typically presents with fever and tender lymphadenopathy.

Imaging Imaging has an important role in diagnosis, because signs and symptoms can be nonspecific. Early diagnosis and prompt treatment are critical to decrease mortality and morbidity.

Splenic abscesses can be solitary, multiple, or multilocular, depending on the source of infection. Microabscesses are seen most commonly, especially with a fungal infection such as candidiasis. If they are large enough, the microabscesses may be seen on sonograms,[53] contrast-enhanced CT, or MRI (Fig. 95-14); CT may be more sensitive than ultrasound in detecting candidal infection.[54] Larger, solitary abscesses also may occur with candidiasis. They may be seen as hypoechoic areas on ultrasound, as low-attenuation areas on CT, and as T2-hyperintense lesions without peripheral enhancement.[55] In rare instances, calcification may be seen on CT.

MRI can be used for the evaluation of microabscesses, which eliminates ionizing radiation exposure but may require patient sedation. MRI demonstrates a high diagnostic

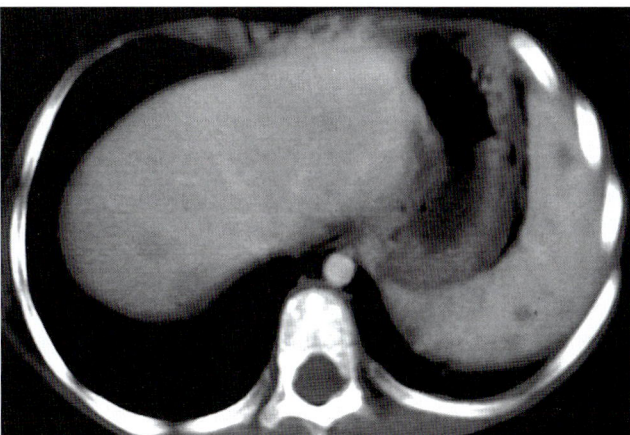

Figure 95-15 Cat scratch fever in a child with fever and abdominal pain. A contrast-enhanced computed tomography scan reveals several well-circumscribed, round and oval, low-attenuation lesions in the spleen. Similar larger foci are seen in the liver. (Courtesy Sharon M. Stein, Nashville, TN.)

accuracy for hepatosplenic fungal disease detection[56] and likely surpasses CT in its ability to detect small fungal lesions.[55]

In persons with cat scratch disease, ultrasound may show hypoechoic lesions ranging from well-defined and homogeneous to indistinct and heterogeneous, whereas contrast-enhanced CT may show hypoattenuating lesions, isoattenuating lesions, or lesions with marginal enhancement (Fig. 95-15). On MRI, lesions demonstrate low signal intensity on T1-weighted sequences and high signal intensity on T2-weighted sequences.[57-59]

Hydatid cysts may demonstrate calcifications, which can be visible on plain films. The cysts generally are anechoic, although the presence of daughter cysts and membranes may manifest with septations and internal echoes. CT shows a focal lesion of lower attenuation than the surrounding splenic tissue, and it is the best modality to show rim calcification.[60]

Tuberculosis, histoplasmosis, and coccidioidomycosis may produce multiple splenic granulomas, which almost always are associated with diffuse organ involvement as a result of hematogenous spread (e-Fig. 95-16). Splenic granulomas also may be detected in patients with chronic granulomatous disease of childhood.

Treatment When results of imaging studies are normal and candidiasis is suspected, laparoscopy is recommended to obtain a histopathologic diagnosis. Laparoscopy is justified by the risk of failure to diagnose and start appropriate therapy and by the potential adverse effects of empiric amphotericin B therapy. A needle biopsy may result in false-negative results because the fungal elements are difficult to isolate.[53] Cat scratch disease is usually self-limited and typically does not require antibiotic therapy.

Benign Cysts and Neoplasms

Benign lesions of the spleen are most commonly cystic. Most splenic cysts are the result of parasitic infection, most commonly in countries where hydatid disease is endemic. Nonparasitic splenic cysts are relatively rare and are usually

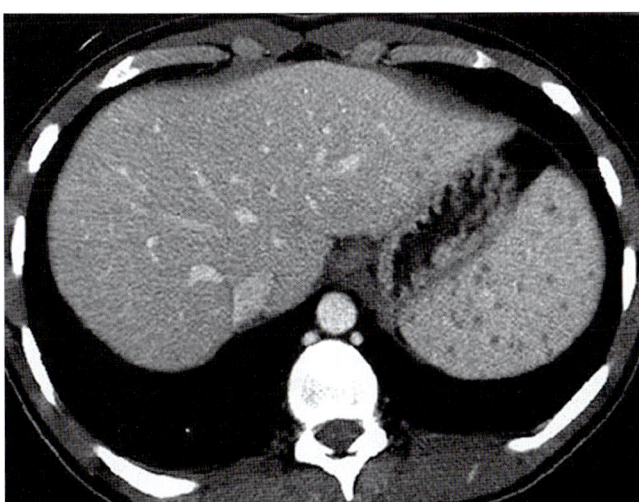

Figure 95-14 Candidiasis in an immune-suppressed child. A contrast-enhanced computed tomography scan of the abdomen shows multiple tiny, low-attenuation lesions diffusely distributed in the spleen. Two additional lesions are seen medially in the liver.

benign. Primary splenic cysts may be of epithelial origin, such as epidermoid, dermoid, or transitional cell cysts, or of endothelial origin, such as lymphatic malformations and hemangiomas. Acquired cysts may be posttraumatic or infectious.

Several classification schemes have been proposed to reflect the etiology, histology, and gross anatomic appearance of splenic cysts.[61,62] These classifications typically differentiate between parasitic and nonparasitic splenic cysts but further differentiate nonparasitic splenic cysts into two categories: (1) "true" (primary) and (2) "pseudocysts" (secondary), based on the presence or absence of epithelium. In these schemes, pseudocysts largely are ascribed to antecedent trauma. A more recent classification[63] modified for the pediatric population[64] proposes that nonparasitic splenic cysts with mesothelial, transitional, or epidermoid epithelial linings are congenital in origin, with antecedent history of trauma only incidental. These authors posit that many cysts labeled posttraumatic pseudocysts are actually congenital and have lost their epithelial lining or become desquamated after intracystic hemorrhage as a result of repeated trauma, infarct, or intrasplenic hemorrhage.[65] This phenomenon results in a "shaggy, hemorrhagic interior, which is totally different from the glistening, shiny white interior of a typical nonparasitic splenic cyst."[63,64] Both gross and microscopic features should be evaluated to discriminate between a posttraumatic pseudocyst and a hemorrhagic congenital cyst.

EPIDERMOID CYSTS

Overview   Epidermoid cysts are the most common noninfectious focal space-occupying lesions of the spleen, accounting for approximately 10% of all nonparasitic splenic cysts worldwide. Familial occurrence of epidermoid cysts has been reported.[66,67]

Etiology   These cysts are thought to be either congenital or posttraumatic, as previously discussed.

Clinical Presentation   Splenic cysts frequently are discovered incidentally on physical examination or during imaging after abdominal trauma. However, sufficiently large cysts can present as splenomegaly, renal compression with hypertension, varicocele, or complications such as peritonitis, intracystic hemorrhage, or rupture. Some patients may present with pain in the abdomen or left shoulder.[63]

Imaging   Epidermoid cysts frequently are large enough to visibly enlarge the spleen on plain radiographs; they are seen as a left upper quadrant mass displacing the stomach and colon (Fig. 95-17, A). A rim of calcification may be seen. On ultrasound, the cysts are characteristically anechoic and sharply demarcated from the surrounding normal splenic tissue. However, hemorrhage, inflammatory debris, or internal fat droplets may cause the cyst to contain internal echoes, at times resembling a hypoechoic solid mass (Fig. 95-17, B). Real-time scanning may show movement of the internal material, and Doppler interrogation reveals no internal blood flow. Liver-spleen scintigraphy demonstrates a focal photopenic defect. On CT and MRI, an uncomplicated epidermoid cyst appears as a rounded, sharply demarcated, nonenhancing mass with cystic imaging characteristics (Fig.

95-17, C and D). If it is complicated by hemorrhage, the internal signal intensity of the lesion on MRI reflects the chemical state of the hemoglobin within it. Calcifications are best identified on CT. Posttraumatic cysts may be difficult to distinguish radiologically from other cysts, but they may have irregular walls and internal echoes from debris.

Treatment   Imaging (especially ultrasound) can be used to guide percutaneous drainage. Follow-up imaging demonstrating reduced size of the cyst can indicate improvement. Surgical options for symptomatic cysts include total splenectomy, hemisplenectomy,[68] or total cystectomy.[65]

HEMANGIOMAS

Overview   Splenic hemangiomas are the most common primary neoplasm of the spleen when all ages are considered.[69-72] Hamartomas are considered to be slightly more common in children.[73]

Etiology   Splenic hemangiomas, which arise from the sinusoidal epithelium, are likely congenital in origin. Histologically they contain a proliferation of vascular channels lined with a single layer of epithelium.[69] They may be single, multiple, or may occur as part of a generalized angiomatosis.[72]

Clinical Presentation   Most splenic hemangiomas in children are asymptomatic, although larger lesions have the possibility of rupture or the development of hypersplenism.[73,74]

Imaging   The lesions are predominantly solid but may show cystic components. On ultrasound, the solid lesions are typically well marginated with variable echogenicity and internal vascular flow. Calcifications may be seen.[69] On noncontrast CT, hemangiomas are well-defined hypoattenuating or isoattenuating masses with contrast enhancement.[69,70,72] On MRI, splenic hemangiomas are hypointense to isointense on T1-weighted images and hyperintense on T2-weighted images. Variable enhancement patterns can be seen after administration of contrast material.[72]

Treatment   A splenectomy is curative for patients with symptomatic lesions, although other therapies, such as medical treatment with steroids, have been tried with success in some cases.[74]

HAMARTOMAS

Overview   Hamartomas, also known as splenomas or nodular hyperplasia of the spleen, are rare, nonneoplastic malformations of the spleen, with an incidence of 3 in 200,000 splenectomies.[75]

Etiology   It is proposed that splenic hamartomas result from "remote ischemic or infectious/inflammatory and reparative injury to the spleen."[76] Gross pathologic inspection reveals that they are bulging, spherical masses of dark red tissue resembling adjacent spleen parenchyma, with no surrounding capsule. Histologically, splenic hamartomas are composed of splenic sinusoidal tissue with no lymphoid follicles (red pulp) and display variable chronic inflammation with macrophages,

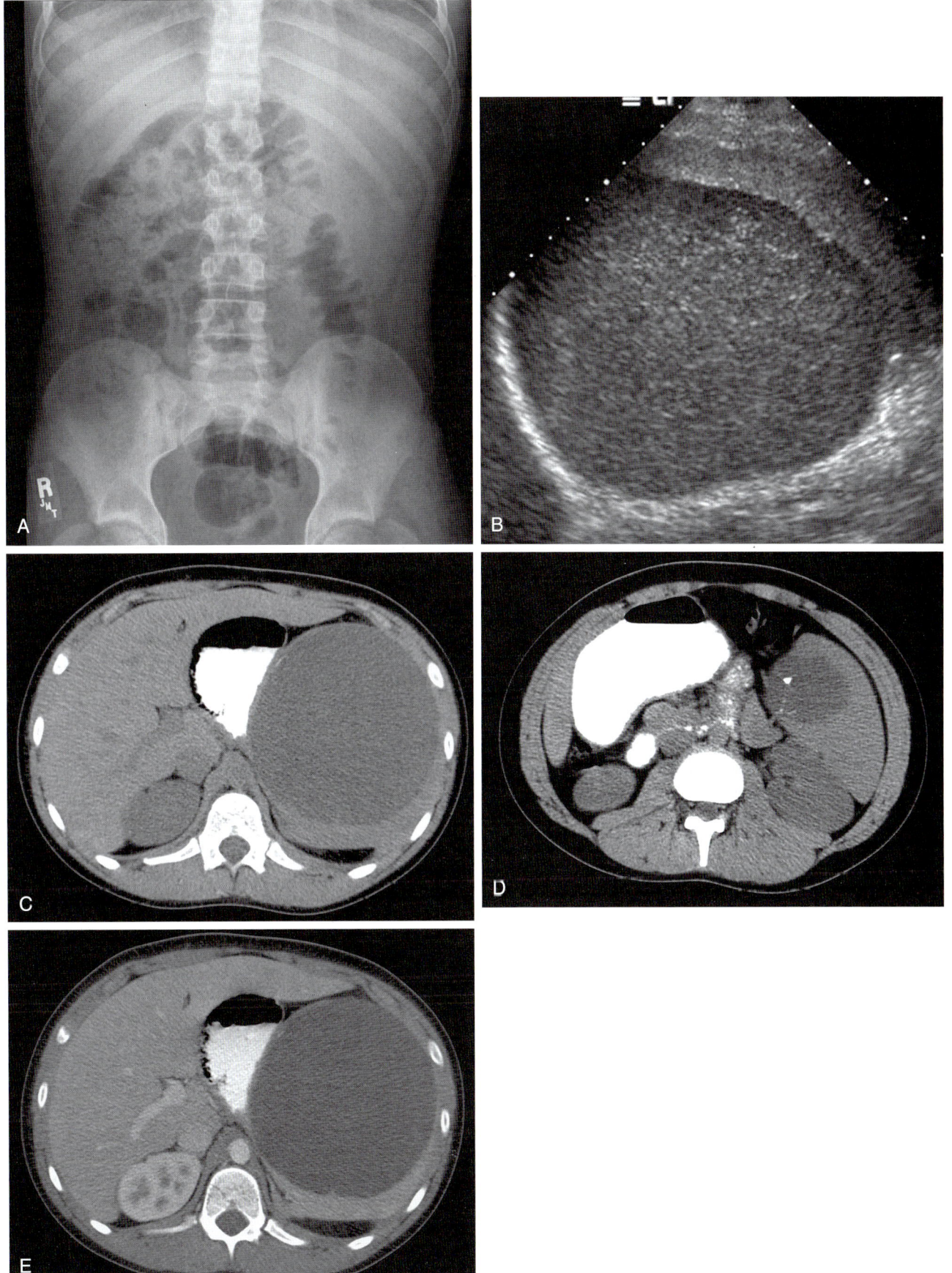

Figure 95-17 A 12-year-old boy with an epidermoid cyst. **A,** A left upper quadrant mass was discovered incidentally on a plain film obtained during the workup of hematuria. **B,** A sagittal ultrasound image of the spleen shows a large, well-circumscribed lesion with internal echoes. **C** and **D,** Computed tomography (CT) images without intravenous contrast show the intrasplenic cyst with focal, punctate calcification. **E,** A CT scan after intravenous administration of contrast material shows a well-circumscribed, nonenhancing mass of fluid attenuation enlarging and distorting the spleen and displacing the stomach medially. (Courtesy Henrique Lederman, MD, Sao Paulo, Brazil.)

lymphocytes, plasma cells, extramedullary hematopoietic cells, fibrosis, hemosiderosis, and calcification.[69,76]

Clinical Presentation Most patients are asymptomatic, and the lesion is found incidentally; if it is large, the potential exists for rupture and hemoperitoneum. Many patients have associated hematologic abnormalities, including anemia, thrombocytopenia, or pancytopenia.[76] Hamartomas may occur in association with tuberous sclerosis and hamartomas elsewhere, as well as with hematologic conditions, including refractory microcytic anemia, sickle cell anemia, hereditary spherocytosis, and dyserythropoietic hemolytic anemia.[76]

Imaging Because they are composed of splenic tissue, hamartomas may not be detected with ultrasound unless they alter the contour of the spleen, producing a focal bulge. Hamartomas that are identified by ultrasound are most commonly well-circumscribed, solid and homogeneous, or partly cystic and heterogeneous. They have variable echogenicity.[69,77-79] The variety of described morphologic patterns is likely derived from the preponderant growth of one or another of several histologic components. Hamartomas typically reveal increased blood flow on Doppler interrogation.[69]

On CT, splenic hamartomas show similar or decreased attenuation relative to spleen on precontrast images, and they show dense and prolonged enhancement after administration of intravenous contrast material.[75] Hamartomas are isointense to normal splenic parenchyma on T1-weighted MRI, heterogeneously hyperintense on T2-weighted images, and demonstrate diffuse heterogeneous enhancement on postcontrast imaging, with more uniform enhancement on delayed images.[52,72] On ^{99m}Tc sulfur colloid scintigraphy, they may have radiopharmaceutical uptake greater than that in the surrounding normal spleen.[77]

Treatment Resection is indicated when the lesion is symptomatic or if a definitively benign diagnosis cannot be made through imaging.[75,76]

LYMPHATIC MALFORMATIONS

Overview Lymphatic malformations are rare, benign tumors that are diagnosed in children more commonly than in adults. They may be single or multiple and may cause splenic enlargement. Splenic lymphangiomatosis usually is associated with lymphangiomas found elsewhere; thus it has been recommended that if splenic lymphangiomas are identified, the diagnostic search should be extended beyond the spleen.[69]

Etiology It is believed that splenic lymphatic malformation may represent a hamartomatous versus neoplastic lesion or a congenital developmental defect as part of the spectrum of cystic hydroma.[69]

Clinical Presentation Clinical manifestations range from an asymptomatic incidental finding to a large, symptomatic mass that may cause symptoms from compression of adjacent structures. Specific symptoms include left upper quadrant pain, nausea, and abdominal distension.[69] Larger lesions may cause bleeding, consumptive coagulopathy, hypersplenism, and portal hypertension.[69] Diagnostic evaluation should

include extrasplenic organs; multiple-organ involvement indicates lymphangiomatosis, with possible involvement of the liver, pericardium, mediastinum, lung, and bone.

Imaging On ultrasound, CT, and MRI, lymphatic malformations are most commonly septated, nonenhancing cystic lesions. Although typically anechoic on ultrasound, they occasionally may demonstrate internal echoes as a result of hemorrhage or infection. On CT they appear as single or multiple thin-walled, low-density masses with sharp margins in the subcapsular regions, and they demonstrate no significant contrast enhancement. Curvilinear mural calcifications may be present. The cysts generally have low signal intensity on T1-weighted images and high signal intensity on T2-weighted images (e-Fig. 95-18); however, they may have high signal intensity on T1-weighted images as a result of internal hemorrhage or proteinaceous fluid. Lymphatic malformations often involve the capsule and trabeculae of the spleen, where lymphatics are concentrated. In cases of lymphangiomatosis, the spleen may be diffusely replaced by expanding lesions.

Treatment Typically, with solitary small or asymptomatic lesions, no surgical intervention is required. Symptomatic lesions may be treated with a splenectomy or partial splenectomy, although sclerotherapy may be an option for some patients.

PELIOSIS

Overview Peliosis is an uncommon entity that is characterized by multiple blood-filled spaces without an endothelial lining; it typically is associated with peliosis hepatis.[69]

Etiology Peliosis consists of multiple blood-filled spaces within the spleen and is associated with hematologic disorders, use of anabolic steroids, and cachexia.

Clinical Presentation Many cases of peliosis are asymptomatic and discovered incidentally; however, if peliosis occurs along the periphery of the spleen, the potential exists for rupture and hemoperitoneum.[80,81] Cases of life-threatening intraperitoneal hemorrhage have been reported.[82]

Imaging On ultrasound, splenic peliosis may reveal an echogenic mass with poorly defined foci of varying echogenicity.[69] The condition also may demonstrate multiple well-defined hypoechoic lesions of varying size and occasionally fluid-fluid levels within the nodules. On CT, splenic peliosis appears as multiple lesions of low attenuation without calcification.[83]

Treatment Surgery usually is required for definitive diagnosis and treatment.[69]

Malignant Neoplasms

Malignant neoplasms of the spleen usually are related to multifocal neoplastic disorders such as leukemia and lymphoma or, rarely, metastatic disease. Angiomatous tumors include littoral cell angiomas, hemangiopericytomas, and angiosarcomas.

ACUTE LEUKEMIA

Overview   Leukemia is the most common form of childhood malignancy. It results from an accumulation of abnormal white blood cells in the bone marrow, liver, spleen, skin, or central nervous system. Acute lymphocytic leukemia (ALL) is significantly more common than acute myelogenous leukemia and accounts for approximately 75% of all childhood leukemias. Chronic myeloid leukemia constitutes the remaining childhood leukemias.[84,85]

Etiology   The etiology of childhood leukemia is unclear. Epidemiologic studies have evaluated various risk factors for the development of childhood leukemias, including environmental, genetic, and infectious risk factors. Ionizing radiation is the only environmental risk factor that has been significantly linked to ALL or acute myelogenous leukemia.[86]

Clinical Presentation   The clinical diagnosis of acute leukemia typically is made by physical examination, where lymph node, liver, or spleen enlargement may be detected, as well as evaluation of the blood count and peripheral smear. ALL and other childhood leukemias usually are accompanied by splenomegaly as a result of diffuse infiltration of the spleen. Chronic myelogenous leukemia is rare in children but frequently is accompanied by massive splenomegaly.

Imaging   Imaging studies of the spleen are rarely performed in children with leukemia because the diagnosis is made by other means, and the results of splenic imaging have no impact on staging or prognosis. Moreover, organ function is usually preserved, even with massive leukemic infiltration. However, the spleen often is involved during the hematologically active stages of acute pediatric leukemia, and it frequently serves as a sanctuary site during hematologic remission. Ultrasound may be useful in detecting occult visceral involvement and relapse, monitoring tumor response to chemotherapy, and assessing the complications of chemotherapy. In one retrospective study, sonograms were reviewed and correlated with clinical, hematologic, and autopsy studies. Patterns of organ involvement included hepatosplenomegaly (41%), isolated splenomegaly (20%), and panorganomegaly (16%). Altered internal splenic architecture was demonstrated in all cases.[87]

Treatment   When specific abnormalities are found, such as infectious complications of chemotherapy, antibiotic or antifungal agents are used; evidence of tumor relapse may alter chemotherapy regimens.

LYMPHOMA

Overview   Accurate imaging of splenic lesions is critically important in children with lymphoma because it can alter staging, treatment protocols, and overall prognosis. Additionally, other nonmalignant conditions may mimic tumor involvement and lead to an erroneous diagnosis.

Etiology   Pediatric lymphoma is a heterogeneous group of malignancies that are derived from the immune system and characterized by enlargement and proliferation of lymph nodes and secondary lymphoid tissues. The spleen is affected in 20% of patients with non-Hodgkin lymphoma (NHL), whereas the spleen is involved in 30% to 40% of persons with Hodgkin disease (HD) at presentation.[88] Organ size should not be used to assess splenic involvement, because the spleen can be normal in size with tumor infiltration, and it may be enlarged without neoplastic involvement.

Clinical Presentation   Clinical presentation varies according to the underlying lymphoma, with splenic involvement diagnosed during physical examination or at subsequent imaging.

Imaging   NHL often has a similar appearance to leukemic infiltration but also may have focal lesions large enough to be seen on ultrasound as ill-defined hypoechoic areas, especially in patients with a high-grade malignancy at histologic examination. On CT, the low-attenuation lesions do not show appreciable contrast enhancement compared with adjacent parenchyma. HD also can cause diffuse splenic infiltration that may or may not be detectable as focal splenic masses. If the only subdiaphragmatic site of involvement is the spleen, detection in the spleen is important for purposes of staging and prognosis.[52] However, ultrasound, CT, and MRI can result in false-negative examinations because these modalities depend on morphologic changes of enlargement or discrete nodules to detect lymphomatous involvement, whereas the imaging tissue characteristics of splenic lesions in persons with HD lesions may be similar to those of normal spleen when it is diffusely infiltrated.[52,89]

Metabolic imaging with fluorine-18 (^{18}F) fluorodeoxyglucose (FDG) positron emission tomography (PET) is superior to ultrasound, CT, and MRI in identifying splenic involvement with lymphoma and detecting active disease (Fig. 95-19). ^{18}F-FDG PET/CT detects lymphomatous involvement of the spleen by identifying elevated glucose metabolism in tumor cells, regardless of whether gross morphologic changes have occurred. A meta-analysis reported sensitivity and specificity of ^{18}F-FDG PET for the initial staging and restaging of NHL and HD as 90.3% and 91.1%, respectively.[90] ^{18}F-FDG PET/CT is superior to separate CT and ^{18}F-FDG PET in the staging and restaging of lymphoma, and it is the study of choice for staging and follow-up of HD and aggressive NHL.[89,91]

Treatment   Treatment options for splenic involvement with lymphoma include chemotherapy, radiotherapy, radioimmunotherapy, and splenectomy.

LITTORAL CELL ANGIOMA

Overview   A littoral cell angioma is an uncommon tumor characterized by anastomosing vascular channels that may anastomose with normal splenic sinuses at the interface with normal parenchyma; some cases have demonstrated malignant features.[92] The lesion can occur at any age, but it is more common in adults than in children.[69,93]

Etiology   The entity arises from the littoral cells lining the splenic red pulp.

Clinical Presentation   Patients may present with splenomegaly, thrombocytopenia, and systemic symptoms. This entity

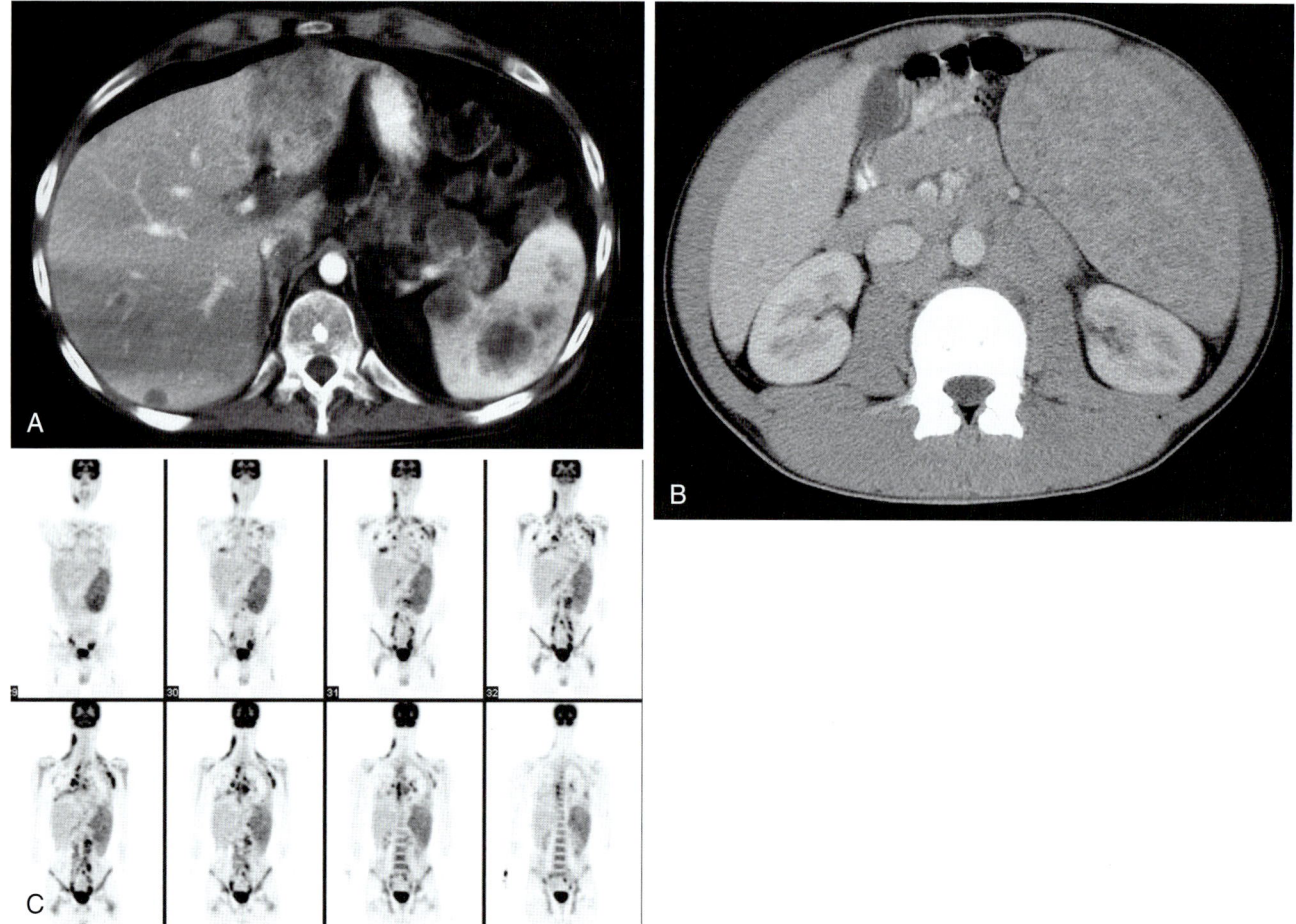

Figure 95-19 **A,** A contrast-enhanced abdominal computed tomography (CT) scan in a 19-year-old with multiple episodes of relapsing disease and new left upper quadrant pain. The examination reveals multiple large, round, hypodense, nonenhancing masses in the spleen. Note additional foci of disease in the liver. **B,** Contrast-enhanced CT performed as part of a staging evaluation in a 14-year-old boy with Hodgkin disease shows splenomegaly with numerous low-attenuation lesions throughout the spleen. **C,** Coronal images from a fluorine-18 fluorodeoxyglucose (FDG) positron emission tomography examination of a 15-year-old reveal marked enlargement of the spleen with moderate to marked increased FDG uptake. Note also nodal disease in the neck, supraclavicular regions, mediastinum, lungs, porta hepatis, retroperitoneum, iliac and inguinal regions, and the bone marrow.

presents as multiple lesions within an enlarged, heterogeneous spleen. The diagnosis should be considered in cases of multiple splenic lesions and hypersplenism.

Imaging Littoral cell angiomas are heterogeneously hypoechoic on ultrasound and initially are of low attenuation on CT but typically become progressively isodense on delayed images after contrast enhancement.[69,93] On MRI, the lesions are well circumscribed and are predominantly T1 hypointense. On T2-weighted images, they may appear hyperintense or they may remain hypointense against the normal bright spleen parenchyma, presumably because of hemosiderin within the lesions.[69] The lesions show progressive contrast enhancement after administration of gadolinium.[92]

Treatment Treatment includes supportive therapy for the coagulopathy and endovascular embolization of the spleen to increase platelet count; when these approaches fail, a splenectomy may be indicated. Ertan and colleagues[93] have published a thorough review of the pathogenesis, clinical course, imaging appearance, and treatment of this very rare pediatric tumor.

HEMANGIOPERICYTOMA

Overview A hemangiopericytoma is a rare vascular tumor that most commonly originates in the soft tissues of the extremities; it is even less common as a primary tumor of the spleen, and most often occurs in young adult patients.[69]

Etiology Hemangiopericytomas originate from the pericytes of the capillary networks. Cytogenetic analysis of some tumors show evidence of break points and translocations, and some investigators have suggested that the karyotype of hemangiopericytomas arising in soft tissues may differ from that of the spleen.[94]

Clinical Presentation The tumor has variable biologic behavior and high potential for malignancy.[69] When it occurs in the spleen, patients may be asymptomatic or they may present with splenomegaly. Reported presentations have included massive hemorrhage and splenic abscess, presumably as a result of superinfection.[94]

Imaging In the spleen, hemangiopericytomas may appear as a single large mass with smaller lesions within the parenchyma. Multiple hypoechoic lesions may be seen on ultrasound. Calcifications may be seen in the lesions on CT, along with contrast enhancement of the solid portions and septations. The lesions demonstrate hypointensity on T1-weighted MR sequences and hyperintensity on T2-weighted sequences.

Treatment The treatment for splenic hemangiopericytoma is surgical excision/splenectomy. Careful long-term follow-up is required because of its aggressive behavior and a recurrence rate of 50%.[69,94]

ANGIOSARCOMA

Overview Angiosarcomas are rare, highly malignant neoplasms that can occur at any age but are less common in children than in adults. They have no gender predilection and are considered the most common malignant tumor of the spleen outside of hematologic or lymphatic malignancies.[69]

Etiology Some of these tumors are believed to occur in preexistent lesions, such as after chemotherapy for lymphoma, or arise from otherwise benign lesions, such as splenic hemangiomas.[95]

Clinical Presentation The presentation may include left upper quadrant pain, fever, fatigue, weight loss, anemia, and thrombocytopenia. Splenomegaly is common.[95] In older patients, angiosarcomas of the spleen are associated with previous chemotherapy for lymphoma and radiation therapy for breast cancer.[69]

Imaging Ultrasound images most commonly reveal a complex heterogeneous mass with hypoechoic cystic areas, likely reflecting areas of hemorrhage and necrosis. Solid echogenic regions display increased flow on color Doppler imaging. On CT the lesions are ill-defined, with lower attenuation than the surrounding spleen, and they demonstrate heterogeneous contrast enhancement and areas of necrosis.[69] Metastases are most common in the liver, lungs, bone, and lymph nodes.

Treatment Because chemotherapy typically is ineffective, a splenectomy is performed. The prognosis is very poor.

SPLENIC METASTASES

Splenic metastases from solid primary tumors are less common with childhood tumors than with adult tumors. The most common primary tumors are lung, melanoma, breast, and testicular germ cell tumors, particularly choriocarcinoma. Metastases may be single or multiple and frequently do not cause splenomegaly (e-Fig. 95-20). Splenic metastases portend a poor prognosis.

✓ WHAT THE CLINICIAN NEEDS TO KNOW

- Spleen size
- Sonographic echogenicity of spleen parenchyma
- Presence of congenital anomaly
- Presence of splenic mass
- Any change from prior examinations

Key Points

Sonography is the primary imaging modality for evaluating splenic size, shape, location, and multiplicity.

Radionuclide imaging with ^{99m}Tc sulfur colloid helps in the assessment of splenic congenital anomalies.

Transient heterogeneous splenic enhancement patterns are commonly encountered during rapid bolus techniques on contrast-enhanced CT.

Splenomegaly is usually a manifestation of an underlying systemic condition.

Hypersplenism is a syndrome of sequestration of blood elements within an enlarged spleen.

Hamartoma and hemangioma are the most common primary tumors of the spleen.

Lymphoma is the most common malignancy of the spleen.

Suggested Readings

Abbott RM, Levy AD, Aguilera NS, et al. From the archives of the AFIP: primary vascular neoplasms of the spleen: radiologic-pathologic correlation. *Radiographics.* 2004;24:1137.

Applegate KE, Goske MJ, Pierce G, et al. Situs revisited: imaging of the heterotaxy syndrome. *Radiographics.* 1999;19:837.

Elsayes KM, Vamsidhar RN, Mukundan G, et al. MR imaging of the spleen: spectrum of abnormalities. *Radiographics.* 2005;25:967-982.

Hilmes MA, Strouse PJ. The pediatric spleen. *Semin Ultrasound CT MRI.* 2007;28:3-11.

Paterson A, Frush DP, Donnelly LF, et al. A pattern-oriented approach to splenic imaging in infants and children. *Radiographics.* 1999;19:1465.

References

Full references for this chapter can be found on www.expertconsult.com.

Chapter 96

The Pancreas

PARITOSH C. KHANNA and SUMIT PRUTHI

Embryology, Anatomy, and Physiology

The pancreas (from the Greek words *pan,* meaning "all," and *kreas,* meaning "flesh") arises from two anlagen that develop from the endodermal lining of the duodenum. Before 28 days of gestation, the dorsal part develops from a diverticulum from the dorsal aspect of the duodenum caudal to the hepatic diverticulum. It grows upward and backward into the dorsal mesogastrium to form part of the head and the entire body and tail. The ventral pancreatic bud develops between 30 and 35 days of gestation as a diverticulum from the primitive bile duct that forms part of the head and uncinate process. The ventral pancreas rotates counterclockwise posterior to the duodenum at day 37 of gestation, and the two portions fuse at about the sixth week of embryonic life. The ductal systems fuse, and the duct from the dorsal bud becomes the accessory pancreatic duct (of Santorini); the duct from the ventral bud enlarges to become the main pancreatic duct (of Wirsung), after it fuses with the distal two thirds of the dorsal duct. The opening of the accessory duct is often obliterated.

Developmental deviation from this embryologic pattern can give rise to variants. The usual ductal configuration is most commonly bifid, formed by the ducts of Wirsung and Santorini (60% of cases). Less common configurations include a rudimentary duct of Santorini (30%); a dominant duct of Santorini (1%); and *ansa pancreatica,* in which the duct of Santorini curves as it courses to the duct of Wirsung. Ductal narrowing can be seen at the site of fusion of the dorsal and ventral ducts. The absence of proximal dilation allows differentiation of this normal variant from a true stricture. Duodenal obstruction, pancreatobiliary maljunction pancreatitis, and biliary cysts occur secondary to developmental variants. Pancreatobiliary maljunction is associated with congenital common bile duct webs.[1]

The pancreas grows substantially in the first year of life, and growth slows from year 1 through 18. The gland is relatively larger in children than in adults, and the overall ratio of gland size to patient body size decreases with age (Table 96-1). The pancreatic head is more prominent in children compared with the body and tail. The diameter of the pancreatic duct also varies with age (Table 96-2). Enlarged ducts (>1.5 mm at 1 to 6 years, >1.9 mm at 7 to 9 years, and >2.2 mm at 13 to 18 years) are associated with pancreatitis.

The pancreas lies transversely in the retroperitoneum. It is divided into the head, body, and tail (Fig. 96-1). The head is to the right of midline, situated within the "C-loop" of the duodenum. At the junction of the inferior and left margins of the pancreatic head is an extension of the gland called the *uncinate process.* The anterior surface of the pancreatic head is in contact with the transverse colon, gastroduodenal artery, and loops of small intestine. The anterior surface of the uncinate process is in contact with the superior mesenteric artery and vein. The posterior surface of the head is adjacent to the inferior vena cava, common bile duct, renal veins, and the abdominal aorta.

The pancreatic body is in contact with the stomach anteriorly and superiorly. Its posterior portion abuts the abdominal aorta, splenic vein, left kidney, adrenal gland, and origin of the superior mesenteric artery. Loops of jejunum and ileum lie inferiorly. The tail may be more bulbous in children than the head or body and is narrower in adults. The pancreatic tail lies in the phrenicolienal ligament in contact with the gastric surface of the spleen and the splenic flexure of the colon.

Pancreatic function is both exocrine and endocrine. Exocrine functions are directed toward digestion, with secretions exiting through the pancreatic duct into the duodenum. The islets of Langerhans represents endocrine tissue that contains several types of hormone-producing cells (insulin, glucagon, somatostatin, etc.) that help regulate blood glucose levels and digestive function. The B cells produce insulin; A cells, glucagon; G cells, gastrin; D cells, somatostatin; and D_1 cells, vasoactive intestinal peptide (VIP) and secretin.

Imaging the Pancreas in Children

The pancreas itself is not seen on plain radiographs, although calcifications in patients with chronic pancreatitis or cystic fibrosis may be identified on abdominal radiographs (Fig. 96-2). In acute pancreatitis, dilated loops of bowel and fluid levels within the upper midabdomen may suggest localized ileus. A pancreatic mass may be sufficiently large to displace adjacent gas-filled portions of the gastrointestinal (GI) tract.[2]

Table 96-1

Normal Sonographic and Computed Tomographic Dimensions of the Pancreas			
Age	Head	Body	Tail
Ultrasound (Mean ± SD, cm)			
<1 month	1.0 ± 0.4	0.6 ± 0.2	1.0 ± 0.4
1 month to 1 year	1.5 ± 0.5	0.8 ± 0.3	1.2 ± 0.4
1-5 years	1.7 ± 0.3	1.0 ± 0.2	1.8 ± 0.4
5-10 years	1.6 ± 0.4	1.0 ± 0.3	1.8 ± 0.4
10-19 years	2.0 ± 0.5	1.1 ± 0.3	2.0 ± 0.4
CT (Mean ± SD, mm)			
20-30 years	28.6 ± 3.8	19.1 ± 2.1	18.0 ± 1.6
21-40 years	26.0 ± 3.4	18.2 ± 2.4	16.5 ± 1.8
41-50 years	25.2 ± 3.6	17.8 ± 2.2	15.8 ± 1.7
51-60 years	24.0 ± 3.6	16.0 ± 2.0	15.1 ± 1.9
61-70 years	23.4 ± 3.5	15.8 ± 2.4	14.7 ± 1.8
71-80 years	21.2 ± 4.3	14.4 ± 2.7	13.0 ± 2.1

Modified from Heuck A, Maubach PA, Reiser M, et al. Age-related morphology of the normal pancreas on computed tomography. *Gastrointest Radiol.* 1987;12:18-22; and Siegel MJ, Martin KW, Worthington JL. Normal and abnormal pancreas in children: US studies. *Radiology.* 1987;165:15-18.

Ultrasonography (US) is the primary screening tool to evaluate the pediatric pancreas.[3] The pancreas is most easily seen if the stomach and duodenum are not distended with gas. Ingestion of water devoid of gas bubbles may improve visualization. The distal body and tail may also be imaged in the prone position using the left kidney as an acoustic window. Age-matched normal dimensions of the pancreas are given in Table 96-1.[3] Pancreatic size is best measured at its body, but individual variation is sufficient to warrant caution when determining pancreatic size. Enlargement of the pancreas should be diagnosed when the anteroposterior dimension of the pancreatic body is greater than 1.5 cm.[4] The normal duct may be seen as a single- or double-track echogenic line anterior to the junction of the splenic and mesenteric veins (see Fig. 96-1). The pancreas has a spectrum of echogenicity relative to that of the liver, but in most children, the pancreas is hypoechoic or nearly isoechoic with the liver. However, in neonates, particularly in premature infants, the pancreatic gland is more echogenic.[5] US is also helpful for image-guided biopsy and in aligning radiotherapy.[6]

Computed tomography (CT) of the pancreas[7] is indicated less frequently than US, but it is valuable in certain conditions, particularly pancreatitis, tumors, and pseudocysts with uncommon features. The pancreas is best visualized during bolus injection of intravenous (IV) contrast material, which readily identifies the adjacent vessels, and with meticulous administration of GI contrast to opacify the adjacent stomach and duodenum. The pancreas is hypodense compared with the liver, both with and without intravenous contrast. The contours of the pancreas are commonly smooth but may be slightly lobulated. Because the pancreas in children is oblique to the axial plane, multiple thin sections may be necessary for optimal visualization; in-plane reconstructions, particularly from axial volumetric data obtained with multidetector equipment, can image the pancreas in its own oblique plane.

Imaging of the pancreatic head may be optimized by scanning the patient in the right lateral decubitus position soon after ingestion of GI contrast material. With this technique, the optimally opacified duodenal C-loop outlines the pancreatic head, and opacified proximal jejunal loops outline the remainder of the gland. CT is the best modality for assessing neoplasms, pancreatic trauma, and pancreatitis and its complications and for further evaluation of abnormalities on US. Thin collimation volumetric CT coupled with curved planar reformations produces quality imaging of pancreatic and peripancreatic tissues.[8]

Magnetic resonance imaging (MRI) of the pancreas[9,10] is more difficult in children than in adults because of adjacent gas-filled loops of intestine and motion artifact from peristalsis and respiration.[11] Nevertheless, MRI is a powerful tool for imaging pediatric developmental abnormalities. The pancreas normally has signal intensity equal to that of liver on T1- and T2-weighted spin echo images with midfield strength magnets. Pancreatic images produced with high-field strength magnets may have greater signal intensity than those of the liver. To some degree, signal varies with age. Although normal children do not have as much intrapancreatic macroscopic fat as adults, adolescents have more fat in the pancreatic septa than do preadolescent children, and the amount of intrapancreatic fat may be increased in children with cystic fibrosis. The value of MRI is enhanced by the use of breath-holding techniques (generally not possible in younger children), fat suppression, contrast enhancement, and respiratory gating.

Table 96-2

Normal Diameter of the Pancreatic Duct by Ultrasound and Computed Tomography	
Age (Years)	Diameter (Mean ± SD, mm (Range))
Ultrasound	
1-3	1.13 ± 0.15 (0.9-1.3)
4-6	1.35 ± 0.15 (1.0-1.5)
7-9	1.67 ± 0.17 (1.3-1.9)
10-12	1.78 ± 0.17 (1.5-2.2)
13-15	1.92 ± 0.18 (1.6-2.4)
16-18	2.05 ± 0.15 (1.8-2.4)
Computed Tomography	
18-29	1.5 ± 0.5
30-39	1.6 ± 0.5
40-49	1.9 ± 0.3
50-59	2.0 ± 0.5
60-69	2.1 ± 0.4
70-81	2.0 ± 0.5

Modified from Siegel MJ, Martin KW, Worthington JL. Normal and abnormal pancreas in children: US studies. *Radiology.* 1987;165:15-18; Heuck A, Maubach PA, Reiser M, et al: Age-related morphology of the normal pancreas on computed tomography. *Gastrointest Radiol.* 1987;12:18-22; Chao HC, Lin SJ, Kong MS, et al. Sonographic evaluation of the pancreatic duct in normal children and children with pancreatitis. *J Ultrasound Med.* 2000;19:757-763; and Glaser J, Hogemann B, Krummenerl T, et al. Sonographic imaging of the pancreatic duct. New diagnostic possibilities using secretin stimulation. *Dig Dis Sci.* 1987;32:1075-1081.

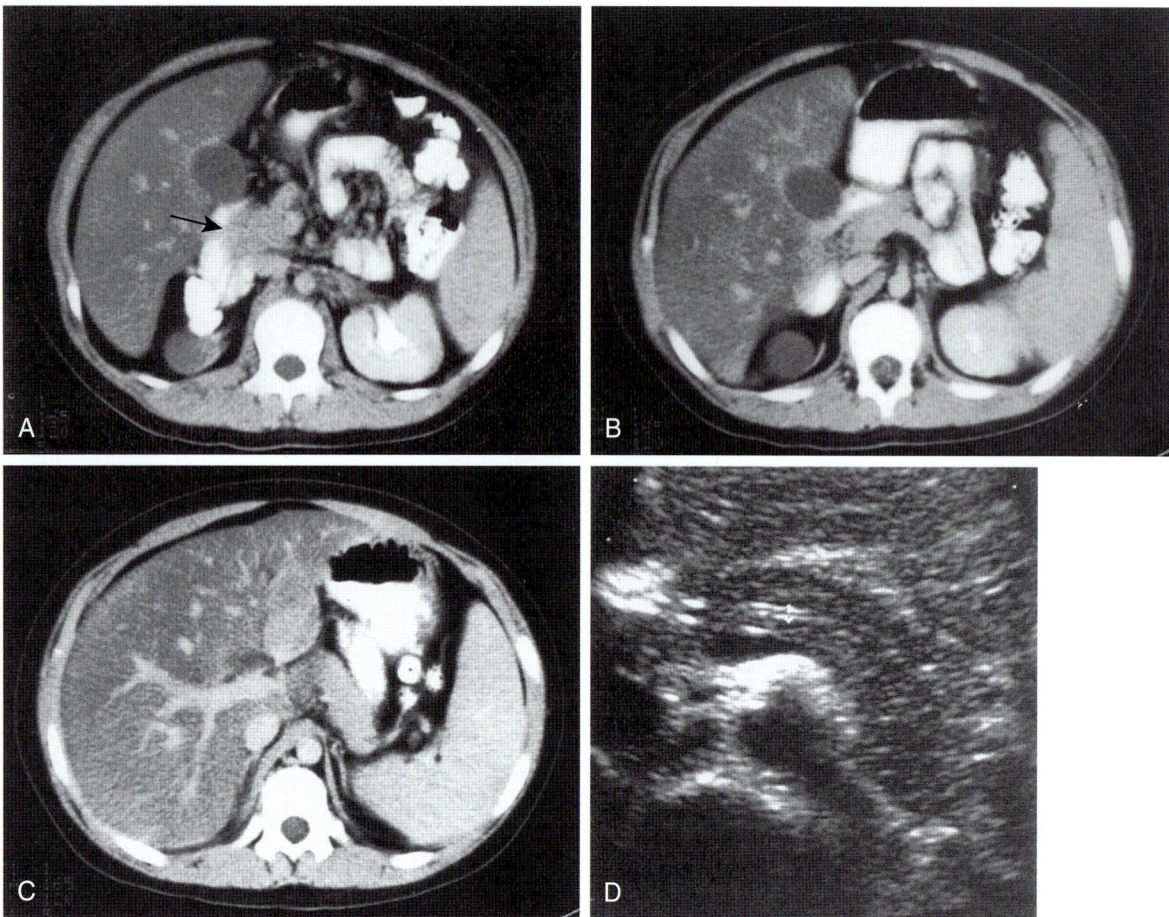

Figure 96-1 Normal pancreas in an 11-year-old boy. **A** to **C,** Computed tomography (CT) sections of the pancreas. The head of the pancreas (*arrow* in *A*) is slightly bulbous and distinct from the contrast-filled duodenal sweep. The body of the pancreas (**B**) is narrower than the head or tail and is seen anterior to the aorta, from which the superior mesenteric artery arises. The tail of the pancreas (**C**) is thicker in children than in adults and extends to the spleen. **D,** Transverse ultrasound shows the double track of a normal pancreatic duct.

Because of its noninvasive nature, magnetic resonance cholangiopancreatography (MRCP)[12] may be more useful than endoscopic retrograde cholangiopancreatography (ERCP)[13,14] in children (Fig. 96-3). Reported sensitivity, specificity, and accuracy are 87%, 90%, and 89% respectively

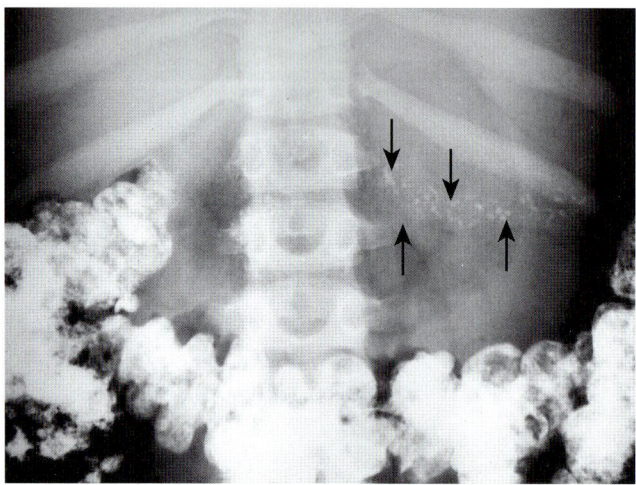

Figure 96-2 Cystic fibrosis in a 9-year-old girl. Multiple pancreatic calcifications (*arrows*) are seen on radiography.

for stones; 100%, 98%, and 98% for cholangitis; 92%, 97%, and 96% for bile duct tumors; and 89%, 96%, and 95% for periampullary stenosis.[15] MRCP is also useful in certain congenital abnormalities, such as pancreas divisum, and after pancreatic trauma to identify duct of Wirsung transections. Although intravenous CT cholangiography is superior to MRCP in delineating postoperative anatomy after choledochal cyst repair, MRCP is highly accurate (84%) in depicting the anastomotic site, intrahepatic biliary tree, and reconstructed bowel, and it clearly demonstrates pancreatobiliary maljunction, residual distal common bile duct, common channel,[16] and pancreatic duct.[17] Similarly, MRCP accurately depicts the postoperative anatomy and complications after orthotopic liver transplantation.[18] A normal MRCP may obviate the need for ERCP or percutaneous transhepatic cholangiography, and abnormalities visualized with MRCP can direct the modality and route for further intervention. An overview of MRCP pitfalls has been provided by Van Hoe and colleagues.[19]

Secretin stimulation with MRCP further enhances the imaging information obtained, because it gives additional, valuable, functional and anatomic information about the pancreatic duct and pancreatic excretory capacity. Secretin-enhanced MRCP has been described in detail in recent years[20-23] and has been found useful for detection

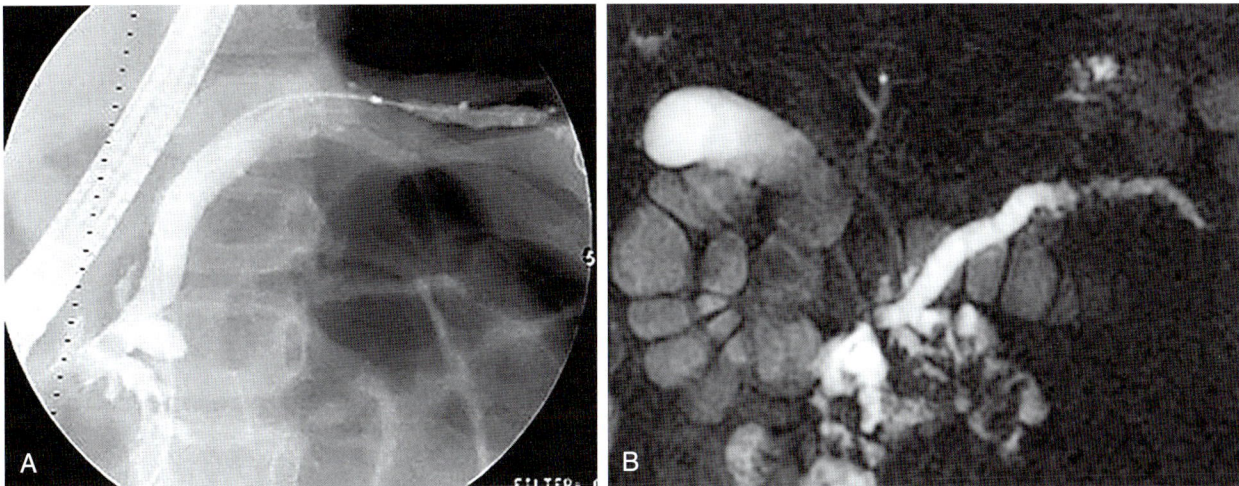

Figure 96-3 Endoscopic retrograde cholangiopancreatography (ERCP) and magnetic resonance cholangiopancreatography (MRCP) in a 9-year-old with recurrent pancreatitis and stones. **A,** Anteroposterior image from ERCP shows abnormal dilation of the proximal pancreatic duct and narrowing, irregularity, beading, and an undulating caliber distally. **B,** Anterior MRCP image of the same patient similarly defines the abnormal caliber and irregularity of the pancreatic duct, consistent with recurrent pancreatitis. The common bile duct is normal. (Courtesy Dr. Kimberly Applegate, Indianapolis, IN.)

and diagnosis of a variety of congenital, inflammatory, and neoplastic pancreatic conditions.[24] Secretin causes temporary dilation of pancreatic ducts, principally by increasing pancreatic exocrine secretions, thus it allows better visualization of the ducts during MRCP.

Congenital and Hereditary Pancreatic Abnormalities

CONGENITAL PANCREATIC ABNORMALITIES[25,26]

Pancreas Divisum

Overview Pancreas divisum occurs when the dorsal and ventral ducts fail to fuse, although the pancreas is otherwise anatomically normal. This anomaly has been described in 4% to 14% of the population, depending on the method of evaluation.

Clinical Presentation In such cases, the accessory ampulla drains the major portion of the gland. It has been suggested that the incidence of pancreatitis is higher, although recent literature refutes this.

Imaging CT in children with pancreas divisum and pancreatitis demonstrates enlargement of both ducts, in addition to the characteristic findings of pancreatitis. Further enlargement of the ducts can be provoked with secretin stimulation.[27,28] Increased thickness of the pancreatic head has also been described.[29] Zeman and colleagues[30] reported that thin-section CT demonstrated the unfused ducts in 5 of 12 patients (Fig. 96-4), and two distinct pancreatic moieties separated by a fat cleft was seen in 4 patients. Pancreas divisum may be

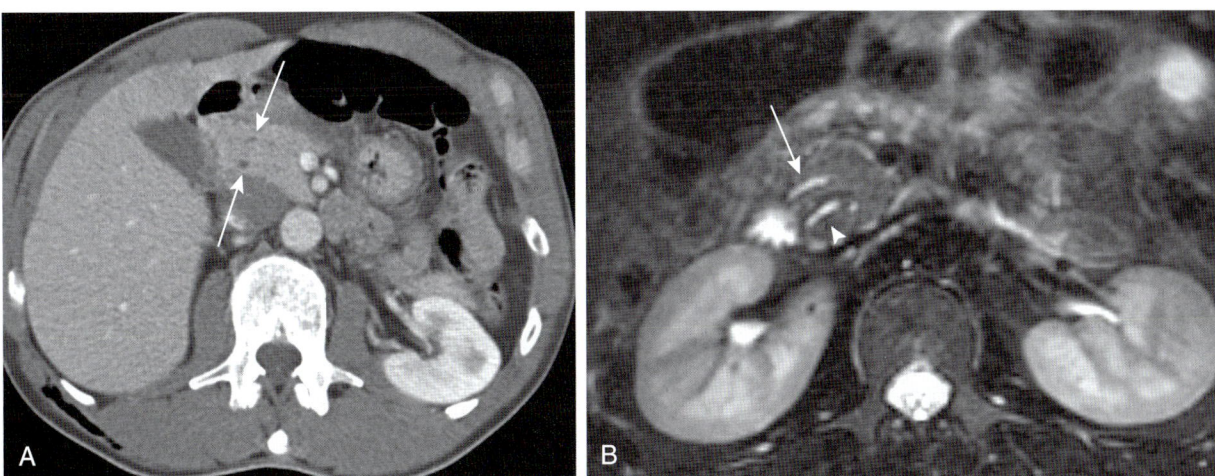

Figure 96-4 Pancreas divisum. **A,** Axial contrast-enhanced computed tomography shows two pancreatic ducts (*arrows*). **B,** Axial fast spin-echo T2-weighted magnetic resonance image from a teenager with recurrent pancreatitis shows separate ducts of Santorini (*arrow*) and Wirsung (*arrowhead*) in the pancreatic head. (Courtesy Dr. Marilyn Siegel, St. Louis, MO.)

associated with minor papilla adenoma beyond the childhood years.

Treatment   Pancreas divisum in symptomatic individuals varies and has not been well established. Minor papilla sphincterotomy to facilitate normal egress of pancreatic enzymes and duct stenting has been attempted.[31]

Congenital Short Pancreas

Overview   Congenital short pancreas, also known as *agenesis of the dorsal pancreatic anlage*,[32] occurs when the portion of the pancreas derived from the dorsal embryonic bud is absent, and only the smaller portion, derived from the ventral anlage, is present. Thus, the pancreatic neck, body, and tail are absent. This anomaly has been described in patients with polysplenia syndrome, or it may be a sporadic finding.

Clinical Presentation   Variable symptoms of abdominal pain and epigastric discomfort and diabetes may be present.[33]

Imaging   Only a globular pancreatic head can be identified on CT (Fig. 96-5). Size is variable, and some patients show an enlarged or prominent pancreatic head, whereas others may show a normal sized or even mildly atrophic and small pancreatic head. The diagnosis of agenesis of the dorsal pancreas is inconclusive without demonstration of the absence of the dorsal pancreatic duct, either with MRCP or ERCP. Patients with this abnormality have an increased risk of developing diabetes mellitus[34] because of the paucity of islet cells, most of which are located in the distal pancreas. This condition may also be associated in later life with pancreatic tumors[35] such as intraductal papillary mucinous neoplasms.

Treatment   Treatment is supportive and is directed at the abdominal pain, pancreatitis, and diabetes.

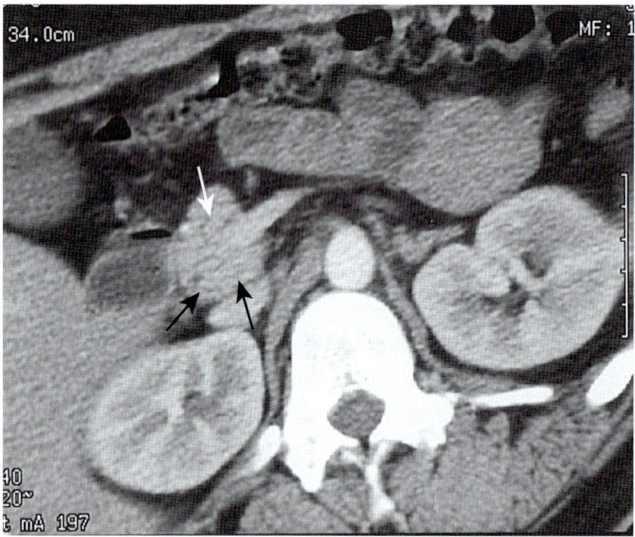

Figure 96-5 Congenital short pancreas. Axial contrast-enhanced abdominal computed tomography shows a congenital short pancreas, with only a bulbous pancreatic head present (*arrows*). (Courtesy Dr. George Taylor, Boston, MA.)

Ectopic Pancreas

Overview   Ectopic pancreatic tissue[36] is an aberrant rest of normal pancreatic tissue remote from the pancreatic body that occurs in 1% to 13% of the population. The vast majority of pancreatic rests (about 70%) are located in the stomach,[37] duodenum, and jejunum, but they can occur elsewhere, such as omphaloenteric duct rest.[38] An association with Beckwith-Weidemann syndrome has been reported.[39]

Clinical Presentation   Most pancreatic rests are incidental findings and are asymptomatic.

Imaging   Besides the findings described above, a noncommunicating gastric duplication cyst has been described that contained ectopic pancreatic ducts and islets without acini.[36,40]

Treatment   Laparoscopic gastric wedge resection is a safe and effective treatment for symptomatic pancreatic rests located in the stomach.

Annular Pancreas

Overview   Several theories of embryonic dysgenesis have been proposed for annular pancreas, but most suggest some form of rotational anomaly of the ventral bud, which may be bifid. The pancreatic annulus, or the portion surrounding the duodenum, frequently has a separate duct entering the duodenum opposite the ampulla of Vater. Duodenal contents may reflux through this duct into the annulus. Affected patients may have associated duodenal stenosis or atresia and may come to medical attention with duodenal obstruction in infancy. Many other associated abnormalities have been described, the most common being intestinal malrotation, tracheoesophageal fistula, anal atresia, and cardiac abnormalities.

Clinical Presentation   Annular pancreas is frequently diagnosed in infancy because of associated duodenal obstruction. However, in approximately half the cases, the diagnosis is made beyond infancy (Fig. 96-6). The associated abnormalities described above are most common in patients who also have trisomy 21. Annular pancreas has also been described in de Lange syndrome, with heterotaxy, and as a cause of extrahepatic biliary obstruction.[41] Pancreatitis that solely affects the annulus of an annular pancreas has been reported in adults.[14]

Imaging   MRI has advantages over CT in the diagnosis of annular pancreas, because with MRI it is easier to detect and characterize the tissue surrounding the duodenum as pancreatic. Diagnosis by US has also been described.[42] ERCP and MRCP are used to investigate ductal anatomy. Coincidence of congenital short and annular pancreas with gallbladder agenesis and splenic malrotation is rare.[43]

Treatment   Treatment usually is through a bypass of the obstructed segment of duodenum by duodenoduodenostomy or gastrojejunostomy.[44]

Congenital Pancreatic Cysts

Overview   Congenital cysts of the pancreas are rare and are often confused with choledochal,[45] omental, or mesenteric

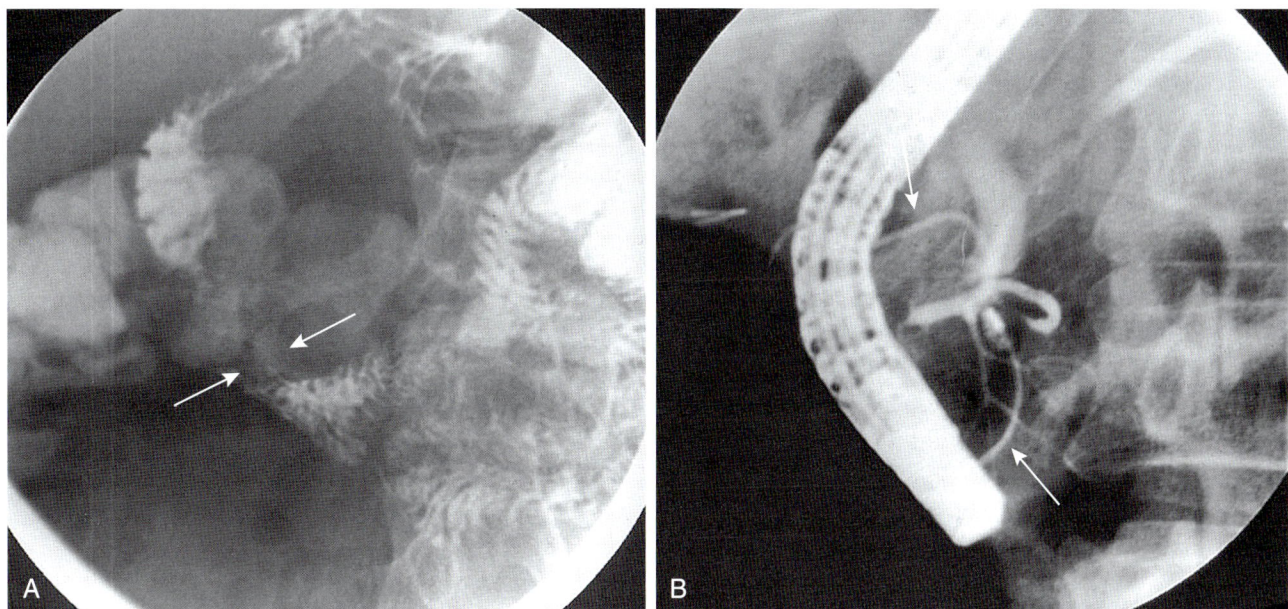

Figure 96-6 Annular pancreas. **A,** Oblique view during an upper gastrointestinal series shows extrinsic narrowing of the duodenal C-loop (*arrows*). **B,** Endoscopic retrograde cholangiopancreatography confirms the presence of small ducts (*arrows*) encircling the duodenum, consistent with an annular pancreas. (Courtesy Dr. George Taylor, Boston, MA.)

cysts (e-Fig. 96-7). Single congenital pancreatic cysts are very rare and occur predominantly in females.[46]

Clinical Presentation Congenital pancreatic cysts are usually asymptomatic, but when symptoms do occur, they are related to mass effect and compression of adjacent structures.

Imaging Congenital cysts are anechoic by US; they are usually unilocular, located in the pancreatic tail, and range in size from microscopic to 5 cm.[47] Rarely, they may communicate with the ductal system. In contrast to single congenital pancreatic cysts, multiple congenital cysts may be associated with a polycystic disorder such as von Hippel–Lindau disease.[48] Juxtapancreatic GI duplication cysts occur as abnormalities of the developing foregut and therefore usually have an alimentary tract epithelial lining. Most of these cysts arise from the stomach or duodenum but may rarely be sequestered within the pancreas.[49]

Treatment Surgical removal is usually only necessary for symptomatic cysts or those concerning for neoplasia.

HEREDITARY SYSTEMIC CONDITIONS WITH PANCREATIC INVOLVEMENT

Cystic Fibrosis

Overview Cystic fibrosis (CF) leads to exocrine pancreatic insufficiency in 80% of affected patients. The pancreatic ductules contain goblet cells that produce abnormally thick mucus, leading to obstruction of enzyme egress pathways and associated pancreatic changes.

Clinical Presentation Patients have pancreatic insufficiency, mainly exocrine, with failure to thrive, abdominal distension,

steatorrhea, and occasional rectal prolapse. Patients with pancreatic cystosis (see below) are usually asymptomatic.

Imaging In young patients with cystic fibrosis (CF), US[50] shows a normal pancreas or pancreatic enlargement, but chronic obstruction ultimately results in shrinkage of the gland with fatty infiltration and fibrosis. On US, these histopathologic changes are visualized as increased echogenicity of the gland. CT shows a shrunken pancreas with reduced attenuation secondary to fatty infiltration. Fibrosis without fatty infiltration is found infrequently. Unenhanced scans may show pancreatic calcifications, ductal dilation, and pancreatic cysts (Fig. 96-8).[51] MRI findings are variable but can accurately depict the changes of fatty infiltration, fibrosis, and atrophy.[52-54]

Cystic transformation of the pancreas, or *pancreatic cystosis,* in children and young adults with CF has been described.[55,56] This is an unusual form of pancreatic involvement with CF, in that the pancreas is replaced by macrocysts that are rarely more than 1 cm in diameter. This can be imaged with US, CT (Fig. 96-9), and MRI. These are true, epithelium-lined cysts that result from the accumulation of inspissated mucus, produced as a result of residual exocrine secretory function in the acinar cells, proximal to ducts obstructed from inflammation.

Treatment Exocrine pancreatic insufficiency is treated by supplementation with pancreatic enzyme products. Treatment otherwise is supportive and directed toward the underlying CF.

Shwachman-Diamond Syndrome

Overview and Clinical Presentation Shwachman-Diamond syndrome is an autosomal-recessive disorder that results in

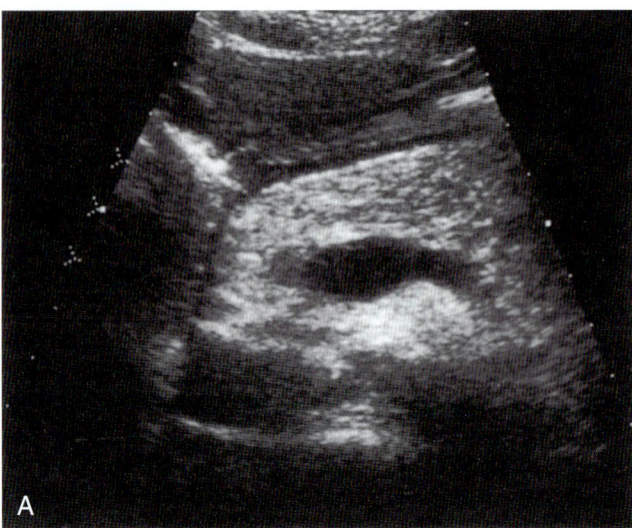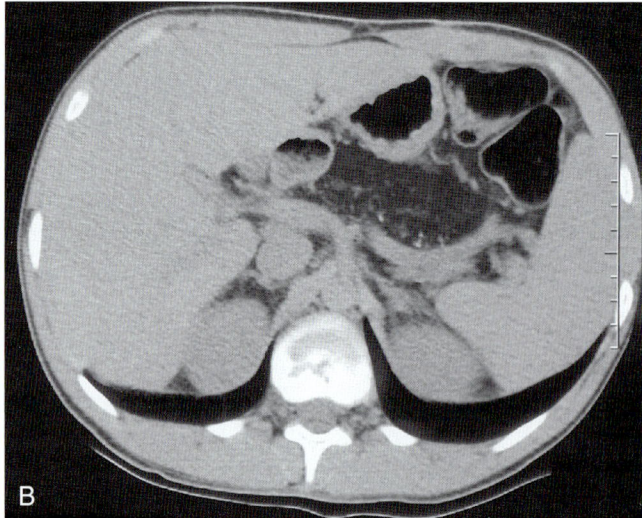

Figure 96-8 Cystic fibrosis (CF) with diffuse fatty replacement of the pancreas. **A,** Markedly hyperechoic pancreas on US in an 18-year-old woman with CF and fatty infiltration of the pancreas. **B,** Axial noncontrast abdominal computed tomography shows diffuse fatty replacement of the pancreas with multiple tiny calcifications. (Courtesy Dr. Robert Kaufman, Memphis, TN.)

short stature, exocrine pancreatic insufficiency, metaphyseal chondrodysplasia, and bone marrow dysfunction.

Imaging US and CT evaluations of the pancreas demonstrate fatty replacement (pancreatic lipomatosis)[57] as described earlier in patients with CF (e-Fig. 96-10). Other causes of pancreatic lipomatosis include chronic pancreatitis, prolonged steroid use, obesity, Cushing syndrome, hemochromatosis, obstruction of the duct of Wirsung, and Johanson-Blizzard syndrome.

Treatment Exocrine pancreatic insufficiency is treated by supplementation with pancreatic enzyme products. Other current treatment strategies include surgery for skeletal

deformities, granulocyte colony stimulating factor for neutropenia, and bone marrow transplantation for marrow failure.

von Hippel–Lindau Disease

Overview and Clinical Presentation von Hippel–Lindau disease (VHL) is an autosomal-dominant disorder characterized by hemangioblastoma in multiple organs, especially the retina and central nervous system; skin lesions and cysts of numerous organs, including the pancreas. Pancreatic involvement is seen in approximately 21% of patients.[58] Up to 75% of these multiple pancreatic lesions (e-Fig. 96-11) likely originate from progenitor cells, not mature endocrine cells as previously thought.[59]

Imaging VHL-associated cysts are typically anechoic on US and have reduced attenuation on CT compared with the surrounding pancreatic tissue. Multiple cysts—as well as serous and mucinous cystadenomas of the pancreas, carcinoma, adenocarcinoma, and islet cell tumors—are also associated with VHL.[60] Adenocarcinoma occurs in affected adults, and pancreatic calcifications can be seen on unenhanced CT scans.

Treatment Although symptoms are rare, specific treatment of pancreatic lesions is required in selected patients, mainly those with large neuroendocrine tumors that require surgical resection.[61]

Autosomal-Dominant Polycystic Disease

Overview Autosomal dominant polycystic disease is a hereditary disorder with 100% penetrance but variable expressivity.

Clinical Presentation Symptoms of large pancreatic cysts include abdominal pain, jaundice, and fever.

Figure 96-9 Cystic fibrosis with pancreatic cystosis. Axial contrast-enhanced computed tomography in an 18-year-old man demonstrates multiple macrocysts of varying sizes that nearly completely replace the pancreatic parenchyma. The patient was asymptomatic, and no further imaging was obtained.

Imaging Renal cysts are the dominant feature, but cysts may also be found in the liver, spleen, adrenal glands, and pancreas. Pancreatic cysts are present in about 10% of patients, and the gland is typically less involved than the kidneys or liver.

Treatment Large, symptomatic pancreatic cysts may require surgical or percutaneous intervention.

Hereditary Pancreatitis

Hereditary pancreatitis is an autosomal-dominant disease in which patients have recurrent episodes of pancreatitis. This condition is discussed later in the chapter.

Beckwith-Wiedemann Syndrome

Overview and Clinical Presentation Beckwith-Wiedemann syndrome (BWS) is a relatively frequent overgrowth syndrome with an incidence estimated at 1 in 14,000 births. It is probably an autosomal-dominant disorder with variable transmission. The BWS gene has been identified on the short arm of chromosome 11 (11p15.5). The syndrome is characterized by visceromegaly, hemihypertrophy, and development of malignant tumors in 10% to 15% of affected patients; benign tumors are also found.

Imaging Cross-sectional imaging studies may show nonspecific pancreatic enlargement. Patients may develop pancreatoblastoma or nesidioblastoma, as discussed later under Pancreatic Neoplasms. Because of this risk, routine US screening is initiated at an early age.

Treatment Surgical intervention is required for pancreatic tumors.

Hemochromatosis

Overview Hemochromatosis is an autosomal-recessive disorder that manifests as iron accumulation mainly in the liver, pancreas, and heart secondary to excessive iron reabsorption from the intestine, which leads to organ dysfunction.

Clinical Presentation Symptoms referable to the pancreas may be absent or nonspecific, such as malaise and fatigue, or they may be those of insulin resistance that result from pancreatic damage from iron deposition and culminates in diabetes.

Imaging The pancreatic changes from hemochromatosis are better appreciated with MRI, rather than CT, because of the magnetic susceptibility effects of iron. The liver and pancreas appear diffusely hypointense on T2*- and T2-weighted sequences. Distinction should be made from acquired transfusional iron overload (hemosiderosis), in which iron accumulates in the reticuloendothelial cells and leads to T2 hypointensity in the liver and spleen; with the exception of very severe cases, the pancreas is usually normal.

Treatment Treatment is directed toward the resultant diabetes, and supportive treatment—such as phlebotomy, desferrioxamine mesylate iron chelation therapy, and restriction of oral intake of iron-rich foods and beverages—is undertaken to prevent further damage from iron overload.

Pancreatitis

ACUTE PANCREATITIS

Overview Acute pancreatitis manifests as mild, moderate, severe, or necrotizing disease. It is uncommon in childhood, possibly because the most common predisposing factors in adults, alcohol and cholelithiasis, are seldom encountered in children. In a series of 61 children with acute pancreatitis, the most common cause was multisystem disease, including Reye syndrome, which is now uncommon; sepsis; shock; hemolytic uremic syndrome; and viral infection, specifically with mumps.[62] Other causes included blunt trauma in 15% of patients, congenital anatomic abnormalities in 10%, metabolic diseases in 10%, and drug toxicity in 3%. No cause was identified in 25% of patients. MRCP is useful in identifying unsuspected abnormal ductal anatomy in patients with idiopathic pancreatitis.[63]

Anatomic abnormalities associated with pancreatitis include pancreas divisum, congenital choledochal dilation, cysts with pancreatobiliary malunion/maljunction (40% to 50%),[64] duodenal web, and congenital pancreatic cyst. An anomalous pancreatobiliary ductal junction may also cause pancreatitis, because the abnormal insertion of the common bile duct into the pancreatic duct may facilitate reflux of bile into the pancreas.[65-67] The frequency of acute pancreatitis in children with a choledochal cyst is reportedly as high as 68%. Associated metabolic disorders include hypercalcemia, hyperlipidemia, and CF; the drugs implicated most frequently are L-asparaginase (e-Fig. 96-12), steroids, and acetaminophen. A reported increased incidence of biliary sludge in adult patients with pancreatitis suggests that biliary sludge may be the probable cause in as many as 70% of patients with idiopathic pancreatitis.[68]

Traumatic acute pancreatitis may be accidental or otherwise. This includes blunt abdominal trauma, such as bicycle handlebar injuries and motor vehicle accidents. Pediatric pancreatic trauma is distinct from that in the adult population, because the child's abdominal muscles are underdeveloped, which makes them more susceptible to pancreatic injury. Further, pediatric pancreatic injury is not usually associated with multiorgan injury as it is in adults.

Clinical Presentation Patients with nontraumatic acute pancreatitis typically come to medical attention with abdominal pain, most frequently in the epigastrium. Nausea and vomiting are common associated symptoms. Elevation of serum concentrations of pancreatic enzymes—amylase, lipase, and trypsinogen—is common. Although abnormal laboratory values are typically considerably more sensitive than imaging in identifying pancreatitis, imaging studies may be useful to confirm the diagnosis and to determine the extent of associated inflammatory changes and complications. Very rarely, pancreatitis may be the presenting symptom of a pancreatic malignancy in children and adolescents.

Imaging Abdominal radiographic findings are nonspecific, but certain findings are suggestive. Reactive ileus or "sentinel loops" from nearby GI structures may lead to abnormal air-fluid levels in the stomach and duodenum, focal dilation of the duodenal sweep, and dilation of the transverse colon that ends abruptly at the splenic flexure; left pleural effusion may also occur. Although ascites is common, the amount is rarely sufficient to be appreciated on abdominal radiographs.

US may be the initial imaging procedure for the evaluation of possible pancreatitis. Semierect and coronal scans, as well as the standard scanning planes, may improve evaluation of an abnormal pancreas.[69] The edema that accompanies acute pancreatitis often results in a diffusely enlarged hypoechoic gland. A minority of affected patients have increased pancreatic echogenicity (see e-Fig. 96-12), and some have a normal-appearing pancreas. The pancreatic duct may be dilated,[70] but this is an inconsistent finding; this is especially true when the gland is markedly swollen, because this causes compression of the duct. When the duct is dilated, there is a correlation with serum lipase in the acute and healing phases of the disease. Masses may be identified in the pancreas that represent focal areas of fluid, hemorrhage, or phlegmon formation, seen as a focal, inflammatory, hypoechoic mass. Ascites is usually identified on US.

The presence of peripancreatic fluid collections is evidence of acute pancreatitis. The most commonly involved areas are the lesser sac, anterior pararenal space,[71] transverse mesocolon, and perirenal space. US is excellent in demonstrating these fluid collections. Fluid collections may be found as far from the pancreas as the mediastinum and the inguinal regions, and inflammation may involve the adjacent splenic vein and may result in thrombosis.

CT may show pancreatic abnormalities to better advantage than US. The findings mirror those seen with US and include pancreatic swelling, ductal dilation, mass effect from phlegmon or hemorrhage, peripancreatic fluid collections, thickening of adjacent fascial planes, and ascites. Abscesses and necrosis are particularly well delineated on CT, especially with dynamic CT.[72] Patients with necrosis have higher rates of morbidity, mortality, and complications.

ERCP is seldom needed in children, but it is useful to evaluate complicated or recurrent pancreatitis[73] and in cases of unusual pseudocyst formation. The findings range from mild irregularity of the duct to ductal narrowing with wall ectasia and acinar enlargement, which has been likened to a "string of beads." Marked ductal ectasia is usually not seen in acute pancreatitis. MRCP[74] may replace ERCP in the evaluation of childhood pancreatitis because of its noninvasive nature (see Fig. 96-3). Secretin administration may help to optimize MRCP visualization of the pancreatic duct and its radicles, and it increases the sensitivity for identifying structural abnormalities.

Pseudocyst formation is a potential complication of pancreatitis, regardless of cause. Although most pseudocysts are in the region of the pancreas itself (Fig. 96-13; see e-Fig. 96-12), they can appear nearly anywhere in the abdomen and in the mediastinum (e-Figs. 96-14 and 96-15).[75,76] In adults, approximately 5% of patients with acute pancreatitis develop pseudocysts. Although most pseudocysts resolve spontaneously within an average of 5 months,[77] some persist and require intervention.[78,79] Features associated with spontaneous resolution include a pseudocyst diameter less than 7.5 cm, absence of internal debris, and total pseudocyst volume less than 250 mL.

Imaging is indicated when a pseudocyst is suspected. They frequently cause mass effect on adjacent structures, especially the stomach and duodenum, and this may be seen on radiographs or upper GI studies performed for unexplained abdominal pain. Pseudocysts are typically anechoic, although some may contain debris. Their effect on adjacent organs may be identified on US but is seen to better advantage with CT. ERCP usually shows the irregular ductal dilation of chronic inflammation (see Fig. 96-3, A, and e-Fig. 96-15, G). Skeletal changes, particularly bone marrow infarcts, have long been recognized as a complication of pancreatitis, possibly related to increased levels of circulating lipase and to generalized enzymatic dysfunction of the pancreas.[80]

Treatment Primary treatment includes analgesia and bowel rest with parenteral nutrition.[81-85] Postpyloric enteral feeds may be begun prior to oral refeeding to prevent relapse and to provide nutritional support while preventing gut mucosal atrophy. Antibiotic use is recommended for necrotic pancreatitis, and ERCP can reduce morbidity and mortality in select cases. Surgery and interventional procedures are indicated for infected necrotic pancreatitis and complications such as pseudocyst and abscess formation, splenic artery and vein thrombosis, hemorrhage, and pseudoaneurysms.

CHRONIC PANCREATITIS

Overview Chronic pancreatitis in children is less common than acute pancreatitis. Although it occurs as a sequela of the acute disease, chronic pancreatitis can also be found in association with other entities, such as CF. Familial hereditary pancreatitis is an autosomal-dominant disease that usually presents in childhood or during the teenage years.

Clinical Presentation Patients with chronic pancreatitis usually come to medical attention with persistent abdominal pain; some have constant, debilitating pain, whereas others have pain related to food intake, especially fats and protein-rich meals. Steatorrhea as a result of fat malabsorption is common, and weight loss is attributed to malabsorption and a reduction in food intake secondary to pain and food aversion. Diabetes may result from chronic pancreatic damage, and chronic pancreatitis may result in obstructive jaundice secondary to biliary strictures.[86]

Imaging Ductal dilation, pseudocysts, and calcifications are the most common imaging abnormalities in chronic hereditary pancreatitis,[87] and pancreatic atrophy may also occur. Chronic fibrosing pancreatitis is characterized by bands of collagen enclosing normal acini[88]; the resulting mass simulates a tumor.

Treatment Pancreatic enzyme supplementation is used for treatment of malabsorption and steatorrhea. Dietary fat restriction, analgesics and opiates for pain, and insulin for diabetes are other treatment strategies. Therapeutic endoscopy and surgery may also be used.[89,90]

TRAUMA

Overview Pediatric pancreatic trauma manifests in several ways besides the acute pancreatitis discussed above.

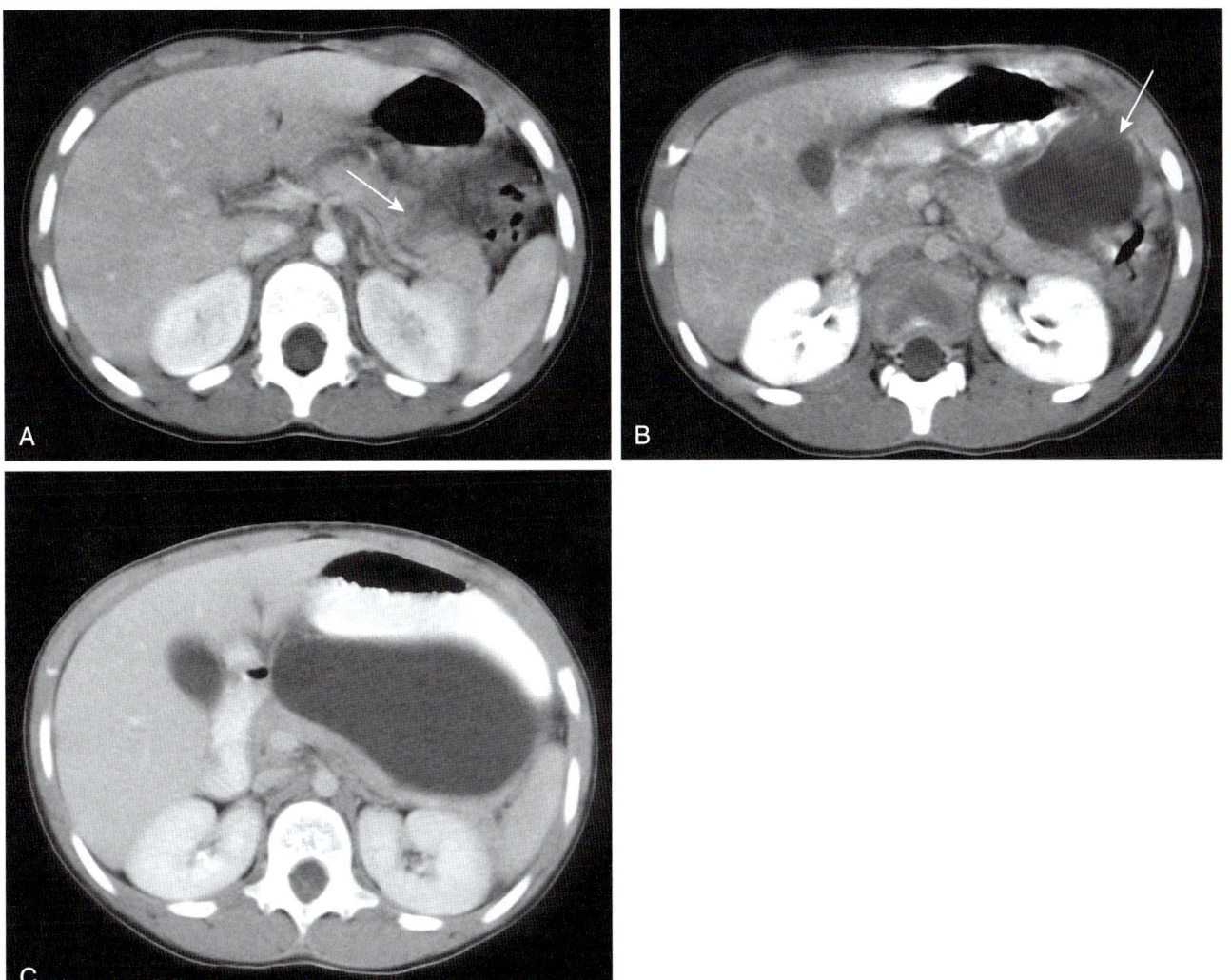

Figure 96-13 Posttraumatic pseudocyst in a 7-year-old. Ten days after blunt epigastric trauma, the patient continued to have vomiting and rising amylase levels. **A,** Axial contrast-enhanced abdominal computed tomography shows a pancreatic laceration (*arrow*) in the midbody. Pseudocyst formation (*arrow*) is shown on follow-up imaging 10 days (**B**) and 20 days (**C**) after the initial study. (Courtesy Dr. Robert Kaufman, Memphis, TN.)

Clinical Presentation Features of trauma, shock, and acute pancreatitis are seen.

Imaging At US, posttraumatic contusions may appear as a focal or diffusely enlarged, hypoechoic gland. However, because abdominal pain may be due to the trauma itself and associated acute pancreatitis, US may be limited. CT is the best imaging modality in these cases and demonstrates focal or diffuse hypoattenuation and enlargement of the gland, heterogeneous attenuation, peripancreatic fat stranding or frank fluid collections, abscesses, and pseudocyst formation. Fluid between the pancreas and splenic vein is a secondary sign of pancreatic injury. Pancreatic laceration, transection, and comminution are direct signs of injury and appear as hypoechoic or hypoattenuating areas that may be subtle in the early stages of injury. Duodenal hematomas are often associated and can serve as pointers to pancreatic trauma. These and pancreatic hematomas also may obstruct the pancreatic duct and biliary tree. CT may demonstrate pancreatic hypoenhancement, and associated CT features of shock bowel and the hypoperfusion complex may also be present.

ERCP is the gold standard for evaluation of the ductal system in trauma, particularly if stent placement is anticipated. Noninvasive MRCP may be used preceding ERCP but is often limited because of distorted anatomy from posttraumatic edema and hematoma.

Treatment Treatment is supportive and directed at the dominant pancreatic abnormality resulting from the trauma. Disruption of the pancreatic duct is treated surgically or by therapeutic endoscopy with stent placement, whereas injuries without duct involvement are usually treated nonsurgically.[91-93]

PANCREATIC NEOPLASMS

Primary pancreatic tumors, both benign and malignant, are very rare in childhood and adolescence (Table 96-3). Pancreatic tumors that occur in pediatric patients include solid-cystic pseudopapillary tumor (Frantz tumor), pancreatoblastoma, and islet cell tumors; carcinomas are rare. Other tumors that typically occur elsewhere, but can arise within the pancreas, include lymphoma[94,95] and rhabdomyosarcoma

Table 96-3

Classification of Common Pancreatic Tumors of Childhood

Location	Benign	Malignant
Exocrine pancreas	Pancreatic cysts	Pancreatoblastoma
	Papillary-cystic tumor	Duct cell adenocarcinoma
	Duct adenoma	
	Mucinous cystadenoma	Acinar cell carcinoma
	Serous cystadenoma	
	Intraductal papilloma	
Connective tissue	Hemangioendothelioma	Sarcoma
	Lymphangioma	Lymphoma
	Teratoma	Leiomyosarcoma
Secretory/ endocrine	Islet cell hyperplasia	Insulinoma (10%)
	Insulinoma (90%)	Gastrinoma (60%)
	Gastrinoma (40%)	Gastrinoma (60%)

Modified from Enríquez G, Vázquez E, Aso C, et al. Pediatric pancreas: an overview. *Eur Radiol.* 1998;8:1236-1244.

and rare cases of pancreatic neuroblastoma. Secondary involvement of the pancreas by adjacent tumor, especially neuroblastoma, may be difficult to distinguish from a primary pancreatic tumor.

Solid-Cystic Papillary Tumor

Overview   Solid-cystic papillary tumor is also known by many other terms: Frantz tumor, solid pseudopapillary tumor, papillary epithelial neoplasm (PEN), solid and papillary epithelial neoplasm (SPEN), solid and cystic acinar cell tumor, papillary and solid neoplasm, papillary-cystic epithelial neoplasm, papillary-cystic carcinoma, solid and cystic tumor, solid and papillary neoplasm, papillary cystic tumor, and low-grade papillary neoplasm.[96] Solid-cystic papillary tumor is histologically low grade, with a reported 5 year survival of 97%. It accounts for about 0.2% to 2.7% of all nonendocrine pancreatic tumors.

Clinical Presentation   This tumor seems to have a predilection for women[97] and for persons of Asian extraction; it is probably the most common pancreatic tumor in Asian children. Although the median age at diagnosis is 26 years, approximately 20% of cases have been reported in children. Children usually have a better prognosis than adults, owing to less frequent metastatic disease. Abdominal pain is the presenting symptom in about one third of cases, and a palpable abdominal mass is typically present; jaundice is extremely rare.

Imaging   CT findings include a large, well-defined, solid mass with varying degrees of cystic components that usually represent necrosis but are unrelated to tumor size (Figs. 96-16 and 96-17).[98-100] Calcifications may also be present. On T1-weighted MR sequences, a low signal rim may represent either a fibrous capsule or compressed pancreatic parenchyma; central high-signal areas that represent debris or hemorrhagic necrosis have also been reported. Almost half of all lesions occur in the pancreatic head. Invasion of adjacent structures occurs and is often associated with liver and lymph node metastases.[101-103]

Pancreatoblastoma

Overview   Pancreatoblastoma, or pancreaticoblastoma,[104,105] arises from the pancreatic acinar cells, usually in the head or tail of the gland. The cells of these tumors represent persistence of the fetal anlage of the pancreatic acinar cells. Pancreatoblastoma is one of the most common exocrine tumors in pediatric patients and represents about 0.5% of all pancreatic epithelial tumors.

Clinical Presentation   These tumors are found in boys twice as often as in girls. Incidence of pancreatoblastoma in East Asia is relatively high. Serum α-fetoprotein is elevated in 25% to 55% of cases, and an association with Beckwith-Wiedeman Syndrome has been reported. A review of 153 patients with pancreatoblastoma found that the median age at presentation was 5 years, although this tumor has been diagnosed in patients as old as 68 years.[106] The liver is the most common site of metastatic disease (88% of metastatic sites), which was found in 17% of the patients in this series. Factors associated with a worse prognosis include metastatic or nonresectable disease and age older than 16 years at diagnosis. Pancreatoblastomas are often large at presentation, up to 12 cm, and areas of central necrosis are sometimes present.

Imaging   US and CT findings of pancreatoblastoma are often indistinguishable from those of pancreatic adenocarcinoma. Masses are typically hypoechoic and heterogeneous on US.[106] On CT, pancreatoblastoma is hypodense and appears to be multiloculated with enhancing septa (Fig. 96-18). Calcifications are not uncommon. When vascular encasement is present, it usually involves the inferior vena cava or mesenteric vessels. Despite the typically large size of pancreatoblastomas, obstruction of the biliary system is infrequent. Although variable, MRI characteristics include typically low signal intensity compared with the liver on T1-weighted spin echo images and isointensity to hyperintensity on T2-weighted images; enhancement varies.[107] Although findings are nonspecific as to tumor type, imaging suggests the malignant nature of the tumor and can clearly exclude the kidney and adrenal glands as organs of origin.

Islet Cell Tumors

Overview   Hormonally active tumors arise from the islet cells and may be benign or malignant. Islet cell tumors are named after the hormone produced, and insulinoma is the most common islet cell tumor in children (Fig. 96-19 and e-Fig. 96-20). *Diffuse adenomatosis* (nesidioblas*tosis*) refers to diffuse adenomatous islet cell hyperplasia, and *focal adenomatous hyperplasia* (nesidioblas*toma*) refers to focal involvement.[108]

Clinical Presentation   Patients with insulinoma are seen initially with hypoglycemia, which typically manifests in children as erratic behavior and seizures. Patients with nesidioblastosis can also be seen initially with hypoglycemia. In a series of 12 pediatric patients, only 3 patients with profound hypoglycemia had identifiable islet cell tumors; the others had islet cell hyperplasia or nesidioblastosis on histologic examination of specimens obtained after partial pancreatectomy.[108] Tumors that secrete vasoactive intestinal polypeptide (VIP), so-called VIPomas, are associated with the

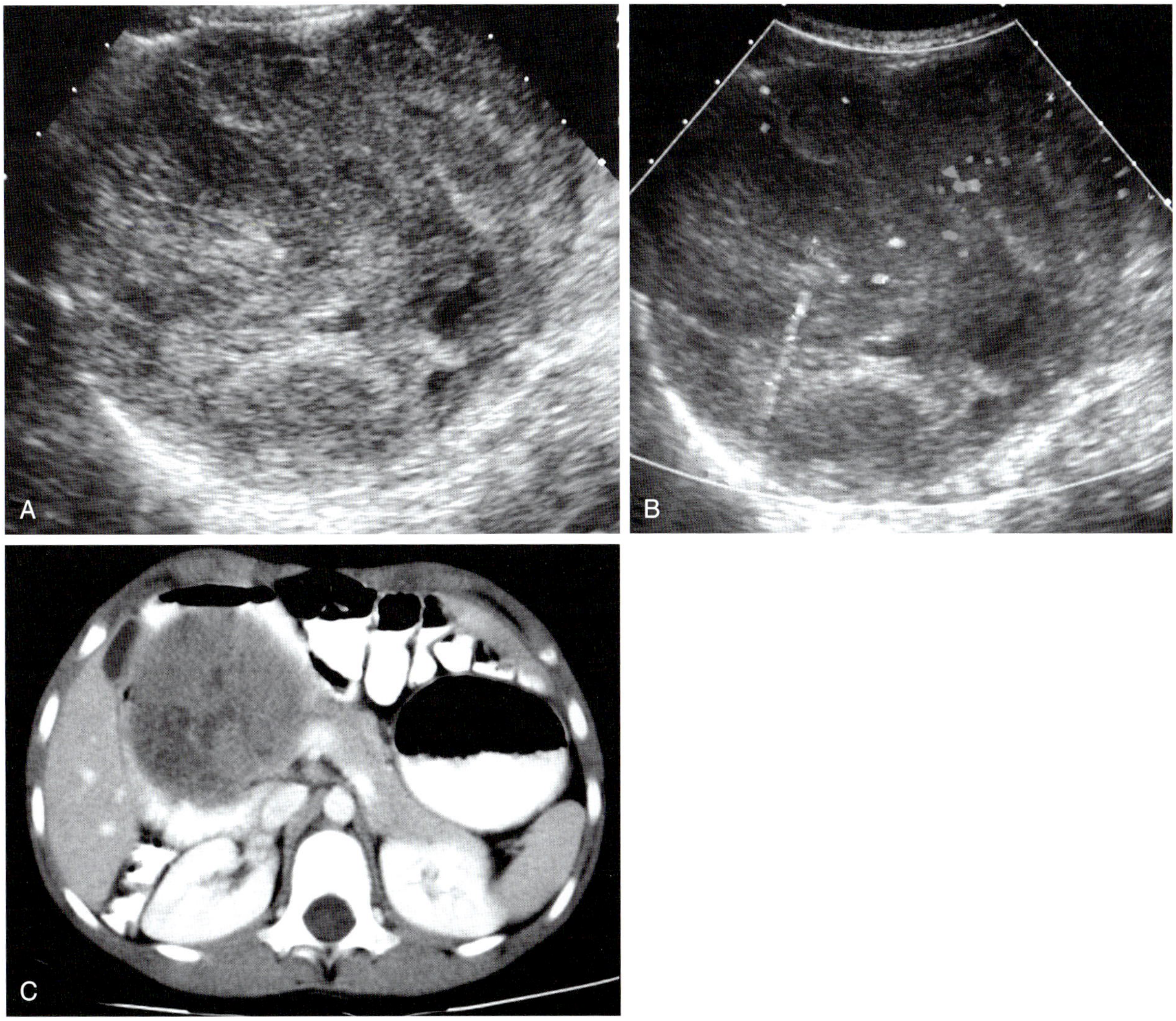

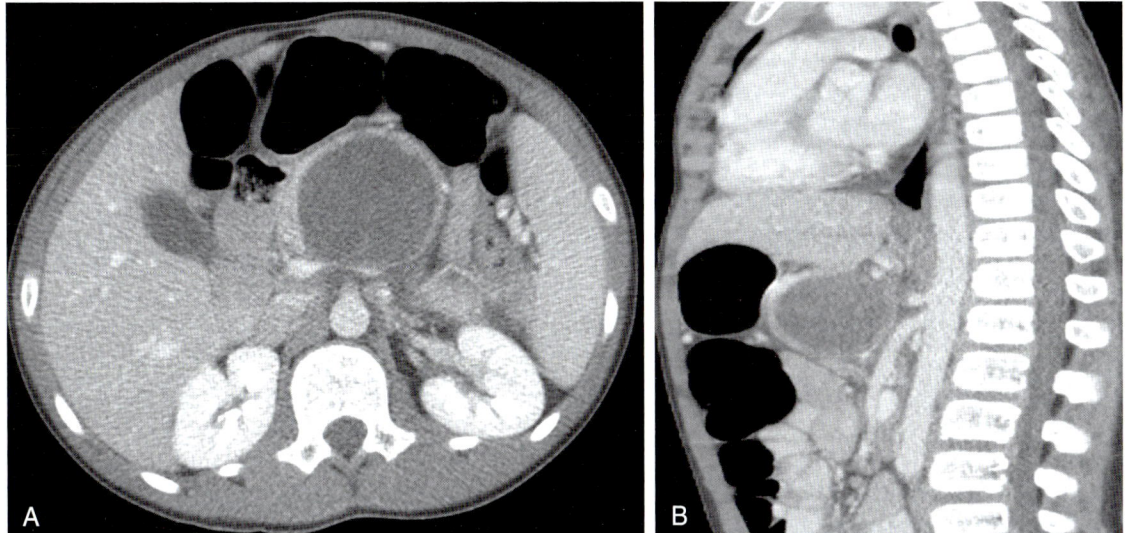

Figure 96-16 Solid-cystic papillary tumor (Frantz tumor). **A,** Axial ultrasound through the midabdomen shows a large, heterogeneous, solid mass that arises from the pancreatic head. **B,** The mass is mildly vascular, as shown with gray scale depiction of the color Doppler image. **C,** Axial contrast-enhanced computed tomography through the midabdomen shows the mildly heterogeneous enhancement pattern of the mass and its origin from the head of the pancreas, widening and displacing the duodenal loop.

Figure 96-17 A solid-cystic papillary tumor that was causing abdominal pain in a 12-year-old boy. **A,** Axial computed tomography through the upper abdomen shows a large, centrally necrotic, peripherally solid enhancing mass centered in the pancreatic body. Axial (**A**) and sagittal (**B**) images demonstrate that the mass abuts the celiac axis posteriorly and protrudes into the lesser sac anteriorly.

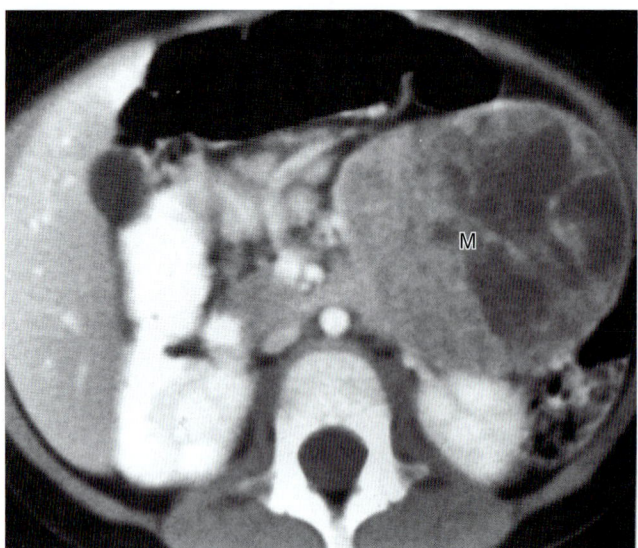

Figure 96-18 Pancreatoblastoma. Axial contrast-enhanced computed tomography in a child shows a large, heterogeneously enhancing mass (M) arising from the pancreatic tail. (Courtesy Dr. Marilyn Siegel, St. Louis, MO.)

syndrome of secretory diarrhea, hypokalemia, and achlorhydria. VIPomas are rare, functioning tumors with an estimated annual incidence of 0.2 to 0.5 per million population.

Imaging The most common site for islet cell tumors is in the pancreatic head.[109] These tumors are round or oval and are well circumscribed on US. They are hypoechoic but may have a hyperechoic rim; isoechoic and hyperechoic lesions have also been described in children and young adults. Tumors may be located superficially or may be deep within the pancreas. On CT, contrast may cause marked tumor enhancement, particularly in the arterial phase (see Fig. 96-19). Because these tumors are hypervascular, arteriography may be necessary in high-risk patients in whom US and CT are nondiagnostic, although magnetic resonance angiography (MRA) may replace this invasive technique. Intraoperative US has been used successfully to locate functioning islet cell tumors in children.[110,111] Selective venous sampling in children with hyperinsulinism can also help diagnose and localize tumors.[112] Indium-111-pentetreotide (Octreoscan) scintigraphy may also be useful in the diagnosis of primary or metastatic tumors.[109]

Other islet cell tumors are rare in children, but they may be found in association with tumors in other organs as part of the multiple endocrine neoplasia (MEN) syndromes. Type 1 (MEN 1) is an inherited condition characterized by synchronous or metachronous tumors of the parathyroid glands, anterior pituitary, pancreas, GI tract, and other less commonly involved organs. Patients usually seek medical attention in their twenties and thirties, and rarely, in familial cases, in childhood. Pancreatic involvement is in the form of multiple islet cell tumors.[108] Gastrinomas may be found in children with Zollinger-Ellison syndrome. In one series, 2 of 56 reported cases of VIP-producing tumors in children were islet cell tumors; neurogenic tumors generated the hormone in the other patients.[113] Glucagonomas and somatostatinomas have not been reported in children.

Other Pancreatic Tumors

Overview The exocrine tissues of the pancreas give rise to benign and malignant tumors that are hormonally inactive, such as cystadenoma, adenocarcinoma, and adenosarcoma.

Clinical Presentation The most common presenting symptoms include abdominal pain in 55.8%, nausea or vomiting in 32.6%, fatigue in 25.6%, and an abdominal mass in 23.3%.[114] Cystadenomas and adenocarcinomas of the pancreas occur in children and have been described in infants as well.[115] Pancreatic adenocarcinoma has been described in an adolescent boy with Peutz-Jeghers syndrome,[116] and there is a hundredfold increased risk of pancreatic adenocarcinoma in patients with this syndrome.[117]

Imaging On US, solid tumors are typically hyperechoic, and cystic lesions are anechoic or hypoechoic. Adenocarcinomas may have cystic or hemorrhagic areas that result in mixed echogenicity. CT usually identifies a pancreatic mass of variable size, often causing biliary obstruction. In a recent study, pancreatic duct adenocarcinomas were identified in only 3 patients younger than 20 years among a total cohort of 439 cases, corresponding to an incidence of 0.1% in this age group.[118] Such tumors are often associated with a genetic predisposition. Because the diagnosis of pancreatic carcinoma is so rare in children (only about 50 cases have been reported), imaging evaluation is often delayed, and vascular invasion and metastases to lymph nodes and liver may be noted on imaging.

Rhabdomyosarcoma may arise primarily in the pancreas (e-Fig. 96-21), as may lymphoma (Fig. 96-22). Neuroblastoma has been reported in the pancreas either as a primary (e-Fig. 96-23) or secondary to direct extension. A single case of abdominal desmoid tumor presenting in the pancreas was reported in a 17-year-old boy with familial adenomatous polyposis syndrome.[119]

Lymphatic malformations of the pancreas are extremely rare and account for less than 1% of cases.[120] They may occur in any portion of the pancreas at any age and are more frequent in females. On imaging, lymphatic malformations appear as septated, fluid-filled masses. Clinical presentation is nonspecific and includes nausea, vomiting, vague abdominal pain, and a palpable mass.

Exceptionally rare tumors of the pancreas include anaplastic large cell lymphoma,[94] infantile myofibromatosis,[121] and mature cystic teratoma.[122] Cystic teratoma of the pancreas has been reported in at least seven pediatric patients, who ranged in age from 2 to 16 years. These tumors arise from pluripotent cells of ectodermal cell lines and, like other extragonadal teratomas, likely originate from aberrant germ cells. Such tumors may be indistinguishable from other cystic abdominal masses.

Pancreatic involvement with metastatic disease is also rare but includes malignant melanoma, lymphoma (e-Fig. 96-24), rhabdomyosarcoma (Fig. 96-25), acute lymphoblastic leukemia, and osteosarcoma (e-Fig. 96-26).[123]

Treatment of Pancreatic Neoplasms Most pancreatic tumors are treated primarily with pancreatic resection and pancreatoduodenectomy. Resection is complete for aggressive and advanced tumors; partial pancreatectomy[124] and enucleation may be indicated for less aggressive or small neoplasms.

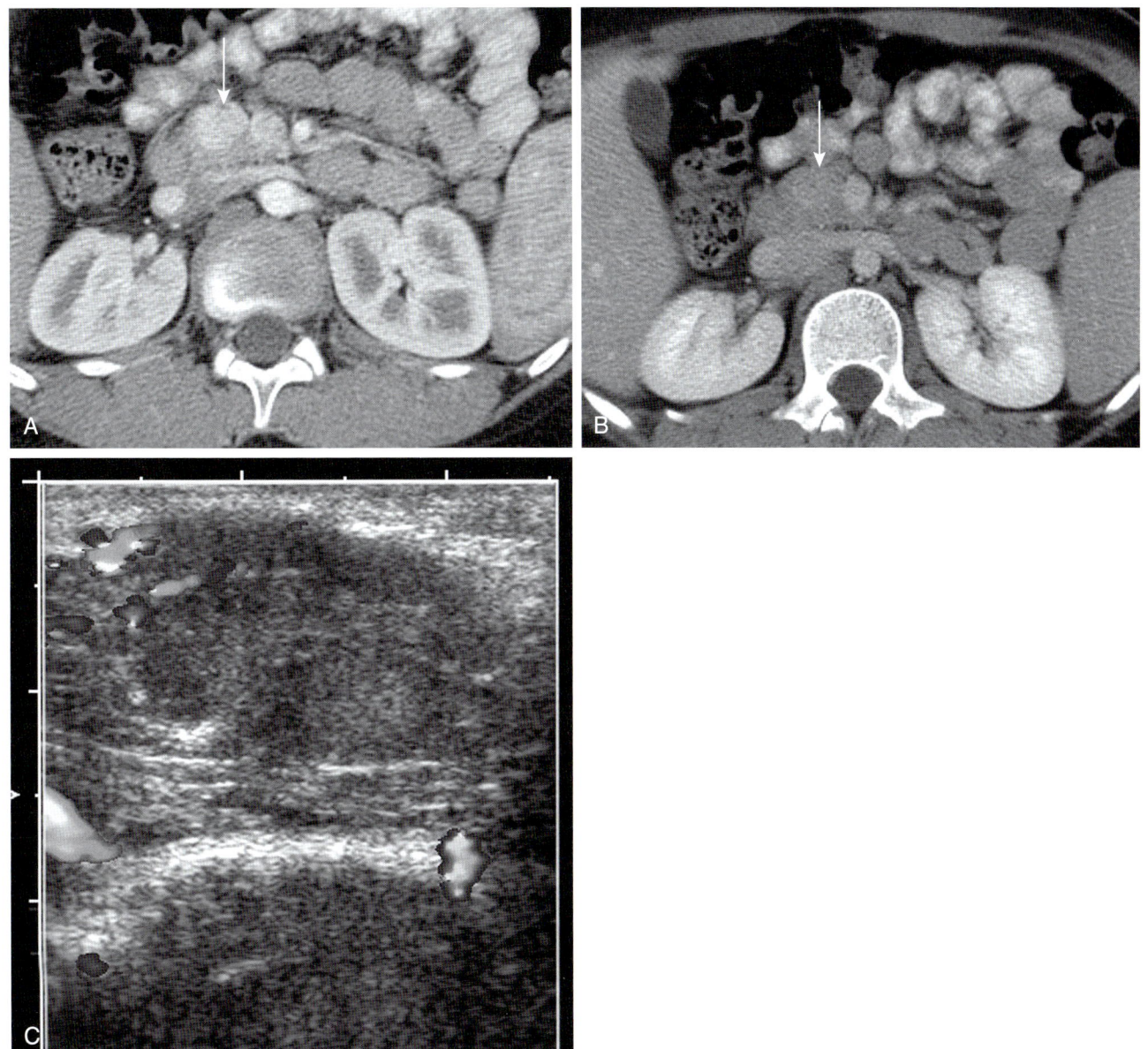

Figure 96-19 Insulinoma. Axial contrast-enhanced computed tomographic images through the pancreas during the arterial (**A**) and venous (**B**) phases show a well-defined, ovoid, enhancing mass at the junction of the head and body of the pancreas (to the left of the superior mesenteric vein; *arrows*) that is particularly conspicuous on the arterial phase. **C,** Intraoperative ultrasound confirms the mass as a well-defined lesion of intermediate echogenicity within the pancreas. (Courtesy Dr. George Taylor, Boston, MA.)

Radiotherapy or chemotherapy is less frequently indicated in the pediatric population.[108] Supportive medical therapy may be indicated, such as IV glucose for insulinoma- or adenomatosis-induced hypoglycemia and for gastrinoma-induced Zollinger-Ellison syndrome.

Pancreatic Infections

HYDATID DISEASE

Overview Pancreatic hydatid disease, or echinococcosis, is extremely rare and can result from parasitic infestation with *Echinococcus granulosus,* a parasite that affects humans and other mammals, most notably dogs and sheep. The disease manifests as cysts in the affected organ; only rarely is the pancreas the only organ involved.[125]

Clinical Presentation Jaundice and abdominal pain may be the first symptoms of hydatid disease of the pancreas, and hydatid disease may also be a rare cause of recurrent pancreatitis.[126]

Imaging Abdominal CT demonstrates a complex, cystic pancreatic mass, most commonly in the pancreatic head.[125] Larger cysts may have smaller "daughter" cysts within them.

Treatment Conservative therapy with albendazole and surgical procedures such as subtotal cystectomy, distal

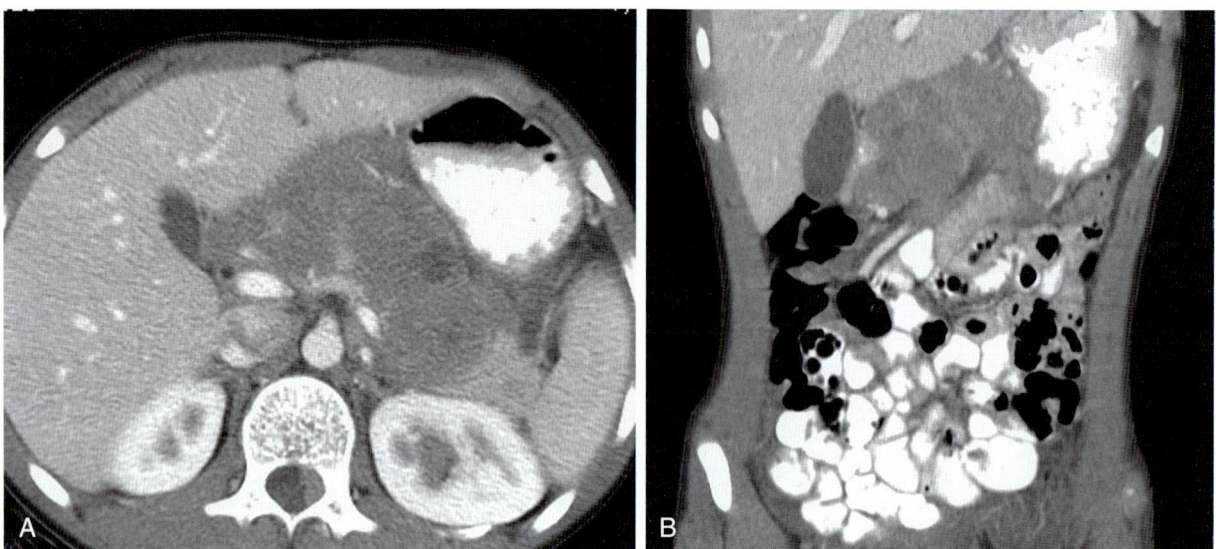

Figure 96-22 Primary pancreatic non-Hodgkin lymphoma. Axial (**A**) and reconstructed coronal (**B**) contrast-enhanced computed tomographic images through the abdomen show diffuse enlargement of the pancreas with focal low-density regions suggestive of necrosis. Mass effect on the stomach from this primary pancreatic Burkitt lymphoma is best seen on the coronal reconstruction. (Courtesy Dr. George Taylor, Boston, MA.)

pancreatectomy, cystoenteric anastomosis, Whipple resection, marsupialization, and external drainage have been used.[127]

TUBERCULOSIS

Overview and Clinical Presentation   Patients with abdominal tuberculosis are either human immunodeficiency virus positive or otherwise immune compromised, or they are from areas endemic for tuberculosis.

Imaging   Abdominal tuberculosis (Fig. 96-27) can result in focal pancreatic parenchymal lesions or tuberculous abscesses, usually with one or more calcified components and imaging evidence of abdominal tuberculosis elsewhere (retroperitoneal adenopathy that is usually matted and may or may not be centrally necrotic or calcified; tuberculous ascites; matting of bowel loops or omentum, so-called omental cake; and intraperitoneal adhesions).[128]

Treatment   Antituberculous multidrug therapy is recommended for up to 1 year; three to four drugs are given for the first 2 months, and then two drugs are given for up to 10 months. Surgical intervention is used for complicated cases.

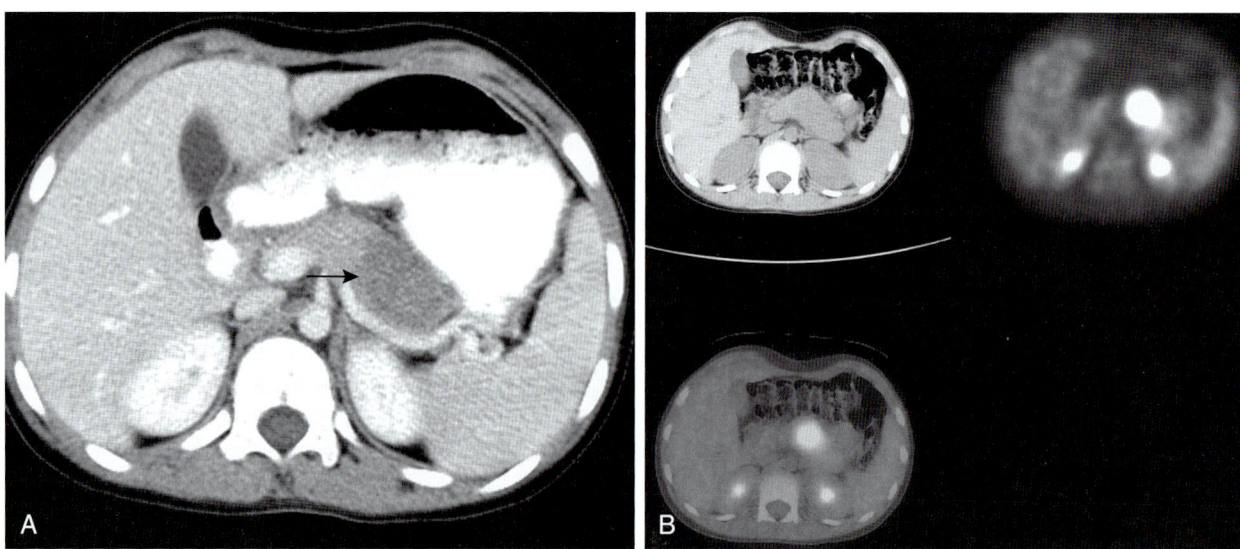

Figure 96-25   Recurrent rhabdomyosarcoma metastatic to the pancreas. Three years earlier, this 10-year-old girl had been treated for alveolar rhabdomyosarcoma of the calf. **A,** Axial contrast-enhanced abdominal computed tomography (CT) shows a well-defined low-density mass in the pancreas (*arrow*). **B,** Axial fluorodeoxyglucose positron emission tomography CT image shows the lesion as a focal mass with intense uptake of radiopharmaceutical in the midbody of the pancreas.

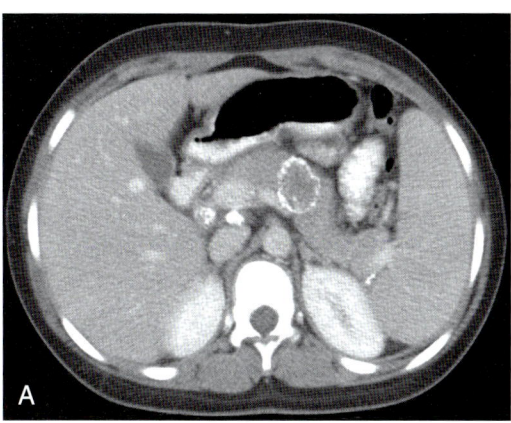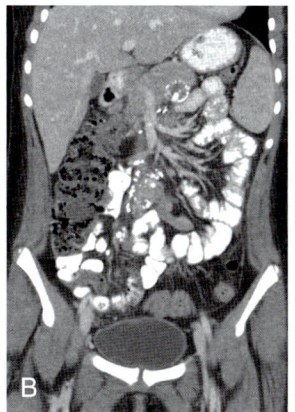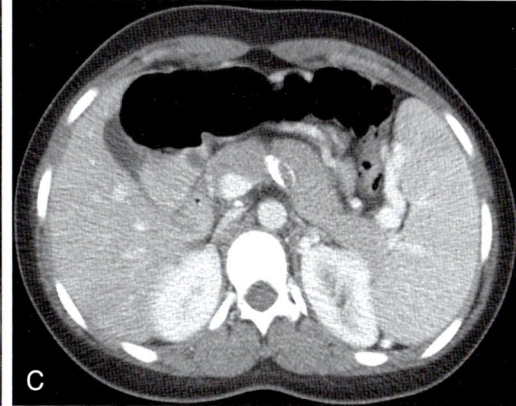

Figure 96-27 Pancreatic tuberculosis in an HIV-positive teen. **A,** Axial computed tomography (CT) through the upper abdomen shows a large, peripherally calcified, relatively hypodense lesion in the pancreatic body. **B,** Coronal CT image through the abdomen demonstrates this lesion again; both axial and coronal images demonstrate calcified retroperitoneal lymph nodes. This patient was on multidrug therapy for abdominal tuberculosis. **C,** Axial CT through the upper abdomen 2 years later demonstrates interval shrinkage of the peripherally calcified pancreatic body lesion; calcific foci appear more coarse and chunky as a result.

WHAT THE CLINICIAN NEEDS TO KNOW

Pancreatic sizes that include the head and uncinate process, isthmus, body, and tail

Pancreatic configuration (normal, annular, pancreas divisum, etc.)

Echogenicity, density, and intensity of the parenchyma

Imaging appearance of peripancreatic tissues and the pancreatic bed

Whether pancreatic and common bile duct dilation are present

Whether pancreatic or peripancreatic collections are present

Whether a pancreatic mass or other focal lesion is present

Any change from prior examinations

Trauma: Direct evidence at imaging includes contusion, transection, laceration, and comminution. Indirect findings include pancreatic and peripancreatic edema, fluid between the splenic vein and pancreas, phlegmon, abscess, pseudocyst, duodenal hematoma, and superimposed features of pancreatitis.

Common neoplasms: Pseudopapillary tumors are usually in the pancreatic head and are mixed solid-cystic tumors with a peripheral fibrous capsule and central necrosis, sometimes with hemorrhage, and calcifications. This may invade adjacent structures and metastasize to liver or nodes. Pancreatoblastomas are heterogeneous, predominantly hypoechoic or hypodense, with septations and calcifications. Encasement and obstruction of the IVC, mesenteric vessels, and biliary tree may also be evident.

Key Points

Congenital and hereditary conditions: Apart from specific morphologic imaging features, pancreas divisum may have imaging features of pancreatitis, and annular pancreas manifests with duodenal obstruction. Imaging of patients with CF may reveal a spectrum of findings, from a normal to mildly enlarged pancreas in early stages of the disease to complete fatty replacement with calcification or "pancreatic cystosis" in advanced stages.

Pancreatitis: Acute pancreatitis manifests with regional bowel ileus (so-called sentinel loops on radiographs) and ascites; the pancreas itself may appear normal on imaging or may demonstrate edema, necrosis, pancreatic duct dilation, peripancreatic edema, hemorrhage, phlegmon, or abscess. Other complications evident by imaging include pseudocysts, splenic artery pseudoaneurysms, and hemorrhage from or thrombosis of splenic vessels. Chronic pancreatitis manifests as ductal dilation and calcification and, rarely, with tumorlike masses in chronic fibrosing pancreatitis.

ACKNOWLEDGMENTS

We acknowledge and thank Dr. Sue C. Kaste for her conceptualization of the original chapter and contributions to the current one.

Suggested Reading

Chung EM, Travis MD, Conran RM. Pancreatic tumors in children: radiologic-pathologic correlation. *Radiographics.* 2006;26(4):1211-1238.

Nijs E, Callahan MJ, Taylor GA. Disorders of the pediatric pancreas: imaging features. *Pediatr Radiol.* 2005;35:358.

Nijs EL, Callahan MJ. Congenital and developmental pancreatic anomalies: ultrasound, computed tomography, and magnetic resonance imaging features. *Semin Ultrasound CT MR.* 2007;28(5):395-401.

Shimizu T, Suzuki R, Yamashiro Y, et al. Magnetic resonance cholangiopancreatography in assessing the cause of acute pancreatitis in children. *Pancreas.* 2001;2:196.

To'o KF, Raman SS, Yu NC, et al. Pancreatic and peripancreatic diseases mimicking primary pancreatic neoplasia. *Radiographics.* 2005;25:949.

References

Full references for this chapter can be found on www.expertconsult.com.

Chapter 97

Congenital and Neonatal Abnormalities

JAYNE M. SEEKINS, WENDY D. ELLIS, and HENRIQUE M. LEDERMAN

Overview

Severe congenital esophageal malformations are usually diagnosed in the neonate; other congenital lesions, such as isolated tracheoesophageal fistulae (TEF) and duplications cysts, may remain elusive or even asymptomatic and are seen more often in the older child.

Esophageal Atresia with and Without Tracheoesophageal Fistula

Overview   First described in 1670, esophageal atresia was a universally fatal anomaly until late in the fifth decade of the twentieth century, when pediatric surgeons began successfully treating these children. Esophageal atresia with and without TEF is part of a heterogeneous spectrum of anomalies that ranges from isolated esophageal atresia to isolated TEF. Lesions are typically classified according to the association and location of the fistulous connection between the esophagus and the airway (Fig. 97-1). The incidence of esophageal atresia is approximately 1 in 4500 births in the United States and 1 in 3500 births worldwide, with a tendency to occur more commonly in boys, although the gender difference varies with the type of lesion. Maternal risk factors include white race, first pregnancy, and advanced age. There is also an increased risk in the siblings of patients with esophageal atresia.[1,2]

Etiology   The development of esophageal atresia is poorly understood and still debated. Dominant theories in the past have been based on the model of a tracheoesophageal septum, a lateral ridge of tissue believed to separate the foregut into a dorsal component (the esophagus) from a ventral component (the trachea) in a caudocephalic direction. However, further investigation has suggested that this process does not occur in humans.[1,3] Kluth and Fiegel[3] suggest that the formation of the esophagus and trachea is the result of "a system of folds" in the cranial and caudal ends of the tracheoesophageal space that move toward each other, thus separating the space into the ventral trachea and dorsal esophagus. Following this theory, esophageal atresia with fistula results from an abnormally ventral position of the dorsal fold; isolated esophageal atresia is attributed to a vascular accident rather than abnormal separation of the alimentary and respiratory canals.[3,4] The association of the esophageal atresia complex with conotruncal anomalies and anomalies associated with DiGeorge syndrome suggests that abnormal development of pharyngeal arches may be related to this malformation.[1]

Further research with animal models concerns the investigation of genes that influence the temporal and spatial sequence of expression of molecular and genetic pathways, including retinoic acid receptors, and sonic hedgehog pathway effectors. Human teratogens that have been associated with this anomaly include abnormal maternal hormonal milieu (including estrogen, progesterone, and thyroid hormones), intrauterine exposure to thalidomide and diethylstilbestrol, and maternal diabetes.[1]

Clinical Presentation   Patients with esophageal atresia with or without fistula typically come to medical attention prenatally or soon after birth. Patients with isolated esophageal atresia are most likely to be seen with maternal polyhydramnios and to be identified at prenatal evaluation. Esophageal atresia and TEF may have been suspected during pregnancy, but neonates generally come to medical attention in the first few hours of life with excessive salivation and drooling, choking and regurgitation during feeds, and sometimes with cyanosis and/or respiratory distress.[1]

The incidence of associated congenital anomalies has been reported to be between 50% and 70% and is most common in infants with isolated esophageal atresia and least common in children with isolated TEF.[5] The most common associated anomalies, in descending order of frequency, include cardiac, genitourinary, gastrointestinal, musculoskeletal, and neurologic anomalies. Approximately half of the children with esophageal atresia who have associated anomalies can eventually be classified as having a known syndrome, either chromosomal or named, such as VACTERL (*v*ertebral anomaly, *a*norectal atresia, *c*ardiac lesion, *t*racheoesophageal fistula, *r*enal anomaly, *l*imb defect), (Fig. 97-2) CHARGE (*c*oloboma, *h*eart malformation, choanal *a*tresia, mental *r*etardation, *g*enitourinary and *e*ar malformations), Fanconi anemia, Opitz and Goldenhar syndromes.[6,7] In particular, patients with isolated esophageal atresia have an increased incidence of trisomy 21 (11%) and duodenal atresia (10%).

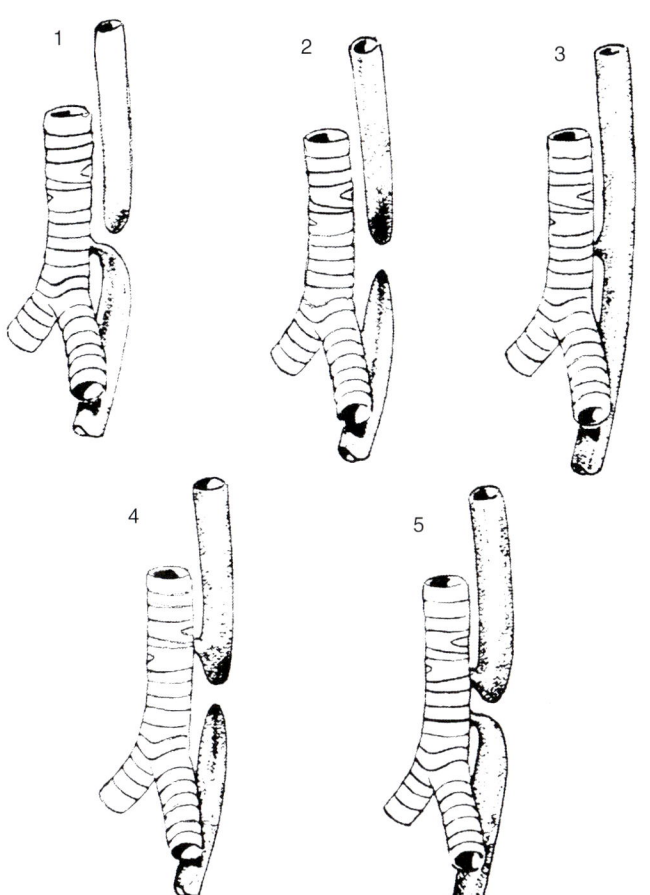

Figure 97-1 Types of esophageal atresia, with and without tracheo-esophageal fistula. *Type 1* represents esophageal atresia with a distal fistula and is the most common form, occurring in approximately 84% of patients. *Type 2* illustrates esophageal atresia without a fistula, seen in about 6%. *Type 3* is an isolated H-type fistula (4%), and *type 4* describes esophageal atresia with the fistula arising from the proximal pouch (5%); *type 5*, with fistulae arising from both the proximal and distal pouch, is the least common (~1%).[1]

Imaging Imaging is used in both the prenatal and neonatal diagnosis of esophageal atresia. Esophageal atresia is a cause of polyhydramnios. Fetuses with esophageal atresia may also have an absent or small stomach bubble. Unfortunately, these ultrasound findings alone lack specificity, with a reported 20% to 40% positive predictive value.[8] Accuracy in diagnosis is improved when a blind-ending pouch is visualized in the fetal neck, and newer data suggest that fetal magnetic resonance imaging (MRI) may play an increasingly important role in prenatal diagnosis.[9,10] More commonly, the diagnosis is made in the immediate neonatal period. If the diagnosis of esophageal atresia is suspected in the first few hours of life, placement of a flexible feeding tube or enteric tube should be attempted. Introduction of contrast into the pouch is not typically necessary for confirmation of the diagnosis, although introduction of air into the pouch may improve its identification. Introduction of contrast into the pouch may reveal the rare patient who has a proximal fistula with or without atresia, although today this is typically diagnosed endoscopically.

On radiographs of the abdomen, absence of bowel gas indicates esophageal atresia without a distal TEF (Fig. 97-3).

In this setting, a TEF from the proximal pouch cannot be excluded with chest radiographs and requires endoscopy for diagnosis. Likewise, the presence of bowel gas on abdominal radiographs in a patient with esophageal atresia indicates the presence of a distal TEF (Fig. 97-2 and 97-4).[1] In patients who are intubated, air may be forced into the stomach through the fistula, resulting in gastric overdistension, which may result in perforation. In addition, approximately 2.5% of patients will have a right-sided aortic arch that should be identified on preoperative echo or ultrasound since esophageal repair is performed on the side opposite the arch.[1,11,12]

Treatment/Follow-up Surgical repair is typically undertaken within 1 to 2 days, after the clinical workup is complete, including treatment of more emergent medical issues. Open or thoracoscopic division/ligation of the fistula and primary esophageal anastomosis is the treatment of choice. For long-gap atresia, a gastrostomy tube can be placed for palliation, while mechanical efforts are made to elongate the proximal and distal pouches prior to primary repair. Alternatively, if these procedures fail, an esophageal substitute (usually colon or ileocolon) can be interposed between the proximal and distal segments. Isolated esophageal atresia is typically associated with a small proximal pouch and almost no thoracic esophagus (see Fig. 97-3), and patients are typically palliated

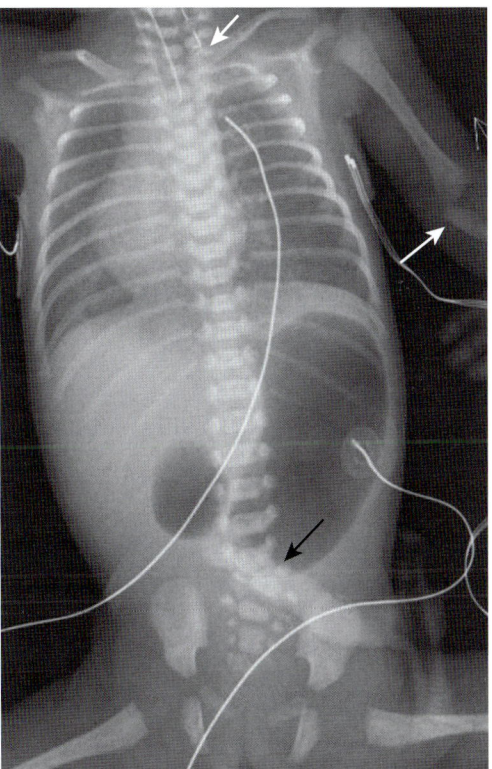

Figure 97-2 VACTERL (*vertebral anomaly, anorectal atresia, cardiac lesion, tracheoesophageal fistula, renal anomaly, limb defect*) syndrome. Newborn girl born at 32 weeks gestation demonstrates the abnormalities seen with the VACTERL association. The patient is intubated because of the lung disease of prematurity. The enteric tube (*short white arrow*) ends just above thoracic inlet in the proximal esophageal pouch, and abdominal bowel gas indicate a distal tracheoesophageal fistula, whereas a "double bubble" sign, and absence of distal bowel gas indicate duodenal atresia. There are 13 pairs of ribs, and a hemivertebra between L5 and S1 (*black arrow*). Note the absent radius in the left arm (*white arrow* points to the ulna).

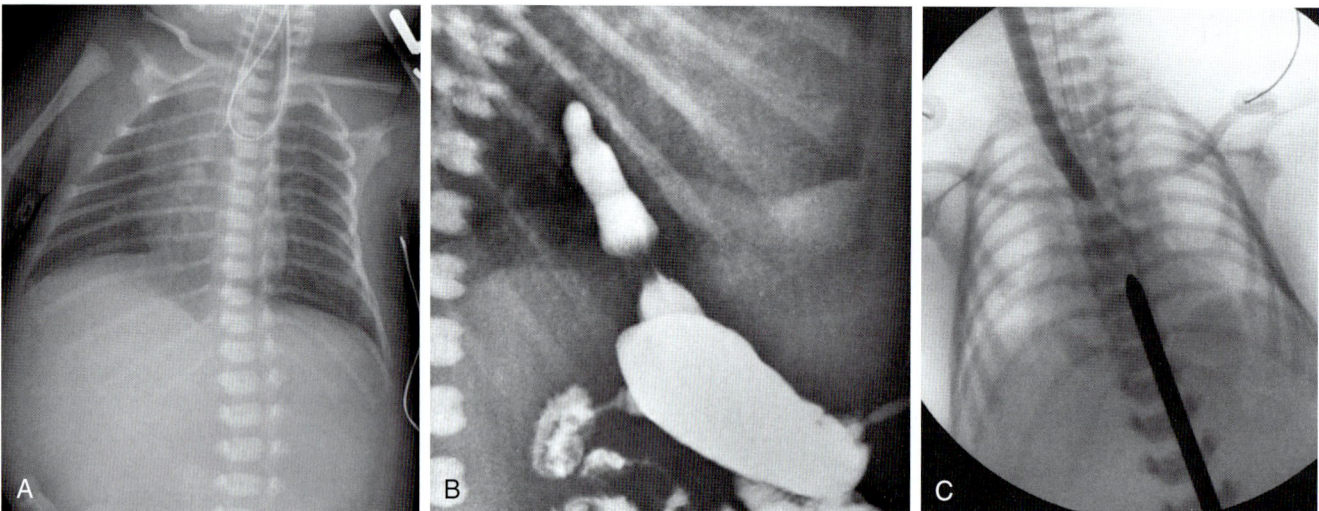

Figure 97-3   Isolated esophageal atresia. **A,** Newborn boy born at 37 weeks gestation with isolated esophageal atresia. The enteric tube turns cephalad in the blind-ending proximal esophageal pouch, and abdominal bowel gas is absent. **B,** Gastrostomy injection with reflux into the short distal esophageal segment in a patient with esophageal atresia without a distal fistula. **C,** Esophageal atresia with the gap between the segments confirmed at surgery. Frontal view reveals bougies in both the proximal and distal segments, showing a long gap between them.

with a gastrostomy tube in the first 24 to 48 hours of life, followed by delayed repair.[1]

Imaging also plays an important role in the evaluation of early and late complications of esophageal atresia repair. Complications include anastomotic leak, anastomotic stricture, and recurrent TEF; these are evaluated with esophagram (e-Fig. 97-5). Because standard esophageal contrast studies

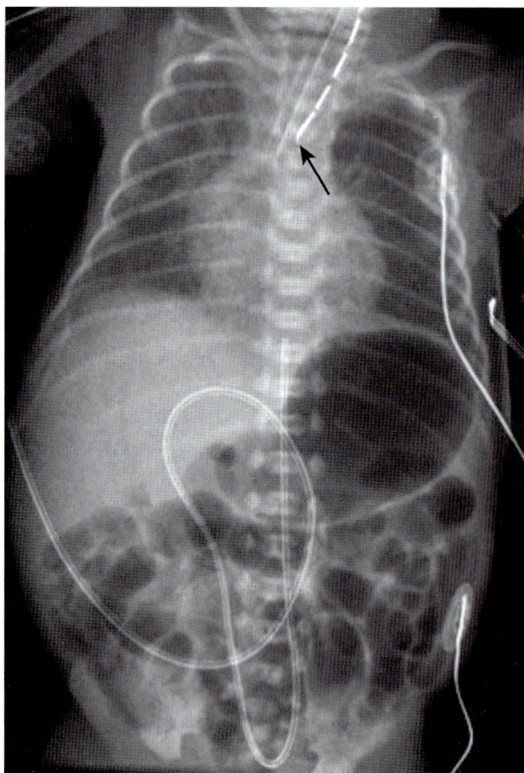

Figure 97-4   Esophageal atresia with tracheoesophageal fistula. Radiograph of a newborn preterm girl shows that the enteric tube (*arrow*) ends in the proximal esophageal pouch, and the distal bowel gas pattern is abundant.

miss a reported 50% of recurrent fistulae, bronchoscopy may also be required if recurrent fistula is suspected.[1]

Isolated Tracheoesophageal Fistula

Overview   Congenital, isolated TEF without atresia (type 3 in Fig. 97-1) is often termed an *H-type fistula,* and it differs significantly from the other types of tracheoesophageal malformations in its presenting spectrum and features. This type of fistula can be difficult to identify, both clinically and radiographically.[13] Large fistulae usually present very early in life and are relatively easy to see on an esophagram (Fig. 97-6). More commonly, the fistulae are small, inconstantly patent, and may require repeated examinations to identify. A major reason for inconstant patency of a fistula is that normal esophageal mucosa can be redundant, which can transiently occlude the esophageal side of the fistula.[14] Although rare, multiple fistulae can be present.[15]

Rarely, a bronchus originates directly from the esophagus, resulting in an anomaly termed *esophagotrachea* or *esophageal bronchus* (Fig. 97-7). This anomaly leads to severe respiratory distress with feeding and may be associated with esophageal atresia, TEF, or both.[16] Bronchoesophageal fistula between the esophagus and a normal bronchial tree has also been described.[17]

Clinical Presentation   These patients typically come to medical attention with recurrent episodes of coughing or choking and may progress to recurrent pneumonias, either in infancy or later in childhood.[18,19] Patients with unexplained, intermittent respiratory distress and recurrent pneumonia should always be considered at risk for the presence of a TEF, and radiographic examination is warranted.

Imaging   This is often termed an *H-type fistula* because of its appearance on an esophagram: it connects to the trachea

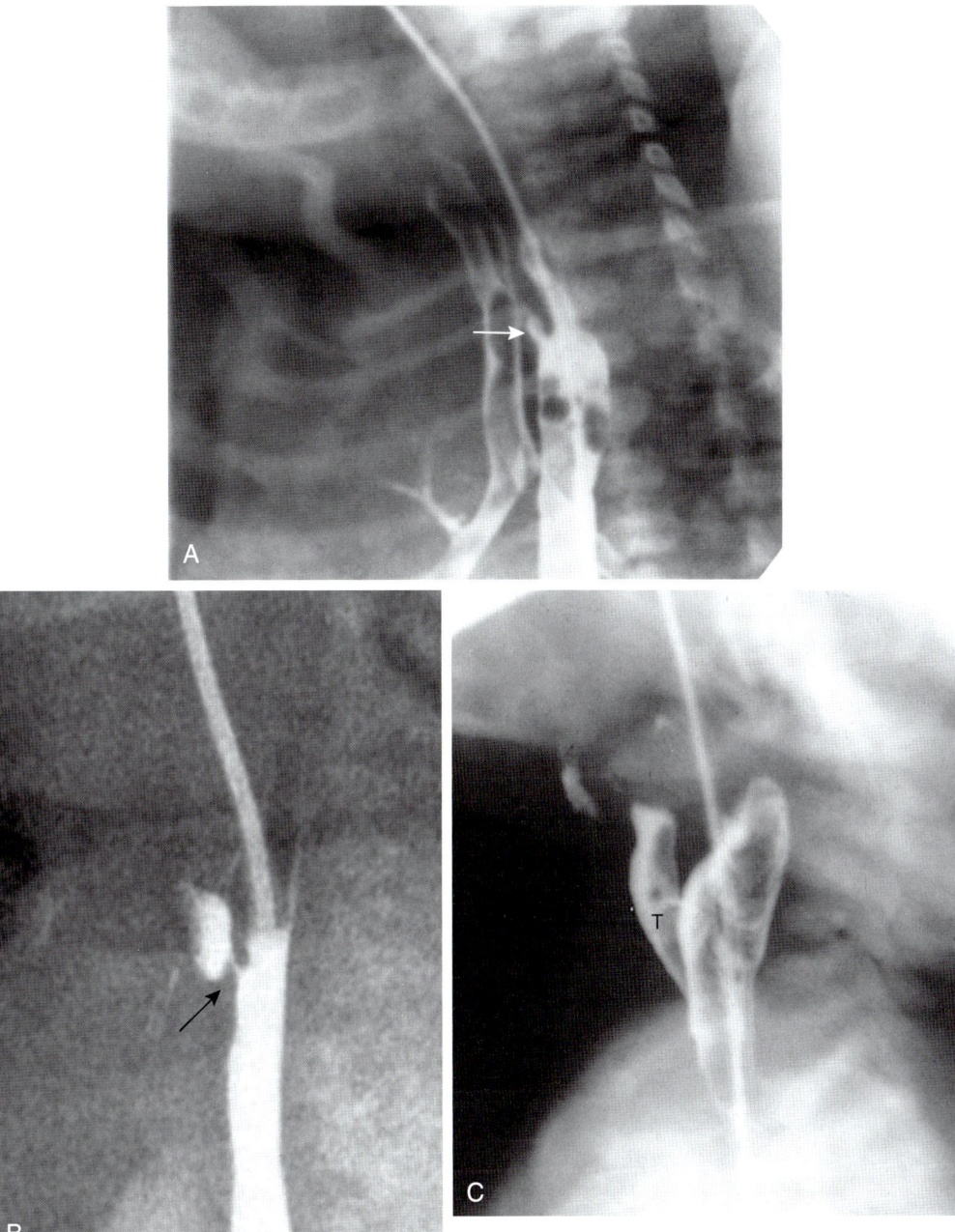

Figure 97-6   H-type fistula. **A,** Tracheoesophageal fistula (*arrow*) in a 7-day-old boy with imperforate anus. **B,** Demonstration of another H-type fistula (*arrow*) from the upper cervical esophagus to the trachea, using the technique of contrast injection through a feeding tube with very careful volume control. **C,** Large H-type fistula from the upper cervical esophagus to the trachea (*T*).

posteriorly and to the esophagus anteriorly as it courses cephalad from the esophagus to the trachea (see Fig. 97-6).

The examination should begin with a single contrast esophagram using digital, pulsed fluoroscopy in the right lateral to slightly right anterior oblique position. The position should be optimized during the examination to allow the best view of the anterior wall of the esophagus and posterior wall of the trachea. One of the keys of this examination is achieving full distension of the esophagus, because this is important to optimize filling and visualization of the fistula. If no abnormality is detected while the patient is swallowing, an esophageal catheter may be placed under fluoroscopic guidance, particularly in patients with normal prior examinations, in

whom a fistula remains suspect, or in those in whom contrast is seen within the trachea from an unclear source.[20] The examiner slowly withdraws the catheter from the distal esophagus in the cephalic direction, while carefully injecting contrast material with enough velocity and volume to distend the esophagus maximally under constant fluoroscopic monitoring. The catheter should have an end hole, without more proximal side holes, for adequate control of the contrast infusion. Even if a fistula is noted, the injection should continue until the catheter is withdrawn into the hypopharynx, but care must be taken not to allow contrast material to spill over into the trachea. Although there is a danger of spilling contrast material into the airway with injection of the high

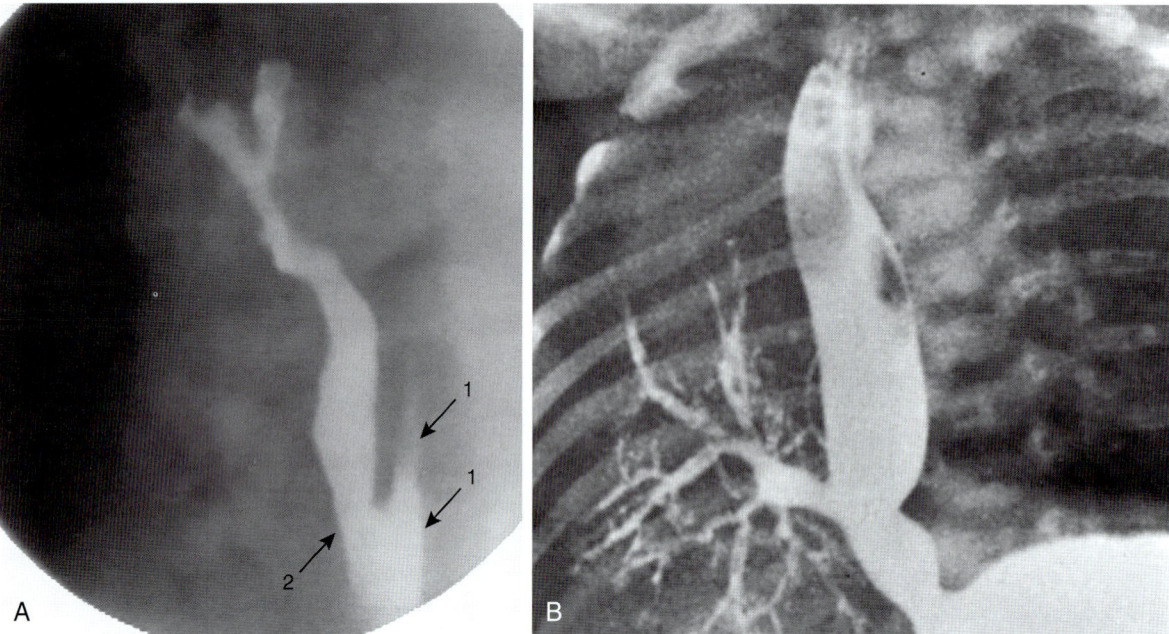

Figure 97-7   Connections between esophagus and airway. **A,** Congenital esophagobronchial fistula. Oblique view shows esophagus (*arrows* with 1) and bronchus to right upper lobe (*arrow* with 2). **B,** Esophageal bronchus. Frontal view from an esophagram demonstrates the origin of the right main bronchus from the distal esophagus.

cervical esophagus, it is important to examine this area, because many fistulae occur at the level of the lower cervical or upper thoracic spine (see Fig. 97-6, C).[21] Slow retraction of the catheter and careful fluoroscopic monitoring allow constant visualization and help to prevent overflow into the trachea.[22]

Treatment/Follow-up   Surgical correction of the fistula is the treatment of choice. Endoscopic, thoracoscopic, and open thoracotomy surgical techniques can be used.[23,24]

Fistula identification can be elusive at times, and repeat examination can be undertaken if clinical suspicion remains high. This also applies to those children who have been previously repaired, because a previously unseen fistula can be present, or the child may have failed primary therapy.[15]

Laryngotracheoesophageal Clefts

Overview   Laryngotracheoesophageal clefts occur in approximately 1 in 10,000 to 20,000 live births and consist of fistulous communications between the alimentary canal and the airway, either confined to the hypopharynx and larynx (Fig. 97-8) or extending inferiorly to include the esophagus.[25] Several related classifications have been proposed based on the extent of the communication between the respiratory and alimentary pathways.

Pettersson[26] originally described three types in 1955, with a fourth type identified by Ryan and colleagues[27] in 1991: type I is limited to the larynx, type II extends beyond the cricoid lamina to include the cervical trachea, type III forms an esophagotrachea and extends to the carina; and type IV extends beyond the carina to involve part of one or both mainstem bronchi.

More recently, other investigators have made modifications to the original classifications, to include therapeutic implications. The classification of Benjamin and Inglis,[28] as modified by Sandu and Monnier,[29] takes into account the degree of involvement of the cricoid cartilage in a cleft and extension into the cervical trachea and beyond. In this classification, type 0 refers to a submucosal cleft; type I is a cleft confined to the supraglottic region, type II extends below the vocal cords into the cricoid cartilage, type IIIa extends through the cricoid cartilage, type IIIb extends beyond the cricoid cartilage into the cervical trachea, and type IV extends into the thoracic trachea for a variable length.[25,28,29]

Etiology   The larynx forms from the endoderm of the foregut caudally and from the mesenchyme of branchial arches four and six cranially.[25] Incomplete separation and/or incomplete midline fusion of these concurrent processes during early gestation is believed to result in the persistent midline defect with varying extent and severity.

Clinical Presentation   The clinical presentation varies with the extent of the cleft, with varying degrees of respiratory distress aggravated during feeding, that begins early in infancy with choking, stridor, aspiration, recurrent pneumonia, and cyanosis.[25] In some patients, esophageal mucosa herniates into the defect and offers some protection against aspiration, but symptoms of respiratory distress secondary to compromise of the airway increase.[25] Anomalies such as esophageal atresia and VACTERL association may occur in patients with laryngotracheoesophageal clefts and other abnormalities, such as anal atresia, bronchial or tracheal stenosis and pulmonary hypoplasia, hypospadias, and coarctation of the aorta. Laryngotracheoesophageal clefts also occur as part of syndromes such as CHARGE, Opitz G/BBB (laryngeal malformations, craniofacial anomalies, genitourinary anomalies, and

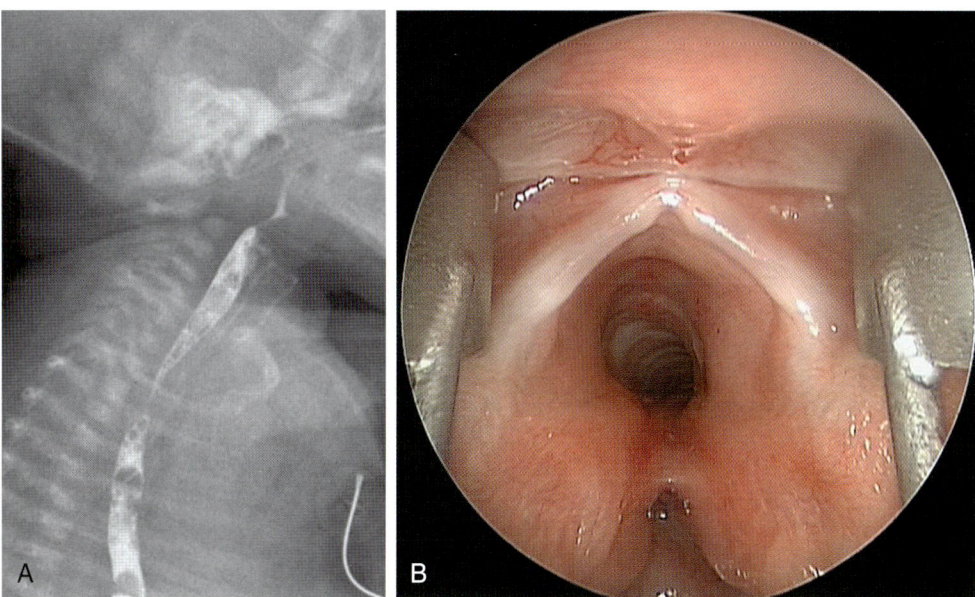

Figure 97-8 Laryngotracheal cleft. **A,** Laryngotracheoesophageal cleft. Contrast swallow demonstrates large-volume aspiration from a posterior laryngeal wall defect. **B,** Endoscopic photograph from the same patient shows a posterior laryngeal wall defect and type 2 or 3 laryngotracheal cleft.

ventral midline anomalies), and Pallister-Hall (laryngeal, GI, cardiopulmonary, limb, and neurologic malformations) syndromes.[25]

Imaging Diagnosis is usually made by laryngoscopy. On contrast esophagram (see Fig. 97-8, *A*), contrast is seen within the airway, although this can be confused with aspiration or with TEF. If computed tomography (CT) is performed, a common tracheoesophagus may be seen in extensive lesions, containing both the endotracheal and orogastric tubes.[30]

Treatment Follow-up The goal of treatment is to maintain the airway and ventilation while minimizing aspiration and allowing adequate nutrition. Endoscopic surgical therapy can be used to repair some of the less extensive clefts, and it has been reported with success in type IIIa and IIIb clefts. Types III and IV are usually corrected with an open surgical approach,[29] and extensive clefts may require both cervical and thoracic approaches.[1,25] Postoperative survival rates range between 50% and 75%, depending on the extent of the cleft and severity of associated anomalies. Late complications include anastomotic leaks, pharyngeal and esophageal dysfunction, and gastroesophageal reflux.[1]

Acquired Pharyngoesophageal Perforation

Overview Perforation of the pharynx or upper esophagus occurs in approximately 0.1% of neonatal intensive care unit discharges and is typically secondary to manipulation, such as attempted intubation; the imaging findings of this injury overlap with those of esophageal atresia.

Etiology This injury is more common among premature infants. The mechanism of injury is believed to relate to passage of a catheter, or even the obstetrician's finger, against

reflexive contraction of the cricopharyngeus muscle and narrowing of the esophageal introitus as it is compressed against the cervical vertebrae with hyperextension of the infant's neck. This leads to formation of a retroesophageal tract, which descends along the posterior mediastinum. The path of the catheter, or that of subsequently inserted catheters, may follow the perforation and enter the blind-ending tract in the prevertebral space; this resembles the appearance of esophageal atresia on radiographs.

Alternatively, the catheter may pass into the right pleural space, presumably as the tube passes above the cricopharyngeal "roll bar" (the posterior and transverse hypopharyngeal portions of the cricopharyngeal muscle) and is deflected to the right by the brachiocephalic vessels. Saliva, formula, and gas collect in the pleural space.

Imaging On chest radiographs, the findings of air or of a coiled enteric tube over the cervicothoracic junction resemble the findings in esophageal atresia. Distinguishing features include an unusually long blind pouch and irregularity of the outline of the false lumen. On esophagram, contrast extravasates into the newly created retroesophageal space (e-Fig. 97-9). Introduced contrast material is not easily aspirated into the syringe, and with time, the contrast dissipates along adjacent tissue planes (contrast should be water soluble and nearly iso-osmolal). Coexisting pneumomediastinum and pneumothorax or hydropneumothorax are helpful signs in detecting this complication and in differentiating it from esophageal atresia (see e-Fig. 97-9).

Clinical Findings The initial clinical presentation may be relatively silent, but patients manifest increased secretions with episodes of choking and cyanosis associated with feeding, and the development of crepitus and clinical deterioration follows, along with the inability to easily pass a feeding catheter.

Treatment/Follow-up Once the injury has been recognized, the majority of these patients can be managed conservatively, with withdrawal of enteral feedings, institution of antibiotics, and drainage of pleural effusion or pneumothorax if present. This management is successful in the vast majority of patients, and surgical treatment is reserved for complications, such as mediastinal abscess.

Esophageal Stenosis

Overview Congenital esophageal stenosis is a rare condition that occurs in 1 in 25,000 to 50,000 live births.[1,31] The three histologic subtypes are fibromuscular stenosis, membranous web, or tracheobronchial remnants.

Membranous stenosis is considered one of the rarest forms of this rare lesion and is usually located in the middle or distal third of the esophagus; it typically demonstrates an eccentric opening and is covered with squamous epithelium. Fibromuscular stenosis demonstrates subepithelial proliferation of smooth muscle and fibrosis. Stenosis associated with tracheobronchial remnants demonstrates cartilaginous tissue proliferation that partially or completely encircles the esophagus—usually in the lower third, within 3 cm of the gastroesophageal junction—and is often associated with esophageal atresia and TEF.[1,31,32]

Etiology The etiology of fibromuscular stenoses is uncertain, whereas that of membranous stenoses may be similar to that of membranous stenosis elsewhere in the GI tract. Stenoses as a result of tracheobronchial rests are thought to arise from incomplete separation of the tracheoesophageal septum during gestation with sequestration of the tracheal cartilage in the esophageal wall; this is carried distally by the growth of the esophagus.[1,32,33]

Clinical Presentation The typical presentation is that of dysphagia later in infancy, especially after introduction of solids,[34] or in older patients who may present with regurgitation, choking, vomiting, and failure to thrive.[35] The child may also come to medical attention with retention of a foreign body outside of the cervicothoracic junction, the aortic arch, the left bronchial crossing, or the gastroesophageal junction, which are the typical locations in which foreign bodies lodge in the normal esophagus.

Imaging Esophagram in patients with esophageal stenosis demonstrate an area of narrowing with partial obstruction (Fig. 97-10). Stenoses secondary to web or to fibromuscular hypertrophy may be seen in the upper or mid portion of the esophagus. Stenoses secondary to tracheobronchial remnants appear as a discrete narrowing of the esophagus along its distal portion, typically within 3 cm of the gastroesophageal junction and particularly in a patient with esophageal atresia. There may be impaction of food material, therefore a filling defect appears on esophagram proximal to the stenotic site. The diagnosis may be confirmed by endoscopy and histopathology.[34]

Because of the rarity of congenital esophageal stenosis, the findings at esophagram may be misinterpreted as stricture, such as secondary to gastroesophageal reflux, or as achalasia, if located very close to the gastroesophageal junction.[33,35] In such cases, manometric studies may be helpful in excluding the diagnosis of achalasia.[35]

If the diagnosis is delayed, cross-sectional imaging may demonstrate marked thickening of the wall of the esophagus, resembling esophageal leiomyomatosis.[35]

Treatment/Follow-up It is essential that a stricture as a result of gastroesophageal reflux be excluded prior to the diagnosis of esophageal stenosis.[1] Endoscopic balloon dilatation can be used as a primary and therapeutic procedure and is most successful in those patients without a true cartilaginous component of the stenosis.[36,37] Membranous stenoses are amenable

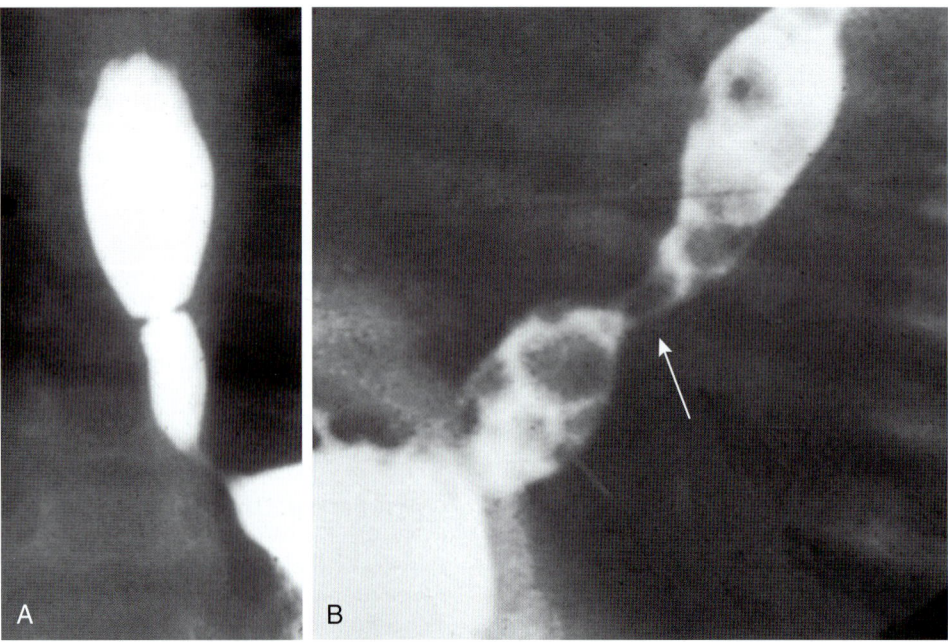

Figure 97-10 **A,** Weblike narrowing of the distal esophagus with proximal dilatation secondary to esophageal cartilaginous rests. The diagnosis is suggested by the location of the narrowed segment. **B,** Esophagram demonstrates stenosis in the distal portion of the esophagus (*arrow*) secondary to cartilaginous remnants. (Courtesy Dr. E. Afshani, Buffalo NY.)

to endoscopic dilation and resection, although surgical resection of the stenotic segment is reserved for strictures that are not amenable to one or more treatments with dilation or that recur after dilation.[38] Follow-up esophagram can be performed to assess for perforation, recurrent stenosis, or stricture after dilation or surgical resection.

Esophageal Duplication Cysts

Overview Duplication cysts of the esophagus represent part of the spectrum of foregut duplication cysts: they include *bronchogenic cysts,* which typically include mural cartilage or respiratory glands[39]; *neurenteric cysts,* which communicate with the spinal canal through a vertebral defect; and *esophageal duplication cysts* that may occur in the neck, associated with the cervical esophagus, or in the thorax, or they may involve the thorax and the upper abdomen as in a thoracoabdominal duplication cyst. Approximately two thirds occur in the right side of the mediastinum secondary to dextrorotation of the stomach during embryogenesis.[40]

Esophageal duplication cysts comprise approximately 20% of alimentary tract duplications and represent the most common site of duplications after the ileum[41,42] and approximately 10% of mediastinal masses in children.[43] Diagnostic criteria met by esophageal duplication cysts include attachment to the esophagus, two muscular layers enveloping the cyst, and lining by squamous, columnar, cuboidal,

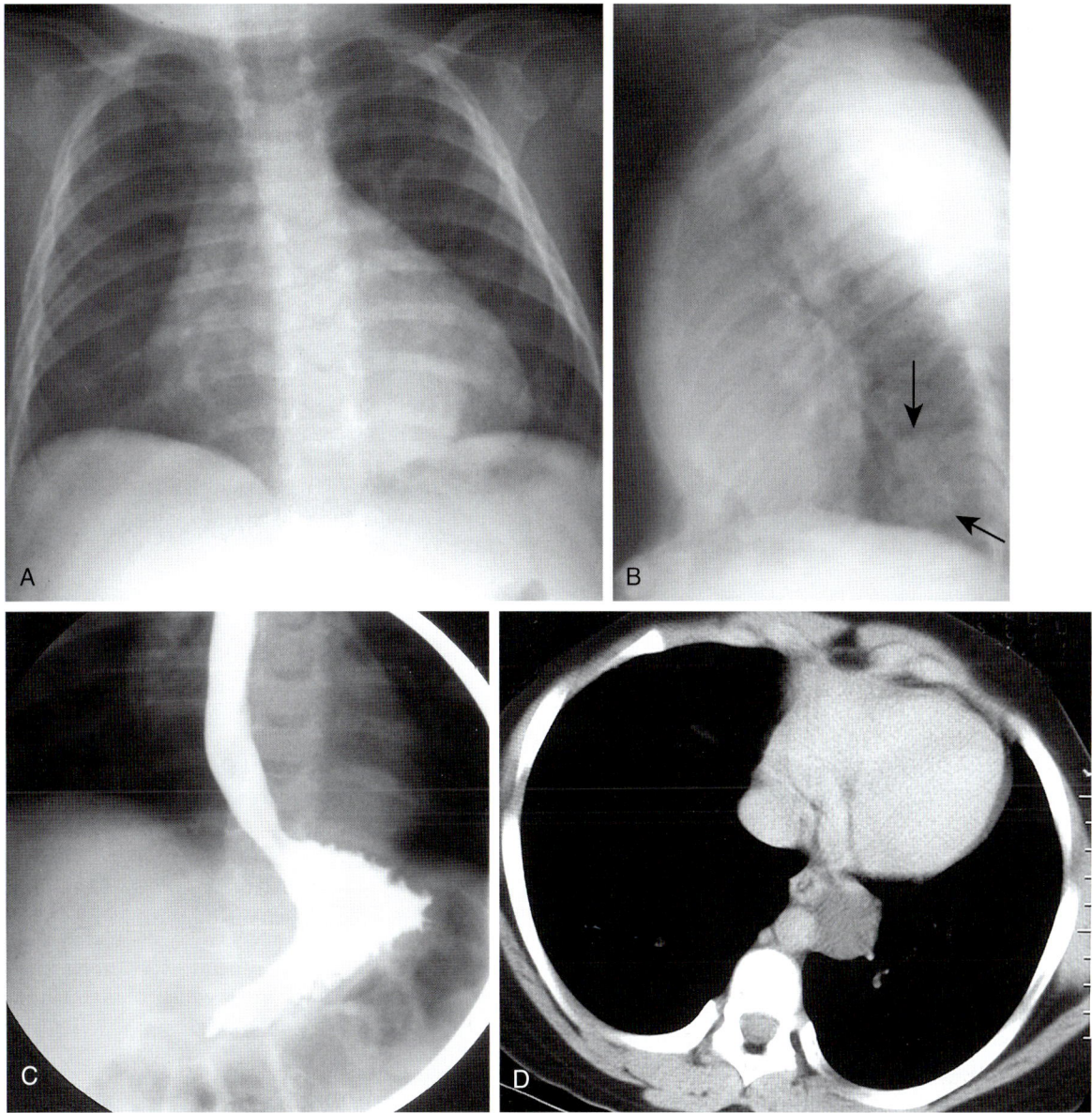

Figure 97-12 **Esophageal duplication cysts. A,** Frontal chest radiograph reveals a paraspinal retrocardiac mass at the left base. **B,** Lateral image confirms the posterior location of the lesion (*arrows*) with a positive spine sign. **C,** Esophagram shows deviation of the esophagus by the mass, confirming its posterior mediastinal location. **D,** Computed tomographic scan with intravenous contrast material demonstrates the persistently low attenuation of the duplication and its relationship to the esophagus.

pseudostratified or ciliated epithelium, or epithelium that "demonstrates some level of the gastrointestinal tract."[40] True tubular duplications of the esophagus are rare. These cysts may extend below the diaphragm to involve the stomach, and they may communicate with the stomach or esophagus.

Neurenteric cysts are duplication cysts that communicate with the spinal canal, and they differ in etiology from the classic type of duplication cyst. The archetype of this spectrum of anomalies is the dorsal enteric fistula, a patent communication between the gut and the dorsal midline skin surface that traverses the vertebral body (or interspace), the spinal canal and its contents, and the posterior vertebral elements. These are discussed in Chapter 43.

Etiology Esophageal duplication cysts are believed to be the result of a budding error of the dorsal portion of the foregut between the third and sixth weeks of gestation. These cysts arise from the posterior portion of the foregut and contain mucosa that, by histologic examination, is usually gastric or, more rarely, intestinal.[40] True tubular esophageal duplications likely develop from faulty recanalization of the esophageal lumen during the tenth week of gestation.[39,41,44] They may or may not communicate with the esophageal lumen.

Clinical Presentation Cervical duplication cysts are usually symptomatic very early in life, and patients come to medical attention with respiratory distress. Potential for respiratory compromise may be evident in fetal life, and an ex utero intrapartum treatment may be needed at delivery.[40] Large thoracic duplication cysts that occur in the superior mediastinum may manifest with respiratory distress or dysphagia because of compression of adjacent structures, or they may be found incidentally (e-Fig. 97-11).[42] Duplication cysts that occur in the lower esophagus are often asymptomatic and are discovered incidentally (Fig. 97-12), although they may become symptomatic as a result of inflammation, if they contain gastric mucosa, or as a result of superinfection or hemorrhage.[46]

Neurenteric cysts may present with back pain and progressive neurologic deficit if not diagnosed prenatally or in early infancy.[47] Infants may be brought to medical attention with meningitis. These defects are typically associated with midline vertebral lesions such as spina bifida, other dysraphic defects, or scoliosis (e-Figs. 97-13 and 97-14 and Fig. 97-15).

The combination of esophageal duplication with other anomalies, such as spinal defects, should prompt a search for additional duplications along the alimentary tract, which can be found in up to one third of cases.[42]

Imaging Radiographs may demonstrate a sharply demarcated middle or posterior mediastinal mass and associated vertebral anomalies in cases of neurenteric cyst (see e-Fig. 97-14, *A*).

Esophagrams (see e-Fig. 97-14, *B*) will suggest an intramural mass, but typically no connection between the two structures is seen, except in cases of communication of the lumen in long, tubular duplications.[44] Ultrasound can confirm the cystic nature of the mass in utero but is rarely utilized in these chest lesions after birth.[48] CT and MRI are the modalities of choice to confirm the cystic nature of the mass and to best delineate the abnormality. The cyst fluid typically has

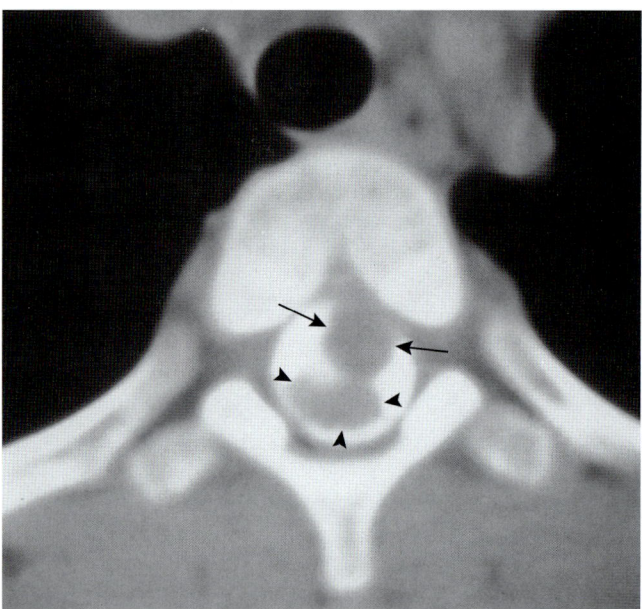

Figure 97-15 Intraspinal neurenteric cyst. Axial computed tomographic section with intrathecal contrast demonstrates an intraspinal mass (*arrows*) anterior to the compressed spinal cord (*arrowheads*) surgically proven to represent an intraspinal neurenteric cyst. Note the associated congenital cleft in the vertebral body.

the attenuation and signal characteristics of water, although this can be affected by hemorrhage or infection.

For neurenteric cysts, CT myelography (see Fig. 97-15) can demonstrate the extent of the lesion and any associated vertebral anomaly. MRI, however, is the study of choice to evaluate the presence and extent of intraspinal abnormalities.[49] These lesions are usually intradural and extramedullary.[50] Those enteric cysts that contain gastric mucosa with acid and pepsin secretion can be identified by nuclear imaging and are at risk for hemorrhage.[51]

Treatment/Follow-up Complete surgical resection is recommended.[45] Even if asymptomatic at discovery, esophageal duplication cysts are at risk for development of bleeding, infection, and cancer.[39]

Key Points

Patients with esophageal atresia and distal fistula will have air in the abdomen, whereas patients without a distal fistula will not have abdominal gas.

Approximately 2.5% of patients with esophageal atresia have a right-sided aortic arch, which is important to identify preoperatively.

The majority of patients with esophageal atresia complex have associated anomalies, although this decreases to approximately 25% among those with isolated or H-type fistulae.

Distinguishing features between esophageal atresia and traumatic pharyngoesophageal perforation include an unusually long pouch, irregularity of its lumen, presence of pneumomediastinum, and contrast on esophagram that outlines both true and false lumens.

The clinical and radiographic diagnosis of an isolated TEF can be elusive, and repeat examination can be considered in difficult cases.

Laryngotracheoesophageal clefts may be confused with TEFs or mistaken for aspiration during esophagram.

Congenital esophageal stenosis with tracheobronchial remnants is typically located in the distal esophagus, and when abutting the esophagogastric junction, can be mistaken for achalasia.

Suggested Readings

Berrocal T, Torres I, Gutiérrez J, et al. Congenital anomalies of the upper gastrointestinal tract. *Radiographics.* 1999;19(4):855-872.

Ioannides AS, Copp AJ. Embryology of oesophageal atresia. *Semin Pediatr Surg.* 2009;18(1):2-11.

Jones DW, Kunisaki SM, Teitelbaum DH, et al. Congenital esophageal stenosis: the differential diagnosis and management. *Pediatr Surg Int.* 2010;26(5):547-551.

Kluth D, et al. The embryology of foregut malformations. *J Pediatr Surg.* 1987;22:389-393.

Laffan EE, Daneman A, Ein SH, et al. Tracheoesophageal fistula without esophageal atresia: are pull-back tube esophagograms needed for diagnosis? *Pediatr Radiol.* 2006;36(11):1141-1147.

Leboulanger N, Garabedian EN. Laryngo-tracheo-oesophageal clefts. *Orphanet J Rare Dis.* 2011;6:81.

References

Full references for this chapter can be found on www.expertconsult.com.

Chapter 98

Disorders of Swallowing

JAYNE M. SEEKINS and HENRIQUE M. LEDERMAN

Phonation and coordinated movement of liquid and food are the result of complex, integrated, and intact neuromuscular function. When a person's swallowing function is abnormal because of a structural anomaly, neuromuscular deficit, or postsurgical change, a swallowing function study can be performed. Most swallowing disorders in infants and children are a result of neurologic abnormalities, of which cerebral palsy is the most common.[1,2]

General Examination Principles

Specialized radiographic studies of deglutition can be performed in the radiology department in association with occupational therapists or speech pathologists, depending on the institution. Usually a videofluoroscopic swallow study (VFSS) is performed.

The history related to feeding and associated clinical conditions of the patient must be detailed and should include data about the acuity of the clinical complaint, the child's feeding history, the ability to suck, the use of utensils, positioning and irritability during and after feeding, usual appetite, and signs of fatigue during feeding.

The initial step in the swallowing evaluation is to assess the competence of the velopharyngeal mechanism. First, the patient is observed during quiet breathing and phonation. During feeding, the patient is placed in the true lateral position and is fed contrast material of varying thickness with a bottle with a nipple initially, while swallowing is evaluated in real time with video fluoroscopy, including examination from the mouth to the carina. Either a single image or a sweeping image down to the carina and back to the mouth may be obtained.[3-6] Imaging in the frontal projection using a basal or Towne view[6] may be performed after lateral imaging; this view permits evaluation of lateral wall movement and correlation with nasopharyngoscopy (e-Fig. 98-1).[3,7]

If the infant will not take contrast material from the nipple, the contrast material can be introduced into the baby's mouth carefully with a blunt-tipped syringe (between the cheek and the lateral aspect of the teeth or gums), or a feeding tube can be inserted through the nipple into the baby's mouth and contrast material can be introduced in a controlled manner under fluoroscopic guidance to initiate swallowing (e-Fig. 98-2). The contrast medium is mixed with increasingly thicker food mixtures, beginning with thin liquids and progressing to solid food if such food is age appropriate. Evaluation of the patient's ability to handle food with different textures aids in planning an appropriate diet to meet nutritional needs and in planning future therapy. If the patient requires a special diet or only eats certain foods, this food can be brought to the examination and used for the study.

Causes of Swallowing Dysfunction

The most common causes of swallowing dysfunction in pediatric patients include central neurologic dysfunction, congenital anomalies with anatomic abnormalities and mechanical interference in the swallowing apparatus, congenital and acquired retropharyngeal processes, and connective tissue disorders.

CENTRAL NEUROLOGIC DYSFUNCTION

Overview Cerebral palsy is the most common cause of swallowing dysfunction in infants and children. Other neuromuscular disorders are brainstem dysfunction, cranial nerve abnormalities, intracranial neoplasms, meningomyelocele, muscular dystrophies, and myasthenia gravis. Familial dysautonomia (Riley-Day syndrome) leads to autonomic dysfunction with esophageal dysmotility and frequent aspiration pneumonias. Abnormality of the neuromuscular mechanism elevating the soft palate may lead to reflux of contrast material into the nasopharynx, with subsequent pooling of contrast in the pharynx and potential airway aspiration. Abnormalities of other muscle groups lead to defective function of the epiglottis and upper esophageal sphincter, with aspiration into the airway being common[1] (Fig. 98-3; Videos 98-1 and 98-2).

Etiology Swallowing dysfunction is related to dysfunction in one or more of the three phases of swallowing: the oral phase, with the inability to deliver food into the mouth (e.g., poor suck); the pharyngeal phase, with failure to move the food through the pharynx, elevate the soft palate, and close the epiglottis; and/or the upper esophageal phase, with abnormal coordination of relaxation and contraction of the upper esophageal sphincter.[1] Swallowing coordination is mediated through the cranial nerves responsible for both sensation and motor function, as well as osseous and muscular structures supplied by both the autonomic and voluntary nervous system. Thus swallowing dysfunction may be due to

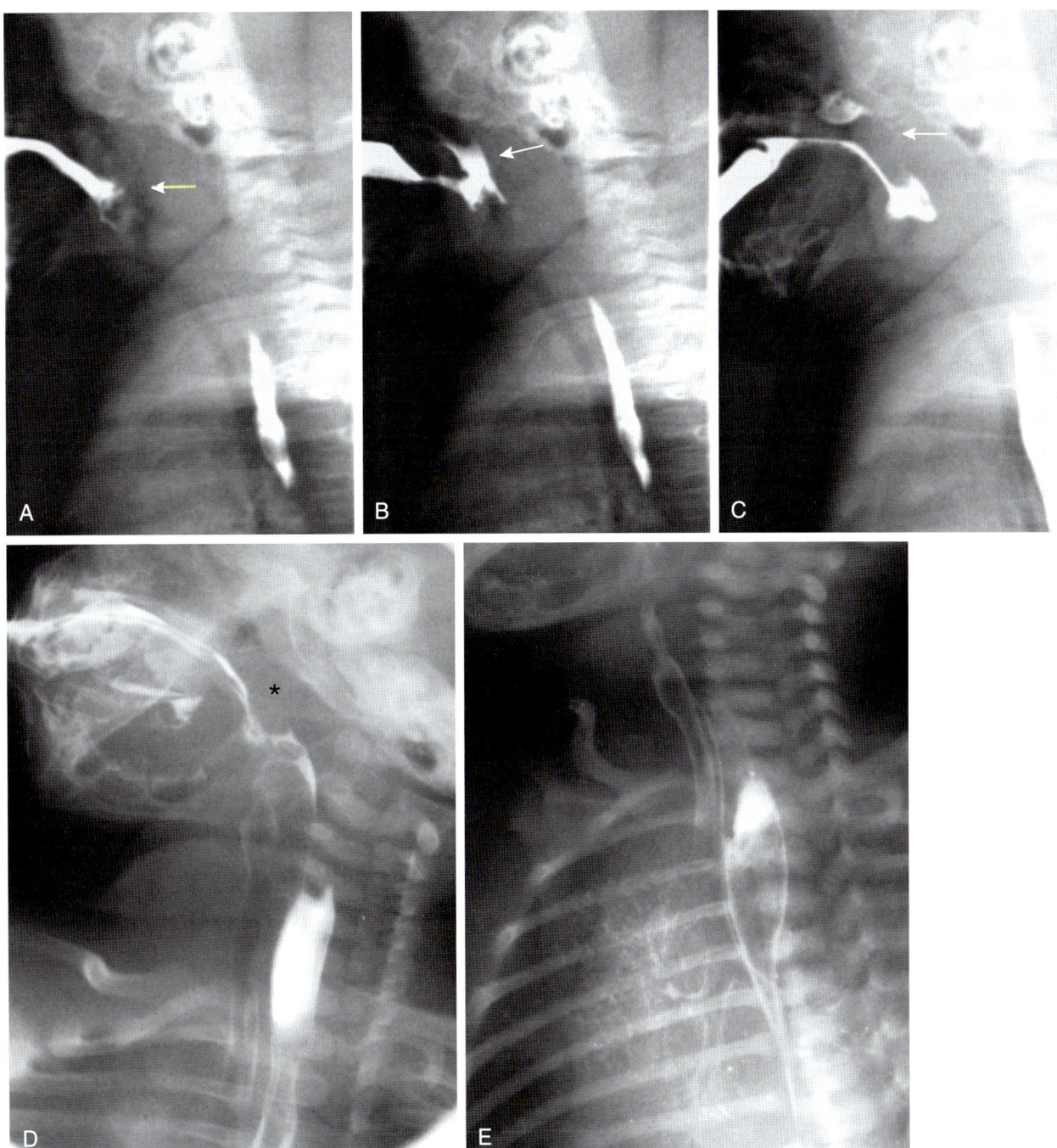

Figure 98-3 Swallowing. **A,** As the nipple is inserted into the infant's mouth, the tongue and soft palate are relaxed and the nasopharynx opens (*arrow*). **B,** Normally, the tongue elevates, pushing the nipple to the roof of the mouth, and the soft palate elevates. In this example, the soft palate did not elevate and close off the nasopharynx, resulting in nasopharyngeal reflux (*arrow*). **C,** The infant finally did close the nasopharynx by elevation of the soft palate against the adenoid tissue (*arrow*). Contrast material remains in the nose and in the hypopharynx. **D,** During this barium swallow study, complete closure of the nasopharynx occurs and no nasopharyngeal reflux is present (*asterisk*), but aspiration of contrast into the larynx and trachea occurs. **E,** An oblique view in the same patient as shown in part **D** reveals extensive airway aspiration during a routine barium swallow study as a result of a lack of coordination during swallowing. Barium coating of the lung parenchyma is present.

a large number of conditions that affect any of the mechanical and functional processes necessary for normal swallowing and phonation.

Clinical Presentation The severity of disordered swallowing and the resultant degree of aspiration will vary with the level of neurologic deficit. Depending on the specific neurologic defect, any or all components of the swallowing mechanism may be affected. Symptoms include nasopharyngeal regurgitation, gagging, coughing and choking during feedings, recurrent pneumonia, malnutrition, and failure to thrive.[1,8] However, in some patients at risk for disordered swallowing and aspiration, the gagging and coughing reflex itself may be defective, and these patients are subject to silent aspiration.

Because of the risk of silent aspiration in these patients, VFSS should be performed to aid nutritional management and to help reduce aspiration when possible.[9]

Imaging During VFSS, contrast material can be seen within the nasopharynx or trachea, with disordered swallowing. Dysfunction in the pharyngeal phase may be related to a mechanical problem such a cleft palate, or weak pharyngeal contraction or lack of coordination may be noted, resulting in inadequate passage of pharyngeal contents, with findings resembling cricopharyngeal achalasia.[1,10] It also is important to note whether the patient can spontaneously clear the contrast from an abnormal location and if the cough reflex is present, diminished, or absent (silent aspiration).[9]

Treatment and Follow-up Treatment can range from thickening liquids adequately to prevent aspiration to complete oral restriction with enteric tube feeding or total parenteral nutrition. The swallow study can be repeated as the patient matures, or as requested, to assess the effect of any interval medical or surgical treatment.

CONGENITAL ANOMALIES

Overview Multiple congenital anomalies can lead to abnormal swallowing. Mechanical problems such as those seen in persons with the Robin sequence who have a small mandible can lead to significant feeding difficulties. Macroglossia, as is seen in patients with Beckwith-Wiedemann syndrome, can present with similar problems. Disorders of the mouth and jaw such as cleft lip and cleft palate likewise can lead to difficulties with swallowing.[7] These disorders are usually readily physically apparent or diagnosed prenatally.

Etiology The etiologies of the various congenital anomalies that can result in abnormal swallowing obviously are quite different. As an example, cleft palate is a result of the partial or total lack of fusion of the palatal shelves between the eighth and twelfth weeks of gestation.[13]

Micrognathia may be seen alone or as part of a syndrome such as the Robin sequence and is usually due to incomplete mandibular maturation or failure of normal mandibular development as a result of external causes.[14,15]

Clinical Presentation Symptoms correlate with the anatomic abnormality and therefore can vary widely, but they usually include choking, pneumonia, or repeated pneumonitis. Cleft lip and cleft palate occur with varying severity, are usually clinically obvious, and can lead to feeding difficulties by interfering with normal sucking.

Imaging Conditions such as cleft lip/palate, micrognathia, and macroglossia are not routinely imaged postnatally beyond evaluation of the functional difficulties they produce.[11,12]

Treatment and Follow-up Cleft lip/palate are corrected surgically in infancy. Follow-up is usually with endoscopy. Mild micrognathia may be relieved with prone positioning and a nasopharyngeal airway until the infant grows. More severe mandibular hypoplasia that does not respond to conventional treatment may be treated with a distraction osteotomy.[14]

Macroglossia is treated clinically or surgically with partial, anterior wedge lingual resection to allow for the return of normal swallow function.[16]

RETROPHARYNGEAL PROCESSES—CONGENITAL AND ACQUIRED

Overview Retropharyngeal processes can be congenital or acquired. Cricopharyngeal spasm or achalasia is most often associated with an underlying neuromuscular disorder, but it can rarely occur as a primary abnormality.[10] Masses, both benign and malignant, are rare causes of dysphagia and range from those that can be seen in utero, such as lymphatic malformation and cervical esophageal duplication, to lesions acquired postnatally, such as foreign bodies, infectious diseases, and trauma.

Etiology In patients with cricopharyngeal achalasia, the normal relaxation of the cricopharyngeus muscle in response to contraction of the middle and inferior pharyngeal constrictors does not occur, resulting in a varying degree of obstruction to propulsion of the bolus into the esophagus.[10] The swallowing abnormality in patients with a retropharyngeal process is related to the effect of the mass interfering with the coordinated peristalsis needed to effect proper swallowing.

Clinical Presentation Symptoms of dysphagia vary in presentation according to the underlying abnormality. Congenital masses may have been noted on prenatal imaging, and in some cases, such as lymphatic malformations, they may be visible on physical examination. Onset of dysphagia in conjunction with fever or other signs of infection suggests the presence of a retropharyngeal abscess or superinfection of a preexistent lesion. Prior trauma, such as orogastric tube insertion or caustic or foreign body ingestion, also may produce dysphagia and disordered swallowing.

Imaging Radiographs of the neck are helpful in assessing whether the airway is narrowed, a mass is pressing upon the airway, or a foreign body is present. In patients with a retropharyngeal process, radiographs demonstrate increased density with mass effect, anterior bowing and displacement, and narrowing of the airway (e-Fig. 98-4). A swallow study demonstrates similar findings for the esophagus.

Ultrasound, CT, and MRI all have roles in the evaluation of neck masses. If these masses are present prenatally, imaging may guide any immediate intervention needed at birth.

In patients with cricopharyngeal spasm or achalasia, VFSS demonstrates the posterior impression of the cricopharyngeus muscle (Fig. 98-5).

Treatment and Follow-up In patients with cricopharyngeal achalasia, waiting may allow time for maturation, particularly when it is found in premature infants who are otherwise normal. In patients with primary cricopharyngeal achalasia, balloon dilatation has been advocated; surgical management remains controversial.[10] Infectious masses are treated with appropriate antibiotics and drainage if necessary. Masses typically are resected, although lymphatic malformations may be treated with sclerotherapy.

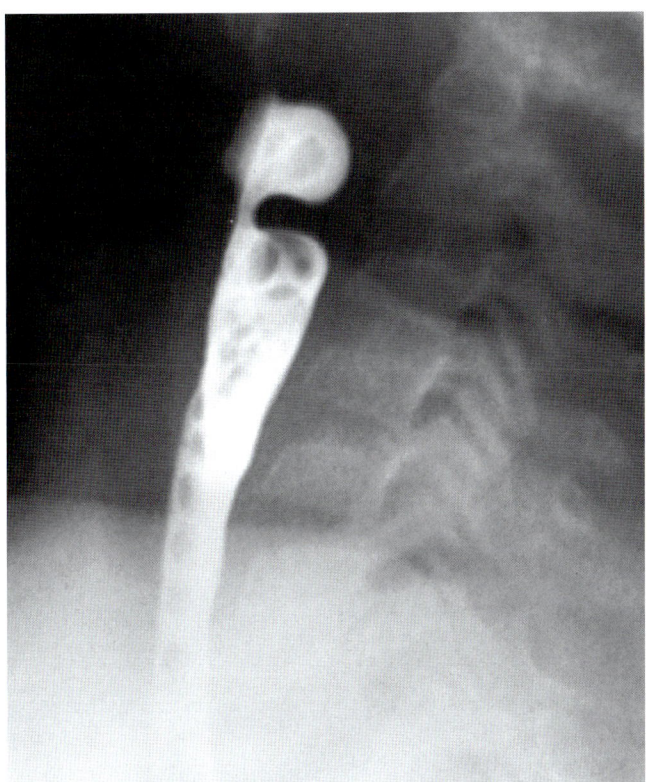

Figure 98-5 Cricopharyngeal achalasia. A posterior impression on the esophagus as a result of persistent contraction of the cricopharyngeal muscle in a patient with dysphagia.

CONNECTIVE TISSUE DISORDERS

Overview Scleroderma and mixed collagen disorders usually occur in adolescents and adults and are rare in children. Pharyngeal and upper esophageal function is usually normal. Esophageal dysmotility typically begins at the level of the aortic arch. At this level, the esophageal muscle changes from striated to smooth muscle, which is affected more in patients with scleroderma.[17] Poor to absent primary peristalsis occurs in the distal two thirds of the esophagus. Secondary gastroesophageal reflux, with or without esophagitis and reflux stricture, may occur.

Dermatomyositis is an inflammatory myositis that primarily affects the striated muscle of the pharynx and upper esophagus. Dilatation of these structures with disordered peristalsis occurs frequently, as does nasopharyngeal reflux of ingested material. The associated vasculitis may result in esophageal ulceration and perforation.[18]

Etiology In patients with scleroderma, swelling of endothelial cells occurs, with an adventitial periarterial fibrotic cuff.[19] Dermatomyositis is associated with a complement-mediated microangiopathy.[20]

Clinical Manifestations The esophagus is involved in nearly all patients with scleroderma, and approximately 50% to 90%

have clinical symptoms of esophageal dysfunction, most commonly dysphagia and dyspepsia.[19] Dermatomyositis involves the pharynx and upper esophageal sphincter, thus interfering with the appropriate direction of the food bolus into the esophagus. In addition to dysphagia and the inability to swallow without the aid of gravity, patients exhibit hoarseness, nasal speech, and nasal regurgitation.[20]

Imaging In older children and adolescents, a chest radiograph may aid the initial workup. The radiograph may demonstrate a dilated esophagus and possibly an air–fluid level. Associated findings of connective tissue disease may be noted, such as interstitial lung disease.

Evaluation of swallowing in persons with scleroderma usually demonstrates a normal swallow mechanism but abnormal distal esophageal motility and dilation (Fig. 98-6). Distal stricture formation usually is related to gastroesophageal reflux as a result of the incompetent lower esophageal sphincter.

Dermatomyositis can cause disordered swallowing of the pharynx and upper esophagus. Reflux of barium into the nasopharynx may be seen.[20]

Treatment and Follow-up Treatment of the underlying disease is the primary goal. Initially, findings and symptoms of reflux can be addressed medically.[19,20] Distal esophageal strictures may respond to balloon dilatation; a myotomy may be required in severe cases.

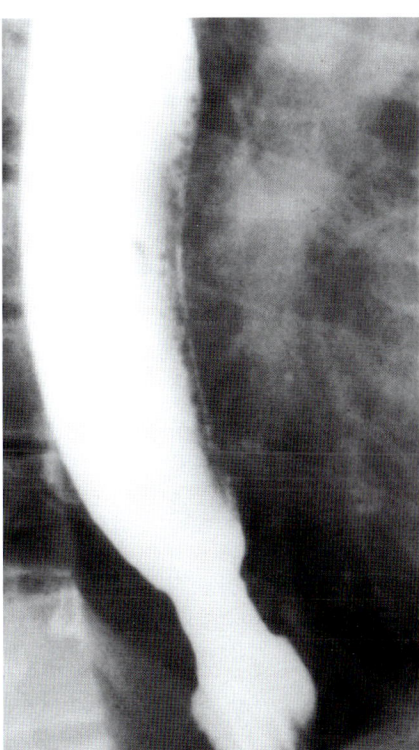

Figure 98-6 Scleroderma. Dilatation of the distal esophagus, which was associated with slowed and delayed emptying, and decreased peristaltic activity, in a patient with scleroderma.

Key Points

Swallowing abnormalities can be due to a central neurologic disorder or an anatomic disorder of the tongue, mouth, jaw, or esophagus.

The video fluoroscopic assessment of swallow function is usually performed in collaboration with a speech pathologist or occupational therapist.

Suggested Readings

Derkay CS, Schechter GL. Anatomy and physiology of pediatric swallowing disorders. *Otolaryngol Clin North Am.* 1998;31(3):397-404.
Fisher SE, Painter M, Milmoe G. Swallowing disorders in infancy. *Pediatr Clin North Am.* 1981;28:845.
Kramer SS. Radiologic examination of the swallowing impaired child. *Dysphagia.* 1989;3:117.
Tuchman DN. Cough, choke, sputter: the evaluation of the child with dysfunctional swallowing. *Dysphagia.* 1989;3:111.

References

Full references for this chapter can be found on www.expertconsult.com.

Chapter 99

Acquired Esophageal Disorders

ALEXANDER J. TOWBIN and LINCOLN O. DINIZ

Overview

The esophagus is a muscular tube that transports food and oral secretions from the mouth to the stomach via coordinated peristalsis of striated and smooth muscle.[1] A number of acquired disorders prevent the esophagus from functioning normally. These disorders generally present with symptoms such as dysphagia, food sticking, or food bolus impaction. In addition, a number of self-inflicted, accidental, or iatrogenic injuries are common in the pediatric esophagus.

Acquired abnormalities of the esophagus can be separated into several broad categories: gastroesophageal reflux (GER); trauma, including ingestion of foreign bodies; inflammatory conditions; infections; motility disorders; postsurgical changes; neoplasms; and other conditions. Disorders in each of these categories will be discussed in this chapter.

Imaging

An esophagram or an upper gastrointestinal (UGI) series is the most common method used to image the esophagus directly. The two fluoroscopic studies differ in that an UGI provides a more complete evaluation of the upper gastrointestinal tract, extending from the mouth through the proximal jejunum, whereas an esophagram typically focuses on the upper gastrointestinal tract between the mouth and body of the stomach. Both studies allow the radiologist to evaluate the anatomy and function of the esophagus by watching a contrast bolus move through the esophageal lumen (see Chapter 98 for a more complete description of the technique).

Computed tomography (CT) and magnetic resonance imaging (MRI) are rarely used as primary methods of imaging the esophagus; however, both CT and MRI have the advantage of allowing the radiologist to visualize the esophageal wall and lesions extrinsic to the esophagus.[2] Use of cross-sectional imaging to evaluate the esophagus has several major limitations that prevent their use as a primary imaging modality: first, neither CT nor MRI provides functional information of esophageal motility; second, the esophagus is not able to be distended reliably to evaluate wall thickness accurately; third, and neither study is able to provide mucosal detail.

Gastroesophageal Reflux

Overview GER is defined as the retrograde passage of gastric contents into the esophagus.[3] When symptoms or lesions occur as a result of GER, it is referred to as gastroesophageal reflux disease (GERD).[4] The primary mechanism of GER is transient relaxation of the lower esophageal sphincter. This relaxation can be triggered by vasovagal reflex initiated by gastric distension or cardiopulmonary receptors or by a swallow that does not trigger esophageal peristalsis.[3] In children, severe GERD has several known risk factors, including neurologic disorders such as spastic quadriplegia and cerebral palsy, esophageal atresia, chronic lung disease such as cystic fibrosis, and hiatal hernia.[5,6]

Clinical Presentation GER is ubiquitous in infants, occurring in 100% of 3-month-olds, 40% of 6-month-olds, and 5% to 20% of 1-year-olds.[4,6] In children and adolescents, GERD increases in incidence with age. Symptoms of GERD are reported to occur on a weekly basis in 2% of 3- to 9-year-olds and 5% to 8.2% of children aged 10-17 years.[7]

The symptoms of GERD depend on age. In infants, symptoms include irritability, feeding difficulty, poor weight gain, and sleep disturbance. In older children, symptoms include heartburn, abdominal pain, regurgitation or vomiting, and dysphagia.[3] Extraesophageal symptoms of GERD also can occur and include chronic cough, asthma, apnea, bradycardia, sore throat, dental erosions, and recurrent otitis or sinusitis.[3] When compared with adults, children report fewer episodes of heartburn, dysphagia, and chest pain and more episodes of vomiting and regurgitation.[4]

GERD often is diagnosed on the basis of symptoms and a trial of acid-reduction therapy. When symptoms are not specific or are atypical, confirmatory testing can be performed. Intraesophageal pH monitoring traditionally has been thought of as the gold standard because of its ability to measure the pH in the esophagus over a long period. The main limitation of this technique is that patients may have abnormal esophageal acid exposure without symptoms of GERD or retrograde bolus movement in the esophagus.[3,8] To evaluate for the retrograde passage of gastric contents and esophageal acidity, combined pH/impedance probes are used.[8]

Imaging UGI imaging often is performed in the setting of GER to evaluate for an anatomic abnormality; however, it should not be used as the primary method of diagnosing GER or GERD. UGI has multiple limitations in diagnosing GER, including its nonstandard technique, lack of correlation with symptoms, and use of ionizing radiation. Methods used to provoke reflux such as the Valsalva maneuver, positional changes, abdominal compression, or leg lifting may increase the sensitivity of detecting GER but lower the specificity.[3] Because more sensitive diagnostic tests are available and the radiologic findings do not correlate with symptoms, the collaborative practice guideline set forth by the American College of Radiology and the Society for Pediatric Radiology do not recommend provocative maneuvers or prolonged fluoroscopy for the detection of GER.[9]

Even though UGI imaging should not be prolonged to identify GER, GER often is present (Fig. 99-1). The percentage of patients who have GER on UGI imaging decreases with age from 80% of infants <18 months to 30% of adolescents between 12 and 18 years.[3] It should be noted that although the height of reflux often is reported as a surrogate for its severity, no correlation exists between the height of GER on UGI imaging and symptoms of GERD.[3]

Technetium-99m sulfur colloid also can be used to diagnose GER. Although scintigraphy is a sensitive method of detecting GER, it has many of the same limitations as UGI mainly, the presence of GER does not correlate with symptoms of GERD. In addition to this limitation, scintigraphy also requires the use of ionizing radiation. A limitation unique to scintigraphy is its inability to diagnose some of the complications of GERD. Scintigraphy is thus reserved for cases in which pH monitoring is not able to be performed or when evaluation of gastric motility also is required.

Esophageal complications of GERD include esophageal strictures and Barrett esophagitis. Esophageal strictures, also known as peptic strictures when they are caused by GERD, typically occur in the lower third of the esophagus and are a result of acidic injury. They are cited as being present in up to 15% of children with GERD and can occur at any age.[10] Many patients who experience strictures have an associated comorbidity, with 25% having a neurologic impairment.[10]

Barrett esophagus is defined as metaplasia of cells in the distal esophagus from squamous to columnar epithelium. Its prevalence in children with GERD ranges from 0.25% to 4.8%.[6,11] Risk factors for the development of Barrett esophagus in children include severe chronic GERD, congenital abnormalities, neurologic impairment, hiatal hernia, and family history.[6] Although it is associated with a thirtyfold increase in esophageal adenocarcinoma in adults, the risk of developing adenocarcinoma is not defined in children.[6]

Treatment Multiple options exist for treating GERD, depending on the patient's age, comorbidities, and severity of symptoms. Generally, lifestyle changes and pharmacotherapy are first-line options. Lifestyle changes include avoidance of overfeeding, thickening feeds, upright positioning during sleep, and avoidance of second-hand smoke.[3] A goal of medical therapy is to decrease the acidity of the refluxed gastric contents, which is generally performed by using proton pump inhibitors and histamine receptor antagonists.[3] In patients with continued severe GERD after pharmacotherapy or other comorbidities such as neurologic impairment, antireflux surgery such as Nissen fundoplication is performed. Strictures are treated with esophageal dilation and fundoplication. In a small percentage of patients, severe and recurrent strictures will require extensive and repeated dilatations and may require surgical resection or replacement of the esophagus.[10]

Trauma

Esophageal injury can occur via several different mechanisms. Because the esophagus connects the mouth to the remainder of the gastrointestinal tract, it often is the structure injured by ingested noxious materials.

FOREIGN BODIES

Ingested foreign bodies are common in children, with most occurring in children younger than 3 years.[12] The American Association of Poison Control Centers reported approximately 125,000 foreign body ingestions in pediatric patients in 2009.[13] This number is only a fraction of the actual number of foreign bodies ingested because it represents only the ingestions that are reported to poison control centers.

Coins

Overview In the United States and Europe, coins are the most commonly ingested foreign body.[12] It is estimated that 4% of all children swallow a coin.[14] Although most coins spontaneously pass through the gastrointestinal tract, they can

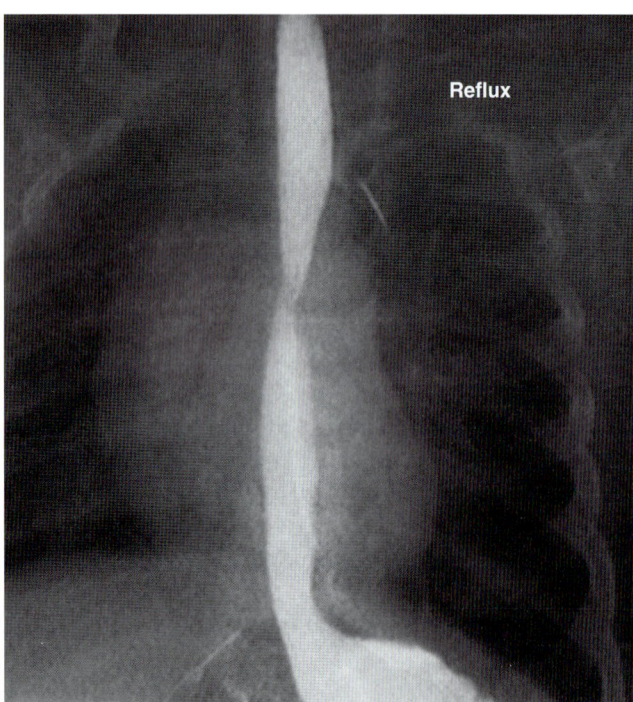

Figure 99-1 Gastroesophageal reflux. Image from an upper gastrointestinal examination shows retrograde flow of contrast from the stomach into the esophagus. Note the wide-open esophageal sphincter.

lodge in the esophagus. Coins typically lodge in one of three locations: the thoracic inlet (60% to 70%), the mid esophagus at the level of the aortic arch (10% to 20%), and just above the lower esophageal sphincter (20%).[12]

Clinical Presentation Symptoms of chronic foreign body impaction include respiratory distress, asthma symptoms, cough, nausea, vomiting, and dysphagia. Respiratory symptoms are a result of local inflammation surrounding the foreign body.[14] Patients with chronic foreign body impaction are at risk of esophageal perforation.

Imaging Radiographs are useful to identify the location of the coin and to look for signs of chronic impaction. Coins generally are described as oriented in the coronal plane when they are located in the esophagus on the frontal radiograph, although reports have been made of sagittally oriented coins in the esophagus.[15] Inflammatory changes that develop in patients with chronic foreign body impaction can be visualized as thickening of the space between the esophagus and trachea on lateral chest radiographs (e-Fig. 99-2, *A* and *B*); these changes therefore are useful in patients in whom the episode was not witnessed and the time course is not known. An esophagram often is performed in patients with a chronic foreign body impaction to evaluate for perforation or development of a tracheoesophageal fistula.

Treatment Coins, like other esophageal foreign bodies, can be removed via Foley catheter balloon extraction or endoscopy. Foley catheter extraction has been used as a safe and effective method of coin removal in children older than 1.5 years before esophageal edema has developed.[16] Despite its history of safe extractions and lower cost, Foley balloon extraction has fallen from favor because of concerns about patient safety related to airway compromise or esophageal

injury.[17] Endoscopy is now the preferred method for extraction at most centers.

Batteries

Overview Button battery ingestion by children is increasing in frequency.[18] Button batteries often are found in objects such as watches, calculators, toys, and hearing aids. Management of battery ingestion is different than that of coins, because batteries lodged in the esophagus can cause severe damage in as little as 2 hours.[18] Tissue damage is caused by one of three mechanisms: leak of alkaline contents, pressure necrosis, and generation of a current causing electrolysis of tissue fluids at the battery's negative pole.[18]

Clinical Presentation If ingestion is witnessed, extraction should occur before the development of symptoms. If symptoms develop, they include drooling, chest discomfort, choking, gagging, and airway obstruction. Damage can include esophageal perforation or creation of a fistula to the trachea or to a major blood vessel, leading to exsanguination.[18]

Imaging Batteries can be distinguished on radiographs by their characteristic halo appearance with a circle of lucency just within the outer border (Fig. 99-3 and e-Fig. 99-4). An esophagram with water-soluble iso-osmolal contrast can be performed after removal to evaluate for the presence of complications, such as esophageal perforation or a tracheoesophageal fistula.

Treatment If a battery is lodged in the esophagus, the clinician who requested the imaging study should be contacted immediately to arrange emergent extraction. Follow-up imaging may be indicated, as previously discussed.

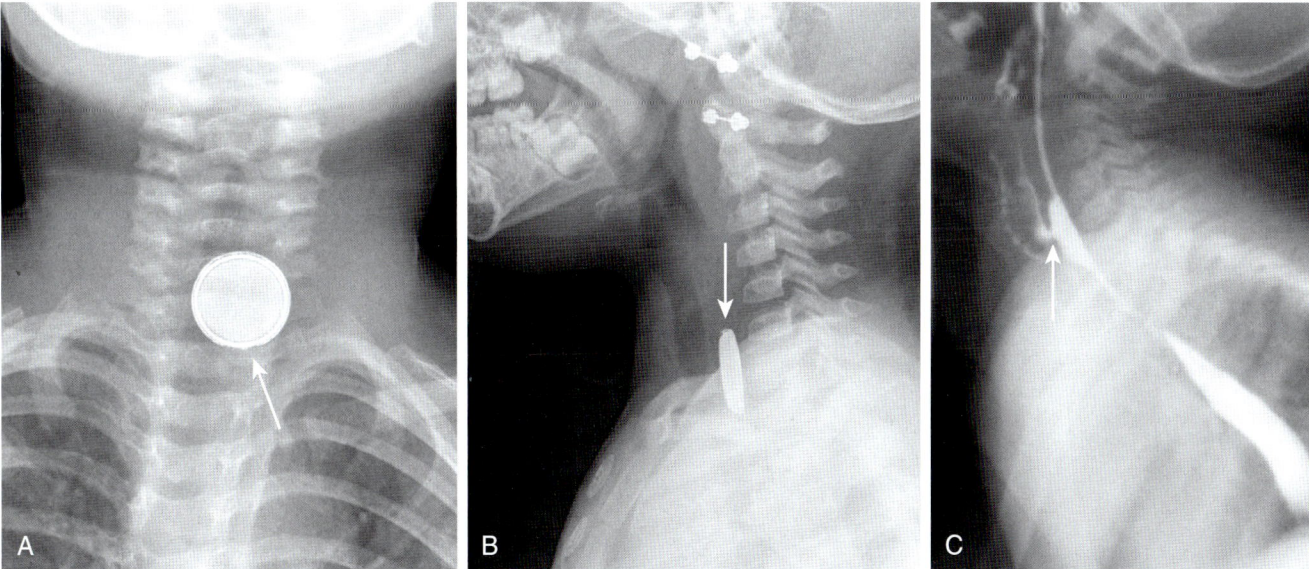

Figure 99-3 A swallowed battery. **A,** A frontal radiograph of the airway shows a button battery (*arrow*) lodged in the proximal esophagus. The inferior margin of the battery is eroded and has an irregular edge. Note that the battery has a characteristic appearance with alternating dense and lucent bands. **B,** A lateral radiograph of the airway shows the button battery (*arrow*) lodged in the proximal esophagus. On the lateral view, the edge of the battery has a beveled appearance. **C,** A lateral view from an esophagram after removal of the battery shows a tracheoesophageal fistula (*arrow*) at the site where the battery was lodged.

FOOD BOLUS IMPACTION

Overview Impacted food boluses are relatively infrequent in children but may be the initial presenting symptom of eosinophilic esophagitis, peptic stricture, achalasia, vascular rings, or an extrinsic mass.[19,20] Eosinophilic esophagitis is the major cause of food bolus impaction in children, accounting for >50% of all cases. The most common remaining cause of food bolus impaction in children is an area of narrowing in a patient with prior esophageal atresia repair or Nissen fundoplication surgery.[21]

Clinical Presentation Acute impaction of food typically leads to symptoms of dysphagia and drooling; difficulty swallowing may lead to aspiration.

Imaging On UGI imaging, an impacted food bolus appears as a persistent filling defect in the esophagus (Fig. 99-5). The impacted food can completely obstruct the esophagus, which is seen on UGI imaging as a standing column of contrast that does not pass beyond the food bolus.

Treatment When a food bolus is identified, it is removed endoscopically. An esophagram can be performed after extraction or passage of the food bolus to evaluate for the underlying cause, if it is not already known. An esophageal biopsy is recommended in patients diagnosed with food bolus impaction, particularly if they do not have a history of prior esophageal surgery.

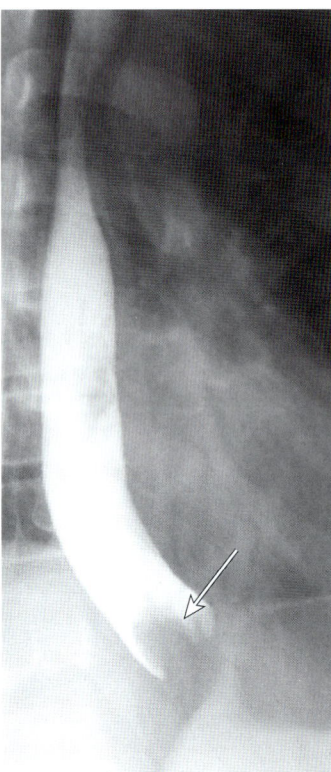

Figure 99-5 Food impaction. An esophagram shows a persistent filling defect (*arrow*) in the distal esophagus. The patient underwent endoscopy to remove the food bolus. The biopsy obtained during endoscopy confirmed a diagnosis of eosinophilic esophagitis.

CAUSTIC INGESTION

Overview Ingestion of caustic materials remains relatively common in childhood. In 2009, a total of 212,263 ingestions of household cleansers were reported to the American Poison Control Centers, more than 75% of which occurred in children.[13] The age group at highest risk for caustic ingestion is children younger than 5 years,[13] with a peak around 2 years of age when children are learning to explore their home but are not yet able to distinguish between harmless and harmful substances.[22]

Whereas caustic ingestion is usually accidental in children, in adults or adolescents it is usually purposeful. The extent and severity of injury depends on several factors: the corrosiveness of the ingested substance, the quantity ingested, the physical state of the substance, the duration of the contact time of the substance with the esophagus, and subsequent secondary infection.[22,23]

A variety of substances can cause a caustic injury, including alkalis (pH up to 12) and acids (pH as low as 2). In contrast to acidic substances, which are sour, alkalis have a relatively innocuous taste, leading to ingestion of a greater volume.[22] Further, alkaline agents produce liquefaction necrosis and rapid penetration, leading to more severe injury.[23]

Clinical Presentation After caustic ingestion, patients with severe injury typically present with pain, drooling, and airway symptoms; more visible signs of tissue damage include lip swelling, mouth ulcers, and erythema of the tongue.[22] Esophageal stricture is an important late complication of caustic ingestion, occurring in 2% to 63% of patients[23]; it can form in as little as 3 weeks after injury.[24]

Imaging Initial management of patients with caustic ingestion includes a radiograph of the chest and lateral neck to evaluate for pneumomediastinum. An esophagram is not indicated in the acute phase because it delays endoscopy and does not reveal mucosal injuries.[22]

When strictures develop, they can be diagnosed on the basis of symptoms and confirmed with an esophagram (Fig. 99-6 and e-Fig. 99-7). Caustic strictures can be focal or can occupy a long segment of the esophagus depending on the substance ingested; acid ingestion typically causes a focal or short segment stricture, whereas alkali substances cause a long segment stricture.[24] Strictures most commonly occur in the upper or mid esophagus. Multiple strictures also can occur.

Treatment Acutely, patients are treated with steroids, proton pump inhibitors, and antibiotics. Endoscopic evaluation is performed to assess the extent of damage and to grade the injury. Strictures are first treated with balloon dilation under fluoroscopy. The advantage of balloon dilation over dilation using a bougie is that balloons dilate strictures in a radial direction rather than in a longitudinal direction. This is thought to be less likely to cause an esophageal perforation.[22] After the balloon is inflated and the waist is seen to disappear, an esophagram is performed to evaluate for a leak that occurs in 4% to 30% of patients.[24] If balloon dilation fails, operative treatment with either stricture resection or esophageal replacement is performed.

Patients with a history of caustic ingestion are at risk of developing squamous cell carcinoma of the esophagus. Given

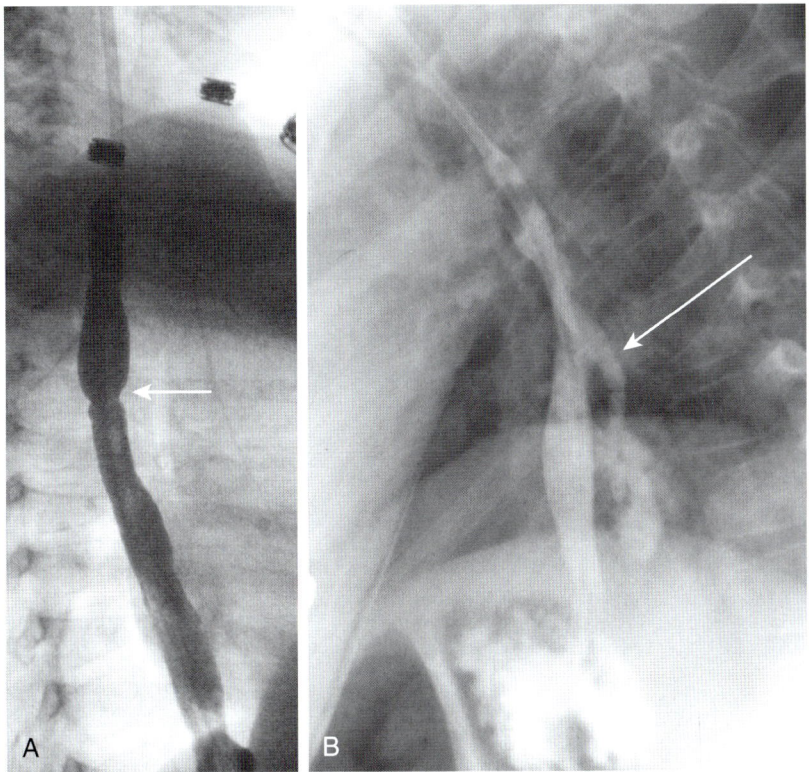

Figure 99-6 Caustic ingestion. **A,** An esophagram in a patient with a recent history of lye ingestion shows an irregular contour of the esophagus and a focal area of narrowing (*arrow*). **B,** An esophagram in the same patient 3 months later and immediately after dilation of an esophageal stricture shows an esophageal perforation with leakage of contrast (*arrow*).

this risk, these patients should undergo surveillance with endoscopy as adults.[22]

PILL ESOPHAGITIS

Overview Pill esophagitis is an esophageal injury caused by medications; the drugs most frequently implicated are doxycycline and alendronate.[25] Other drugs reported to cause esophageal injury include nonsteroidal antiinflammatory drugs, potassium chloride, ferrous sulfate, phenytoin, and quinidine.[25] Characteristics of medications that are more likely to cause esophageal injury include the acidity of the medication and a capsule formulation that renders it more likely to stick in the esophagus.[26] Pill esophagitis is also more likely to occur in patients with delayed esophageal transit time. Factors that delay esophageal transit include taking a pill with little or no water immediately before going to bed, decreased saliva production, and anatomic areas of narrowing.[26]

Clinical Presentation Patients with pill esophagitis typically present with dysphagia, odynophagia, and chest pain. Pill esophagitis often can be diagnosed by history alone.

Imaging UGI imaging is not commonly performed due to the classic history but can show a circular area of ulceration. If endoscopy is performed, a circular ulceration is identified with normal surrounding mucosa. The ulceration typically occurs at an anatomic area of narrowing such as at the level of the aortic arch, left mainstem bronchus, or gastroesophageal junction.[26]

Treatment Pill esophagitis is treated by changing pill-taking habits (e.g., taking pills with more water or taking pills long before going to bed), crushing pills, taking a liquid suspension, or switching medications.

IATROGENIC TRAUMA

Overview Iatrogenic trauma is the most common cause of esophageal perforation in children, representing 75% to 85% of all cases.[27] Esophageal perforation can be life-threatening because the esophagus lacks a serosa. The surrounding loose areolar connective tissue is unable to prevent the spread of infection; thus oral flora and digestive enzymes are able to spread to the mediastinum.[27] The most common cause of iatrogenic perforation in children is from stricture dilation. Other causes include complications of nasogastric tube placement, endotracheal intubation, endoscopy, pedicle screw placement, and sclerotherapy of esophageal varices.[28-30] The typical location of perforation depends on the age of the patient. In neonates, perforation typically occurs in the cervical esophagus at the pharyngeal/esophageal junction.[27]

Clinical Presentation Neonates often present after a difficult intubation with nonspecific symptoms, including drooling, choking, or coughing with feedings. In older children, perforation is more common in the thoracic esophagus. They typically present with respiratory distress, chest pain, or subcutaneous emphysema.[27]

Imaging The initial diagnostic examination is often frontal and lateral radiographs of the chest. Findings on the chest

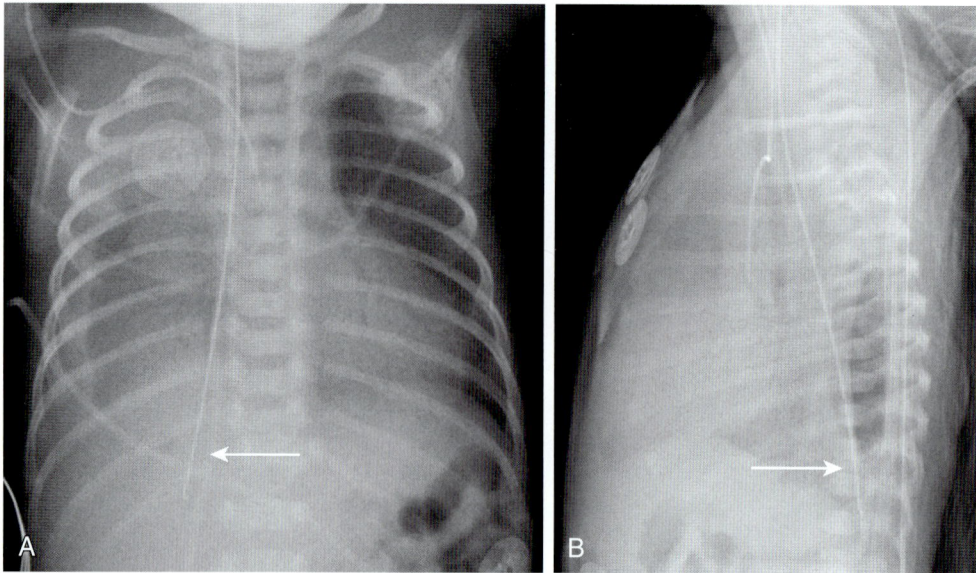

Figure 99-9 Nasogastric tube perforation. **A,** A frontal radiograph of the chest in the patient shown in Figure 99-8 one day after the initial radiograph shows a new, abnormal course of the nasogastric tube (*arrow*). The tip of the tube is now overlies the right upper quadrant, and there is a new right pleural effusion. **B,** A lateral radiograph of the chest shows an abnormal posterior course of the nasogastric tube (*arrow*). The tip of the tube projects over the right posterior costophrenic sulcus.

radiograph include pneumothorax, pneumomediastinum, and pleural effusion. If the event was caused by nasogastric tube placement, an abnormal course of the tube may be seen (e-Fig. 99-8 and Fig. 99-9).[27] The location of the perforation often can be determined from the radiograph. Left-sided pneumothorax and effusion are more likely to occur in the setting of an upper thoracic perforation, whereas right-sided findings are more likely to occur with perforations in the distal esophagus.[27]

UGI imaging can be useful in diagnosing and locating a perforation. If UGI is performed, water-soluble iso–osmolal contrast should be used first. If no contrast extravasation is noted, barium can then be used because it is more sensitive in the detection of an esophageal leak.[27] Three patterns of perforation have been described on esophagrams: first, a local cervical leak is identified if there is a retropharyngeal pocket of contrast; a submucosal leak appears as a linear tract posterior and lateral to the esophagus; finally, free perforation appears as contrast flowing into the pleural space.[27]

CT generally is not used to diagnose an esophageal perforation, but in a complex, acutely ill patient, CT may be the first study performed. Signs of esophageal perforation on CT include pneumomediastinum, mediastinal fluid, esophageal wall thickening, and a catheter extending beyond the esophageal lumen.

Treatment Treatment usually consists of expectant medical management with broad-spectrum antibiotics, pleural drainage via a chest tube, and nutritional support with total parenteral nutrition or gastrostomy; a nasogastric tube may be placed beyond the perforation under direct visualization. Operative exploration is considered in patients in whom the aforementioned more conservative management fails.[27]

BLUNT ESOPHAGEAL TRAUMA

Overview The esophagus is rarely injured after chest trauma because of its flexibility and ability to decompress via the mouth and stomach.[31] Reported causes of esophageal injury include handlebar injury, crush injury, opening a bottle of a carbonated drink in the mouth, and child abuse.[32-35] A tracheoesophageal fistula is an even rarer complication of trauma.

Clinical Presentation Patients usually present with coughing induced with swallowing. Other findings include subcutaneous emphysema, pneumothorax, dysphagia, dyspnea, and hoarseness.

Imaging A chest radiograph or CT may show pneumomediastinum and pleural effusion in a child presenting with blunt trauma. UGI can be used to confirm the diagnosis. An esophagram can be performed to diagnose a suspected tracheoesophageal fistula.[36]

BOERHAAVE SYNDROME

Overview Boerhaave syndrome is defined as spontaneous rupture of the esophagus, often after vomiting. The rupture typically involves the distal portion of the thoracic esophagus. Boerhaave syndrome is rare in children. When it does occur, nearly 50% of cases occur in neonates.[37]

Clinical Presentation Patients typically present with vomiting, lower thoracic pain, and subcutaneous emphysema.

Imaging In most children the rupture occurs on the right side, in contrast to adults, in whom the rupture is usually left sided,[37] and therefore a chest radiograph in an infant will demonstrate a right-sided pneumothorax and pleural effusion. Diagnosis is confirmed with an esophagram and/or endoscopy; however, insufflation during endoscopy may lead to a life-threatening pneumothorax.

Treatment Although children and neonates are more likely to have a better prognosis than adults, surgery remains the treatment of choice for persons with Boerhaave syndrome. A conservative approach can be used in patients with small tears and is used in patients with presentation or diagnosis greater than 24 hours.[37]

Inflammatory Conditions

EOSINOPHILIC ESOPHAGITIS

Overview Eosinophilic esophagitis is a chronic inflammatory disease characterized by dense esophageal eosinophilia. During the past decade, awareness of the disease has increased along with an increase in the number of cases diagnosed. Currently it is thought that eosinophilic esophagitis occurs with an incidence of up to 1:10,000 children per year.[38] Eosinophilic esophagitis is three to four times more common in males and can occur at any age.[39] To be diagnosed with eosinophilic esophagitis, patients must have both the histologic and clinical features of the disease. Histologically, eosinophilic esophagitis is characterized by an esophageal mucosal biopsy with more than 15 eosinophils per high-power field.

Clinical Presentation Patients present with esophageal symptoms that mimic GERD. Older children tend to present with

vomiting and abdominal pain, although in infants the presentation is more likely feeding difficulties; diagnosis in infants younger than 6 months is rare. Patients often have other signs of atopy, including dermatitis, food allergies, and asthma.[39]

Imaging Because the symptoms of eosinophilic esophagitis are protean and simulate those of GERD, diagnosis often is delayed. UGI frequently is performed as part of the diagnostic workup of patients because of their esophageal symptoms. On UGI imaging, the most common finding is a normal esophagus.[40] The most common positive findings are GER, irregular contractions, esophageal dysmotility, esophageal strictures, esophageal rings, small caliber esophagus, and food bolus impaction (Fig. 99-10).[40]

Treatment Eosinophilic esophagitis is thought to represent an allergic response to food and is usually treated with attempts to identify and eliminate the offending agent(s), or with an elemental diet. Steroids also may be used alone or combined with diet therapy.[39]

EPIDERMOLYSIS BULLOSA

Overview Epidermolysis bullosa is a rare group of hereditary blistering disorders caused by mutations in genes expressed at the dermal-epidermal junction. More than 100 distinct genotypes and 20 phenotypes of disease of varying severity have been described.[41]

Clinical Presentation Patients often experience skin blistering and erosions with minor mechanical trauma. Repeated

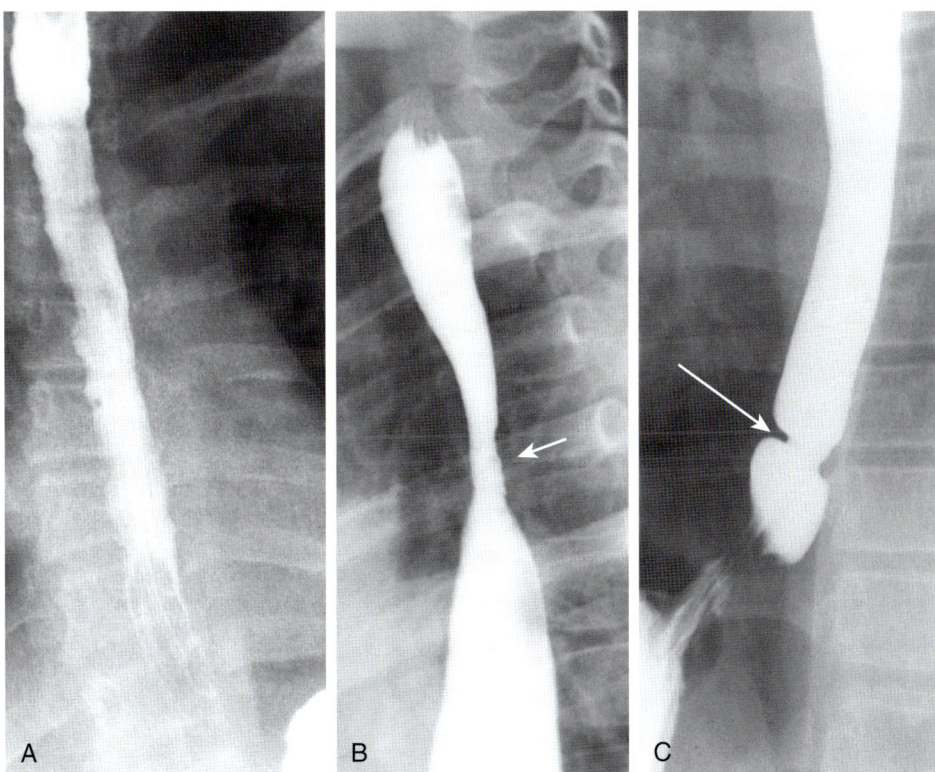

Figure 99-10 Eosinophilic esophagitis. **A,** An esophagram shows diffuse irregular contractions of the esophagus. **B,** An esophagram shows a stricture (*arrow*) of the mid esophagus. **C,** An esophagram shows a Schatzki ring (*arrow*) of the distal esophagus.

blistering leads to scar formation and causes symptoms such as contractures. Extracutaneous sites also can be affected and include the esophagus, bowel, rectum, anus, bladder, urethra, and trachea.[41]

Imaging   In the esophagus and oropharynx, scar formation leads to dysphagia and esophageal strictures. Any segment of the esophagus may be involved, although approximately half of strictures occur in the cervical esophagus.[42]

Treatment   The initial treatment of choice for esophageal strictures in children is balloon dilation under fluoroscopic or endoscopic visualization (Fig. 99-11 and e-Fig. 99-12).[41,42] Patients often require multiple dilations to treat recurrent or persistent strictures.[42]

CROHN DISEASE

Overview   Crohn disease is a chronic inflammatory disease of the gastrointestinal tract characterized by waxing and waning symptoms, transmural inflammation of the bowel wall, and skip lesions. It can affect any portion of the gastrointestinal tract from the mouth to the anus, but it most commonly affects the small bowel and colon in children. Esophageal symptoms of Crohn disease are uncommon; however, endoscopic and histologic findings are more frequent and occur in 7.6% and 17.6%, respectively.[43]

Clinical Presentation   Dysphagia is the most common symptom of esophageal Crohn disease followed by odynophagia, chest pain, nausea, and vomiting.[44]

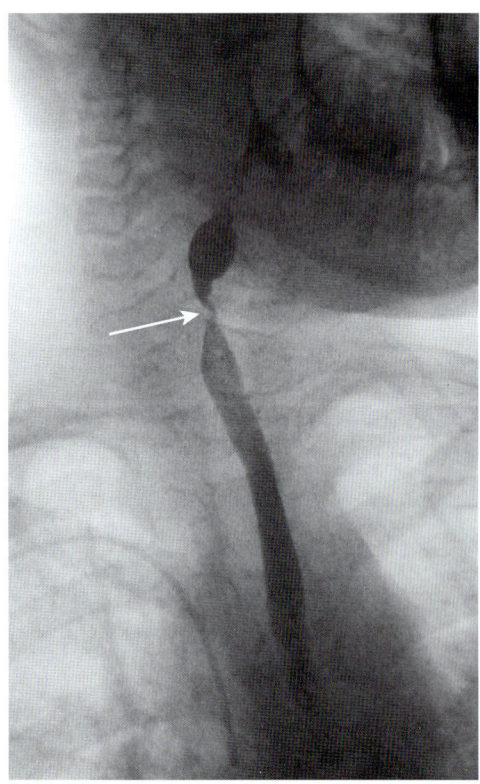

Figure 99-11   Epidermolysis bullosa. An esophagram shows a tight stricture (*arrow*) in the cervical esophagus.

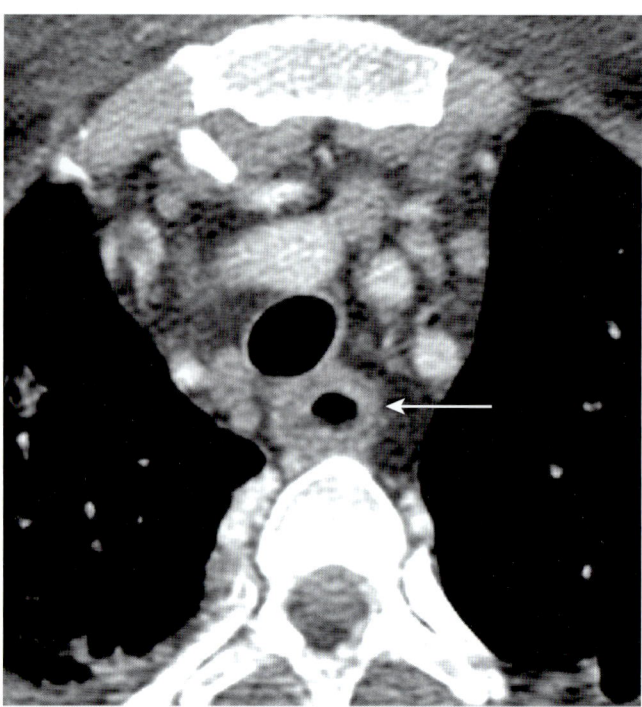

Figure 99-13   Chronic granulomatous disease. Axial contrast-enhanced computed tomography shows thickening of the wall of the proximal esophagus (*arrow*).

Imaging   Although the esophagram often is normal, esophageal Crohn disease can manifest with mucosal irregularity, aphthous ulcers, or stricture.[43]

CHRONIC GRANULOMATOUS DISEASE

Overview   Chronic granulomatous disease is an uncommon primary immunodeficiency characterized by recurrent bacterial and fungal infections occurring at epithelial surfaces. Gastrointestinal manifestations are present in most patients with chronic granulomatous disease. Any portion of the gastroesophageal tract may be involved from the mouth to the anus. Esophageal involvement is uncommon.

Clinical Manifestations   The symptoms overlap those of other entities affecting the esophagus and include vomiting, dysphagia, heartburn, and odynophagia.[43]

Imaging   In the esophagus, dysmotility and strictures have been seen on UGI.[45] CT of the chest can demonstrate esophageal wall thickening (Fig. 99-13).[46]

BEHÇET SYNDROME

Overview   Behçet disease is an immune-mediated systemic vasculitis that affects multiple systems. It likely represents an exaggerated inflammatory endothelial response. The entity is more prevalent in Mediterranean and Middle Eastern countries, as well as Japan and Southeast Asia.

Clinical Manifestations   Behçet syndrome is a multisystem disorder characterized by pyoderma, gastrointestinal and genital mucous membrane ulceration, uveitis, and central nervous system vasculitis.[47] Oral ulcerations often are the first manifestation of disease. Because these ulcerations are non-specific, diagnosis often is delayed until abnormalities of the genitals, gastrointestinal system, or central nervous system develop. Patients also are at risk of experiencing venous thrombosis and arterial aneurysms, which can be life threatening.

Imaging In the esophagus, dysmotility, ulceration, and stricture have been described on UGI imaging.[47] These findings often are difficult to distinguish from Crohn disease. Diagnosis is made by the presence of mouth ulcers in association with two other major criteria, including skin lesions, recurrent genital ulcerations, or the presence of an excessive dermal inflammatory response termed "pathergy."

Treatment Treatment is geared at reducing the overactive inflammatory response and includes corticosteroids, azathioprine, and interferon.[45]

INFECTIOUS ESOPHAGITIS

Overview Infectious esophagitis typically is seen in immunocompromised children. Affected children may have a congenital or acquired immunodeficiency. Children receiving immunosuppressive therapy such as chemotherapy or post-transplant immunosuppression also may be affected.

Imaging Endoscopy has replaced UGI imaging as the method of diagnosing infective esophagitis because of its ability to visualize the abnormality directly and to obtain a tissue sample for culture. If UGI is performed for infectious esophagitis, the double-contrast technique is preferred, if possible, to visualize mucosal detail.

CANDIDA ESOPHAGITIS

Overview *Candida albicans* is the most common infective agent causing esophagitis.[48] Oropharyngeal candidiasis is the strongest risk factor for the development of esophagitis in patients with neutropenia or human immunodeficiency virus (HIV) infection.

Clinical Manifestations Patients typically present with odynophagia, dysphagia, and chest pain.

Imaging On endoscopy, the appearance of esophageal candidiasis varies from a few small, raised white plaques to confluent plaques with hyperemia and ulceration.[48] An esophagram is less sensitive than endoscopy in making the diagnosis.[48] On esophagram, severe infection is characterized by a shaggy appearance of the esophagus as a result of multiple ulcers and nodular plaques.

Treatment Treatment is with antifungal medications, including fluconazole and nystatin. Caspofungin and amphotericin are reserved for systemic cases and cases resistant to therapy. Prophylactic therapy is used in immunocompromised patients.

CYTOMEGALOVIRUS ESOPHAGITIS

Overview Cytomegalovirus (CMV) is common in the population at large and is one of the more common opportunistic infections in immunocompromised patients. When it affects the GI tract, CMV most commonly involves the esophagus and the colon.

Clinical Manifestations Patients with CMV involving the GI tract present with chronic diarrhea, abdominal pain, bleeding, perforation, odynophagia, peritonitis, and bowel obstruction.[49]

Imaging Esophagitis is the second most common gastrointestinal manifestation of CMV infection after colitis.[49] Endoscopy is the diagnostic method of choice; however, UGI imaging can demonstrate the large, shallow ulcers characteristic of CMV infection.

Treatment The most effective treatment for CMV infection in immunocompromised patients is restoration of immunocompetence, such as the use of antiretroviral agents in patients with HIV.[49]

HUMAN IMMUNODEFICIENCY VIRUS ESOPHAGITIS

Overview Giant esophageal ulcers can occur in patients with HIV infection. Ulcers in these patients have several different causes, including CMV, *Candida albicans*, mycobacteria, and herpes simplex virus.[50] The ulcer is called an HIV-related or idiopathic giant ulcer when the cause of the ulcer cannot be attributed to a known pathogen.

Clinical Presentation Patients present with esophageal symptoms of odynophagia, dysphagia, and retrosternal chest pain and may experience hematemesis. Complications include bleeding, strictures, and fistulas into the tracheobronchial tree.[51]

Imaging Idiopathic giant ulcers typically occur in the middle to distal third of the esophagus. Smaller satellite ulcers also may be present.[50] Idiopathic giant ulcers are difficult to distinguish from ulcers caused by CMV infection, although idiopathic giant ulcers are said to be larger and have overhanging edges.[50]

Treatment Treatment is geared to the infectious agent that is identified. If the ulcer is idiopathic, treatment is with steroids; thalidomide also may be added.[51]

TUBERCULOSIS

Overview Involvement of the esophagus by tuberculosis is rare, occurring in 0.15% of patients. Several reports have been made of esophageal erosion with formation of a tracheoesophageal fistula in patients with tuberculosis.[52,53] Esophageal perforation is thought to occur by one of three methods: rupture of a mediastinal abscess into the esophagus, formation of a traction diverticulum as a result of tuberculous mediastinitis, or erosion as a result of pressure necrosis of adjacent lymph nodes.[52]

Clinical Presentation Symptoms depend on the complications; patients with esophagotracheal or esophagobronchial fistulas may experience extensive coughing after the ingestion of fluids, along with hematemesis.[54]

Imaging   When a perforation occurs, an esophagram shows extraluminal extension of contrast into the mediastinum or through the fistula. On CT, large, low-density mediastinal lymph nodes are observed in addition to pneumomediastinum.

Treatment   Treatment is geared to addressing the complications in addition to use of antituberculous medications.

Esophageal Motility Disorders

Primary esophageal motility disorders are uncommon in children. Esophageal dysmotility usually is most commonly seen in patients with prior esophageal surgery or as a result of an underlying inflammatory condition such as GERD.

ESOPHAGEAL ATRESIA

Overview   Esophageal atresia is a congenital malformation occurring in 1 in 2500 births (see Chapter 97, Congenital and Neonatal Abnormalities). It is corrected via surgical repair in the early neonatal period. The repair has several potential complications: recurrent tracheoesophageal fistula, esophageal strictures at the site of anastomosis, and food bolus impaction (Fig. 99-14).

Esophageal dysmotility is nearly ubiquitous in patients with a history of esophageal atresia. Two potential theories for the etiology of esophageal dysmotility have been proposed: primary dysgensis of the esophageal nerve supply, or postoperative damage to the esophageal nerve supply after the initial repair.[55]

ACHALASIA

Overview   Achalasia is a primary motor disorder characterized by failure of the lower esophageal sphincter to relax with swallowing.[56] Achalasia typically presents with dysphagia, chest pain, vomiting, regurgitation, or symptoms of GER.[57] Diagnosis can be made via manometry, upper endoscopy, or UGI imaging. Manometry is the gold standard for diagnosis and shows aperistalsis of the smooth muscle of the esophagus, incomplete relaxation of the lower esophageal sphincter, and elevated resting pressure in the lower esophageal sphincter.[58] Biopsy confirms the diagnosis of achalasia with hypertrophy of the muscularis and absent ganglion cells.

Clinical Presentation   Patients present with progressive dysphagia, regurgitation, chest pain, nocturnal cough, and heartburn.[58] Aspiration pneumonia, esophageal perforation, or esophageal cancer can develop in patients with untreated achalasia.

Imaging   On the chest radiograph, the esophagus can appear dilated and filled with air (Fig. 99-15). This appearance is often unusual and can mimic a medial pneumothorax. UGI

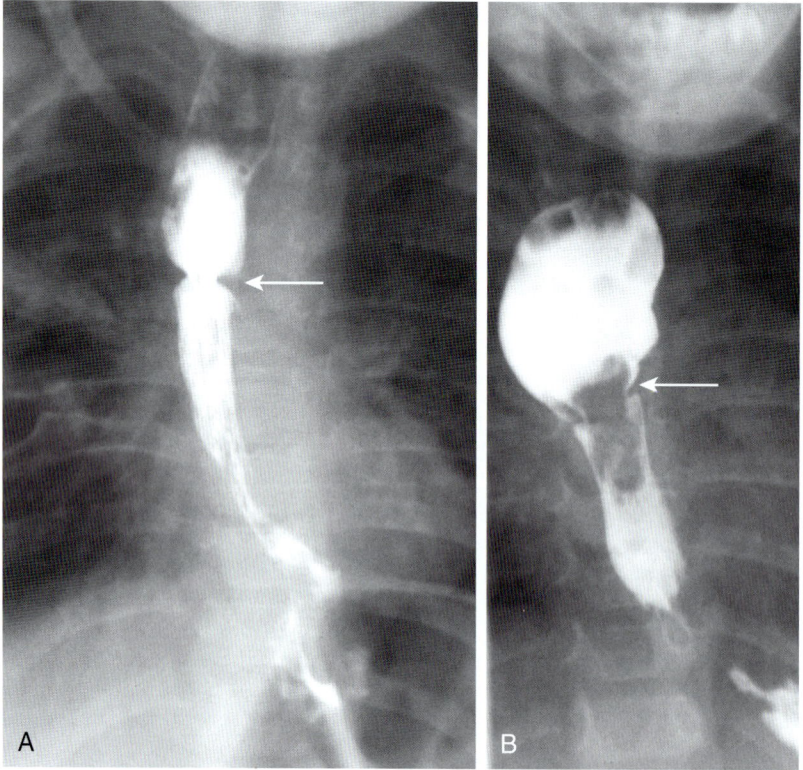

Figure 99-14   Repaired esophageal atresia and tracheoesophageal fistula. **A,** An esophagram shows a stricture (*arrow*) at the esophageal anastomosis site and typical dilatation of the upper esophageal pouch. **B,** An esophagram in a different patient shows a persistent filling defect (*arrow*) at the site of the esophageal anastomosis representing impacted food. The proximal esophagus is dilated as a result of a history of esophageal atresia and the partial obstruction.

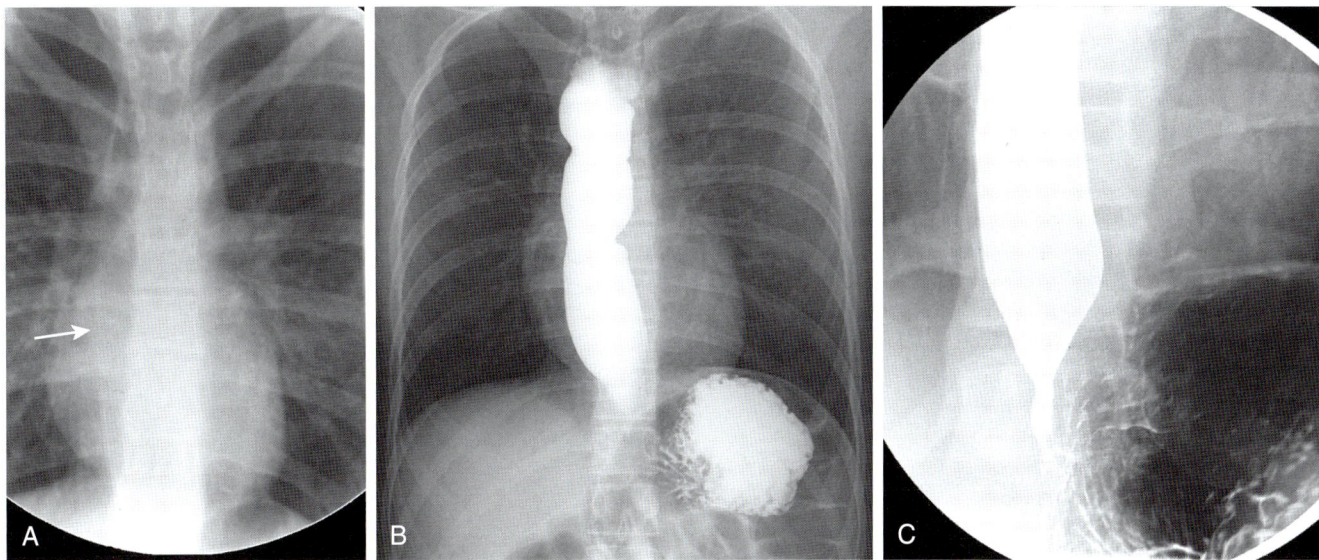

Figure 99-15 Achalasia. **A,** A frontal radiograph of the chest in a patient with achalasia shows a linear density representing the lateral wall of the dilated, air-filled esophagus (*arrow*) in the right paraspinal region. **B,** An overhead radiograph of the chest after completion of an esophagram shows a dilated and irregular esophagus with a narrowed gastroesophageal junction. **C,** A spot image from the esophagram shows the dilated distal esophagus coming to a point at the gastroesophageal junction. The distal narrowing gives the characteristic bird's beak appearance of achalasia.

imaging shows dilation of the proximal esophagus, lack of peristalsis, and smooth tapering of the distal esophagus with a bird's beak appearance near the gastroesophageal junction.[58] This appearance of the distal esophagus also can be seen on sonography[58] and should be recognized if it is captured incidentally during abdominal ultrasound imaging.

Treatment Achalasia can be treated with balloon dilation or Heller myotomy.[57]

Esophageal Masses

LEIOMYOMAS

Overview Although they are rare, leiomyomas are the most common esophageal tumor in children. In contrast to adults, the lesions in children are more likely to be multiple or diffuse.[59] Diffuse esophageal leiomyomatosis is a rare hamartomatous condition in which proliferation of the smooth muscle of the esophagus occurs. Esophageal leiomyomatosis can be associated with leiomyomas at other sites or with Alport syndrome (i.e., nephropathy, astigmatism, and myopia).[60]

Clinical Presentation Isolated leiomyomas may be an incidental finding, or patients may present with progressive symptoms of dysphagia, vomiting, regurgitation, weight loss, and retrosternal pain.[60]

Imaging Two potential findings on a chest radiograph are a tubular posterior mediastinal mass and rightward deviation of the azygoesophageal stripe.[59,60] Findings on an esophagram can mimic achalasia and demonstrate a dilated tortuous esophagus with decreased peristalsis, tapered narrowing, and deviation from midline caused by the intramural masses.[60] If cross-sectional imaging is performed, it can show diffuse circumferential wall thickening of the esophagus; a discrete soft tissue mass protruding from the esophagus also may be present.[60]

Treatment Diffuse esophageal leiomyomatosis generally is treated with an esophagectomy and gastric pull-through.

MALIGNANCIES

Esophageal malignancies are very rare in children. Several conditions place patients at a higher risk for malignancy, including GERD with Barrett esophagitis, caustic ingestion, and achalasia. Esophageal carcinoma is more common in certain regions of the world because of a nutritional deficiency of trace elements, consumption of pickled moldy foods, nitrosamines, and thermal injury. Areas with endemic human papilloma virus infection also have a higher incidence of esophageal carcinoma.[61]

Extraesophageal tumors can abut the esophagus. The most common thoracic tumors to affect the esophagus are thoracic neuroblastomas and plexiform neurofibromas[62] (Figs. 99-16 and 99-17). These tumors can cause mass effect on the esophagus but rarely invade it. Depending on the degree of mass effect, the patient can present with dysphagia.

Other Esophageal Lesions

ESOPHAGEAL VARICES

Overview Esophageal varices are seen in the setting of portal hypertension. Varices primarily occur around the esophagus, stomach, spleen, and retroperitoneum. When portal hypertension is suspected, endoscopy is the best method to screen for varices.

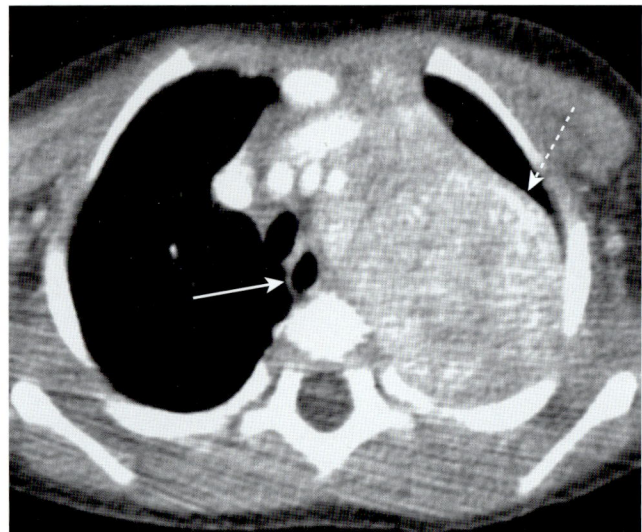

Figure 99-16 Neuroblastoma. Axial contrast-enhanced computed tomography shows a large, partially calcified left paraspinal neuroblastoma (*dashed arrow*) displacing the esophagus (*arrow*) toward the right.

Clinical Presentation Patients present with symptoms of portal hypertension; varices themselves are silent until an episode of bleeding ensues. Variceal bleeding is the most serious complication of portal hypertension and is associated with a mortality of up to 30%.[63]

Imaging Varices can be identified on contrast-enhanced CT as dilated serpiginous vessels (Fig. 99-18). On UGI imaging, they appear as a lobulated filling defect in the distal esophagus.

Treatment Varices typically are treated with sclerotherapy, banding, or placement of a portosystemic shunt.

ESOPHAGEAL DIVERTICULA

Overview Esophageal diverticula are uncommon in children. They can be associated with stricture, prior esophageal atresia repair, prior injury such as with a chronic foreign body, and connective tissue disorders such as Ehlers-Danlos syndrome.[64-66]

PLUMMER-VINSON SYNDROME

Overview Plummer-Vinson syndrome is an uncommon disease that typically occurs in middle-aged white women, although it can occur in the pediatric age group.

Clinical Presentation Plummer-Vinson syndrome is characterized by dysphagia, iron deficiency anemia, and esophageal webs. It is associated with celiac disease and increased menstrual blood loss.[67]

Imaging The esophageal webs are best seen on esophagram or UGI where they typically occur in the proximal esophagus. They are characterized by one or more thin, horizontal membranes in the esophageal lumen.[67]

Treatment Patients are treated for the underlying cause of anemia along with iron supplements and esophageal dilation. Esophageal or pharyngeal cancer occurs in 3% to 15% of patients with Plummer-Vinson syndrome.[67]

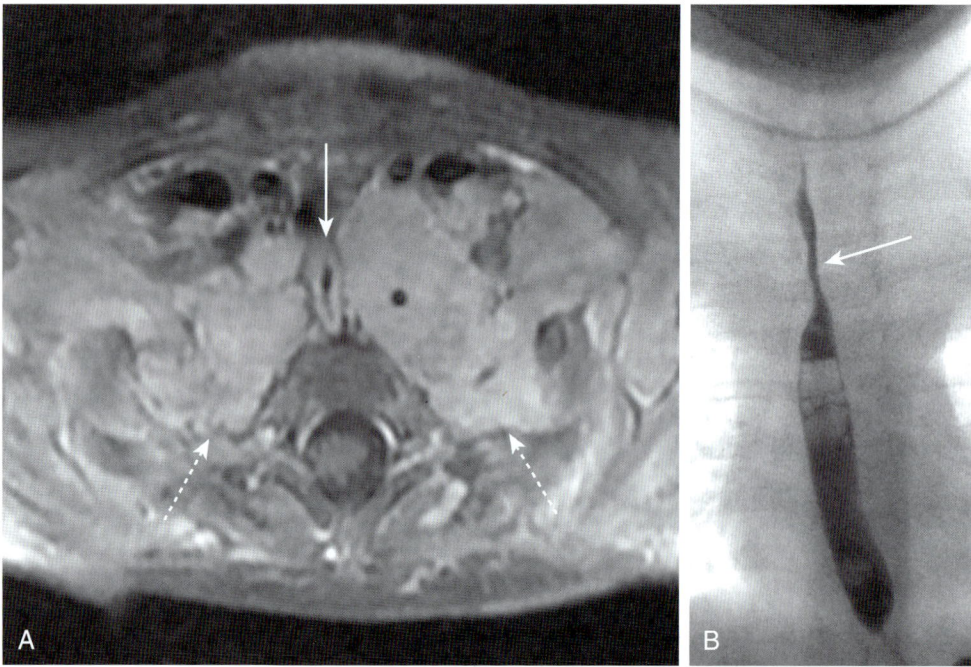

Figure 99-17 Neurofibromatosis. **A,** T1-weighted postcontrast image of the upper chest in a patient with type 1 neurofibromatosis show bilateral plexiform neurofibromas (*dashed arrows*) occupying the lung apices and extending to the axillae. The masses are compressing the esophagus (*arrow*). **B,** An esophagram in the same patient shows narrowing of the proximal esophagus (*arrow*) as it passes between the plexiform neurofibromas; the density from the masses extending to the thoracic apices also can be appreciated.

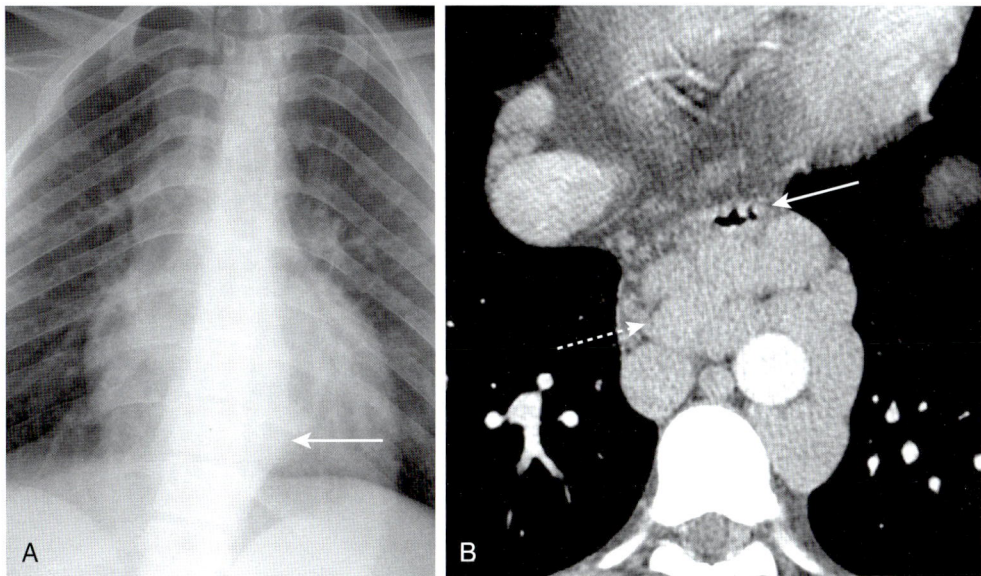

Figure 99-18 Portal hypertension and esophageal varices. **A,** A frontal radiograph of the chest in a patient with portal hypertension shows a soft tissue mass (*arrow*) in the left paraspinal region. **B,** Axial contrast-enhanced computed tomography in the same patient shows multiple dilated paraesophageal varices (*dashed arrow*) displacing the esophagus anteriorly (*arrow*).

Key Points

The symptoms of GERD depend on age.

When compared with adults, children with GERD report fewer episodes of heartburn, dysphagia, and chest pain and more episodes of vomiting and regurgitation.

Provocative maneuvers or prolonged fluoroscopy is not recommended for the detection of GER.

Coins are the most commonly ingested foreign body.

Button batteries lodged in the esophagus should be removed emergently.

Food bolus impaction is associated with eosinophilic esophagitis.

Iatrogenic trauma is the most common cause of esophageal perforation in children.

Infectious esophagitis typically is seen in immunocompromised children.

Suggested Readings

Boyle JT. Gastroesophageal reflux disease in 2006. The imperfect diagnosis. *Pediatr Radiol.* 2006;36(suppl 2):192-195.

Callahan MJ, Taylor GA. CT of the pediatric esophagus. *AJR Am J Roentgenol.* 2003;181:1391-1396.

Fordham LA. Imaging of the esophagus in children. *Radiol Clin North Am.* 2005;43:283-302.

Staton RJ, Williams JL, Arreola MM, et al. Organ and effective doses in infants undergoing upper gastrointestinal (UGI) fluoroscopic examination. *Med Phys.* 2007;34:703-710.

References

Full references for this chapter can be found on www.expertconsult.com.

Chapter 100

Congenital and Neonatal Abnormalities

NANCY R. FEFFERMAN and SUDHA P. SINGH

Although they are relatively rare, congenital and neonatal abnormalities of the stomach may present in a clinical spectrum ranging from asymptomatic to complete gastric obstruction. These abnormalities include such entities as duplication cysts, diverticula, microgastria, and anomalies involving the antropyloric region.

Gastric Duplication Cyst

Overview Duplication cysts may occur anywhere along the gastrointestinal tract, from the mouth to the rectum. They typically occur on the mesenteric surface of the viscus to which they are attached. More than 80% are spherical and do not communicate with the lumen, whereas approximately 18% are tubular and may communicate with the lumen of the adjacent bowel. Duplication cysts are named by the segment of gut to which they are attached, not by the type of mucosa lining the lumen, which may include representatives of all portions of the gastrointestinal tract, including the pancreas.[1] Gastric duplication cysts are rare and comprise approximately 4% to 7% of intestinal duplications.[1,2]

Although the cysts usually are located along the greater curvature of the stomach, they may occur in other regions of the stomach, including the pylorus,[3-5] in addition to ectopic sites.[6] Most gastric duplication cysts are spherical and typically do not communicate with the gastric lumen. Histologically, the cysts usually are lined with gastric mucosa.[2] Ectopic pancreatic tissue has been reported in approximately 37% of cases,[1,7,8] with rare reported communication with the pancreatic ductal system.[7]

Etiology The etiology remains controversial. Several hypotheses have been postulated to explain the embryology of gastrointestinal tract duplications because no single theory is sufficient to explain the characteristics of all types of duplication cysts. These theories include abnormal luminal recanalization, intrauterine ischemia, abortive twinning, bronchopulmonary foregut malformation, and persistence of an embryologic diverticulum.[1,9-13]

Clinical Presentation Gastric duplication cysts occur more frequently in females at a ratio of 2:1.[14] If it is not discovered prenatally on ultrasound,[15,16] postnatal clinical presentation usually occurs during the first year of life[17] with symptoms including intestinal obstruction, a palpable mass, gastrointestinal bleeding, abdominal pain, and hematemesis[18,19] or melena.[20] Uncommon complications of gastric duplication cysts include pancreatitis as a result of ectopic pancreatic tissue with perforation and pseudocyst formation[21] and gastric outlet obstruction simulating hypertrophic pyloric stenosis.[4,22,23]

Imaging Although gastric duplication cysts may be evident on plain radiography as a masslike density in the upper abdomen,[18] the low sensitivity and specificity limits the utility of plain radiography. Gastrointestinal contrast examination may demonstrate an effect of the mass on the adjacent hollow viscus by the cyst (Fig. 100-1), and uncommonly it may demonstrate communication between the stomach and the cyst. Ultrasonography using a high-frequency transducer is an excellent imaging modality for characterization of these cystic masses, which often demonstrate the "gut signature" or "double-wall" sign, representing the inner hyperechoic mucosal layer and peripheral hypoechoic muscle layers typical of the gastrointestinal tract (Figs. 100-1, *B*, and 100-2); free fluid may be found in cases of perforation (Fig. 100-3). Cysts may be completely anechoic or may contain septations and internal echoes representing proteinaceous material, blood products, or debris related to infection[24] (see Fig. 100-2). Computed tomography (CT) demonstrates a well-circumscribed homogeneously low-attenuating mass in the left upper quadrant. Peripheral enhancement, wall thickening, and heterogeneous attenuation of the cyst wall may be present if complicated by inflammation. On magnetic resonance imaging (MRI), the cysts exhibit fluid characteristics at T1 and T2 weighting, but the signal may increase on T1-weighted sequences in the presence of hemorrhage or other proteinaceous material. Imaging with technetium 99m–pertechnetate is very helpful when gastric mucosa lines the cysts.[25] Meticulous technique is necessary to differentiate the duplication cyst from the adjacent stomach; multiple views may be required. Single photon emission tomography CT may be useful in defining the abnormality.

Treatment Treatment of both symptomatic and asymptomatic gastric duplication cysts entails surgery with complete

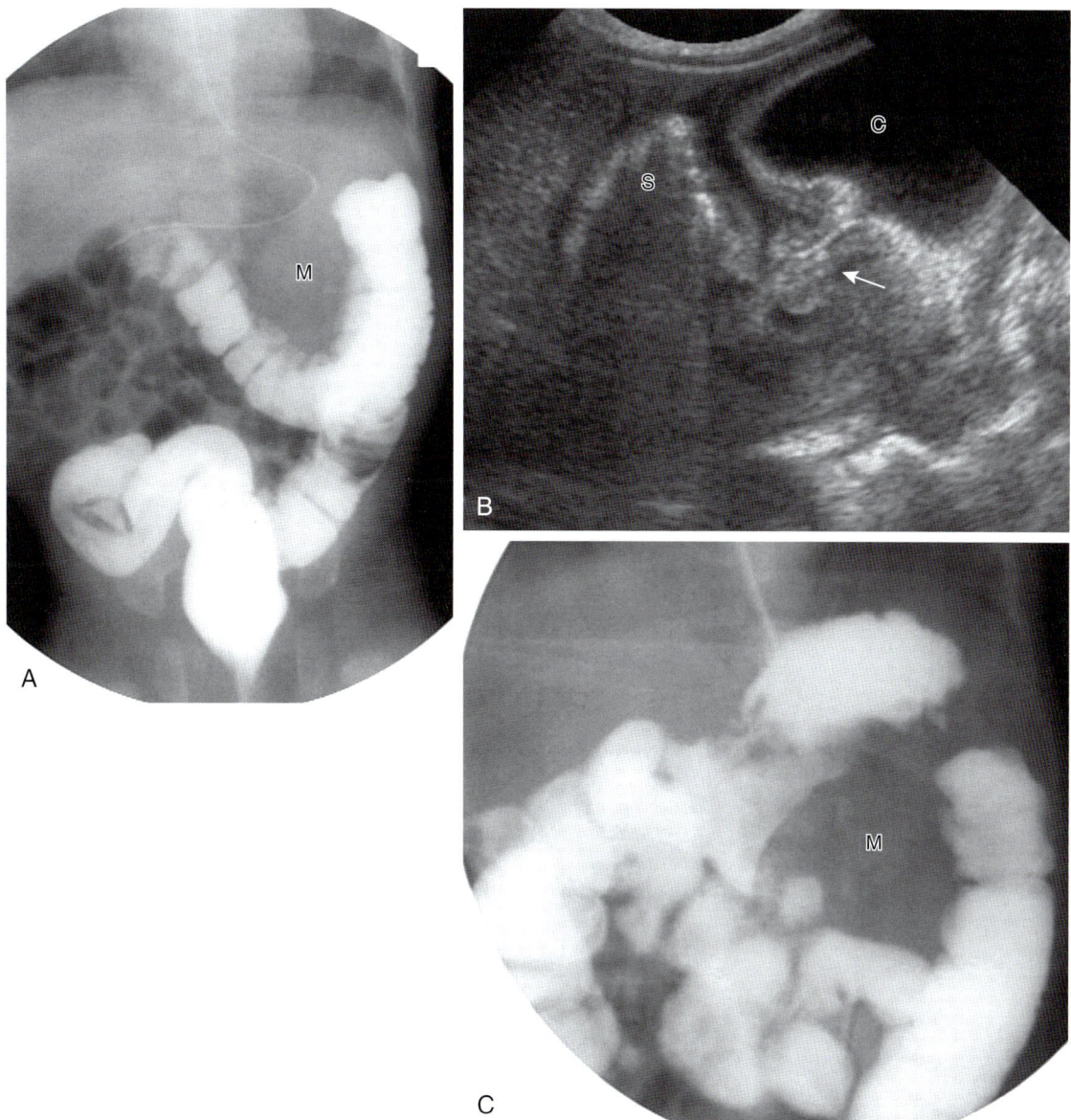

Figure 100-1 Gastric duplication in a 6-week-old infant with hematemesis. **A,** Barium enema study demonstrates a mass (*M*) between the greater curvature of the stomach and the contrast-filled transverse colon. **B,** An ultrasound study demonstrates typical findings of fluid-filled cyst (*C*). The stomach (*S*) contains shadowing gas. The connection of the cyst with the gas-filled stomach is seen (*arrow*). **O,** An upper gastrointestinal study performed after barium enema administration demonstrates mass effect (*M*) on the greater curvature of the stomach. (Courtesy Dr. D. Barlev, New York, NY.)

excision of the cyst. If the cyst cannot be resected without violating the adjacent gastric lumen, a partial gastric resection may be necessary.[7] Laparoscopic resection of gastric duplication cysts also has been described.[26-28]

Gastric Diverticula

Overview Gastric diverticula are rare in the general population, with a reported prevalence of 0.02% to 0.04%; they are even less common in children, with 4% of gastric diverticula occurring in patients younger than 20 years.[29,30]

Gastric diverticula may be congenital or acquired; the congenital form constitutes approximately 72% of all gastric diverticula. Congenital gastric diverticula are true diverticula, containing all three layers of the gastric wall. These diverticula typically involve the posterior wall of the stomach within 2 to 3 cm of the gastroesophageal junction. Acquired gastric diverticula are pseudodiverticula and usually are located near the gastric antrum.[29]

Etiology The cause of congenital gastric diverticula is thought to be related to the division of the longitudinal fibers of the wall of the stomach in such a way that results in a defect in the musculature of the gastric wall, which is affected by arterial perforators and the absence of peritoneal investment of the posterior gastric wall, which contribute to the weakness of the gastric wall.[29] Acquired diverticula, on the other hand, usually are related to peptic ulcer disease or pancreatitis.[29]

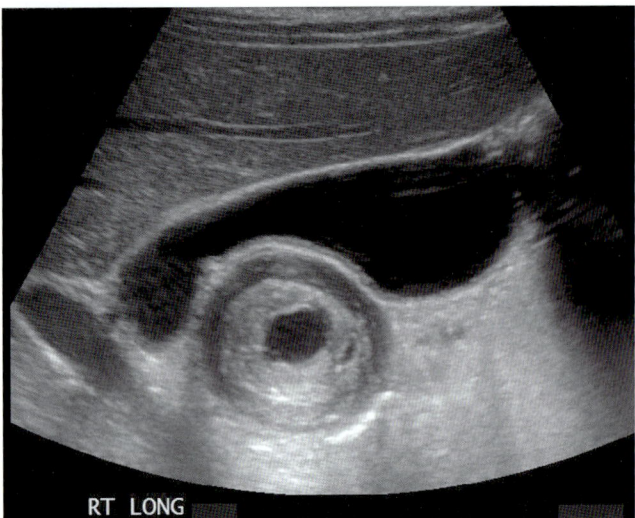

Figure 100-2 **Gastric duplication cyst.** An ultrasound image of the upper mid abdomen along the long axis of the body and antrum of the stomach demonstrates a complex cystic mass contiguous with the greater curvature of the stomach, with a hypoechoic wall suggesting the muscular layer of gut signature.

Clinical Presentation Although most gastric diverticula are clinically asymptomatic, symptomatic lesions in children tend to present in early childhood and adolescence. The symptoms can range from nonspecific complaints such as recurrent abdominal pain, nausea, and vomiting to massive hemorrhage and perforation; such symptoms may relate to the presence of ectopic pancreatic tissue within the diverticula, causing erosions and ulceration.[29,31-33] Large antral partial diverticula can cause partial gastric outlet obstruction by compression or intussusception of the antropyloric region (Fig. 100-4).

Imaging Imaging evaluation of suspected gastric diverticula includes a fluoroscopic contrast upper gastrointestinal series, which demonstrates an outpouching of the gastric wall that communicates with the gastric lumen. Right anterior oblique

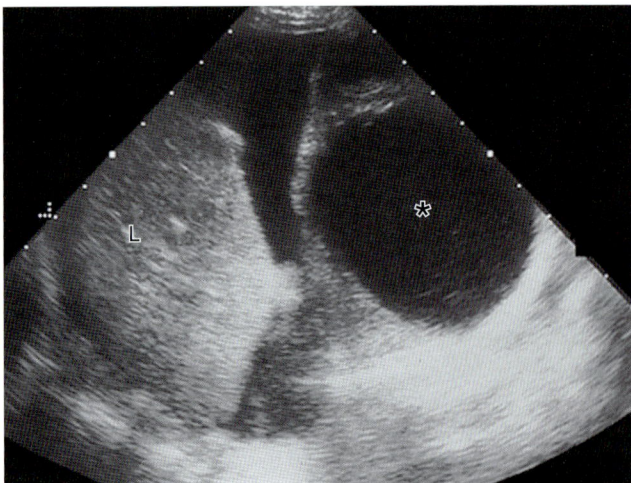

Figure 100-3 **A ruptured gastric duplication cyst.** A sagittal ultrasound image through the medial portion of the right lobe of the liver (L) demonstrates a thin-walled, approximately 4-cm simple cyst (asterisk). Free fluid, complex in its dependent portion, was found at surgery to represent hemorrhage resulting from rupture. (Courtesy Dr. C. Mitchell, Peoria, IL.)

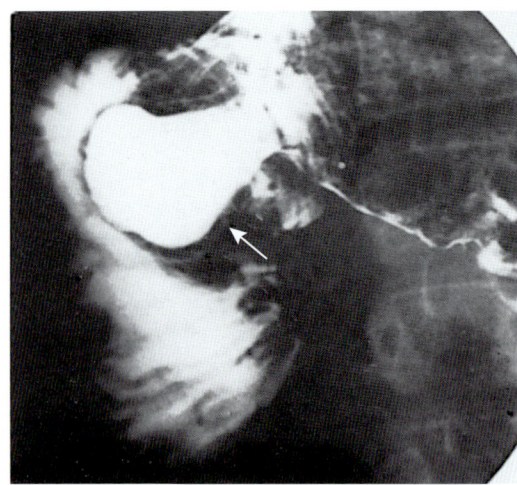

Figure 100-4 **Gastric diverticulum.** The barium-filled diverticulum is seen to be featureless with air-filled antrum (arrow) proximal to it and barium-filled duodenal sweep distal to it. The diverticulum originated at the gastroduodenal junction and was lined with gastric mucosa.

positioning optimizes the sensitivity of this imaging study because of the posterior wall location of most congenital gastric diverticula. Gastric diverticula also may be identified with cross–sectional imaging.

Treatment Symptomatic gastric diverticula may be treated pharmacologically with histamine-2 blockade. Surgical resection is reserved for patients whose symptoms are unresponsive to pharmacotherapy and can be performed with either laparotomy or laparoscopic excision.[31,34]

Congenital Microgastria

Overview Congenital microgastria is a rare anomaly of the pediatric gastrointestinal tract characterized by a small, tubular stomach, typically associated with a distended esophagus. In persons with microgastria the stomach is lined by normal gastric mucosa but the total cell mass is significantly reduced.[35,36] Agastria, or complete absence of the stomach, is the most extreme form of microgastria.

Congenital microgastria is almost always accompanied by other congenital anomalies; isolated congenital microgastria is extremely rare. Associated congenital anomalies include a wide range of entities such as heterotaxy with asplenia and malrotation,[37] congenital diaphragmatic hernia,[38] tracheoesophageal clefts, hiatal hernia,[36] jaw and palate abnormalities,[39] DiGeorge syndrome, primary ciliary dyskinesia,[40] central nervous system abnormalities, and vertebral, cardiac, renal, and limb reduction anomalies (VACTERL association). It has been suggested that microgastria in association with limb reduction defects and central nervous system anomalies may have an autosomal recessive mode of inheritance.[41,42]

Etiology Microgastria is thought to result from impaired foregut development. The embryonic foregut elongates to form the primordial stomach during the fourth week of gestation. Dilatation of the region of the future stomach occurs in the fifth week. Lateral flattening of the stomach and a 90° rotation occur during the sixth week, and the lesser and greater curvatures become established during the sixth and seventh weeks. The growth of the fundus appears during the eighth or ninth week.[35] Early arrest of the process leads to microgastria; the size and the shape of the stomach therefore depends on when the arrest of development occurs.[36] During the fifth week of gestation, the spleen begins to form along the dorsal mesogastrium of the stomach; this association in the development of the stomach and the spleen serves to explain the association of microgastria with asplenia. The association of microgastria with limb reduction anomalies is attributed to impairment of early mesodermal development.[42]

Clinical Presentation The prenatal presentation mimics esophageal atresia. Failure to visualize the fetal stomach in early second trimester scans suggests the possibility of microgastria or esophageal atresia.[37] The presence of the anomalies commonly associated with microgastria on an antenatal scan also should alert one to the possibility of microgastria. Postnatally, the clinical presentation is variable depending on the severity of microgastria and the associated anomalies present. The infant may present with feeding intolerance, severe gastroesophageal reflux, and associated anomalies, which will modulate the clinical presentation and determine overall prognosis and mortality. Rare infants with isolated microgastria may present with failure to thrive, stridor or cyanosis during feeding,[43] feeding intolerance, recurrent aspiration pneumonia, and malnutrition as a result of severe gastroesophageal reflux. Pernicious anemia may be present as a result of decreased intrinsic factor production because of the decreased gastric cell mass.

Imaging Chest and abdominal radiographs may show a very dilated or megaesophagus outlined by air. The stomach bubble may be absent. An upper gastrointestinal (UGI) series shows a small midline tubular stomach (less than 25% of the normal size) associated with severe gastroesophageal reflux and a megaesophagus as a result of the overflow from the small capacity stomach (Fig. 100-5). Esophageal motility is ineffectual as a result of the gross dilatation. Additional imaging studies, including spine radiographs, cardiac echo, ultrasound, CT, and MRI can be performed as indicated to identify associated anomalies.

Treatment The treatment for microgastria should be individualized, depending on the severity of the microgastria and associated anomalies. Conservative or medical treatment may be tried initially but usually is not effective in severe cases because the stomach does not enlarge with time. Recent literature suggests that an early operation may be indicated for better growth and development and an improved quality of life overall. Most of the patients are treated with a Hunt-Lawrence pouch (a double lumen roux-en-Y jejunal pouch) for increasing the size of the gastric reservoir with improved growth patterns after surgery.[35]

Pyloric Web, Diaphragm, and Atresia

Overview Complete and partial gastric outlet obstruction in neonates and children have been described with a spectrum

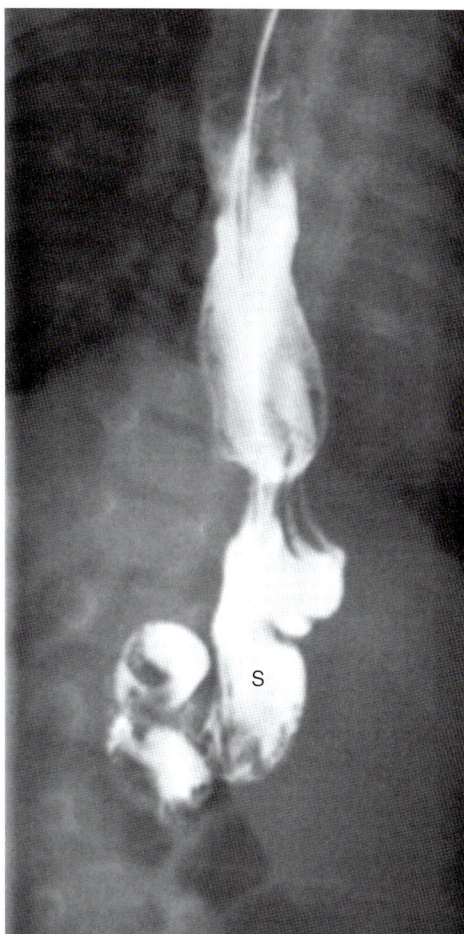

Figure 100-5 Microgastria. A frontal view, which includes the upper abdomen from an upper gastrointestinal series performed with a nasogastric tube, demonstrates a small midline stomach (*S*) with a grossly patent gastroesophageal junction and megaesophagus. The patient also has malrotation of the bowel.

of uncommon morphologic abnormalities that include atresia and webs or diaphragms of the gastric antrum or pylorus. Complete atresias involving the pylorus or antrum are extremely rare, constituting fewer than 1% of all gastrointestinal atresias.[44] Incomplete obstructions as a result of webs or diaphragms are reported to be the more commonly encountered form of this rare abnormality.[45] The webs are thin circumferential membranes measuring between 2 and 4 mm that span the lumen of the stomach, perpendicular to its long axis,[46] typically located 1 to 2 cm from the pylorus, and composed of a central core of submucosa and muscularis mucosae between two layers of gastric mucosa.

Etiology The exact etiology remains controversial; a number of theories have been postulated, including incomplete or abnormal canalization of the foregut during embryologic development or intrauterine mechanical or chemical injury.[44,47]

Clinical Presentation Complete obstruction due to antral or pyloric atresia occurs as a result of obliteration of the antropyloric channel and classically presents in the neonatal period with nonbilious vomiting. The diagnosis also may

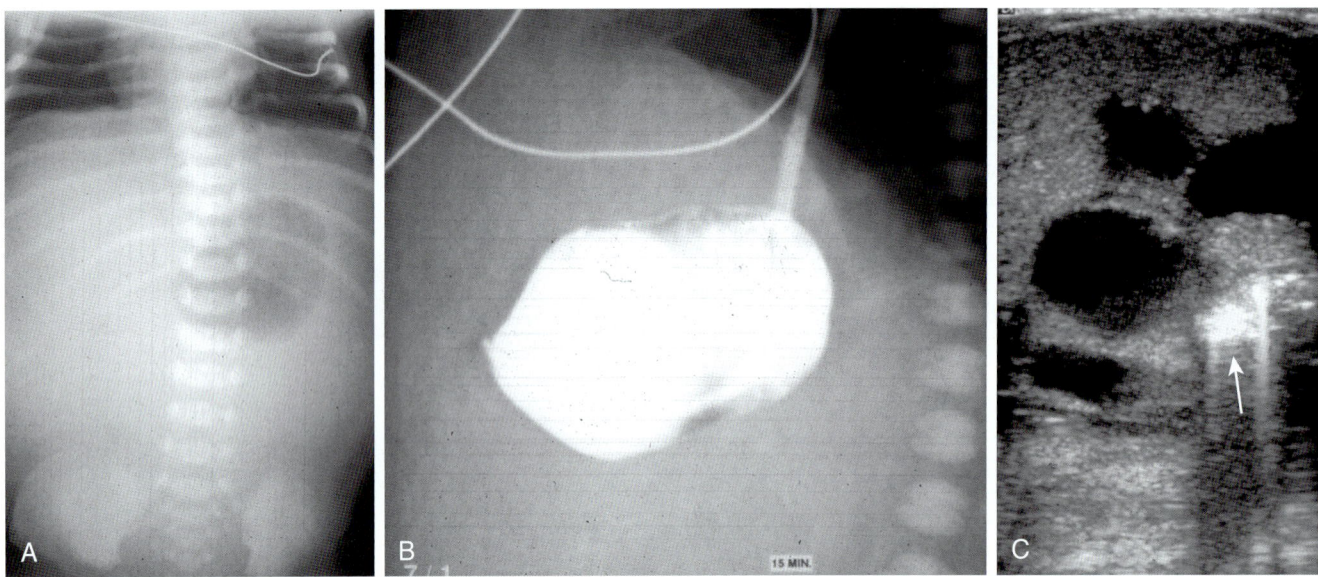

Figure 100-6 An infant with pyloric atresia associated with multiple atresias. **A,** An abdominal radiograph shows some distension of the stomach with gas and otherwise a gasless abdomen. **B,** An upper gastrointestinal image through an orogastric tube shows a blind-ending stomach with no further passage of contrast. **C,** Ultrasound examination shows gas within the blind-ending gastric antrum (*arrow*). Other loops of bowel are distended with fluid because of the multiple atresias and retained gastrointestinal secretions. (Courtesy Dr. Marta Hernanz-Schulman, MD, Nashville, TN.)

be suggested on prenatal imaging by the presence of polyhydramnios and persistent gastric distension with absence of distension of distal bowel loops.[45] Although pyloric atresia may occur as an isolated entity, it can be associated with multiple atresias and with epidermolysis bullosa (EB). According to the Third International Consensus Meeting on Diagnosis and Classification of EB, pyloric atresia is associated with the simplex and junctional forms of EB.[48] Incomplete gastric outlet obstruction due to the presence of antropyloric webs or diaphragms has a variable clinical presentation depending on the size of the orifice, which can range from 2 to 30 mm. Clinical manifestations include vomiting, failure to thrive, and intermittent abdominal pain.[49]

Imaging In patients with pyloric atresia, postnatal imaging findings include an air-filled distended gastric bubble with absence of bowel gas distal to the stomach. Fluoroscopic contrast examination will confirm gastric outlet obstruction. Ultrasound will reveal a blind-ending gastric antrum with no gas distally (Fig. 100-6).

In patients with antral web or diaphragm, fluoroscopic imaging evaluation of the stomach may demonstrate a double bulb appearance representing the distended antral segment interposed between the web and the true duodenal bulb, and/or a linear filling defect in the distal stomach outlining the antral membrane (Figs. 100-7 and 100-8). Early filling images of the stomach are recommended because visualization of the filling defect may be obscured by dense contrast. Failure to achieve maximal distal antral distension may be associated with presence of a diaphragm or web that may not be visualized.[47] Sonographic demonstration of antropyloric webs also has been described in the literature.[50] Sonography requires meticulous technique and a fluid-filled stomach; sonographic findings include gastric distension, the presence of persistent linear echogenic structure projecting into the

distal gastric lumen, and delayed gastric emptying. Definitive diagnosis is made endoscopically.

Treatment Treatment depends on clinical symptoms. Complete obstruction related to atresia requires surgical intervention to bypass the obstruction and create a patent lumen.[44] Incomplete outlet obstruction related to presence of a pyloric web may require surgical resection if the patient is clinically symptomatic. Endoscopic transection of pyloric webs has been described.[51]

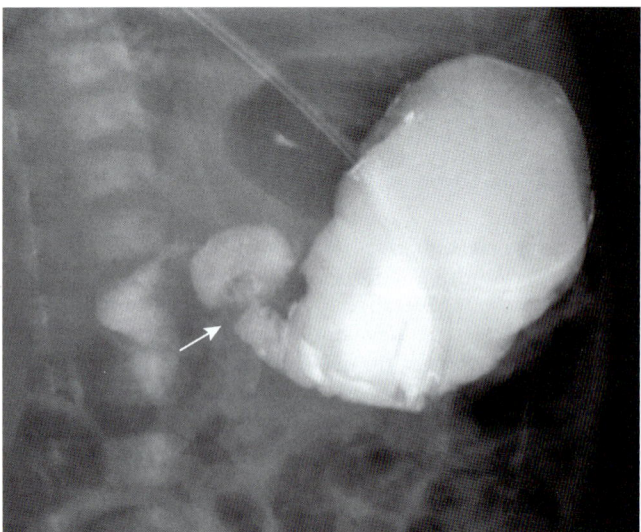

Figure 100-7 A pyloric web in an infant who presented with vomiting since birth. Introduction of barium via a nasogastric tube demonstrates a circular band or indentation in the distal antrum (*arrow*). Endoscopy demonstrated a pyloric web. (Courtesy Dr. Stuart C. Morrison, Cleveland, OH.)

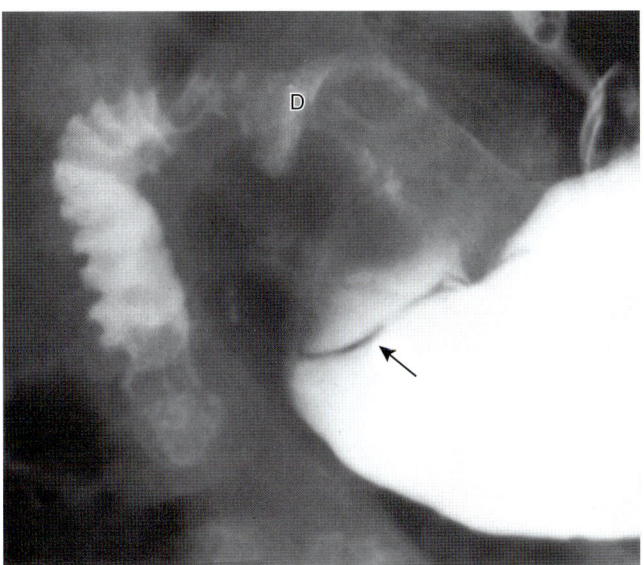

Figure 100-8 Antropyloric web. A spot image from an upper gastrointestinal series demonstrated barium in the antrum with a thin radiolucent band (*arrow*) representing a web in an older child who presented with a long history of intermittent vomiting. *D*, Duodenal bulb.

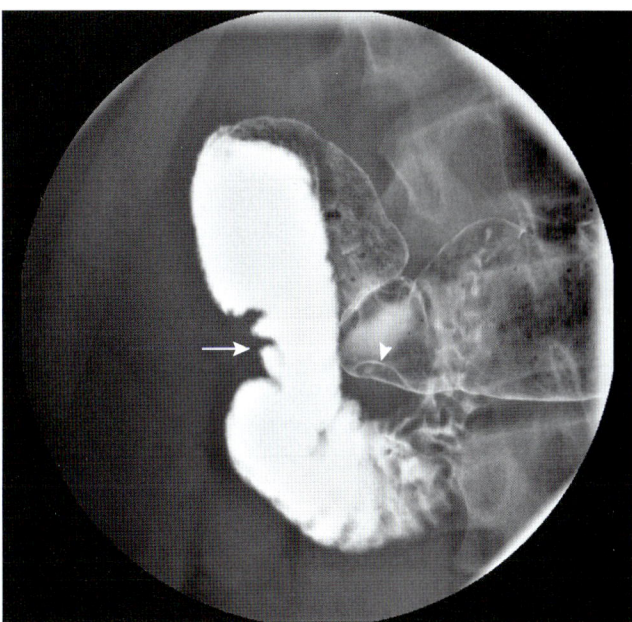

Figure 100-9 Ectopic pancreas in a teenage girl with chronic vomiting. An air contrast upper gastrointestinal series demonstrates a small mass in the pylorus with central umbilication, which was proven at surgery to represent an ectopic pancreas (*arrowhead*). Annular pancreas/duodenal stenosis also was diagnosed, as demonstrated by narrowing along the second portion of the duodenum, which also was confirmed at surgery (*arrow*).

Ectopic Pancreas

Overview An ectopic pancreas is defined as the presence of pancreatic tissue outside its normal location, with no anatomic and vascular connection with the pancreas proper.[52] It is the most common heterotopia in the gastrointestinal tract. The incidence varies widely and has been reported to be between 0.6% and 13.7% at autopsy[53] and 0.2% of laparotomies.[52] The male to female ratio is approximately 2:1. Most of the ectopic pancreas occur in the proximal gastrointestinal tract: duodenum (28%), antropyloric region of the stomach (26%), and jejunum (16%).[54] Rare sites reported include the ileum, gallbladder, Meckel diverticulum, mediastinum, umbilicus, spleen, esophagus, omentum, fallopian tubes, common bile duct, colon, urachus, adrenal gland, and ileal and jejunal diverticula.[52]

Etiology The exact etiology of ectopic pancreas is unclear. Several theories have been put forward, such as metaplasia of the pluripotential cells of the embryonic foregut or separation of pancreatic cells during early embryonic development and transplantation to other organs.[55] The ectopic pancreatic tissue may be normal with well-formed acini and ducts, may have no identifiable acini with disorganized pancreatic ducts admixed with smooth muscle (adenomyomas), or may be a combination of the two.

Typically, ectopic pancreas is an incidental finding.[56] However, the patient may present with symptoms referable to the location of the ectopic pancreatic tissue, such as abdominal pain, gastrointestinal bleeding, obstruction, and intussusception in the GI tract; if in the mediastinum, presentation may include chest pain and shortness of breath in the mediastinum. A correlation between the presence of symptoms, lesion size, and extent of mucosal involvement has been suggested. The ectopic pancreas can develop disease processes such as acute/chronic pancreatitis, pancreaticolithiasis, cysts, and tumors that involve normal pancreatic tissue.

Imaging UGI imaging typically demonstrates an intramural mound of tissue projecting into the gastric lumen in the prepyloric region along the greater curvature with a characteristic central umbilication (representing an attempt at duct formation). Diagnosis can be suggested only if the central umbilication is seen (Fig. 100-9). Endoscopic ultrasound demonstrates nonspecific findings, such as a submucosal solid mass with intermediate echogenicity.[54] CT may demonstrate localized wall thickening of the bowel or a small mass with an enhancement pattern similar to pancreatic tissue and overlying mucosal thickening. Distending the bowel lumen with negative oral contrast may be helpful.[53] MR imaging may help localize the ectopic pancreatic tissue by demonstrating an area with signal characteristics and enhancement similar to pancreatic tissue on all sequences; demonstration of ducts in the tissue or mass on MR cholangiopancreaticography is pathognomic for ectopic pancreas.[54] A preoperative definitive diagnosis of this condition is rarely made because of its rarity and nonspecific imaging findings.

Treatment An ectopic pancreas diagnosed incidentally does not require treatment. Cases with symptoms or suspicion of malignancy are treated by surgical resection of the involved segment.[54]

Key Points

Gastric duplication cysts are rare among the gastrointestinal duplications and most commonly are located along the greater curvature of the stomach.

Microgastria usually is associated with other congenital anomalies, such as the VACTERL association.

The imaging hallmark of microgastria is a small midline stomach with significant reflux into a megaesophagus.

Complete atresias involving the pylorus or antrum are extremely rare, constituting fewer than 1% of all gastrointestinal atresias. Incomplete obstructions due to webs or diaphragms are the more commonly encountered form of this rare abnormality.

Suggested Readings

Andriessen MJG, Matthyssens LE, Heij JA. Pyloric atresia. *J Pediatr Surg.* 2010;45:2470-2472.

Barlev DM, Weinberg G. Acute gastrointestinal hemorrhage in infancy from gastric duplication: imaging findings. *Emerg Radiol.* 2004;10:204-206.

Granata C, Dell'Acqua A, Lituania M, et al. Gastric duplication cyst: appearance on prenatal US and MRI. *Pediatr Radiol.* 2003;33:148-149.

Jones VS, Cohen RC. An eighteen year follow-up after surgery for congenital microgastria—case report and review of literature. *J Pediatr Surg.* 2007;42:1957-1960.

Mortelé KJ, Rocha TC, Streeter JL, et al. Multimodality imaging of pancreatic and biliary congenital anomalies. *Radiographics.* 2006;26:715-731.

Rodeberg DA, Zaheer S, Moir CR, et al. Gastric diverticulum: a series of four pediatric patients. *J Pediatr Gastroenterol Nutr.* 2002;34:564-567.

References

Full references for this chapter can be found on www.expertconsult.com.

Chapter 101

Hypertrophic Pyloric Stenosis

MARTA HERNANZ-SCHULMAN

Overview

Hypertrophic pyloric stenosis (HPS) is the most common surgical entity affecting infants during the first 6 months of life.[1] It has an incidence of approximately 2 to 5 per 1000 births among children of European descent, but its incidence is much lower in other populations—approximately 0.7 per 1000 births among children of African American or Asian extraction. The preponderance among male infants is well known, variably cited as 2.5 to 5.5:1.[2] Its incidence is inversely proportional to birth order, with odds ratio to birth order cited as 1, 2, 3, 4+ being roughly equivalent to increased risk levels of 1.9, 1.5, 1.3, and 1.0.[3] The condition demonstrates a familial predisposition, suggesting a polygenic inheritance with greater penetrance in males; thus among children of affected fathers, the risk is approximately 5% for sons and 2.5% for daughters, whereas among children of affected mothers, the corresponding risk is 20% for boys and 7% for daughters. Proband concordance in monozygotic twins is cited as between 0.25 and 0.44, whereas in dizygotic twins it is reduced to 0.05 to 0.10, which is very similar to that of nontwin siblings.[3]

Hirschsprung originally described the entity postmortem in two patients[4] and incorrectly assumed that HPS is congenital. Although some exceptions may exist, as discussed later in this chapter, data indicate that HPS is not present at birth, and its symptoms and characteristic anatomic changes typically present between 3 and 12 weeks of age. Rollins et al.[5] examined 1400 neonates who had normal ultrasound findings at birth; HPS later developed in nine of these subjects. These findings and others lend credence to the belief that the disease evolves over a course of days to weeks.[6-8] Occasional case reports indicate that the diagnosis of HPS is made earlier in life, but documentary proof often is incomplete.[9]

Anatomy

NORMAL

The stomach is divided by the incisura angularis into the body and fundus proximally and the antrum distally. The latter is further subdivided by the sulcus intermedius into a pyloric vestibule proximally and a pyloric antrum or pyloric canal distally, which is approximately 2.5 cm in length and terminates at the pyloric sphincter and orifice, which lead into the duodenum[10] (Fig. 101-1).

ABNORMAL

In infants with HPS, the pyloric antrum is no longer distensible and therefore is no longer clearly demarcated from the pyloric sphincter. The entire complex presents as one elongated canal with thickened muscular walls and filled with edematous mucosa. The thickened muscular walls are unable to relax, thus preventing the normal distensibility of the canal, and the lumen is obstructed by redundant, thickened, and hyperemic folds of mucosa (Fig. 101-2, A and B).[6,11,12]

Etiology

Although the diagnosis and surgical treatment of HPS have undergone a remarkable evolution during the past century, its cause remains unknown. The final common pathway seems to be one of work hypertrophy of the circular muscle of the pylorus, as if it were under constant stimulation, and it becomes unable to relax; the mucosa also becomes edematous and hypertrophied, sometimes markedly, simulating a polypoid mass.[13,14]

Because of a lack of an obvious etiologic agent or process, associated findings have been linked to etiology—for example, to a paucity of omentum (likely due to emaciation) and to "higher development of the nervous system" in children of the "intellectual classes"[18] in the eighteenth and early twentieth centuries. More recently, attention has centered on the hypertrophied muscle. The thickened muscle is depleted of inhibitory peptides (such as vasoactive polypeptide); synaptic vesicles, presynaptic terminals, and neural cell adhesion molecules; markers for enteric glia; interstitial cell of Cajal; and nitric oxide synthetase activity at the messenger ribonucleic acid level, with increases in insulin-like and platelet–derived growth factors. Immunoreactivity studies evaluating desmin content suggest immaturity of the intermediate filaments in the hypertrophied pyloric muscle.[19-29] The mucosa is thickened and edematous, and both muscle and mucosa are hyperemic when evaluated with color and spectral Doppler imaging.[6,13] Despite the extensive anatomic and biochemical changes documented in persons with HPS, as early as 4 months after surgery, the anatomic changes and assays for nerve growth factor, interstitial cells of Cajal, and nitric oxide synthase activity revert to normal.[27,30]

Prostaglandin E2 generation in the gastric mucosa and increased concentration in the gastric secretions of patients

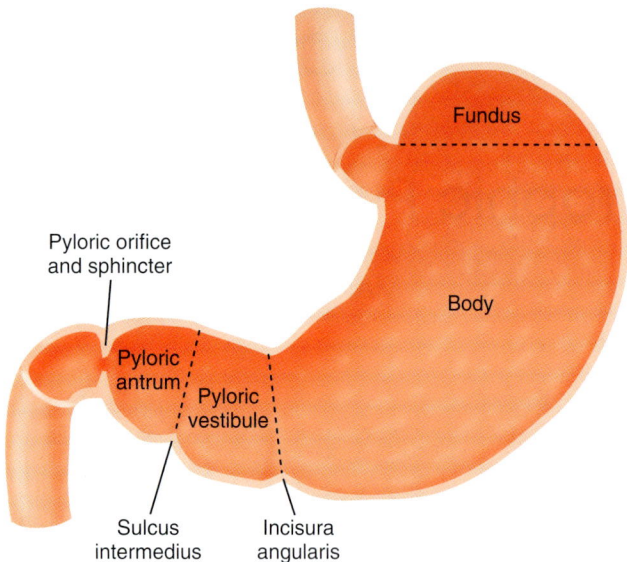

Figure 101-1 Schematic illustration of gastric segmental anatomy.

with HPS have been reported.[31] Prostaglandin E1 and E2 have been reported to induce proliferation of gastric mucosa[32] and are related to muscle contraction in the human gastrointestinal tract[23]; prostaglandin therapy has preceded the development of HPS requiring surgery.[33] The macrolide antibiotic erythromycin is a prokinetic agent and has been associated with increased risk of developing HPS in some series, particularly when the infants are exposed very early in life; however, further studies have determined that the link, if it exists, is weak and the potential risk is very small.[3] More recently, genetic susceptibility loci have been identified, including chromosomes 16p12-p13 and 11q14-q22 and genes encoding neuronal nitric oxide synthase on chromosome 12q.[15-17]

It is very difficult to extricate an initiating event from the multiplicity of associated abnormalities; the inciting event(s) of HPS remain obscure, and whether any or all of the multiple reversible abnormalities represent cause or effect of the initial condition remains intriguing and uncertain.

Clinical Presentation

Babies with HPS typically present with a history of forceful nonbilious vomiting, often described as "projectile," that may be relatively sudden in onset or preceded by initially mild symptoms consistent with gastroesophageal reflux. If the diagnosis is not made promptly, protracted vomiting leads to dehydration and to the development of hypochloremic metabolic alkalosis, with paradoxical aciduria as renal mechanisms designed to maintain intravascular volume supervene, conserving sodium at the expense of hydrogen ions. Starvation can exacerbate the effect of the diminished hepatic glucuronyl transferase activity, leading to indirect hyperbilirubinemia in a small number of infants. In patients who present after significant weight loss and who are thin and dehydrated, peristaltic waves may be seen on the wall of the scaphoid abdomen, progressing from the left upper quadrant across the epigastrium, flanked by a protuberant rib cage.[11] Currently, most infants present earlier, with less severe physical findings and laboratory abnormalities. Investigators have emphasized the changing pattern of presentation of infants with HPS; most infants presenting today do not have evidence of metabolic abnormalities, and it has been suggested that the increased availability of ultrasound may be a factor in earlier diagnosis.[34-36]

Diagnosis and Imaging

PHYSICAL EXAMINATION

Physical examination in experienced hands often is diagnostic through palpation of the "olive" or "pyloric tumor," terms often used to designate the tactile findings in persons with HPS. This examination requires a calm infant and a committed examiner willing to dedicate 15 minutes or longer to the examination, which may require decompression of the overdistended stomach via a nasogastric tube.[37] If the olive is palpable, the examination is diagnostic. The sensitivity of abdominal palpation varies with the experience of the examiner and ranges between 24% and 99%; specificity ranges between 92% and 99%.[37-41] False-positive results do occur and have been reported to be as high as 14%, with anatomic variants such as unusual extensions of the left lobe of the liver

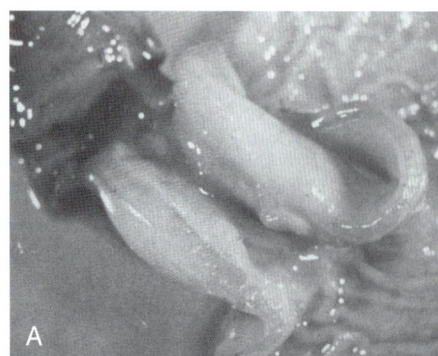
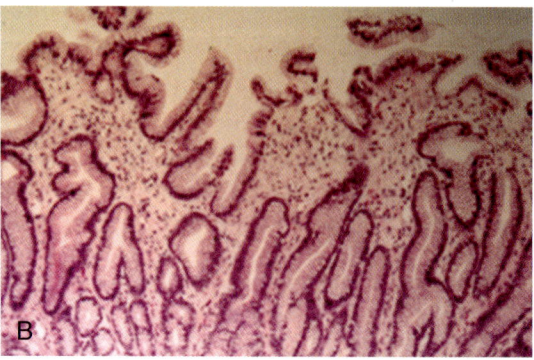

Figure 101-2 Histopathologic anatomy. **A,** A gross postmortem specimen of hypertrophied pylorus in an infant who succumbed to this condition. Note the thickened muscle and the thickened mucosa, which would fill and obstruct the lumen of the unsectioned antropyloric canal. **B,** A histologic specimen of antropyloric mucosa in an infant with pyloric stenosis with typical presentation, operative findings, and postoperative recovery. The hematoxylin and eosin stain shows mucosal hyperplasia with elongated, branched, and mildly distorted pits and abundant edematous lamina propria.

and congenital abnormalities such as malrotation and duplication cysts.[42,43]

The documented accuracy of ultrasound diagnosis has generated a trend toward reliance on imaging rather than on the potentially more protracted physical examination. Although the loss of clinical skills may be lamentable in some respects, and some persons have argued that imaging increases the financial cost of the workup of HPS, other investigators have recognized that, despite "fading skills," the rapidity and accuracy of ultrasound diagnosis can result in "better patients," that is, better surgical candidates at the time of diagnosis.[34,35]

RADIOGRAPHIC STUDIES

Radiography

Plain radiographs may strongly suggest the diagnosis, revealing a markedly distended stomach, particularly if several peristaltic waves are seen, with little gas distally (Fig. 101-3),[44] although absence of these findings does not negate the diagnosis. In rare instances, HPS has been reported in association with isolated gastric pneumatosis that resolves after the stomach is decompressed (e-Fig. 101-4).[45]

Upper Gastrointestinal Series

Before the advent of real-time ultrasound imaging, the contrast upper gastrointestinal (GI) series was used for diagnosis and still may be more widely used than ultrasound by radiologists with limited pediatric sonographic experience. When ultrasound shows a normal antropyloric canal, the upper GI series also sometimes is used to evaluate and document other potential causes of the patient's symptoms, such as reflux. Barium or a water-soluble agent may be used as oral contrast material; if the latter is chosen, it is important to use a low-osmolality contrast medium approximating physiologic serum osmolality, because the child may vomit and aspiration may occur. To obtain a technically satisfactory contrast study, it may be necessary to pass an enteric tube into the stomach to decompress it, because a large amount of preexistent gastric contents will dilute the contrast medium and also increase the chance of vomiting and aspiration during the examination itself. If an enteric tube is used, placing it distally and introducing the contrast material with the patient in the prone right oblique position tends to require less contrast material to outline the gastric outlet.

In addition to a delay in the passage of contrast material from the stomach, several other radiographic signs are present in infants with HPS. The pyloric channel is narrowed, and as contrast material begins to enter the narrowed channel, it may appear as a "beak" that evolves into a "string" or a "double tract" sign as contrast material courses between the interstices of the luminal mucosa, compressed by the thickened, unrelaxing antropyloric muscle, which typically is curved upward and posteriorly (Fig. 101-5). The enlarged muscle mass encroaches upon the lumen of the antrum proximally, resulting in the "shoulder sign"; when the duodenal base is also deformed by the thickened muscle, the appearance may resemble an "apple core" lesion. The "pyloric tit" occasionally can be seen along the lesser curve just proximal to the impression of the pyloric mass; it represents contrast material trapped within the lumen of the stomach, compressed between a peristaltic wave and the impression of the pyloric muscle upon the adjacent, more distal portion of the stomach. Virtually all of the aforementioned signs can be seen transiently in most infants. The study should document the persistence of the findings to ensure the diagnosis of HPS.

ULTRASONOGRAPHY

Ultrasound was first applied to the diagnosis of HPS in five cases described in 1977 utilizing B-mode sonography.[46] Since that time, ultrasound has become the modality of choice in the diagnosis of HPS in most pediatric centers and is considered the "gold standard" by many investigators.[11,35,37] Unlike the upper GI test, this examination does not require contrast material to traverse the obstructed canal for diagnosis, and thus the diagnosis can be made quickly, without the need for additional distension of the stomach and without radiation exposure to the infant, which can be prolonged in infants with a high degree of obstruction.

The examination typically is performed with linear transducers operating at a frequency of 7.5 MHz or higher. The time of the last feeding may be annotated on the image, and the degree of gastric distension related to the last feeding can give an initial clue as to the presence or absence of gastric outlet obstruction.

The examination is begun with the patient in the supine position. The transducer is placed in the transverse plane over the gastroesophageal junction, which is constant in location anterior to the aortic hiatus, and the transducer is then swept

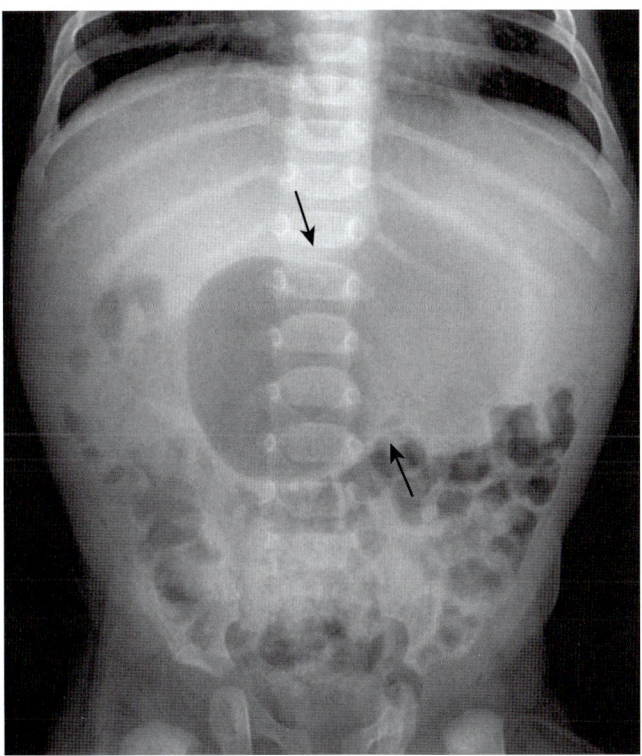

Figure 101-3   An abdominal radiograph in an infant with pyloric stenosis. An abdominal radiograph demonstrates a distended stomach with a peristaltic wave (*arrows*), with normal to mildly decreased distal gas. In the appropriate clinical setting, these findings are highly suggestive of pyloric stenosis.

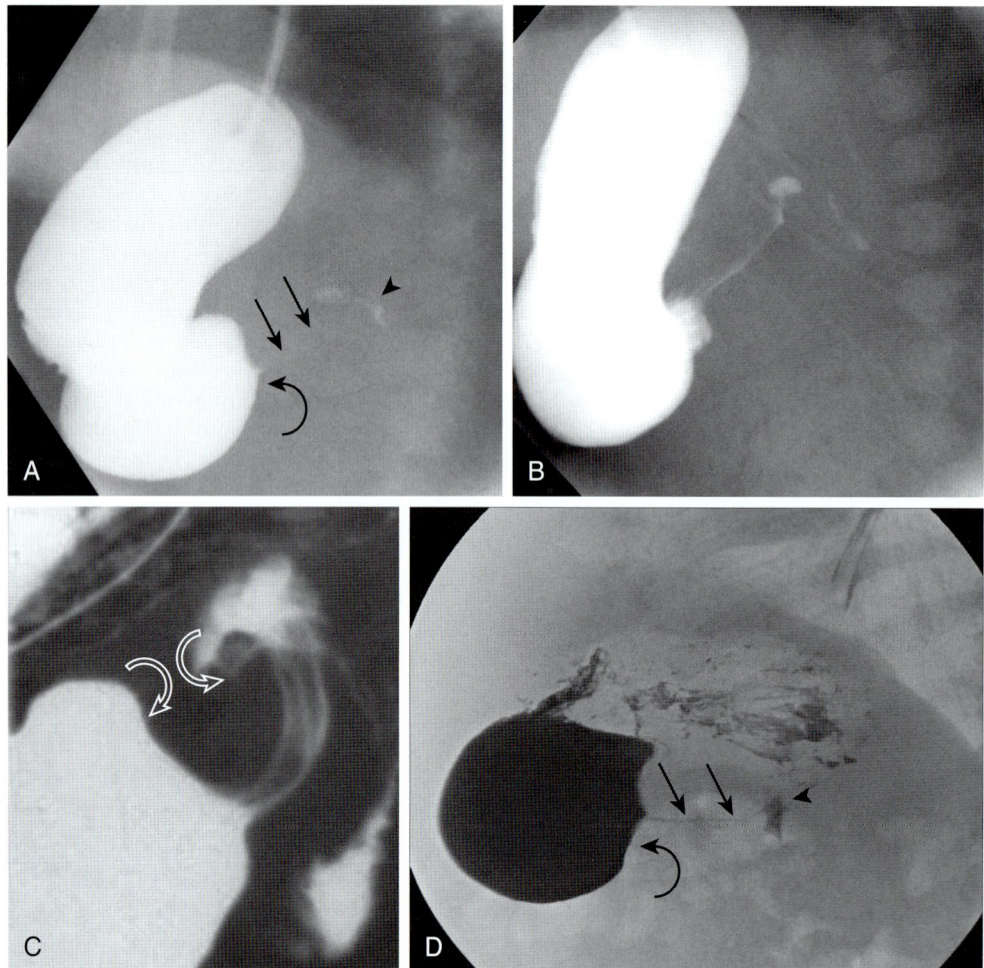

Figure 101-5 Upper gastrointestinal series in patients with pyloric stenosis. **A,** An orogastric tube was used to evacuate the stomach, and barium was instilled under fluoroscopic control. The image shows a peristaltic wave and a small amount of contrast entering the narrowed canal, demonstrating both a beak (*curved arrow*) and string sign (*straight arrows*). The arrowhead points to the duodenal bulb. **B,** Shortly after the image shown in part **A,** additional contrast material egressed into the pyloric channel, now outlining a double tract proximally. **C,** An oblique radiograph in another infant with pyloric stenosis shows mass impression upon the proximal antrum and the distal duodenal base (*curved arrows*), spanned by the upwardly and posteriorly directed antropyloric canal with three contrast tracts coursing through the intraluminal mucosal folds. **D,** An oblique radiograph of the same infant shown in Fig. 101-8, **C**. *Curved arrows* point to the mass impression of the pyloric muscle on the gastric antrum, or "shoulder sign."

along the length of the stomach until the distal antrum and duodenal cap are identified; once the duodenal bulb is identified, the immediately proximal antropyloric canal can be evaluated for morphology and relaxation, thus identifying either HPS or a normal antropyloric canal (Fig. 101-6). The abnormal pylorus is typically, but not invariably, found just medial to the gallbladder, anterior to the right kidney.

Much emphasis has been placed on the measurements used to diagnose HPS. Certainly, these measurements are helpful and necessary, but they can be confusing because they vary among different patients, in the same patient, and among various series published over three decades, paralleling an increase in operator experience and equipment resolution. The initial and seminal report of static B-mode ultrasound in HPS by Teele and Smith, published in the *New England Journal of Medicine* in 1977,[46] used a pyloric diameter of 1.8 to 2.8 cm (mean, 2.5 cm) for diagnosis. Muscle thickness became more important in subsequent reports with real-time capability.

A 1986 prospective study of 200 infants with HPS who underwent scanning with a mechanical sector transducer operating at 7.5 MHz found a mean muscle thickness of 3.4 mm (range, 3 to 5 mm) and a mean pyloric length of 22.3 mm (range, 18 to 28 mm) that discriminated between normal and abnormal patients with a 100% success rate.[43] A subsequent study of 323 patients found that mean muscle thickness was 4.8 mm (range, 3.5 to 6 mm) and mean pyloric length was 17.8 mm (range, 11 to 25 mm)[47]; these investigators found muscle thickness to be the most helpful discriminant, with an accuracy of 99.4%. In a 1991 series by O'Keeffe et al.,[7] who reported on 145 consecutive patients, a muscle thickness of 3 mm or greater was determined to be diagnostic of HPS, with muscle thickness less than 1.5 mm in 98% of normal patients. These results were validated in a 1993 series by Hernanz-Schulman et al.,[48] who evaluated 152 infants and found that a persistent muscle thickness of 3 mm or greater was diagnostic of HPS, with no false-positive examinations.

In younger and previously premature infants, the tendency exists for pyloric measurements to be smaller at presentation than in full-term, older infants.[48,49] In a more recent review of these patients, a significant association was found between

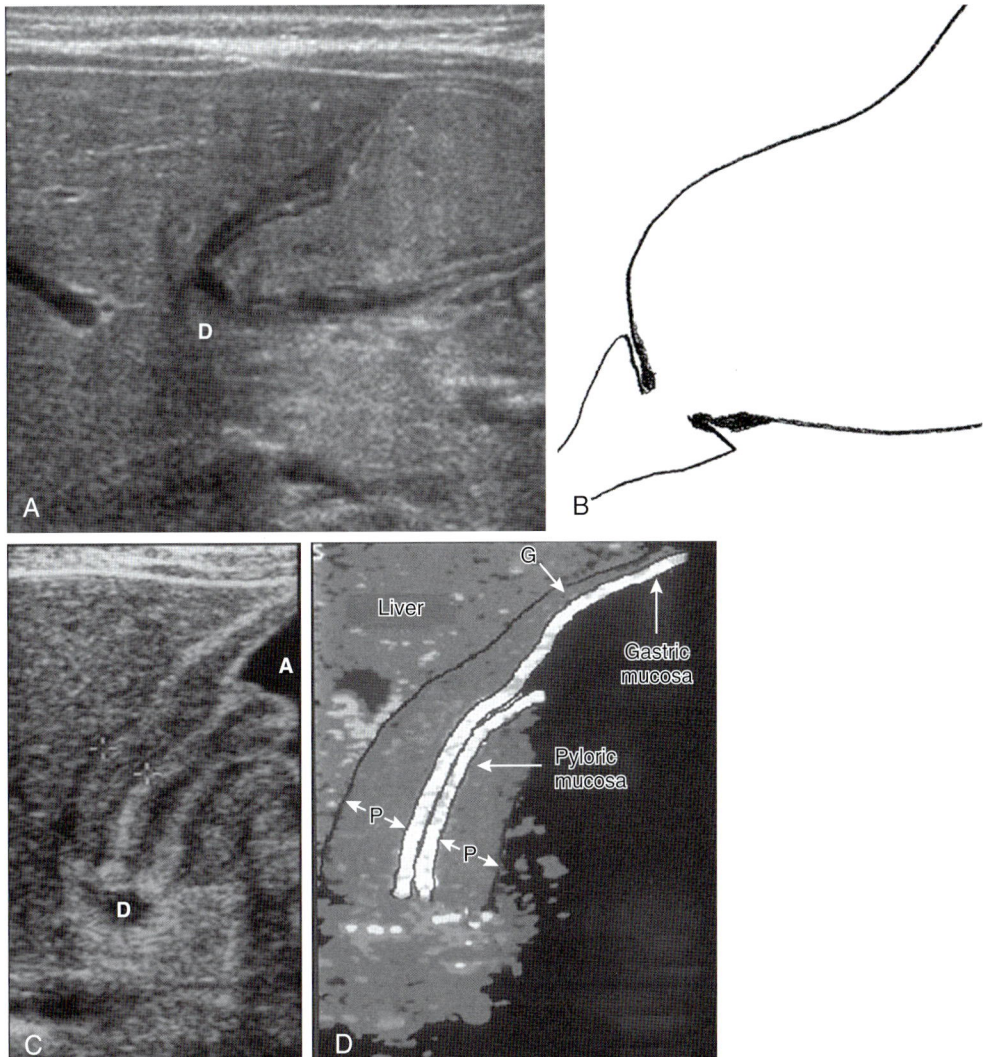

Figure 101-6 Antropyloric canals with schematic drawings. **A,** Ultrasonogram in an infant with a normal pylorus. The stomach is distended with formula ingested just prior to the examination. The pylorus is normal. D, Duodenal bulb. **B,** A schematic drawing of findings in part **A**. **C,** Ultrasonogram in a child with pyloric stenosis. The pyloric muscle (between crosshairs) is thickened, measuring >3 mm; the mucosa is hypertrophied, filling the lumen and protruding into the fluid-filled antrum (A). D, Duodenal bulb. **D,** A schematic drawing of the findings in part **C**. G, Gastric wall muscle; P, pyloric muscle.

pyloric dimensions and patient age and weight; however, these changes did not have an impact on their existing diagnostic criteria for HPS: a muscle thickness of 3 mm or greater and length 15 mm or greater.[50]

A normal antropyloric channel has a sonographic appearance similar to that at upper GI, with a relaxed, open lumen directly adjacent to the duodenal bulb via the pyloric orifice (see Figs. 101-6, A, and 101-7).

The abnormal antropyloric canal, on the other hand, shows persistent thickening of the muscle and mucosa to variable degree (Fig. 101-8). The length of the hypertrophied canal is variable, ranging from as little as 14 mm to greater than 20 mm. The lower limit of persistent muscle thickness is 3 mm, without evidence of relaxation of the antropyloric canal throughout the examination.[11] Evaluation of the patient over time is important. Increased but transient contractions of the pylorus, or pylorospasm, may mimic HPS in both appearance and measurement if the examination is performed quickly (Fig. 101-9).[51] The hypertrophied pyloric muscle and

mucosa typically show abundant flow as seen on color and spectral Doppler interrogation (e-Fig. 101-10). Although the patient might not have been fed for hours, the stomach typically is distended. However, it is important to realize that despite the lack of relaxation of the abnormal antropyloric canal, some gastric contents will pass through in many patients during the period of observation. HPS is not a complete obstruction; diagnosis by an upper GI examination is obviously based upon this fact (e-Fig. 101-11, Video 101-1). In some patients, for reasons that are not yet clear and with an unknown temporal relationship to the development of this condition, the muscle is very active, and visible contractions temporarily shorten and thicken, as well as lengthen and thin, the pyloric muscle as seen on real-time ultrasound. The appearance suggests that more proximal muscle that has not lost its ability to relax and return to normal is being actively recruited, an intriguing finding when considering the development and etiology of HPS (e-Fig. 101-12, Video 101-2).

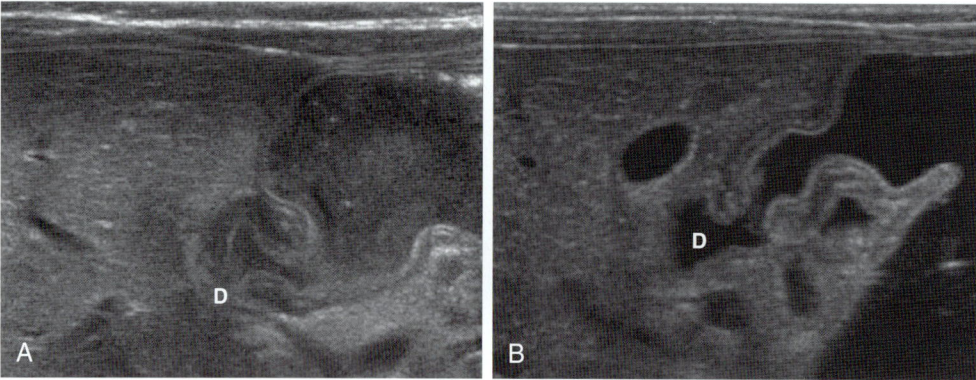

Figure 101-7 A normal antropyloric canal in two infants. **A,** The stomach is filled with formula. Note that the antropyloric muscle is mildly thickened, but the mucosa is normal, and the antropyloric canal is distensible and filled with gastric contents. *D,* Duodenal bulb. **B,** The stomach is filled with Pedialyte. Again, the antropyloric muscle is mildly thickened, but the lumen is distensible and filled with gastric contents. *D,* Duodenal bulb.

Pitfalls

The normal pylorus might be difficult to visualize because of excessive amounts of overlying bowel gas. In such cases, it is helpful to use the left lobe of the liver as an acoustic window and angle inferiorly to identify the pylorus. If the stomach is empty, the child is unlikely to have HPS; in such cases, the child may be given Pedialyte or glucose water, which will not only improve the ability to identify the pylorus and duodenal bulb, but also will allow definitive documentation of the normal anatomy (Fig. 101-13).[11,48,52]

In patients with HPS, the pylorus may be difficult to identify because a very distended stomach displaces it posterior to the antrum; this displacement is also the cause of one of the false-negative pitfalls in palpation (Fig. 101-14). Some investigators have advocated emptying the stomach with a nasogastric catheter,[53] but we prefer to turn the supine infant toward his or her left side, thus displacing the bulk of the fluid toward the fundus and allowing the hypertrophied pylorus to rise anteriorly for optimal evaluation.

Equivocal examinations occur when, after sufficient observation, the muscle measures between 2 and 3 mm in thickness. In such cases, follow-up examination is indicated if the patient continues to vomit. The rate of evolution of HPS is not known; also unknown are whether the process begins with pylorospasm, potential inciting event(s), and the time course. Therefore in equivocal cases, follow-up sonography is indicated.[7,8,12]

Differential Diagnosis

Other entities that can mimic HPS on sonographic examination are antropyloric gastritis (with or without ulcer disease) and chronic granulomatous disease of childhood. However, these conditions present at a later age and do not typically present a clinical uncertainty.

The most common antropyloric abnormality mimicking HPS on an upper GI series is pylorospasm. Although a spasm

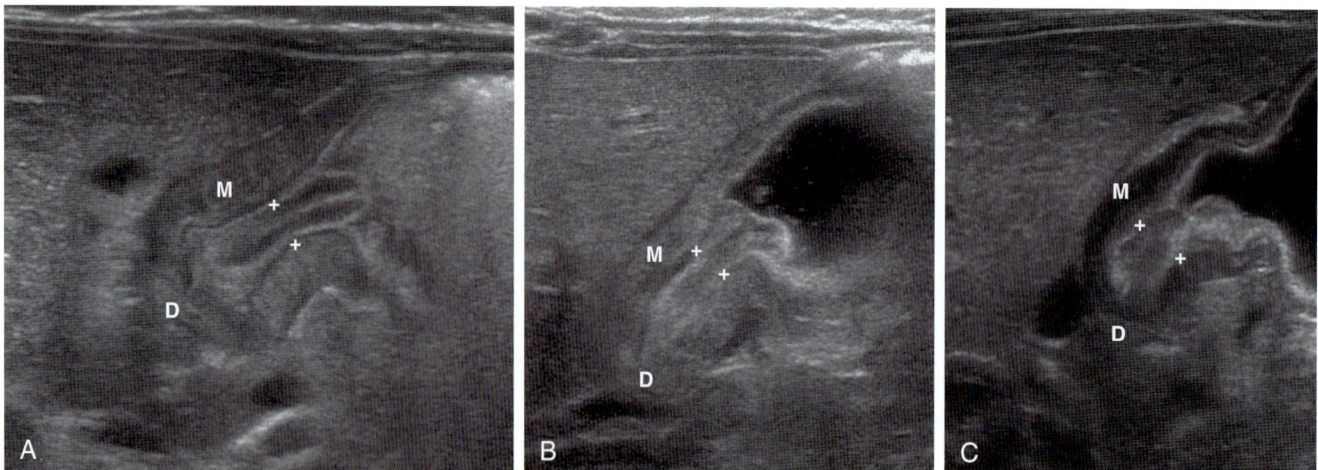

Figure 101-8 Pyloric stenosis in three infants. **A,** An abnormal pylorus shows a double layer of edematous mucosa (between crosshairs) sandwiched within the thickened muscle (*M*), protruding into the gas and formula-filled antrum as the "nipple sign." *D,* Duodenal bulb. **B,** An abnormal pylorus in another infant shows thickened muscle (*M*) and mucosa (between crosshairs) again with protrusion into the proximal antrum. *D,* Duodenal bulb. **C,** An infant with progressive vomiting and poor weight gain. The muscle (*M*) is thickened to >3 mm and the mucosa (between crosshairs) measured 8 mm in thickness, also protruding proximally into the fluid-filled antrum. *D,* Duodenal bulb. The same infant as in Figure 101-5, **D.**

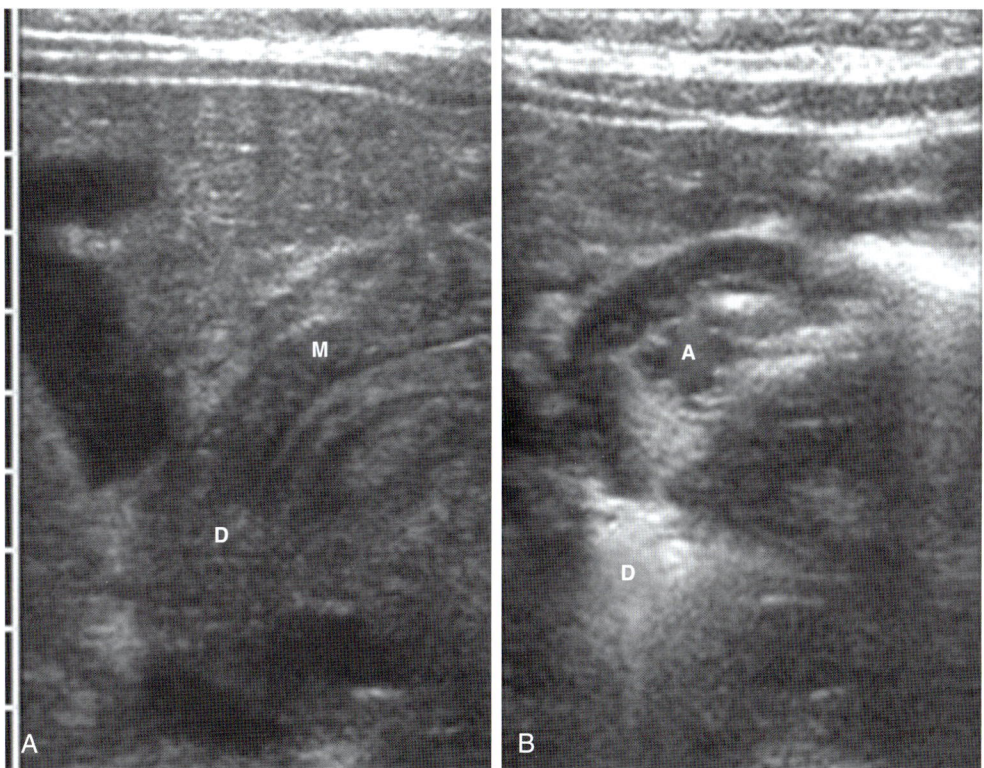

Figure 101-9   Transient ultrasound findings. **A,** The antropyloric channel in an infant with vomiting shows narrowing with thickened muscle that measured up to 4 mm in thickness. *M,* Muscle; *D,* duodenal bulb. **B,** The antropyloric channel in the same infant as depicted in **A,** 4 minutes later. The canal is open. *A,* Open antropyloric canal; *D,* duodenal bulb.

also may cause the pyloric muscle to appear thicker on ultrasound, a spasm is a transient phenomenon usually distinguishable from HPS, or which may necessitate a follow-up examination, as previously discussed. Focal foveolar hyperplasia, a polypoid mucosa in the antropyloric portion of the stomach, usually is associated with a history of congenital heart disease and prostaglandin therapy. The lobulated mucosal mass has been reported to cause gastric outlet obstruction and has developed into full-fledged HPS in some cases.[32,33,54]

Diagnostic Algorithm

Palpation of the pyloric mass is the first diagnostic examination by the physician. In further evaluation and referral, consideration can be given to the investment of time and relative invasiveness of inserting an orogastric tube to evacuate the stomach and for surgical or imaging referral. The cost and time delay of obtaining a surgical consultation/visit versus the cost, time delay, and accuracy of an imaging examination

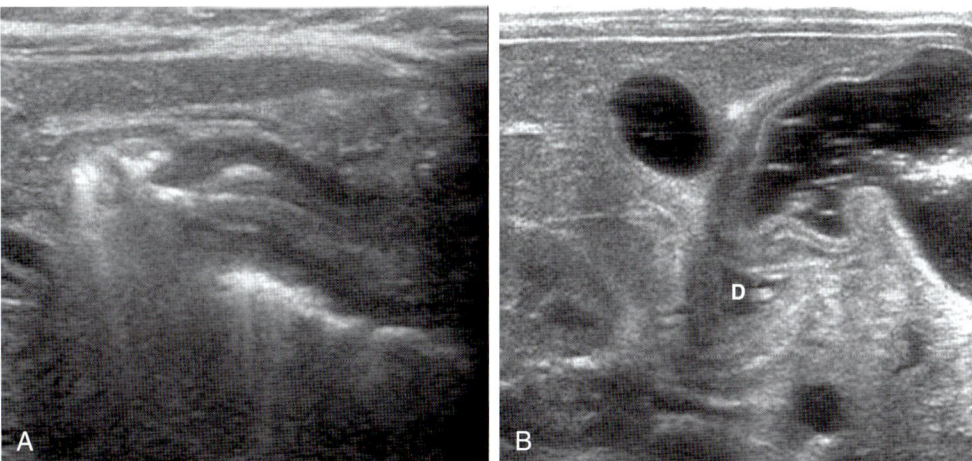

Figure 101-13   An empty stomach mimicking pyloric stenosis. **A,** An 8-week-old girl with vomiting. The stomach initially was empty, which is initial evidence against the presence of pyloric stenosis in most infants. However, the collapsed distal antropyloric canal appears "elongated," thus mimicking some of the findings in pyloric stenosis. The muscle measured between 1.7 and 2.8 mm. **B,** After the infant drank Pedialyte, the antrum distended with a completely normal appearance. *D,* Duodenal bulb.

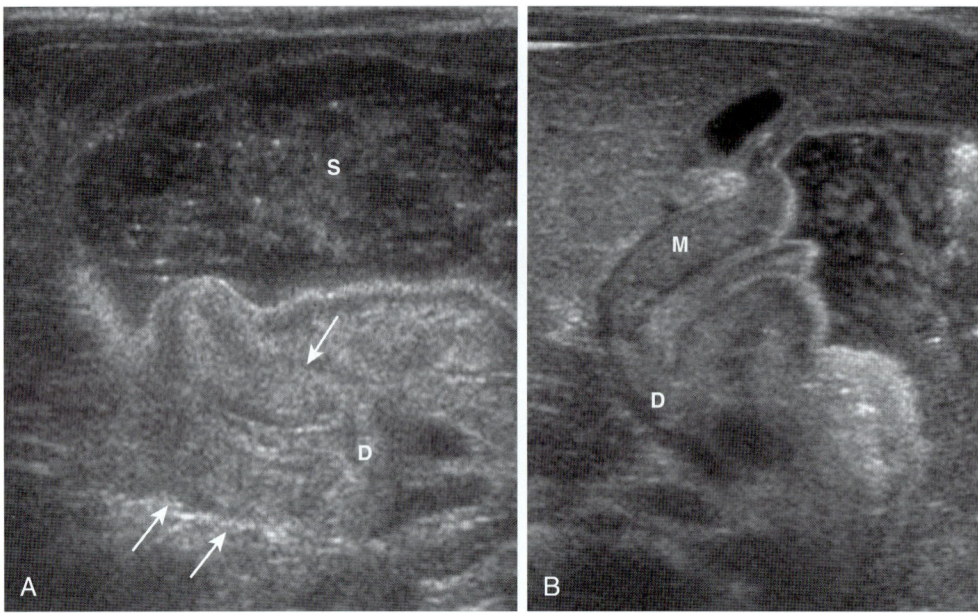

Figure 101-14 A pitfall when scanning an overdistended stomach in an infant with pyloric stenosis. **A,** An image of the overdistended distal stomach in an infant with pyloric stenosis shows the hypertrophied pylorus (*arrows*) folded behind the stomach (*S*). *D,* Duodenal bulb. **B,** When the infant is turned toward a left posterior oblique position, the hypertrophied pylorus is allowed to rise anteriorly and is much more easily detected and detailed. Note the pyloric mucosa protruding into the fluid-filled antrum. *M,* Muscle; *D,* duodenal bulb.

may differ across locations and clinical practices. If the pyloric mass is palpated by the surgeon, no diagnostic imaging is necessary; if it cannot be palpated by the surgeon, imaging should be considered. Waiting and reexamining the patient with prolongation of inpatient care likely is not cost-effective in most settings and may lead to delay in diagnosis and treatment. We do not advocate sedating an infant to increase sensitivity in palpating the pyloric mass, as has been suggested in the past.[38]

Some investigators have advocated use of the upper GI series as the first examination in patients with symptoms of HPS for two reasons: (1) although ultrasound may be quite accurate in the diagnosis of HPS, it is not always diagnostic in infants with vomiting from other causes, and (2) an upper GI series is deemed by some persons to be more cost effective as the first imaging examination compared with ultrasound. Because a follow-up upper GI series may be requested in patients with normal ultrasound findings, a cost savings could be realized if the upper GI series is performed instead of ultrasound.[41,55] However, ultrasound images can be obtained beyond the lumen of the pylorus and can assess the thickness of the muscle, as well as any adjacent masses or other lesions, and there is no need to further distend the stomach with the addition of contrast media. More importantly, because we adopt the "as low as reasonably achievable" approach to pediatric imaging, we believe that ultrasound should be the first imaging examination in patients suspected of HPS, particularly in young infants in whom fluoroscopy could be prolonged.[11,48,56] If the ultrasound shows that the pylorus is normal, vomiting is clearly nonbilious, and the duodenum is normal in caliber, the likelihood is high that the cause of vomiting is gastroesophageal reflux, which initially could be treated empirically or documented with scintigraphy (Fig. 101-15).

Treatment

Surgical pyloromyotomy, introduced by Ramstedt in 1912, is the traditional therapy for infants with HPS. In this procedure, the muscle is incised and the mucosa is allowed to protrude through the incision without resuturing (Fig. 101-16).

Several publications have redirected attention to medical therapy, which is based on the theory that muscle spasm is a contributing factor to the muscular hypertrophy and obstruction. In a prospective trial of infants treated with surgical or medical therapy, the latter was successful in 85% of medical cases, with 2 of 14 requiring a pyloromyotomy;

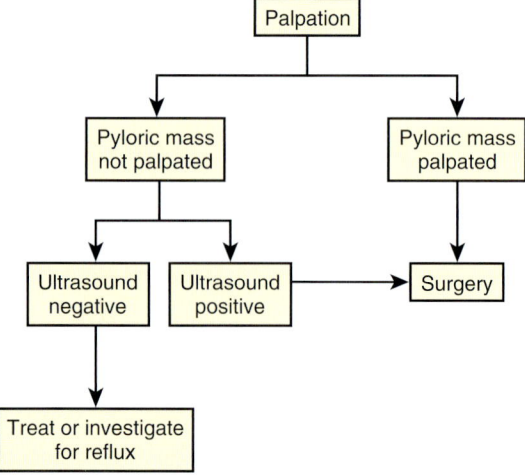

Figure 101-15 A diagnostic algorithm for infants suspected of having pyloric stenosis.

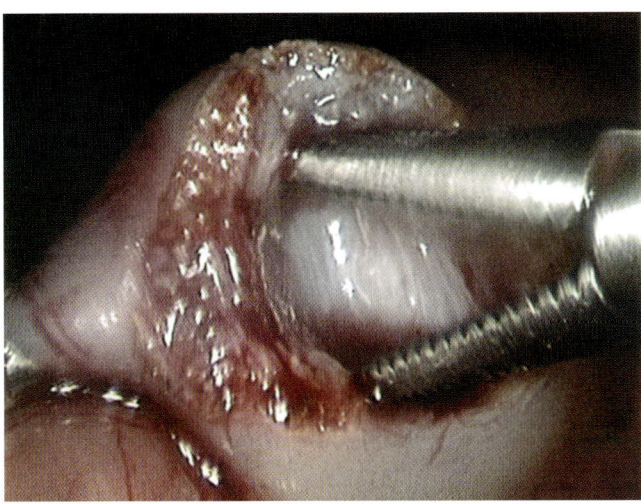

Figure 101-16 An intraoperative photograph of a muscle-splitting Ramstedt pyloromyotomy. (Courtesy Dr. Robert Cywes.)

mean time to full feeds was 2.7 days in the surgical group and 5.3 days in the medically treated group.[57] In a larger prospective trial including 52 medically treated infants, medical therapy had a 87% success rate; the mean hospital stay was 5 days in the surgical group and 13 days in the successfully medically treated group.[58] Another trial reported a 75% success rate of medical therapy, with prolonged resolution of symptoms resulting in some of the parents in the medical treatment group opting for surgery before completion of medical treatment.[59]

Laparoscopic pyloromyotomy, which was first reported in 1991,[60] has been advocated recently by some pediatric surgeons. Metaanalyses and prospective trials suggest that mucosal perforation, a complication of both open and laparoscopic procedures, may be more problematic with laparoscopy, because initially the perforation may not be recognized and thus require reoperation. Wound infection appears to be slightly less frequent with laparoscopy. Although cosmetic results are superior with laparoscopy, the data to date suggest that, once the learning curve for the laparoscopic approach is mastered, little difference exists in the overall outcome between these two procedures, with some prospective studies suggesting that the laparoscopic group shows less postoperative emesis and requires less postoperative analgesia.[61-65]

Balloon dilation has been attempted unsuccessfully in a limited number of patients; however, a potential role after failed pyloromyotomy or recurrent HPS has been investigated with partial success in a very limited number of patients.[66-68]

Key Points

Radiographic findings in persons with HPS may include the following:
- Gastric distension on an abdominal radiograph
- A narrowed, elongated, curved pyloric channel
- Beak sign
- String or double tract sign
- Shoulder sign
- "Pyloric tit" on lesser curve

Ultrasound findings in persons with HPS include the following:
- Retained gastric contents
- Thickened pyloric muscle measuring 3 mm or more
- A narrow, elongated, or curved antropyloric channel that does not normalize
- Redundant mucosa measuring similar to or greater than muscle thickness
- Increased Doppler flow signal of mucosa and/or the muscular layer

References

Full references for this chapter can be found on www.expertconsult.com.

Chapter 102

Acquired Disorders

RICARDO RESTREPO and DIANA V. MARIN

Acquired disorders of the stomach in children are not common and can be conceptualized as disorders with an underlying congenital predisposition (e.g., gastric volvulus), as inflammatory (e.g., peptic ulcer disease), and as tumors or tumor-like conditions. From a radiologic point of view, fluoroscopic contrast studies remain the mainstay of diagnostic examinations for most abnormalities of the stomach. However, depending on the specific concern and underlying clinical conditions, the stomach can also be evaluated with cross-sectional imaging such as ultrasound and computed tomography (CT), as well as nuclear medicine studies.

Gastric Volvulus

Etiology Normally, the stomach is relatively fixed in the peritoneal cavity at the esophagogastric junction, with four additional ligaments: (1) gastrohepatic, (2) gastrosplenic, (3) gastrocolic, and (4) gastrophrenic (Fig. 102-1) *Gastric volvulus* is defined as an abnormal rotation of the stomach of more than 180 degrees around its long (organoaxial) or short (mesenteroaxial) axes (Fig. 102-2, *A* and *B*), causing a closed loop obstruction, with consequences such as incarceration, strangulation, and perforation.[1] Predisposing factors for gastric volvulus include congenital or acquired absence of one or more ligaments as isolated abnormalities or conditions such as asplenia and diaphragmatic defects.

In organoaxial gastric volvulus, an inversion of the position of the greater and lesser curves of the stomach occurs, with the greater curvature positioned to the right and superior to the lesser curvature. In mesenteroaxial gastric volvulus, the stomach folds on its short axis; this leads to reversal of the relationship between the gastroesophageal junction and the pylorus. Clinically, two primary scenarios exist. The first is the acute fulminant presentation, most often encountered in the mesenteroaxial type, with sudden and persistent vomiting and acute abdominal pain.[1] The chronic intermittent presentation is more often associated with the organoaxial type, with less specific symptoms, including recurrent abdominal pain, vomiting, and gastric distension.[2]

Imaging Abdominal radiographs in patients with gastric volvulus typically show marked gastric distension. The stomach becomes spherical, with paucity of distal bowel gas, indicating gastric outlet obstruction (Fig. 102-3, *A*). Other findings include diaphragmatic elevation and the presence of two air-fluid levels in the stomach. Occasionally, the type of gastric volvulus can be inferred by the gastric configuration: a pylorus projecting over the gastric fundus and an unusual nasogastric tube course are suggestive of the mesenteroaxial type, whereas an inversion of the relationship of the greater and lesser curvatures is suggestive of the organoaxial type; mixed types also occur, with combined imaging findings.

Although, in most cases, plain radiographs are highly suggestive of the diagnosis, the upper gastrointestinal (UGI) series remains the diagnostic procedure of choice, demonstrating the type of volvulus and evidence of gastric outlet obstruction. If performed, other imaging modalities such as CT can also be useful in demonstrating the abnormal orientation of the stomach (see Fig. 102-3, *B*) as well as associated anomalies such as heterotaxy or the presence of pneumatosis.[2]

Treatment and Follow-up Gastropexy, which is the treatment of choice, can be performed laparoscopically.[3,4]

Spontaneous Gastric Perforation

Etiology Spontaneous perforation of the stomach is an uncommon event mainly seen in the neonatal period as a cause of pneumoperitoneum.[5] The etiology is unknown, but possibilities include sudden gastric distension with a degree of ischemia attributable to perinatal hypoxia, a more distal bowel obstruction, and congenital focal absence of the muscle of the gastric wall.[6-8] Beyond the neonatal period, perforation is rare and usually secondary to trauma (tubes, catheters), surgery (fundoplication), caustic ingestion, or peptic ulcer.[1] The most common presenting manifestations of perforation include sudden onset of abdominal distension, ileus, respiratory distress, and, less frequently, cyanosis, fever, vomiting, and bloody stool.[9]

Imaging Abdominal radiography is the imaging method of choice when perforation of the gastrointestinal (GI) tract is suspected. As in any other type of GI perforation, abdominal radiographs will typically demonstrate free intraperitoneal air. A reported suggestive sign of gastric perforation is the lack of an air-fluid level in the stomach in a horizontal beam view, and relative paucity of gas in the distal bowel.[10]

Treatment and Follow-up Gastric perforations require surgical repair. At surgery, most of the perforations are linear and are found high in the stomach along the greater curvature.[8]

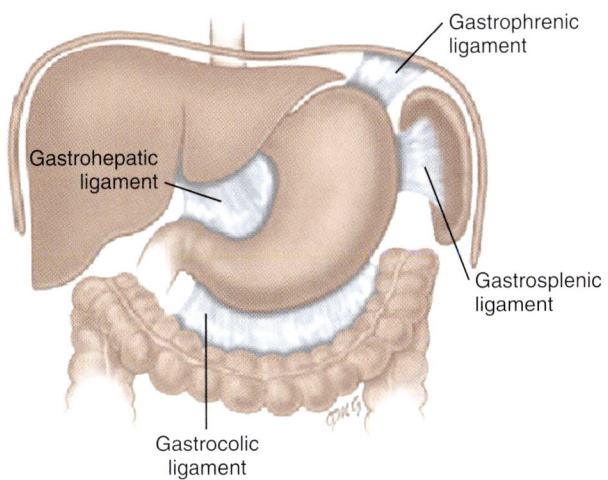

Figure 102-1 Schematic drawing of stomach and its anchoring ligaments. (From Timpone VM, Lattin Jr GE, Lewis RB. Abdominal twists and turns: Part 1, gastrointestinal tract torsions with pathologic correlation. *AJR Am J Roentgenol.* 2011;197(1):86–89. Reprinted with permission from *American Journal of Roentgenology.*)

Gastritis and Gastropathy

Gastritis is a nonspecific term that refers to the presence of inflammatory cells within the gastric wall; the diagnosis is made histologically, as the mucosa may appear normal at endoscopy. It differs from gastropathies, which demonstrate evidence of epithelial damage and regeneration but have little in the way of inflammatory infiltrate, and are often associated with specific conditions such as portal hypertensive gastropathy.

In children, inflammatory changes in the stomach can result from several etiologies, including infections (e.g., secondary to *Helicobacter pylori*), severe stress (e.g., during a serious illness), chemicals (e.g., ingestion of corrosive substance), eosinophilic gastritis, hypertrophic gastropathy (Ménétrier disease of childhood), and secondary to other

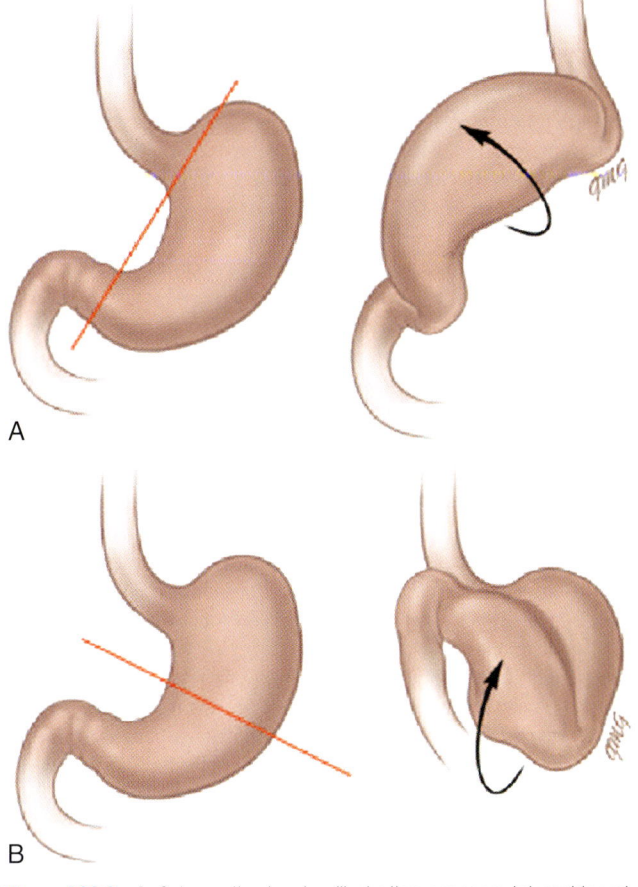

Figure 102-2 **A,** Schematic drawing illustrating organoaxial gastric volvulus. **B,** Schematic drawing illustrating mesenteroaxial gastric volvulus. (From Timpone VM, Lattin Jr GE, Lewis RB. Abdominal twists and turns: Part 1, gastrointestinal tract torsions with pathologic correlation. *AJR Am J Roentgenol.* 2011;197(1):86–89. Reprinted with permission from *American Journal of Roentgenology.*)

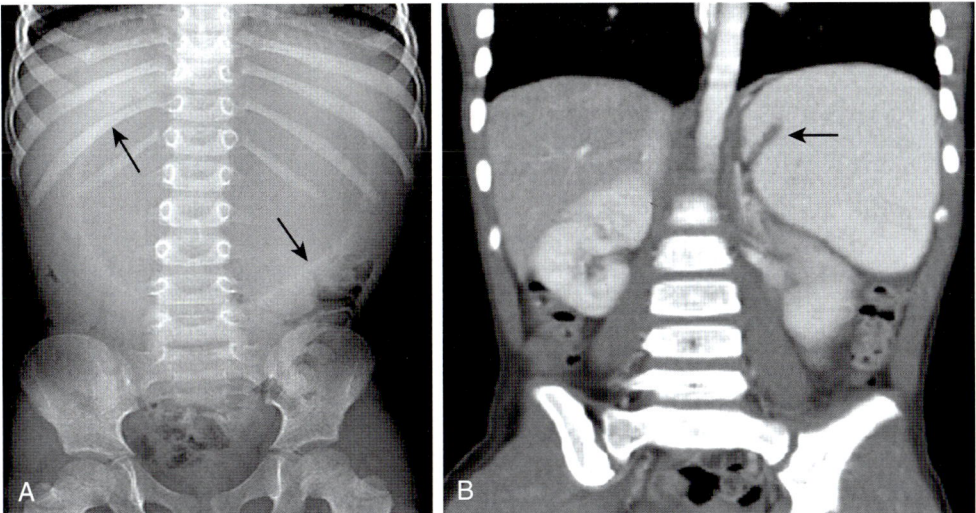

Figure 102-3 Mesenteroaxial volvulus in a 6-year-old girl presenting with acute unremitting vomiting. **A,** Supine abdominal radiograph shows a dilated, spherical gastric bubble (*arrows*) with paucity of distal bowel gas. **B,** The coronal image of a contrast-enhanced computed tomography scan shows a reversal of the axis of the distended stomach with the pylorus superiorly located and inverted (*arrow*).

systemic entities such as Crohn disease and chronic granulo-matous disease.

Peptic Ulcer Disease

Etiology Peptic ulcer disease represents ulceration of the gastric or duodenal mucosa resulting from, on the one hand, an imbalance between the mucosal protective mechanisms and, on the other, the aggressive factors of acid and pepsin production, injury, and infection.[11] The gel layer, a protective bicarbonate and mucous barrier lining the stomach, is approximately 0.2 to 0.5 mm in thickness and consists of 95% water and 5% mucin glycoprotein. Breaches in this gel layer, secondary to *H. pylori* or antiinflammatory drugs, result in a continuum of damage to the underlying mucosa, with ulceration occurring when damage extends to the muscular layer.

Peptic ulcer disease in children may be *primary* or *secondary* (induced by drugs, alcohol, stress, or metabolic disease), with each form having different manifestations and prognostic implications. *H. pylori* has been recognized as a common human pathogen associated with both inflammatory and malignant conditions of the upper gastrointestinal tract, and affects nearly all children with peptic ulcer disease.[12] Primary peptic ulcers are associated with *H. pylori* infection.

In addition to being classified as primary and secondary, peptic ulcers can also be classified according to the site of involvement (*gastric* or *duodenal*). Gastric ulcers are mostly seen in neonates and young children, whereas duodenal ulcers are more common after the neonatal period and tend to be secondary to systemic illness or chronic intake of medications such as non-steroidal antiinflammatory agents. Zollinger-Ellison syndrome causes secondary peptic ulcer disease, often with multiple ulcerations caused by increased acid generated by a gastrin-producing tumor (Fig. 102-4).[11,13]

Symptoms of ulcer disease vary with age; infants and young children present with feeding problems and vomiting. In some patients, the first sign of peptic ulcer disease may be upper or lower GI hemorrhage or acute severe abdominal pain due to perforation. Pain can be nocturnal or occur early in the morning. Unlike in adults, the pain is neither precipitated nor relieved by meals or antacid use.[11]

Imaging Endoscopy has assumed the primary role in the diagnosis of ulcer disease over the past two decades, while the role of the radiologist has dramatically decreased and is now limited to the incidental case, as UGI contrast studies have been demonstrated to have a high false-negative rate for ulcer detection.[14,15] However, these studies, as an initial tool to evaluate the child with abdominal pain and vomiting, may incidentally demonstrate the ulcer. Perforated ulcers may be incidentally identified on CT in the evaluation of a child with acute abdominal pain (Fig. 102-5).

Treatment and Follow-up Current therapy has been proven to be effective and is based on medications that decrease acid production. In the cases of *H. pylori* infection, a combination therapy, including a histamine-2 blocker or proton pump inhibitor, antibiotics, and, bismuth, may be necessary to eradicate the causative organism and prevent both recurrence and malignant complications.[11]

Hypertrophic Gastropathy (Ménétrier Disease)

Etiology Hypertrophy of the gastric rugal folds, in association with protein-losing enteropathy, in childhood is labeled *Ménétrier disease*, or *hypertrophic gastropathy of childhood*.[16] The clinical, pathologic, and etiologic factors of this disease in children differ from those of the adult form. In adults, the disease is chronic and premalignant. In children, the disease is self-limiting, with a peak age of presentation of 5 years. Presentation includes acute vomiting, diarrhea, upper abdominal pain, and anorexia. Peripheral edema is usually present and may be associated with ascites and pleural effusions. Rarely, signs of GI bleeding occur with coexisting ulceration of the gastric rugae. The etiology of the disease remains unknown; however, it has been previously associated with several infectious agents, including cytomegalovirus, *H. pylori*, mycoplasma, herpes virus, and *Giardia lamblia*.

Imaging Diagnosis is most commonly made with UGI contrast studies demonstrating thickened gastric mucosal folds in the fundus and body, sparing the antrum and pylorus, with normal appearance of the small bowel.[17] Ultrasound has also been successfully used in diagnosis.[18] On the CT scan, similar findings of thickened rugal folds in the fundus and body of the stomach can be seen, with sparing of the antrum (Fig. 102-6). Endoscopy confirms the diagnosis. Differential diagnosis includes eosinophilic gastritis, primary gastric lymphoma, gastric carcinoma, inflammatory pseudotumor, gastric varices, Zollinger-Ellison syndrome, lymphangiectasia, and anisakiasis if there is a history of ingestion of raw fish.[16]

Treatment and Follow-up The disease in children is self-limiting, as mentioned above.[16] After correction of hypoproteinemia, complete clinical recovery usually occurs within 2 to 4 weeks, although symptoms found on radiologic and endoscopic assessment may require months to resolve.[19]

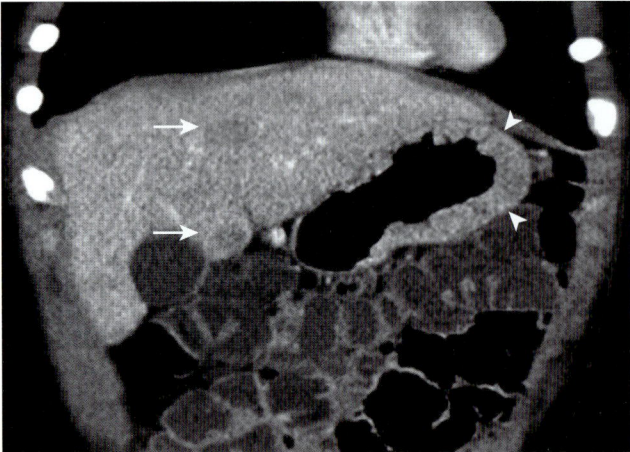

Figure 102-4 Zollinger-Ellison syndrome secondary to a pancreatic gastrinoma in a 10 year-old-boy. The coronal image of a contrast-enhanced computed tomography shows marked segmental thickening of the gastric fundus and body (*arrowheads*). Two hypodense lesion in the liver indicate metastases (*arrows*).

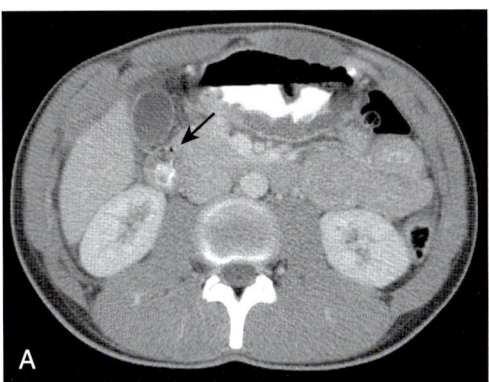 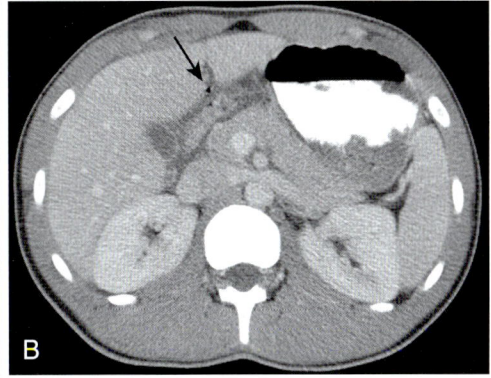

Figure 102-5 Perforated duodenal ulcer in 16-year-old boy on nonsteroidal antiinflammatory regimen for previous knee injury and surgery, presenting with acute onset of abdominal pain while in school. **A,** A contrast-enhanced computed tomography scan shows marked thickening of the duodenal wall and small amount of free air (*arrow*). **B,** The slightly more cephalad image shows fluid about the duodenum and additional free air extending toward the area of the falciform ligament (*arrow*).

Chronic Granulomatous Disease

Etiology Chronic granulomatous disease (CGD) of childhood is a hereditary disorder of neutrophil function, which is typically inherited as an X-linked recessive disorder, but three autosomal recessive defects have also been identified. The genetic alteration leads to a defect in activation of the NADPH (nicotinamide adenine dinucleotide phosphate-oxidase) molecule within the phagocyte, preventing the formation of free radical superoxide in the "respiratory burst," and resulting in survival of catalase-positive organisms within the phagocytes, with chronic inflammatory reaction and granuloma formation.[20] In the stomach, narrowing of the gastric antrum is a distinctive manifestation of CGD, occurring in 16% of cases.[21] Gastric outlet obstruction occurs in the X-linked recessive form more commonly than in the autosomal recessive form and presents at a mean age of 44 months, usually with severe vomiting.[22] Histologically, a granuloma forms within the involved antral wall; however,

the etiology of the antral wall thickening is unclear, as an infectious agent is not typically isolated.[23]

Imaging A patient with CGD and signs of gastric outlet obstruction should be initially evaluated with either an ultrasound or a UGI contrast study. The patient's medical history is vital to obtain the correct diagnosis. Ultrasound demonstrates the circumferential antral wall thickening. The UGI contrast study shows concentric antral narrowing and evaluates the degree of gastric obstruction.[21] To detect the gastric wall thickening on CT, the stomach should be distended. Although CT is not the primary modality to assess gastric involvement, it may be helpful in identifying disease in other areas of involvement such as mesenteric adenopathy and hepatic or splenic involvement. The differential diagnosis of gastric antral involvement includes peptic ulcer disease, Crohn disease, (Fig. 102-7), and eosinophilic gastritis.[24,25]

Treatment and Follow-up Most patients respond in a few weeks to conservative medical management with nutritional support, steroids, and antibiotics.[22]

Eosinophilic Gastritis

Etiology Eosinophilic gastroenteritis is a cluster of rare and poorly understood illnesses that share as their hallmark gastric and intestinal eosinophilic infiltration, peripheral eosinophilia, and elevated serum immunoglobulin E and may involve other parts of the GI tract, including the esophagus, duodenum, and colon. Patients may present between infancy and adolescence, with symptoms of abdominal pain, anorexia, failure to thrive, anemia, gastric obstruction, protein-losing enteropathy, and ascites with eosinophilia.[26] Foods most often associated with exacerbations include cow's milk, eggs, and soy. The disease is likely to remit before adulthood in approximately 70% of pediatric patients.

Imaging On UGI or CT a lacy or nodular mucosal pattern is seen in the antrum, with sparing of the body and fundus, corresponding to the eosinophilic infiltration of the layers of the bowel wall, as seen on histology (Fig. 102-8).[27] On ultrasound, the predominantly antral abnormality can mimic

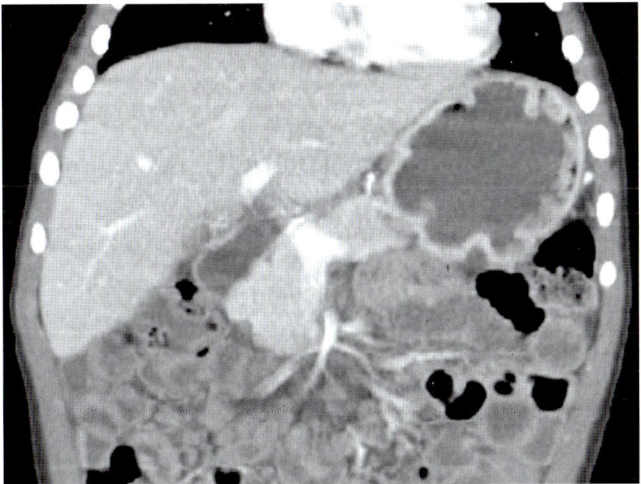

Figure 102-6 **Ménétrier disease.** Contrast-enhanced coronal computed tomography reformation shows the typical thickening of the gastric folds in the fundus of the well distended stomach in a 4-year-old boy presenting with 10 days of vomiting with streaks of blood, palpebral edema, and hypoalbuminemia. Ménétrier disease confirmed with endoscopy and gastric biopsy.

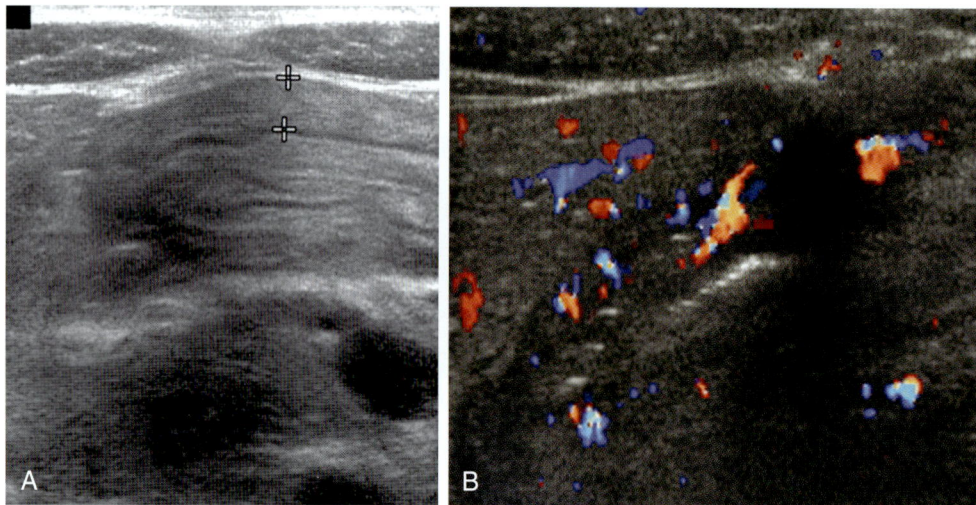

Figure 102-7 Antral involvement in 15-year-old boy with chronic granulomatous disease, presenting with vomiting. **A,** *Ultrasound of the gastric antrum shows marked mural thickening; anterior wall between crosshairs measured 6 mm.* **B,** *Color Doppler evaluation of the same area shows hyperemia.*

findings seen in hypertrophic pyloric stenosis, and this condition should be suspected if such findings are seen in conjunction with eosinophilia.[28]

Treatment and Follow-up Restriction of the offending foods has a variable effect. Other treatments include oral cromolyn, corticosteroids, and amino acid–based elemental diet.[29]

Gastric Tumors and Tumor-Like Conditions

GASTROINTESTINAL FOREIGN BODIES

The ingestion of foreign objects is relatively common in pediatric patients. This is a potentially serious problem, with peak occurrence between 6 months and 3 years of age. However, significant morbidity occurs in only approximately 1% of the patients, with many patients remaining asymptomatic.[30,31] Since some foreign bodies may remain in the stomach, it is important to identify them and be aware of complications that could occur if these foreign bodies are not removed.

Etiology Coins and smooth, blunt objects account for most ingested foreign bodies; however, the materials commonly ingested differ, according to geography and cultural group.[32] In addition to the complications related to the size and shape of the foreign object, some ingested foreign bodies such as batteries can lead to toxicity because of their chemical composition (Fig. 102-9) or to mechanical problems and pressure necrosis, as can occur after ingestion of multiple magnets.

Imaging Approximately 64% of foreign bodies are radiopaque and can be identified on plain films.[30] Non-radiopaque ingested objects include those made of wood or plastic. Images of the neck, chest, and abdomen are indicated when foreign body ingestion is suspected; the child must be imaged from the mouth to the anus. Fluoroscopic studies using water-soluble contrast may be useful in identifying cases of suspected non-opaque foreign body ingestion.[32]

Treatment and Follow-up Although 90% of foreign bodies that have passed through the esophagus do so spontaneously, removal of sharp objects before they enter the duodenum is recommended.[32,33] Once the foreign body has passed through the stomach, caregivers of the child are instructed to review the stool to verify that the object has been expelled. If, after a week, the child has not excreted the object, a radiograph is necessary to locate it; if it is still in the duodenum, endoscopic removal is indicated.[34] Disk or button batteries require special attention and should be endoscopically removed because of the damage caused by their direct corrosive effects. If they are located within the esophagus, button batteries should be removed emergently because of the potential for burns and strictures. Removal from the stomach is more important with larger batteries that are less likely to pass spontaneously.[33,35]

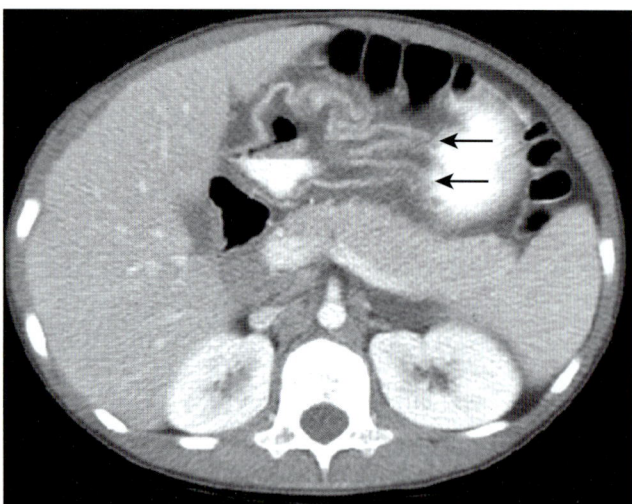

Figure 102-8 Eosinophilic gastritis in a 14-year-old with chronic abdominal pain, failure to thrive, and nausea. Contrast-enhanced computed tomography shows marked thickening of the gastric rugae predominantly in the antrum (*arrows*). There is mural stratification indicating edema. Note the lack of subcutaneous fat in this child with failure to thrive.

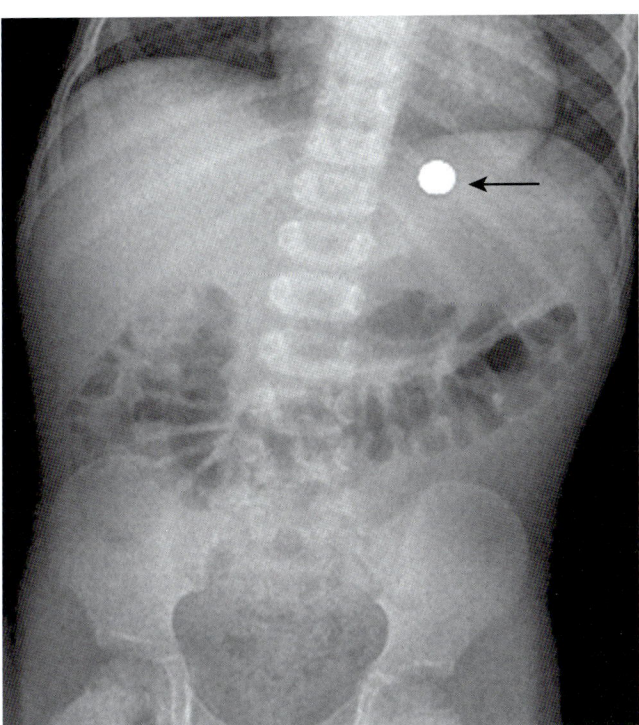

Figure 102-9 Ingested watch battery in a 2-year-old child. Supine view of the chest and abdomen shows the ingested battery (arrow) in the gastric fundus.

BEZOARS

Bezoars are foreign bodies within the stomach or other portions of the GI tract that form from the accretion of nondigestible materials and increase in size over time. The term *bezoar* originates from the Arabic word "badzehr." The original meaning of the Arabic word was "antidote for poisons" because bezoars from animals were thought to have healing or magical powers and were used as homeopathic treatment for a wide variety of maladies such as seizure disorders and bubonic plague.[36]

Patients with bezoars can be asymptomatic or present with relatively nonspecific symptoms such as epigastric discomfort. Other complaints include bloating, nausea and vomiting, early satiety, halitosis, dysphagia, and failure to thrive.

Etiology Patients with developmental delay and psychiatric illnesses such as anorexia nervosa are at increased risk for bezoars. Predisposing factors include prior gastric surgery, diabetes mellitus with gastroparesis, cystic fibrosis, intrahepatic cholestasis, and renal failure.

The three most common bezoar types are (1) *trichobezoars* composed of ingested hair, (2) *phytobezoars* composed of plant matter, and (3) *lactobezoars* composed of undigested milk curds (Box 102-1). Trichobezoars usually result from swallowing of multiple small amounts of hair plucked from the head or fibers from fur, rugs, or garments. The hairs or fibers become lodged in the gastric mucosal folds and over a period, an intraluminal mass develops. The bezoar forms a cast of the lumen of the stomach and a tail may extend into the duodenum as well. Additional bezoars may occur more distally in the bowel (Fig. 102-10) and occasionally may

---

Box 102-1 Types of Bezoar According to the Ingested Material

Phytobezoar: Nondigestible food particles found in fruits (dates, persimmon) and vegetables (cellulose, hemicellulose, lignin)

Trichobezoar: Hair or other fibers; associated with young females and/or patients with psychiatric illnesses who ingest hair, carpet, rope, string, etc.

Lactobezoar: Compact mass of undigested milk concretions traditionally seen in preterm neonates on highly concentrated formula

Pharmacobezoar: Conglomeration of medications or medication vehicles

Other: Mixture of hair, fruit, and fiber

Worms

---

extend throughout the intestine, in which case, it is termed "Rapunzel syndrome."[36]

Phytobezoars are composed of plant matter such as cellulose and fruit tannins. They develop most frequently following the ingestion of high-fiber vegetables and fruits, and in adults, they are seen most frequently in patients who have had prior surgery.

Lactobezoars (Fig. 102-11) occur in pediatric patients with a history of prematurity and who are given a highly concentrated formula; additional risk factors include poor neonatal gastric motility and dehydration.

Imaging In the case of bezoars, the plain radiograph demonstrates a filling defect outlined by gas in the region of the stomach, with gastric distension if gastric outlet obstruction

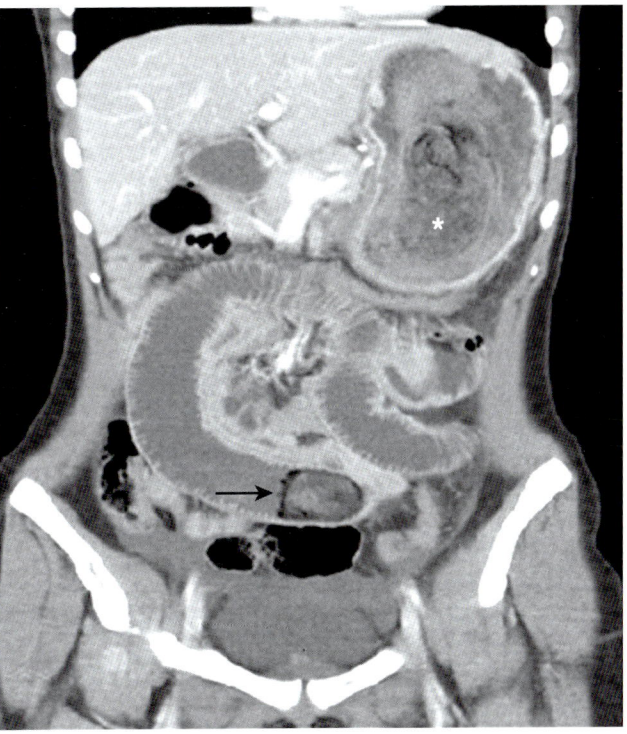

Figure 102-10 Trichobezoar in an adolescent girl with anorexia nervosa. A coronal image of a contrast-enhanced computed tomography scan shows a trichobezoar (*asterisk*) of multiple densities forming a cast within the gastric lumen. An additional trichobezoar in the midjejunum (*arrow*) is causing proximal small bowel obstruction.

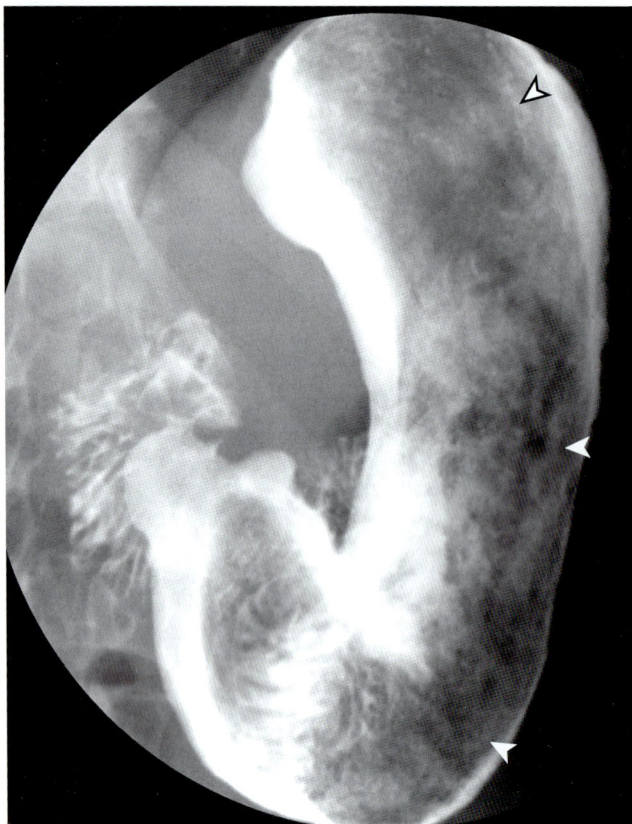

Figure 102-11 Lactobezoar in a 6-month-old infant. Oblique view of an UGI shows a well-defined oval filling defect in the gastric lumen (*arrowheads*), which was confirmed to be a lactobezoar on subsequent endoscopy.

is also present. Fluoroscopic contrast studies will show the mass when the contrast material coats the bezoar and infiltrates within its interstices, producing the characteristic mottled appearance (see Fig. 102-11). A CT scan may also help identify a bezoar, typically without the need for ingestion of contrast material; CT may also help identify additional bezoars (see Fig. 102-10) as well as potential complications such as obstruction or perforation.[1]

Treatment and Follow-up Therapeutic options for treating amenable bezoars include fragmentation and dissolution with enzymatic therapy or, in cases of lactobezoars, gastric lavage with saline, followed by dietary modification. In cases of motility disorders, the administration of prokinetic agents is important to prevent recurrence. Surgical or endoscopic extraction is reserved for trichobezoars or for those instances where the above measures fail.[36]

GASTRIC TUMORS

Etiology Tumors of the stomach, whether primary or metastatic, are rare in children. The differential diagnosis of a gastric mass includes polyps, lymphoma, GI stromal tumor (GIST), leiomyosarcoma, teratoma, and inflammatory pseudotumor.

Polyps, which may occur anywhere along the GI tract, are the most common gastric tumors in children. Isolated gastric polyps are typically benign hyperplastic polyps or are related to pancreatic heterotopia. Polyps can be part of a syndrome such as hamartomatous polyps in Peutz-Jeghers syndrome or adenomatous polyps in Gardner syndrome and familial adenomatous polyposis. Gastric polyps may be seen in up to 60% of patients with familial polyposis syndrome, and lifelong endoscopic surveillance of these patients is warranted because of the potential for malignant transformation of adenomatous polyps.[37] An increased risk of malignancy is also seen in patients with Peutz-Jeghers syndrome.[38-41]

Primary gastric lymphoma can be divided into mucosa-associated lymphoid tissue (MALT) lymphoma and non-MALT lymphoma.[42,43] MALT lesions typically arise in response to a stimulus such as *H. pylori* infection and are rare in children.[44,45] Non-MALT primary gastric lymphomas are also rare and are usually high-grade non-Hodgkin lymphomas of B-cell origin, usually of the Burkitt type.[46]

GIST are mesenchymal neoplasms derived from the muscle wall of hollow viscera in the GI tract and are thought to perhaps be derived from the interstitial cells of Cajal. These tumors are very rare in pediatric patients and are thought to represent a majority of tumors previously carrying the diagnoses of leiomyomas, leiomyosarcomas, and leiomyoblastomas.[47] However, unlike those tumors, GIST neoplasms are positive for c-KIT and PDGFRA kinase protein and gene mutations, although the pathology in pediatric patients may not be as clear.[48-50] These tumors may be found in the gastric antrum or body, are more commonly found in adolescent girls, and may be associated with pulmonary chondroma and extra-adrenal paraganglioma (Carney triad), or neurofibromatosis type-1.[47,50]

Leiomyoma and *leiomyosarcoma* are also mesenchymal neoplasms; unlike GIST, these tumors are c-KIT and PDGFRA negative but do demonstrate smooth muscle markers. They are uncommon in children, the peak age at presentation being the sixth decade. Although polypoid leiomyomas are the most common smooth muscle neoplasm arising in the GI tract, they are very rare outside of the esophagus and rectosigmoid; likewise, the malignant leiomyosarcoma in the stomach is very rare.[51]

Gastric teratomas comprise less than 1% of teratomas in pediatric patients and occur much more frequently in the sacrococcygeal region, the mediastinum, and gonads.[52] Gastric teratomas show a striking male predominance and present early in life in neonates and infants.[53,54]

Inflammatory pseudotumor, also known as *plasma cell granuloma*, is composed of myofibroblasts, fibroblasts, histiocytes, plasma cells, and lymphocytes. It occurs most commonly in the lung but can occur rarely in the stomach. It is associated with microcystic anemia, hypergammaglobulinemia, and elevated sedimentation rate.[55]

Gastric neoplasms have similar presentations, which include palpable mass, GI bleeding, anemia, abdominal pain, and, less frequently, gastric outlet obstruction. In cases of lymphoma, constitutional symptoms can be present.

Imaging Polyps can be seen on UGI contrast study series as pedunculated or sessile smooth mucosal lesions arising from the gastric wall. Adenomatous polyps are usually antral and multiple. The appearance is similar on CT, requiring appropriate gastric distension to secure the diagnosis (Fig. 102-12).[56]

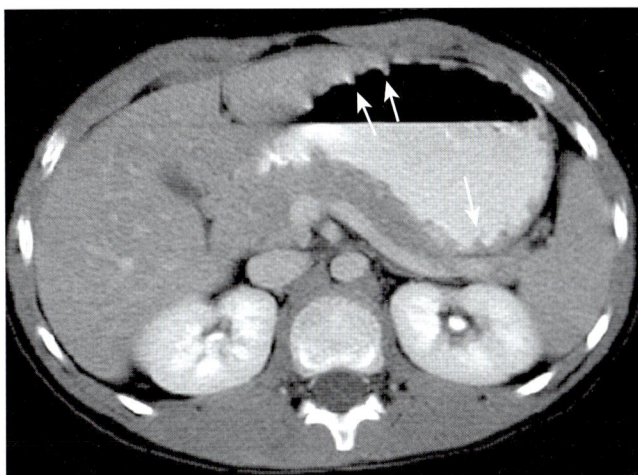

Figure 102-12 Multiple gastric polyps in a patient with Gardner syndrome, status post total colectomy. Contrast-enhanced computed tomography shows multiple tiny polyps arising diffusely from the gastric wall protruding into the lumen (*arrows*), confirmed at endoscopy.

In both the rare primary and the more common secondary gastric lymphomas, CT reveals focal or diffuse mural masses that can protrude into the gastric lumen (Fig. 102-13) or cause mass effect on adjacent structures. Multifocal intestinal involvement can be present, as well as hepatosplenomegaly and regional or distant adenopathy. On UGI, mucosal nodularity, rugal thickening, and masses with or without associated ulceration can be seen.[45] CT–positron emission tomography (CT-PET) is used in the contemporary staging of lymphoma in children and to assess disease activity and involvement of distant sites, particularly in lymph nodes that do not meet size criteria for pathologic involvement.[57,58]

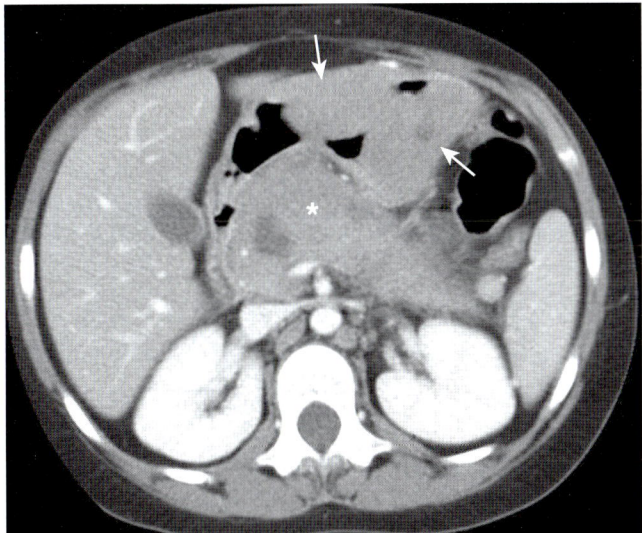

Figure 102-13 Burkitt's lymphoma in a 14-year-old girl presenting with vomiting and fever. Axial image of a contrast enhanced computed tomography scan shows two large smooth and homogeneous masses arising from the gastric wall protruding into the gastric lumen (*arrows*). The masses are isodense to muscle. A large more heterogeneous mass involving the pancreas is also present (*asterisk*).

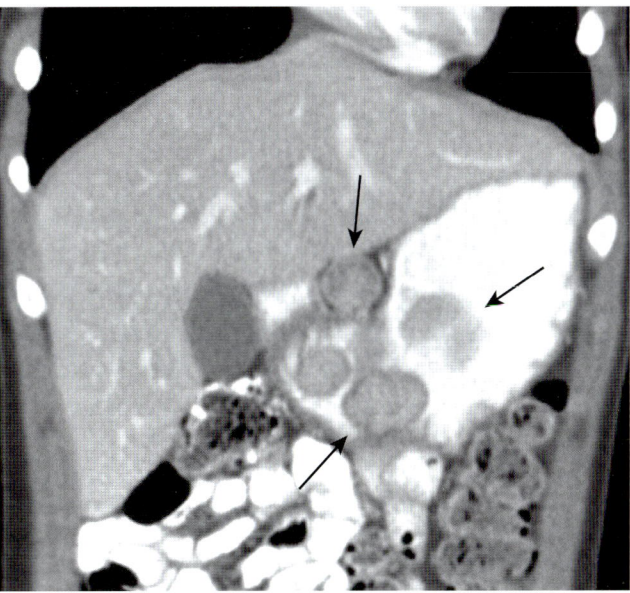

Figure 102-14 Multifocal gastrointestinal stromal tumor in an adolescent girl presenting with chronic abdominal pain and anemia. A coronal image from a contrast-enhanced computed tomography scan shows multiple small, well-defined masses arising from the wall of the gastric antrum (*arrows*).

Other tumors such as GIST are seen as masses extending into the gastric lumen (Fig. 102-14) or as mass effect on adjacent structures. Extension beyond the stomach is best appreciated on cross-sectional imaging such as CT or magnetic resonance imaging. CT-PET is useful in the assessment of distant metastases.[50] When calcifications are present, teratoma may be suspected.[52]

Treatment and Follow-up   Once the diagnosis of a mass has been suggested on imaging studies, it should prompt endoscopic evaluation and biopsy for confirmation. The treatment of gastric lymphoma, which still remains controversial, is usually chemotherapy, but *H. pylori*–eradicating therapy has been also advocated.[59,60] CT-PET is currently used to monitor response to treatment.[57,58]

Resection is the first-line treatment and the only treatment that may lead to full remission in patients with primary GIST and other solid gastric tumors. It may be possible to remove smaller lesions endoscopically. In very advanced inoperable or metastatic disease, chemotherapy with targeted c-KIT tyrosine kinase inhibitors has proven very effective in GIST. CT-PET is the imaging modality of choice for monitoring the response to chemotherapy.[61,62]

WHAT THE CLINICIAN NEEDS TO KNOW

- Types of gastric volvulus, diagnostic imaging, and the possible complications
- Differential diagnosis of gastric wall thickening in children
- Imaging appearance of high-risk GI foreign bodies such as magnets and batteries
- Types of neoplasms in children that involve the stomach and the diagnostic characteristics of these neoplasms

Key Points

The two types of gastric volvulus have different presentations. The *organoaxial type* usually presents with chronic abdominal pain, vomiting, and gastric distension. The *mesenteroaxial type* typically has a sudden presentation, with vomiting and acute abdominal pain.

Once they have reached the stomach, most ingested foreign bodies require no intervention, as they are excreted spontaneously.

Predisposing factors for bezoars include are psychiatric problems, previous gastric surgery, gastroparesis, cystic fibrosis, and renal failure.

Gastric wall thickening in children can be caused by several conditions. When involving the antrum, eosinophilic gastritis and CGD must be considered. When involving the fundus and body, Ménétrier disease is possible.

Suggested Readings

Chen MK, Beierle EA. Gastrointestinal foreign bodies. *Pediatr Ann.* 2001;30:736-742.

Lin C, Lee H, Hung H, et al. Neonatal gastric perforation: report of 15 cases. *Pediatr Neonatol.* 2008;49(3):65-70.

Oh SK, Han BK, Levin TL, et al. Gastric volvulus in children: the twists and turns of an unusual entity. *Pediatr Radiol.* 2008;38:297-304.

Wang L, Lee H, Yeung C, et al. Gastrointestinal polyps in children. *Pediatr Neonatol.* 2009;50(5):196-201.

References

Full references for this chapter can be found on www.expertconsult.com.

Congenital and Neonatal Abnormalities

MARTA HERNANZ-SCHULMAN

Duodenum

Congenital anomalies of the duodenum consist of intrinsic obstructing lesions, such as duodenal atresia and stenosis, or extrinsic lesions that affect the duodenum, such as midgut malrotation with Ladd bands, annular pancreas, preduodenal portal vein, and duplication cysts; intrinsic and extrinsic lesions may coexist in the same patient.

INTRINSIC LESIONS: DUODENAL ATRESIA AND STENOSIS

Overview Duodenal atresia and stenosis represent a spectrum ranging from complete to partial obstruction, presenting from prenatal life to late childhood or even adulthood. The incidence of duodenal atresia or stenosis is cited as approximately 1:7000 live births and represents nearly half of intestinal atresias.[1,2] Similar to atresia of the more distal bowel, duodenal atresia is classified as types I through III. Type I atresias consist of a completely or partially obstructing membrane, type II atresias are connected by a fibrous cord, and type III atresias are separated by a gap. The duodenal diverticulum or "windsock" duodenum is considered a variant of type I atresia.[3]

Etiology The lumen of the duodenum is obliterated during the fourth to sixth weeks of gestation because of rapid cell division and normally recanalizes by the twelfth week. The etiology of duodenal atresia and stenosis is believed to be the result of failure of recanalization of the lumen of the duodenum.[4,5]

Clinical Presentation Presentation may occur prenatally with polyhydramnios, which occurs in approximately 30% to 50% of cases,[3,5] and premature birth is seen in nearly half of patients.[5] Approximately one third of cases of congenital duodenal obstruction presenting in the neonatal period are due to duodenal stenosis.[5] Postnatally, infants with atresia typically present with vomiting within the first 24 hours of life. Because duodenal atresia/stenosis typically occurs distal to the ampulla of Vater, these patients will present with bilious vomiting. However, obstruction occurs proximal to the ampulla of Vater in as many as 23% of patients.[6,7] Such

patients will present with nonbilious vomiting, simulating hypertrophic pyloric stenosis. Because duodenal obstruction is proximal, abdominal distension is not a typical finding, although fullness in the epigastric region may be present as a result of the dilated stomach and duodenum. Patients with duodenal stenosis may present later in life, depending on the degree of obstruction; presentation may be relatively nonspecific (such as failure to thrive), or it may present as pancreatitis as a result of reflux into the pancreatic duct, proximal to the site of obstruction.[8,9] Presentation may be precipitated by ingestion of a foreign body, which fails to pass and may exacerbate the degree of obstruction, leading to abdominal pain and/or vomiting.[10] In patients with a duodenal diaphragm, an intraluminal duodenal diverticulum or "windsock" may be found, and presentation also may be precipitated by ingestion of a foreign body.[11]

Associated anomalies are common in patients with duodenal atresia/stenosis and may be responsible for presenting signs and symptoms. Annular pancreas and malrotation are seen in approximately one third of cases.[5] Trisomy 21 is present in approximately 25% to 40% of infants with duodenal atresia/stenosis; conversely, approximately 4% of infants with Down syndrome have duodenal obstruction.[5,12] Hirschsprung disease has been reported in approximately 1% to 3% of patients with duodenal atresia and Down syndrome.[13,14] Duodenal atresia may be seen in approximately 5% of patients with esophageal atresia with or without a fistula.[15] Heterotaxy with polysplenia has been reported in patients with duodenal diaphragm/intraluminal diverticulum.[8,16]

Imaging Abdominal radiographs are the starting point in the evaluation of a child with suspected obstruction. In the neonate with duodenal atresia, the abdominal radiograph demonstrates the classic "double bubble appearance," representing the dilated stomach and duodenum.[17,18] Because obstruction has been present in utero, the obstructed proximal duodenum is typically large, approximately one half to one third the size of the stomach (Fig. 103-1); at times the pylorus is wide open, and the two bubbles are not distinctly separated (see Fig. 103-1, *B*). This appearance on the abdominal radiograph is diagnostic, and contrast studies to confirm the diagnosis are not needed. Rarely, air can be seen distally in a patient with complete atresia; this occurs when the atresia

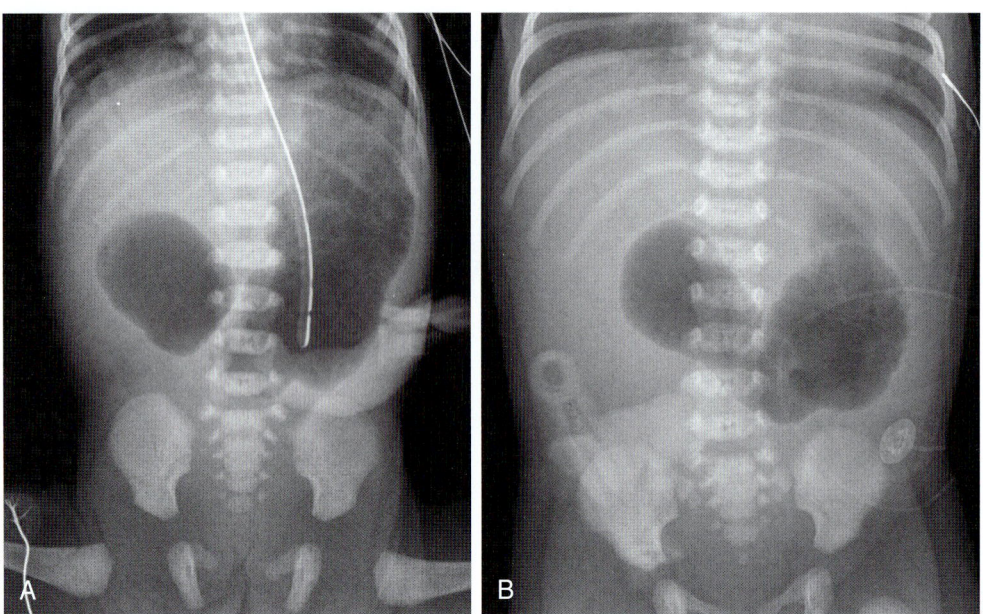

Figure 103-1   Duodenal atresia. **A,** A 1-day-old premature infant born at 32 weeks' gestation with prenatally diagnosed duodenal atresia. The radiograph shows the classic double bubble, with a distended stomach and duodenum and no distal gas. **B,** A full-term infant with a prenatal diagnosis of duodenal atresia. The radiograph shows a gaping pylorus through which there is wide communication between the dilated stomach and the dilated duodenum, with no distal gas. At surgery, an associated malrotation without volvulus was discovered, and a Ladd procedure was performed, in addition to a duodenoduodenostomy.

is flanked by the branches of an anomalous bifid common bile duct, with separate insertions into the duodenum above and below the point of atresia. Air or contrast material may be seen refluxing into the anomalous ducts, which allow the contents of the obstructed proximal duodenum to course into the distal duodenum, bypassing the point of obstruction (Fig. 103-2).[7,19] In patients with duodenal stenosis, dilatation of the stomach and proximal duodenum and decrease in distal gas is seen commensurate with the degree of obstruction. If the stenosis is mild or the stomach is decompressed via an

enteric tube, the plain abdominal radiographs may be nonrevealing (e-Fig. 103-3). In patients with duodenal atresia associated with esophageal atresia with a fistula, plain films are diagnostic (Fig. 103-4).

An upper gastrointestinal (GI) series may be needed in patients with duodenal stenosis or in cases in which differentiation from malrotation is a concern. Furthermore, malrotation can coexist with duodenal stenosis or atresia (e-Fig. 103-5).[20] Therefore if any clinical concern for malrotation exists or if surgery is to be delayed, an upper GI series is

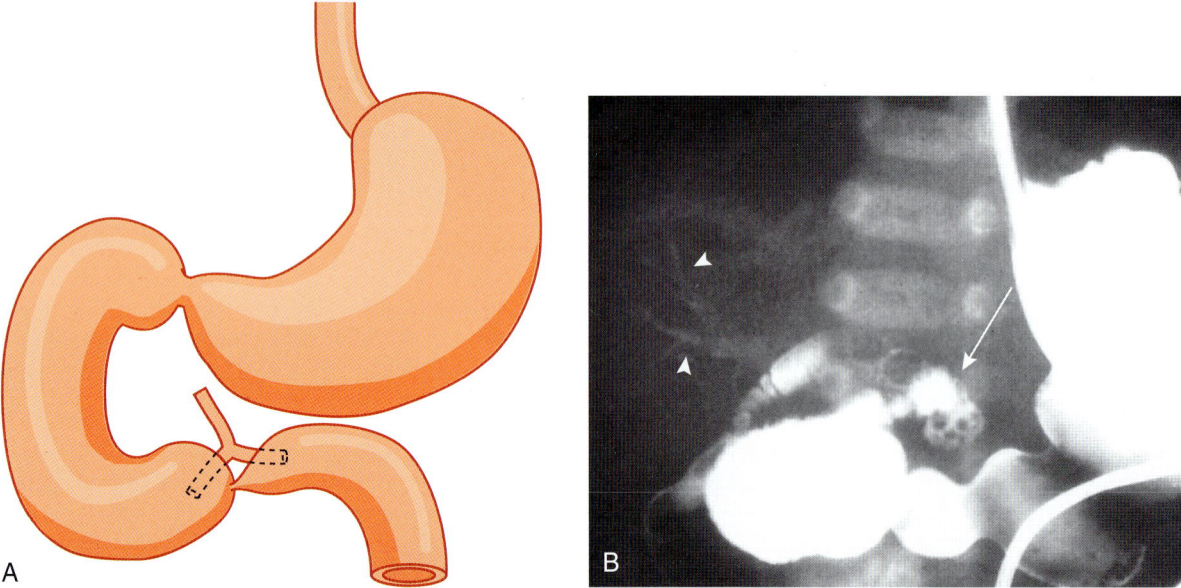

Figure 103-2   Duodenal stenosis with anomalous ducts. **A,** A schematic rendering of duodenal obstruction bypass by dual anomalous ducts. **B,** An upper gastrointestinal series in a neonate with duodenal atresia shows contrast material within the ductal system (*arrowheads*) and within the bowel lumen beyond the site of obstruction.

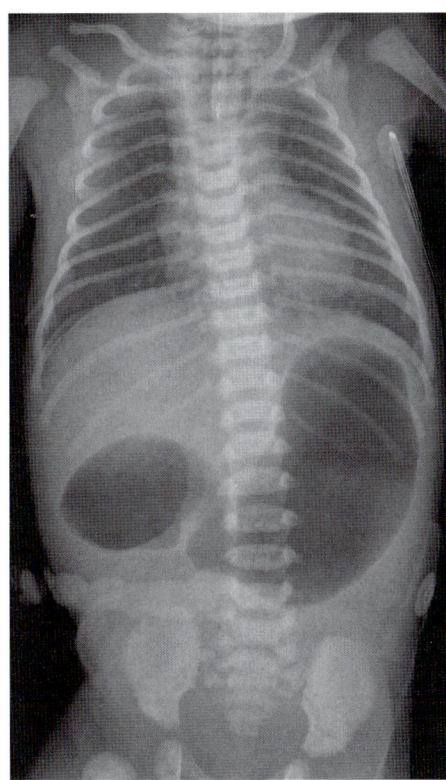

Figure 103-4 A 1-day-old infant with esophageal and duodenal atresia. Note the orogastric tube in the proximal esophageal pouch; abdominal double bubble indicates a distal tracheoesophageal fistula and duodenal atresia.

indicated. In patients with duodenal atresia, contrast enema has been performed in the past to assess the rotation of the bowel, but this examination is not helpful if it is normal or if the cecum is high-riding.[21,22]

In patients with duodenal stenosis, an upper GI series will confirm the partial obstruction (Fig. 103-6); when a web is present, the membrane may be seen as a thin linear filling defect (see Fig. 103-6, *B* and *C*). A duodenal diverticulum is more conspicuous, particularly when underscored by an

ingested foreign body (e-Fig. 103-7). In patients with duodenal atresia simulating duodenal stenosis as a result of bypass of the obstruction by anomalous ducts, contrast may be seen within the ducts, as previously discussed (see Fig. 103-2).

Cross-sectional imaging currently does not have a routine place in evaluation of patients with duodenal atresia or stenosis. However, occasionally a patient with duodenal stenosis proximal to the ampulla of Vater will present with nonbilious vomiting and come to ultrasound with a primary concern of pyloric stenosis. In those cases, ultrasound will reveal an abnormally distended pylorus and dilatation of the duodenal bulb (Fig. 103-8).

Treatment Treatment of duodenal atresia and symptomatic duodenal stenosis is surgical repair. At the time when Ladd reported surgical correction of duodenal obstruction in 1932,[23] the reported mortality rate was approximately 40%.[24] In 1990, Kimura et al. described the technique of diamond-shaped anastomosis, which has become the standard procedure for open repair, with reported mortality of 5% to 10%, largely due to associated anomalies, particularly those involving cardiac lesions.[24,25] More recently, laparoscopic duodeno-duodenostomy has been introduced with increasingly good results and reported improvement in return of bowel function, leading to reduced length of hospital stay.[24,26]

EXTRINSIC LESIONS: ANNULAR PANCREAS, MALROTATION, PREDUODENAL PORTAL VEIN, AND DUPLICATION CYSTS

Annular Pancreas

Overview Annular pancreas refers to encirclement of the descending portion of the duodenum by the pancreatic head. The prevalence of annular pancreas is not known, because asymptomatic cases are not always identified. Autopsy prevalence varies between 1 to 15:100,000 adults, whereas endoscopic retrograde cholangiopancreatography (ERCP) studies report 1 to 4:1000 among symptomatic patients.[27,28] In children the incidence is estimated at approximately 1 to 12:15,000 births.[29] Annular pancreas may result in extrinsic duodenal obstruction; however, most cases of duodenal

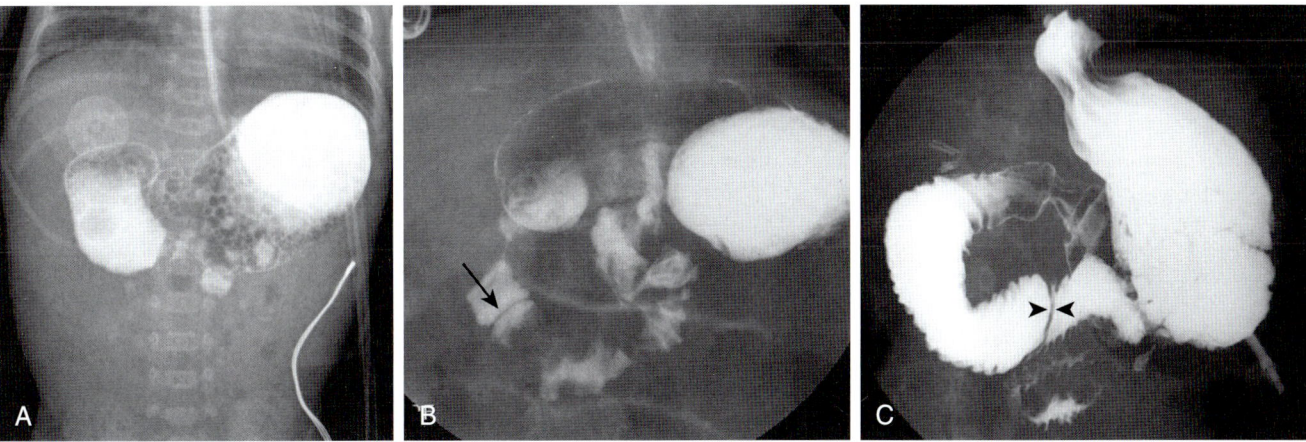

Figure 103-6 Duodenal stenosis. **A,** The same infant as shown in e-Figure 103-3, *A.* A 30-minute radiograph after upper gastrointestinal (GI) examination shows the duodenal obstruction. **B,** The same infant as shown in e-Figure 103-3, *B.* An image from an upper GI examination shows a duodenal web (*arrow*). **C,** Image from an upper GI examination in a 9-month-old girl demonstrates a thin duodenal web (*arrowheads*).

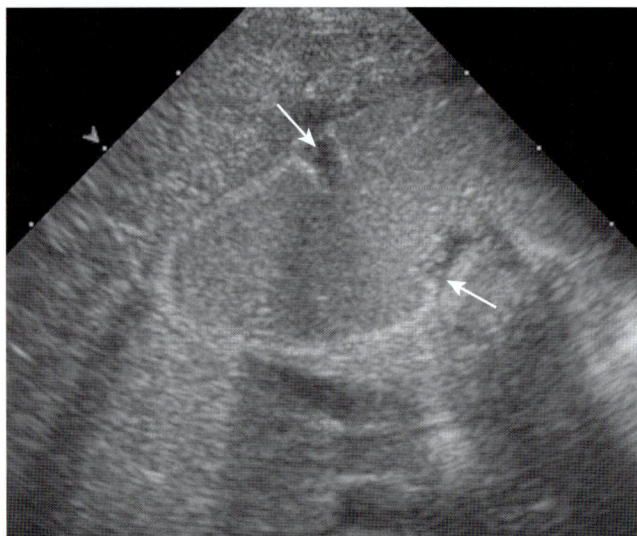

Figure 103-8 Duodenal stenosis. An ultrasound image of a 4-week-old girl with nonbilious vomiting and suspected pyloric stenosis. The image shows a widely dilated pylorus (*arrows*) and duodenal bulb. The diagnosis of duodenal stenosis was confirmed at subsequent surgery.

obstruction with annular pancreas are most likely the result of an associated intrinsic duodenal abnormality.[3]

Etiology The pancreas arises as a small ventral and a larger dorsal bud from the duodenum. Normally the ventral bud rotates and fuses with the dorsal bud. When the ventral bud becomes tethered to the duodenum prior to rotation, or if the ventral bud fails to rotate completely before fusion, the result is an annular pancreas.[3,28,30] The pancreatic annulus, the portion surrounding the duodenum, frequently has a separate duct entering the duodenum, opposite the ampulla of Vater. Duodenal contents may reflux through this duct into the annulus.

Clinical Presentation Annular pancreas may be asymptomatic, and adult presentation has been reported (median age of 47 years) with signs and symptoms consistent with neoplasm, jaundice due to obstruction of the common bile duct, or pancreatitis, because duodenal contents may reflux through a separate pancreatic duct into the annulus.[28,31] Pediatric patients typically present at a median age of 1 day at diagnosis with findings related to duodenal obstruction, which are either revealed at prenatal sonography or manifested as vomiting or feeding intolerance soon after birth.[28] Older pediatric patients can present with pancreatitis and jaundice.

Associated anomalies are common in children and include malrotation, esophageal atresia, anal atresia, and cardiac defects, particularly in patients with trisomy 21 and Cornelia de Lange syndrome[12,28]; annular pancreas also has been reported in patients with heterotaxy.[32]

Imaging Plain radiographs show findings of duodenal dilatation in patients who have an obstruction. An upper GI series will show narrowing of the descending portion of the duodenum (Fig. 103-9, A). Ultrasound may show a ring of pancreatic tissue about the descending portion of the duodenum, although the duodenum might be difficult to follow, and the appearance may resemble a mass at the level of the

head of the pancreas (Fig. 103-9, B). A more definitive diagnosis can be made with computed tomography (CT; Fig. 103-9, C to E). Magnetic resonance imaging (MRI) also may show the ring of pancreatic tissue, but MR cholangiopancreatography will show more definitive findings, outlining the annular course of the pancreatic ducts (see Fig. 103-9 F and G), analogous to the findings seen with endoscopic retrograde cholangiopancreatography (e-Fig. 103-10).

Treatment As in the case of intrinsic duodenal obstruction, treatment is surgical bypass; interruption or division of the pancreatic tissue around the duodenum is not indicated because of the likelihood of postoperative leakage or pancreatitis.[3]

Malrotation

Overview

The term "malrotation" indicates that the normal rotation of the midgut was not completed, thus presenting a spectrum of abnormalities that affect both the duodenojejunal and the cecal poles of the midgut, singly or in unison. The prevalence of malrotation is difficult to determine, inasmuch as asymptomatic cases may not be recognized; it has been quoted as high as 1:500 live births,[33] which seems excessive, as that is similar to the incidence of pyloric stenosis (2 to 5:1000).

The midgut encompasses the portion of the bowel that is supplied by the superior mesenteric artery and that extends from the distal descending duodenum to the distal transverse colon. The embryonic midgut undergoes 270° of counterclockwise rotation (as viewed from the front) through a relatively complex series of steps to achieve its final position.

The gut begins as a straight tube, with the duodenojejunal junction and the cecum along a straight line. As the gut begins to grow, it forms a primary loop about the axis of the superior mesenteric artery, with the apex at the omphalomesenteric duct; the proximal portion is the prearterial (duodenojejunal) limb, and the distal portion is the postarterial (ileocecal or cecocolic) limb. Initially, the duodenum and cecum rotate 90° counterclockwise, such that the duodenojejunal junction comes to lie in the right upper quadrant and the cecum comes to lie in the left lower quadrant. At approximately 6 weeks of gestation, continued growth of the intestinal tube results in herniation of the bowel into the umbilical cord and a second counterclockwise turn of 90° at the duodenojejunal junction. By the tenth week of gestation, the bowel begins its return into the abdominal cavity, beginning with the prearterial segment, and the duodenum undergoes its final 90° of rotation to terminate in the left upper quadrant and undergo fixation at the ligament of Treitz; the cecum undergoes its final 180° of rotation to terminate in the right lower quadrant and undergo fixation to the posterior peritoneum, through shortening and resorption of its dorsal mesentery.

The bowel is thus suspended from a mesentery that is attached to the posterior abdominal wall and that extends from the left upper to the right lower quadrants (Fig. 103-11). The configuration of the duodenal C-loop mirrors the 270° of rotation that it has undergone.[21,34-37] The final steps in bowel rotation and fixation involve resorption of the dorsal mesenteries of the ascending and descending colon and elongation of the ascending colon with descent of the cecum, processes that are ongoing until several months of postnatal

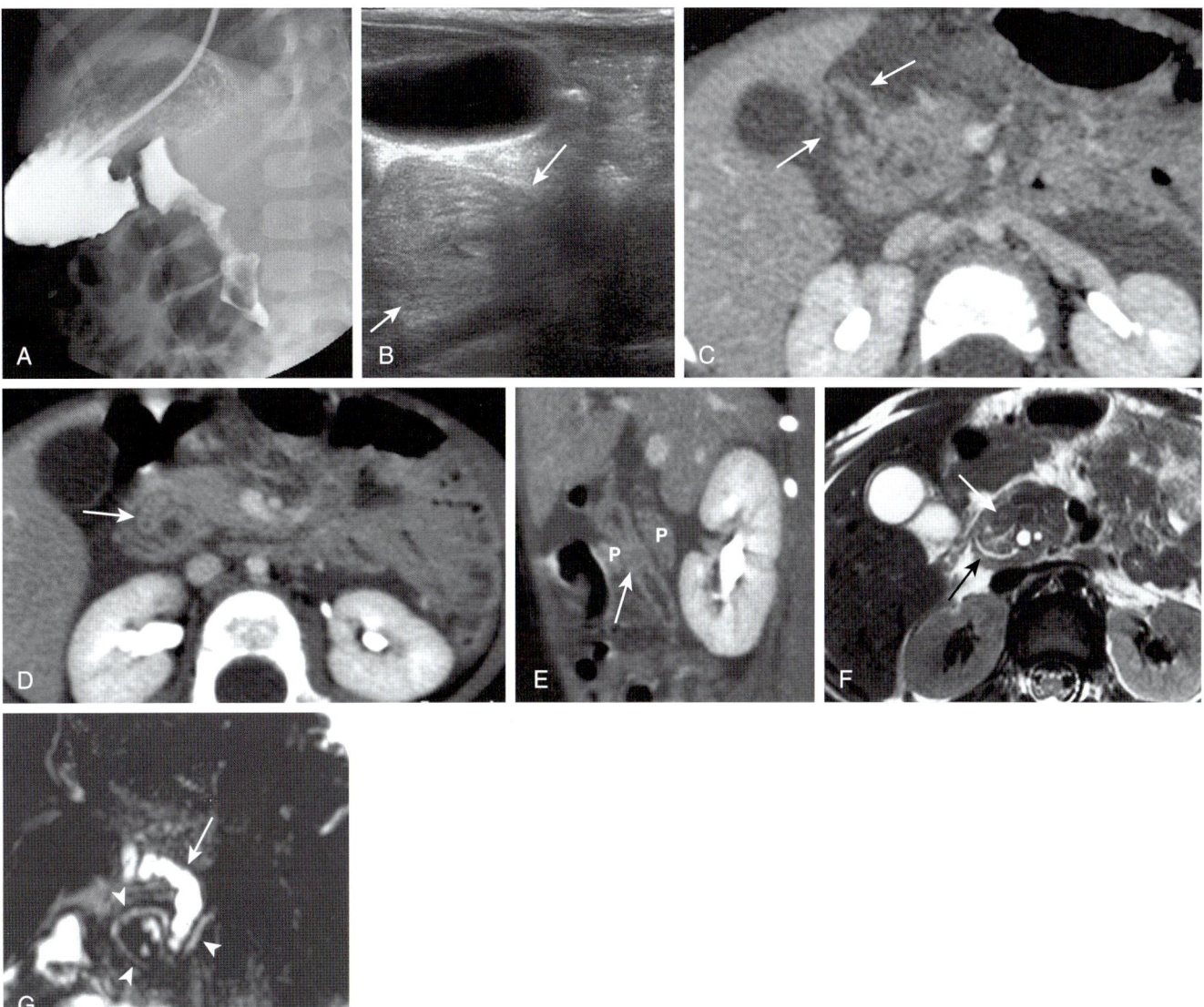

Figure 103-9 Annular pancreas. **A,** An upper gastrointestinal (UGI) examination in a 2-year-old girl with annular pancreas demonstrates a circumferential impression upon the descending duodenum. The patient had presented with pancreatitis; the UGI examination was performed after her symptoms had subsided, to assess for an underlying element of duodenal obstruction. **B,** Ultrasound at the time of initial presentation shows a thickened head of the pancreas (*arrows*); the central duodenum was not identified. **C-E,** Abdominal computed tomography images. **C,** The duodenum (*arrows*) is seen entering the head of the pancreas. **D,** The duodenum (*arrow*) is again seen within the head of the pancreas, just lateral to the common bile duct. **E,** Sagittal reformat shows the duodenum (*arrow*) with pancreatic tissue (*P*) anterior and posterior to its descending portion. Free fluid is secondary to pancreatitis. **F,** Abdominal T2-weighted magnetic resonance (MR) shows the duodenum (*white arrow*) within the head of the pancreas, with circumferential pancreatic tissue, outlined by a portion of the encircling pancreatic duct dorsally (*black arrow*). **G,** MR cholangiopancreatography delineates the pancreatic duct (*arrowheads*) and its circumferential course at the head of the pancreas. The arrow points to the dilated common bile duct. (Courtesy Melissa A. Hilmes, Nashville, TN.)

life.[33] The Meckel diverticulum is the demarcation point between the embryonic prearterial and postarterial limbs.

Etiology

The aforementioned background is important in the understanding of the clinical problems that arise with malrotation and malfixation of the bowel.

Malrotation arises when the process of normal rotation is arrested, which can occur at any point along the rotation of the duodenojejunal or cecal segments. If it is arrested after the initial 90° of counterclockwise rotation, the duodenojejunal junction and the small bowel will be located on the right side of the abdomen, and the cecum and the remainder of the colon will be located in the left side of the abdomen. Despite the fact that the initial 90° of counterclockwise rotation have occurred in both the duodenojejunal junction and the cecum, this arrangement is nevertheless known as nonrotation, a specific variant of malrotation, characterized by a relatively long mesenteric pedicle.[38]

Progression of the rotation process beyond the nonrotation stage brings the duodenojejunal junction and the cecum into proximity, and arrest along this portion of the spectrum typically results in a shorter mesenteric pedicle from which the bowel is suspended (Fig. 103-12), believed to increase the risk for subsequent volvulus. Reversed rotation is a rare form of malrotation in which the gut undergoes 90° of clockwise rotation, instead of the normal 270° of

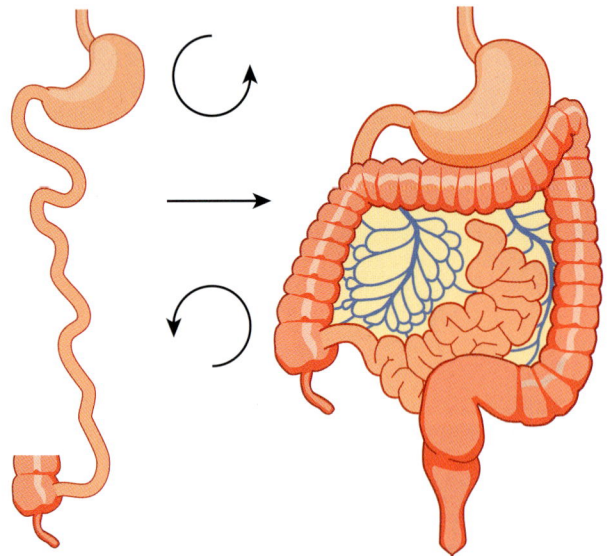

Figure 103-11   Normal rotation of midgut. The midgut starts as a straight tube; 270 degrees of counterclockwise rotation of the duodenojejunal junction places it in the left upper quadrant, whereas 270 degrees of counterclockwise rotation of the cecum places it in the right lower quadrant. Normal fixation of the bowel after rotation is completed results in the midgut being suspended from a broad-based mesentery, with retroperitoneal attachment at both ends.

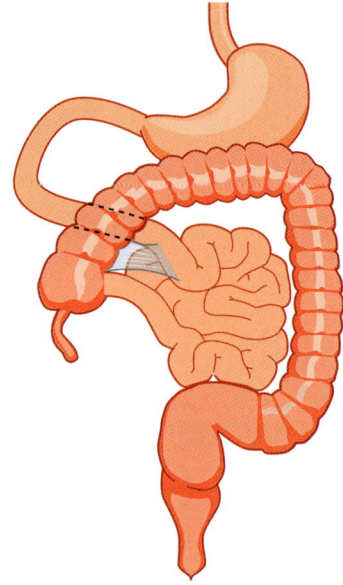

Figure 103-12   Malrotation. As the gut rotation is arrested between the initial 90 degrees ("nonrotation") and the normal 270 degrees, the duodenojejunal junction and the cecum approximate, resulting in suspension of the midgut from a narrow mesenteric pedicle without normal attachments. This arrangement is at high risk for midgut volvulus.

counterclockwise rotation. Starting from the initial straight tube, this rotation results in the location of the duodenojejunal junction in the left upper quadrant and of the cecum in the right lower quadrant. However, in these cases, the ceco-colic loop returns into the abdomen first, which results in the transverse colon, not the duodenum, being located between the aorta and the superior mesenteric artery.[39,40]

Several disorders of fixation also commonly occur in patients with malrotation. Ladd bands are the result of abnormal mesenteric attachments that are formed in patients in whom the rotational process is incomplete. These bands, named after Dr. William E. Ladd, typically extend from the edge of the liver to the malrotated cecum, crossing over and causing obstruction and kinking of the duodenum (Fig. 103-13); however, they can rarely occur more distally, in the jejunum or ileum.[34]

Internal hernias are the result of abnormal or incomplete fixation of the ascending (right paraduodenal or mesocolic) or descending portions of the colon, resulting in a defect through which the bowel can herniate. Herniation into the defect in the ascending colonic mesentery results in a right paraduodenal or mesocolic hernia, whereas herniation into the defect in the descending colonic mesentery results in a left paraduodenal or mesocolic hernia.[34,37] In persons with a normally rotated bowel, abnormal or incomplete fixation of the ascending colon, cecum, or sigmoid colon can result in volvulus of these structures, which typically does not occur until late adult life.

Clinical Presentation

The presentation of patients with malrotation depends on whether obstruction is present, and if so, whether the obstruction is acute or chronic, as well as on associated malformations. Presentation may occur in utero, and the infant may be born with short bowel as a result of in utero bowel necrosis and resorption, or with the apple-peel type of atresia.[41,42] In asymptomatic patients malrotation may be discovered in the course of evaluation for other clinical concerns.

Acute Volvulus   In persons with volvulus, the duodenum rotates, typically clockwise, about the axis of the superior mesenteric artery (Fig. 103-14) and is obstructed at its third portion, distal to the ampulla of Vater. Because approximately 60% to 80% of patients with volvulus present in the first month of life,[33,34,38,43,44] the typical presentation is that of a previously well neonate who experiences the sudden onset of bilious vomiting. The infant may experience crampy abdominal pain, which could be confused with colic. If the obstruction is significant, the abdomen may become initially scaphoid after distal intestinal contents are evacuated. Vascular compromise may lead to intraluminal bleeding and hematochezia, seen in 10% to 15% of patients with volvulus.[37] As ischemia of the midgut supervenes, the abdomen becomes distended and firm, with physical signs of peritonitis, and the patient will present in shock with cardiovascular collapse.[34]

Chronic Volvulus   Partial or intermittent volvulus tends to present more insidiously, with an average duration of symptoms of 28 months or greater before the correct diagnosis is made.[34] The patient usually has a history of abdominal pain, which can be severe but often is vague and intermittent, and often is associated with intermittent vomiting and/or failure to thrive. Impairment of venous and lymphatic flow leads to signs and symptoms of malabsorption.[45,46] The correct diagnosis is frequently delayed, with interim diagnoses including central or psychogenic vomiting, milk or other food allergies, and various malabsorption syndromes, such as celiac disease.[20,34,47,48]

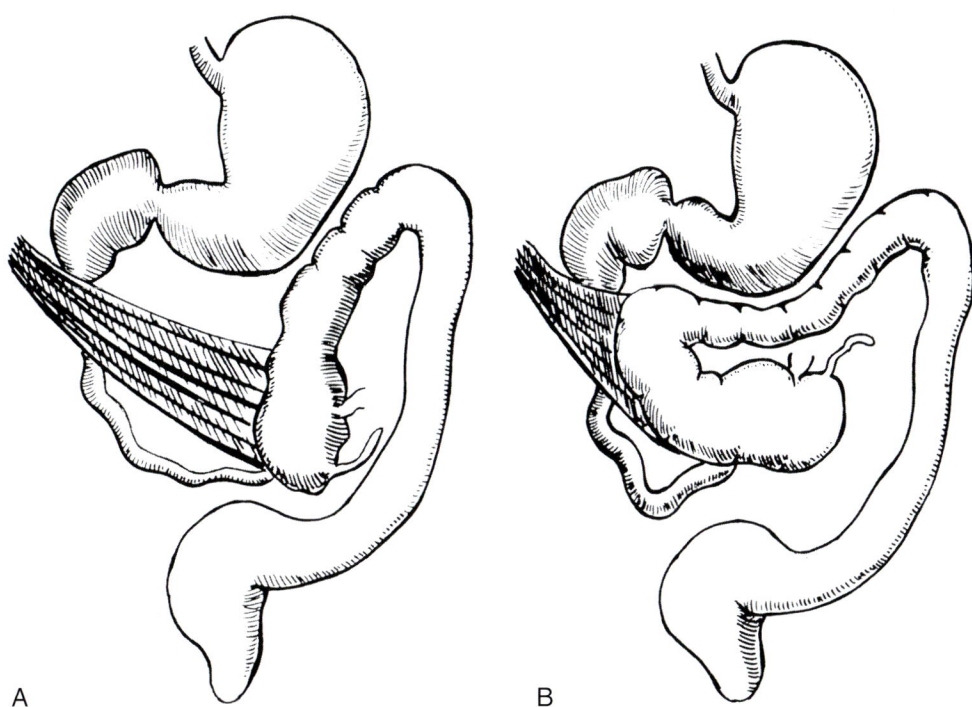

A   B

Figure 103-13 **Ladd bands.** Illustration of two instances in the spectrum of malrotation, demonstrating dense peritoneal bands (Ladd bands) extending from the cecum to the right upper quadrant, crossing over and obstructing the duodenum. These bands must be divided after reduction of the volvulus to relieve the obstruction.

Other Presentations

Ladd Bands Patients with duodenal obstruction as a result of Ladd bands may present acutely, with sudden onset of bilious vomiting, or they may present with more chronic symptoms, with failure to thrive and intermittent abdominal pain.[34]

Internal Hernias Either right or left mesocolic or paraduodenal hernias produce symptoms by entrapment of bowel,

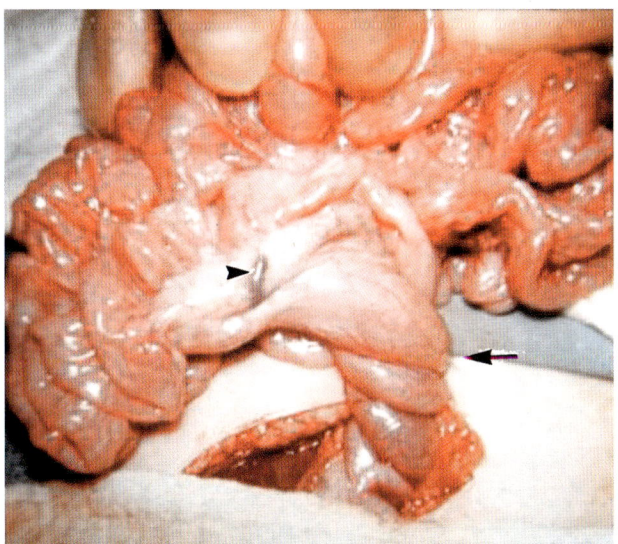

Figure 103-14 **Acute midgut volvulus.** Surgical findings of midgut volvulus. The duodenum is corkscrewed inferiorly *(arrow)* and the superior mesenteric vein *(arrowhead)* is engorged.

which can produce partial or complete obstruction and may progress to ischemia and necrosis of bowel. Symptoms therefore consist of abdominal pain and vomiting.

Associated Conditions

Multiple malformations and conditions are associated with malrotation and are reported to occur in 30% to 60% of patients with malrotation.[34,38] Intrinsic duodenal stenosis and annular pancreas have been discussed previously, and other intestinal atresias also occur.[5,38] Other abnormalities include Hirschsprung disease and anorectal malformations, cloacal extrophy, Eagle-Barrett (prune belly) syndrome, megacystis-microcolon-intestinal hypoperistalsis or Berdon syndrome, Cornelia de Lange syndrome, Marfan syndrome, and Meckel syndrome.[21,37,38,49] Malrotation also is found in some patients with trisomy 13, 18, and 21, in whom malrotation is cited as being 25 times more common than in the general population.[21,50] Malrotation is part of anomalies in which the gut is unable to achieve its normal rotation—gastroschisis, omphalocele, and Bochdalek diaphragmatic hernia—and is also extremely common in patients with heterotaxy.[51-53]

Imaging

Plain abdominal radiographic findings in patients with malrotation without obstruction or volvulus may show an abnormal distribution of stool, with absence of stool pattern in the right lower quadrant, which has been termed the radiologic "Dance's sign."[48] In patients with nonrotation, all colonic stool may be seen as confined to the left half of the abdomen.

In patients with volvulus, the radiographs may be completely normal at the onset of the bilious vomiting (Fig.

103-15, *A*). As distal bowel contents are evacuated and greater obstruction supervenes, the radiographs may show distension of the stomach, with relatively minor or subtle distension of the duodenum (Fig. 103-15, *B* and *C*). It is important to note that in malrotation with volvulus, the duodenum is not typically markedly distended, as is the case with duodenal stenosis or atresia; obstruction with Ladd bands is more likely to lead to an appearance more resembling that of the double bubble. The lack of marked bowel distension in an infant with volvulus may lead to a false sense of security or to the suspicion of a more common condition such as pyloric stenosis, if the significance of the bile-stained vomitus is not appreciated.

Ominous plain radiographic findings of ischemia in patients with volvulus include abdominal distension, separation of bowel loops, tubular appearance of bowel loops, fold thickening, and thumbprinting. Diffuse fluid and gaseous distention of the bowel is a finding that suggests gangrenous bowel and a poor prognosis (Fig. 103-15, *D*).

Upper GI Series An upper GI series is at present considered the standard examination to evaluate for malrotation and for its complications, particularly volvulus.

Documentation of normally rotated bowel can be challenging, and technique is very important. In pediatric patients, documentation of the normally rotated C-loop needs to be

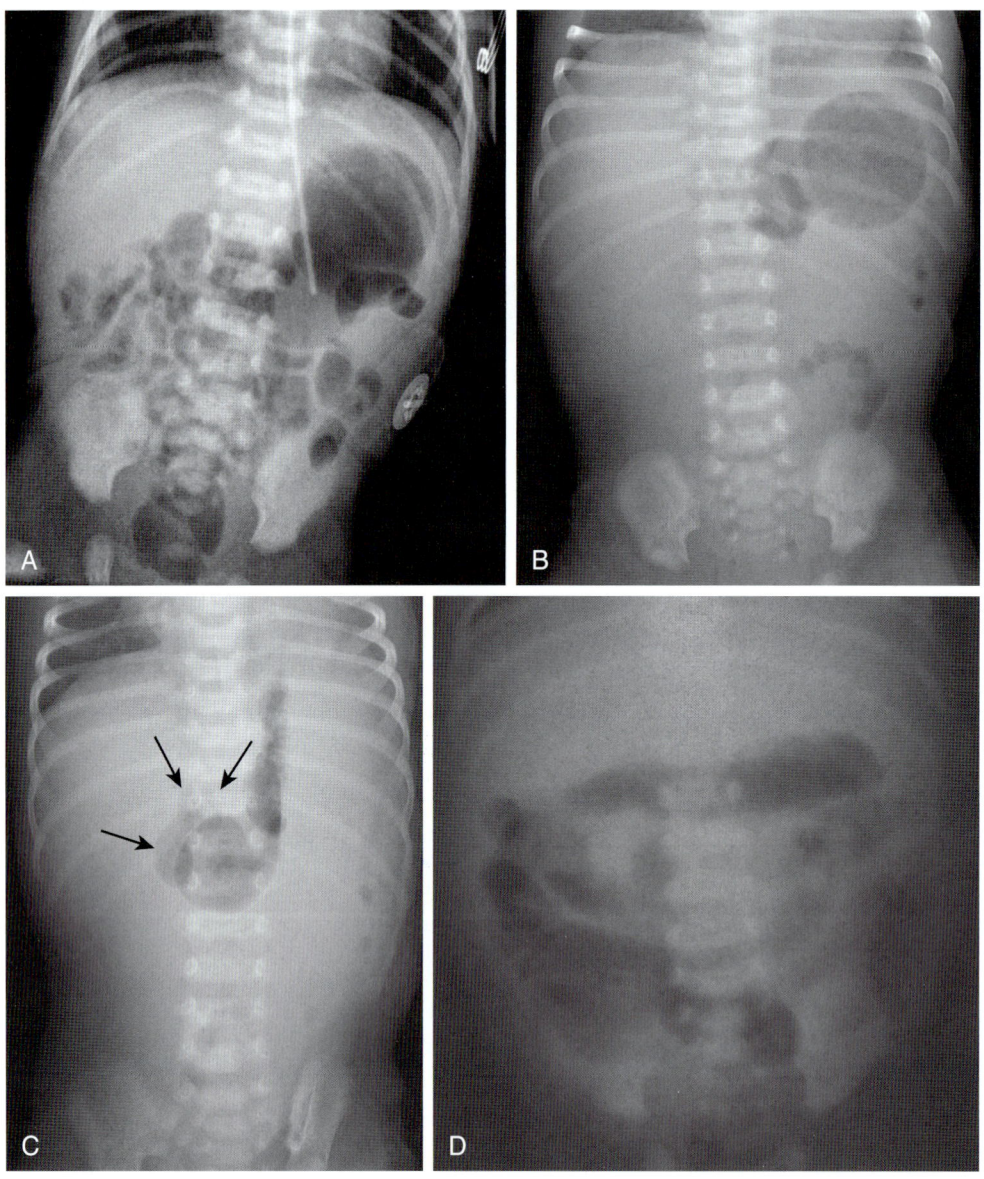

Figure 103-15 **Acute midgut volvulus.** Abdominal radiographic findings. **A,** An abdominal radiograph in 2-day-old infant with bilious vomiting and midgut volvulus. The bowel gas pattern is easily interpreted as within normal limits. **B** and **C,** Supine (**B**) and left decubitus (**C**) radiographs in a 7-day-old infant with bilious vomiting and midgut volvulus. The bowel gas pattern is abnormal, with very little gas distal to the stomach, and a scaphoid abdomen. No distension of the duodenum is appreciated, and the stomach is normal in size, but there is discrepancy between the size of the stomach and the marked lack of gas distally. On the decubitus radiograph, distension of both the stomach and the duodenum (*arrows*) is appreciated, with remarkable paucity of distal gas. **D,** A 2-week-old infant with bilious vomiting for several days. The radiograph shows a severe ileus pattern with abdominal distension and fluid and gas distending loops of bowel throughout the abdomen. The bowel was necrotic at subsequent surgery, and the infant died.

made on passage of the first bolus of contrast from the stomach; missing this opportunity can result in confusing and misleading findings. The course of the duodenum must be documented in both frontal and lateral projections, because the lateral view is essential to document the retroperitoneal position of both ascending and descending portions.[37,54] The duodenojejunal junction, recognized by an acute flexure as the duodenum returns to the peritoneal cavity, should be located to the left of the left pedicle at the same craniocaudal level as the duodenal bulb. The lateral view should show ascending and descending portions entirely superimposed anterior to the spine; anterior deviation of the descending limb is abnormal. The technique is discussed in Chapter 85. When malrotation with volvulus is suspected, we typically will use a low-osmolality water-soluble agent and position an enteric tube distally within the stomach to improve control over the first bolus. The fluoro-grab function of most current fluoroscopes allows movielike documentation of the progress of the first bolus through the duodenum without additional radiation dose, and it can be very helpful in confirming normal rotation, as well as in sorting out difficult cases and normal duodenal variants. The radiologist should be familiar

with normal variants such as duodenum inversum, in which the duodenum shows a parallel ascending and descending course to the right of the spine, before crossing to the left and emerging into the peritoneal cavity at a normally positioned ligament of Treitz (Fig. 103-16, Video 103-1).[55] Conversely, it is imperative that an abnormal course of the duodenum in patients without volvulus be recognized, including abnormal location of the duodenojejunal junction on the frontal image (see Fig. 103-16, *C*) and an abnormally anterior course of all or part of the duodenum on the lateral view. Abnormal location of the duodenojejunal junction—"excessive redundancy of the duodenum to the right of the spine"—may be indicative of malrotation[55] and other findings, such as position of the duodenum on the lateral view, position of the cecum, and cross-sectional imaging may need to be considered.

In symptomatic patients with malrotation, the upper GI examination may reveal the volvulus itself, presenting a spiral twisting of the duodenum (classically described as a "corkscrew") as it wraps around the axis of the superior mesenteric artery (see Fig. 103-16, *D*). When complete obstruction is present, the contrast column may terminate in

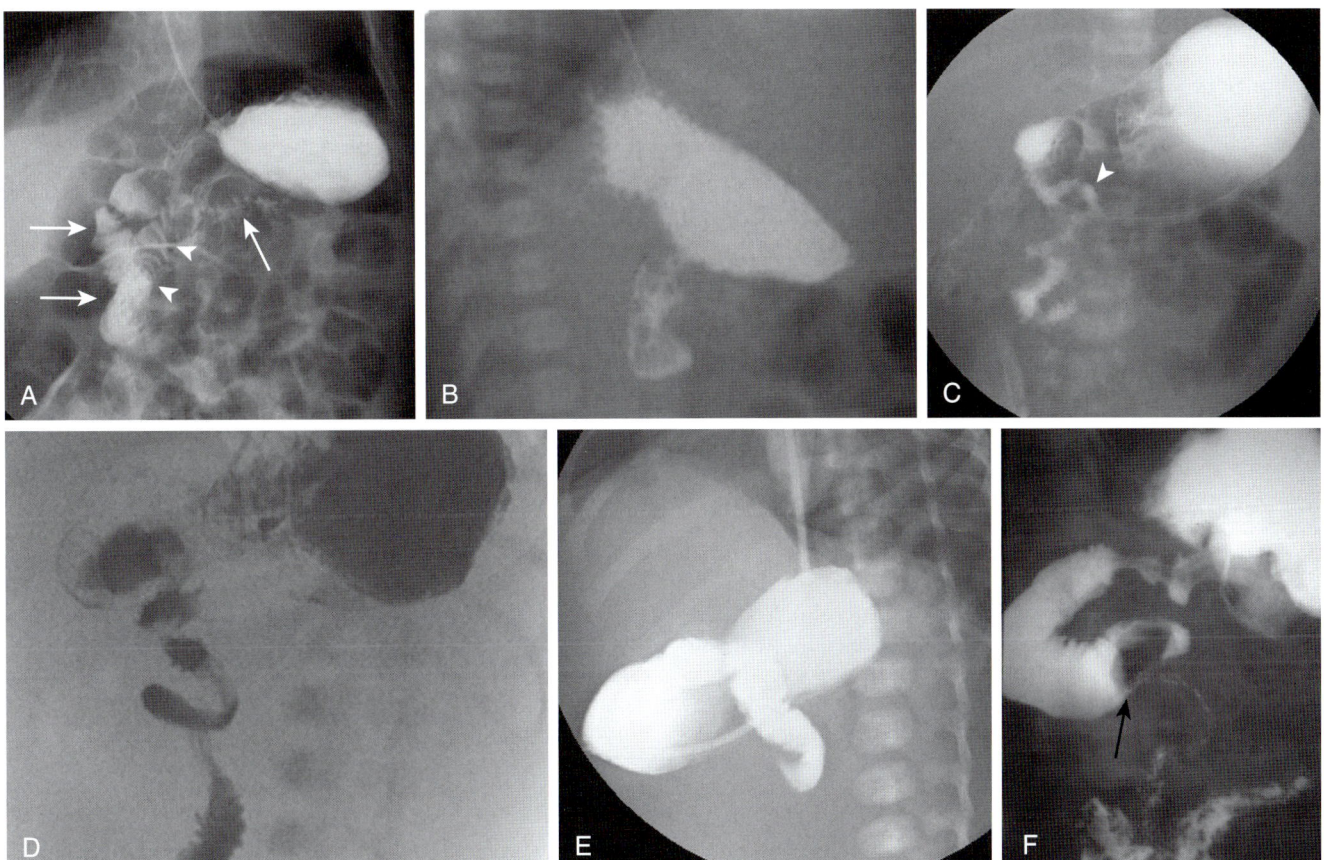

Figure 103-16 Upper gastrointestinal imaging (UGI) of the duodenum. **A** and **B,** Normal variant of duodenum inversum. A frontal image (**A**) of an infant with duodenum inversum. Note that after the vertical course of the duodenum on the right (*left, parallel arrows*), it ascends (*arrowheads*) before crossing the midline to a normally positioned duodenojejunal junction at the ligament of Treitz (*right arrow*). A lateral view (**B**) in a patient with duodenum inversum shows normal posterior position of the duodenal course. **C,** Malrotation in an infant without volvulus. A frontal image demonstrates that the presumed duodenojejunal junction (*arrowhead*) is low and to the right of the midline. **D,** A fluoro-grab image obtained during UGI in the same 7-day-old patient illustrated in Figure 103-15, **B** and **C**. Note the classic corkscrew configuration of the duodenum as it wraps around the twisted mesenteric pedicle. **E,** A UGI on another 7-day-old infant with a 1-day history of bilious vomiting and dehydration. The duodenum was completely obstructed, terminating in a configuration resembling a beak. **F,** Ladd bands in a 2-month-old girl with malrotation. A left posterior oblique spot UGI from a series demonstrates a dilated proximal duodenum as a result of crossing bands at the level of the third portion of the duodenum. The presumed duodenojejunal junction is abnormal. Note the kinking of the duodenum (*arrow*).

a beaklike configuration as the contrast is propelled into the entrance of the spiral but cannot proceed further (see Fig. 103-16, *E*).

In patients with obstruction resulting from Ladd bands, the duodenum may demonstrate a kinked configuration (see Fig. 103-16, *F*) that at times resembles a Z-shape instead of the normal C-loop. The Z-shape is the result of tacking down and kinking of the duodenum by the abnormal attempts at fixation and at times may be very difficult to differentiate from volvulus.

Contrast Enema Barium enema had been advocated by surgeons and radiologists in the investigation of patients suspected of malrotation and volvulus, in the belief that cecal position would define the presence or absence of malrotation while avoiding introduction of barium contrast proximal to the obstructed duodenum.[20,56] However, with the understanding that up to 30% of patients with malrotation and its complications could have a normally rotated cecum, and with the realization that a high-riding cecum in a neonate may in fact be normally rotated,[20,57,58] the contrast enema is no longer considered the main fluoroscopic diagnostic tool in the investigation of these patients. Follow-through small bowel to evaluate the cecum when the upper GI series shows confusing findings has been advocated and may be helpful in some cases, but the previous problems are not obviated. The cecum itself may be very difficult to define if the appendix does not fill, and a colonic segment in the right lower quadrant may be mistaken for the cecum. However, a clearly abnormal cecal position, especially in children with an equivocal location of the duodenal-jejunal flexure, is diagnostic of malrotation.

Challenging Cases

Overview A clearly abnormal course of the duodenum renders the diagnosis of malrotation straightforward (see Fig. 103-16, *C*). Unfortunately, subtle cases exist that lead to false-negative interpretations, and as previously discussed, normal variants may lead to false-positive results. In a retrospective review of 163 patients with surgically proven malrotation, upper GI examination had a sensitivity of 96%, with seven false-negative examinations.[59] On the other hand, a 15% false-positive diagnosis by upper GI examination, as demonstrated on subsequent surgical findings, also has been reported.[60] The frontal course of the duodenum may be misleading if the duodenojejunal flexure occurs over rather than to the left of the pedicle of the spine, if it occurs below the plane of the duodenal bulb, or if abnormal redundancy of the course of the duodenum occurs. The duodenojejunal junction also can be displaced by postoperative changes after liver transplantation,[61] peritoneal masses, or abnormal, dilated bowel loops.[62] Limitations of the lateral view include the fact that the aorta and the superior mesenteric artery are not visualized, and therefore true retroperitoneal position of the duodenum cannot be ascertained unequivocally, despite the parallel course of its ascending and descending portions anterior to the spine.[22]

Interpretative Errors False-positive interpretations usually result from failure to recognize normal variants or from displacement of a normal ligament of Treitz. Position of the proximal small bowel in the right upper quadrant, as an isolated finding, is not indicative of malrotation.[55,59] We know that the neonatal duodenum is mobile.[58] Therefore in patients in whom there is internal traction upon the duodenum, such as infants with dilatation of bowel, the duodenojejunal junction may appear abnormally located on the upper GI examination.[62] Normal variants of duodenal course, such as duodenum inversum (see Fig. 103-16, *A* and *B*, and Video 103-1) or redundant duodenum, also may lead to false-positive interpretations, although marked redundancy of the duodenum also can be a sign of malrotation.[55] Analysis of the true lateral view, or correlation with cross-sectional information, may be needed in some of these cases. A high position of the cecum or a mobile cecum, particularly in a neonate, also are typically normal findings but make evaluation for malrotation particularly challenging in individual patients.

Potential false-negative outcomes may result from suboptimal technique, such as failing to delineate the course of the duodenum on the first bolus of contrast from the stomach or from misinterpretation of the subtle finding of malrotation, such as kinking of the duodenum along its course or location of the duodenojejunal junction abnormally low or to the right of the left pedicle of the spine.[21,37,54,58,59] A proposed scoring system whereby the presence of three of nine potential findings would indicate malrotation, whereas one of nine was considered normal and two of nine was considered indeterminate, has not met with universal success.[55,58]

Cross-Sectional Imaging

Although cross-sectional imaging is not usually the first type of examination performed in patients in whom malrotation is a concern, it nevertheless may be the first examination performed for a given patient. The radiologist needs to be familiar with the findings of malrotation, particularly if it is associated with volvulus. The findings can be categorized as follows: (1) abnormal relationship of the superior mesenteric artery and vein; (2) volvulus; and (3) abnormal course of the duodenum.

Ultrasound On ultrasound, as with other cross-sectional imaging, the relationship of the superior mesenteric artery and vein is readily evaluated. The superior mesenteric artery has a smaller size and surrounding hyperechoic halo and is located posterior and to the left of the superior mesenteric vein; identification can be confirmed with brief Doppler interrogation. This relationship was noted to be abnormal in patients with malrotation[63] but it is neither highly sensitive nor highly specific for malrotation with or without volvulus.[64]

The "whirlpool" sign in patients with volvulus refers to a whirlpool-like appearance of the duodenum and superior mesenteric vein wrapped clockwise around the axis of the superior mesenteric artery.[65] In patients with this condition, a dilated duodenum can be followed as it enters into the volvulus (Fig. 103-17, *A* and *E*, and Video 103-2). It should be noted that this sign encompasses rotation of the duodenum, as well as the mesenteric vein. The sensitivity and specificity of the sonographic whirlpool sign has not been

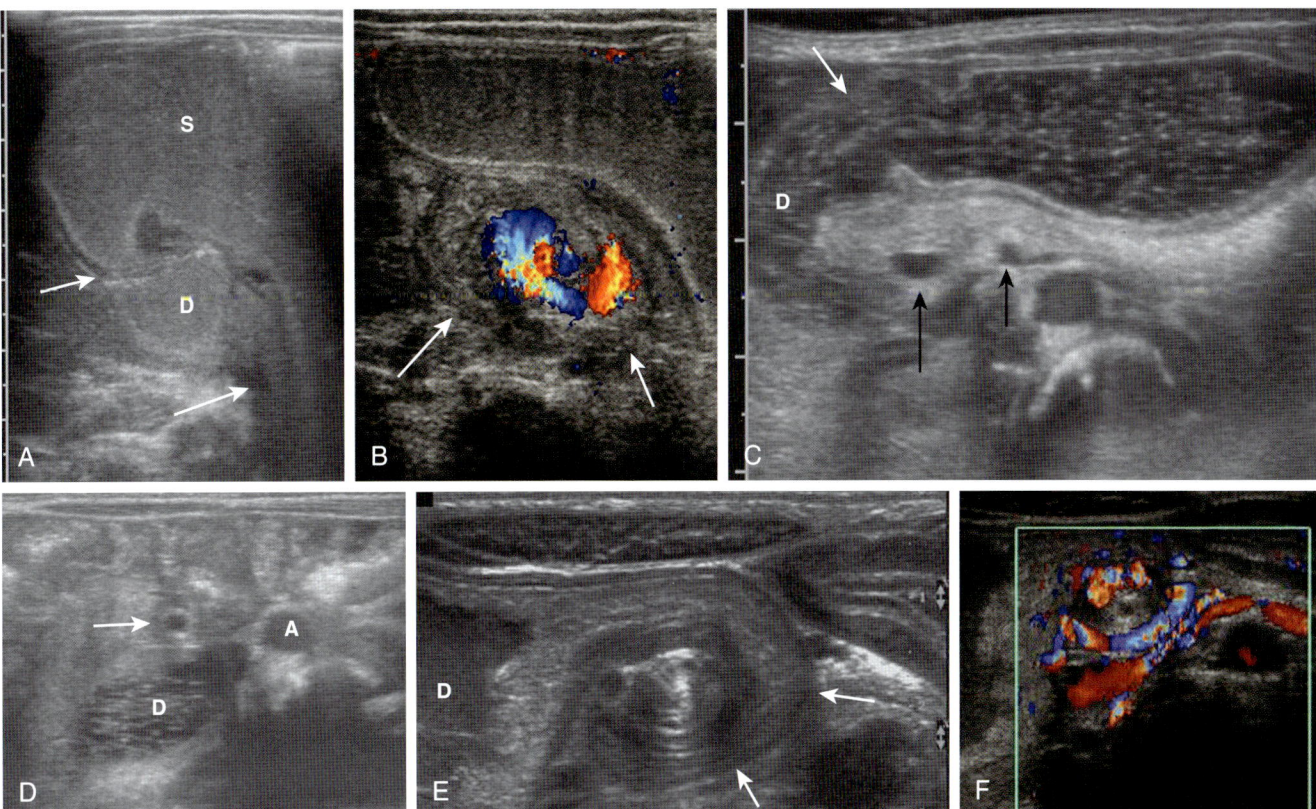

Figure 103-17   Acute and chronic midgut volvulus. **A** and **B,** An 18-day-old boy with a history of vomiting since birth, which had recently become "projectile" and was "occasionally yellow." Ultrasound was requested to assess for pyloric stenosis (see Video 103-2). **A,** An ultrasound image shows a dilated stomach (*S*) and duodenum (*D*), with the latter deviated medially as it enters into the volvulus (*long arrow*). The pylorus (*short arrow*) is widely open. **B,** A subsequent image shows the duodenum at the outer edge of the twist (*arrows*), with the twisting superior mesenteric vein and the centrally located superior mesenteric artery. The patient subsequently had surgical detorsion and lysis of Ladd bands. **C** and **D,** A 7-day-old girl presenting with history of 36 hours of vomiting (see Video 103-3). **C,** A transverse sonogram demonstrates a distended pylorus (*white arrow*) leading to a dilated duodenum (*D*), which curves medially around the superior mesenteric artery (SMA) (*short black arrow*) and superior mesenteric vein (*long black arrow*). **D,** A slightly more caudal image shows the dilated duodenum (*D*) terminating in a beak between the aorta (*A*) and the SMA (*arrow*). **E** and **F,** A 5-year-old boy who weighed 15 kg at presentation with a long history of vomiting, a 14-lb weight loss during the previous 3 weeks, and on a gluten-free diet for a recent diagnosis of gluten enteropathy (see Video 103-4). **E,** A transverse sonogram of the upper abdomen shows a markedly dilated duodenum (*D*) narrowing as it enters into the volvulus (*arrows*). **F,** Color Doppler imaging at a similar level as **E** shows the mesenteric vein around the twist. Detorsion of a 720-degree twist and division of Ladd bands was accomplished at surgery.

studied in large numbers of patients, but reports on smaller cohorts suggest that it is sensitive and specific for malrotation with volvulus.[66,67] It should be noted that this sign is not present in patients with malrotation without volvulus at the time of the examination and that it can be relatively subtle (Fig. 103-17, *C* and *D*, and Video 103-3). In older patients presenting with chronic volvulus, the sonographic findings are similar, although the duodenum may be considerably larger, because it has had a longer time to become dilated (Fig. 103-17, *E* and *F*, and Video 103-4).

The normal retroperitoneal course of the duodenum posterior to the superior mesenteric artery is an indication of normal rotation of the bowel; this course can be seen in cross-sectional imaging and has been underscored recently as an important finding on abdominal ultrasound.[22]

CT is not the procedure of choice in evaluation of malrotation, but if it is performed for other reasons, the course of the duodenum and the position of the cecum should be assessed, and volvulus should be recognized if it is present (Fig. 103-18).

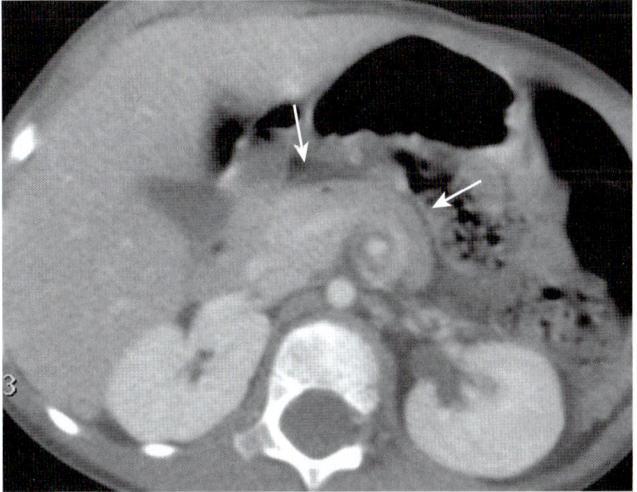

Figure 103-18   Chronic midgut volvulus. A computed tomography (CT) scan in a 2-year-old child with long history of intermittent abdominal pain and emesis. The CT image demonstrates volvulus with the duodenum (*arrows*), which contains small bubbles of gas, entering into the twist.

Treatment The treatment for malrotation with volvulus consists of surgical detorsion, identification and lysis of Ladd bands, straightening of the duodenum along the right abdomen, and placement of the cecum in the left lower quadrant, thus broadening the base of the mesentery and creating a separation between the duodenojejunal junction and the cecum resembling nonrotation, with incidental appendectomy. This procedure, which bears his name, was described by Dr. Ladd, and remains the standard for patients with malrotation.[23,68] A laparoscopic Ladd procedure can be performed, but it may be very difficult to perform in an acutely ill neonate with volvulus; it has also been suggested that fewer postoperative adhesions in laparoscopic surgery may predispose to recurrent volvulus, although insufficient comparative data are available at this time.[69,70] When accompanied by volvulus, the surgery is emergent, and correction of existing metabolic and electrolyte derangements must be undertaken. When malrotation in the absence of volvulus is found in the older child or adult, surgery is indicated if the patient is symptomatic. The role of surgery versus conservative management in asymptomatic older patients with malrotation without volvulus, such as patients with heterotaxy,[71] remains controversial.[72]

Preduodenal Portal Vein

Overview The portal vein forms at the junction of the superior mesenteric and splenic veins, and its normal course is retropancreatic and retroduodenal. The preduodenal portal vein, first reported in 1921, courses anterior to the pancreas and duodenum; it is important because of its associated anomalies, but its major significance is surgical.[73]

Etiology A preduodenal portal vein is the result of abnormal resorption of segments of the paired embryonic vitelline veins and their connections (e-Fig. 103-19). Normally the upper communicating branch between the left and right vitelline veins persists, with resorption of the cephalad segment of the left vitelline vein, the caudal segment of the right vitelline vein, and of the lower communicating branch, resulting in the duodenum coursing ventral to the portal vein. The preduodenal portal vein results when the upper communicating branch is resorbed, with persistence of the lower communicating branch, which courses ventral to the duodenum; there is resorption of the left vitelline vein and persistence of the cranial portion of the right vitelline vein.[74,75]

Clinical Presentation The preduodenal portal vein is associated with conditions that cause duodenal obstruction, including duodenal web, annular pancreas, and malrotation. Therefore the major presenting symptom of patients with a preduodenal portal vein is duodenal obstruction, as a result of the associated anomaly in most cases.[76,77] A preduodenal portal vein is highly associated with heterotaxy, particularly polysplenia.[53,78] Besides obstruction, the most important concern is inadvertent injury during surgery.[77,79] A preduodenal portal vein should be identified before surgery whenever possible, particularly in patients at risk for this anatomy, such as patients with polysplenia and biliary atresia.[51,53,80]

Imaging The preduodenal portal vein is well visualized with cross-sectional imaging. On ultrasound, the sagittal course of the superior mesenteric vein can be followed as it moves ventrally, over the pancreas, to enter the liver, ventral to both pancreas and duodenum (Fig. 103-20).[53,81] On CT and MRI, the findings are similar (Fig. 103-21).[82]

Treatment No treatment is necessary for an asymptomatic preduodenal portal vein. When the vein is associated with obstruction, bypass of the obstruction or correction of malrotation or Ladd bands is indicated.[83]

Small Bowel

CONGENITAL/NEONATAL ANOMALIES OF THE SMALL BOWEL

Small Bowel Atresia and Stenosis

Overview Atresia and stenosis affect the jejunum and ileum more commonly than any other portion of the abdominal

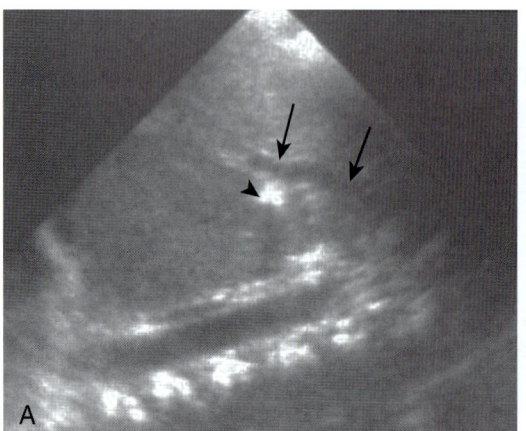
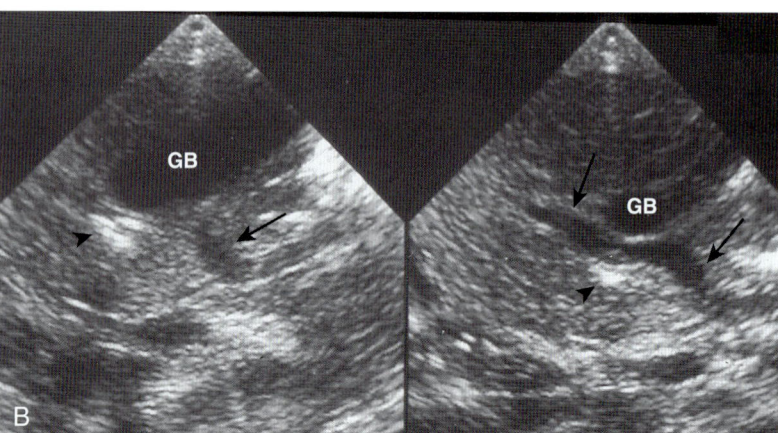

Figure 103-20 A preduodenal portal vein. **A,** A sagittal sonogram in a child with asplenia shows the superior mesenteric vein (SMV)/portal vein continuation (*arrows*) into the liver passing anterior to the duodenum, outlined by a small amount of gas (*arrowhead*). **B,** Sequential sagittal sonograms in a child with polysplenia demonstrate the course of the SMV (*arrows*) coursing over the pancreas and the duodenal bulb (*arrowheads*), again outlined by a small amount of air. *GB* indicates a midline gallbladder.

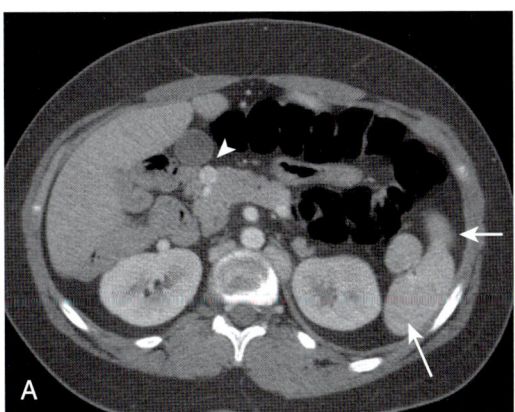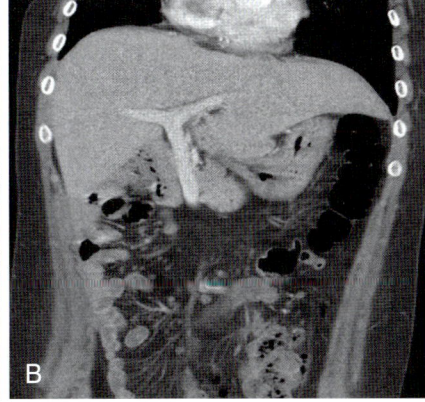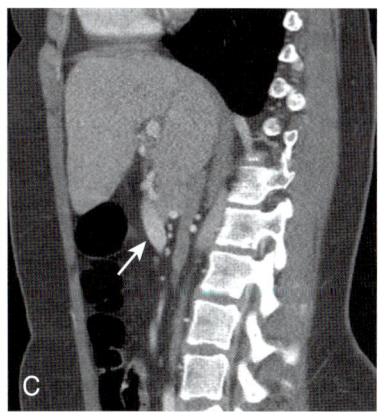

Figure 103-21 A preduodenal portal vein. **A,** A computed tomography scan in a child with polysplenia (*arrows*) shows a preduodenal portal vein (*arrowhead*). The superior mesenteric artery is in normal position anterior to the aorta. The inferior vena cava was duplicated below the level of the renal hila. **B,** Coronal reformatting shows the abnormal course of the portal vein as it courses to the liver. **C,** Sagittal reformat shows the anterior course of the portal vein (*arrow*).

gastrointestinal tract: approximately 51% involve the jejunum and ileum, compared with the duodenum in 40% and the colon in approximately 9%.[84] The incidence of jejunoileal atresia ranges between one and three cases per 10,000 live births, depending on geographic location, with the incidence being greater in persons of European and African-American descent than in persons from Latin America. Small bowel atresias in the ileum occur distally in nearly two thirds of cases. In the jejunum this ratio is reversed, with nearly two thirds occurring proximally and one third distally. Atresia is much more common than stenosis, which accounts for only approximately 5% of cases,[85] particularly in the ileum.

Jejunoileal atresias have been subdivided into five types and subtypes[84,86] (Fig. 103-22). Type I represents mucosal or membranous atresia, which is limited to luminal discontinuity. In type II, the blind ends of the bowel are connected by a fibrous cord, with continuity of the underlying mesentery. Type IIIa indicates discontinuity between the bowel ends with an adjacent mesenteric defect, whereas IIIb is long-segment atresia with a wide mesenteric defect, typically described as "apple peel," "Christmas tree," and "maypole" mesentery because of the appearance of the residual distal small bowel coiled around its tenuous vascular supply through retrograde flow via the ileocolic, right colic, or inferior mesenteric arteries.[87] Type IV refers to multiple atresias (e-Fig. 103-23).

Etiology Unlike the duodenum, in which the etiology of atresia and stenosis is believed to be failure of recanalization, the most likely and accepted etiology in the jejunum, ileum, and colon is a vascular accident, the location and extent of which governs the location and severity of the resultant defect. Experimental data in multiple species undergoing prenatal ligation of mesenteric branches resulting in corresponding bowel atresias gives credence to this theory.[85,88] More circumstantial evidence in humans includes the findings of lanugo and bile pigments distal to the point of atresia, indicating patency of the intestinal lumen beyond the point when recanalization of the gut had been completed.[89]

Conditions that can result in prenatal gut ischemia include gastroschisis, intrauterine volvulus, intussusception, and internal hernias.[90] Atresias are found in patients who have undergone significant compression of bowel segments, such as

incarceration in omphalocele or in tight gastroschisis defects. Signs of peritonitis have been found in up to 48% of patients with atresia.[85] Extensive "apple-peel" small bowel atresia is postulated to occur as a result of occlusion of the superior mesenteric artery distal to the origin of the right colic and ileocolic arteries (Fig. 103-24).

Clinical Presentation Patients with intestinal atresia may present prenatally with polyhydramnios or postnatally with bilious vomiting, upper or generalized abdominal distension, jaundice, and abnormalities in passage of meconium.

The percentage of infants with polyhydramnios increases with more proximal atresia, because less bowel surface area is present to absorb swallowed amniotic fluid, and polyhydramnios is present in approximately 38% of patients with jejunal atresia. The percentage of patients presenting with bilious emesis postnatally also increases with more proximal atresia, seen in approximately 84% of patients with jejunal atresia. Jaundice occurs more often in patients with jejunal (32%) than ileal (20%) atresia. Most patients, though not all, fail to pass meconium in the first 24 hours of life. Patients with more proximal atresias may show some distension of the upper abdomen, but abdominal distension due to dilatation of multiple loops of bowel is the rule in patients with distal atresias. Infants with the apple-peel variant of intestinal atresia tend to be premature and have a low birth weight, and more than half are shown to have malrotation of the midgut.[85]

Other anomalies outside of the gastrointestinal system may be present in nearly one third of patients, more often in patients with jejunal than with ileal atresia.[91] Although duodenal atresia shows a high association with trisomy 21, this is not the case with jejunoileal atresia, which is seen in approximately 0.55% to 3% of patients with Down syndrome. Multiple atresias and the apple-peel variant of intestinal atresia can show a genetic pattern in some families, and apple-peel atresias have been reported with a constellation of other anomalies, including ocular abnormalities and microcephaly.[95]

Imaging Plain radiographs in patients with bowel obstruction will differ from the normal appearance of the bowel (Fig. 103-25). Patients with proximal atresias will show

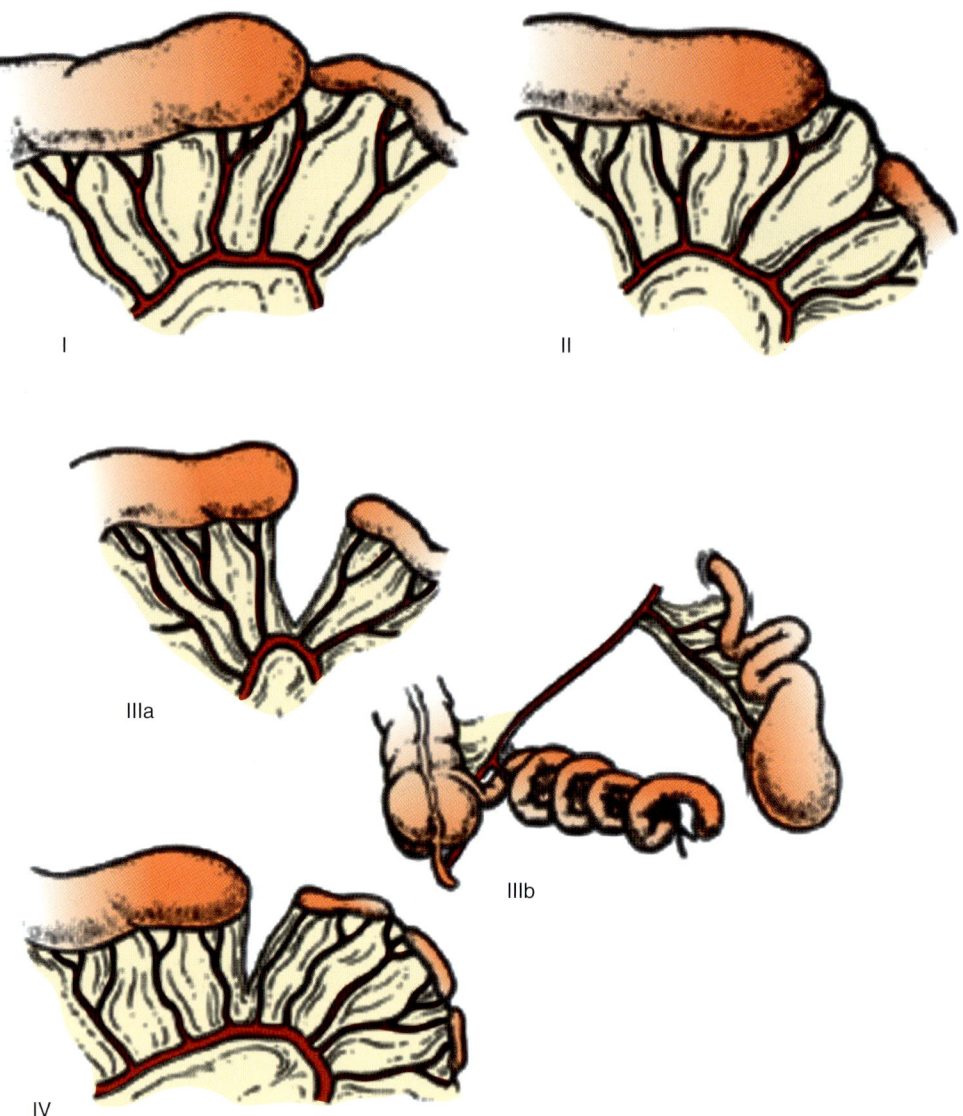

I

II

IIIa

IIIb

IV

Figure 103-22 Classification of jejunoileal atresias. Type I is a mucosal or membranous atresia, in which only the lumen is atretic, with continuity of outer wall and mesentery. In type II atresia, the atretic segment is connected to the distal bowel by a fibrous cord, with an intact mesentery. Type IIIa indicates discontinuity between the atretic segment and the distal bowel, with an associated mesenteric defect. In type IIIb the mesenteric defect is large, with absence of a portion of the bowel; the remaining distal bowel is wrapped in "Christmas tree" or "apple-peel" fashion around a remnant arterial supply. Type IV refers to multiple atresias. (From Grosfeld JL, Ballantine TV, Shoemaker R. Operative mangement of intestinal atresia and stenosis based on pathologic findings. *J Pediatr Surg.* 1979;14(3):368-375.)

dilatation of the stomach, duodenum, and jejunum to the point of atresia, although the degree of dilatation may be decreased if decompression occurs via the enteric tube (Fig. 103-26). In patients with ileal atresia (Fig. 103-27), abdominal radiographs will reveal dilatation of multiple gas-filled loops of bowel, often with protuberance of the flanks and elevation of the hemidiaphragms. Unlike older infants and adults, in neonates it is not possible to distinguish small from large bowel, and dilated loops of small bowel distributed along the expected location of the colon can mimic a dilated colon.[92] However, gas will not be found in the rectum (Fig. 103-27), a finding that can be optimized by obtaining a prone cross-table lateral radiograph. Patients with jejunal apple-peel atresia will have findings of proximal atresia (e-Fig. 103-28). In patients with jejunal stenosis, the findings will be similar, with distal gas and proximal dilatation dependent upon the

degree of stenosis (e-Fig. 103-29). Ileal stenosis is much less common.

In patients with proximal jejunal atresia, plain films with the aforementioned findings are usually diagnostic. Upper GI examination will demonstrate the dilated stomach, duodenum, and small bowel to the point of first atresia (see Fig. 103-26). In patients with plain film findings of distal obstruction, fluoroscopic diagnosis is accomplished with contrast enema. In patients with distal obstruction, use water-soluble contrast material diluted to a near iso-osmolal concentration (see Chapter 85 for additional information on technique). In patients with ileal atresia, the contrast enema will reveal a very small, unused colon, known as a microcolon, whose lumen has not been distended by swallowed material or succus entericus. The differential diagnosis of microcolon is that of distal small bowel obstruction, ileal atresia, or

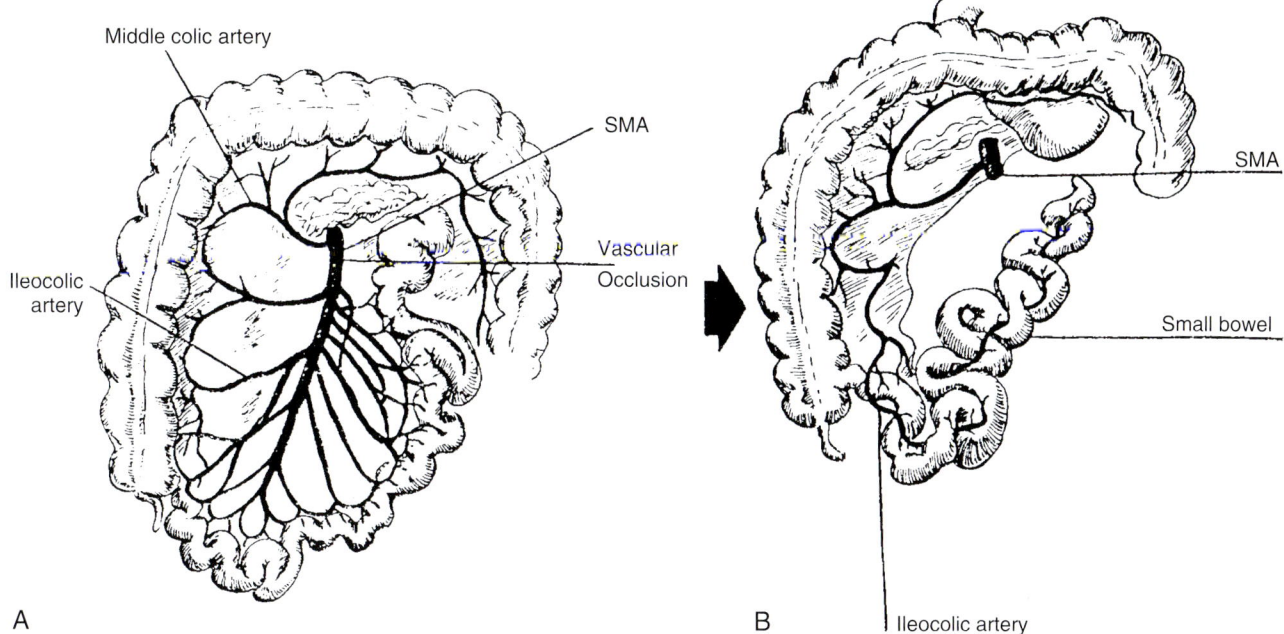

Figure 103-24 **Apple-peel variant of intestinal atresia. A,** A schematic drawing of the normal distribution of the superior mesenteric artery (*SMA*) and its branches. If there is prenatal occlusion at the point indicated, part of the jejunum and the accompanying dorsal mesentery will involute. **B,** Sequelae of **A,** with collateral supply of the residual distal small bowel via ileocolic branches of the distal superior mesenteric artery that are supplied by connections to the inferior mesenteric artery. The residual distal ileal loops wrap around their collateral supply, resembling an apple peel.

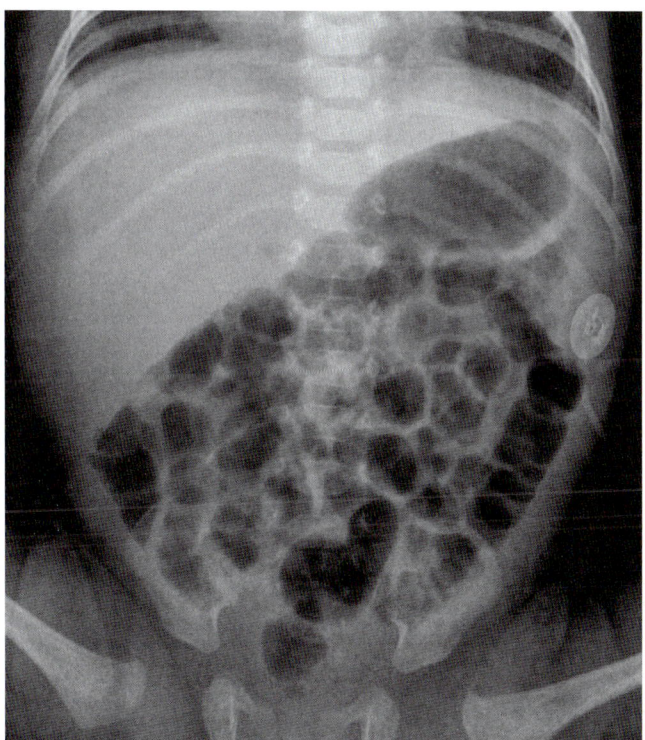

Figure 103-25 **Normal neonatal bowel gas pattern.** A supine abdominal radiograph in a female neonate outlining a normal bowel gas pattern, with multiple rounded and polyhedral gas bubbles of similar size distributed throughout the abdominal cavity, and gas in the rectum.

meconium ileus. The differential overlaps with some cases of long-segment Hirschsprung disease. Meconium pellets typically are absent from the microcolon in patients with ileal atresia (see Fig. 103-27).

Treatment The treatment and management of patients with jejunal and ileal atresia or stenosis is surgical. Although considerable morbidity still plagues the survivors of these abnormalities,[90] the prognosis of these infants has undergone revolutionary improvement. Survival has improved from approximately 1% to 10% in the first half of the twentieth century to 95% currently, related to improvement in surgical techniques, perioperative care, and nutritional support.[90]

Meconium Ileus

Overview Meconium ileus is responsible for approximately 20% of neonatal intestinal obstruction and denotes an obstruction in the terminal ileum as a result of inspissated meconium.[93] Meconium ileus is the initial presentation in approximately 15% to 20% of patients with cystic fibrosis (CF). Although most patients who present with meconium ileus will be diagnosed with CF, exceptions have been reported, including patients with pancreatic insufficiency and patients with very long segment Hirschsprung disease encompassing the small bowel.[94-97] More recent reports suggest that a greater percentage of infants with meconium ileus might not have CF, but the underlying cause of distal small bowel obstruction in such infants is unknown.[95,98]

Etiology Patients with CF have a defect in the gene sited in locus q31.2 of chromosome 7, which encodes for the CF transmembrane conductance regulator (CTFR) protein and renders it ineffective in the regulation of chloride transport

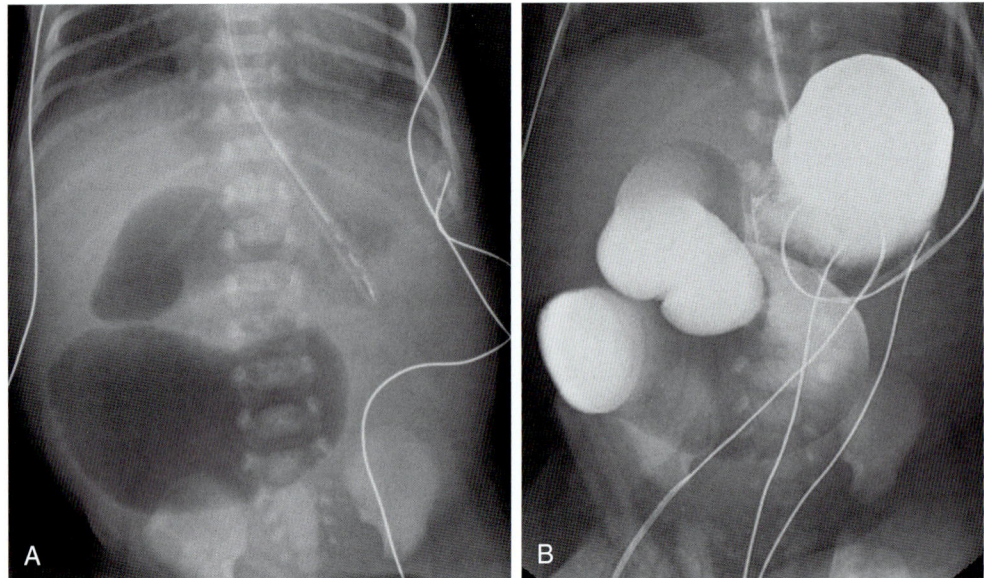

Figure 103-26 Jejunal atresia. **A,** Abdominal radiograph in an infant boy on his first day of life. An orogastric tube has decompressed the stomach, but markedly dilated proximal loops are identified, with no distal gas. Note that despite the marked distension of the obstructed bowel, the flanks are not protuberant, and there is no elevation of the hemidiaphragms, confirming the decompressed state of the more numerous distal bowel loops. **B,** An upper gastrointestinal examination, with water-soluble iso-osmolal contrast material in the same infant. Contrast fills the dilated proximal loops to the point of atresia. Notice the correlation with the abdominal radiograph in **A.**

across cell membranes in lungs, liver, pancreas, skin, digestive, and reproductive tracts. In the fetal gut, abnormal secretory products of the intestinal epithelium result in meconium with an abnormal electrolyte environment and increased concentration of protein (particularly albumin), which interacts with other components of meconium, such as mucopolysaccharides, to form abnormally viscid and tenacious meconium. Degradation of this material is impeded by abnormal concentration of pancreatic enzymes, which also is the result of a defective CTFR protein.[99,100] The meconium inspissates within the distal small bowel lumen, causing high-grade small bowel obstruction (Fig. 103-30).

Clinical Presentation The presentation of infants with meconium ileus is one of distal bowel obstruction, which may be complicated by an in utero event leading to prenatal perforation. Patients with uncomplicated or simple meconium ileus may have been identified prenatally with abdominal distension, dilatation of bowel loops, and hyperechoic bowel.[101-103] Approximately 20% of the infants demonstrate polyhydramnios in utero, more frequently in the subgroup with complicated meconium ileus. Postnatally they will present with abdominal distension, failure to pass meconium, and bilious vomiting.

Complicated meconium ileus occurs in approximately 40% to 50% of cases[95,104] and results from an in utero event: the weight of the tenacious meconium can lead to a segmental volvulus, which in turn can lead to perforation with meconium peritonitis, resulting in a loculated meconium cyst or a small bowel atresia. The prenatal perforation may seal over in utero or may persist postnatally. By the age of 6 months, prognosis is similar to patients who did not present with meconium ileus.[104]

Patients with CTFR G542X mutations have been reported to have a higher incidence of meconium ileus than do patients with other mutations, whereas complicated meconium ileus has been reported more frequently in patients homozygous for the classic ΔF508 mutation. Modifier genes located on chromosomes 4q35.1, 8p23.1, 11q25, and 19q13 also have been reported to affect the clinical presentation of infants with CF and the development of meconium ileus.[98]

Meconium peritonitis is not specific to meconium ileus; it occurs in patients in whom an intrauterine perforation is present for any reason. Occasionally a child is born with intraperitoneal calcifications consistent with meconium peritonitis, in whom the perforation has sealed over, and who is otherwise well, with no definable clinical sequelae (Fig. 103-31, *A*).

Imaging Radiographs of infants with complicated meconium ileus, in addition to signs of distal bowel obstruction, may show intraperitoneal calcifications consistent with meconium peritonitis and/or mass effect consistent with a meconium cyst (see Fig. 103-31, *B* to *F*). Patients with such signs of complicated meconium ileus are not candidates for contrast fluoroscopic evaluation of either the upper or lower GI tracts. However, ultrasound is useful in some infants with complicated meconium ileus to document the location and size of a suspected meconium cyst. Hyperechoic bowel loops, described in the fetus,[101-103] also may be seen postnatally (see Fig. 103-31, *D*).

In infants with no evidence of complicated meconium ileus, abdominal radiographs will show abdominal distension and multiple dilated loops of bowel, consistent with a distal obstruction (Fig. 103-32). In patients with meconium ileus, the ileal loops are packed with meconium, which often renders a characteristic "soap bubble" appearance, originally described by Neuhauser in 1946.[105] Air-fluid levels tend to be less conspicuous than in patients with ileal atresia,[106] although their presence does not negate the diagnosis.

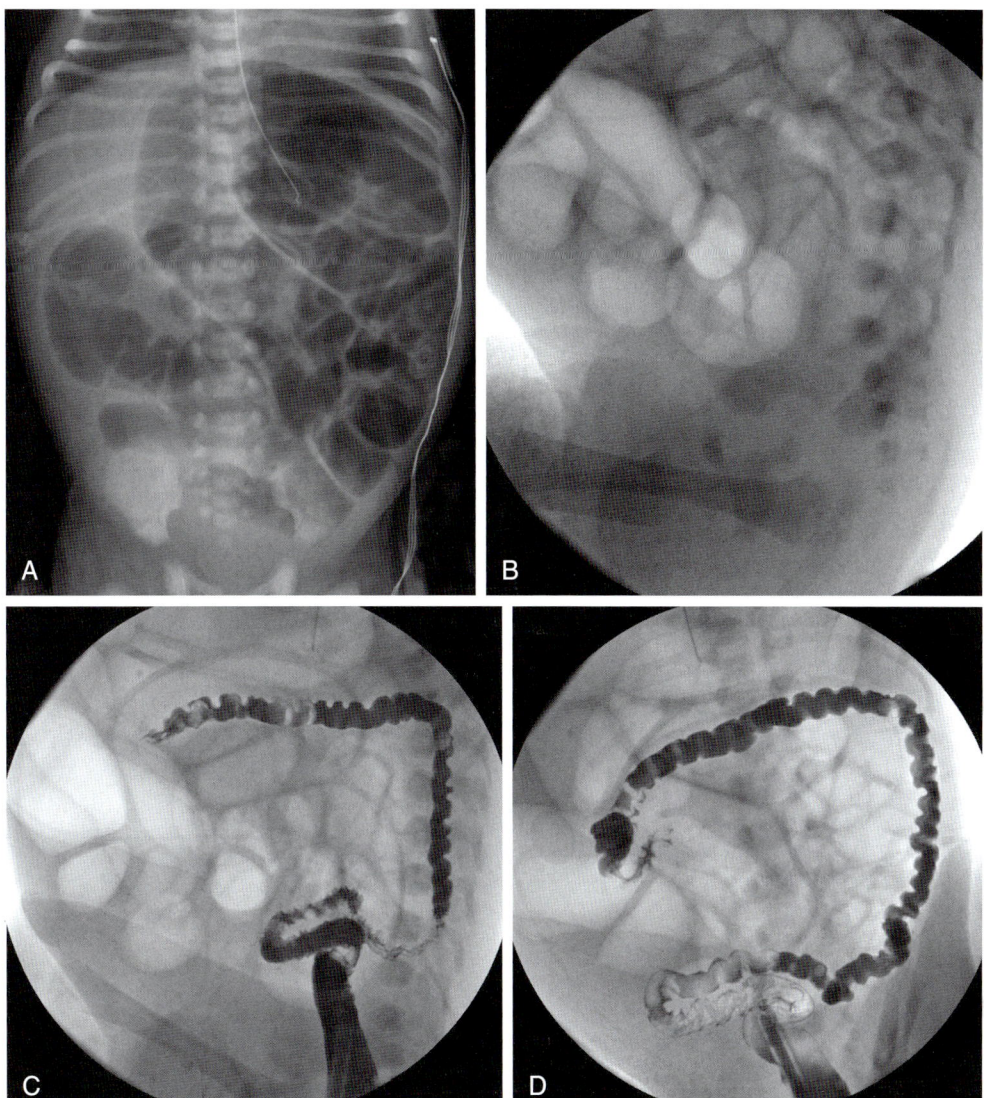

Figure 103-27 Ileal atresia. **A,** An abdominal radiograph in an infant boy demonstrates multiple dilated loops of bowel filling the abdomen. Some distension of the flanks and elevation of the diaphragms is seen, despite orogastric tube decompression. **B,** A lateral radiograph prior to a contrast enema demonstrates absence of distal gas. A catheter is present in the distal rectum. **C** and **D,** Consecutive images from a contrast enema demonstrate a microcolon, outlined by introduced contrast and air; the colon is otherwise empty, without evidence of meconium pellets.

Similar to patients with ileal atresia, diagnostic imaging evaluation starts from below with contrast enema. As previously discussed, the diagnostic examination begins with water-soluble contrast material diluted to a near iso-osmolal concentration. Barium is not recommended because barium inspissated within the tarry meconium is unlikely to prove helpful, and it is not necessary for diagnosis. Hyperosmolal material likewise will not be helpful if the diagnosis proves to be Hirschsprung disease (see Chapter 85 for additional information on technique). The examination will reveal a small colon, known as a microcolon, similar to that seen in patients with ileal atresia. However, in patients with meconium ileus, in whom the distal ileum is impacted with tarry, tenacious meconium, small meconium pellets may be seen within the microcolon (see Fig. 103-32, *B*). If contrast material refluxes into the distal ileum, meconium pellets may be identified; if contrast material reaches into the dilated loops of bowel, ileal atresia is excluded. However, contrast material may not reflux readily into the dilated bowel loops in patients

with meconium ileus because of the inability to traverse the segments containing inspissated meconium; in such cases, final diagnosis is made at surgical intervention.

Treatment Patients with complicated meconium ileus as revealed on clinical evaluation, findings of calcifications on abdominal radiographs or free intraperitoneal air, are managed surgically. An enema procedure has no role in these patients.

The mainstay of treatment for patients with simple meconium ileus initially was surgery, with enterotomy and intraoperative irrigation of the bowel to solubilize, disimpact, and remove the inspissated obstructing meconium.[107] Since the initial description by Noblett in 1969, the therapeutic Gastrografin contrast enema often is the initial treatment in patients with uncomplicated meconium ileus. Its success has been attributed to the hyperosmolarity of the medium (1900 mOsm/L), as well as to the surfactant properties of polysorbate 80 (Tween 80).[108] Expected complications related to hyperosmolarity of the agent and subsequent fluid shifts

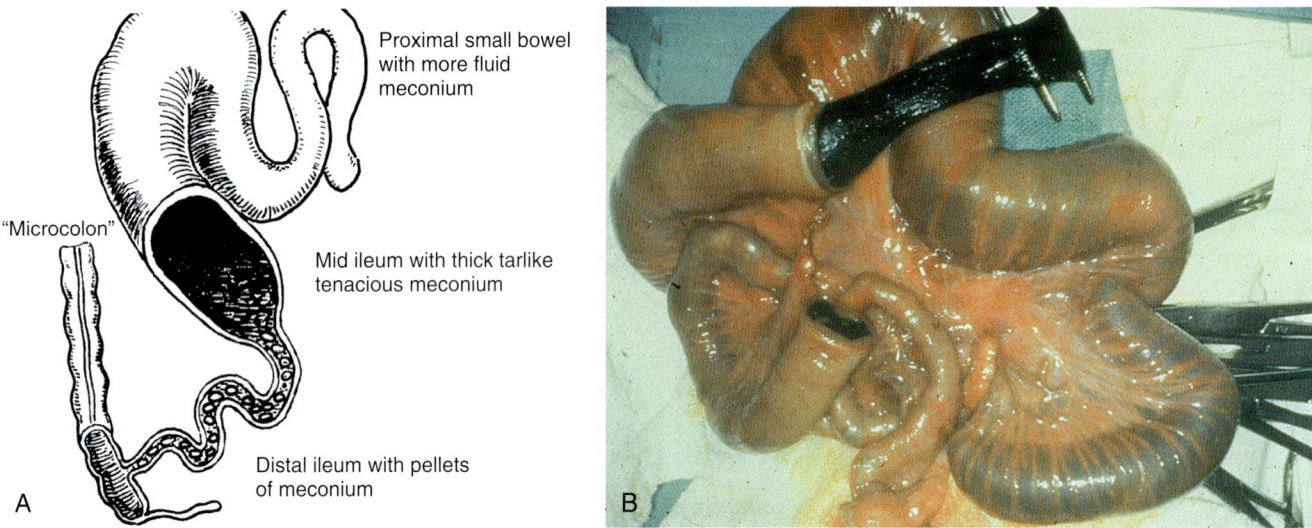

Figure 103-30 Meconium ileus. **A,** A schematic drawing of an uncomplicated meconium ileus. Pellets of inspissated meconium fill the terminal ileum proximal to a microcolon. Several loops of more proximal ileum contain thick, tenacious meconium. **B,** An intraoperative radiograph shows an enterotomy of proximal bowel and the nature of the thick and tenacious meconium. Note the dilated proximal loops of bowel filled with meconium and the progressively small caliber of the distal bowel leading to the microcolon. (**A,** Leonidas JC, et al. Meconium ileus and its complications. A reappraisal of plain film roentgen diagnostic criteria. *Am J Roentgenol Radium Ther Nucl Med.* 1970;108(3):598-609. **B,** Courtesy Dr. Wallace W. Neblett III, Nashville, TN.)

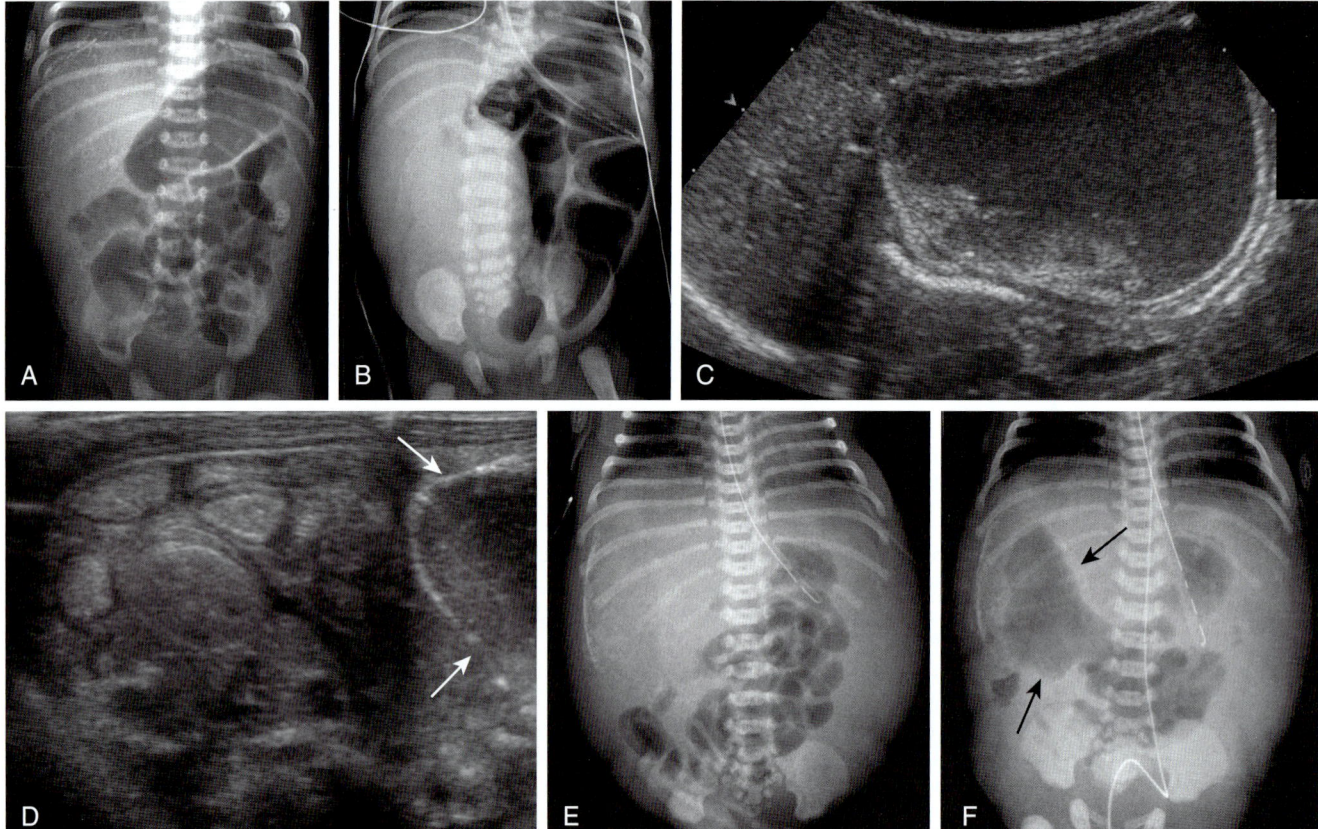

Figure 103-31 Spectrum of meconium peritonitis and meconium cyst. **A,** An abdominal radiograph of a 2-day-old infant with extensive intraperitoneal calcifications consistent with in utero perforation and meconium peritonitis. The child did well, without evidence of persistent perforation or obstruction, and after appropriate observation, was discharged home. **B,** A 2-day-old female infant with abdominal distension and bilious aspirates. Abdominal radiograph shows markedly dilated loops of bowel, absence of bowel gas in the right abdomen, and a partly calcified mass. **C,** Ultrasound images from the same infant in part **B** demonstrate the subhepatic, partly calcified mass with internal debris and a fluid-fluid level. **D,** An additional ultrasound image from the same infant in part **B** showing a portion of the cyst wall (*arrows*) and multiple, abnormal, hyperechoic loops of bowel. **E,** Another infant boy with bilious aspirates and abdominal distension on day 1 of life. Abdominal radiographs demonstrate marked distension of the flanks and localized calcification in the right upper quadrant consistent with a meconium cyst; this diagnosis was confirmed upon subsequent ultrasound imaging. **F,** An abdominal radiograph on the same patient as shown in part **E**, obtained a few hours later. The radiograph shows a persistent perforation, with extraluminal air (*arrows*) extending into the site of the meconium cyst.

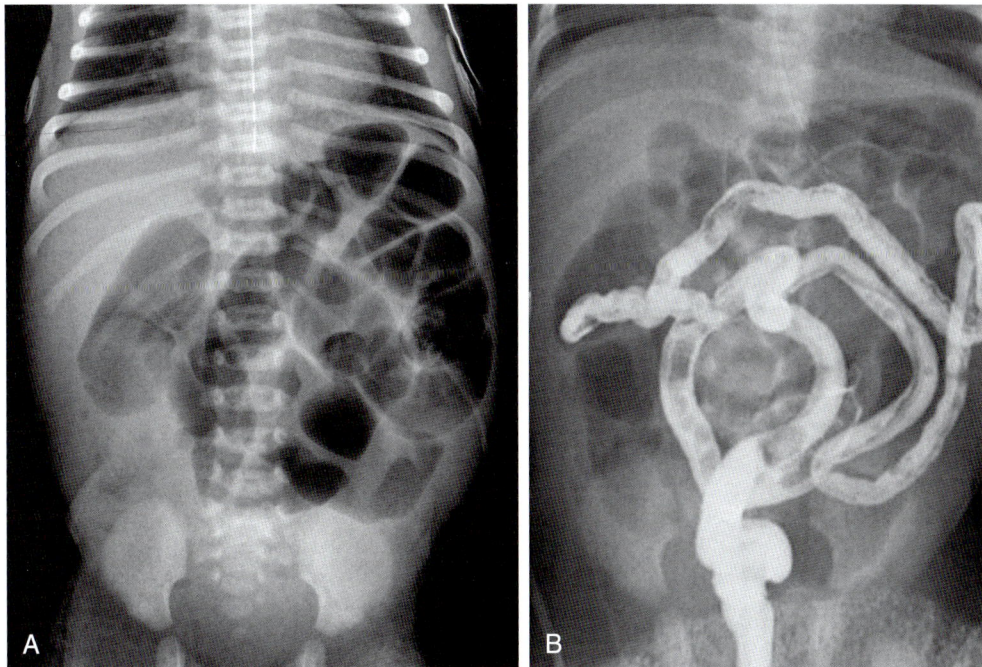

Figure 103-32   A meconium ileus. **A,** An abdominal radiograph in a 3-day-old infant with abdominal distension and bilious aspirates shows dilatation of multiple loops of bowel. No calcifications are seen on the radiograph. **B,** Contrast enema on the same infant as shown in part **A** demonstrates a microcolon with multiple tiny meconium plugs, consistent with the diagnosis of meconium ileus. Compare to Fig. 103-27, *C* and *D*.

can be managed with careful fluid and electrolyte monitoring and replacement after the enema procedure. Before the procedure, the patient likewise should be prepared for the enema with adequate fluid and electrolyte replacement, and surgical consultation and standby are imperative.

Subsequent investigators have reported problems with bowel necrosis after administration of the Gastrografin enema,[41] ascribed to the polysorbate component, which has been found experimentally to cause mucosal damage and necrosis in experiments on animals.[109] For these reasons, many pediatric radiologists avoid use of Gastrografin and instead use other moderately hyperosmolar media. A survey of pediatric radiologists in North America, published in 1995, showed a higher success rate when an additive such as N-acetylcysteine (Mucomyst) was used but showed no correlation of success rate with osmolarity of the contrast medium used; the reported perforation rate was 2.75%, with a higher risk of perforation in cases in which balloon occlusion of the rectum was used.[110]

A therapeutic enema may need to be repeated for definitive resolution of the obstruction. Success may be dependent at least partly on the perseverance of the operator, because the contrast material does not easily advance beyond the obstructing meconium into the dilated loops of bowel. The overall success can vary between 0 and 100% in specific institutions[110] but is reported to be between 50% and 65%.[104]

Surgery is indicated for patients for whom the therapeutic enema is unsuccessful at relieving the bowel obstruction.

MECKEL DIVERTICULUM

Overview   Meckel diverticulum is named after Johann Friedrich Meckel the younger, who was the first to report extensively on its embryology, anatomy, and clinical manifestations in the early nineteenth century. Meckel diverticulum is found in approximately 1% to 4% of the population and is located within 100 cm from the ileocecal junction.[111]

Etiology   The Meckel diverticulum is a remnant of the vitelline or omphalomesenteric duct, the communication between the embryonic gut and the yolk sac. This duct normally obliterates by the fifth to seventh week of gestation. Approximately 25% of diverticula may have a persistent attachment to the abdominal wall, considered to represent a remnant of the left omphalomesenteric artery. In addition to a Meckel diverticulum with or without persistent attachment to the abdominal wall, remnants of the omphalomesenteric duct include patency of the duct presenting as an umbilicoileal fistula and fibrous vitelline cords connecting the ileum to the umbilicus, with or without a vitelline cyst along the length of the cord.[112,113]

Clinical Presentation   Most Meckel diverticula remain asymptomatic, with complication rates estimated at 4% to 6%, decreasing with age.[113,114] Although the prevalence of diverticula is similar in both genders, symptoms are more likely to occur in males and in younger patients.[113,114] The most common clinical presentation is that of painless rectal bleeding. Meckel diverticulum accounts for approximately 50% of lower GI bleeding in infants and toddlers, typically occurring as a complication of gastric mucosa within the diverticulum. The incidence of gastric mucosa within bleeding Meckel diverticula is estimated at 23% to 80%.[112,113] Heterotopic pancreatic tissue is found in 5% to 16% of cases.[113] In addition to bleeding, gastric and pancreatic mucosa can lead to inflammation of the diverticulum, with abdominal pain mimicking appendicitis, and which similarly can evolve into perforation and/or obstruction.[112,115,116]

Meckel diverticulum can present as distal small bowel obstruction through a variety of other mechanisms. The diverticulum may invert into the ileal lumen and serve as a lead point for intussusception. If the diverticulum remains attached to the umbilicus, it can serve as an anchor for a segmental volvulus, or the fibrous cord can promote a bowel obstruction as an adhesion or as a closed loop obstruction. Volvulus also can occur with very large or "giant" diverticula. The Meckel diverticulum can become incarcerated in an inguinal hernia, known as a Littre hernia.[113] Patients with obstruction present with abdominal pain and vomiting, which is complicated by bleeding in cases of intussusception.

Meckel diverticula also can present with neoplasia, typically in adult patients; the tumors are most commonly carcinoids, and complications include luminal obstruction and intussusception. Meckel diverticula may contain enteroliths and also may present with parasitic infections, such as ascariasis, and lodged ingested foreign bodies.[112]

Imaging   Plain films are not particularly helpful in the diagnosis of Meckel diverticula except as indicators of some of its complications, such as obstruction. Fluoroscopic examination such as small bowel follow-through requires very careful technique and may be able to demonstrate the antimesenteric saccular outpouch from the distal ileum, particularly when enteroclysis is performed, or when the diverticula are larger, such as the "giant" diverticula that measure greater than 5 to 6 cm in diameter and up to 15 cm in length.[113] However, small diverticula may be inconspicuous and difficult to subtract from the multiple bowel loops in the background.

The most well-known imaging examination for detection of Meckel diverticula is the technetium pertechnetate abdominal scintigram (see Chapter 85).[117] This examination is dependent upon the presence of gastric mucosa, with a reported sensitivity of 80% to 90%, a specificity of 95%, and accuracy of 90% in pediatric patients,[118] although accuracy may be lower in patients who present with a hemoglobin <11 g/dL.[117] Use of single photon emission CT has been reported to identify the Meckel diverticulum in some patients in whom conventional planar imaging is unsuccessful.[113] Duplication cysts with gastric mucosa are part of the differential diagnosis of a positive scan but often can be differentiated clinically or with other cross-sectional imaging modalities.

In patients with inflamed diverticula, ultrasound and CT can detect the inflamed diverticulum, which appears as a blind-ending structure, surrounded by inflammation. On cross-sectional imaging the findings may be very difficult to distinguish from appendicitis in some cases; however, in other cases, a much larger size and periumbilical location may suggest the correct diagnosis preoperatively (Fig. 103-33). In patients in whom intussusception is present, the intussuscepted diverticulum is outlined by air during air enema reduction.[119] Both ultrasound and CT may identify the intussuscepted, thick-walled, fluid-filled diverticulum within the intussusceptum complex.[113,120,121]

Treatment   The treatment of complicated Meckel diverticula is surgical resection. However, the treatment of diverticula that are asymptomatic and incidentally discovered during surgery for another reason is less clear; the potential for the development of complications needs to be weighed against the potential for postsurgical complications, reported as 1% to 2% for patients with incidental resection, with a mortality rate of 0.001%.[112] Some authors advocate a judicious approach to this problem, taking into consideration higher risk factors for complications, such as younger age and male gender.[122] Laparoscopic diagnosis and resection of symptomatic diverticula is currently advocated, with some investigators suggesting that laparoscopy can replace the Meckel technetium scan in patients with a high clinical suspicion of Meckel diverticulum as the bleeding source.[112,123]

DUPLICATION CYSTS

Overview   Duplication cysts of the GI tract are characterized by contiguity with and adherence to a segment of the alimentary tract, by a smooth muscle coat and mucosal lining including one or more types of cells found within any portion of the alimentary canal, and by a shared a blood supply with native GI structures.[124] They can occur anywhere along the length of the entire GI tract from the mouth to the anus and are most common near the terminal ileum.[125] Duplication cysts occur along the mesenteric border of the involved

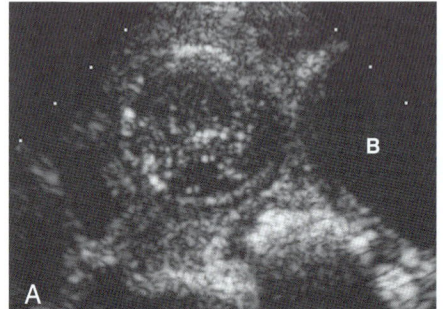 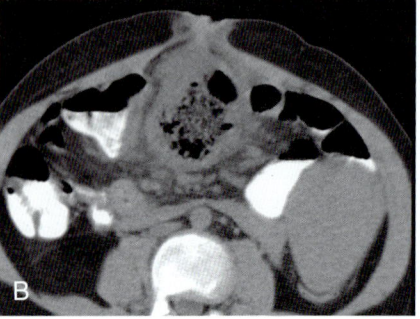 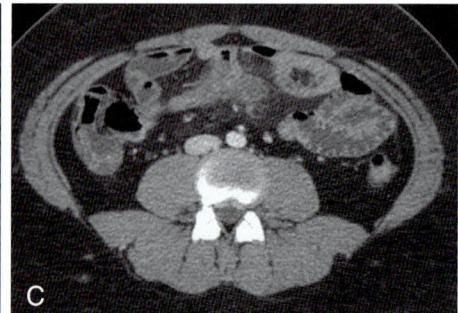

Figure 103-33   Meckel diverticulum. **A,** A sagittal ultrasound image along the midline in a 2-year-old girl outlines a round structure with intestinal contents and a gut signature located above the bladder (*B*) fundus, with surrounding echogenicity; an inflamed Meckel diverticulum was identified at subsequent surgery. **B,** A computed tomography (CT) image of an adolescent boy with abdominal pain demonstrates a large, inflamed loop of bowel in close association with the umbilicus, representing an inflamed Meckel diverticulum. **C,** A CT image in another adolescent shows a smaller Meckel diverticulum in the periumbilical region, with associated inflammation demonstrated by fat stranding.

bowel loop, and therefore in the duodenum they are found medial to the descending limb or along its third portion; duodenal duplications account for approximately 6% of the total and thus are uncommon.[126] Most duplication cysts do not communicate with the intestinal lumen.

Etiology   The etiology of alimentary tract duplications is not certain, and no one single theory satisfactorily explains all instances of duplication anomalies. One theory holds that duplication cysts are the result of incomplete attempts at twinning, a theory that also suggests an explanation for duplications of other organs, such as the bladder and urethra. The split notochord theory suggests that there is herniation of a diverticulum of the foregut through a gap in the notochord; this theory is helpful in understanding duplications that are associated with anomalies of the spine. A third possibility theorizes that these anomalies are the result of diverticula that form during the recanalization stage of the bowel. A fourth hypothesis suggests that environmental factors, such as trauma or hypoxia, can induce the events that can result in an enteric duplication.[126]

Clinical Presentation   The presentation of duplication cysts is usually related to their size, thus presenting with mass effect, palpable mass, obstruction, or localized volvulus, or to the type of mucosa in its lining because cysts containing gastric mucosa can ulcerate, bleed, and lead to inflammatory changes. Patients present with abdominal pain and vomiting. Mass effect by duplication cysts can lead to bilious or nonbilious vomiting, or the patients may present with weight loss and failure to thrive. Duodenal duplication cysts can lead to pancreatitis, possibly related to compression of the pancreatic duct,[127] and also have been reported to cause fluid accumulation within the lesser sac.[128] Duplication cysts may act as a fulcrum for segmental volvulus.[125] Those located in the terminal ileum and ileocecal valve may act as a lead point in intussusception and should be suspected when intussusception occurs in infants within the first 3 months of life.

Imaging   Plain radiographs are usually noncontributory but may demonstrate a soft tissue mass or evidence of obstruction if the cyst is large, particularly if it is located along the distal aspect of the stomach or the duodenum.

An upper GI series could be the first study obtained in a child presenting with vomiting; in cases of duplication cysts of the duodenum, the examination reveals a filling defect along the mesenteric wall of the duodenum or extrinsic compression (Fig. 103-34). Compression of the gastric outlet or of the first portion of the duodenum by the cyst has been described as a "beak" sign.[129] If focal communication occurs between the cyst and the duodenum, contrast material will enter the duplication.

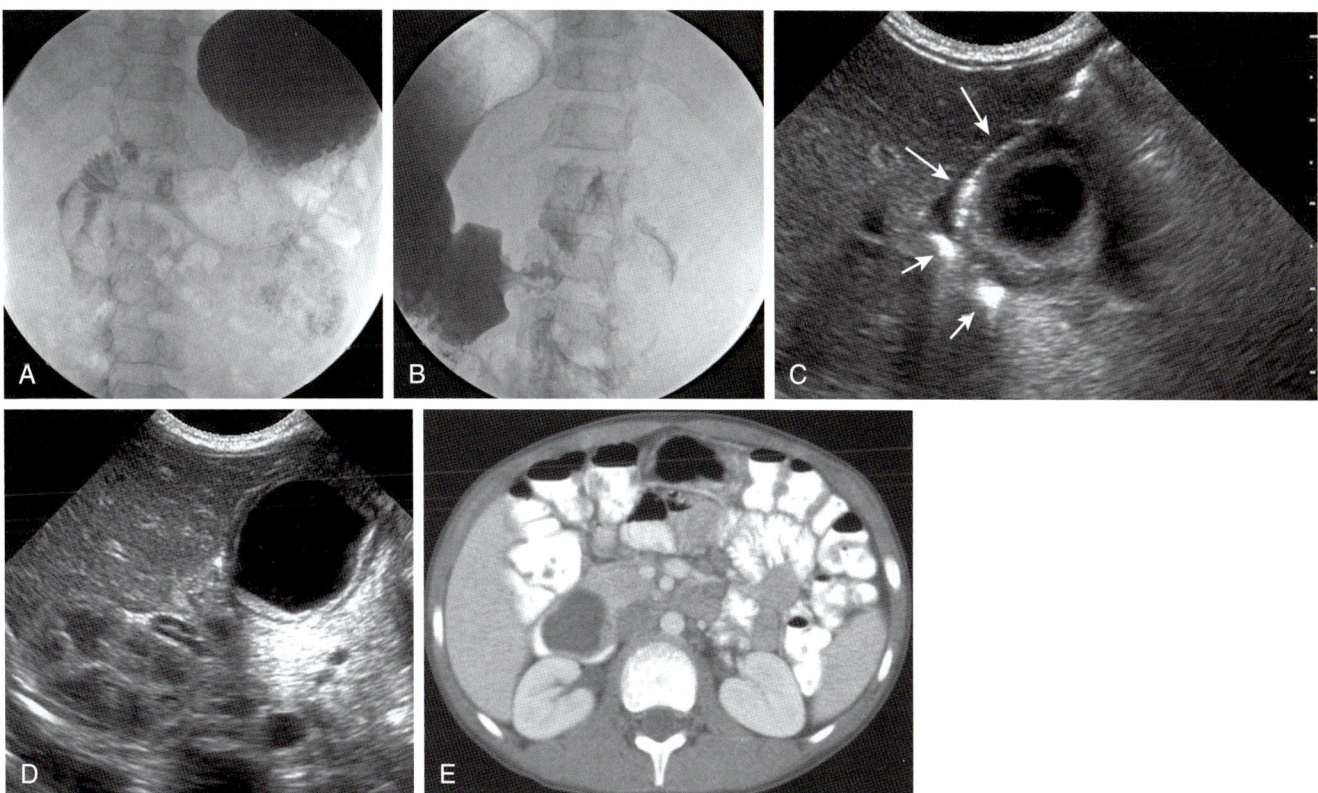

Figure 103-34   A duodenal duplication cyst. **A** and **B,** Two images from an upper gastrointestinal examination in an 11-year-old boy demonstrate intramural mass effect upon the mesenteric border of the duodenum. **C** and **D,** A 1-day-old infant with a prenatal diagnosis of an abdominal cyst resected at 2 weeks of age. **C,** The sonogram shows the cyst to be intimately related to the distal antrum (*long arrows*) and the descending duodenum (*short arrows*). **D,** An additional image shows the typical double layer of a duplication cyst, indicative of gut signature. **E,** A computed tomography image on the same patient as in parts **A** and **B** illustrates clearly the location of the mass along the medial border of the duodenum.

Small bowel duplication cysts beyond the duodenum may present with obstruction, inflammation, intussusception, or a combination (e-Fig. 103-35; also see Chapter 108). Cross-sectional imaging can confirm the diagnosis of a duplication cyst suspected from a prior study, or it may be the initial imaging modality used. Ultrasound typically reveals an anechoic cyst, but the fluid may contain debris if there has been infection or hemorrhage from associated ectopic gastric mucosa and ulceration. The typical "bowel wall signature" of an enteric duplication cyst is usually present.[130-132] The presence of bowel wall signature may help to differentiate a duodenal duplication cyst from a pancreatic pseudocyst. However, the gut signature is not completely sensitive or specific to duplication cysts; the gut signature may be obliterated by superimposed inflammatory changes and may be seen in other conditions, such as mesenteric cyst, cystic teratoma,[133] and ovarian cysts.

CT demonstrates a discrete fluid-filled cyst on the mesenteric border of the involved bowel segment, often with contrast enhancement of the cyst wall. On MRI, hemorrhage or infection can alter the signal characteristics of the cyst on water-sensitive sequences. MRI is particularly helpful in cases of duodenal duplication cyst, where MR cholangiopancreatography can demonstrate the relationship of the cyst to the duodenal wall, the pancreatic head, and the pancreatic and biliary ductal systems, which is important preoperative information for the surgeon.[126]

Treatment The most common treatment for duplication cysts is resection, although marsupialization with internal drainage also may be performed. Cysts with gastric mucosa should be excised or stripped of the mucosal lining; complex cases may require more extensive surgical excision.[126]

LYMPHATIC MALFORMATION, MESENTERIC, AND OMENTAL CYSTS

Overview Abdominal lymphatic malformations can be located in the mesentery or omentum as mesenteric or omental cysts. Lymphatic malformations have only an endothelial lining, are usually multiloculated, and may contain chyle. Most lymphatic malformations occur in the mesentery rather than the omentum because of its richer lymphatic content, most commonly in the ileal mesentery.[134,135] Such cysts of lymphatic origin are lined by flat endothelial cells and contain lymphoid tissue within their walls.

Mesothelial cysts, on the other hand, occur in the small bowel, the mesentery, and the mesocolon and are the result of accumulation of fluid between mesothelial layers. They are lined by mesothelium, without mural muscle fibers or lymphatic structures.[136] Nonpancreatic pseudocysts also may occur in the mesentery, or more often in the omentum, and are believed to result from prior trauma or infection, with no inner cellular lining on histology.

Etiology The etiology of lymphatic malformations and lymphatic mesenteric and omental cysts is not known; hypotheses include failure of embryonic lymphatic spaces to develop normal connections and drainage into the venous system, and benign proliferation of ectopic lymphatics sequestered from the venous system.[134]

Clinical Presentation Abdominal lymphatic malformations are rare, representing approximately 5% of all such malformations, and with a quoted prevalence of approximately 1 per 20,000 admissions at a children's hospital, with a lower incidence in African Americans.[134,137] In children, presentation is more common in boys, although in adults the presentation is more common in women, through a putative estrogenic effect.[138] These lesions may be asymptomatic and discovered incidentally, or they may present as a result of size or complications of the lesion. Mass effect can result in the development of partial obstruction over time or acutely as a result of acute enlargement of the cyst secondary to hemorrhage. Abdominal pain can occur through torsion of the cyst or one of its components (Fig. 103-36) or torsion of adjacent bowel loops with the cyst acting as a fulcrum. Cysts can become infected, producing fever, abdominal pain, or sepsis.[134,135]

Imaging Plain radiographs may show a large mass displacing intestinal loops. Dilated loops may be seen in patients with obstruction. Upper GI contrast studies show displacement of bowel with no communication. Ultrasound demonstrates the multilocular nature of the mass with fine septations (see Fig. 103-36). Most of the mass is anechoic, but some of the loculated spaces may have internal echogenicity, depending on the chyle or blood content.[139] On CT the attenuation values of the fluid range from near fat to near water, depending on its composition. On CT, septa and loculations are usually demonstrated, unless their attenuation value merges with that of the surrounding fluid in scans performed without contrast material; septa may enhance with injection of intravenous contrast material. Fine calcifications may be present in some cases.[134] MRI of lymphatic malformations shows characteristics of the cyst ranging from fluid with low-intensity signal on T1-weighted images to fat with high-intensity signal.[140]

Treatment Traditional treatment is surgical resection with complete extirpation of the cyst, although percutaneous drainage and sclerotherapy is a reasonable alternative in some cases. In children with mesenteric cysts, treatment is more likely to require segmental bowel resection than in adults (50% to 60% vs. 33%).[134] If complete resection is not possible, marsupialization of the cyst with sclerosis of the lining can be performed. A surgical classification of mesenteric cysts, based on operative management, includes four types: type 1 is on a pedicle, and easily removed, although more likely to undergo torsion. Type 2 is sessile and restricted to the mesenteric boundaries, whereas type 3 has retroperitoneal extension, representing an increased surgical challenge. Type 4 refers to multicentric cysts.[137]

Laparoscopic resection is possible; however, this technique is best approached with caution because of relatively limited experience, if the diagnosis is not certain preoperatively, or if the procedure will necessitate segmental bowel resection.[141-143]

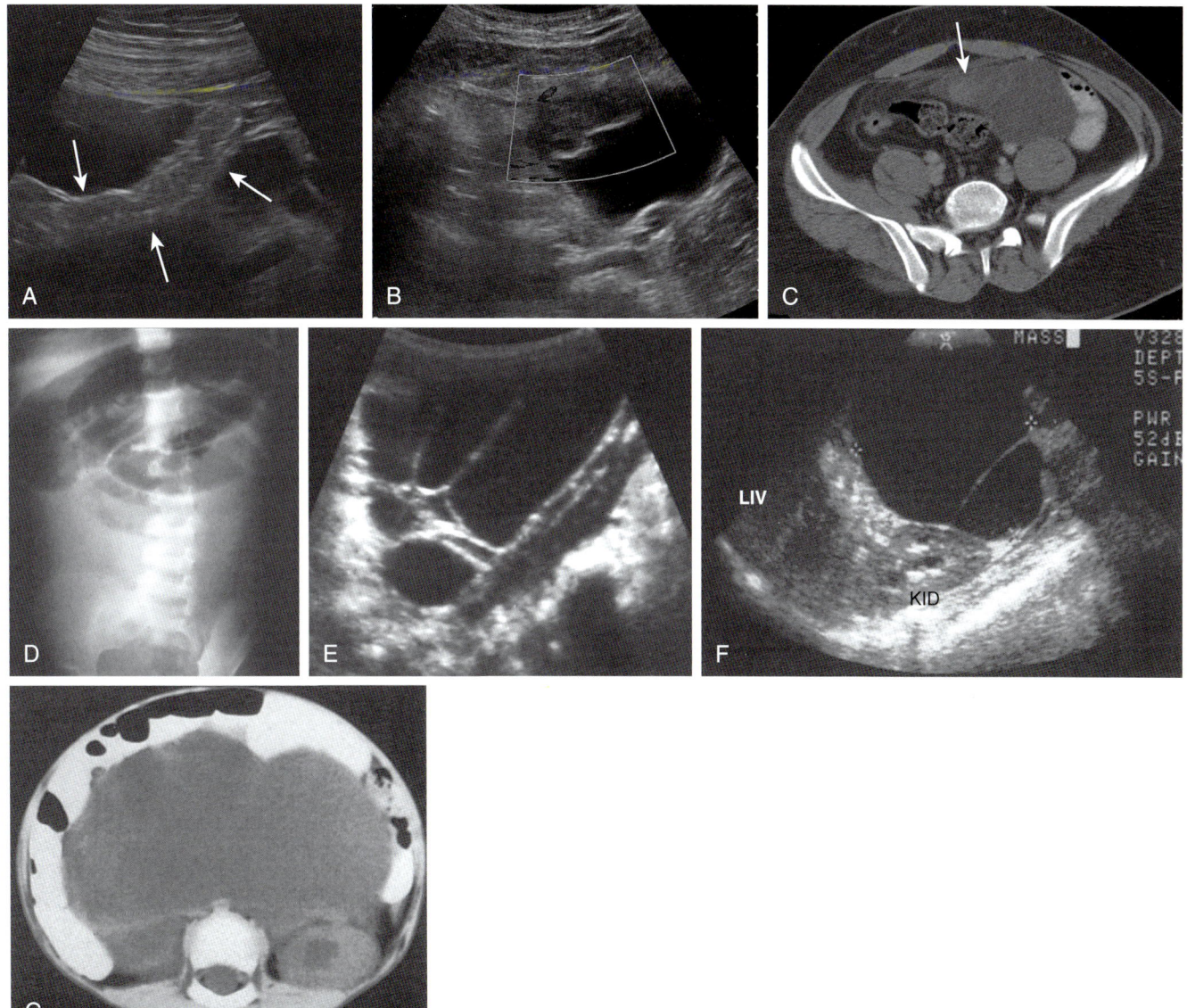

Figure 103-36 Mesenteric lymphatic malformations. **A,** A 14-year-old boy presented with abdominal pain and dysuria. An ultrasound image of the left midabdomen reveals a multiseptated cystic mass with an intervening dumbbell loop of small bowel (*arrows*). **B,** A color Doppler image obtained more inferiorly in the supravesical area shows an avascular solid-appearing component to the cystic lesions, with surrounding hyperechogenicity consistent with inflammation and edema. **C,** A computed tomography (CT) an shows the solid-appearing component (*arrow*) corresponding to the avascular structure noted in part **B** and surrounding inflammation with fat stranding in the supravesical area. At surgery, a loculated mesenteric cyst was removed, with volvulus and infarction of a supravesical component, leading to the presenting symptoms and imaging findings. **D,** An abdominal radiograph from a different patient presenting with vomiting with clinical concern for intussusception. The radiograph demonstrates dilated loops of bowel, displaced into the upper abdomen. **E,** A longitudinal sonogram along the right flank in the same patient as shown in part **D** demonstrates a multiseptated cystic mass occupying the lower portion of the abdomen, representing a cystic lymphangioma. **F,** A longitudinal ultrasound scan through the upper abdomen in another patient shows a septated, hypoechoic mass abutting the liver (*LIV*) and right kidney (*KID*). **G,** A CT scan of shows the same patient as shown in part **F** confirms the massive fluid-filled structure displacing contrast-filled loops of bowel.

Key Points

The finding of a double bubble on a plain film is diagnostic of duodenal atresia/stenosis, and contrast studies are not required for confirmation.

Associated anomalies in patients with duodenal atresia/stenosis include trisomy 21, Hirschsprung disease, esophageal atresia, and heterotaxy.

Malrotation can lead to midgut volvulus because of the lack of normal bowel fixation and the short mesenteric pedicle.

The normal position of the ligament of Treitz may be altered in children with a normal rotation who have other abnormalities, such as masses or dilated loops of bowel.

Microcolon refers to an unused colon and is associated with distal small bowel obstruction.

Conditions that can result in prenatal gut ischemia and atresia include gastroschisis, intrauterine volvulus, intussusception, and internal hernias.

Meconium ileus is the result of tarry, tenacious meconium impacted in the distal small bowel, causing distal small bowel obstruction.

Calcifications in abdominal radiographs of infants with meconium ileus are a sign of complicated meconium ileus and meconium peritonitis. Such patients are operative candidates without further imaging or attempts at nonoperative treatment.

Painless rectal bleeding is the most common presentation of Meckel diverticulum.

Gut signature is a suggestive diagnostic finding of a duplication cyst on sonography, but it is not completely specific.

Duplication cysts are most common in the ileum, where they can act as lead points for intussusception.

Lymphatic cysts are lined by endothelial cells. Mesothelial cysts are the result of accumulation of fluid between mesothelial layers and are lined by mesothelium.

Suggested Readings

Applegate KE, Anderson JM, Klatte EC. Intestinal malrotation in children: problem-solving approach to the upper gastrointestinal series. *Radiographics*. 2006;26(5):1485-1500.

Cheng G, et al. Sonographic pitfalls in the diagnosis of enteric duplication cysts. *AJR Am J Roentgenol*. 2005;184(2):521-525.

Gorter RR, et al. Clinical and genetic characteristics of meconium ileus in newborns with and without cystic fibrosis. *J Pediatr Gastroenterol Nutr*. 2010;50(5):569-572.

Lampl B, et al. Malrotation and midgut volvulus: a historical review and current controversies in diagnosis and management. *Pediatr Radiol*. 2009;39(4):359-366.

Losanoff JE, et al. Mesenteric cystic lymphangioma. *J Am Coll Surg*. 2003;196(4):598-603.

Sagar J, Kumar V, Shah DK. Meckel's diverticulum: a systematic review. *J R Soc Med*. 2006;99(10):501-505.

Stollman TH, et al. Decreased mortality but increased morbidity in neonates with jejunoileal atresia; a study of 114 cases over a 34-year period. *J Pediatr Surg*. 2009;44(1):217-221.

Strouse PJ. Disorders of intestinal rotation and fixation ("malrotation"). *Pediatr Radiol*. 2004;34(11):837-851.

Yousefzadeh DK. The position of the duodenojejunal junction: the wrong horse to bet on in diagnosing or excluding malrotation. *Pediatr Radiol*. 2009;39(suppl 2):S172-S177.

References

Full references for this chapter can be found on www.expertconsult.com.

Chapter 104

Acquired Abnormalities

MARTA HERNANZ-SCHULMAN

Duodenal Obstruction

Acquired abnormalities of the duodenum that result in obstruction include superior mesenteric artery syndrome and posttraumatic obstruction, as well as obstruction such as duodenal intussusception, due to complications of feeding catheters.

SUPERIOR MESENTERIC ARTERY SYNDROME

Overview First described at autopsy by von Rokitansky in 1861,[1] the term superior mesenteric artery (SMA) syndrome refers to obstruction of the third portion of the duodenum at its crossing between the aorta and the SMA. It also is known by other terms, including cast syndrome and Wilkie syndrome after David Percival Wilkie, who termed it "chronic duodenal ileus" in his description of 75 patients in 1927.[2] The overall prevalence is cited to be between 0.013% and 0.3% of patients undergoing upper gastrointestinal (UGI) examinations.[3-6]

Etiology The normal angle between the aorta and the SMA is between 25 and 60 degrees, and the normal aorto–SMA distance is 10 to 28 mm,[3] parameters that have been found to be significantly correlated to adult body mass index, particularly in females.[7] The etiology of SMA syndrome has been ascribed to an abnormally low angle between the aorta and the SMA, bringing them in close apposition at the crossing of the third portion of the duodenum. The abnormally low angle and decreased distance between the aorta and the SMA is thought to occur because of an abnormally low origin of the SMA or an abnormally high position of the duodenojejunal junction at the ligament of Treitz, so that the third portion of the duodenum is located nearer to the origin of the SMA.[1,7,8]

Although asthenic individuals, particularly after acute weight loss, are most susceptible to the development of SMA syndrome, in a series by Biank et al., it was found that this presentation occurred in only approximately 50% of their patients. In their study population, the body mass index ranged between the 3rd and 97th percentile for age, with a mean at the 39th percentile. Premorbid conditions included Nissen fundoplication, cerebral palsy, traumatic brain injury, and posterior spinal fusion.[6] Other persons predisposed to SMA syndrome include burn victims and patients with lumbar hyperlordosis or who are in spinal traction or a spinal cast.[9] According to one report the syndrome occurred in several members of one family, raising the question of genetic predisposition.[10]

Clinical Presentation The clinical syndrome occurs more commonly in females between the ages of 10 and 39 years, although it has been described rarely in neonates.[11-13] The most common clinical presentation includes abdominal pain, vomiting, nausea, early satiety, and anorexia[6,14]; acute presentation may follow one of the aforementioned premorbid conditions.

Imaging Plain radiographs may show gastric dilatation, but the stomach may be decompressed by vomiting or by an enteric tube. Contrast UGI study shows dilatation and partial obstruction of the third portion of the duodenum, terminating in a straight line at the expected location of the crossing of the SMA, with active but poorly effective peristalsis across the point of obstruction (Fig. 104-1, A). A useful maneuver to confirm that the obstruction is a consequence of SMA syndrome is to place the patient in a left side down decubitus position, which tends to relieve SMA obstruction.

Ultrasound has been used to measure both the angle and the distance between the aorta and the SMA but may have difficulty outlining their relationship to the duodenum unless the latter is fluid-filled. Computed tomography (CT) (Fig. 104-1, B and C) and magnetic resonance imaging (MRI) are able to assess the dilatation of the duodenum, as well as its relationship to the SMA.

Treatment Nonoperative treatment centers on weight gain with high-calorie enteral nutrition either by mouth or transpyloric tube feedings beyond the point of obstruction, or with hyperalimentation; such nonoperative intervention is successful in most patients.[6] Medical treatment is most likely to be successful when the syndrome is of acute onset.[15]

Operative treatment is reserved for patients in whom medical management fails and typically consists of a duodenojejunostomy.[16] Some authors advocate obtaining a biopsy specimen of the duodenum and jejunum before undertaking surgery to exclude infection, an infiltrative or neoplastic process, or intestinal pseudoobstruction as a cause of the duodenal dilatation.[1]

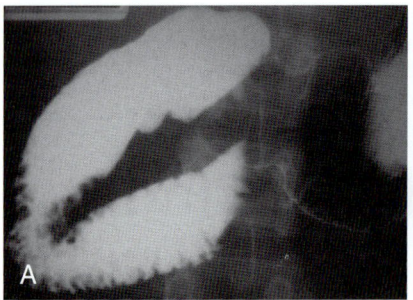 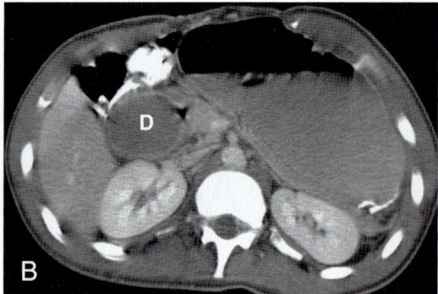 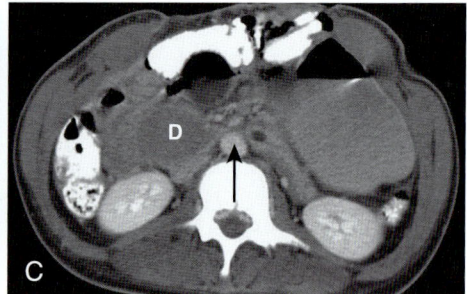

Figure 104-1 Superior mesenteric artery syndrome. **A,** A 15-year-old girl with rapid weight loss. An anteroposterior spot image from an upper gastro-intestinal examination demonstrates complete obstruction at the third portion of the duodenum. **B** and **C,** Two images from a computed tomography scan in a 22-year-old who had sustained a gunshot wound, resulting in paraplegia. The stomach and duodenum (*D*) are dilated. The arrow points to the compression of the duodenum at the crossing of the superior mesenteric artery, with resolution of dilatation of the duodenal lumen beyond the point of compression.

DUODENAL HEMATOMA

Overview A duodenal hematoma is an infrequent injury in pediatric patients, occurring in fewer than 3% of children with abdominal injuries, and usually is associated with blunt abdominal trauma, both accidental and nonaccidental. The hematoma often extends beyond the ligament of Treitz into the proximal jejunum as a duodenojejunal hematoma.[17] In a series of 33 children with a blunt duodenal injury, nonacci-dental trauma was the most common cause of duodenal injury (24%), followed by motor vehicle crashes, handlebar injures, sports injuries, and other forms of direct trauma.[18]

Etiology The retroperitoneal duodenum contains a vascular submucosal and subserosal plexus and lies relatively fixed against the rigid spine, thus facilitating injury after blunt abdominal trauma. Bleeding is contained within the submu-cosa and subserosa and encroaches into the lumen of the duodenum. In children, this injury typically occurs after directed blunt trauma such as a direct punch or kick to the epigastrium, or as a result of handlebar injuries. Motor vehicle injuries such as those involving sudden deceleration forces also can produce a shearing injury and result in an intramural hematoma.[17,19] Duodenal hematomas also have been reported in patients with coagulation abnormalities after a relatively minor trauma, after undergoing an endoscopic duodenal biopsy,[19-23] or when pancreatitis develops, with the latter postulated to be a result of disruption of the intramural vas-culature by pancreatic enzymes.[24,25]

Clinical Presentation The clinical presentation includes abdominal pain and vomiting, which typically is bilious. When a duodenal hematoma occurs after blunt trauma, pan-creatitis related to an associated pancreatic injury may develop. A luminal obstruction sufficient to produce symptoms may not occur immediately after injury, and the child may not present until several days after the traumatic event. When a duodenal hematoma occurs after significant trauma such as a motor-vehicle accident, the CT examination may show the diagnosis before symptom onset. One should always remem-ber that this injury, in the appropriate clinical setting, should raise the concern for inflicted trauma.[17,20,26]

Imaging Plain radiographic films may be the initial modality in a child presenting with epigastric abdominal pain, tender-ness, and vomiting. Depending on the degree of obstruction and the severity of vomiting, the radiographs may show dis-tension of the stomach and duodenum, with paucity of distal bowel contents (Fig. 104-2, *A*).

Findings of a UGI examination depend on the ability of some of the contrast material to traverse the obstructed portion of the duodenum. If no or very little contrast material moves through, the luminal border of the distended duode-num may show a lobulated contour. As contrast material passes through the obstruction, the lobulated contour of the filling defect will outline the column of contrast across the duodenum (Fig. 104-2, *B*). Smaller hematomas may demon-strate more subtle findings, such as some thickening of the duodenal folds.[17]

Ultrasound (Fig. 104-2, *C*) typically shows a distended first portion of the duodenum, with a filling defect encroach-ing upon and obliterating its lumen.[27,28] The echogenicity of the hematoma is variable, depending on the status of the clot; the clue to the diagnosis is the fact that the mass follows the course of the duodenum. On Doppler interrogation, the lesion has no flow.

CT demonstrates similar findings, with dilatation of the duodenum and a nonenhancing mass that follows the course of the duodenum, obliterating its lumen (Fig. 104-2, *D* and *E*).

MRI often is not performed in children with duodenal hematomas. If it is performed, it again will show a mass fol-lowing the course of the duodenum, obliterating its lumen, with signal characteristics consistent with an evolving hema-toma that may appear in concentric layers of differing signal intensity.[29]

Treatment Patients with duodenal perforation need emergent surgery, but the treatment for a duodenal hematoma generally consists of decompression of the stomach and duodenum via a nasogastric tube and maintenance of hydration and nutrition with total parenteral nutrition until the hematoma resolves. In one series of 27 children with a duodenal injury who were treated conservatively, the mean time to resolution of symp-toms ranged between 12 and 16 days.[18,30] If complete obstruc-tion is present without improvement, it may be necessary to evacuate the hematoma surgically.[18]

DUODENAL INTUSSUSCEPTION

Overview Duodenal intussusception may be seen in both antegrade and retrograde directions, typically around a gas-trojejunal (GJ) tube.

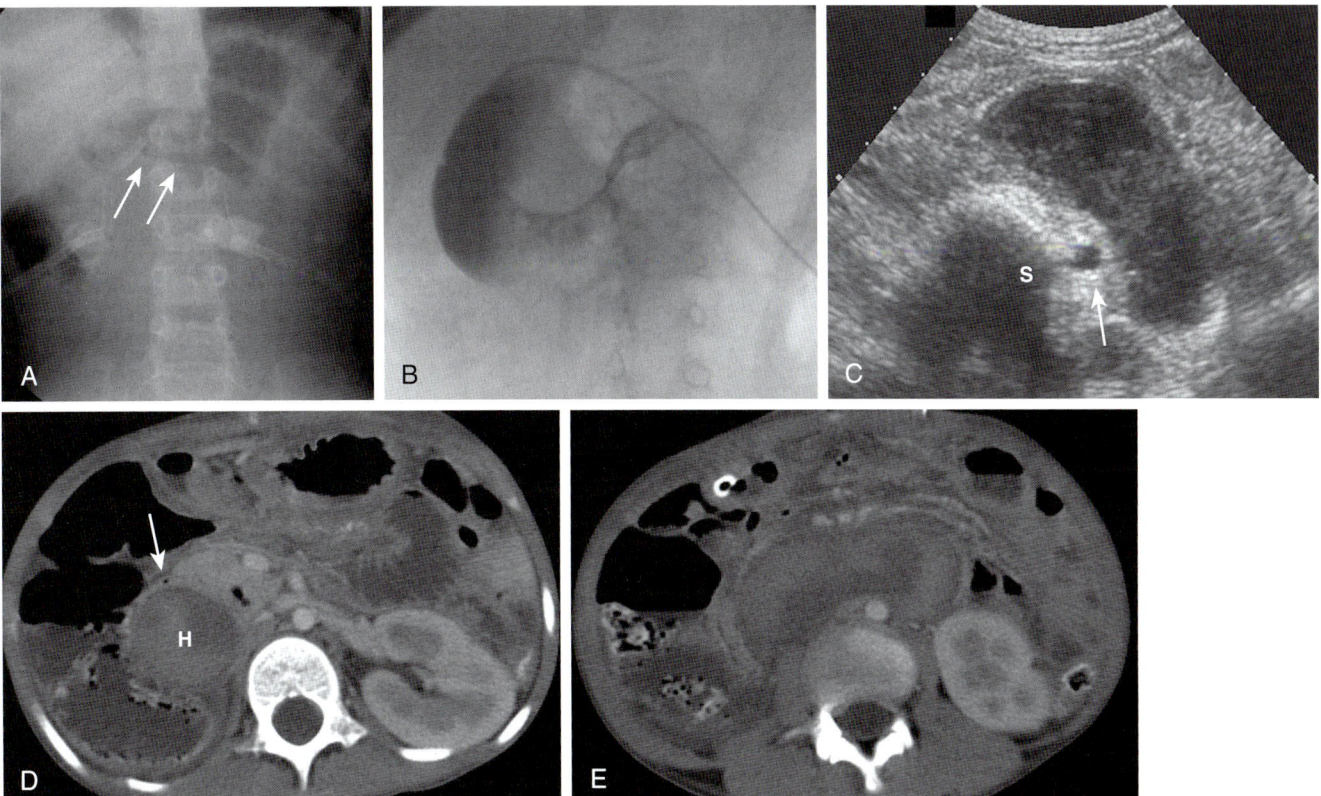

Figure 104-2 Duodenal hematoma. **A,** An 8-year-old with agenesis of the corpus callosum who had undergone an upper endoscopy with a duodenal biopsy and subsequently developed persistent bilious vomiting. The abdominal radiograph shows a polypoid density (*arrows*) encroaching upon the gas along the inferior border of the antrum. Gaseous distension of the duodenum is seen with very little gas distally. **B,** An upper gastrointestinal examination from a 10-year-old boy with cerebral palsy and mental retardation who presented with dehydration and inability to tolerate feedings. Introduction of contrast material into the duodenum during an unsuccessful attempt at gastrojejunal tube placement shows an obstructing duodenal hematoma as a filling defect upon the third and distal second portions of the duodenum. **C,** An abdominal ultrasound on the same patient shown in part **A** demonstrates the heterogeneous duodenal hematoma, following the course of the third portion of the duodenum. *S,* Spine. Arrow points to the aorta. **D,** A computed tomography (CT) image at the level of the junction of the second and third portions of the duodenum in the same patient in parts **A** and **C** shows the large heterogeneous hematoma (*H*) obliterating the duodenal lumen. The arrow points to the duodenal wall and gas bubble in the residual obliterated lumen. **E,** A more distal CT section through the third portion of the duodenum (an analogous section to ultrasound in part **C**) shows again the heterogeneous hematoma, which is obliterating the lumen of the third portion of the duodenum.

Etiology Antegrade duodenojejunal intussusception is a relatively common complication of the placement of postpyloric GJ tubes, because the tube acts as a lead point for the intussusception. Children with GJ tubes have a 16% to nearly 50% rate of antegrade intussusception.[31,32] It is believed that intussusceptions are more likely in boys, in younger patients, in patients with larger bore tubes and tubes with a distal pigtail that may act as a lead point, and when prokinetic agents are administered.[32,33] Intussusception also can occur around a weighted nasojejunal tube.[34]

Retrograde intussusception, on the other hand, is much less common and is believed to occur as a tube with an inflated terminal balloon, which has migrated distally as a result of peristalsis, is pulled back toward the stomach.[35,36]

Clinical Presentation The presentation typically is the onset of vomiting, which is bilious in approximately half the cases[31] and may be accompanied by abdominal pain/irritability. However, sometimes these intussusceptions are asymptomatic and are discovered at the time of a routine tube check,[37] and therefore they may be transient. Hematemesis or bloody

gastric aspirates typically are described in patients with retrograde intussusceptions.[35,36]

Although it bypasses the duodenum, retrograde intussusception also occurs after gastric surgery, such as a gastrojejunostomy. The intussuscepted jejunum may be gangrenous; obstruction and hematemesis are typical in acute presentations.[38]

Imaging Abdominal radiographs and ultrasound are helpful in making the diagnosis (e-Fig. 104-3). Radiographs may reveal gastric outlet obstruction, and in cases of retrograde intussusception, gas within the stomach will demonstrate the distal mass protruding into the gastric antrum. Ultrasound demonstrates the classic appearance of bowel within bowel at the gastric outlet[31,35,39] and may show a balloon as a lead point. Particularly in retrograde intussusception, upper GI examination will demonstrate the classic "coiled spring" appearance as the contrast material passes into the intussusception; the amount of contrast material may be small and the findings relatively subtle, and thus a high index of suspicion is helpful in arriving at the correct diagnosis.[39] On a CT image, the intussusception will be seen extending along the course of the duodenum, and it is seen particularly well when it is outlined by air or contrast medium.[40]

Treatment   Introduction of air or saline solution through the tube has been successful in reducing intussusception,[31] although antegrade intussusceptions can be treated by replacement of the GJ tube over a wire.[33] This complication can be prevented by changing to a smaller bore GJ tube, using a catheter without a pigtail, or shortening the length of GJ tube.[41] If the intussusception occurs around a nasojejunal tube, the tube should be removed.[37]

Retrograde intussusception is usually managed by deflation of the balloon,[35] although in some cases of supervening bowel ischemia, surgical resection may be necessary.[42]

Duodenal Inflammatory Conditions

This section discusses inflammatory conditions that affect the duodenum specifically, such as ulcer disease, as well as duodenal manifestations of other inflammatory conditions.

DUODENAL ULCER DISEASE

Overview   Ulcer disease can involve the duodenum and, as in the stomach, it is associated with *Helicobacter pylori* infection, a pathogen that is estimated to colonize or infect approximately half the world's population.[43] The prevalence of ulcer disease is lower in children than in adults, but duodenal ulcers are more common than gastric ulcers in children after the neonatal period.

Etiology   Duodenal ulcerations result when the inherent defense mechanisms are overwhelmed, including epithelial cell renewal and regeneration, duodenal bicarbonate production, preservation of mucosal blood flow, and production of prostaglandins.[44] The understanding of peptic and duodenal ulcer disease in both adults and children has changed dramatically since the elucidation of the role of *H. pylori* infection (then known as *Campylobacter pyloridis*) in its development by Warren and Marshall in 1984,[45,46] for which they were awarded the Nobel Prize in 2005. Because *H. pylori* is trophic for gastric epithelium, duodenal ulcers related to *H. pylori* are believed to occur at sites of gastric metaplasia[47] and thus are related to increased acid secretion and decreased bicarbonate output by the duodenum, resulting in lower luminal pH and precipitating bile acids, which otherwise would exert an inhibitory effect on the growth of *H. pylori*. Acid hypersecretion additionally promotes the activation of pepsinogen to pepsin, facilitating mucosal ulceration.[47]

A higher rate of *H. pylori* infection has been reported in children with duodenal ulcers (62%) than in those with peptic ulcers (20%), although other sources do not always confirm this relationship.[48] Transmission of *H. pylori* is mainly by the oral-oral or fecal-oral route and requires contact with intestinal secretions; light contact, such as kissing, is not believed to be effective.[49,50] Colonization with this pathogen has greater prevalence in locations with suboptimal sanitary infrastructure.[50] Childhood is the primary period of colonization by *H. pylori*, with cases often clustering within families as a

result of intrafamilial transmission.[50] In Western nations the prevalence of *H. pylori* colonization is decreasing and has been reported in as few as 27% of children from Western European centers, although it is thought that some underreporting may be occurring because the specimens are being cultured from the stomach rather than the duodenum.

With eradication of *H. pylori*, particularly in Western countries, the proportion of duodenal ulcers that are not related to *H. pylori* increases. Other causes of duodenal ulcer disease include therapy with nonsteroidal antiinflammatory drugs (NSAIDs). These agents promote ulceration by inhibition of cyclooxygenase 1 and 2 enzymes, which have a role in maintaining the integrity of the gastric epithelium and its mucous barrier, as well as in the response to inflammatory processes. NSAIDs also may increase the production of inflammatory mediators such as leukotrienes.

Clinical Presentation   Children with duodenal ulcer disease may present with epigastric tenderness, pain that wakes the child from sleep at night, hematemesis, melena, anorexia, poor weight gain, and vomiting.[48,51] Other manifestations include failure to thrive with growth disturbance and poor weight gain, iron deficiency anemia, and idiopathic thrombocytopenic purpura.[50]

Imaging   Fluoroscopy and upper GI examinations largely have been supplanted in the diagnosis of duodenal ulcer disease by upper endoscopy, which has become the gold standard for diagnosis, in addition to allowing biopsy and culture of detected abnormalities. When upper GI examination is performed, double contrast is more sensitive in the detection of ulcer disease, although this procedure is much more difficult to perform in younger patients and impossible to perform in infants.

Despite the shift to endoscopy, duodenal ulcers should be detected during upper GI examination if they are present. Duodenitis, which can be a result of ulcer disease, is manifested by thickening of the duodenal folds, and this finding has a sensitivity of 45% in detecting duodenal inflammation (e-Fig. 104-4).[51] Free peritoneal air may be seen if perforation has occurred (Fig. 104-5, *A*). Barium is the usual contrast agent, but contrast material that has a high iodine concentration and low osmolality and is water soluble should be used if perforation is a concern. The imaging appearance of duodenal ulcers in children is similar to that in adults. The most common finding in an acute ulcer is contrast within an ulcer crater (Fig. 104-5, *B*). Radiating folds that represent surrounding mucosal edema also may be seen. When the ulcer is on the nondependent wall of the duodenum, air will fill the ulcer outlined by barium. Chronic duodenal ulcers may lead to a scarred and deformed duodenum, but this appearance is less common in children than in adults. So-called "giant duodenal ulcers" are rare and occur more commonly in association with NSAIDs, in patients with end-stage renal disease, and in patients with Crohn disease.[47]

Ultrasound typically is not performed in patients with known duodenal ulcer disease. Thickening of the bowel wall has been described, as well as surrounding fluid and gas in cases of perforation.[52]

On CT, thickening of the duodenal wall may be detected, along with contrast material within an ulcer crater.[53] In cases

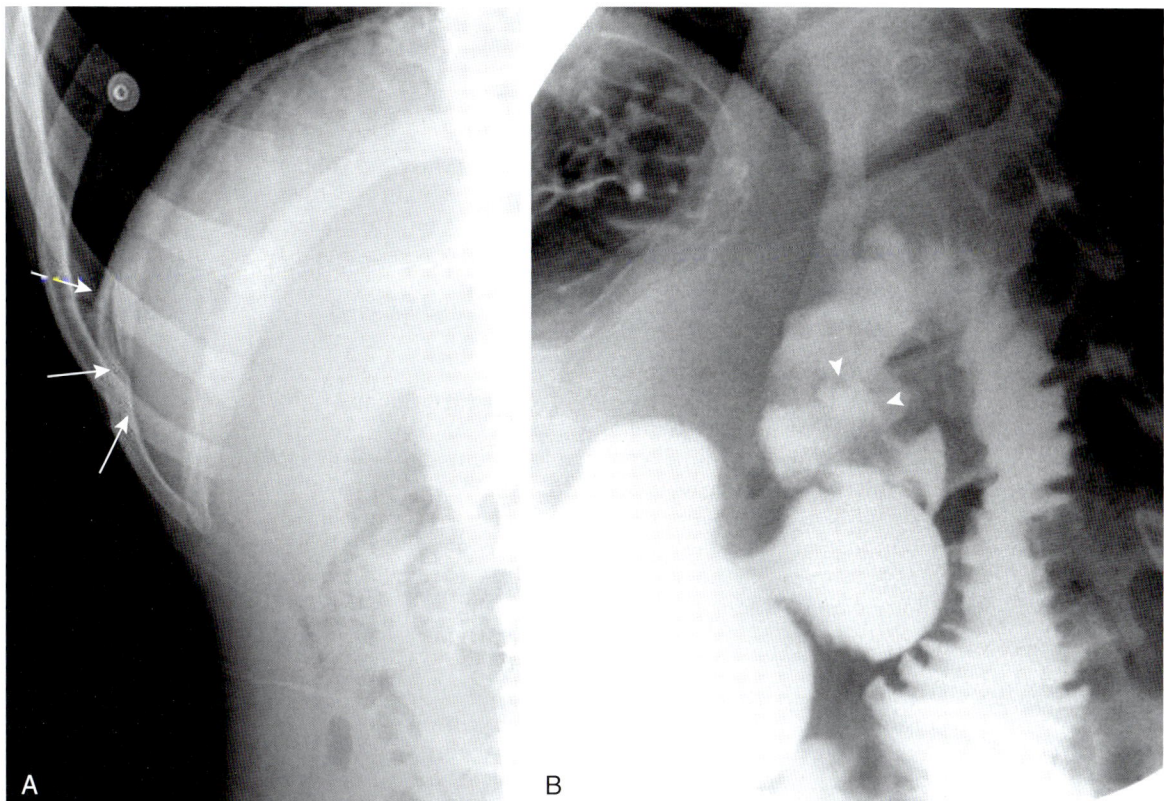

Figure 104-5 A duodenal ulcer. **A,** A left lateral decubitus radiograph in a boy with a 1-week history of abdominal pain demonstrates pneumoperitoneum lateral to the liver (*arrows*). **B,** A spot image of the duodenal bulb from an upper gastrointestinal (UGI) examination with water-soluble contrast material for the same patient shown in part **A** reveals a collection of contrast in the ulcer crater (*arrowheads*). (**B,** Courtesy Dr. Tamar Ben-Ami, Chicago, IL.)

of perforation, periduodenal fluid and retroperitoneal and intraperitoneal free air may be identified[24] (Fig. 104-6).

Treatment Although the initial reports by Marshall and Warren indicated that the pyloric *Campylobacter* organisms were sensitive to multiple antibiotics,[54] not all current strains demonstrate similar wide susceptibility. Eradication of *H. pylori* in symptomatic patients requires triple therapy with a proton pump inhibitor and two antibiotics for a 2-week treatment course.[50]

ZOLLINGER-ELLISON SYNDROME

Overview The Zollinger-Ellison syndrome refers to autonomous oversecretion of the hormone gastrin by a gastrinoma, resulting in unusually severe and refractory ulcer disease, typically accompanied by diarrhea. The condition is rare, with an incidence quoted as one to three new cases per million population.[55] Gastrinomas and the Zollinger-Ellison syndrome can occur sporadically or, in approximately 15% to 38% of cases, as part of the multiple endocrine neoplasia type

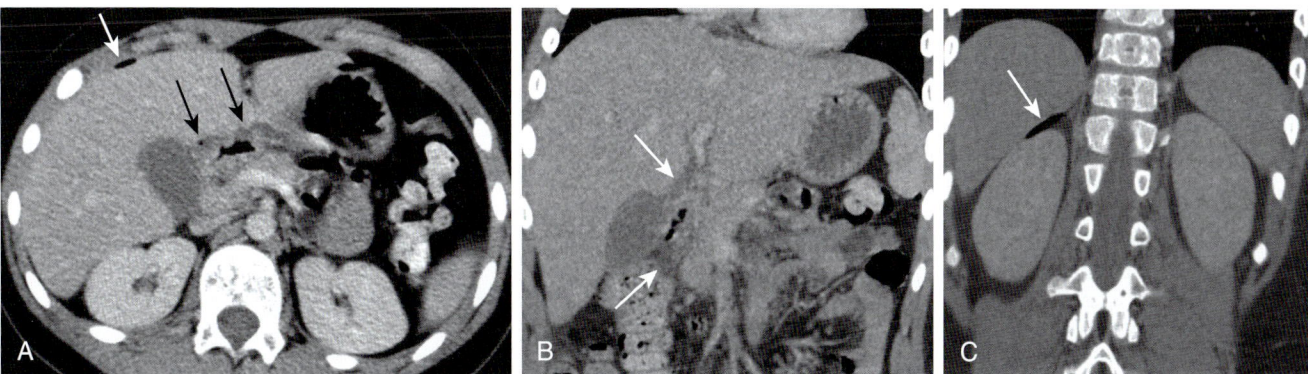

Figure 104-6 A perforated duodenal ulcer. **A,** A computed tomography scan in a 9-year-old boy with a 2-day history of abdominal pain, fever, and decreased activity shows thickening of the duodenum, with a small amount of periduodenal fluid and air (*black arrows*), and free air anterior to the liver (*white arrow*). **B,** A coronal reformatted image again shows thickening of the duodenum and periduodenal fluid (*arrows*). **C,** A more posterior coronal reformatted image shows additional free air (*arrow*) superior to the right kidney.

1 (MEN-1) syndrome[55-57]; conversely, the Zollinger-Ellison syndrome occurs in approximately 21% to 70% of patients with MEN-1.

The Zollinger-Ellison syndrome is typically diagnosed in the fifth decade, with approximately 90% of cases presenting between the ages of 20 and 60 years.[57] Approximately 8.6% occur in children, about four times more commonly in boys, and typically no earlier than the second decade, with the youngest case reported in a 5-year-old girl.[56,58,59] The syndrome tends to present at a younger age when it is part of the MEN-1 syndrome.

Most gastrinomas are located in the wall of the duodenum or in the head of the pancreas, but they also can be located in more distant regions, including the heart, ovary, kidneys, and mesentery. Tumors can be both small and multiple, presenting a challenge to diagnosis.[60-62] However, most gastrinomas occur in the so-called gastrinoma triangle, which is located to the right of the SMA and bounded superiorly by the confluence of the cystic and common bile ducts, the junction of the second and third portions of the duodenum inferiorly, and medially by the junction of the head and body of the pancreas.[60,63]

Etiology   The etiology of the syndrome is the autonomous neoplastic overproduction of gastrin, resulting in acid hypersecretion and extensive ulcer disease. The cause of sporadic gastrin-secreting tumors is not known; however, MEN-1 is the result of an autosomal-dominant mutation in the 10 exon tumor suppressor gene *MEN-1*, encoding the 610 amino acid protein MENIN. Parathyroid hyperplasia, pancreatic endocrine tumors (of which gastrinoma is the most common), pituitary adenomas, and adrenal adenomas occur in this syndrome. Patients also are prone to the development of carcinoid tumors, gastric, thymic, and bronchial lesions, lipomas, and skin lesions, including melanomas.[57]

Clinical Presentation   Patients may present with a triad of abdominal pain, weight loss, and diarrhea in conjunction with ulcer disease, which typically is negative for *H. pylori*. This constellation of symptoms is highly suggestive of Zollinger-Ellison syndrome. Patients also may present with hematemesis, tarry stools, and anemia. Patients with gastrinoma and Zollinger-Ellison syndrome should undergo further investigation for MEN-1.[57,58] Some patients with MEN-1 may present initially with evidence of hyperparathyroidism, such as urolithiasis; manifestation of gastrinoma may follow, sometimes up to 25 years later.[64] Approximately 60% of gastrinomas are malignant, and 50% have metastasized at diagnosis.[60,65]

The primary ulcer site is the duodenum, and ulcers can occur in the distal duodenum as well as the jejunum, sites that should raise concern for gastrinoma. In a pediatric series of patients with Zollinger-Ellison syndrome, the primary ulcer site was the duodenum in 72% and the jejunum in 28%.[58]

Successful initial treatment with proton pump inhibitors may delay the diagnosis by assuaging the symptoms.[55,57] The diagnosis is made by demonstration of hypersecretion of gastrin, determined by measurement of fasting gastrin levels and acid secretion. However, in patients who are treated with proton pump inhibitors, fasting serum gastrin levels may be sufficiently elevated to overlap with those seen in patients with Zollinger-Ellison syndrome[57]; in such cases, proton

pump inhibitors should be withdrawn for approximately 1 week before repeating the test.[55] In addition to fasting gastrin levels, provocative tests also are used, utilizing secretin, calcium, and meal stimulation.[57]

Imaging   The classic finding on upper GI examination is the presence of ulcers in the duodenum, particularly the distal duodenum, or in the jejunum, as well as thickening of duodenal and gastric folds.[57] Ulcer disease is now more often evaluated endoscopically; up to 94% of patients with Zollinger-Ellison syndrome are reported to have thickened gastric folds.[55]

Ultrasonography has not been found to be sensitive in detecting gastrinomas either inside or outside the liver and pancreas, showing a sensitivity of approximately 19%.[65] With CT, identification of hypervascular pancreatic gastrinomas is optimized with the rapid bolus technique, with thin collimation and reformatted images. With 10-mm collimation, CT has a sensitivity of 38%,[65] although much better performance could reasonably be expected with today's rapid scanners and thin collimation. With MRI, detection is optimized by a high field strength magnet, water-sensitive sequences, and administration of contrast material; MR sensitivity is quoted as 45%.[65] On the other hand, somatostatin receptor scintigraphy using [^{111}In-DTPA-DPhe^1] octreotide was found to be 70% sensitive in the detection of the tumors.[57,65] In a later publication of 151 patients with gastrinomas,[61] diagnostic sensitivity of imaging was similar: 24% for ultrasound, 39% for CT, 46% for MRI, and 79% for somatostatin-receptor scintigraphy. In approximately one third of patients, all imaging studies are negative.[61] Imamura has described a venous sampling technique that is helpful in detecting more than 90% of gastrinomas that are <5 mm. The technique involves venous sampling after selective arterial injection of secretin or calcium to elicit gastrin release from the gastrinoma, termed the selective arterial secretagogue injection test (SASI).[62,66]

Treatment   Control of hyperacidity is one of the key elements in survival.[57,67] At one time, control of hyperacidity was achieved with gastrectomy; today, acid suppression is achieved medically with proton pump inhibitors. Thus the management of patients is geared toward treatment of the gastrinoma itself and other manifestations of the MEN-1 syndrome if it is present. Although most gastrinomas demonstrate slow growth, 25% show more rapid growth, and approximately 60% to 90% demonstrate malignant behavior.[61] In a study of 151 patients, more than half of the patients with sporadic gastrinomas were free of disease after surgery, and most of these patients were able to achieve a long-term cure; this approach is preferred in patients with sporadic gastrinoma.[61] In patients with MEN-1 and gastrinoma, some authors advocate a pancreas-preserving total duodenectomy to achieve a cure in some of the patients.[62]

INFLAMMATORY BOWEL DISEASE

Overview   Crohn disease most commonly involves the distal small bowel and colon and will be discussed in Chapters 105 and 107.

Although involvement of the duodenum with Crohn disease is nearly universally accompanied by ileal or ileocolic disease,[68,69] there is a wide difference in the reported percentage of patients with Crohn disease who have duodenal involvement, with increasing prevalence in more recent reports.[70] This finding is likely related to the more frequent use of endoscopy for the diagnosis, along with the fact that a large percentage of patients with endoscopic and histologic disease do not have clinical symptoms separable from those of the more distal involvement.[69,71,72] The duodenum is the most frequently affected segment in both pediatric and adult patients with upper tract Crohn disease.[72]

Etiology The etiology of Crohn disease remains unknown, although a genetic predisposition is underscored by familial occurrence and concordance of the disease in monozygotic twins (44% to 58%).[73] Other factors that affect the development of the disease include immune dysfunction, gut flora, and environmental factors such as active or passive cigarette smoking, appendectomy, diet, perinatal infections, and measles infection.[73]

Clinical Presentation Patients with duodenal involvement tend to present at a younger age than do patients with distal involvement,[74] typically with nonspecific abdominal pain and general malaise and weight loss.[75]

Complications related to duodenal involvement include involvement of the ampullary region of the duodenum, leading to biliary and pancreatic obstruction.[76] Pancreatitis may occur, although it is attributed to other causes such as medications used to treat the primary disease.[77] Fistula formation also occurs, although it is believed that fistulas between the duodenum and small bowel or colon usually originate in the latter, rather than in the duodenum.[69]

Imaging Just as the diagnosis of Crohn disease has shifted from radiography to endoscopy, the imaging modalities have shifted from radiography to cross-sectional imaging, including ultrasound with color or power Doppler, CT, and MRI. However, if upper GI examination is requested in a patient with abdominal pain and weight loss, the diagnostic findings should be appreciated.

The typical imaging findings on upper GI examination in patients with Crohn disease are similar to those found in the distal bowel. Double-contrast studies are more sensitive than single-contrast examinations in identifying the aphthous lesions that characterize the early stages of the disease. These lesions typically will be found in the antrum, pylorus, and duodenum. Duodenal fold thickening, luminal narrowing, wall thickening, and fistula and sinus tract formation are also findings seen at upper GI examination (Fig. 104-7).

Ultrasound is able to detect bowel wall thickening, and Doppler is able to detect the hyperemia characteristic of active Crohn disease, similar to terminal ileal disease.[78-81]

CT is helpful in identifying involved bowel segments and surrounding pathology, such as abscess and fistula formation, and is most helpful in patients who are acutely ill, patients with bowel obstruction, and other patients who are unable to tolerate MRI because of procedure length and other requirements such as sedation in younger patients. Duodenal findings include fold thickening, increased enhancement, and stricture formation.[24,53,82]

MR enterography is becoming the ideal modality in the routine imaging evaluation of patients with Crohn disease. The findings in the duodenum are similar to those in other bowel segments.[83,84]

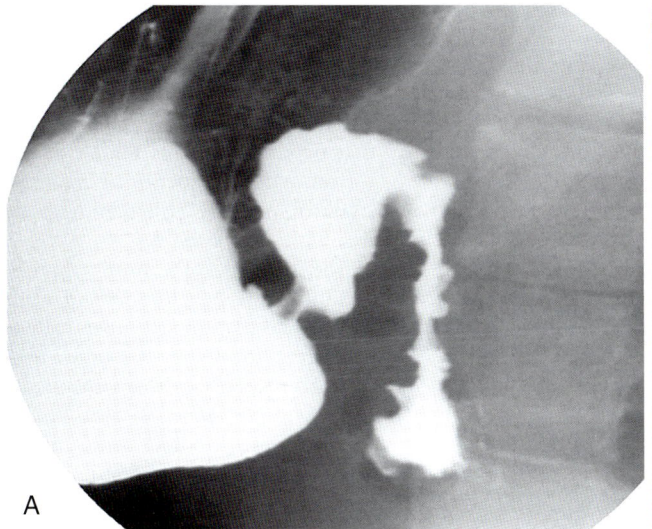

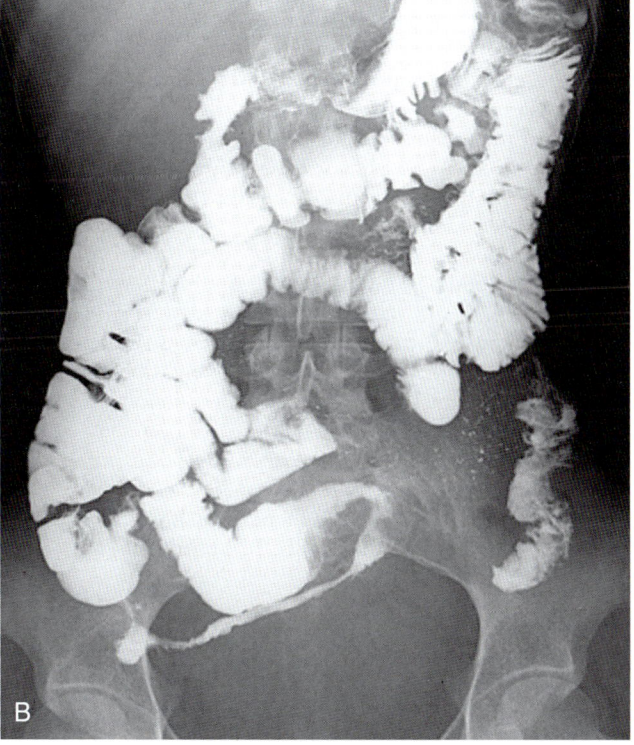

Figure 104-7 Crohn disease. **A,** A right anterior oblique upper gastrointestinal spot image demonstrates duodenal mucosal fold thickening. **B,** A small bowel follow-through again identifies the duodenal changes, as well as typical involvement of the terminal ileum with luminal narrowing and spiculation. (Courtesy Lakshmana Das Narla, Richmond, VA.)

Treatment Therapy for duodenal Crohn disease typically includes exclusion of *H. pylori*. Treatment then consists of proton pump inhibition to inhibit gastric secretion and promote ulcer healing, as well as corticosteroids. Azathioprine and 6-mercaptopurine are used to maintain remission. Strictures may be amenable to endoscopic balloon dilatation. Patients who do not respond to medical management, or in whom a massive gastrointestinal hemorrhage develops, may need surgical intervention.[69]

CYSTIC FIBROSIS

Overview Cystic fibrosis has multiple manifestations in the gastrointestinal tract; those affecting the small bowel and colon are covered in Chapters 103 and 105. Duodenal involvement includes duodenal fold thickening, ulceration, and stricture formation.[85]

Etiology Duodenal and gastric ulceration has been reported in as many as 10% of autopsy reports of pediatric patients with cystic fibrosis.[86] The etiology of these duodenal abnormalities is thought to be related to impaired secretion of bicarbonate by the duodenum and pancreas, which curtails the ability to buffer gastric acid.[87] Thickening of the duodenal folds is believed to be related to hyperacidity, abnormal mucus production, and hypertrophy of Brunner glands.[86] A hyperacid duodenal environment also leads to precipitation of bile salts and decreased fat absorption.

Inflammatory changes in the gut of patients with cystic fibrosis have been found through identification of T-cell activation products[88] and output of inflammatory proteins.[89] The etiology of inflammatory changes in the duodenal mucosa may include factors such as increased antigenic load as a result of pancreatic insufficiency, defective digestion of luminal contents,[88] and altered intestinal flora.[90]

Clinical Presentation Patients usually present with abdominal pain; hematemesis may occur if ulcer disease is present.[86] Patients also may manifest symptoms of severe gastroesophageal reflux, which is thought to be partly related to gastrointestinal dysmotility and the need for frequent postural drainage.[91]

Imaging The findings on upper GI examination typically demonstrate thick and coarse duodenal folds (e-Fig. 104-8), particularly along the first and second portions; ulceration[86]; or frank stricture formation.[85,87] Distortion and kinking of the duodenal contours at times simulates a mass lesion.[92]

Treatment Patients are treated with proton pump inhibitors or histamine-2 (H_2) receptor antagonists to decrease the acidity of the duodenal environment, which helps prevent ulceration and increases the ability to absorb fats and fat-soluble vitamins.[93,94]

Duodenal Neoplasms

Duodenal neoplasms are uncommon. The frequency of benign tumors of the small bowel at autopsy has been reported as being 0.16%, and of these, approximately 18% are located in the duodenum. Fewer than 2% of malignant gastrointestinal tumors arise in the small bowel.[95,96] Neoplasms that are characteristic to the duodenum include lesions related to Brunner glands, adenomas associated with polyposis syndromes, and duodenal carcinoid tumors. Brunner gland hyperplasia has been described as being of three types: diffuse through the duodenum; circumscribed and confined to its first portion; and Brunner gland adenoma, which refers to lesions larger than 1 cm.[95] Brunner gland hyperplasia and duodenal polyps may be seen in approximately 15.2% of uremic patients of all ages undergoing upper GI examination, compared with approximately 0.3% of nonuremic patients.[95]

Duodenal polyps are reported in approximately 0.4% of children undergoing upper endoscopy.[97] Most duodenal polyps not associated with Brunner glands are associated with polyposis syndromes. Familial adenomatous polyposis (FAP) is the most commonly associated systemic abnormality in patients with duodenal adenomatous polyps; conversely, adenomatous duodenal polyps occur in approximately 90% of patients with FAP.[96,97] In an endoscopic study of 24 pediatric patients with FAP, periampullary adenomas were found in 41%.[98] Children with Peutz-Jeghers syndrome develop hamartomatous polyps in the duodenum,[97] although adenomatous changes develop in 3% to 6% of hamartomas.[96] Brunner gland hypertrophy develops in patients with juvenile polyposis,[97] but cancers of the duodenum also have been reported in this population.[96]

Duodenal carcinoids are associated with the Zollinger-Ellison syndrome, particularly in association with MEN-1 (G-cell carcinoids, of which approximately one third manifest as Zollinger-Ellison syndrome) and with neurofibromatosis type 1 (D-cell carcinoids that produce somatostatin). Approximately two thirds of duodenal carcinoids are G-cell gastrin tumors, whereas somatostatin-producing D-cell tumors represent approximately one fifth of duodenal carcinoids, nearly exclusively located in the periampullary region.[99]

Etiology The hyperplasia of Brunner glands that occurs in uremic patients is thought to be related to elevated gastrin levels and hyperacidity that occur in patients with end-stage renal insufficiency.[95,100,101] Brunner gland adenomas are associated with chronic renal failure, chronic pancreatitis, peptic ulcer disease, and infection with *H. pylori*.[102]

Mutations that render the product of tumor suppressor genes ineffective are important in the development of malignancy. Patients with FAP have a mutation within the adenomatous polyposis coli (*APC*) gene located in the long arm of chromosome 5 at 5q21. Peutz-Jeghers has been mapped to the serine threonine kinase 11 (*STK*) gene on chromosome 19 p13.3. Genetic loci in separate kindred with juvenile polyposis have been reported in the *SMAD4* gene located on chromosome 18q21.1 and the *PTEN* gene on chromosome 10q23.

Clinical Manifestations Patients with Brunner gland hyperplasia typically are asymptomatic. When symptoms occur, patients tend to present with bleeding, obstruction, pain, vomiting, and diarrhea.[95] Large lesions such as Brunner gland adenoma can present with gastric outlet obstruction, biliary obstruction, and pancreatitis when affecting the periampullary region.[102]

Duodenal carcinoids may manifest as Zollinger-Ellison syndrome. However, D-cell somatostatin-producing tumors

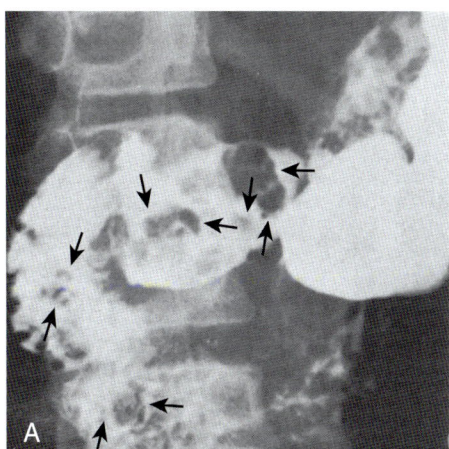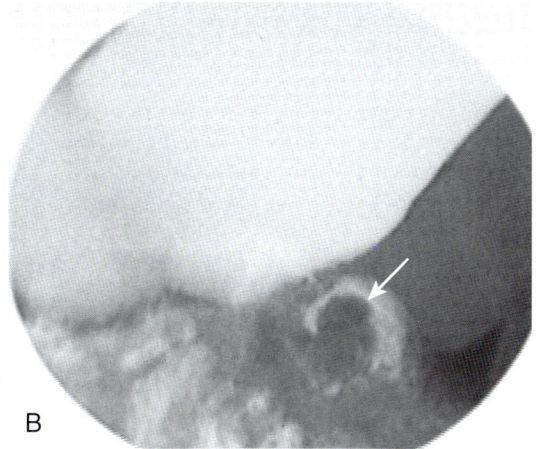

Figure 104-10 Peutz-Jeghers syndrome with duodenal polyps. **A,** Multiple polyps in the duodenum (*arrows*) in a 12-year-old boy with Peutz-Jeghers syndrome. He also had polyps in the stomach, colon, and the remainder of the small intestine. **B,** A 9-year-old boy with Peutz-Jeghers syndrome presenting with symptoms of intermittent obstruction. An upper gastrointestinal spot image of the proximal jejunum demonstrates a filling defect (*arrow*) due to duodenojejunal intussusception. A hamartomatous duodenal polyp was found to be the lead point at endoscopy. (Courtesy R. Paul Guillerman, Houston, TX.)

arising in the duodenum are usually too small to produce clinically apparent symptoms related to hormone overproduction; such symptoms are present in less than 10% of cases and typically include abdominal pain, diarrhea, steatorrhea, and weight loss. Unlike carcinoids occurring in other parts of the small bowel, those that occur in the duodenum are not associated with serotonin overproduction and thus do not produce symptoms of the carcinoid syndrome.[99]

Imaging On upper GI examination, a filling defect within the duodenal bulb may be demonstrated (e-Fig. 104-9). On ultrasound and CT, large or prolapsing lesions may present a confusing picture and be mistaken for a pancreatic mass, which can have significant surgical implications if the true nature and location of the lesion are not documented preoperatively. A giant Brunner gland adenoma may demonstrate gastric outlet obstruction on abdominal radiographs.[102] Multiple polyps, such as are seen in patients with FAP or Peutz-Jeghers syndromes, appear as multiple filling defects, at times complicated by intussusception (Fig. 104-10). Duodenal carcinoids have been described as intraluminal or mural filling defects, sometimes with ulcerations, and occasionally producing obstruction by intussusception; duodenal folds may be thickened in a small number of patients. On CT, duodenal carcinoids have been described as lesions with marked contrast enhancement in the arterial phase, decreased enhancement in later phases, and possible invasion into the adjacent pancreas. On MRI they have been described as having low signal on T1 weighting, with a heterogeneously high signal on water-sensitive sequences, and positive gadolinium enhancement.[99]

Treatment Brunner gland hyperplasia does not require specific treatment if the patient is asymptomatic. Conservative treatment consists of control of gastric acidity with proton pump antagonists and H₂ blockers. Brunner gland adenomas may be amenable to endoscopic removal, although larger or more diffuse lesions may require more extensive surgical polypectomy or segmental or more extensive duodenal resection.[102] Patients with FAP undergo periodic endoscopic

screening, even pediatric patients starting at the time of initial screening colonoscopy. In children, upper gastrointestinal symptoms are present in only a small number of patients and are not predictive of the presence of duodenal adenomas. Management of complicating periampullary adenocarcinoma includes pancreaticoduodenectomy. Endoscopic ampullectomy may be helpful in some patients with early lesions.[98]

Key Points

SMA syndrome is thought to be caused by an abnormally small angle and reduced distance between the aorta and the SMA. Predisposing conditions include Nissen fundoplication, cerebral palsy, traumatic brain injury, posterior spinal fusion, burns, lumbar hyperlordosis, and spinal traction/cast.

Causes of duodenal hematoma include nonaccidental trauma and other blunt injuries to the epigastrium, such as handlebar injuries, motor vehicle crashes, and sports injuries. An injury may precede signs of duodenal obstruction by several days after an assault or other traumatic event.

Duodenal intussusception is a relatively common complication of postpyloric GJ tubes, which act as a lead point.

Duodenal ulcer disease is associated with infection by *H. pylori*, which is estimated to colonize/infect approximately half the world's population.

Zollinger-Ellison syndrome refers to autonomous oversecretion of gastrin by a gastrinoma, resulting in unusually severe and refractory ulcer disease, accompanied by diarrhea. Approximately 15% to 38% of cases occur as part of MEN-1.

Continued

Duodenal involvement in patients with Crohn disease is identified more frequently with endoscopic evaluation.

Duodenal ulceration in patients with cystic fibrosis is related to impaired secretion of bicarbonate and increased acid production, producing an acidic duodenal environment.

Most pediatric duodenal polyps that are not associated with Brunner gland hyperplasia are associated with polyposis syndromes.

Duodenal carcinoids are associated with the Zollinger-Ellison syndrome but not with the carcinoid syndrome, because they do not produce serotonin.

Suggested Readings

Agrons GA, et al. Gastrointestinal manifestations of cystic fibrosis: radiologic-pathologic correlation. *Radiographics*. 1996;16(4):871-893.

Attard TM, Abraham SC, Cuffari C. The clinical spectrum of duodenal polyps in pediatrics. *J Pediatr Gastroenterol Nutr*. 2003;36(1):116-119.

Ellison EC, Johnson JA. The Zollinger-Ellison syndrome: a comprehensive review of historical, scientific, and clinical considerations. *Curr Probl Surg*. 2009;46(1):13-106.

Gaines BA, et al. Duodenal injuries in children: beware of child abuse. *J Pediatr Surg*. 2004;39(4):600-602.

Hughes UM, et al. Further report of small-bowel intussusceptions related to gastrojejunostomy tubes. *Pediatr Radiol*. 2000;30(9):614-617.

Kalach N, et al. Frequency and risk factors of gastric and duodenal ulcers or erosions in children: a prospective 1-month European multicenter study. *Eur J Gastroenterol Hepatol*. 2010;22(10):1174-1181.

Levy AD, et al. Duodenal carcinoids: imaging features with clinical-pathologic comparison. *Radiology*. 2005;237(3):967-972.

Long FR, et al. Duodenitis in children: correlation of radiologic findings with endoscopic and pathologic findings. *Radiology*. 1998;206(1):103-108.

Mashako MN, et al. Crohn's disease lesions in the upper gastrointestinal tract: correlation between clinical, radiological, endoscopic, and histological features in adolescents and children. *J Pediatr Gastroenterol Nutr*. 1989;8(4):442-446.

Merrett ND, et al. Superior mesenteric artery syndrome: diagnosis and treatment strategies. *J Gastrointest Surg*. 2009;13(2):287-292.

References

Full references for this chapter can be found on www.expertconsult.com.

Chapter 105

Acquired Lesions of the Small Intestines

GRACE S. PHILLIPS and SUMIT PRUTHI

This chapter discusses the various acquired entities that affect the pediatric jejunum and ileum. The entities discussed include small bowel obstruction (SBO) and pseudoobstruction, infections and inflammatory conditions, and functional, infiltrative, and neoplastic entities.

Small Bowel Obstruction

OVERVIEW

SBO as a result of acquired conditions may be due to intrinsic or extrinsic abnormalities and is relatively uncommon among the pediatric population, particularly in infants younger than 1 year, in whom congenital anomalies are far more common causes of obstruction. Some causes of acquired obstruction actually result from complications of congenital anomalies, such as herniation and incarceration of bowel through an inguinal hernia.

Abnormalities that mimic obstruction include *chronic intestinal pseudoobstruction* (CIPO), defined by a consensus group as a "rare, severe disabling disorder characterized by repetitive episodes or continuous symptoms and signs of bowel obstruction, including radiographic documentation of dilated bowel with air-fluid levels, in the absence of a fixed, lumen-occluding lesion."[1,2] Dilation of various parts of the gastrointestinal (GI) tract, including the small bowel, is characteristic of intestinal pseudoobstruction; these entities are further discussed in Chapter 106.

ETIOLOGY

The most common acquired causes of obstruction in children are adhesions, hernias, tumors, inflammatory bowel disease (IBD), and volvulus.

Adhesions

Adhesions are a common cause of obstruction in patients who have undergone prior abdominal surgery. Obstruction secondary to adhesions is more common in neonates, particularly after surgery for repair of abdominal wall defects such as gastroschisis. In older children, adhesive obstruction occurs most often after pelvic surgery, usually after appendectomy.[3] The postappendectomy incidence does not seem to be related to positive versus negative appendectomy, but some data suggest that it is decreased after a laparoscopic versus an open procedure.[4]

Incarcerated Hernia

Several types of hernias can lead to bowel obstruction in children, and overall they are responsible for approximately 10% of bowel obstructions.[3]

Inguinal hernias are a relatively common condition in children, with an overall incidence between 0.8% and 4.4%.[5] The vast majority of inguinal hernias in children are indirect hernias related to a patent processus vaginalis.[6] The incidence of inguinal hernia is 10 times higher in boys than in girls.[7] Inguinal hernias have both a higher incidence (~ 30%) and a higher risk of incarceration (31%) in premature infants.[8]

Other hernias that can lead to SBO include mesocolic (right or left paraduodenal) hernias (see Chapter 103) and herniation of bowel around an incompletely fixated falciform ligament.

Tumors

Tumors may cause bowel obstruction as extrinsic lesions or as intrinsic lesions, such as intussusception secondary to polyps or to lymphoma, typically Burkitt lymphoma. Tumors are further discussed at the end of this chapter.

Omphalomesenteric Duct Remnants

Omphalomesenteric remnants are the residua of the embryologic yolk stalk, and they become apparent in several ways, depending on the type of abnormality and ensuing complications (see also Chapter 103). Normally, the entire attachment regresses. The lumen may be obliterated, but a fibrous cord may persist, with or without cystic remnants within it. Attachment of the mid small intestine to the anterior abdominal wall via a persistent cord may lead to distal SBO in a manner similar to an adhesion; or the remnant may predispose to volvulus of a bowel loop about the fibrous cord.

Adynamic Ileus

Adynamic ileus can cause bowel distension and may mimic mechanical obstruction. Adynamic ileus occurs invariably following major abdominal operations, and if prolonged, it may be difficult to differentiate from an early postoperative or recurrent obstruction.[3] In addition, adynamic ileus may also occur in the setting of burns, trauma, and certain medications. The pathophysiology of postoperative ileus remains incompletely understood, but the disruption of the normal autonomic gastrointestinal (GI) motility is multifactorial and related to pharmacologic, inflammatory, hormonal, metabolic, and neuropsychologic influences.[9]

CLINICAL PRESENTATION

The degree of abdominal distension depends on the level of obstruction; more distal levels are associated with greater distension. SBO in children usually presents with persistent bilious vomiting and abdominal pain.[10] Infants and young children may also come to medical attention with irritability and refusal to eat. The presence of fever is concerning for ischemia and bowel compromise, particularly if accompanied by unremitting pain unresponsive to proximal decompression.

IMAGING

Patients with long-standing complete obstruction will demonstrate dilated loops of bowel with differential air-fluid levels on horizontal-beam images and absence of stool and gas in the colon (Fig. 105-1, A and B). In partial obstruction, gas and stool may be present in the colon; however, a caliber difference between proximal loops of dilated bowel and bowel distal to the obstruction should remain evident.

Conventional radiographs may reveal the level of obstruction, but in many cases, they may show less specific changes of incomplete obstruction or adynamic ileus. The level and, at times, the cause of obstruction may be more readily demonstrated on CT. Small bowel follow-through (SBFT) may also be done, more often in young infants.

Although adynamic ileus can simulate mechanical obstruction on plain radiographs, some signs, if present, are useful in distinguishing the two entities. Supine radiographs of the abdomen show dilated loops of bowel in both conditions; however, mechanical obstruction usually causes proximal dilation with reduced caliber of the distal bowel, whereas adynamic ileus typically causes uniform dilatation of the entire small and large bowel. In neonates, it is not possible to differentiate small and large bowel; in those cases, a prone cross-table lateral view of the rectum can be very helpful in assessing the caliber of the distal bowel when obstruction is suspected. Supine views are much less helpful, because the rectum may not be visible as a result of proximal obstruction, or it may be filled with fluid that layers dependently within the posterior rectum.

Decubitus views are frequently more successful in revealing the scattered air-fluid levels of adynamic ileus than are upright images, and they are of course more helpful in neonates and infants, who are unable to stand. Decubitus views are also important in evaluating for free intraperitoneal air.

CT can be helpful in revealing the level and occasionally the cause of the obstruction. Administration of oral contrast is not always necessary (see Fig. 105-1, C), and only water-soluble agents should be administered if bowel perforation is a potential complication. CT may be particularly helpful in the diagnosis of a closed-loop obstruction and obstruction related to adhesions, with dilated bowel loops seen proximally and collapsed bowel distal to the point of obstruction. The level of obstruction may also be demonstrated by SBFT.

The diagnosis of an incarcerated hernia is typically established by history and physical exam, although radiographs (Fig. 105-2) or ultrasound may occasionally be used to confirm the diagnosis.

TREATMENT

The treatment for obstruction depends on its cause, but treatment is often surgical. Patients with partial obstruction who lack fever, leukocytosis, or unremitting pain can be observed with bowel decompression; in postadhesive obstruction, this treatment is successful in the majority of cases. However, patients with evidence of complete obstruction, fever, leukocytosis, and unremitting pain require prompt surgical intervention.[11]

In the absence of peritoneal signs, the treatment of choice for an incarcerated inguinal hernia is manual reduction, which has a success rate of 80%, followed by repair 24 to 48 hours after reduction.[7] Surgical repair is also typically suggested for umbilical hernias that persist in children older than 4 years of age because of the increasing risk of incarceration with age.[12]

Treatment of postoperative ileus has traditionally consisted of bowel rest and decompression via nasogastric tube. More recently, investigators have advocated early enteral nutrition; nonsteroidal antiinflammatory drugs to decrease inflammation; minimally invasive surgical techniques, such as laparoscopy when feasible; and minimization of narcotic use for control of postoperative pain.[9]

The treatment of CIPO depends on the underlying cause and may include prokinetics; surgery in the form of

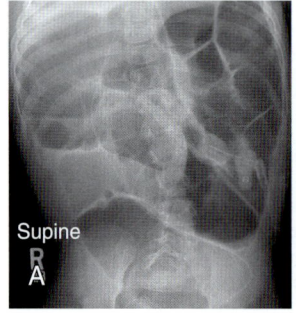
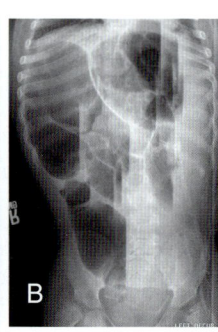
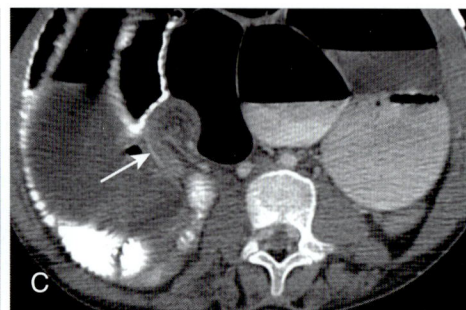

Figure 105-1 Small-bowel obstruction caused by adhesions. **A,** Supine radiograph of the abdomen in an 8-year-old boy with a history of multiple abdominal operations and increasing abdominal distension shows dilated, gas-filled loops of bowel. **B,** Horizontal-beam left lateral decubitus image demonstrates multiple differential air-fluid levels. **C,** Axial computed tomography image shows a transition zone (*arrow*) between dilated proximal bowel loops and collapsed distal bowel loops. Adhesions resulting in a small-bowel obstruction were lysed at surgery.

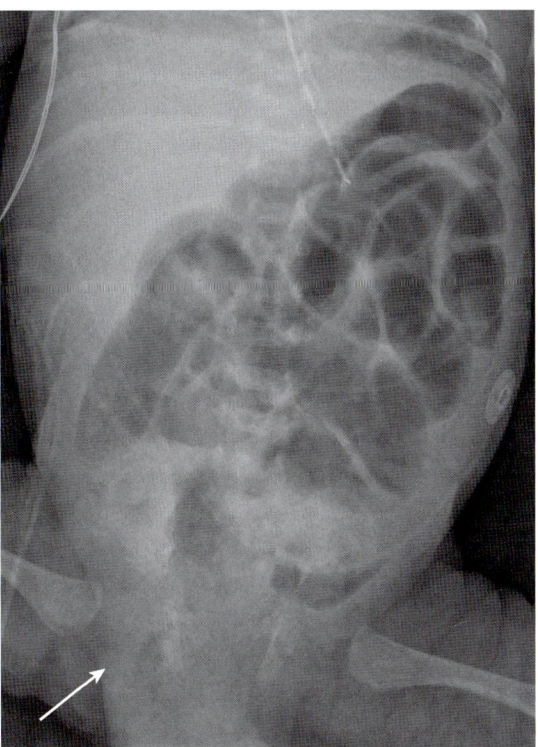

Figure 105-2 Small-bowel obstruction caused by inguinal hernia. Supine radiograph of the abdomen in a 1-month-old boy, former 26-week gestational age, who presented with a distended abdomen and a right inguinal hernia demonstrates dilated, gas-filled loops of bowel. Bowel gas is seen within the right inguinal hernia (*arrow*). Obstructive symptoms improved after manual reduction of the hernia.

gastrostomy, jejunostomy, and/or loop enterostomy; and total parenteral nutrition (TPN).[2] Intestinal transplantation may be considered in patients with life-threatening complications from TPN.

Inflammatory Conditions of the Small Bowel

INFECTIOUS DISEASES

Overview

Infectious diarrhea is a major source of childhood mortality and accounts for approximately 2.5 million deaths per year worldwide.[13] Viruses, bacteria, and parasites are potential causative agents of acute gastroenteritis in children, and viruses are the most common cause of pediatric intestinal infection in the United States.[14]

Etiology

Viral Infection

Gastroenteritis secondary to viral agents is one of the most common causes of *acute infectious diarrhea,* defined as acute onset of at least three loose stools per day.[15] In the United States, viral gastroenteritis is most common secondary to rotavirus, adenovirus, and norovirus (*Caliciviridae*).[15,16]

Bacterial Infection

Bacterial pathogens are estimated to cause between 2% and 10% of infectious diarrhea cases in developed countries.[16-18] *Shigella, Salmonella, Escherichia coli,* and *Campylobacter* are the most commonly identified bacterial agents in the United States.[16] Infections with *Yersinia enterocolitica, Vibrio* species, *Aeromonas,* and *Plesiomonas* are more commonly found in patients in developing countries.[16] *Clostridium difficile* can be isolated from the intestine of up to 50% of normal neonates, and this rate decreases to less than 5% by 2 years of age.[16] Illness-associated *C. difficile* infection is often associated with decreases in other intestinal flora secondary to exposure to broad-spectrum antibiotics, such as penicillin, clindamycin, and cephalosporins; this results in antimicrobial-associated diarrhea or pseudomembranous colitis.[16]

Parasitic Infection

The most common intestinal parasites in the United States are *Giardia lamblia* and *Cryptosporidium*.[16] Although humans are the major reservoir of infection, *Giardia* can infect domesticated animals, such as dogs and cats, and fecal-oral transmission occurs through contaminated water or food. *Cryptosporidium* may be spread by person-to-person transmission or through contaminated water, such as in swimming pools. People may also be infected through livestock, birds, and reptiles.

Helminths, or parasitic worms, include the nematodes or roundworms—ascarids, hookworms, and pinworms—and also the *Platyhelminthes,* or flatworms, such as schistosomes and tapeworms. One or more of these parasitic agents are estimated to infect approximately one third of the impoverished populations of developing countries.[19] Among these, children and adolescents tend to harbor the largest helminthic loads, which leads to both physical and cognitive impairment in this vulnerable population.[19]

Human Immunodeficiency Virus (HIV)

Approximately 2.5 million children are infected with HIV worldwide, often in conjunction with other endemic conditions, such as malaria and helminthic infection.[19,20] Although antiretroviral therapy has decreased the prevalence of vertical mother-to-child transmission and perinatal HIV in developing countries, approximately 420,000 children are still infected annually, primarily through mother-to-child transmission.[20]

Clinical Presentation

Viral Infection

Viral gastroenteritis commonly manifests with vomiting followed by severe watery diarrhea, nausea, abdominal pain, headaches, and low-grade fever.[21] Associated upper respiratory symptoms are common and may precede the GI presentation.

Bacterial Infection

Considerable overlap occurs in clinical symptoms of viral and bacterial enteritis. However, high fever, shaking chills, and bloody stools are more commonly seen with bacterial enteritis than with viral gastroenteritis.[16] Diagnosis may be established by the presence of stool leukocytes and positive stool culture.

Parasitic Infection

Clinical symptoms after *Giardia* infection are variable, and some patients may be asymptomatic. Children may have foul-smelling diarrhea with flatulence, abdominal distension, and anorexia.[16] Diagnosis may be established by microscopic smear examination or immunofluorescence antibody testing of stools.

Cryptosporidium infection is usually self-limited in the immunocompetent child and may be asymptomatic or may be confused with viral gastroenteritis. Common symptoms include diarrhea, fever, and emesis.[22] In immunocompromised patients, including those with HIV, the infection may have a protracted course with severe, chronic diarrhea and subsequent malnutrition and dehydration, which may result in death.[16,22]

Human Immunodeficiency Virus

Persistent diarrhea from a variety of pathogens may be a presenting symptom of HIV. Enteritis may be caused by the viruses, bacteria, and parasites described above. In addition, the child with HIV may be susceptible to opportunistic infections such as cytomegalovirus, *Mycobacterium avium-intracellulare,* and fungi, especially *Candida albicans.*[20] HIV enteropathy can also occur as a direct effect on the bowel and is manifested as a diarrheal disease, with an incidence estimated to be between 30% and 40%. This is considered a diagnosis of exclusion, after other infectious and noninfectious causes are excluded.[23]

Imaging

Imaging studies are not generally indicated for diagnosis of infectious diarrhea in children. However, symptoms may sometimes mimic abdominal conditions, such as appendicitis or intussusception, and abdominal radiographs are occasionally requested to exclude other potential causes of the patient's symptoms. Depending on the time course and the degree of motility disturbance, nonobstructive dilation of bowel loops may occur. The most common radiographic findings are fluid-filled loops of distended bowel with multiple scattered air-fluid levels on horizontal-beam radiography, in contrast to differential air-fluid levels characteristic of obstruction. Absence of stool throughout the colon is commonly seen, along with air-fluid levels in the rectum. Pneumatosis intestinalis may rarely be seen.[24]

Cross-sectional imaging is not indicated in patients with clinically obvious gastroenteritis, but it is sometimes requested when other entities are being considered. US or CT may demonstrate small-bowel wall thickening, fluid-filled distended bowel loops (e-Fig. 105-3),[25,26] and intraabdominal and retroperitoneal lymphadenopathy.[27] Real time US may reveal transient small-bowel intussusception during periods of hyperperistalsis.

The terminal ileum and the cecum are often involved in bacterial enteritis, such as with *Yersinia*; this may be termed *infectious ileocecitis*. On imaging, inflammatory changes such as bowel wall thickening are typically apparent (Fig. 105-4). Involvement of the more distal colon may be variable. Right lower quadrant lymphadenopathy may also be seen.[21,28]

If contrast studies are performed in children with parasitic enterocolitis, they may show dilution of barium from fluid retention, minimal thickening of mucosal folds, and rapid or delayed transit time, depending on the chronicity of the disease. Disordered peristalsis is commonly seen. Certain specific findings can be seen, depending upon the underlying causative organism. On barium studies, *Giardia* produces thickened mucosal folds in the duodenum and jejunum that are associated with rapid transit time and dilution of contrast material (e-Fig. 105-5).[29]

Among the helminthic organisms, *Ascaris lumbricoides* causes the most striking and specific radiographic abnormalities. The disease results from swallowed larvae that grow into adult worms within the intestinal tract. Barium studies outline the organisms, which may appear singly or in clumps. The live worms may ingest barium, permitting visualization of their intestinal tracts.

Nonspecific edema of the affected intestine is the most frequently found abnormality on barium studies in patients with HIV enteropathy. Effacement of the mucosal pattern is common,[27] especially with *Cryptosporidium* infection.

Treatment

Treatment is dependent upon the underlying causative agent. Viral gastroenteritis is typically a self-limited condition. Oral and intravenous (IV) rehydration therapies are effective supportive interventions in cases of infectious diarrhea, particularly with viral infections. The treatment of bacterial enterocolitis also includes supportive therapy. Antimicrobial therapy is not always necessary for certain pathogens, such as *Salmonella*, although even in those cases, it may be needed, depending on the underlying immunocompetence of the host. Agents such as metronidazole and nitazoxanide are active against *Giardia* and *Cryptosporidium*, respectively. The pharmacopeia available for treatment of helminthic infections is relatively limited, particularly when considering the global ubiquity of these infections, and it includes diethylcarbamazine and newer agents such as albendazole and praziquantel.[16,19,22]

Inflammatory Bowel Disease

IBD comprises two major disorders: Crohn disease and ulcerative colitis. Crohn disease can involve any part of the GI tract, whereas ulcerative colitis only affects the colon and is discussed in Chapter 107.

CROHN DISEASE

Overview

The peak incidence of Crohn disease is in young adulthood, but 25% of patients come to medical attention during childhood or adolescence.[30] Crohn disease is characterized by segmental transmural granulomatous inflammation of the intestine. The mucosal layer is extensively destroyed, and ulcers are usually present. The intestinal lumen is often

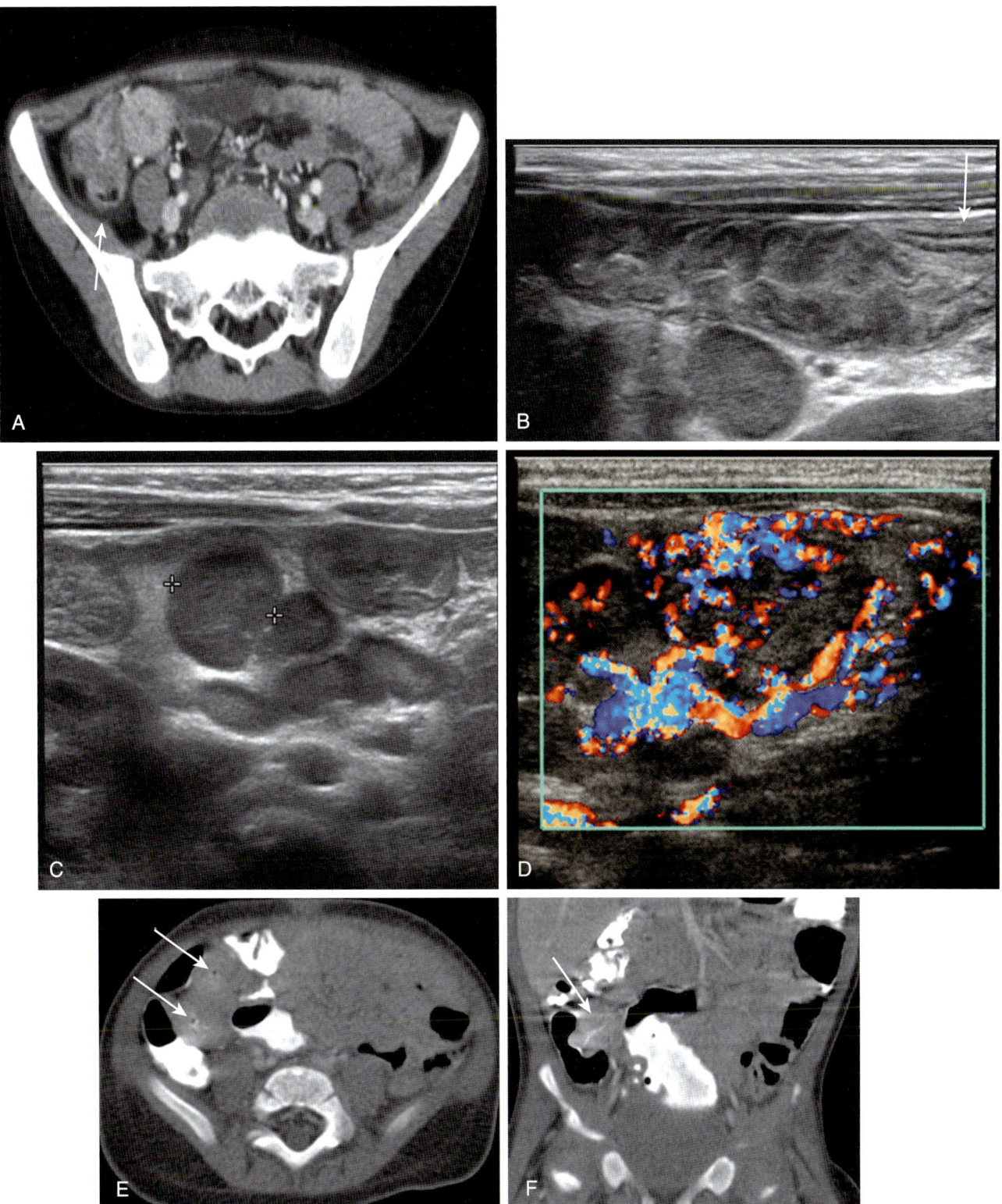

Figure 105-4 Bacterial enterocolitis. **A,** *Shigella* enteritis. Contrast-enhanced computed tomography (CT) reveals concentric thickening and enhancement of the terminal ileum and cecum, along with a small amount of pericecal fluid (*arrow*). *Shigella sonnei* was cultured from the stool. **B,** For a 5-month-old with mucous diarrhea and abdominal pain, ultrasound was requested to assess for suspected intussusception. A transverse sonogram of the right lower quadrant shows a markedly thickened terminal ileum, along with a visible transition to normal bowel (*arrow*) more proximally. A large lymph node is seen deep to the terminal ileum. **C,** Transverse image in same infant as shown in *B,* obtained slightly more cephalad, reveals a large nodal aggregate medial to the ascending colon and anterior to the lower pole of the right kidney (*calipers* outline one of the nodes). **D,** Color Doppler image in the same infant shows marked hyperemia in the thick-walled terminal ileum and in the surrounding mesentery and lymph nodes. **E,** *Yersinia* enteritis. CT in a 9-month-old boy who had a 10 day history of fever, emesis, and voluminous diarrhea demonstrates pronounced thickening and luminal narrowing of the terminal ileum (*arrows*). **F,** Coronal reformat of the CT scan in same patient as shown in *E* demonstrates similar findings. Stool cultures were positive for *Yersinia enterocolitica.*

narrowed by spasm and by edematous and fibrotic thickening of the wall. The small bowel is involved in approximately 80% of cases, and isolated small-bowel disease, without colonic involvement, occurs in approximately 30% to 40% of patients.[31] The terminal ileum is most frequently involved, but the disease has been described anywhere along the GI tract, from the mouth to the anus, and may occur without terminal ileal involvement.[32,33] In children, the terminal ileum is involved in 50% to 70% of cases, and 10% to 15% have diffuse small-bowel disease.[34]

Etiology

The exact cause of Crohn disease remains unknown, but recent work suggests that failure of intestinal immune homeostasis, with inflammatory mediators directed against gut flora, may be implicated, along with an underlying genetic susceptibility.[35] The *NOD2* (formerly *CARD 15*) gene, located on chromosome 16, regulates the immune response to bacterial products and is abnormal in 20% to 30% of pediatric patients with Crohn disease.[34] T-cell activation and increased activity of proinflammatory cytokines—such as interleukins (IL) 1, 6, and 12—with decreased antiinflammatory cytokines, such as IL-4 and IL-10, are found in the mucosa of patients with Crohn disease.[34,36] Approximately 30% of affected individuals have a positive family history, and there is a 50% concordance between monozygotic twins.[35]

Clinical Presentation

Clinical presentation and severity of disease manifestations are highly variable. Most children with Crohn disease come to medical attention with insidious onset of GI symptoms, including diarrhea, abdominal pain, anorexia, and weight loss with growth retardation at times preceding other abdominal symptoms by months or years.[34] Other clinical findings include abdominal mass, pain, and perianal fistula. Some patients have symptoms that manifest acutely with right lower quadrant pain and fever, mimicking appendicitis. Crohn disease in pediatric patients may be more severe at presentation and may demonstrate a more complicated course than

in adult patients.[35] Extraintestinal manifestations may accompany or precede GI symptoms and include fever, aphthous stomatitis, arthralgias, arthritis, sacroiliitis, erythema nodosum, and digital clubbing. Arthritis is the most common extraintestinal condition in the pediatric population.[34]

The diagnosis of Crohn disease may be suggested by history and clinical exam and is further supported by radiologic exams and endoscopic and histopathologic correlative data. Endoscopic examination with biopsy is an essential step in confirming the diagnosis, excluding other entities, and differentiating between Crohn disease and ulcerative colitis in the 20% of patients with exclusively colonic involvement.[31] Capsule endoscopy is a more recent but well-established technique to assess the small bowel in Crohn disease, particularly in patients whose disease is inaccessible to routine endoscopic procedures.

Imaging

The main role of imaging in patients with Crohn disease is to detect the areas of involvement and further segregate disease into inflammatory, obstructive, and fistulizing disease and to assess response to therapy.

Abdominal radiographs in patients with IBD may be normal. However, the most common finding is absence of stool in the involved portions of the colon.[37] During an acute disease exacerbation, abdominal radiographs are more likely to show abnormalities such as ileus, bowel wall thickening, or obstruction.

Upper GI examinations with SBFT have been frequently used to evaluate jejunoileal manifestations of Crohn disease. One of the earliest changes seen on contrast radiographic examinations is the formation of aphthous ulcers, which are present in both small bowel and colon; these represent shallow erosions surrounded by a radiolucent halos that represent edema. Other findings include nodular irregularity with linear and transverse ulceration. Extensive ulceration can lead to a spiculated or "rose thorn" appearance, which results from deep ulcers that extend into the thickened bowel wall (Fig. 105-6). The intersection of multiple linear and transverse ulcers leads to a cobblestone appearance, also

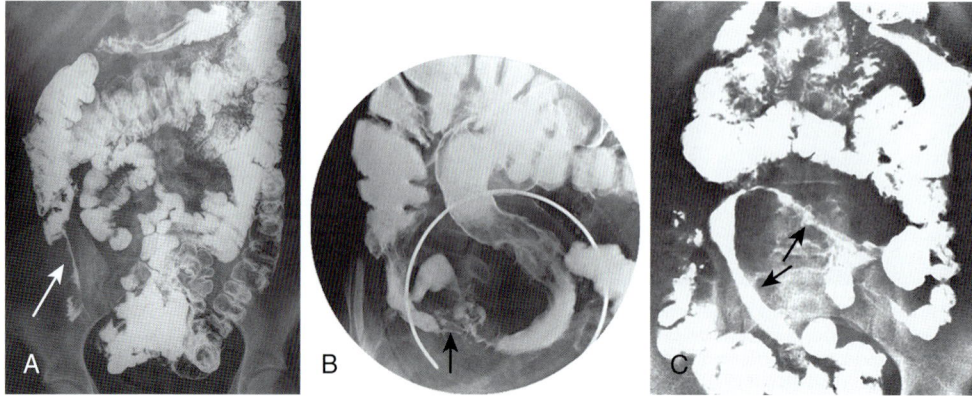

Figure 105-6   Crohn disease. A, Frontal abdominal radiograph from small bowel follow-through in a 17-year-old girl with a history of worsening abdominal pain, fever, fatigue, and decreased appetite shows pronounced luminal narrowing of the terminal ileum (*arrow*) with a "string sign," which indicates a markedly narrowed segment. Displacement of adjacent bowel loops is evident. **B,** Spot film of terminal ileum in an adolescent with Crohn disease. Examination reveals extensive involvement and ulceration of the terminal ileum with a "rose thorn" appearance and spasm. Involvement of the cecum is also apparent, and the appendix is incidentally noted at the cecal tip (*arrow*). **C,** Small bowel series in a 14-year-old girl reveals a markedly narrowed and rigid loop of mid small bowel (*arrows*). The upper arrow points to a "string sign."

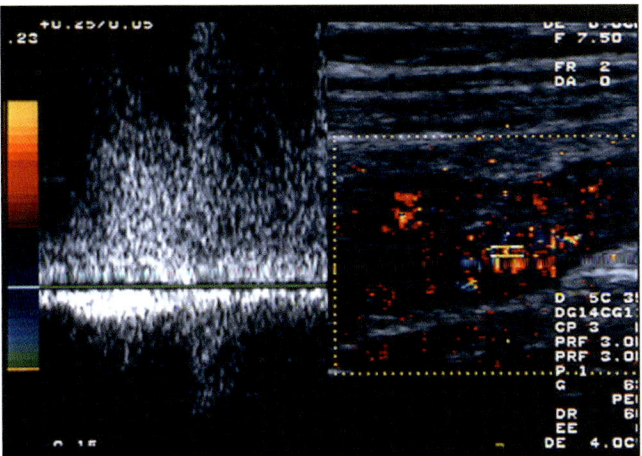

Figure 105-7 *Crohn disease.* Transverse image through the right lower quadrant of an adolescent boy with Crohn disease. Color and spectral Doppler image shows the terminal ileum, which is markedly thickened. Flow to the wall of the terminal ileum is increased, along with venous and high diastolic arterial flow. (Courtesy Marta Hernanz-Schulman MD, Nashville, TN.)

known as *pseudopolyps,* areas of spared mucosa surrounded by adjacent denuded areas. Spasm of involved segments is frequently seen, and intermittent fluoroscopic observation is required to differentiate spasm from stricture. Narrowing of the intestinal lumen secondary to edema and fibrosis is known as the "string sign." The mesentery becomes inflamed, thickened, and fibrotic, which causes separation and retraction of bowel loops.[31,38] The sensitivity and specificity of SBFT has been estimated at approximately 90% and 96%, respectively.[39]

US is an excellent modality in the evaluation of patients with Crohn disease. The involved bowel segment shows a thickened wall with visible transition to uninvolved bowel. Often bowel loops are separated by intervening mesenteric fat, and small lymph nodes are seen. Bowel wall hyperemia has been noted to correlate with disease activity (Fig. 105-7).[40-41] Small abscesses may be missed on US, and it is possible that remote areas of disease may be missed because of overlying bowel gas.

CT is now widely used and has largely replaced SBFT in many centers. CT readily identifies bowel wall thickening, mesenteric changes such as lymphadenopathy, fibrofatty proliferation (Fig. 105-8), luminal narrowing and stricture, and phlegmon formation. CT enterography entails introduction of negative bowel contrast to distend the bowel without obscuring mural enhancement. These techniques may improve identification of complications of disease, such as sinus tracts, fistulae, and strictures. Volumen (E-Z-EM, Inc., New York) is a commonly used commercial product, but whole milk (4% fat) has been reported as a useful substitute.[42] The radiation dose delivered in CT versus SBFT varies, depending on the CT technique and the amount of fluoroscopy and number of radiographs obtained in the SBFT. In either case, the chronic nature of this disease and the need for repeat imaging clearly point to a nonradiation modality as preferrable for monitoring disease activity.[43]

Magnetic resonance imaging (MRI) has become more common for the evaluation of IBD with improved visualization of transmural and extraluminal disease. As with CT, MR enterography demonstrates mural hyperenhancement, bowel wall thickening, stratification and homogenous or striated wall enhancement, and stricture formation—provided adequate bowel distension is achieved (Fig. 105-9). Bowel is considered thickened when it measures greater than 3 mm.[44] Stricture may be suspected if the proximal bowel is greater than 3 cm in diameter, or if there is greater than 10% luminal narrowing in the absence of proximal dilatation.[45] As with CT, luminal contrast agents should be of low signal intensity to allow detection of mural enhancement, which is the most sensitive imaging finding of active disease.[46] Enlarged mesenteric vessels, the so-called "comb" sign, are often seen about affected, hyperenhancing bowel loops on both MR and CT. These findings have been found to correlate with other markers of disease activity, such as elevated levels of C-reactive protein and erythrocyte sedimentation rate.[46] Additional extraluminal findings include lymphadenopathy, fibrofatty proliferation, phlegmon, and abscess. MR enterography has better contrast resolution compared with CT, as well as the added benefit of avoiding radiation exposure, but it cannot be used in patients with MRI-sensitive devices.[47] MR enterography is increasingly advocated for both the initial and follow-up evaluations for patients with Crohn disease.[48]

Prospective studies to compare MR enterography to CT enterography using state of the art techniques have revealed similar sensitivity for detection of active inflammation in the terminal ileum.[32,49] MRI is considered superior to CT for assessment of perineal disease and its complications,

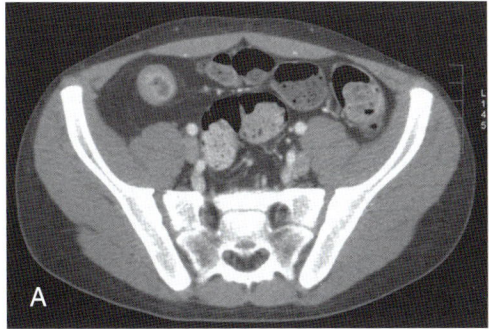
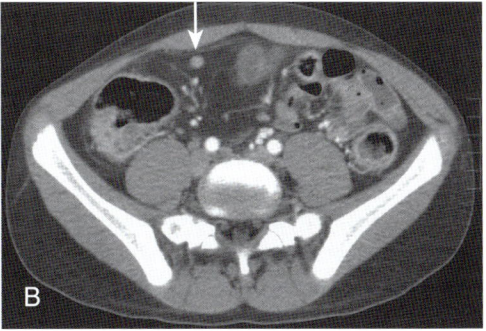

Figure 105-8 *Crohn disease.* **A,** Contrast-enhanced computed tomography through the pelvis of an adolescent boy with Crohn disease illustrates the thickened wall of the terminal ileum, hyperemic mucosa, and characteristic circumferential fat deposition, leading to increased separation of bowel loops. **B,** A section slightly more cephalad in the same patient shows a milder inflammatory change in a more proximal portion of the ileum and again shows fat accumulation, along with a tiny lymph node that is located just deep to the right rectus muscle (*arrow*).

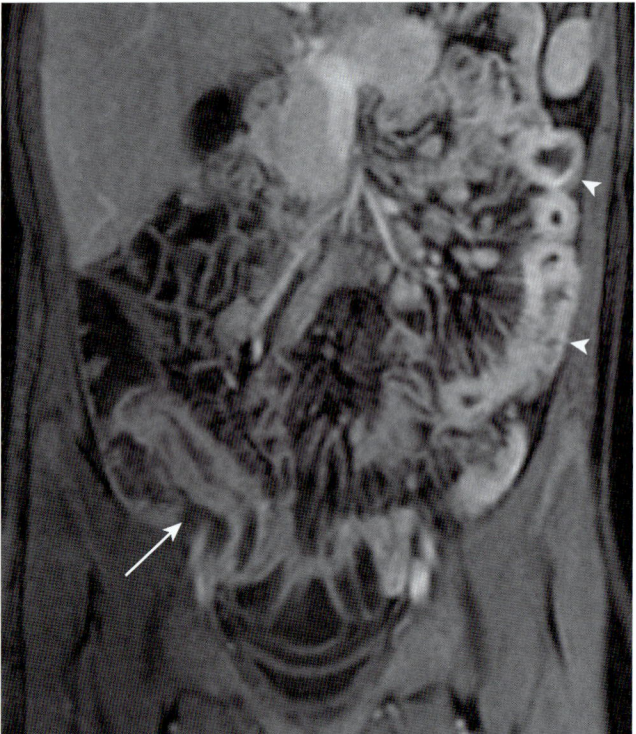

Figure 105-9 **Crohn disease.** Coronal contrast-enhanced T1-weighted image from a magnetic resonance enterography study in an 11-year-old girl with Crohn disease shows a thickened and enhancing terminal ileum (*arrow*). Abnormal enhancement and thickening of jejunal loops in the left abdomen is also apparent (*arrowheads*) with prominence of the vasa recta in the adjacent mesentery (comb sign).

particularly fistulae and sinus tracts.[44] Dedicated contrast-enhanced pelvic MRI can detect perianal fistulae with an accuracy of approximately 90% and can be used to further classify these into various subtypes based on their relationship with the internal and external anal sphincter.[46]

The use of a particular modality in a patient may vary and depends on a variety of factors, including the need for data that would modify therapy, potential radiation dose, need for sedation, as well as local availability and expertise. Because of the chronic nature of Crohn disease, it is important that care be taken to follow the ALARA (as low as reasonably achievable) principle with respect to radiation exposure in this population. When feasible, modalities such as US and MRI should be selected. Radiographs—and in particular fluoroscopic exams and CT, which have the potential for larger patient radiation doses—should be used judiciously with protocols that minimize radiation exposure.

BEHÇET SYNDROME

Overview

Behçet syndrome is an uncommon, immune-mediated vasculitis. This chronic, relapsing condition involves multiple organ systems, including the GI tract and neurologic and cardiovascular systems. The disease is more prevalent in Mediterranean countries, the Middle East, Japan, and Southeast Asia. Prevalence in Asia is reported at approximately 30 per 100,000 population, whereas in North America, it is reported as approximately 7 per 100,000.[50] Patients with this syndrome are at risk for venous and, less commonly, arterial thrombosis; complicating arterial aneurysms, including those of the pulmonary arterial system, may also occur. GI involvement with inflammation and ulceration is reported in 5% to 60% of patients, with the ileocecal area most commonly affected.[51]

Etiology

Behçet syndrome appears to result from vascular endothelial dysfunction and an excessive inflammatory response, termed *pathergy,* which occurs variably as a reaction to nonspecific injury.

Clinical Presentation

Disease onset is typically in the third decade; childhood onset is rare.[52] Males are at two to five times greater risk compared with females.[51] No specific diagnostic test is available for the syndrome; diagnosis is made by detection of recurrent mouth ulcers in association with at least two other major criteria that comprise ocular involvement, skin lesions, recurrent genital ulcerations, and the presence of pathergy.

Imaging

Involvement of the bowel with Behçet disease is characterized by ulcerations—which on GI contrast studies appear as deep, "collar-button" ulcers—and thickening of adjacent mucosal folds.[50] The deep ulcerations can result in perforation and formation of fistulae, which are more easily detected with cross-sectional imaging, including CT and MRI. The esophagus, terminal ileum, and right colon are most commonly affected. GI ulcerations may be confused with other inflammatory bowel diseases that share extraintestinal features.

Treatment

Corticosteroids and other immunosuppressants are indicated during disease exacerbations. Surgical resection of severely involved segments can result in recurrence, with a rate that ranges between 40% and 80%; these typically are seen within 2 years of surgery, often located near the initial anastomosis.[50]

Functional and Infiltrative Diseases

A number of different entities may affect the small intestine with focal or generalized intestinal dilation and with abnormalities of mucosal folds. Entities to be considered in this section include cystic fibrosis (CF), protein-losing enteropathy, graft-versus-host disease (GVHD), and Henoch-Schönlein purpura (HSP).

CYSTIC FIBROSIS

Overview

CF is an autosomal-recessive condition caused by a faulty CF transmembrane conductance regulator (*CFTR*) protein, that results from a variety of mutations mapped to locus q31.2 of chromosome 7. This protein is involved in the regulation of Cl^- transport across cell membranes, not only in the lungs, but also in the digestive system, reproductive tract, and skin. Approximately 3.3% of whites in North America are carriers of a *CFTR* mutation, with a homozygous prevalence of approximately 1 in 3500 whites.[53]

Clinical Presentation

GI involvement in patients with CF includes meconium ileus in the newborn period (see Chapter 103). Older children may show duodenal abnormalities such as dilatation, thickened folds, and ulcerations (see Chapter 104). In older children, the most common intestinal abnormality is the *distal intestinal obstruction syndrome* (DIOS), formerly known as *meconium ileus equivalent*. This syndrome occurs in approximately 15% of patients[54] and is more common among older children and adolescents. Patients come to medical attention with colicky abdominal pain and a palpable right lower quadrant mass that represents impacted fecal material in the ileocolic region. Because mild to severe constipation is a common

concomitant condition, the DIOS diagnosis is reserved for those patients who have signs and symptoms of SBO.

Imaging

Radiographs show small-bowel dilatation with air-fluid levels; bubbly fecal material may also be present, particularly in the right lower quadrant.[55] If CT is performed, dilated small-bowel loops can be followed to the site of impaction in the distal ileum (Fig. 105-10).

Patients with CF may have malabsorption with dilated intestinal loops with thickened folds. The appendix in patients with CF is typically distended by mucoid contents, and although its contents may be expressible with compression, appendiceal diameter alone is not a reliable criterion for diagnosis of appendicitis in these patients; periappendiceal findings therefore become particularly important.[56,57]

Intussusception is found in approximately 20% of CF patients who come in with obstruction, with an inspissated fecal mass acting as a lead point.[58] Mean age at presentation is 10 years. Clinical symptoms tend to be milder than those

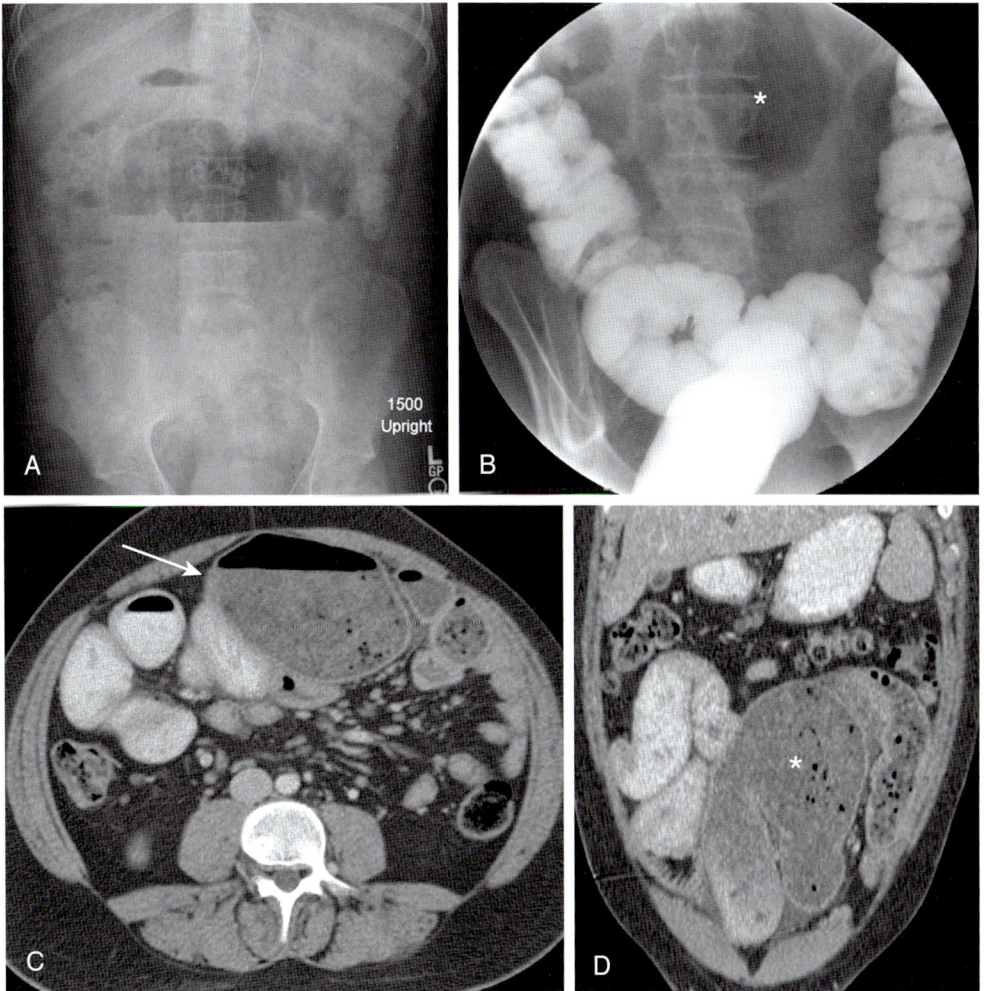

Figure 105-10 Distal intestinal obstructive syndrome. **A,** A 7-month-old boy with cystic fibrosis and increasing abdominal distension, pain, and emesis. Upright abdominal radiograph shows a dilated, gas-filled bowel loop in the central abdomen with an increased air-fluid level. **B,** Contrast enema image shows no substantial reflux into the terminal ileum and persistence of the abnormally dilated bowel loop in the midabdomen (*asterisk*). **C,** Axial contrast-enhanced computed tomography shows flocculent material in a dilated midabdominal bowel loop (*arrow*). **D,** Coronal reformat confirms the axial findings. Flocculent material dilating the small bowel is again seen (*asterisk*). Distal ileal obstruction was confirmed at laparotomy.

in idiopathic intussusception in the younger child, but radiographic findings are similar.[55]

Treatment

Although most patients with DIOS respond to enemas that include mucolytic agents, water-soluble contrast enemas given under fluoroscopic control also may be effective. For best results, reflux into the terminal ileum is necessary. Repeated attempts over a 24 to 48 hour period may be required to completely relieve the impaction. Surgical management may be needed in patients who do not respond to nonsurgical techniques. Treatment of intussusception is with fluoroscopic enema reduction.[55]

PROTEIN-LOSING ENTEROPATHIES

Overview

Protein loss through the GI tract may be related to a range of underlying abnormalities, including immune-mediated dysfunction, such as celiac disease, or to lymphatic obstruction, such as in intestinal lymphangiectasia. In this section we will discuss celiac disease, Whipple disease, and intestinal lymphangiectasia.

Etiology

Celiac Disease

Celiac disease is the most common cause of intestinal malabsorption in childhood. The disease is also known as *nontropical sprue* or *gluten enteropathy,* because the cause is gluten intolerance. Gluten is a protein that is present in wheat and related species, including barley and rye. The disease is more prevalent in Western Europe and North America, where it may affect as many as 1 of every 80 to 300 persons.[59] The hypersensitivity to gluten is related to the tissue transglutaminase (TTG) enzyme, which acts as the autoantigen in celiac disease. Diagnostic tests include measurement of IgA antibody to human recombinant TTG, as well as quantitative serum IgA evaluation. Diagnosis is made when small-bowel biopsy documents villous atrophy. The disorder is associated with type 1 diabetes mellitus; Down, Turner, and Williams syndromes; and IgA deficiency.[59]

Whipple Disease

Whipple disease is caused by *Tropheryma whipplei,* and it is identified at postmortem examination in approximately 0.1% of individuals. It is much more common in men and typically presents in middle age; rarely, the disease is reported in children, most often those from developing areas with poor sanitation. Whipple disease is characterized by the presence of macrophages that persist even after eradication of the initiating organism. Although phagocytosis is normal, macrophages from affected patients appear to be unable to effectively handle the bacterial antigens.[60,61]

Intestinal Lymphangiectasia

Intestinal lymphangiectasia is characterized by dilation of intestinal lymphatics that results in protein loss as lymph leaks into the lumen of the intestine. Intestinal lymphangiectasia may be primary or secondary. *Primary intestinal lymphangiectasia* is associated with developmental abnormalities of the intestinal lymphatics and may be associated with abnormal lymphatics elsewhere in the body. *Secondary intestinal lymphangiectasia* has been found in patients with diseases such as sarcoid or lymphoma that cause obstruction of the intestinal lymphatics.[62] Secondary disease may also be seen when there is an increase in intralymphatic pressure because of an increase in venous pressure, such as with constrictive pericarditis; or increased right atrial pressures, such as in Fontan physiology after single ventricle repair; or congestive heart failure.[59,62]

Miscellaneous Protein-Losing Enteropathies

Patients with immunodeficiency syndromes may have a clinical and radiographic picture similar to that seen in patients with celiac disease. Other causes of protein-losing enteropathy include allergic gastroenteropathy, IBD, infectious mononucleosis, and polyarteritis nodosa.

Clinical Presentation

Celiac Disease

Most children affected with celiac disease come to medical attention between 4 and 24 months of age with failure to thrive, abdominal distension, and diarrhea. Diarrhea is considered one of the hallmarks of the disease, although it is not present in 10% of patients; in fact, some children may rarely come to medical attention with constipation. Children may experience anemia with iron and folate deficiency, hypertransaminemia, arthritis, and behavioral disturbances. Adolescents have delayed puberty, anorexia, and clinical findings related to the hypocalcemia and hypoproteinemia of malabsorption.[59]

Whipple Disease

Patients may seek medical attention with fever and extraintestinal manifestations, particularly migratory arthritis that typically involves larger joints, blood-culture negative endocarditis, central nervous system involvement, and hyperpigmentation resembling Addison disease. These findings may precede the GI manifestations.[60,61]

Intestinal Lymphangiectasia

Several syndromes are associated with intestinal lymphangiectasia, such as neurofibromatosis type 1 (NF1), Turner, Noonan, Klippel-Trénaunay, and Hennekam. Patients with either primary or secondary intestinal lymphangiectasia typically have diarrhea and edema related to hypoproteinemia, failure to thrive, and other symptoms related to malabsorption.[62]

Imaging

The first step in the evaluation of the patient with protein-losing enteropathy is to exclude common etiologies such as malnutrition and liver and renal disease. After excluding other causes, the diagnosis is made by documentation of enteral protein loss by determining the clearance of alpha$_1$-antitrypsin (A1AT) from plasma.[63]

99m-Technetium–labeled human serum albumin (99mTc-HSA) scintigraphy has also been used to document enteral protein leakage. Because of the intermittent nature of the protein loss and the need for serial scanning for up to 24 hours, many centers now utilize A1AT testing. However, 99mTc-HSA scintigraphy has a distinct advantage of localizing the site of protein loss (i.e., large and/or small bowel or stomach).[64]

Abdominal radiographs in patients with celiac disease may show nonspecific small-bowel distension, which can help differentiate it from Whipple disease, in which small-bowel distension is lacking.

Classic imaging findings described on SBFT in celiac disease consist of luminal distension, thickened mucosal folds, and contrast flocculation and segmentation. The last two findings, however, are uncommonly seen with modern-day barium preparations. The mucosal folds may show reversal of the mucosal patterns of jejunum and ileum. The duodenum may exhibit mucosal erosions or thickened nodular folds. Similar thickening of small-bowel folds is seen without dilatation in Whipple disease (e-Fig. 105-11), and barium studies may also show mild bowel dilatation and thickened folds in patients with intestinal lymphangiectasia (Fig. 105-12). However, a substantial number of affected children may have normal barium examination findings.

Patients with immunodeficiency syndromes may have a clinical and radiographic picture similar to that seen in patients with celiac disease. Some affected patients have radiographic findings of lymphoid hyperplasia, particularly in the distal ileum.[65]

When obtained in patients with celiac disease, CT or US imaging may reveal distended loops of jejunum and mesenteric or retroperitoneal lymphadenopathy with dilution of oral contrast. These findings resolve when a gluten-free diet is instituted. There is a high incidence of lymphoma in patients with celiac disease, and any significant mesenteric adenopathy in celiac disease should raise a suspicion for lymphoma.

In Whipple disease, abdominal CT may show additional findings of low-density lymphadenopathy. Lymph nodes usually have a high fat content that results in a low CT attenuation value, usually between 10 and 20 Hounsfield units (HU). Hepatosplenomegaly and ascites also may be present.[66]

In intestinal lymphangiectasia, US and CT findings are related to edema and include intestinal and gallbladder wall thickening, ascites, and a thickened mesentery. Lymphatic malformations may also be present. The absence of adenopathy helps to differentiate this entity from other enteropathies, such as celiac or Whipple disease.

Treatment

Therapeutic approaches for protein-losing enteropathy vary depending on the underlying etiology; the goal of the treatment is to correct the underlying abnormality with supplementation of lost protein and nutrients.

The treatment for celiac disease is a life-long gluten-free diet. Prolonged antibiotic treatment is required for Whipple disease, with monitoring needed because of the risk of recurrence.

In patients with lymphangiectasia, treatment includes a low-fat diet primarily consisting of medium chain triglycerides and high protein. In secondary lymphangiectasia, additional attention is paid to the primary problem.

GRAFT-VERSUS-HOST DISEASE

Overview

Graft-versus-host disease (GVHD) can result from hematopoietic stem cell transplantation. GVHD occurs when the donor lymphocytes react with the tissues of the host, with an inflammatory cascade that often begins in the GI tract.[67,68] Three conditions are generally required for the development of GVHD: 1) the graft must contain immunologically competent cells; 2) the host must possess important transplant alloantigens that are lacking in the donor graft, so that the host appears foreign to the graft; and 3) the host must be incapable of mounting an effective immunologic reaction against the graft.[69,70]

Etiology

GVHD results from donor T-cell epithelial damage in the host target organs.[70] Pathophysiology of GVHD includes pretransplant host tissue injury secondary to preparative ablative radiation and chemotherapy, activation of donor T-lymphocytes, and cytotoxicity against target host cells through the effected inflammatory cascade mediated through

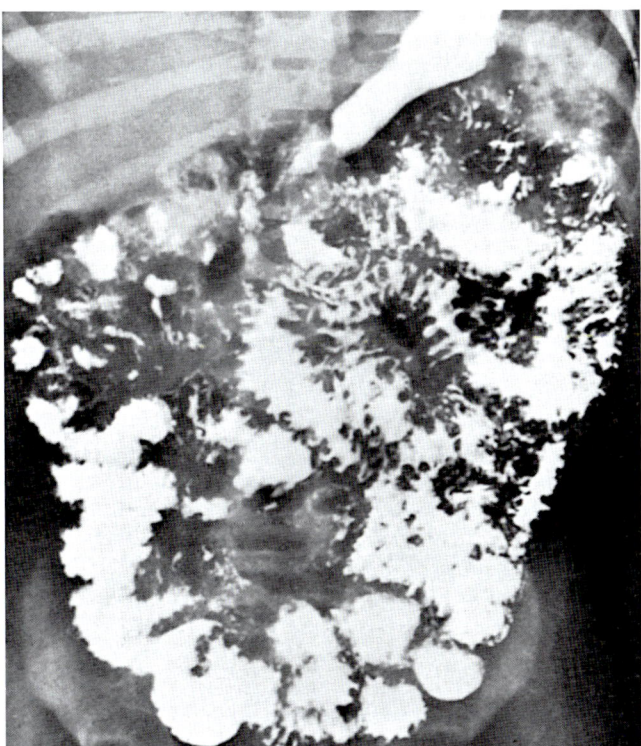

Figure 105-12 Intestinal lymphangiectasia. Small-bowel series in a 3-year-old girl with intestinal lymphangiectasia shows marked coarsening and thickening of the mucosal folds.

histocompatibility antigens.[67,68] The most important elements in the development of GVHD relate to the degree of human leukocyte antigen mismatch.[68]

Clinical Presentation

Acute GVHD occurs within the first 100 days, and commonly within 30 to 40 days, after transplantation.[70] Patients usually come to medical attention with a combination of dermal, hepatic, and GI abnormalities. Dermatitis is manifested as a pruritic, maculopapular rash that may proceed to desquamation. Hepatitis results from involvement of the biliary epithelium and may progress to coagulopathy, encephalopathy, and liver failure. GI manifestations include severe diarrhea, hematochezia, crampy abdominal pain, and ileus. Other organs, including the esophagus and conjunctiva, may also be involved.

Chronic GVHD is defined as occurring at or beyond 100 days after transplant, either as a de novo development or after a variable period of acute disease. The majority of patients have skin abnormalities that include desquamation and vitiligo, which may progress to scleroderma-like changes. Severe mucositis and chronic cholestatic liver disease may occur. Involvement of the hematopoietic system may lead to thrombocytopenia, and this—along with progressive onset, elevated bilirubin, and lichen planus—points to a poor prognosis.[70]

Imaging

Patients receiving bone marrow transplantation are at risk not only for GVHD but for other complications. These include direct toxicity from pretransplant ablative chemotherapy and radiation and also infectious complications with similar clinical presentations. Therefore, imaging may be required to narrow the differential diagnosis in some of these patients.

Radiographs show a pattern of adynamic ileus with separation of bowel loops, thickening of the bowel wall, and air-fluid levels. Less commonly seen are pneumatosis intestinalis and ascites. On occasion the abdomen may be completely gasless (e-Fig. 105-13, A). Contrast studies are usually not necessary but may show severe edema of the bowel wall, with either poor or persistent coating of the mucosa. Some patients have luminal narrowing that leads to a "ribbon" or "toothpaste" appearance of the bowel loops.[71,72]

US reveals loss of stratification of the bowel wall, with variable mural thickening that involves both small bowel and colon.[73] Doppler demonstrates a markedly hyperemic bowel wall with a "hyperdynamic" circulation as assessed by elevated velocities in the superior mesenteric artery (SMA). Supervening ischemic changes may be identified in patients with undetectable mural flow and decreased SMA velocities, which is associated with a poor prognosis.[74]

CT findings in GVHD can be striking (see e-Fig. 105-13, B and C). Bowel loops are variably distended with fluid, and contrast enhancement of the mucosa is marked.[75] Oral contrast is poorly tolerated by these children, and positive luminal contrast actually obscures the important finding of striking mucosal enhancement.[75] These findings mirror the increased flow seen on US. Engorgement of the vasa recta is the most common extraintestinal finding seen on CT and is indicative of hyperdynamic circulation. Other findings include ascites, periportal edema, pericholecystic fluid, and gallbladder wall enhancement.[76]

HENOCH-SCHÖNLEIN PURPURA

Overview

Henoch-Schönlein purpura (HSP) is the most common vasculitis of childhood and affects the small vessels in the skin, joints, GI tract, and kidneys. The incidence of HSP is approximately 10 to 20 per 100,000 population and is most common in children between 2 and 6 years of age.[77,78]

Etiology

Pathophysiology of HSP remains incompletely understood, although it is known to represent an immune complex–mediated vasculitis with multifactorial elements that include genetic predisposition and antigenic stimulation. A significant percentage of patients have antecedent antigenic exposure to infectious agents, such as Group A beta-hemolytic streptococcus, *Mycoplasma,* and adenovirus, among others. Upper respiratory tract infections precede HSP in as many as 50% of cases.[78]

Clinical Features

Arthralgias and GI symptoms may precede the characteristic rash in 30% to 43% of patients.[77] The presence of the characteristic palpable purpuric skin rash is essential for diagnosis, and it occurs along the extensor surfaces with a predilection for the lower extremities.[78] GI symptoms are seen in approximately 50% to 75% of patients and include nausea, vomiting, colicky abdominal pain, and hematochezia.[79] In the small intestine, the disease manifests with bleeding into the bowel wall, which can lead to enteroenteric intussusception. These most often reduce spontaneously, although this is not always the case, and complications from the intussusceptions may ensue that include ischemia of the involved bowel segment (Fig. 105-14).

Imaging

Cross-sectional imaging may show bowel wall thickening with skip areas of abnormality (e-Fig. 105-15); bowel dilation and mesenteric edema may also be seen.[80] Findings on fluoroscopic contrast studies include segmental dilatation and stenosis, bowel wall thickening with separation of bowel loops, filling defects, and coarsening and loss of the normal mucosal fold pattern. Strictures may occur as a late sequela of the disease, likely from vasculitis with secondary focal areas of ischemia.

Treatment

GI manifestations of HSP generally require no treatment, although administration of corticosteroids has been reported to improve symptoms and shorten the symptomatic period.[78,79] Patients with small bowel intussusception require

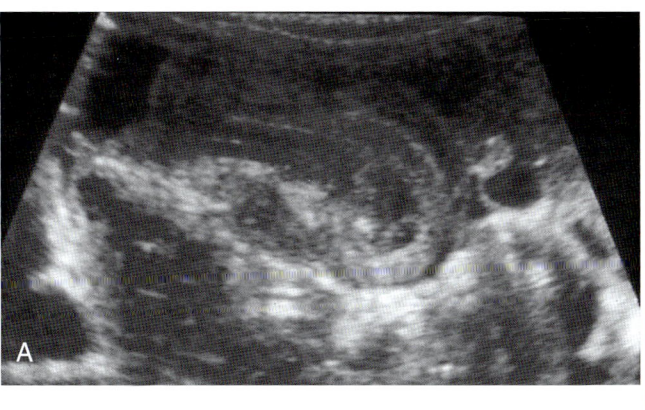
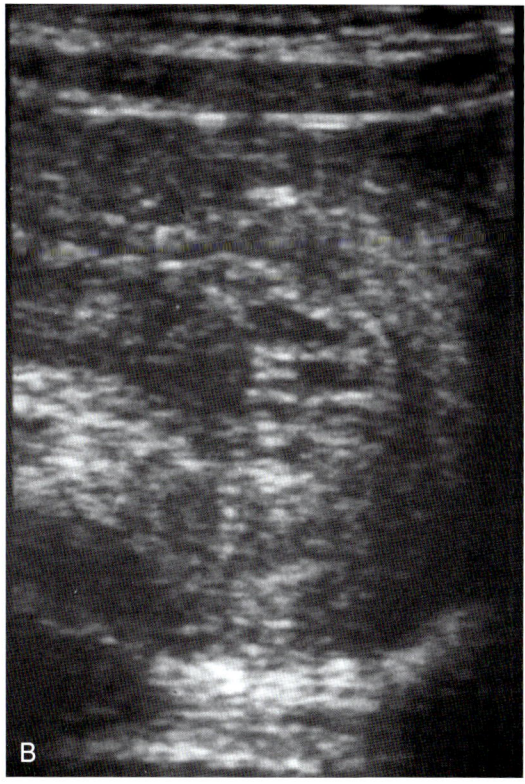

Figure 105-14 Henoch-Schönlein purpura with intussusceptions. **A,** Transverse sonogram of the left lower quadrant in a 6-year-old girl with acute abdominal pain reveals a thick-walled small-bowel loop with intussusception. **B,** Linear transducer image of the tip of the intussusception shows thick-walled bowel layers and sonolucent spaces in the intussuscepted mesentery consistent with edema. At surgery several hours later, an irreducible ileoileal intussusception was identified, which needed segmental bowel resection; the typical petechial rash appeared the following day. (Courtesy Marta Hernanz-Schulman MD, Nashville, TN)

monitoring, because in a minority, the intussusception may not reduce spontaneously, and obstruction and ischemia may supervene.

SMALL-BOWEL INTUSSUSCEPTION

Overview

Intussusceptions in young children are typically ileocolic or ileoileocolic; these are discussed in Chapter 108. Small bowel intussusceptions are more frequently identified with the widespread use of cross-sectional imaging, in which they are often an incidental finding.

Etiology

Small bowel intussusceptions are typically short segment, transient, and asymptomatic. Exceptions include those caused by a lead point such as Meckel diverticulum and polyps in patients with such entities as Peutz-Jeghers syndrome, small-bowel hemangiomas, and lymphoma. Small bowel intussusceptions may also be seen in patients with bowel distension, wall thickening, or abnormal motility, as may be seen in gastroenteritis, Henoch-Schönlein purpura, or celiac disease. In addition, small bowel intussusceptions may occur with the use of gastrojejunostomy tubes or during the postoperative period.

Clinical Presentation

The child with small bowel obstruction may have gastroenteritis and may be imaged for abdominal pain, with the intussusception noted incidentally; these are usually transient and are not found with repeat imaging. Patients with a small bowel intussusception secondary to a lead point that does not not reduce spontaneously, present with abdominal pain and bowel obstruction.[81]

Imaging

As with any other intussusception, imaging findings show bowel within bowel. However, findings that indicate the presence of a transient intussusception include short length (< 3 cm), thin diameter (< 2.5 cm), and location within the small bowel. The findings are similar on US and CT (see Chapter 108, e-Fig. 108-2).[81-83] Findings that suggest a pathologic phenomenon include evidence of bowel obstruction or an identifiable lead point or mesenteric nodes within the complex.

Treatment

Small bowel intussusception in the absence of a lead point or bowel obstruction should be treated symptomatically. Repeat US examination may be performed to document spontaneous resolution when necessary. Pathologic small bowel obstructions are not amenable to fluoroscopic enema reduction and require surgical management.

Tumors

BENIGN TUMORS

Polyps

GI polyps in children may be a solitary and isolated finding, or they may occur in association with a polyposis syndrome. The colon is the primary site of involvement for most of the polyposis syndromes; these are reviewed in Chapter 109. One exception is Peutz-Jeghers syndrome, in which the small bowel is the most commonly involved location with hamartomatous polyps.

Peutz-Jeghers Syndrome

Overview

Peutz-Jeghers syndrome (PJS) is an autosomal-dominant syndrome with incomplete penetrance characterized by mucocutaneous pigmentation and hamartomatous polyps of the GI tract. The estimated prevalence of PJS is approximately 1 per 100,000 individuals.[84]

Etiology

PJS has been attributed to mutations in the *STK11* gene (serine/threonine kinase 11, alias *LKB1*) on chromosome 19p13.3, which was identified in 1998.[84]

Clinical Presentation

The characteristic mucocutaneous pigmentation usually precedes polyp formation and is seen in approximately 95% of patients. This pigmentation is caused by the accumulation of pigment-laden macrophages and consists of brown or black pigmentation of the lips, buccal mucosa, face, palms, and soles that typically presents during early childhood and often fades at adolescence.[84]

Polyps occur most commonly in the small bowel, followed by the colon and stomach, sparing the esophagus. Patients may become symptomatic and may come to medical attention with abdominal pain, intussusception, or bleeding within the first three decades of life. A diagnosis of intussusception will be made in nearly half the patients over their lifetime.

Patients with PJS have an 18-fold increased risk of malignancy compared with the unaffected population.[85] Associated malignancies most commonly involve the GI tract; extraintestinal malignancies may involve the breast, pancreas, reproductive organs, and less frequently the thyroid, gallbladder, and biliary tree.[85] The risk for development of malignancy in PJS patients has been estimated at 2% by age 20, steadily rising to reach 85% by age 70, with a cumulative risk of developing any malignancy estimated at 93%.[84]

Imaging

The polyps usually vary in size and shape and are seen in decreasing frequency in the small bowel, colon, and stomach.

Polyps can be detected on SBFT and on cross-sectional imaging. They usually appear as multiple, large, pedunculated masses scattered throughout the GI tract. Diagnosis is usually made based on the combination of mucocutaneous rash and on biopsy of the polyp. Small bowel intussusceptions occurring in these patients can be easily diagnosed on US or CT, whether simple and transient, or complex (e-Fig. 105-16). Imaging can be used to diagnose and assess other malignancies associated with this condition.

Treatment

Monitoring of polyp burden can be done through imaging techniques such as MRI or through capsule endoscopy, which is considered more sensitive than radiographic studies. Polypectomy can be performed endoscopically. Experimental agents for chemoprevention, such as rapamycin, are being developed and tested.[84] Cancer surveillance is part of the patients' lifelong care.

Other Benign Neoplasms

Overview

Other benign neoplasms that occur in the small intestine of children include hemangiomas, vascular malformations, neurofibromas, fibromas, leiomyomas, GI stromal tumors (GISTs), lipomas, and lipoblastomas. Most benign small-bowel tumors manifest with GI bleeding or intussusception.

Etiology

Hemangiomas can be solitary or multiple and may occur as an isolated finding or in association with a syndrome. Patients with Klippel-Trénaunay syndrome are seen with visceral and cutaneous hemangiomas. Telangiectasias, dilated superficial blood vessels, may occur in the small intestine in Osler-Weber-Rendu syndrome. Vascular malformations that involve the small intestine have also been reported in association with other soft tissue vascular malformations.[86]

Neurofibromas may occur in isolation or as a manifestation of NF1 and are reported to be the most frequent neoplastic lesion arising in the bowel in patients with NF1, seen in approximately 10% to 25% of patients.[87]

GISTs are uncommon in children; the incidence is estimated at 6.5 to 14.5 per million per year, and among these, 0.5% to 2.7% occur in patients younger than 21 years. Pediatric GISTs occur more commonly in girls.[88-90] These tumors are believed to arise from the interstitial cells of Cajal and may exhibit benign or frankly malignant behavior. Although previously confused with rarer smooth muscle tumors, GISTs are differentiated from these tumors, and from neural tumors such as neurofibromas and schwannomas, by the expression of tyrosine kinase growth factor receptor (*KIT,* alias CD117). Whether sporadic, familial, or syndromic, GISTs are the most common mesenchymal neoplasm of the GI tract, and smooth muscle tumors, such as leiomyomas and leiomyosarcomas, arise very rarely.

GISTs are associated with other syndromes, particularly NF1 but also with the Carney triad (gastric GIST, extraadrenal paraganglioma, and pulmonary chondroma), Carney-Stratakis syndrome (paragangliomas and GIST), and familial GIST.[88-92]

Fat-containing tumors that occur in the small intestine include lipomas and lipoblastomas. These appear primarily within the intestinal wall or in the adjacent omentum or retroperitoneum. Lipoblastomas are rare tumors related to embryonal fat, they occur almost exclusively in children, and 90% come to medical attention within the first 3 years of life.[93,94]

Clinical Features

Hemangiomas may manifest with GI bleeding, with obstruction as a lead point for intussusception, or perforation.[86] Neurofibromas that involve the small bowel are often asymptomatic, however, they may be seen initially with GI bleeding or with obstruction secondary to intussusception or segmental volvulus.[87] GISTs most frequently manifest with GI bleeding and at times with secondary anemia. Vomiting, abdominal pain, and obstruction are additional but nonspecific presenting features. Lipomas may ulcerate when larger than 2 cm and may lead to intestinal bleeding or may serve as the lead point for intussusception,[95] and lipoblastomas, although benign, may recur locally in as many as 25% of cases.[93]

Imaging

In patients with small-bowel tumors, abdominal radiographs may reveal a mass effect, if the lesion is sufficiently large, or obstruction, if the lesion has acted as a lead point for intussusception. Fluoroscopic contrast studies may reveal a luminal filling defect or a mural mass. US may be helpful to assess for a lead point, if the lesion is complicated by intussusception. GISTs may be located external to the serosa, and the small-bowel origin may not be readily apparent; contrast attenuation may be uniform, or it may demonstrate internal areas of hemorrhage or necrosis. A similar pattern of enhancement is seen with IV gadolinium on MRI.[92] Lipomas and lipoblastomas demonstrate characteristic low density on CT and fat attenuation on MR.[93,95]

Treatment

Neurofibromas that are symptomatic typically undergo surgical excision,[96] whereas GISTs in pediatric patients tend to have an indolent course, and therapy consists of chemotherapy and evaluation for surgical resection.[90] Lipoblastomas are treated by complete resection, and mesenteric lipoblastomas may require resection of adjacent intestinal loops.[93,94]

MALIGNANT TUMORS

With the exception of lymphoma, malignant tumors of the small intestine in children are exceedingly rare. The tumors discussed in the preceding section, such as GISTs, have both benign and malignant subgroups. Also as discussed previously, patients with PJS may develop GI malignancies. Other polyposis syndromes that largely affect the colon are further discussed in Chapter 109.

Burkitt Lymphoma

Overview

Burkitt lymphoma is the most frequent subtype of non-Hodgkin lymphoma that occurs in children, with a median age of presentation at 8 years; more than one third of the cases occur in children between 5 and 9 years of age.[97]

Etiology

Burkitt lymphoma is a monoclonal B-cell lymphoma that occurs in three principal forms: endemic, sporadic, and immunodeficient. The *endemic form,* as initially identified in Uganda in 1958, occurs in equatorial Africa and Papua New Guinea, with a 95% association with the Epstein–Barr virus (EBV). The *sporadic form* is seen in North America, Northern and Eastern Europe, and the Far East, and its association with EBV is 15%. The *immunodeficient form* is associated with immune-compromised states, particularly with HIV infection, congenital deficiencies, and iatrogenic immunodeficiencies such as occur in allograft recipients.[97]

Clinical Presentation

GI involvement occurs in over half of pediatric patients with Burkitt lymphoma.[98] Terminal ileum, cecum, and appendix are common sites of involvement by Burkitt lymphoma, with the terminal ileum being the most common location secondary to high concentration of lymphatic nodal tissue.[97] Common presenting symptoms include abdominal pain or a palpable abdominal mass, followed by neck swelling.[98] Patients may also come to medical attention with intestinal obstruction related to an intussusception with a pathologic lead point (see Fig. 108-7). Burkitt lymphoma is one of the most rapidly growing tumors, with a doubling time of approximately 24 hours; therefore prompt diagnosis is important.[97]

Imaging

Abdominal radiographs may show evidence of mass effect or obstruction related to an intussusception, or they may appear normal. SBFT may reveal a polypoid mass, strictures or areas of luminal narrowing that resemble IBD, ulceration, or an intussusception.

US in patients with lymphoma typically reveals a mass of low or heterogeneous echogenicity. A hyperechoic center that can be eccentrically positioned represents the apposed mucosal surfaces, and this may be seen when the lymphoma infiltrates the bowel wall (Fig. 105-17, *A*). Intussusception with a hypoechoic lead point may be the initial imaging finding.

CT may also show mesenteric masses and infiltration of the bowel wall (see Fig. 105-17, *B* and *C*) with dilatation of the bowel lumen. The obstruction may be secondary to luminal narrowing or intussusception, because desmoplastic reaction is not commonly seen with Burkitt lymphoma.[97] Ascites may also be present (see Fig. 105-17). The tumor may involve other abdominal sites, and careful evaluation of retroperitoneal organs, liver, and spleen is mandatory. Fluorodeoxyglucose positron-emission tomography may offer additional information during tumor staging.[99]

Treatment

Although it grows rapidly, Burkitt lymphoma is also rapidly responsive to chemotherapy, with an increasingly improving prognosis.[100]

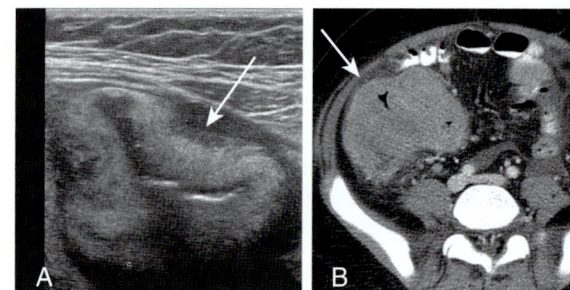 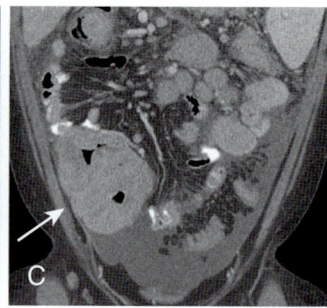

Figure 105-17 Burkitt lymphoma. **A,** Transverse abdominal sonographic image in a 12-year-old boy who presented with abdominal pain, nausea, and diarrhea shows pronounced bowel wall thickening (*arrow*). **B,** Correlative contrast-enhanced CT confirms thickening of bowel in the right lower quadrant (*arrow*) and moderate ascites. **C,** Coronal reformat again shows the involvement of the bowel with tumor (*arrow*) and additionally demonstrates ascites. Burkitt lymphoma was diagnosed on biopsy.

Carcinoid

Overview

Carcinoid is a rare neuroendocrine neoplasm that occurs in the digestive tract in up to 95% of cases.[101] Most commonly found in young adults, carcinoid tumors are rare in children, with a reported prevalence of 0.08% among pediatric tumors treated at a large pediatric cancer hospital.[102]

Etiology

Carcinoid tumors arise from neuroendocrine enterochromaffin or Kulchitsky cells. Although most lesions arise de novo, carcinoid tumors are associated with multiple endocrine neoplasia types 1 and 2 as well as NF1.[103]

Clinical Presentation

Unlike the rapidly growing Burkitt lymphoma, carcinoid tumors have a slow growth rate and indolent course, with a relatively long asymptomatic period.[101] Presentation may mimic acute appendicitis; patients otherwise come to medical attention with intermittent abdominal pain, vomiting, bleeding, and bowel obstruction. In adults, metastases are seen at diagnosis in approximately one fourth of patients.[101] Metastases and the carcinoid syndrome are uncommon in children.[102]

Imaging

On abdominal radiographs, carcinoid tumors are not typically detectable unless complicated by a secondary process such as intussusception and obstruction. Rarely, a calcified appendiceal carcinoid may mimic a fecalith.[103] Carcinoids may be detected on fluoroscopic contrast studies if of sufficient size. On cross-sectional imaging, associated mesenteric desmoplastic reaction or hepatic metastases may be more readily identifiable than the primary tumor. On CT, negative luminal contrast may aid in detection. On MRI, carcinoids may be seen as a subtle, asymmetric mural thickening that is isointense on T1- and mildly hyperintense on T2-weighted sequences.[103]

Treatment

Surgical removal is the first line of treatment for carcinoids, with additional medical treatment that combines antineoplastic chemotherapeutic agents with other agents, such as somatostatin analogs and interferon-α.[103] Tumors less than 2 cm in diameter at diagnosis have a favorable prognosis.[102]

Key Points

The most common causes of acquired small-bowel obstruction in children are adhesions, tumors, and hernias.
Infectious gastroenteritis is most commonly caused by viruses, and imaging generally plays little or no role in the evaluation of the disease.
ALARA principles should be followed with respect to imaging children with Crohn disease.
CT and MRI have largely replaced the fluoroscopic examination of the bowel in the assessment of IBD and have comparable sensitivities and specificities.
MRI is the imaging modality of choice for assessing perianal disease and fistulae in patients with Crohn disease.
Burkitt lymphoma often involves the GI tract in children and is a common lead point for intussusception for older children.

Suggested Readings

Ammoury RF, Croffie JM. Malabsorptive disorders of childhood. *Pediatr Rev.* 2010;31(10):407-415.

Dennehy PH. Acute diarrheal disease in children: epidemiology, prevention, and treatment. *Infect Dis Clin North Am.* 2005;19(3):585-602.

Jacobsohn DA. Acute graft-versus-host disease in children. *Bone Marrow Transplant.* 2008;41(2):215-221.

Levy AD, et al. Gastrointestinal stromal tumors: radiologic features with pathologic correlation. *Radiographics.* 2003;23(2):283-304, 456.

Mattei P, Rombeau JL. Review of the pathophysiology and management of postoperative ileus. *World J Surg.* 2006;30(8):1382-1391.

Ruemmele FM. Pediatric inflammatory bowel diseases: coming of age. *Curr Opin Gastroenterol.* 2010;26(4):332-336.

Tolan DJ, et al. MR enterographic manifestations of small bowel Crohn disease. *Radiographics.* 2010;30(2):367-384.

References

Full references for this chapter can be found on www.expertconsult.com.

Chapter 106

Congenital and Neonatal Disorders

MARTA HERNANZ-SCHULMAN

Overview

In the neonatal period, congenital colonic abnormalities typically present with clinical signs of obstruction. Neonatal anatomic obstruction includes imperforate anus and colonic atresia. Functional lesions that produce obstruction include the spectrum of meconium plug and small left colon syndrome, as well as Hirschsprung disease and neuropathic and myopathic pseudoobstruction syndromes. Some of these conditions, such as Hirschsprung disease, anorectal stenosis, duplication cysts, and chronic intestinal pseudoobstruction (CIPO), can present later in life.

Colonic Atresia and Stenosis

Overview The colon is the least involved segment in intestinal atresias; colonic atresia constitutes between 1.8% and 15% of intestinal atresias, with an overall incidence of approximately 1 in 20,000 births. Colonic stenosis is very rare, with fewer than 15 cases reported in the literature. It typically consists of stricturelike stenosis, although membranous stenosis also has been reported. The anatomic descriptive classification of small intestinal atresias (see Chapter 103) also is applied to colonic atresias.[1,2]

Colonic atresia is associated with other colonic abnormalities, as well as extracolonic and extraintestinal abnormalities. Approximately 22% of patients also may have Hirschsprung disease or hypoganglionosis.[3,4] Extraintestinal anomalies include the musculoskeletal system, heart, abdominal wall, eyes, and central nervous system.[5]

Etiology The etiology of colonic atresia is thought to be similar to that of small bowel atresias, that is, related to an ischemic event in utero that leads to resorption of the involved bowel and discontinuity of the proximal and distal segments.[6] More recently, mutations involving fibroblast growth factor 10 or its receptor have resulted in intestinal atresia in mice, which suggests that genetic determinants also may play a role.[7]

Clinical Presentation Infants with colonic atresia present with abdominal distension, vomiting, and failure to pass meconium. Polyhydramnios is uncommon, because the atresia is sufficiently distal to allow resorption of swallowed amniotic fluid. The onset of vomiting may be delayed compared with more proximal atresias and may become feculent.[5,8] Patients with colonic stenosis demonstrate similar findings proportionate to the degree of stenosis.

Imaging Abdominal radiographs in patients with colonic atresia show distal obstruction with multiple dilated loops of bowel and abdominal distension with flank protuberance and diaphragmatic elevation. However, the proximal colon characteristically is dilated far more than the other loops of bowel (Fig. 106-1, *A*). This disproportionate dilatation is due to competence of the ileocecal valve, which allows intestinal contents forward into the proximal colonic segment but does not allow decompression proximally. Air-fluid levels are seen on horizontal beam radiographs, and prone images show no gas in the rectum (Fig. 106-1, *B*).

A contrast enema performed on these patients demonstrates a microcolon that terminates blindly, devoid of the filling defects characteristic of a meconium ileus (Fig. 106-1, *C*).

Treatment The treatment of colonic atresia is surgical. Because 15% to 20% of patients with colonic atresia also have proximal intestinal atresia, the proximal bowel should be evaluated. Hirschsprung disease should be excluded with suction biopsy before reestablishing intestinal continuity, and coexisting extraintestinal anomalies should be identified.[5]

Anorectal Malformations

Overview Anorectal malformations encompass the spectrum of anal atresia and stenosis, with an incidence of approximately 1:5000 live births worldwide. Approximately one third of patients have isolated lesions, but two thirds of patients are affected by other abnormalities encompassing the gastrointestinal tract and multiple other systems. Approximately 95% of patients have a fistula to the urethra (males), vagina (females), or the perineum; however, 95% of patients with Down syndrome and anorectal malformation have no fistula.[9]

Anatomically, anorectal malformations are classified as high, intermediate, or low lesions, depending on whether the atresia lies above or below the levator sling. Some authors object to this classification because the anomaly is a spectrum,

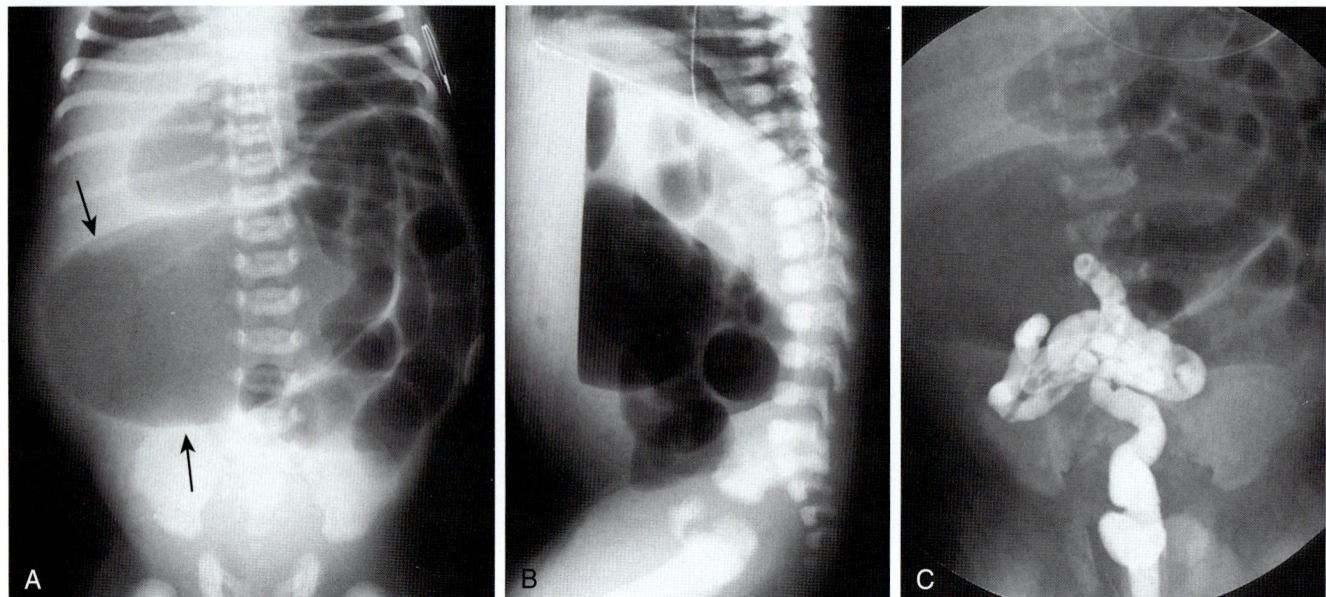

Figure 106-1   Colonic atresia. A, A supine abdominal radiograph of a neonate with abdominal distension and bilious vomiting demonstrates protuberance of the flanks and elevation of the diaphragms. Gas-filled dilated loops of bowel are present, but one loop is dilated far more than other loops, and represents the atretic proximal colonic segment *(arrows).* An orogastric tube decompresses the stomach. **B,** A prone cross-table lateral radiograph shows a large air-fluid level located within the atretic proximal colonic segment. No gas is present in the rectum. **C,** A contrast enema shows a microcolon terminating blindly at the atretic segment.

rather than three separate and distinct types. The classification system of Levitt and Peña (Table 106-1) provides both prognostic information and implications for optimal surgical management.[9] These authors note that girls with high lesions with a high rectovaginal fistula who later present with a persistent/unrepaired urogenital sinus abnormality actually represent girls with a persistent cloaca, which are classified by the length of the persistent cloacal canal.[10]

Rectal atresia often is discussed among the anorectal malformations, although patients with rectal atresia have a normal anal canal and external physical findings. The rectum is atretic 1 to 2 cm above the anus.[10]

Etiology   Anorectal atresia with rectourethral or rectovaginal fistulas may be the result of failure of the urorectal septum to descend to the cloacal membrane and the eventual site of the perineal body; if the cloaca is too small, the hindgut may then terminate anteriorly, entering either the urethra in the male or the vagina in the female. Rectoanal atresias are thought to be related to vascular accidents, similar to the atresias that occur in the small bowel and colon. Imperforate anus is due to failure of breakdown of the anal membrane.[11]

No single genetic abnormality is associated with anorectal malformations. The most common chromosomal abnormalities are trisomy 21 and a microdeletion at chromosome 22q11.2, although abnormalities in multiple chromosomes have been identified.[12] Approximately 15% of patients with rectovestibular or rectoperineal fistulas, which are indicative of low lesions, have a positive family history for anorectal malformations. Genetic studies in both animals and humans have implicated defects in the sonic hedgehog, *Wnt5a,* and *Skt* genes. These studies suggest that the pathogenetic mechanisms of high and low fistulas differ and that fistula formation may be due to a genetic mutation rather than obstruction.

Clinical Manifestations   Anorectal malformations are clinically apparent at birth, with the exception of patients with rectal atresia, who have a normal external appearace. Physical examination may reveal a perineal or vestibular fistula, although the possibility of such a fistula is best evaluated after 24 hours, because meconium may not appear in the perineum before this time. If fecal material appears in the urine, a rectourethral fistula may be inferred. Patients who demonstrate a "flat bottom" (i.e., the buttock crease is not visible) have poor development of pelvic musculature and a more guarded prognosis.[9] Girls with a single perineal orifice have a cloacal malformation (Fig. 106-2).

The best known group of anomalies associated with anorectal malformations is the VACTERL association (vertebral anomalies, anal atresia, cardiac abnormalities, esophageal atresia with or without tracheoesophageal fistula, and renal and limb abnormalities). Associated genetic syndromes include

Table 106-1

Classification of Anorectal Malformations	
Males	**Females**
Perineal fistula	Perineal fistula
Rectourethral fistula	Vestibular fistula
Bulbar	Persistent cloaca
Prostatic	≤3 cm common channel
Recto-bladder neck fistula	>3 cm common channel
Imperforate anus without fistula	Imperforate anus without fistula
Rectal atresia	Rectal atresia
Complex defects	Complex defects

From Levitt M, Peña A. Anorectal malformations. In: Coran A, et al. eds. *Pediatric surgery.* Philadelphia, Mosby; 2012.

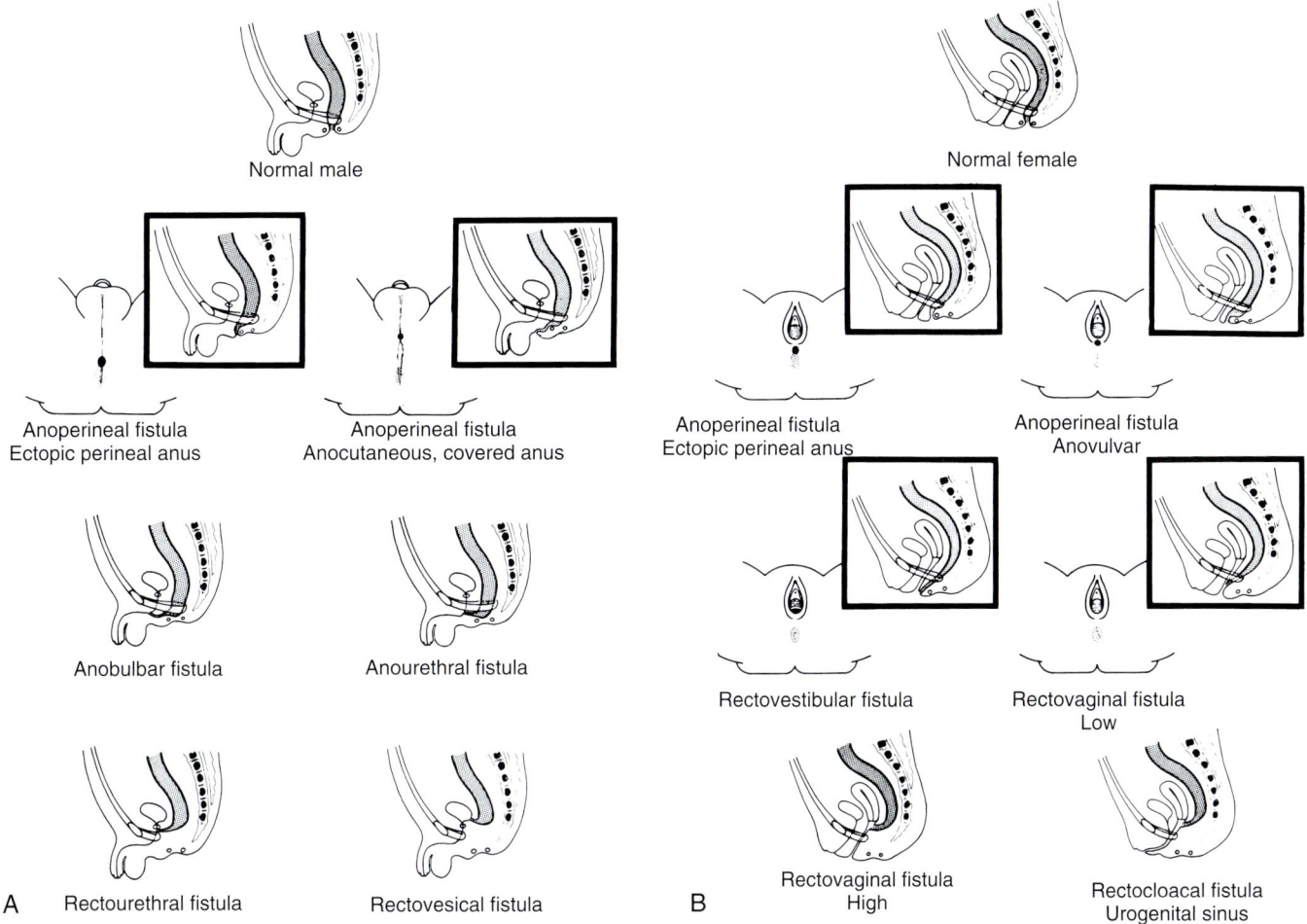

Figure 106-2 Physical examination findings in boys and girls with anorectal malformations. **A,** A schematic diagram of normal and ectopic termination of the hindgut in the male. **B,** A schematic diagram of normal termination and common sites of ectopic termination of the hindgut in the female. (From Santulli TV. In: Mustard WT, et al, eds. *Pediatric surgery.* ed 2. St Louis: Mosby–Year Book; 1969.)

trisomy 21, trisomy 8, and fragile X syndrome.[12] Cardiovascular abnormalities are seen in about one third of patients, most commonly atrial septal defect and persistent ductus arteriosus, followed by tetralogy of Fallot and ventricular septal defect.[9] Vertebral anomalies occur in approximately one third of patients (Fig. 106-3, *A* and *B*), and their severity may be correlated with the complexity of the anorectal lesion. Coronal clefts often are seen in patients with imperforate anus and have been reported as being nine times more common in boys than in girls.[13] Esophageal atresia with tracheoesophageal fistula is seen in approximately 10% of patients, and abnormalities affecting the duodenum (atresia or malrotation) are found in 1% to 2%. Hirschsprung disease, although reported in these patients, is rare.[14] Genitourinary anomalies are common, presenting in one third to one half of cases, again correlated with increasing complexity of the defect. These anomalies range from reflux to renal dysplasia or agenesis, with cryptorchidism and hypospadias seen in male patients. Females may demonstrate müllerian abnormalities, including duplications and obstructions, particularly in the setting of cloacal abnormalities.[9,10]

Imaging The goal of imaging is to elucidate associated anomalies and to determine fistulous anatomy. The sacral

ratio[9] quantifies the degree of sacral hypoplasia by measuring the distance between the iliac crests and the inferior border of the sacroiliac joints (A-B) and the distance between the inferior border of the iliac joints and the tip of the sacrum (C-D); the CD/AB ratio should be >0.77. An increase in the ratio to approach 1.0 indicates better sacral development and better prognosis.

In addition to urinalysis, radiographs of the spine normally are obtained, and patients normally undergo cardiac echocardiography and ultrasound of the kidneys, spinal canal, and pelvis (in girls).

Several imaging methods have been used for evaluation of the atretic anatomy in patients without a perineal fistula. The invertogram relies on visualizing the gas-filled rectum and relating its termination to pelvic bony landmarks—particularly extension below the coccyx, which would classify it as a low lesion.[9] However, problems such as meconium distal to gas and movement of the rectum with infant straining and crying often render this examination inexact and problematic. Voiding cystourethrography can be useful in visualizing the fistula if contrast material flows retrograde into the atretic distal colon during voiding (Fig. 106-3, *C*). Voiding cystourethrography does not always work because meconium may obstruct the fistula. Instilling water-soluble contrast material

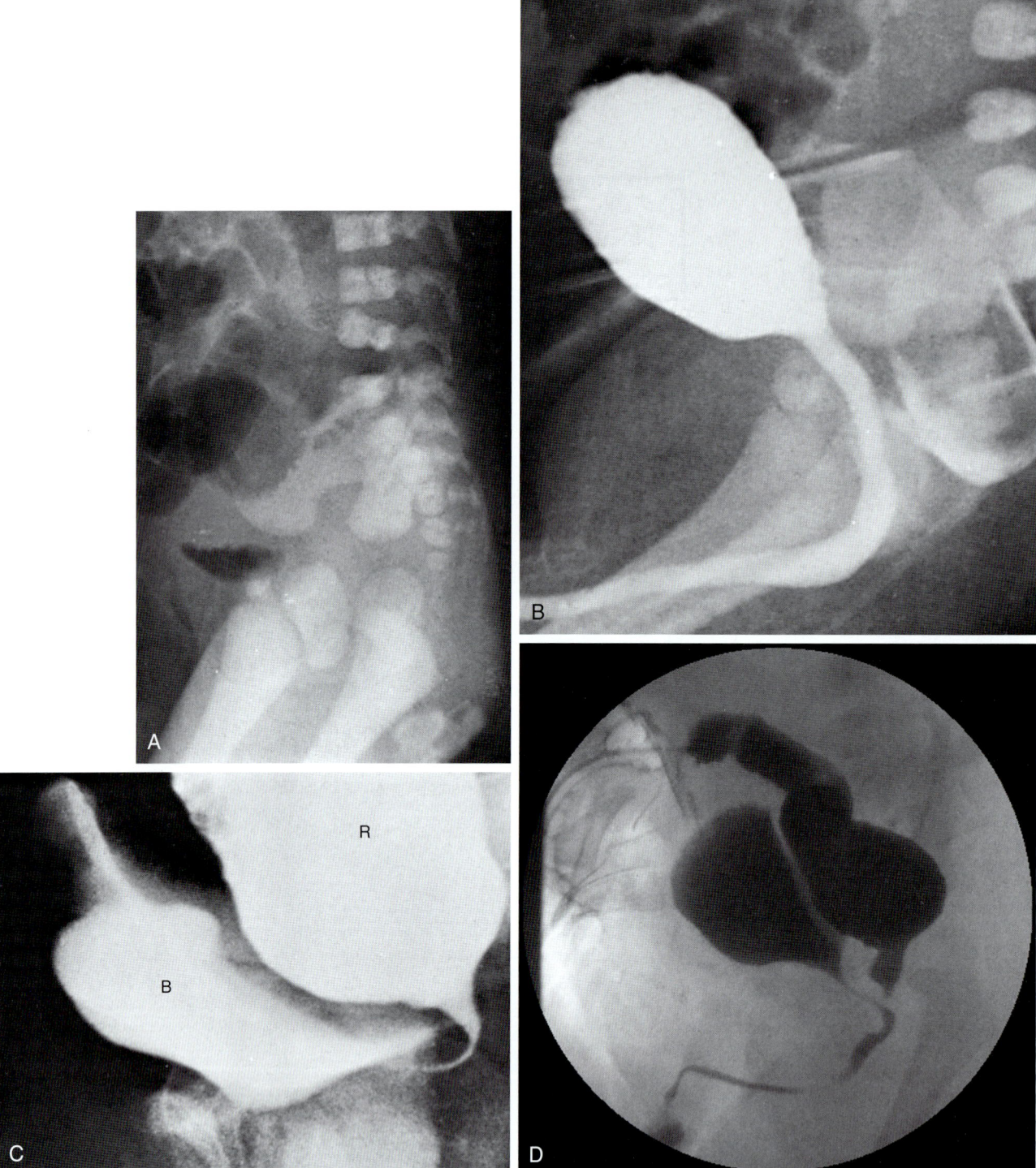

Figure 106-3 High anorectal malformation in a male neonate. **A,** A lateral radiograph of the pelvis and lower abdomen the demonstrating gas in the urinary bladder. In addition, numerous lumbar coronal clefts are identified. **B,** A voiding cystogram demonstrates a rectoprostatic fistula. Note how the rectum bulges inferiorly below the level of the fistula. This accounts for the spuriously small distance sometimes seen between rectal gas and anal marker in such patients, although the bowel edge may lie above the puborectalis sling. **C,** Examination of the rectal pouch with contrast material identifies a rectovesical fistula in a male infant. **D,** Examination of the rectal pouch with contrast material shows the fistulous connection to the posterior urethra in a male infant. (**A,** From Berdon WE, et al. The radiologic evaluation of imperforate anus. An approach correlated with current surgical concepts. *Radiology.* 1968;90(3):466-471.)

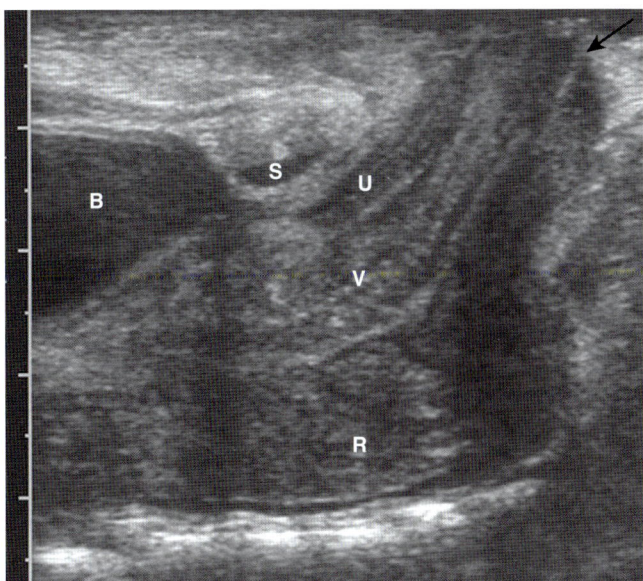

Figure 106-5 Perineal ultrasound of a neonate with a rectovestibular fistula (*arrow*). *B,* Bladder; *U,* urethra; *V,* vagina; *R,* rectum; *S,* symphysis.

into the rectal pouch after a colostomy often is successful in outlining fistulas to the bladder (Fig. 106-3, *D*) or urethra (Fig. 106-3, *E*). Occasionally, gas may outline some of the pertinent anatomy (e-Fig. 106-4).

Ultrasound also is used to evaluate the distal position of the rectum (Fig. 106-5). The meconium in the pouch allows easy visualization of the distal rectum; however, changes in apparent position with straining make it somewhat challenging. Measurements of 10 mm ± 4 correlate with a low lesion, whereas measurements of 24 ± 6 tend to correlate with intermediate and high lesions.[15] Ultrasound can identify the puborectalis musculature; the presence of this musculature correlates with low-type lesions, whereas its absence correlates with high-type lesions.[16]

Magnetic resonance imaging (MRI) also has been used to identify the internal anatomy. High field strengths, small field of view, and sequences without fat suppression, which increase the conspicuity of the muscles of the pelvic floor, are helpful in visualizing the position of the distal rectal pouch with respect to the levator mechanism.[17] MRI also can be used to evaluate the rectum and levator sling after surgery (Fig. 106-6).

Patients with rectal atresia who have normal external anatomy are evaluated with contrast enema. The enema demonstrates a very short distal rectum that terminates blindly (e-Fig. 106-7).

Treatment The treatment of anorectal malformations is surgical but varies with the level and complexity of the lesion. Most boys can undergo repair with a posterior sagittal approach alone, although some with a high lesion also will require an abdominal approach to mobilize a very high rectum. In girls, 30% of cloacas need to be repaired through an abdominal approach. Babies with rectal atresia typically undergo an initial colostomy, with later anastomotic repair of the atretic rectum with the anal canal.[10]

Currarino Association

Overview Although Currarino syndrome initially was described in three infants in 1981 as a triad of anorectal malformation (anorectal stenosis) with rectoperineal fistula,[18] sacral anomaly (classically crescentic abnormality resembling a scimitar), and a presacral mass,[19] this abnormality actually encompasses a much wider spectrum of phenotypic abnormalities and underlying genetic defects.

Etiology Currarino syndrome is an autosomal-dominant disorder with variable penetrance; approximately 50% of the cases are sporadic. A mutation located at 7q36 encoding for the *HLXB9* gene responsible for nuclear transcription factor HB9 plays a role in the dorsoventral separation of the caudal embryo; other genes related to the same differentiation pathway also may exist.[20,21]

Clinical Presentation The patients typically present with constipation and may undergo anorectal dilatation. The presacral

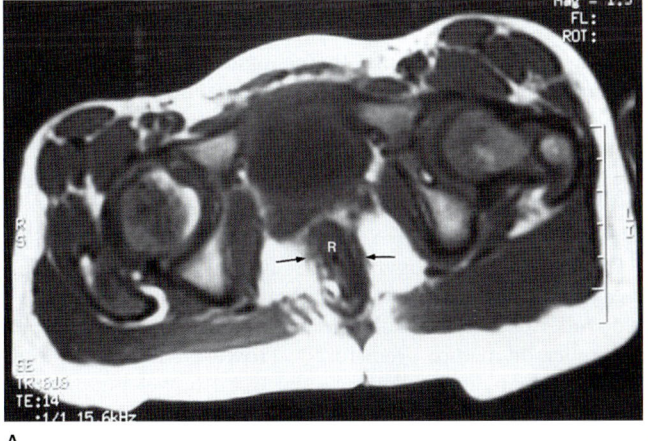

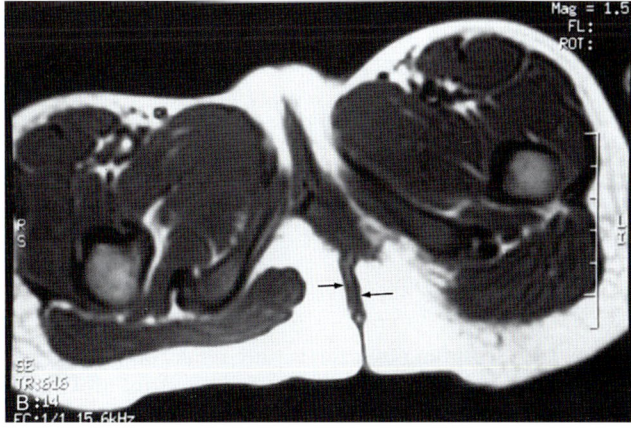

Figure 106-6 Postoperative magnetic resonance after anal atresia repair. **A,** An axial T1-weighted section at the level of the pubic bone shows the rectum (*R*) contained within the puborectalis muscle (*arrows*). **B,** An axial T1-weighted image through the region of the pubic bone on another child after surgery shows that the rectum (*R*) is not enclosed by muscle on the left side. Little puborectalis muscle is seen on the left.

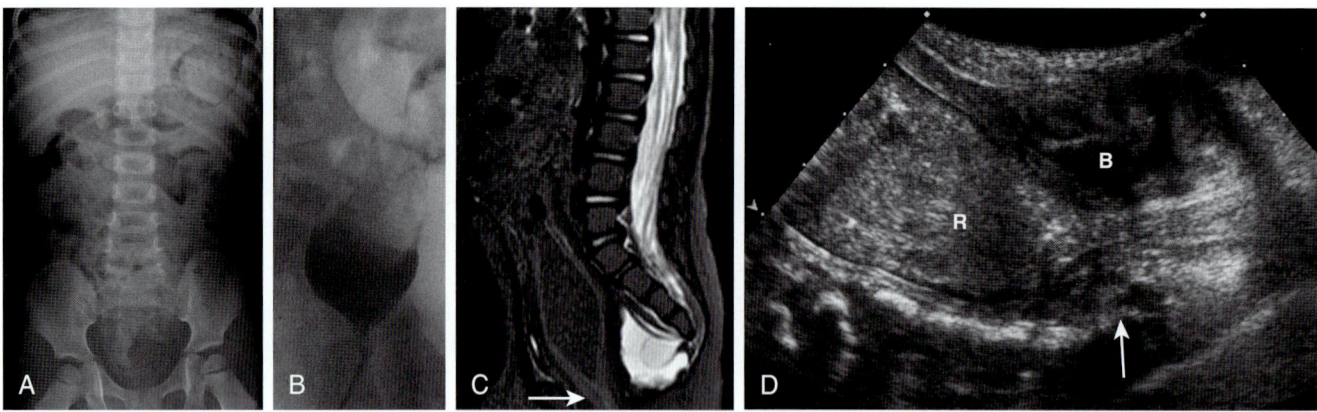

Figure 106-8   Currarino syndrome. **A,** A supine abdominal radiograph in 23-month-old boy with a history of constipation demonstrates an increased amount of stool in the colon and a deletion anomaly along the left side of the sacrum, resembling a scimitar. **B,** A contrast enema demonstrates narrowing of the distal rectum. **C,** A sagittal T2-weighted lumbar spine image demonstrates a cystic retrorectal mass that proved to represent an anterior meningocele. Note the narrowing of the distal rectum (*arrow*). **D,** An anterior sagittal pelvic sonogram of a different male neonate shows a dilated proximal rectum (*R*) distally narrowed and a retrorectal mass (*arrow*) that proved to represent a mature teratoma. *B,* Bladder.

mass is often small and may not be detected unless the syndrome is suspected; an unrecognized presacral mass may present later with complications such as meningitis or development of malignancy.[20-22] The spectrum of presacral masses includes teratoma, rectal duplication cyst, anterior meningocele, leiomyosarcoma, and ectopic nephroblastoma.

Other abnormalities that can be seen in the full spectrum of the syndrome include Hirschsprung disease, dysganglionosis, bladder motility abnormalities, vesicoureteral reflux, rib anomalies, urinary and gynecologic abnormalities, cord tethering and intraspinal lipomas.[18,23]

Imaging   Radiographs of the sacrum may reveal the typical scimitar-shaped sacral abnormality (Fig. 106-8, *A*); other sacral defects, typically deletion abnormalities, may be present. In a minority of patients the sacrum is normal.[21]

Those patients with anorectal stenosis may have a rectoperineal fistula or an anteriorly placed anus and present with constipation, sometimes in early adulthood. Contrast enema shows marked narrowing of the distal rectum, with excessive stool proximally (Fig. 106-8, *B*). If the presacral mass is of sufficient size, it will exert a visible mass effect upon the posterior wall of the distal rectum.

MRI best demonstrates the presacral masses well and provides a window into the spinal canal (Fig. 106-8, *C*). In young infants, the presacral mass often is visible sonographically (Fig. 106-8, *D*).

Treatment   Treatment depends on the phenotypic manifestations of the syndrome on a given patient, and each is treated accordingly. Presacral masses are surgically resected.

Hirschsprung Disease

Overview   Hirschsprung disease is the result of failure of normal bowel innervation as a result of the arrest of proximal to distal migration of vagal neural crest cells, and therefore it is considered a neurocristopathy. As a result of abnormal arrest of migration, a variable length of distal bowel lacks parasympathetic Auerbach (intermuscular) and Meissner (submucosal) plexuses and is unable to participate in normal

peristalsis, resulting in failure of relaxation and functional obstruction. Pathologic evaluation also shows abnormal acetylcholinesterase staining and hypertrophied nerve fibers (e-Fig. 106-9).

Hirschsprung disease occurs in approximately 1 per 5000 live births and is responsible for approximately 15% to 20% of cases of neonatal bowel obstruction, presenting in the newborn period in approximately 80% of cases. The incidence is less among African Americans and Asian Americans, quoted as 2.1 and 2.8 per 10,000 live births, respectively.[24] The transition point between normal and abnormal bowel can occur anywhere and can extend through a variable length of the small bowel; rarely, total intestinal aganglionosis is present.[24] The presence of the transition point at the rectosigmoid is termed short-segment aganglionosis and occurs in approximately 80% to 90% of cases. Males predominate in the incidence of short-segment aganglionosis (the boy : girl ratio is 4 : 1); however, male preponderance diminishes in longer segment involvement.

Hirschsprung disease is most commonly associated with Down syndrome, which is present in approximately 2% to 10% of patients with Hirschsprung disease, with a 5 : 1 boy to girl ratio.[24] Other syndromes associated with Hirschsprung disease include Waardenburg, Shprintzen-Goldberg, McKusick-Kaufman, Bardet-Biedl, Currarino syndrome, and with central hypoventilation (Ondine syndrome), termed *Haddad syndrome*.[24-26] Patients with longer segment aganglionosis are more likely to demonstrate Haddad syndrome than are those with short-segment disease.[27] Between 5% and 30% of patients with Hirschsprung disease have limb, skin, central nervous system, kidney, cardiac, and other malformations.[25]

Etiology   The etiology of Hirschsprung disease is not precisely known. One theory is that the migrating ganglion cells do not reach the distal segment because they are fewer in number or mature prematurely. However, it also is possible that the ganglion cells reach the distal bowel but perish or are unable to proliferate because of a deficient microenvironment.[28] Multiple genetic mutations have been identified, with the most common being the *RET* proto-oncogene located at 10q11, which is found in approximately 15% to 35% of sporadic cases and 50% of familial cases. *EDNRB,* which is located at 13q22, is identified in approximately 5% of cases.[29,30] A positive family history is encountered in a minority of patients (<10%), but this percentage increases to nearly 25% in patients with total aganglionosis, with the degree of risk proportional to the length of the affected segment and the degree of consanguinity.[31,32]

Clinical Presentation Hirschsprung disease in the neonate presents with distal obstruction, including abdominal distension and bilious vomiting. Failure to pass meconium beyond the first 24 hours is seen in up to 90% of patients.[28] Rarely, perforation of the cecum or appendix can occur in neonates, typically in those with long-segment disease.[33,34] In older children, Hirschsprung disease presents with constipation, abdominal distension, and vomiting, with failure to thrive in more severe cases. In late presentations, the zone of transition is typically low.[28]

Hirschsprung-associated enterocolitis is a major cause of morbidity and mortality in patients with Hirschsprung disease, affecting approximately 10% to 50% of patients.[28,35] Clinically it can present either insidiously or abruptly with diarrhea, fever, abdominal distension, colicky abdominal pain, and hematochezia. If the underlying diagnosis is not known, the clinical situation can be confusing, because the expected clinical finding in patients with Hirschsprung disease is constipation rather than diarrhea. The pathogenesis is unknown, but implicated mechanisms include stasis and bowel dilatation, an abnormal epithelial lining, abnormal mucin production, abnormal local immune mechanisms, and viral and bacterial pathogens, notably *Clostridium difficile*, which are promoted by initial intestinal stasis. The incidence of enterocolitis increases with delayed diagnosis, long-segment disease, and comorbid conditions, such as those found in patients with Down syndrome.[35] Postoperative risk factors include development of postoperative intestinal obstruction or development of an anastomotic leak.[35] Contrast enemas generally are not indicated but can be performed carefully with water-soluble iso-osmolal contrast with surgical consultation in cases in which the diagnosis is not certain.

Imaging In neonates, the abdominal radiographs demonstrate distal bowel obstruction (Fig. 106-10). On prone cross-table lateral radiographs, gas usually is noted in the rectum, unlike the situation with small bowel or colonic atresias; however, the caliber of the air-filled rectum is clearly smaller than that of more proximal bowel, and a zone of transition may be identifiable if it is located at the rectosigmoid junction.

Plain radiographs in older children typically do not show findings of bowel obstruction. Evidence of severe constipation is seen, with at times very marked dilatation of the colon. In patients with functional constipation, the rectum typically is the larger portion of the colon, acting as a fecal reservoir. In patients with Hirschsprung disease, the rectum may be normal in size and filled with stool, distending the aganglionic segment; however, the more proximal colon will have the larger diameter.

Radiologic diagnosis is made with contrast enema, which is geared toward identification of the zone of transition (see Fig. 106-10 and e-Fig. 106-11). Routine use of enemas prior to the diagnostic procedure should be avoided, but digital examination in the older age group should not affect the radiographic findings. The study is done with a small catheter, which should be placed as close to the external sphincter as possible in neonates. Water-soluble iso-osmolal agents are preferred in neonates, because hyperosmolal media will lead to increased bowel distension; barium is not optimal if there is another cause of obstruction, such as meconium ileus, nor desirable in case of perforation. In older patients being evaluated for constipation, barium typically is used. Initial images must be obtained in the lateral projection, as soon as the contrast begins to enter the colon, and multiple fluoroscopic stored images are used to document the flow of contrast and the caliber of the colon. Imaging should not be delayed until full colonic distension is achieved because this might obliterate the zone of transition. The enema is terminated when the zone of transition is identified.

The distal, aganglionic colon is typically normal in caliber, with a sharp transition to the dilated proximal colon. The aganglionic segment may exhibit a changing, serrated appearance as a result of aperistaltic contractions of the abnormally innervated bowel. A rectosigmoid ratio <0.9 typically will be present in patients with Hirschsprung disease. However, the rectosigmoid ratio is rarely needed to identify the zone of transition, and it can be misleading in cases of more extensive aganglionosis. Colonic evacuation is impaired in persons with Hirschsprung disease and can be assessed by comparison of a preevacuation image with postevacuation images. Postevacuation and delayed images are helpful in neonates, particularly in those with total colonic aganglionosis. In older children with constipation, delayed images are rarely helpful.

In patients with total colonic aganglionosis, radiographic diagnosis can be problematic. The colon may have a normal appearance, or there can be a pseudotransition zone, sometimes at the splenic flexure, or a microcolon (see e-Fig. 106-11).

In addition, patients with Hirschsprung disease initially can present with meconium plug or with small left colon syndrome (Fig. 106-12); such patients should be monitored carefully, and if normal bowel function does not return, further evaluation such as suction biopsy should be considered.

A definitive diagnosis is made by characteristic biopsy findings, which show absence of ganglion cells, abnormal acetylcholinesterase staining, and hypertrophied nerve fibers (see e-Fig. 106-9). Manometric studies, with failure of relaxation of the internal sphincter with rectal distension, are helpful after the immediate neonatal period.

Abdominal radiographs of patients with Hirschsprung enterocolitis may show dilatation of bowel loops, with an irregular outline consistent with spasm, along with mucosal disruption and ulceration (Fig. 106-13, *A*). Contrast enemas are not indicated, but if performed, they will show ulceration and spasm (Fig. 106-13, *B*).

Treatment Surgical repair of Hirschsprung disease is achieved by resecting the abnormal distal bowel and bringing normally innervated bowel through the sphincteric mechanism. Swenson devised and performed the first successful surgical repair; this procedure consists of resection of the aganglionic segment and anastomosis of normal bowel containing ganglion to the sphincteric mechanism. The Duhamel and Soave procedures are modifications of the Swenson procedure; they are designed to minimize risk of injury to the sphincteric

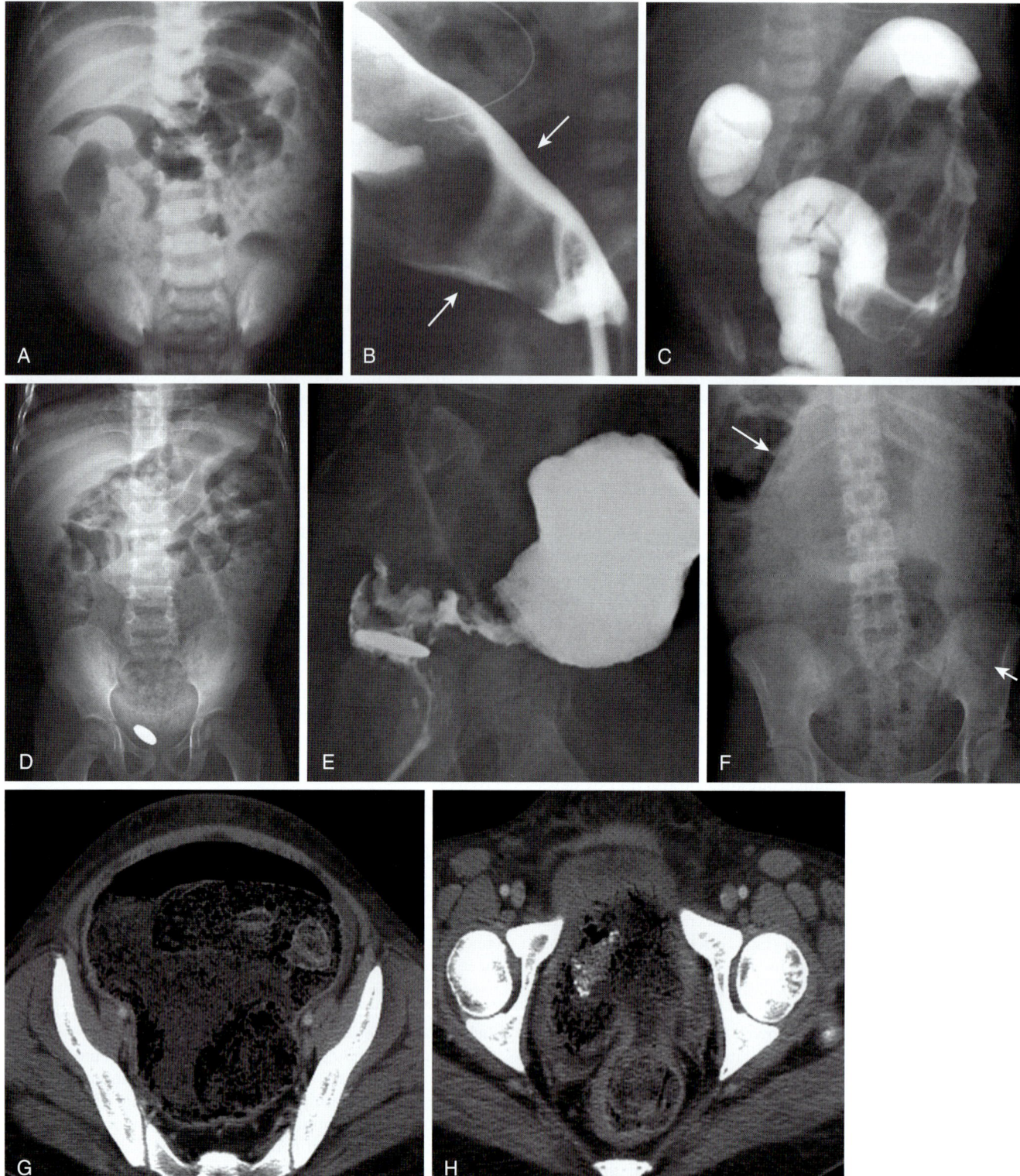

Figure 106-10 Hirschsprung disease. **A,** A supine abdominal radiograph of a 2-week-old baby with abdominal distention and inability to pass stool reveals retention of stool and dilated bowel loops. **B,** A contrast enema in a lateral projection shows the transition zone (*arrows*) at the rectosigmoid junction, which was confirmed surgically. An orogastric tube is incidentally noted. **C,** An abdominal image during a contrast enema in a 2-day-old girl with a positive family history of Hirschsprung disease and signs of distal bowel obstruction. The examination shows an abnormal distal descending colon with an irregular wall resulting from disordered contraction and an apparent transition zone at the splenic flexure. At surgery, Hirschsprung disease with transition zone at the splenic flexure was confirmed. **D,** An abdominal radiograph in a 4-year-old after surgery for repair of an interrupted aortic arch; this child presented with constipation and a retained coin within the rectum for several months. The radiograph shows marked fecal dilatation of the sigmoid, which does not extend into the rectum; the rectum contains a retained coin. **E,** A lateral view of a contrast enema in the same patient as in **D** clearly shows the zone of transition and the retained coin. **F,** An abdominal radiograph of a 15-year-old girl with diabetes and a history of intermittent diarrhea who presented acutely with diarrhea and abdominal distension. The abdominal radiograph shows marked stool burden and colonic dilatation. The sigmoid extends into the abdomen and displaces the transverse colon cephalad (*arrows*). **G,** Computed tomography (CT) for the same patient shown in **F** was requested because of a clinical concern of appendicitis. CT at the upper pelvis shows a dilated sigmoid entering the pelvis. **H,** CT lower in pelvis shows the zone of transition.

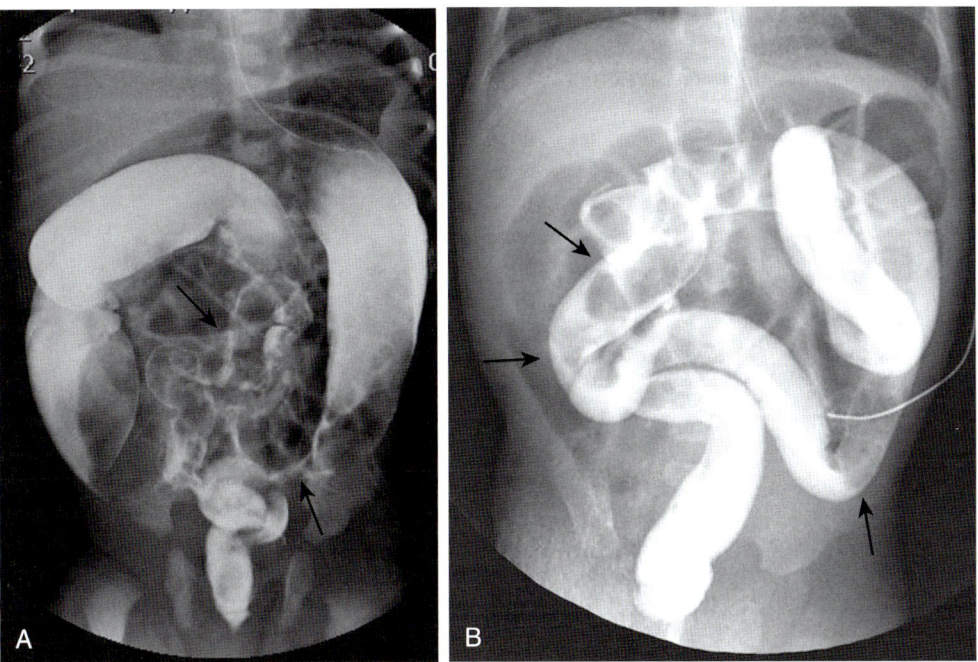

Figure 106-12 Hirschsprung disease simulating small left colon and meconium plug syndromes. **A,** A spot image from a contrast enema on a 2-day-old infant with abdominal distension shows a very small caliber sigmoid and distal descending colon (*arrows*) with a small caliber rectum, suggesting small left colon syndrome. At surgery, Hirschsprung disease was found, with a transition zone at the splenic flexure. **B,** A spot image from a contrast enema in a neonate with distal bowel obstruction demonstrates a uniform caliber colon with multiple filling defects (*arrows*) suggesting meconium plugs. At surgery, Hirschsprung disease was identified involving the entire colon and the distal 20 cm of ileum.

mechanism. The Duhamel procedure involves leaving the anterior portion of the aganglionic rectum in place and anastomosis of ganglion-containing bowel to its posterior wall. The Soave or endorectal pull-through procedure involves resection of the mucosa and submucosa of the aganglionic

bowel and pulling the normal bowel containing ganglion through the muscular rectal sleeve.

Complications include postoperative leaks, strictures, and delayed bowel control. Residual obstruction predisposes to stasis and the consequent risk of enterocolitis. Postoperatively,

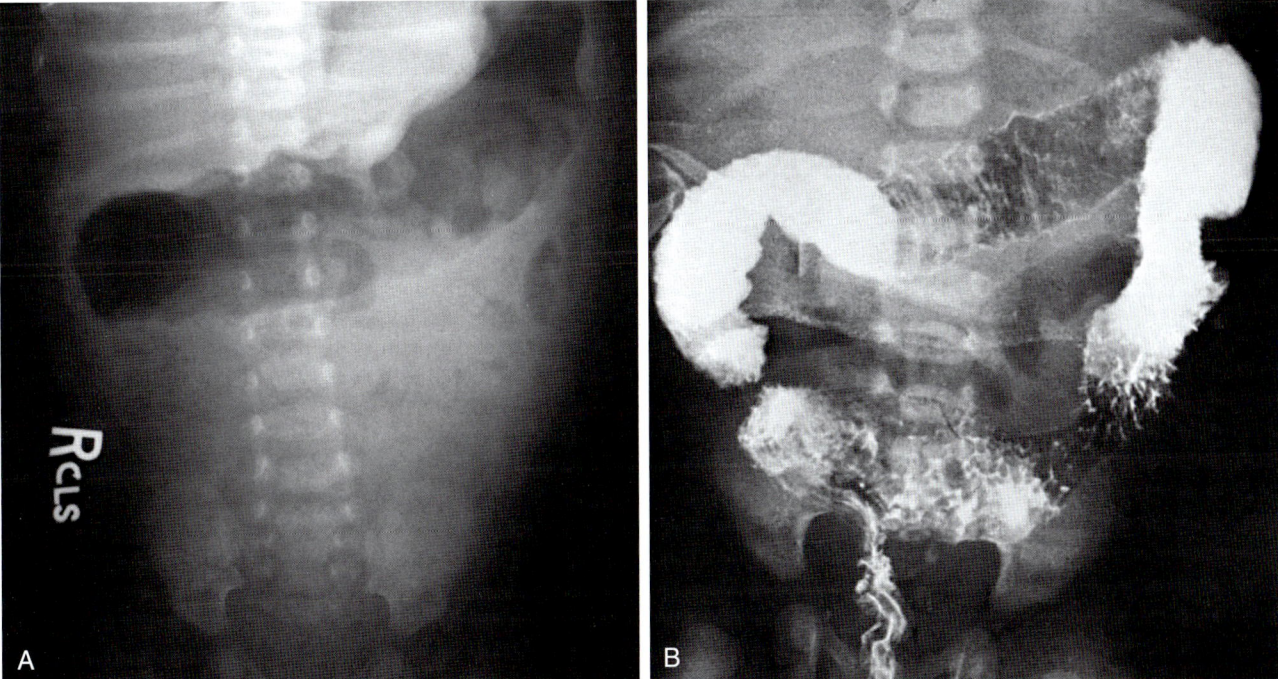

Figure 106-13 Hirschsprung enterocolitis. **A,** An abdominal radiograph of a child with Hirschsprung-associated enterocolitis shows an irregular wall in the gas-filled transverse colon. **B,** Lethal enterocolitis in a 12-day-old boy who presented with fever, foul diarrhea, and shock. A contrast enema (performed elsewhere) shows extensive edema, ulceration, and spasm. The patient died upon arrival at the referral institution.

some narrowing may be seen at the distal muscular sleeve, or the enema may appear normal except for the double density from the retained rectal pouch in patients treated with the Duhamel procedure.

Meconium Plug, Small Left Colon, and Dysmotility of Prematurity

Overview   Meconium plug and small left colon syndromes refer to conditions of colonic dysmotility that present as distal bowel obstruction in neonates and that overlap with each other as well as with Hirschsprung disease. In patients with meconium plug syndrome, a plug of meconium is identified within the colon, which, when evacuated, has a characteristic "white head" (Fig. 106-14, *A*). Small left colon syndrome also may contain meconium plugs within the colon, but in addition a variable portion of the left colon (typically the descending colon and sigmoid) have a characteristically small caliber, resembling a microcolon. In these patients, the

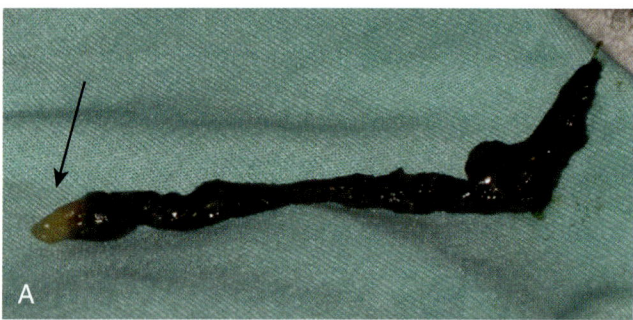

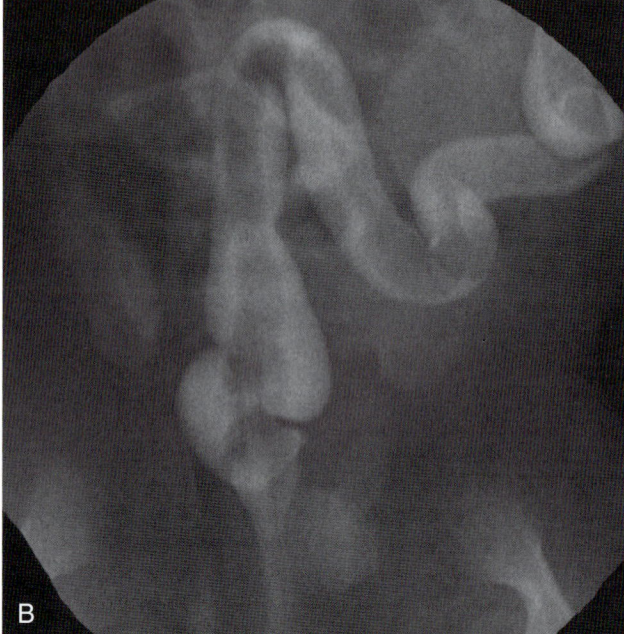

Figure 106-14   Meconium plug. **A,** A meconium plug evacuated after a diagnostic contrast enema demonstrated the distinctive white tip (*arrow*). **B,** A fluorostore image from a contrast enema in a term neonate with vomiting and bowel distension demonstrates the long filling defect characteristic of meconium plug syndrome. The child was relieved of the obstruction after evacuation of the plug, without recurrence of symptoms.

rectum typically is of normal caliber. These conditions also overlap with the failure to pass meconium and at times obstructive symptoms that may be seen in very low or extremely low birth weight infants (<1500 g and <1000 g birth weight, respectively).

Etiology   The etiology of these conditions is believed to be delayed maturation of effective peristalsis and/or abnormally increased water absorption by the colon, leading to a more tenacious meconium. Approximately 40% to 50% of small left colon syndrome cases occur in conjunction with maternal diabetes; conversely, small left colon syndrome has been cited as occurring in approximately 4.7% of infants with a history of maternal diabetes.[36]

Clinical Presentation   Presentation is abdominal distension and bilious vomiting, typically in a term infant. Symptoms may present in very low birth weight and extremely low birth weight patients in the first day of life or later, typically around 10 to 14 days of age, with increasing abdominal distension and failure to pass meconium.[37]

Meconium plug and small left colon syndromes could be the presenting findings in patients with Hirschsprung disease. It is important to monitor these patients closely after initial relief of the obstruction; if symptoms recur or do not abate, a biopsy is necessary to evaluate for Hirschsprung disease.[38]

Imaging   Abdominal radiographs show typical findings of distal obstruction with multiple dilated loops of bowel, although the degree of dilatation tends to be less than that seen in other causes of distal obstruction, such as ileal atresia or meconium ileus.[39] As with other cases of distal bowel obstruction, a diagnostic enema should be performed with water-soluble contrast material with a near iso-osmolal concentration. In cases of meconium plug, the enema demonstrates a colon of normal caliber, typically with a long filling defect caused by the meconium plug (Fig. 106-14, *B*), which the patient may evacuate at the conclusion of the enema. In patients with small left colon syndrome, the examination will reveal a small caliber colon involving a variable length of sigmoid and descending colon, with a typically normal caliber rectum (Fig. 106-15).

Treatment   Patients with meconium plug and small left colon syndrome typically do well after the enema examinations. A biopsy for Hirschsprung disease should be performed in patients who have a protracted recovery or a recurrence of symptoms. In premature infants with obstruction, treatment with enema also is advocated,[37] although the procedure entails more risks in these fragile infants.

Chronic Intestinal Pseudoobstruction

Overview   Chronic intestsinal pseudoobstruction (CIPO) refers to a characteristic, chronically recurring, and at times massive dilatation of the intestinal tract without an identifiable mechanical cause. The term encompasses a heterogeneous group of disorders that affect the enteric nervous system (ENS) and intestinal smooth muscle, resulting in

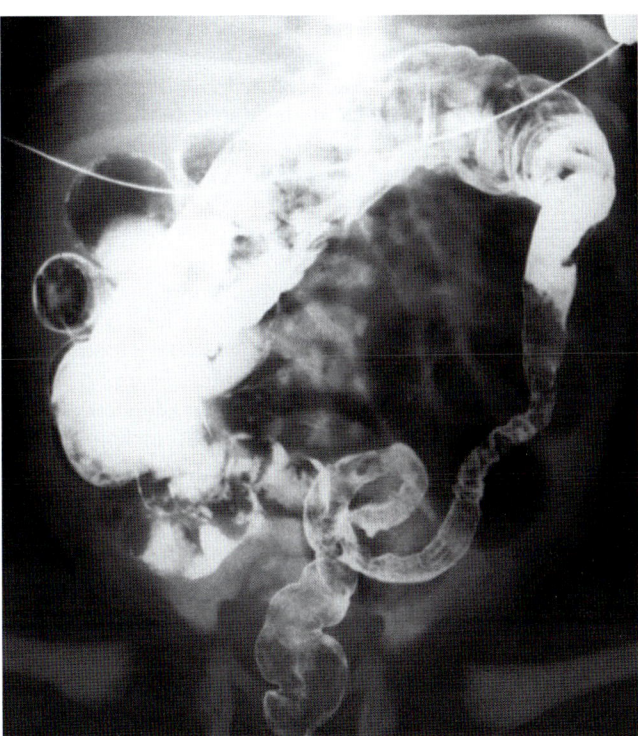

Figure 106-15 Small left colon syndrome. A contrast enema in a term child presenting with distal obstruction demonstrates a normal caliber rectum with diminished caliber of the sigmoid and descending colon, resembling a microcolon.

failure of normal intestinal motility. The condition can be primary (subdivided into neuropathic or myopathic) or secondary, when it occurs in association with various underlying systemic conditions. Patients with the myopathic form of primary disease tend to have involvement of other organ systems, particularly the urinary tract, and may require a vesicostomy.

Primary disease predominates in the pediatric population, with approximately 40% being symptomatic within the first month and 65% within the first year of life. Chronicity is defined as either congenital disease persisting during the first 2 months of life or as persistence for more than 6 months. Histopathology may demonstrate diverse findings such as hypoganglionosis, degenerative changes in smooth muscle fibers, collagen deposition, degeneration of neurons and axons, and proliferation of neurons, nerve fibers, or glial cells.

Neuronal intestinal dysplasia (NID), a form of primary CIPO, is a disorder of intestinal innervation that can be diffuse or localized. NID has two subtypes.[40] Type A consists of aplasia or hypoplasia of sympathetic innervation of the intestine and constitutes less than 5% of cases. Type B accounts for approximately 95% of cases and affects the parasympathetic system, with hyperplasia of the submucosal and myenteric plexus, the presence of dysplastic and ectopic ganglion cells, and increased acetylcholinesterase staining. Type B NID has been found in the proximal intestine of patients with Hirschsprung disease.[41-43]

Secondary disease is associated with multiple conditions, including scleroderma, dermatomyositis, muscular dystrophies, infiltrative diseases such as amyloidosis, nervous system diseases such as myotonic dystrophy, familial dysautonomia, postviral syndromes such as Epstein-Barr, cytomegalovirus,

herpes zoster and rotavirus, fetal alcohol syndrome, and mitochondrial disorders.[44]

Etiology The etiology of intestinal pseudoobstruction and neuronal dysplasia is not known. The ENS generates the rhythmic enteric activity and includes the interstitial cells of Cajal, neurons, and glial cells. The network of interstitial cells of Cajal has been found to be abnormal in some patients with CIPO, and delayed maturation of these cells has been reported in neonates with transient CIPO. Ganglion cells containing nitric oxide synthase, which mediates sphincteric relaxation, have been found to be increased in some patients with CIPO.[44] Most cases of this disease are sporadic, but familial clusters have been reported, particularly in consanguineous families, suggesting possible genetic causes.[23]

Clinical Findings Children present with periodic vomiting, diarrhea, abdominal distension, constipation, pain, and weight loss. Bacterial overgrowth can occur as a result of stasis. NID type A presents in the neonatal period with acute episodes of intestinal spasticity, diarrhea, and hematochezia. NID type B present with chronic constipation and/or pseudoobstruction, typically in the first 3 years of life.[23] Patients in whom small bowel bacterial overgrowth develops as a result of intestinal stasis may exhibit diarrhea, weight loss, and macrocytic anemia.[44]

Multiple anomalies have been documented in patients with primary CIPO. Hirschsprung disease occurs in as many as 10% of cases.[23] Related associations include multiple endocrine neoplasia (MEN) type IIb and neurofibromatosis.[45] Other associations include malrotation, anorectal malformations, congenital short small bowel, and intestinal atresia, as well as extraintestinal problems such as bladder dysfunction, Down syndrome, and histiocytosis.[23]

Imaging Radiographs and cross-sectional imaging demonstrate dilated loops of bowel, particularly the colon; air-fluid levels suggest obstruction but really represent severe adynamic ileus. Megacolon typically is found at contrast enema, without the diagnostic findings of Hirschsprung disease. Contrast small bowel and enema studies show poor motor activity in affected regions but otherwise are not specific. Gut dilatation is common in the colon, the stomach, and the small bowel and can assume massive proportions (e-Fig. 106-16).

Treatment A gastrostomy may be used for feeding (although feeding often is not tolerated) or for venting. Enteral feedings through a jejunostomy are often, but not always, tolerated. Medical management includes use of prokinetic agents and antiemetics. Management of patients with small bowel bacterial overgrowth includes vitamins, antibiotics, and possibly probiotics.[44] Some patients may need intestinal transplantation or combined hepatic and intestinal transplantation if liver failure complicates total parenteral nutrition (TPN).[44]

Megacystis-Microcolon-Intestinal Hypoperistalsis Syndrome

Overview Also known as Berdon syndrome, the megacystis-microcolon-intestinal hypoperistalsis syndrome, or MMIHS, was first described by Berdon and colleagues in 1976.[46] Approximately 182 cases currently have been reported,[41] with an approximately 2:1 female predominance.[47] Malrotation is associated in many patients.[46,47] This syndrome is considered one of the most severe forms of functional intestinal obstruction in the newborn and often is fatal.[47] Without treatment, most patients succumb within the first 6 months of life.[48]

Etiology The etiology of MMIHS is not certain, but case analyses suggest that at least some cases may have an autosomal-recessive inheritance pattern. Histology shows normal ganglion cells in most patients, but the number of these cells is decreased in some patients and increased in others, who show hyperganglionosis as well as giant ganglia.[47] Interstitial cells of Cajal are responsible for generating the electrical slow wave activity that results in coordinated smooth muscle peristaltic activity, and abnormalities in these cells have been found in the urinary bladder[49] and in the intestinal myenteric plexus[50] of patients with MMIHS. In addition, abnormalities of the smooth muscle cells themselves, with evidence of thinning, vacuolar degeneration, and increased connective tissue in both the bowel and bladder, have been found in these patients.[50-52]

Clinical Presentation Infants with MMIHS present with abdominal distension and bilious vomiting as a result of obstruction; abdominal distension is exacerbated by the dilated urinary bladder, and bowel sounds are decreased or absent.

Imaging Abdominal radiographs show marked abdominal distension and a largely gasless bowel, with the markedly distended urinary bladder displacing bowel loops. Ultrasound demonstrates the markedly distended urinary bladder, typically in association with hydroureteronephrosis. Upper gastrointestinal examination demonstrates hypoperistalsis or aperistalsis of the stomach, duodenum, and small bowel. Contrast enema demonstrates a microcolon, with malrotation in more than half of the cases (e-Fig. 106-17).[41]

Treatment Medical treatment with prokinetics and gastrointestinal hormones is usually unsuccessful, and TPN becomes necessary to sustain the infants.[41] Patients who develop complicating hepatic disease become candidates for multivisceral transplantation.[48]

Colonic Duplications

Overview Gastrointestinal duplications are discussed in Chapter 103; in this chapter findings that are characteristic of colonic duplications are discussed. Approximately 17% of all gastrointestinal duplications are colonic,[53] and approximately 5% are rectal; they can be cystic or tubular. Cystic duplications consist of a relatively small segment of duplicated bowel that typically does not communicate with the adjacent lumen. The incidence of gastric mucosa within colonic duplications is reportedly less than in other locations, and therefore they can remain asymptomatic and be discovered incidentally later in life.

Tubular duplications typically connect with the gastrointestinal tract and often drain into the perineum via a fistula, which usually is located anterior to the rectum, or drain to a single or duplicated anus. In an extensive review of 57 cases, Yousefzadeh et al.[54] defined the colon proper as that ending in a perineal anus and the duplicated colon as that ending at a perineal fistula, at a communication with the colon proper, or blindly; however, in some cases both colons end in a duplicated perineal anus or fistulae. The duplications are of variable length and can be classified as extending above or below the peritoneal reflection. If they do not extend below the peritoneal reflection and therefore do not have a perineal opening, communication with the lumen can be at both ends or at a single end. They can extend proximally to involve the cecum, appendix, and terminal ileum.

Approximately 80% of tubular colonic duplications are associated with multiple other anomalies, including renal anomalies, duplication of the genitourinary tract (e.g., uterus, bladder, urethra, or penis), and vertebral and cord abnormalities (e-Fig. 106-18). Rectal duplications are cystic structures located in the presacral space (e-Fig. 106-19).

Etiology The putative etiology of duplications was discussed in Chapter 103; the partial or abortive twinning theory invokes a split in the primitive streak during the embryonic period, with a relatively late split resulting in duplications of the colon.

Clinical Findings Diagnosis of colonic duplication varies with the type and mode of presentation. Duplications may be found incidentally, or secondary to complications. Cystic duplications will show a mass, which may be complicated by bowel obstruction due to volvulus or intussusception. Nausea, vomiting, and abdominal pain are common presenting symptoms. If the duplication has gastric mucosa, patients may become symptomatic as a result of inflammation and ulceration. Obstruction may occur through intussusception, with the duplication cyst as a leading point, or as a result of an acutely enlarging mass, obstructing the colon even if originating in adjacent small bowel (see Fig 103-35, A through C). Finally, colonic and rectal duplications may present as a second opening in the perineum. Rectal duplications can present with constipation as well as urinary obstruction; because they are located behind the rectum, they also may mimic presacral meningoceles or cystic teratomas (e-Fig. 106-19).[53,54] In girls in whom the duplication terminates in a perineal/vaginal opening, the duplication may simulate a rectovaginal fistula.

Imaging Initial suspicion on plain films can be followed up with sonography, computed tomography (CT), or MRI. Tubular duplications with a perineal fistula are best evaluated with contrast enema via both perineal orifices; antegrade contrast studies also may be useful. CT with multiplanar reconstructions and MRI likely will be diagnostic, but their exact role in evaluation remains undefined. Rectal duplications can be identified with plain films and contrast enemas via a mass effect upon the rectum and upon the adjacent genitourinary structures if they are sufficiently large. Sonography and MRI are the best modalities to evaluate noncommunicating cysts (e-Fig. 106-19), although CT also may be diagnostic if it is performed as the initial procedure. When the duplication communicates with the perineum, introduction of contrast material is diagnostic. Investigation of other organ system anomalies should be undertaken with the appropriate imaging modality.

Treatment If a presacral rectal duplication presents as an abscess, drainage is advocated as the initial treatment. Long colonic duplications can be treated by extensive fenestration between the two lumina, with resection of the perineal fistula.

Necrotizing Enterocolitis

Overview Necrotizing enterocolitis (NEC) is a termed coined in 1953[55] to describe an inflammatory condition affecting the gastrointestinal tract of neonates, most commonly premature infants who survive the first few days of life and are receiving enteral nutrition. Despite significant advances in neonatal intensive care, prevention of NEC remains an elusive goal. NEC is considered the most common newborn surgical emergency, and it has greater morbidity and mortality than all other surgical gastrointestinal conditions in this age group combined.[56] Approximately 90% of cases of NEC occur in premature infants. The incidence is inversely proportional to gestational age, with most cases occurring in infants weighing between 500 and 750 g. NEC affects up to 11.5% of infants weighing less than 750 g and 4% of infants weighing between 1250 and 1500 g.[57] Approximately 7% to 13% of cases occur in full-term infants[56]; risk factors include congenital heart disease and other conditions that affect splanchnic blood flow, such as maternal cocaine use and decreased prenatal umbilical blood flow.

A classification of enterocolitis severity based on clinical parameters was suggested in 1978 by Bell and colleagues,[58] and with modifications, it is still used today.[59,60] Stage I is sensitive but nonspecific, as it includes infants in whom NEC is suspected but not definitely diagnosed. Stage IIA is mild but definite NEC, stage IIB is NEC of moderate severity, stage IIIA refers to advanced NEC, and stage IIIB refers to NEC that has advanced to intestinal perforation.

Etiology The most important risk factors for the development of NEC are prematurity and enteral feedings, which have been instituted in 90% of infants in whom NEC develops. Premature neonates have poorly developed intestinal motility that leads to stasis and altered ability to maintain homeostasis between proinflammatory and antiinflammatory compounds, to regulate splanchnic vasoconstriction and blood flow, and to maintain mucosal integrity. Proinflammatory compounds that are upregulated in NEC include platelet activating factor, tumor necrosis factor, and certain types of interleukins, leukotrienes, and oxygen free radicals. Accelerated apoptosis resulting from overproduction of inflammatory compounds has been shown to result in a break at the villus tip of the intestinal mucosal barrier, facilitating bacterial translocation and the inflammatory cascade.[56,57,61]

Clinical Findings In Bell stage I disease, the infant exhibits relatively nonspecific symptoms, including systemic signs such as apnea, bradycardia, and temperature instability and abdominal signs consisting of abdominal distension, hemoccult positive stools, and increased gastric residuals. These signs also could be present in patients with other conditions, such as

sepsis, and therefore they are sensitive but relatively nonspecific. By the time the child reaches stage IIA, clinical findings include abdominal tenderness and grossly bloody stools; by stage IIB, the child has progressed to thrombocytopenia and mild acidosis, as well as abdominal wall edema and tenderness. Infants with severe stage IIIA disease have metabolic and respiratory acidosis requiring intubation and signs of disseminated intravascular coagulation, with worsening abdominal wall erythema, edema, and induration. Patients with stage IIIB disease show clinical evidence of shock and gut perforation.

Complications of NEC in survivors relate to whether short bowel syndrome has developed after resection, with dependence on TPN and its attendant complications. Strictures occur in 9% to 36% of NEC survivors, most often in the colon (70% to 80%), with 21% of these strictures at the splenic flexure. Strictures are more common after medical management and present with failure to gain weight, rectal bleeding, or signs and symptoms of obstruction.[5,56]

Imaging Abdominal radiographs have been the mainstay of imaging NEC, and the Bell criteria therefore have corresponding radiographic findings (Fig. 106-20). Findings of radiographs of infants with Bell stage I disease, similar to the physical findings, are nonspecific, demonstrating a normal bowel gas pattern or a mild ileus. Radiographic findings of stage IIA disease are more specific; an ileus pattern and focal pneumatosis can be seen. As the child's disease progresses to stage IIB, radiographs show extensive pneumatosis with or without portal venous gas and ascites (see Fig. 106-20, *A* and *B*). Stage IIIA demonstrates more prominent ascites and persistent bowel loops, and pneumoperitoneum is the hallmark of stage IIIB disease (see Fig. 106-20, *C*). Periodic imaging is important and is used more frequently in patients who have more advanced disease.

Intramural gas has a characteristic appearance as it wraps around the subserosa of the involved bowel loops. When the lumen is filled with gas, the mucosa and submucosa are outlined as a white line bounded by gas in the lumen centrally and subserosal intramural gas peripherally[62] (see Fig. 106-20, *A*). When perforation is suspected, a horizontal beam radiograph is important to assess for small amounts of free air that may be difficult to detect with routine radiographs taken in the supine position.

Ultrasound has been shown to be useful and often complementary to radiography. Ultrasound can depict intramural and portal venous gas in many cases and can provide additional information about the presence, character and amount of ascites, the presence or absence of peristalsis, thickness of the bowel wall, and blood flow. Early in NEC, the bowel wall is thickened, loses the differential echogenicity of its layers, and becomes hyperemic; as the disease progresses, the bowel wall becomes thin and blood flow can no longer be detected.[62]

Patients in whom strictures develop may be evaluated with fluoroscopic examinations, typically contrast enema; 80% of strictures develop in the colon, and 15% develop in the terminal ileum[56] (Fig. 106-21).

Treatment Initial treatment of patients with NEC is medical, with fluid resuscitation, antibiotics, and TPN. If medical treatment fails, surgery may be indicated. The principal goals

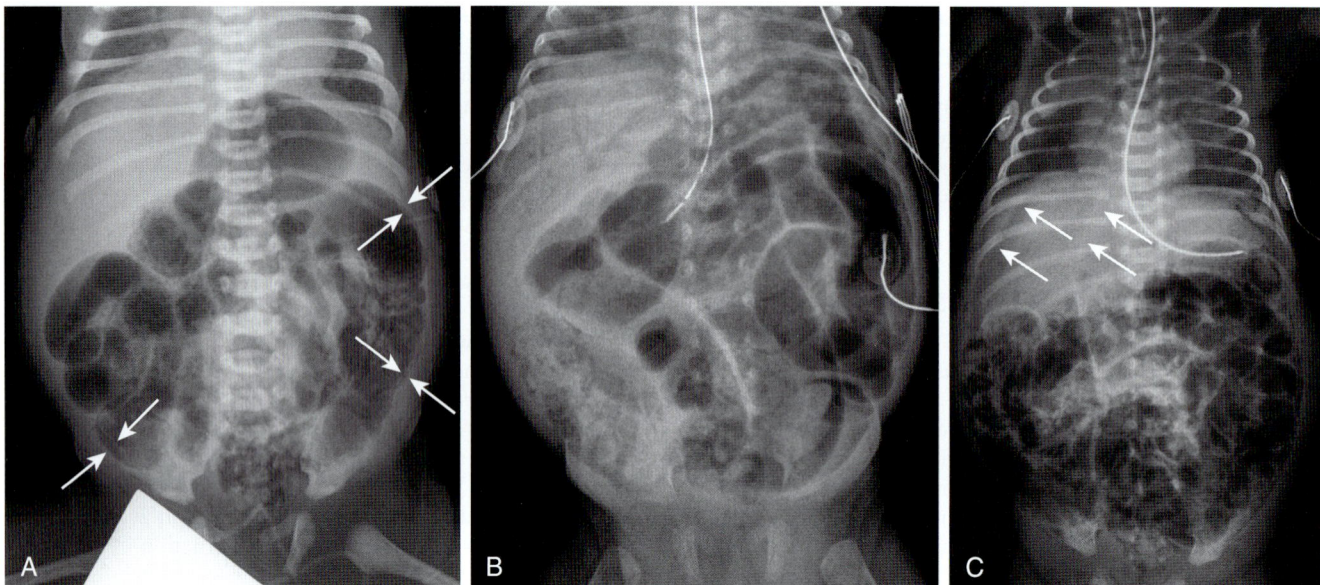

Figure 106-20 Necrotizing enterocolitis—acute. **A,** Supine abdominal radiograph of a 7-day-old male premature infant presenting with abdominal distension and hematochezia demonstrates dilated loops of bowel and extensive pneumatosis. Arrows point to examples of areas in which the mucosa and submucosa are outlined as a white line bounded by luminal and subserosal gas. **B,** A supine abdominal radiograph of a 29-day-old premature infant progressing to acidosis and shock. In addition to marked abdominal distension, there is intramural gas and extensive portal venous gas seen over the liver. **C,** A supine chest and abdomen radiograph of a 10-day-old premature infant with extensive necrotizing enterocolitis progressing to perforation and free intraperitoneal air. Thin arrows point to the edge of the free air overlying the liver, and thicker arrows point to the outline of the falciform ligament. The patient is intubated and shows pulmonary abnormalities consistent with edema and atelectasis.

of surgical intervention are to remove bowel that has become gangrenous while preserving intestinal length. Optimal surgical timing, when the bowel is gangrenous but has not yet perforated, is difficult to define clinically or by imaging.[56] Further, perforation is not always clinically or radiographically obvious; in fact, pneumoperitoneum in infants with surgically proven perforation is present in only approximately 63% of cases.[56] Sonographic findings associated with adverse outcome include focal fluid collections and three or more additional

findings: increased bowel wall echogenicity, bowel wall thickening or thinning, free fluid with internal echoes, absent bowel wall perfusion, and intramural gas.[63] Additional criteria that suggest gangrene prior to perforation include abdominal wall erythema, fixed appearance of intestinal loop(s) on radiography or ultrasound, and clinical deterioration while receiving medical therapy.[56,62] Patients with perforation who are deemed very poor surgical candidates may undergo initial peritoneal drainage.[56,62]

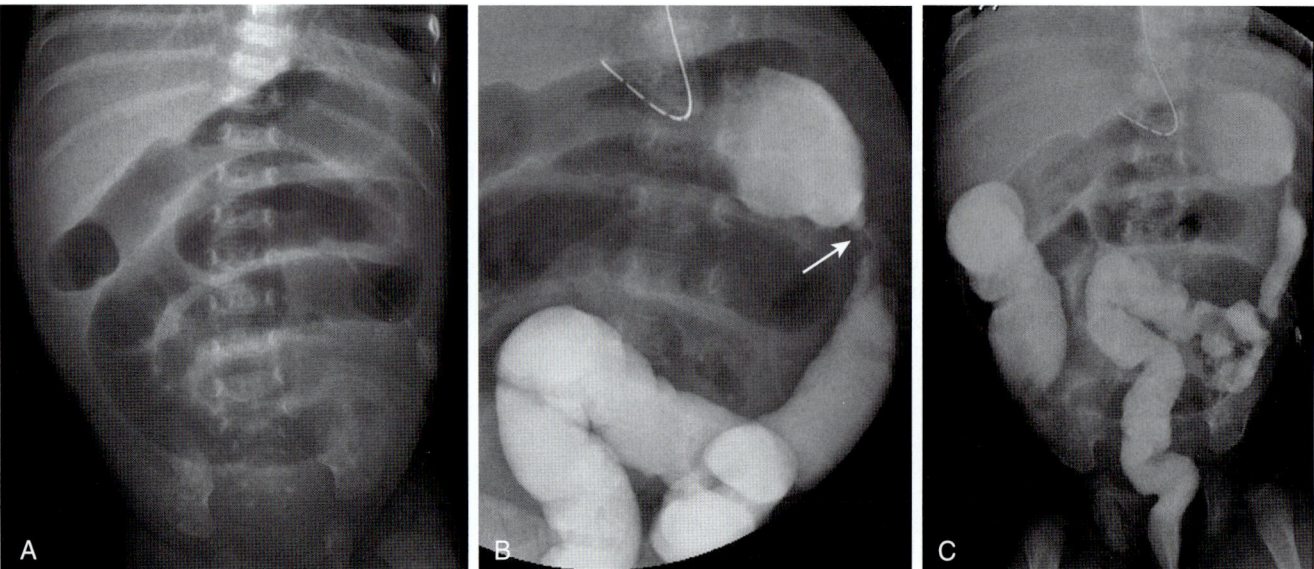

Figure 106-21 Necrotizing enterocolitis (NEC)—development of strictures. **A,** An abdominal radiograph of 7-week-old premature infant with a history of NEC who presents with increasing residuals, vomiting, and abdominal distension shows dilated loops of bowel consistent with a distal, partial obstruction. **B,** A spot image from a contrast enema demonstrates an area of narrowing in the proximal descending colon, consistent with a stricture. **C,** An overhead radiograph confirms the partial obstruction at the site of the post-NEC stricture, which was confirmed surgically.

Key Points

Colonic atresia is uncommon, representing between 1.8% and 15% of all intestinal atresias.

Approximately 95% of patients with anorectal malformations have a fistula to the urethra, vagina, or perineum; however, patients with Down syndrome rarely have fistulae.

The Currarino triad consists of a sacral anomaly, an anorectal malformation, and a presacral mass, but other malformations may coexist.

Histopathologic findings in patients with Hirschsprung disease show absent ganglion cells, hypertrophied nerve fibers, and increased acetylcholinesterase staining.

Findings of patients with Hirschsprung disease when a contrast enema is performed include a zone of transition between aganglionic segment and dilated proximal bowel and an irregular outline as a result of irregular nonperistaltic contractions of the aganglionic segment.

Findings in total colonic aganglionosis include normal findings, microcolon, and apparent zone of transition.

Meconium plug and small left colon syndrome are considered functional obstructions and usually are transient.

Primary CIPO is most common in children and is subdivided into neuropathic and myopathic forms.

MMIHS presents within the first 6 months of life, has a poor prognosis, and malrotation is common.

Unlike other types of duplications, tubular duplications of the colon usually (but not always) connect to the gastrointestinal tract and often drain to the perineum.

NEC is most commonly seen in premature infants who have received enteral nutrition. When full-term infants are affected, comorbidity is usually present, such as congenital heart disease.

Suggested Readings

Cox SG, et al. Colonic atresia: spectrum of presentation and pitfalls in management. A review of 14 cases. *Pediatr Surg Int.* 2005;21(10): 813-818.

Emil S, et al. Meconium obstruction in extremely low-birth-weight neonates: guidelines for diagnosis and management. *J Pediatr Surg.* 2004;39(5): 731-737.

Epelman M, et al. Necrotizing enterocolitis: review of state-of-the-art imaging findings with pathologic correlation. *Radiographics.* 2007;27(2): 285-305.

Levitt MA, Pena A. Anorectal malformations. *Orphanet J Rare Dis.* 2007;2:33.

Martucciello G, et al. Associated anomalies in intestinal neuronal dysplasia. *J Pediatr Surg.* 2002;37(2):219-223.

Puri P, Shinkai M. Megacystis microcolon intestinal hypoperistalsis syndrome. *Semin Pediatr Surg.* 2005;14(1):58-63.

Swenson O. How the cause and cure of Hirschsprung's disease were discovered. *J Pediatr Surg.* 1999;34(10):1580-1581.

References

Full references for this chapter can be found on www.expertconsult.com.

Chapter 107

Inflammatory and Infectious Diseases

KIMBERLY E. APPLEGATE and NANCY R. FEFFERMAN

Inflammatory Bowel Disease

Inflammatory bowel disease (IBD) affects approximately 1 million Americans; the incidence is equal in males and females, and the peak onset is in adolescence or early adulthood. Both ulcerative colitis and Crohn disease represent a chronic inflammatory process without a known specific cause. Ulcerative colitis primarily involves the colon, whereas Crohn disease involves primarily the small intestine. The distinction between ulcerative colitis and Crohn disease defies classification in as many as 10% of patients. In children, the presentation may be nonspecific, leading to a delay in diagnosis that ranges from months to years.[1] Clinical and laboratory markers for active disease are inadequate; therefore repeated imaging is. common, especially in patients with Crohn disease.[2,3]

ETIOLOGY, PATHOPHYSIOLOGY, AND CLINICAL PRESENTATION

Ulcerative Colitis

Chronic ulcerative colitis is an idiopathic inflammatory disease of the colon that typically affects older children and young adults; an infantile form has been described that is devastating and often fatal (e-Fig.107-1). The disease is characterized by mucosal inflammation, edema, and ulceration, and it is accompanied by submucosal edema in the early stages and fibrosis in the later stages. Transmural disease is uncommon. The disease may be localized in the distal colon, or it may spread to involve the entire colon and the terminal ileum. Skip areas are not characteristic, and their presence should raise the diagnosis of Crohn disease.

Fatal outcomes are less common than previously, but they still occur. Bloody diarrhea may appear explosively in as many as one third of affected patients, but the majority come to medical attention with progressive chronic diarrhea. Occasional patients are seen with toxic megacolon, in which marked dilation of the large bowel, primarily the transverse colon, is seen. Many children are first seen with nongastrointestinal symptoms, of which severe growth retardation is the most common and clinically striking. Arthritis may precede the colon symptoms; typically, it is monoarticular or pauciarticular and affects large joints, although seronegative spondyloarthropathy is seen in some affected males. Skin rashes, uveitis, digital clubbing, stomal ulcers, and hepatic dysfunction (primary sclerosing cholangitis and autoimmune hepatitis) occur in a variable number of children, but less frequently than in adults. Patients with ulcerative colitis for 10 years or longer are at risk for colonic carcinomas, which arise in areas of dysplastic mucosa rather than in adenomatous polyps, and may be multiple.

Crohn Disease

Crohn disease that affects the small bowel is discussed in Chapter 105. The disease can affect the colon and the small intestine. Two features that favor the diagnosis of Crohn disease over ulcerative colitis are the frequent sparing of the rectum, and the presence of skip areas in Crohn disease. Colonoscopy is often the initial examination in patients with suspected Crohn colitis, because it allows visualization of early changes and permits biopsy for diagnosis. Capsule endoscopy is commonly used in both adult and pediatric practice to visualize small-bowel abnormalities.[4]

IMAGING

Ulcerative Colitis

Abdominal radiographs are most often nonspecific; typically, they show an absence of recognizable stool from affected colonic segments, and they may show evidence of mucosal edema or "thumbprinting" (Fig. 107-2).[5] Patients with toxic megacolon should not undergo contrast enemas because of the high risk of perforation.

Double-contrast barium enema, formerly the diagnostic imaging procedure of choice, has been replaced by colonoscopy with biopsy.[4,6] Ulcerative colitis always affects the rectum, with contiguous proximal involvement. Skip areas do not occur, although different parts of the colon may not be equally affected. The terminal ileum may become secondarily affected when there is proximal colonic involvement; terminal ileal involvement is known as *backwash ileitis* (e-Fig. 107-3). Ultimately, the colonic wall becomes stiff, shortened, and tubular—the "lead pipe" colon—secondary to fibrosis of the submucosa (e-Fig.107-4). Late-stage disease produces presacral thickening, and retroperitoneal fibrosis is a rare complication.

Computed tomography (CT) or magnetic resonance imaging (MRI) can be performed to investigate disease activity (abdominal pain, fever, or other symptoms), to diagnose complications, or to identify associated liver or biliary disease.[7,8] When ulcerative colitis is active, cross-sectional imaging shows colonic wall enhancement with preservation

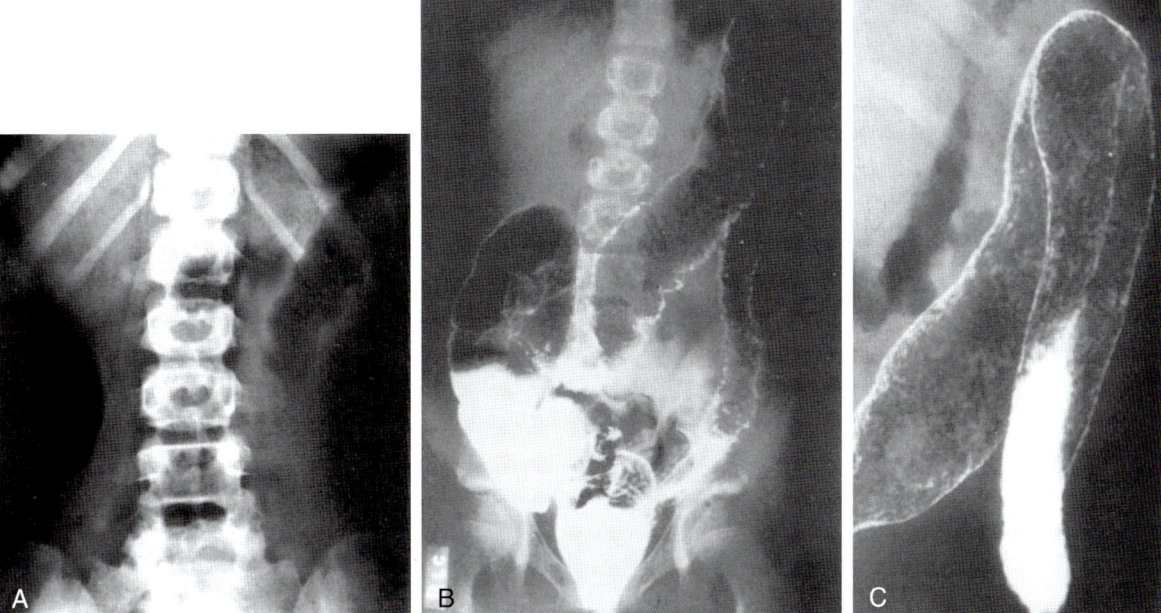

Figure 107-2   Ulcerative colitis in a 14-year-old girl. **A,** Abdominal radiograph shows "thumbprinting" of the distal transverse colon, suggesting submucosal edema. **B,** Double-contrast enema shows granularity and irregularity of the colonic mucosa. Small ulcerations are seen throughout the transverse colon and the descending colon. The entire colon was involved. **C,** Coned-down view of the splenic flexure shows multiple areas of pseudopolyps.

of the smooth outer contour of the bowel (e-Fig.107-5). Surrounding fat stranding, mesenteric adenopathy, ascites, and, when perforation occurs, abscesses may also be evident, but extramural changes are much less common than in Crohn disease. In chronic ulcerative colitis, fatty changes may occur in the submucosa.

Crohn Disease

As with ulcerative colitis, double-contrast barium enemas are seldom used today for diagnosis or monitoring of disease activity. Characteristic aphthous ulcers are small and superficial, seen as an elevated edematous halo with a central umbilication caused by barium in the shallow ulcer crater. Eventually, the inflammation becomes transmural, and the characteristic "rose thorn" configuration develops from deep ulcers that extend into the thickened bowel wall. A "cobblestone" pseudopolyposis pattern, similar to that seen in the small intestine, may be apparent: areas of edematous mucosa separated by areas of denuded mucosa and deep ulcerations.[9] Small-bowel follow-through (SBFT) examinations can identify complications of diseases that affect the colon, and sequelae such as enteric fistulae (Fig. 107-6). Enteroclysis is helpful in unmasking focal areas of disease activity, such as strictures (e-Fig. 107-7). Crohn disease is more likely to lead to colonic strictures than is ulcerative colitis.

CT and MRI are very useful in evaluation of the disease activity and its complications (see Chapter 105). Extent of extramural inflammatory changes and affected loops of bowel can be identified, as can development of abscess or colonic strictures (Figs. 107-8 and 107-9).

Newer imaging techniques include CT or MR enterography and CT or MR enteroclysis, which hold promise in improving the identification of disease activity and its complications. In CT enterography, the patient drinks a negative bowel contrast agent that distends the lumen more than water

or traditional positive contrast and that does not mask vascular mucosal enhancement.[10,11] CT enteroclysis, like small-bowel enteroclysis, is performed by using high-flow contrast introduced via nasoduodenal intubation. It is more invasive than enterography, but it provides a more controlled volume challenge to the bowel in order to define the presence of sinus tracts and fistulae and to differentiate stricture from inflammation of the bowel wall.[12] CT enteroclysis has shown value in both detecting and excluding partial small-bowel

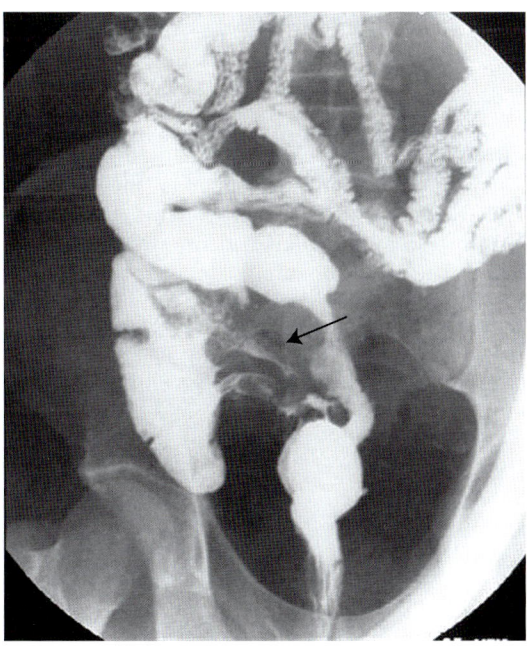

Figure 107-6   Active Crohn disease with fistula formation on small-bowel follow-through. The fistula (*arrow*) extends between the ileum and the medial wall of the cecum.

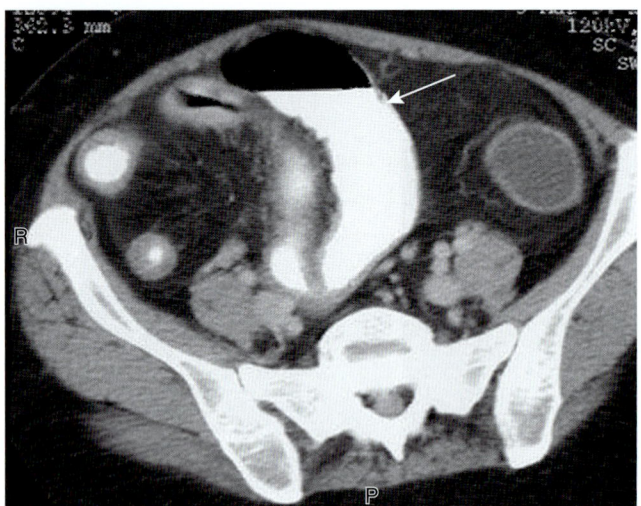

Figure 107-8 Active Crohn disease in a 19-year-old. Computed Tomography shows the distended ileum (*arrow*) proximal to the thick-walled ileal loops and mesenteric stranding and vascular engorgement, resulting from active inflammation. Mural thickening and vascular engorgement of colonic segments is apparent. Positive oral contrast in the lumen interferes with evaluation of mucosal enhancement.

obstruction and to guide specific therapies in these challenging patients.

Increasingly, pediatric centers are using MR imaging, rather than CT to avoid radiation exposure.[2] Magnetic resonance enterography (MRE) yields equivalent images of the small and large intestine and the intraabdominal organs.[13,14] MRE is able to differentiate active inflammation from chronic inflammation in the layers of the bowel wall. Furthermore, CT and MRE are able to identify intraperitoneal complications such as fistulae and abscesses. MRE is also superior to CT for the diagnosis and management of perianal fistulae (Fig. 107-10).[15-17] Some centers will image the entire abdomen and pelvis during these MR studies, because these patients may have inflammatory processes that involve the liver, pancreas, or biliary tree.

TREATMENT

Initial treatment of both ulcerative colitis and Crohn disease is with medical therapy to suppress the inflammation. However, the majority of Crohn patients (up to 80%) and one third of ulcerative colitis patients will end up needing surgery.[18,19] The most common reasons for surgery in Crohn

patients are small-bowel obstructions that do not respond to medical therapy because of bowel stricture or adhesion, and bowel perforation that leads to abscess. The most common reason for surgery in pediatric ulcerative colitis patients is active disease that does not respond to medical management or that leads to complications.

Pseudomembranous Colitis

Pseudomembranous colitis refers to severe colonic disease that occurs in approximately 15% to 25% of patients with antibiotic-associated diarrhea.[20]

ETIOLOGY

The toxins produced by the bacterium *Clostridium difficile* are the most important cause of antibiotic-associated pseudomembranous colitis.[20,21] Other, less common toxins include those produced by *C. perfringens* and *Staphylococcus aureus*. The diagnosis is a clinical and laboratory one, it is more common in adults than in children, and it is rare in infants. Recently, studies have shown an association of recurrent *C. difficile* colitis in patients who had undergone remote appendectomy, suggesting a role of immune protection by the normal appendix.[22,23]

CLINICAL PRESENTATION

Pseudomembranous colitis is characterized by fever, bloody diarrhea, cramping, and colonic mucositis. The condition most commonly follows antibiotic therapy and occurs in hospitalized patients who are often debilitated, immunocompromised, or recovering from surgery. However, it may occur without preceding antibiotic therapy in patients in whom the gut flora has been altered, such as after weaning or surgery. The onset of diarrhea may occur within weeks after cessation of antibiotic therapy.

IMAGING

The radiographic findings are similar to those of the other colitides.[24] Enema is not necessary and should be avoided, particularly in severe cases, to avoid the risk of perforation. Ultrasound (US), MR, or CT findings of pancolitis, with or without ascites, suggest the diagnosis in the appropriate clinical setting.[25,26]

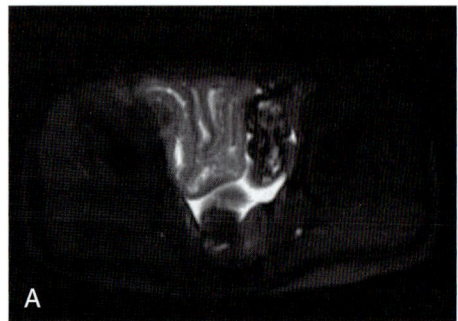
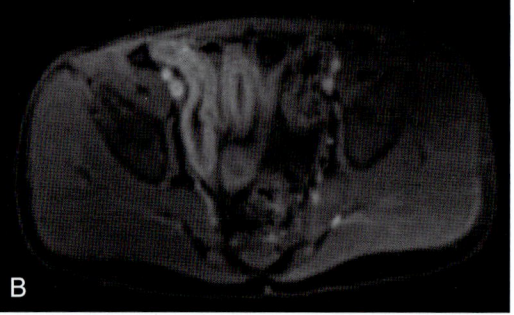

Figure 107-9 Magnetic resonance enterography of active Crohn disease in an 8-year-old boy. **A,** T2-weighted axial image of the pelvis shows several thickened, contiguous loops of terminal ileum that represent active Crohn disease. **B,** After gadolinium administration, bright signal enhancement appears in the bowel wall relative to normal adjacent colon and rectum.

Figure 107-10 Magnetic resonance image (MRI) of perianal fistula in a girl with a new diagnosis of Crohn disease. **A,** Initial axial computed tomography shows of perianal inflammation and small abscesses partially encircling the anus. **B-C,** Axial postcontrast fat-saturated MRI demonstrates the superior image contrast of the findings compared with CT. Exuberant inflammation (*enhancement*) and small abscesses nearly circumscribe the anus. **D,** Perianal abscesses in sagittal view (*arrow*). **E,** Superficial position of the drain (*arrow*) relative to the more deep position of the perianal abscess seen in image *D*. The patient required diverting colostomy to successfully treat her perianal disease. (Reprinted with kind permission of Springer Science+Business Media from Anupindi S, Ayyala R, Kelsen J, Mamula P, Applegate KE. Imaging of inflammatory bowel disease in children. In: Medina LS, Applegate KE, Blackmore CC, eds. *Evidence-based imaging in pediatrics: optimizing imaging in pediatric patient care*. New York: Springer Science+Business Media; 2010.)

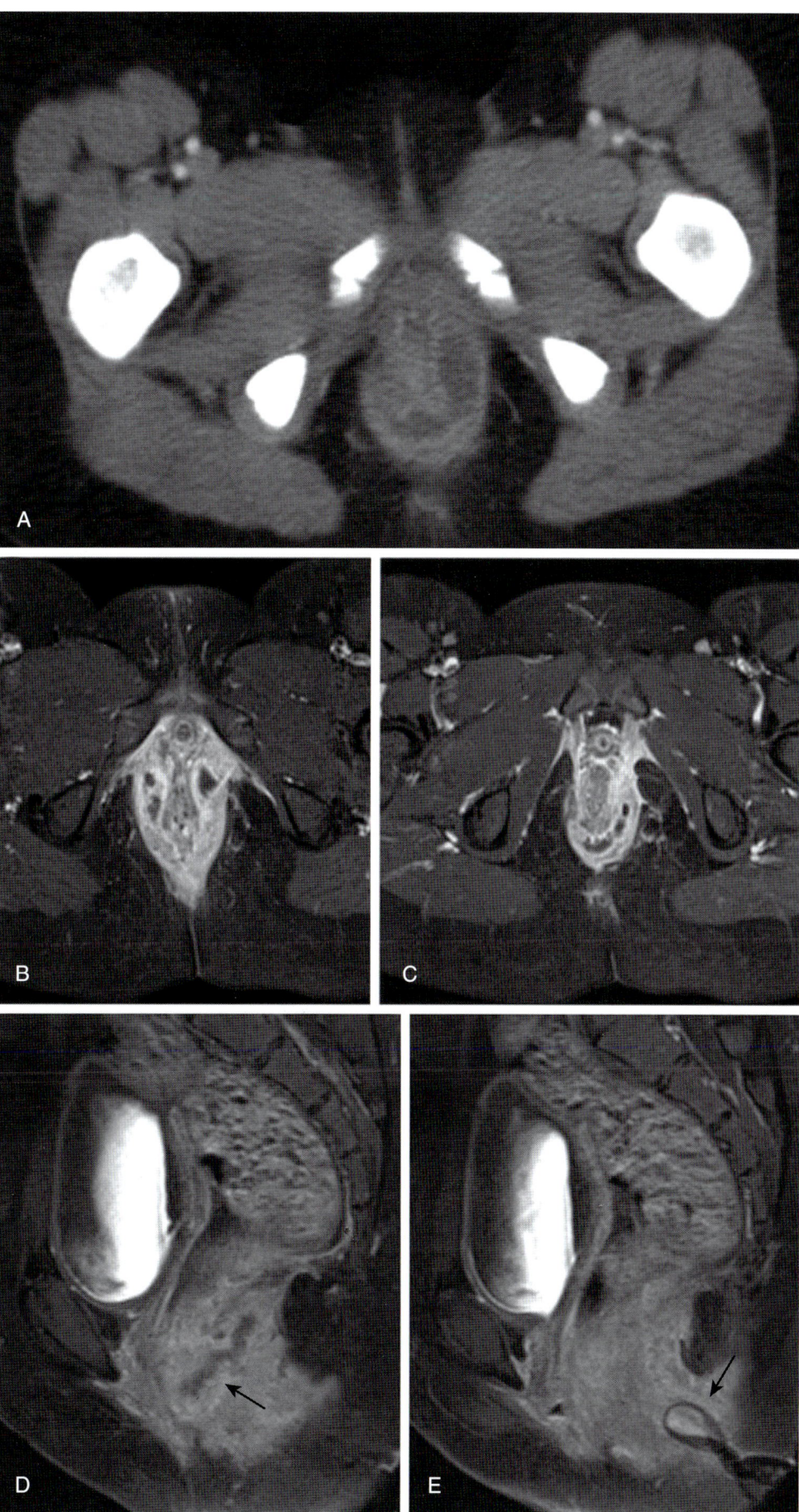

TREATMENT

Preceding antibiotic therapy associated with the colitis should be stopped. The first line of antibiotic treatment is oral metronidazole. Other oral or intravenous (IV) antibiotics may be needed in some patients initially and in the minority who have recurrence.

Hemolytic Uremic Syndrome

The hemolytic uremic syndrome (HUS) is a condition characterized by renal failure and the destruction of red blood cells. In children, it is related to foods such as undercooked meat in 90% of cases. The syndrome has a peak incidence of approximately 6.1 per 100,000 in children aged less than 5 years.[27]

ETIOLOGY

Most cases are caused by a Shiga-like toxin produced by *Escherichia coli* serotype 0157:H7, found in raw or incompletely cooked beef and unpasteurized dairy products. Additional toxins are produced by other bacterial agents and include *Shigella, Salmonella, Yersinia,* and *Campylobacter.* Hemorrhagic colitis is common. Renal and central nervous system complications can markedly affect the course and prognosis of this disease.[28]

CLINICAL PRESENTATION

This syndrome is most common during the summer months in children younger than 5 years of age. HUS usually has a gastrointestinal prodrome of diarrhea that precedes clinical evidence of acute renal failure, fever, anemia, and thrombocytopenia.[28-30] A positive stool culture for the specific Shiga toxin–producing *E. coli* pathogen is definitive when positive. Serologic tests for antibodies to the Shiga toxin or to the lipopolysaccharide 0157 can be done, although these are not widely available.[27]

IMAGING

US, CT, or occasionally contrast enema is generally requested before the correct diagnosis is made. The findings consist of thickening of the wall of the involved bowel segment, more typically the colon, seen as "thumbprinting" on abdominal radiographs or contrast enema, and marked bowel wall thickening on CT or US.[31] The involved segments are typically in continuity without skip lesions, and pancolitis can occur. Fat stranding and free fluid are often seen near the involved segments.[32] Toxic megacolon and colonic perforation have been reported, and colonic strictures can occur as a late complication.[33]

TREATMENT

The treatment for HUS is supportive and may include IV fluids, blood or blood products, and supportive renal dialysis if needed.[34] Children with Shiga-like toxin *E. coli* tend to recover renal function in 55% to 70% of cases.[27]

Radiation Colitis

Ionizing radiation treatment may cause acute inflammation during therapy. Later, chronic symptoms may be related to chronic inflammation or stricture. These changes can occur months to years after exposure and may involve the small bowel, colon, or rectum. Endarteritis, with end-vessel and microvascular circulation compromise, is the hallmark of supervening chronic ischemia.[35]

ETIOLOGY

Radiation injury leads to activation of mucosal cytokines and increased levels of inflammatory mediators such as interleukin (IL)-2, -6 and -8.[36] Factors that affect the development of radiation colitis include patient comorbidities and, most importantly, the total radiation dose and the volume of bowel irradiated; radiation enteritis tends to develop in patients who have received on the order of 45 Gy, but it can occur with doses as low as 5 to 12 Gy.[35,37]

CLINICAL PRESENTATION

Diarrhea, cramping, and sometimes lower intestinal bleeding are the key clinical features of the acute phase, which is usually self-limiting. Eventually, fibrosis may occur, which leads to stiffness and loss of mobility of the affected portions of the colon. Chronic radiation colitis is a progressive, precancerous disease. Additional complications include partial obstruction and fragility of the bowel, which may culminate in perforation.[36] Diarrhea and abdominal pain are additional symptoms in patients with chronic radiation colitis.[36]

IMAGING

Patients with radiation colitis do not usually undergo imaging examinations during the acute phase. Fluoroscopic imaging with either SBFT or contrast enema may delineate the chronic, fibrotic change to the affected colon (e-Fig. 107-11). CT and MR show relatively nonspecific findings of bowel wall thickening; however, the diagnostic finding is the distribution of these changes within the radiation port.[35]

TREATMENT

Treatment is related to symptom relief and includes dietary changes with reduction of fat and lactose intake in addition to medications for nausea and diarrhea. Management of patients with chronic disease can be challenging; as many as 30% of patients my require surgery for fistulae, perforation, or bowel obstruction that does not respond to nonsurgical management.[37]

Neutropenic Colitis

Neutropenic colitis, also known as *typhlitis,* is a necrotizing colitis primarily seen in children with hematopoietic malignancies, although it is also seen in children with solid tumors who undergo high-dosage chemotherapy.[38] There are no definitive diagnostic criteria, although diagnosis is typically made when clinical and imaging findings are suggestive.

ETIOLOGY

Development of the condition is associated with chemotherapy-related low neutrophil counts; acute lymphocytic and myelogenous leukemia are the most common underlying malignancies in pediatric patients.

The disease most often affects the cecum, hence the term *typhlitis*. The appendix may be involved and may produce clinical findings that mimic acute appendicitis.[39] Edema and inflammation of the colon, including the distal ileum, may occur, and pneumatosis, perforation, or abscess may supervene.

CLINICAL PRESENTATION

This condition occurs in less than 5% of children with neutropenia. Abdominal pain, diarrhea, fever, and distended abdomen are the common presenting symptoms.

IMAGING

Radiographs are typically nonspecific and may show a focal ileus in the right lower quadrant. Often, a sentinel loop of dilated terminal ileum may be seen.[40] Because the clinical presentation may mimic acute appendicitis, cross-sectional imaging is a critical diagnostic differentiating tool. US shows a markedly thickened cecal wall that may be either hyperechoic or hypoechoic.[41] Intraluminal fluid and ascites may also be identified. CT shows marked thickening of the affected portions of the colon, which is usually more marked in the cecum; surrounding inflammatory change; and free fluid (Fig. 107-12).[42] Extension of this process may involve the terminal ileum.

TREATMENT

Management most often is conservative and includes antibiotics, but on occasion, bowel resection is necessary. Recovery is more related to the presence and severity of comorbidities than to the neutropenic colitis.[43]

Infectious Colitis

The infectious colitides are usually caused by the same agents that affect the small bowel, discussed in Chapter 105. Imaging studies are rarely needed and, when performed, usually show nonspecific colitis.[31]

Fibrosing Colonopathy

Fibrosing colonopathy was first described in 1994 in patients with cystic fibrosis (CF) who received lipase replacement therapy.[44]

ETIOLOGY

With the introduction of oral, enteric-coated, high-dose pancreatic enzyme medication, clinicians increased the amount of enzyme supplements to many of these patients. Some that

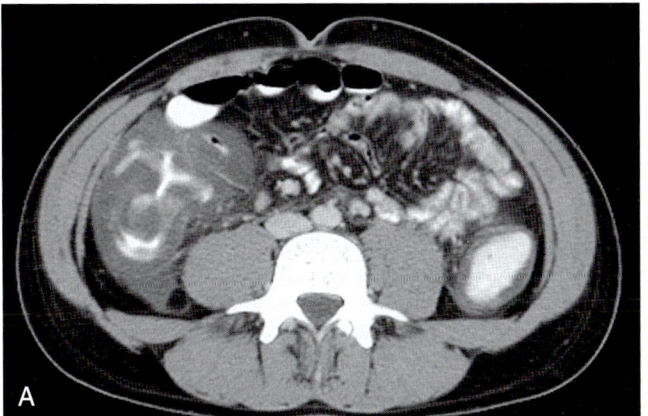
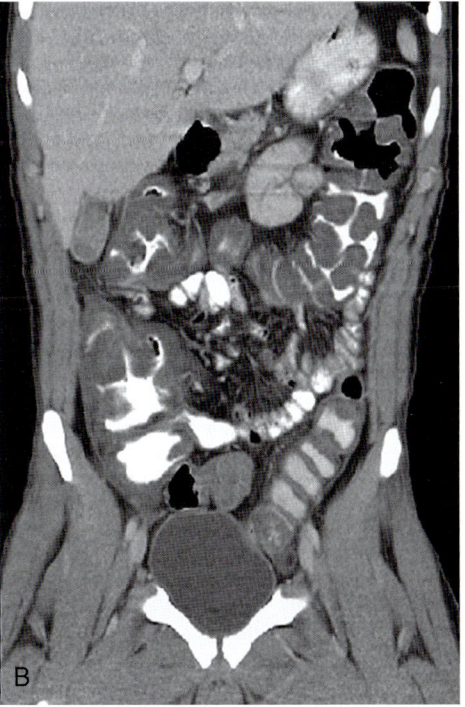

Figure 107-12 Neutropenic colitis. Computed tomography (CT) in an 18-year-old man with acute myelogenous leukemia, fever, and neutropenia. **A,** Axial CT image shows the marked thickening of the cecum and a small amount of free fluid. **B,** Coronal CT reformat shows pancolitis, affecting the right colon to a greater extent.

received particularly high doses later came to medical attention with what has been termed *fibrosing colonopathy*. Children were at higher risk than adults, until strict dosage guidelines were implemented. This entity is now rare because of compliance with appropriate dosage recommendations.[45]

CLINICAL PRESENTATION

The clinical presentation includes abdominal pain, distension, nausea, vomiting, constipation, and occasionally colonic obstruction. Although nonspecific, these signs and symptoms do not respond to medical therapy.

IMAGING

The most common contrast enema findings are colonic strictures, loss of haustra, and colonic shortening.[46] The bowel wall may be thickened, and ascites may be evident on cross-sectional imaging.

TREATMENT

Some of these patients require surgery to relieve the obstruction, and they may also require resection of the fibrotic segment of colon.[45]

Appendicitis

The vermiform appendix—a thin, tubular, intestinal diverticulum attached to the base of the cecum—is often referred to as a *vestigial organ*. Although conventional wisdom has long asserted that the appendix has no known function, there is evidence suggesting that it plays a role in immune function and as a reservoir for normal gut flora.[22,23,47] Inflammation of the appendix remains the most common indication for surgery in both children and adults. Appendicitis in children in the United States approximates 70,000 to 90,000 cases annually with an estimated incidence of 75 to 233 per 100,000 children. The incidence increases with age and peaks in adolescence. Although rare, appendicitis does occur in young children and infants. Boys are affected more frequently than girls by a ratio of 1.4 to 1.0. Classically, appendicitis has been considered a clinical diagnosis with acceptable negative appendectomy rates between 12% and 20%.[48-50] With the marked increase in use of CT and ultrasound during the past decade, these unnecessary surgeries have declined to 5% in many centers.[51]

ETIOLOGY

Appendicitis commonly occurs in the setting of luminal obstruction with subsequent distension of the appendix and ischemic mucosal damage, which leads to bacterial overgrowth and invasion of the wall that in turn results in transmural inflammation and ultimately in perforation. Luminal obstruction may be secondary to the presence of fecaliths, hyperplasia of lymphoid follicles, and foreign bodies that include parasites and carcinoid tumors.[52] The pathophysiology of appendicitis is believed to be a dynamic process that occurs over a 24 to 36 hour period. Although infrequent, subacute appendicitis and spontaneous resolution of acute

appendicitis have been described. Spontaneous resolution of luminal obstruction is the proposed pathophysiology in these cases and has been associated with cystic fibrosis and appendiceal lymphoid hyperplasia.[53,54]

CLINICAL PRESENTATION

Appendicitis can be a challenging diagnosis in children; the clinical presentation is reported to be nonspecific in approximately one third.[55] The classic clinical presentation—early periumbilical pain, followed by migration of localized pain to the right lower quadrant, with associated fever and vomiting—is reported to occur in less than 50% of pediatric patients.[56] More often, the constellation of findings is nonspecific; this is particularly true in younger children who may be unable to communicate symptoms effectively, resulting in delayed diagnosis and higher perforation rates in this cohort of patients. Initial relief of pain and/or more generalized abdominal pain with fever occur after perforation, which usually results in a local abscess adjacent to the appendix; this is because the perforation is usually contained by the omentum, but generalized peritonitis can also occur. Reported perforation rates in children range from 23% to 88%.[55]

IMAGING

Appendicitis demonstrates variable diagnostic findings on various imaging modalities (Box 107-1). Utilization of imaging, particularly CT, is increased in the emergency department for assessment of abdominal pain in children, particularly in those with suspected appendicitis.[57,58] The effectiveness of imaging for suspected appendicitis in children has been debated in the medical literature, which has specifically looked at the impact of imaging on the negative appendectomy and perforation rates. Several studies suggest a stable perforation rate with preoperative imaging,[59-61] whereas others demonstrate a significant decrease in perforation rate, from 35% to 15.5%, with preoperative imaging.[62] However, a decrease in the negative appendectomy rate has been demonstrated in numerous studies.[62-64] When the appendix is normal, the

---

Box 107-1 Imaging Findings in Appendicitis

Plain Radiographs

Ileus, often localized to right lower quadrant
  Scoliosis from splinting
  Appendicolith
  Apparent small-bowel obstruction, most commonly in younger children
  Abscess with mass effect and/or atypical air collection

Ultrasound

Appendiceal diameter > 6 mm
  Noncompressible appendix
Increased flow in wall with color Doppler
Appendicolith with acoustic shadowing
  Periappendiceal fluid, omentum, or abscess
  Perforation that may decompress the appendix
  Abscess

Computed Tomography and Magnetic Resonance

Dilated appendix >7 mm
Wall enhancement and thickening with surrounding fat stranding
Appendicolith
  Abscess

radiologist must evaluate the images for alternative diagnoses, particulary in young children. The most common alternative diagnoses, in decreasing order of prevalence, are mesenteric adenitis, ovarian cyst, pyelonephritis, infectious or inflammatory colitis, omental infarction (e-Fig. 107-13), and urinary system stones.[65,66]

RADIOGRAPHS

Prior to the advent of current cross-sectional imaging modalities, imaging of appendicitis relied on abdominal radiographic findings, which are often normal or nonspecific in approximately 77% of children with appendicitis.[56] The presence of a radiographically visible appendicolith, considered to be the most specific radiographic sign of appendicitis, is only present in approximately 5% to 15% of patients with appendicitis.[56,67] Appendicoliths are seen more frequently on CT, range from 43% to 50%, and are multiple 30% of the time (e-Fig. 107-14).[68,69] Additional nonspecific radiographic findings include a paucity of bowel gas or a soft tissue mass in the right lower quadrant; ileus that may be either focal or diffuse; and less often, small-bowel obstruction.[70] Mild levoconvex curvature of the spine may be present as a result of splinting in response to abdominal pain.

ULTRASOUND

US using a graded compression technique for evaluation of appendicitis was first described in 1986.[70] Since that landmark paper, numerous studies have followed to address the efficacy of US and to evaluate additional sonographic findings.[71-75] The limitations of US relate to several factors that include operator experience, larger patient body habitus, and limited field of view. Optimized technique for US evaluation of suspected appendicitis is fundamental to achieve the sensitivity. The examination is performed with a high-frequency linear transducer that ranges from 9 MHz to 15 MHz, depending on the size of the patient. A linear transducer is necessary not just to obtain the appropriate resolution but also to effect adequate graded compression. Graded compression is essential, because it displaces overlying bowel gas and also helps to decrease the distance between the transducer and the appendix. Additionally, compression helps differentiate normal bowel from an inflamed appendix. The compression is "graded," in that it is exerted slowly, without sudden release, to optimize patient tolerance and prevent rebound tenderness. Transverse and longitudinal scans are performed over the point of maximal tenderness. If the appendix is not identified at this point, additional sonographic interrogation of the right lower quadrant, pelvis, and abdomen is necessary given the variability in location of the appendiceal tip. The most common location of the normal and abnormal appendix is in the midpelvic region over the common right iliac vessels, followed by the retrocecal region, deep pelvic region, and abdomen above the iliac crests.[76]

Sonographic demonstration of the normal appendix is useful in excluding the diagnosis of appendicitis, although in general US is more useful in the diagnosis than in the exclusion of appendicitis. The literature demonstrates wide operator variability with respect to reliable identification of the normal appendix, ranging from 2.4% to 86.2%.[76-80] The higher percentages may reflect the advanced technology,

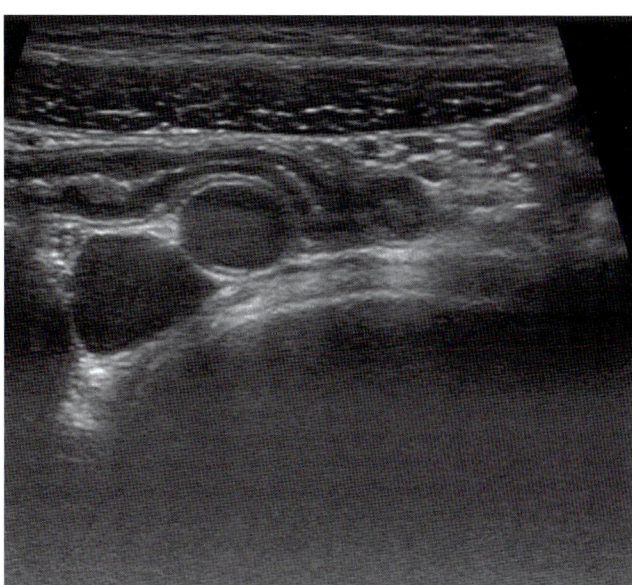

Figure 107-15 **Normal appendix.** Ultrasound image of the normal appendix shows a nondilated, blind-ending tubular structure with a central echogenic line.

improved resolution of US equipment, and improved operator experience. Sonographic findings associated with a normal appendix include a compressible, blind-ending tubular structure without peristalsis; diameter less than 6 mm; absence of wall thickening (less than 3 mm); and presence of a central echogenic line that represents acoustic reflection from the collapsed luminal interface (Fig. 107-15).[74,80,81] The normal appendix can usually be traced to its origin at the base of the cecum (e-Fig. 107-16). Occasionally, the normal terminal ileum, often located just cephalad to the appendix, may be mistaken for a normal appendix, since it is located cephalad of the appendiceal origin. The presence of hypoechoic folds and peristalsis are helpful in differentiating the normal terminal ileum from the appendix.

The single most important US sign of an inflamed appendix is a noncompressible, blind-ending tubular structure with a transverse diameter measuring greater than 6 mm. Additional sonographic signs associated with appendicitis include appendiceal wall thickness greater than 3 mm, wall hyperemia on color Doppler, periappendiceal hypoechoic halo that reflects appendiceal wall edema, periappendiceal hyperechogenicity that reflects periappendiceal edema, and the presence of an appendicolith (Fig. 107-17 and e-Fig. 107-18).[75,77] The secondary sonographic findings vary, depending on the progression of the inflammatory process. Early uncomplicated appendicitis will demonstrate a targetlike appearance with hypoechogenicity centrally as a result of luminal distension with pus or fluid, increased echogencity of the inflamed submucosa, hypoechoic edematous serosa, and increased periappendiceal echogenicity (see Fig. 107-17). As the inflammatory process advances, and suppurative appendicitis ensues, the periappendiceal tissues demonstrate a heterogeneous pattern of increased echogenicity with hyperemia on color Doppler (Fig. 107-19). Increasing appendiceal dilatation, loss of the echogenic submucosal layer, and absence of vascularity with color Doppler are signs of supervening gangrenous change (Fig. 107-20). Although the abnormal appendix may not be visualized with perforated appendicitis, sonographic

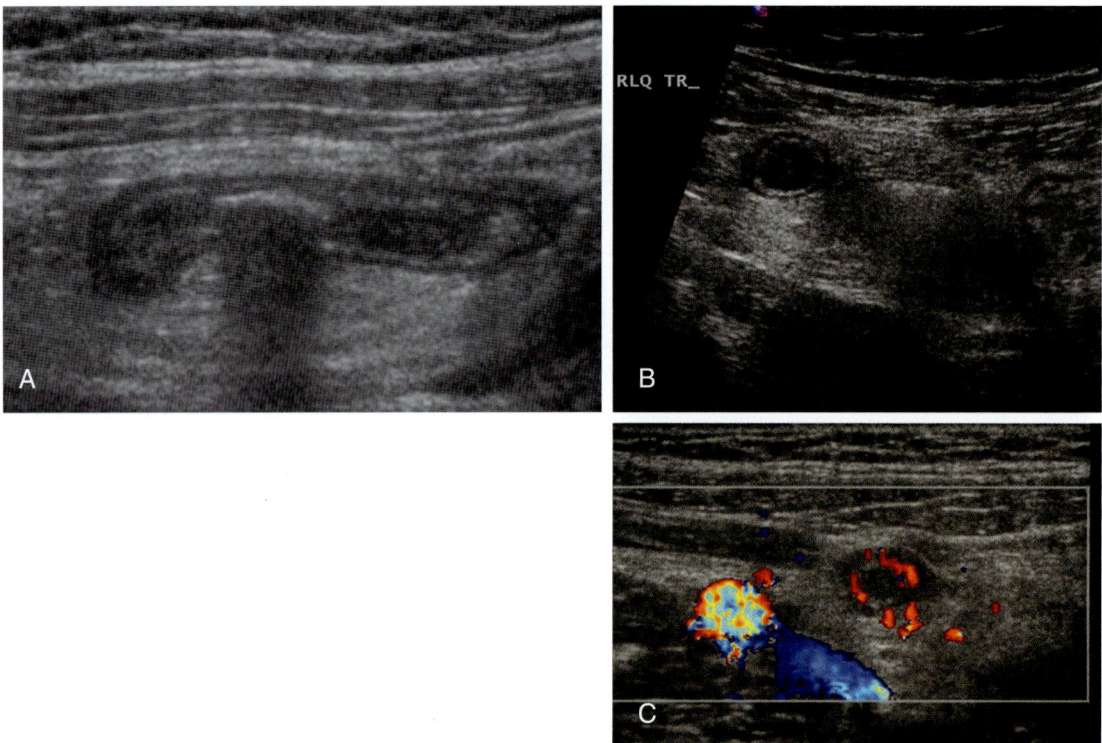

Figure 107-17   Ultrasound (US) of acute appendicitis. **A,** Longitudinal US image of a dilated, noncompressible appendix containing a shadowing appendicolith. **B,** Transverse US image of the appendix demonstrates the characteristic target appearance with increased echogenicity of the surrounding mesenteric fat consistent with periappendiceal inflammation. **C,** Color Doppler interrogation shows hyperemia in the wall of the dilated appendix.

findings suggestive of perforation include phlegmon with poorly defined bowel loops in the right lower quadrant demonstrating overall increased echogencity, a mass of mixed echogenicity, and focal bowel wall thickening, intraperitoneal fluid, loculated fluid collections, or frank abscess.

Absence of visualization of an abnormal appendix in the setting of acute appendicitis may be due to a retrocecal location, obscuration by superimposed bowel gas, or limited US penetration. Additionally, appendiceal inflammatory changes may be confined to the tip of the appendix.[82] If the entire appendix has not been visualized on US, and clinical symptoms suggest appendicitis or other intraperitoneal pathology,

further imaging may be warranted, particularly if there are secondary signs of right lower quadrant inflammation.

COMPUTED TOMOGRAPHY

CT is highly sensitive and specific for the diagnosis or exclusion of appendicitis in children (Table 107-1), and it is often utilized in the setting of a negative or equivocal US or perforated appendicitis. Scanning parameters should be adjusted appropriately for the size of the child to optimize dose. CT protocols vary with respect to the administration of oral, IV, and rectal contrast in addition to focal imaging versus imaging

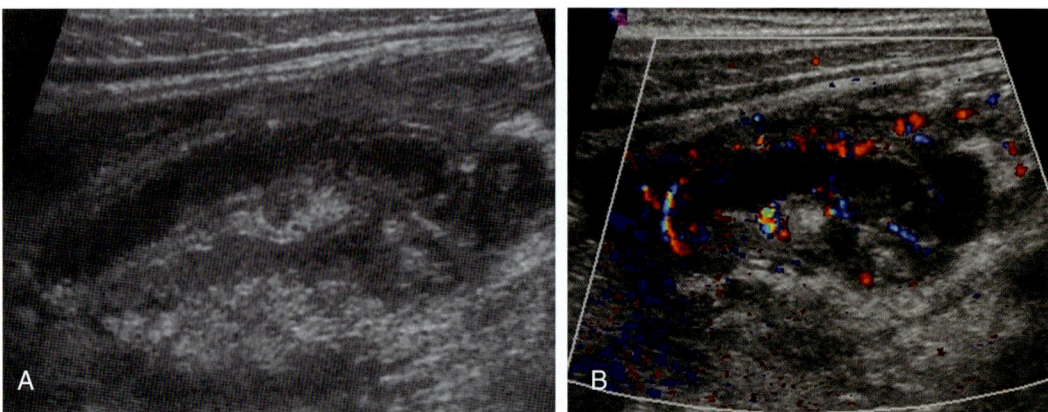

Figure 107-19   Advanced acute appendicitis. **A,** Ultrasound image of an abnormal appendix with increased mixed echogenicity of the adjacent tissues and a small amount of periappendiceal fluid. **B,** Color Doppler interrogation demonstrates hyperemia in the wall of the appendix and in the adjacent soft tissues.

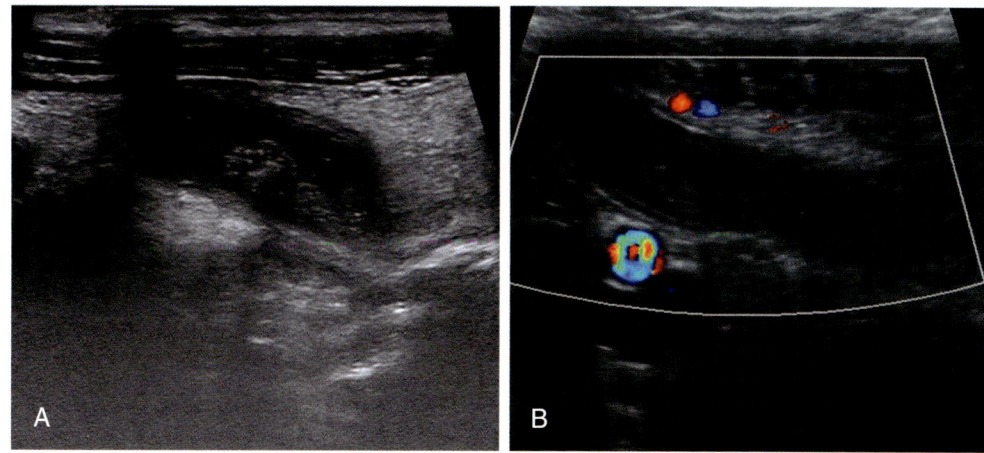

Figure 107-20 Gangrenous appendicitis. Ultrasound images of a dilated appendix with loss of the echogenic submucosal layer and absence of vascularity with color Doppler evaluation.

the entire abdomen and pelvis.[55,81,83-86] A systematic review concluded that IV contrast alone performs as well as or better than CT with IV and positive enteral contrast for the diagnosis or exclusion of appendicitis.[87]

Although the average diameter of the normal appendix typically approximates 6 mm, actual size may vary on CT, from 2 to 11 mm, because the examination is not done with compression, and the appendiceal lumen may distend with gas or feces. The absence of associated CT signs of appendicitis is helpful to confirm a normal appendix. As is the case with US, the appearance of the abnormal appendix varies with the histopathologic stage and severity of the disease process. The inflamed appendix on CT is a dilated, thick-walled tubular structure with centrally decreased attenuation that demonstrates wall contrast enhancement (e-Fig. 107-21 and Fig. 107-22). An obstructing appendicolith may be present in up to 50% of cases (e-Fig. 107-23).[68,69] Adjacent inflammation produces periappendiceal stranding and fluid. Additional nonspecific findings include intraperitoneal free fluid, cecal wall thickening and thickening of adjacent terminal ileum and sigmoid colon, small-bowel obstruction, and mesenteric lymphadenopathy.[88]

With perforation, the appendix may decompress or may even fail to be visualized. Perforation may result in diffuse intraperitoneal inflammation (Fig. 107-24) or, more commonly, in localized phlegmon and abscess formation (e-Figs. 107-25 and 107-26). Diffuse peritonitis is more common in infants younger than age 2 than in older children. Hepatic abscesses and mesenteric or portal pyelophlebitis can also occur. CT is extremely helpful in identifying and

characterizing smaller abscesses and extruded fecaliths that may act as a potential source of recurrent infection.

COMPUTED TOMOGRAPHY AND ULTRASOUND

CT and US are reported to have a nearly equivalent specificity, 95% and 94%, respectively (see Table 107-1).[89] Although CT has a greater sensitivity than US (94% and 88%, respectively although US is much more variable and operator dependent),[89] concerns regarding the potential risks of ionizing radiation exposure associated with CT[90] have prompted increasing use of US in the imaging evaluation of suspected appendicitis. Various imaging algorithms have been described in the literature that include the staged utilization of initial evaluation with US followed by CT for equivocal or non-diagnostic US studies.[51,83,91-93]

MAGNETIC RESONANCE IMAGING

MRI has been reported to yield good results in the evaluation of suspected appendicitis, in both children and adults, using T1- and T2-weighted sequences.[94-98] The sensitivity of MR

Table 107-1

Diagnostic Performance of Ultrasound and Computed Tomography in Children for Clinically Suspected Appendicitis		
	Ultrasound	**Computed Tomography**
Sensitivity (%)	88 (86-90)	94 (92-97)
Specificity (%)	94 (92-95)	95 (94-97)

Values are mean (95% confidence interval).
Doria AS, et al. US or CT for Diagnosis of Appendicitis in Children and Adults? A Meta-Analysis. *Radiology.* 2006;241(1):83-94.

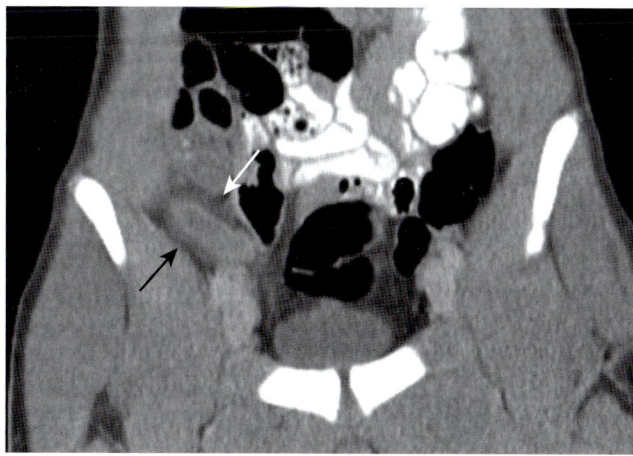

Figure 107-22 Acute appendicitis. Coronal reformatted contrast-enhanced computed tomography image of the pelvis demonstrates a dilated appendix with wall enhancement and periappendiceal inflammation (*arrows*).

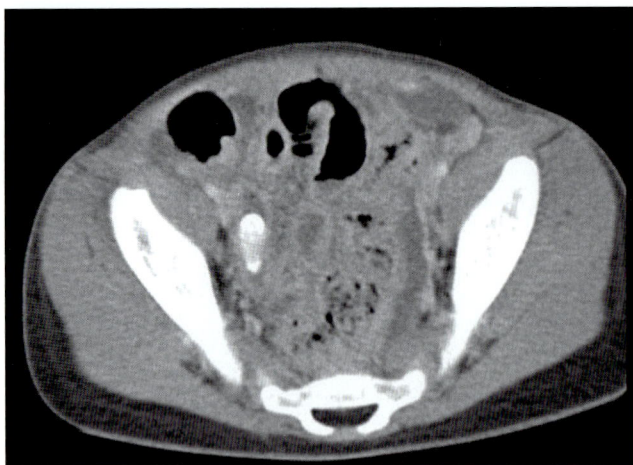

Figure 107-24 **Perforated appendicitis.** Axial contrast-enhanced computed tomography image shows an appendicolith in the right lower quadrant in the remnant of the appendix. Extensive peritoneal inflammation is present with several abscesses.

was 97.6%, and the specificity was 97% in one study using a four-sequence protocol.[99] The abnormal appendix demonstrates thickening of the appendiceal wall with high signal intensity on T2-weighted images, dilated lumen with high signal intensity contents on T2-weighted images, and increased signal intensity of the periappendiceal tissues (Fig. 107-27).[98] Although MRI has the appealing advantage of no ionizing radiation, the current limitations that preclude routine use of MRI for imaging suspected appendicitis in children include relatively long examination time and limited availability compared with CT. The need for sedation in most young infants remains a current limitation, although faster sequence studies with a mean duration of 10 to 14 minutes have been described and performed without sedation in infants as young as 3 years.[99]

TREATMENT

Although appendectomy is the mainstay in the treatment of acute appendicitis, the literature is variable on the management of appendicitis and depends on the institution and the individual surgeon with respect to surgical procedure, timing

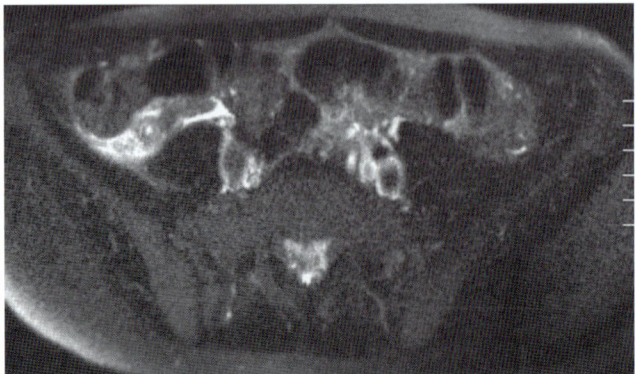

Figure 107-27 **Magnetic resonance imaging of acute appendicitis.** Axial T2-weighted sequence with fat saturation demonstrates a fluid-filled, thick-walled appendix with periappendiceal inflammatory changes. (Courtesy Genevieve Bennett, NYU Langone Medical Center.)

of the surgical procedure, antibiotic therapy, and the clinical presentation of the patient.[100-102] Although open appendectomy is still performed by some surgeons, laparoscopic appendectomy has become a preferred surgical approach.[103] Several studies have suggested that emergent appendectomy may not be necessary, demonstrating that IV antibiotics, along with appendectomies delayed for 12 to 24 hours after presentation, do not significantly increase the rate of perforations, operative time, or length of hospital stay.[104,105] Patients with perforated appendicitis undergo IV antibiotic therapy followed by interval appendectomy several weeks later. If an abscess is present, the child will typically undergo image-guided drainage.[106]

Miscellaneous Disorders

COLONIC VOLVULUS

Colonic volvulus refers to a twisting or torsion of a portion of the colon, such as the cecum or the sigmoid. It is less common in children than in adults. When it occurs in children, the cecum is the most common area to twist; in adults, the sigmoid colon is the most common location.

Etiology

A mobile cecum is a normal variant, seen in as many as 15% of individuals. Cecal volvulus is very rare in the pediatric population and results from dilatation of a mobile cecum, typically in patients with relative immobility, such as that resulting from neurologic impairment; cecal volvulus leads to severe constipation and bowel distension.[107-109] Volvulus of the transverse colon is the least common form reported and is associated with abnormal fixation of the long transverse colon.[110]

Iatrogenic causes of cecal volvulus include the presence of a ventriculoperitoneal shunt (Fig. 107-28) and the Malone antegrade continence enema procedure (e-Fig. 107-29).[111] This procedure provides a catheterizable stoma for colonic enema in patients with chronic constipation, and it may provide a focal point for the bowel to twist. Sigmoid volvulus[112,113] and volvulus of the transverse colon[114] can also rarely occur in children. Predisposing factors are abnormal mesenteric attachments or neurologic impairment, and these lead to hypomobility and severe obstipation.[108]

Clinical Presentation

The clinical presentation for colonic volvulus is that of colonic obstruction with nausea, vomiting, abdominal pain, and distension, although the findings may at times be relatively nonspecific and may be confused with gastroenteritis or some other, much more common condition.[108]

Imaging

Radiographs demonstrate bowel obstruction with marked dilatation of the colonic segment, which may be present in the right lower quadrant or over the midabdomen, if the volvulus involves the right colon (see Fig. 107-28). If a contrast enema is performed, the typical appearance of the site of obstructing volvulus is the "bird beak" sign. On CT

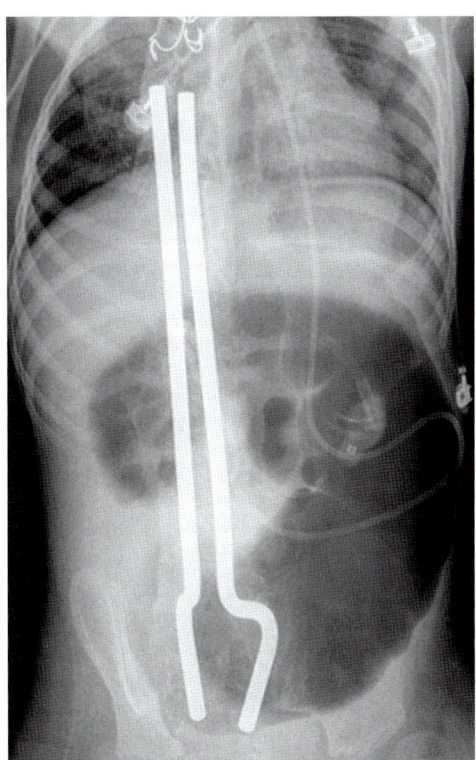

Figure 107-28 Acute cecal volvulus around ventriculoperitoneal shunt tubing. Frontal abdominal radiograph of a teenage boy with developmental delay and chronic constipation, who presented with acute onset of vomiting and abdominal pain. The radiograph shows marked distension of a colonic loop in the left abdomen, which was found at surgery to represent an acutely twisted right colon.

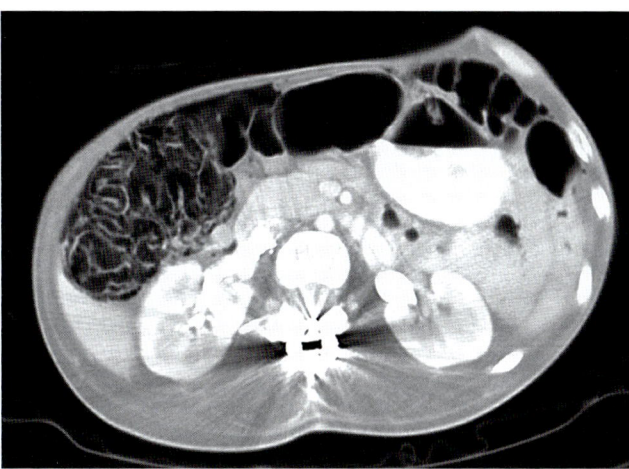

Figure 107-30 Pneumatosis intestinalis. Young adult with Duchenne muscular dystrophy developed pneumatosis, probably as a result of steroid therapy. On lung-windowed axial computed tomography, the air in the wall of the right colon is clearly visualized. It resolved spontaneously.

imaging, enlargement of the twisted portion of the colon is apparent, as is a "whirl sign" at the site of the twist.[110] The markedly enlarged colonic segment may have an enhancing thickened wall (see e-Fig. 107-29). If the bowel becomes ischemic, the wall may not enhance, and pneumatosis may be present.[110]

Treatment

Most children undergo surgical exploration and reduction of the volvulus with resection of necrotic bowel when necessary. There are reports of enema reduction of both cecal and more distal volvulus in children.[115]

PNEUMATOSIS COLI

Overview

Pneumatosis intestinalis, or pneumatosis coli (Fig. 107-30), is a term that refers to the radiographic, US, or CT finding of air in the wall of the intestine, and it may be due to both benign and serious clinical conditions.

Etiology

Pneumatosis is well known to occur in patients with underlying ischemic bowel disease, such as necrotizing enterocolitis (NEC), and in some cases of bowel obstruction. However, it is also described in a wide variety of more benign or chronic conditions, such as Crohn disease, ulcerative colitis, acquired immune deficiency syndrome, in transplant patients, and with viral infections, particularly cytomegalovirus.[116-121] Children are more likely to have pneumatosis than are adults, and depending on the etiology, the condition may generate few symptoms or may be asymptomatic. It is also described as an epiphenomenon probably caused by gas dissection in cystic fibrosis,[119] and in some cases it is related to steroid therapy.

Imaging

When NEC is a clinical concern, abdominal radiography is used for the detection of associated findings that include pneumatosis, ileus, perforation, or portal venous air (see Chapter 106). Repeat radiographs are used when perforation is a concern. In other patients, pneumatosis may be an unexpected finding on radiographs. For the many associated benign conditions, and in those children who are asymptomatic, there is no evidence that serial radiographs are useful.

Sonography may detect pneumatosis of the small or large bowel and may predict outcome in patients with NEC.[122,123]

Treatment

Treatment is directed to the underlying condition, such as NEC or obstruction.

Key Points

Transmural disease is characteristic of Crohn disease but not of ulcerative colitis.

Magnetic resonace enterography is increasingly used for evaluation and monitoring of disease activity.

The toxins produced by the bacterium *C. difficile* are the most important cause of antibiotic-associated pseudomembranous colitis.

Continued

Most cases of HUS are caused by a Shiga-like toxin–producing *E. coli,* serotype 0157:H7, found in raw or incompletely cooked meats and in unpasteurized dairy products.

Radiation colitis can occur months to years after exposure. Endarteritis with end-vessel and microvascular circulation compromise is the hallmark of supervening chronic ischemia.

Neutropenic colitis, also known as *typhlitis,* is a necrotizing colitis primarily seen in children with hematopoietic malignancies.

Sonography is the initial cross-sectional imaging test recommended for appendicitis evaluation, followed by CT if necessary.

CT imaging should be justified and optimized for the clinical indication and size of the child (see www.imagegently.org).

Segmental colonic volvulus occurs in the setting of inanition associated with marked obstipation and distension and deficient supporting ligaments.

Pneumatosis intestinalis occurs in a variety of benign and serious conditions in children.

Suggested Readings

Dillman JR, et al. CT enterography of pediatric Crohn disease. *Pediatr Radiol.* 2010;40(1):97–105.

Doria AS, et al. US or CT for diagnosis of appendicitis in children and adults? A meta-analysis. *Radiology.* 2006;241(1):83–94.

Fike FB, et al. Neutropenic colitis in children. *J Surg Res.* 2011; 170(1):73–76.

Kurbegov AC, Sondheimer JM. Pneumatosis intestinalis in non-neonatal pediatric patients. *Pediatrics.* 2001;108(2):402–406.

Shikhare G, Kugathasan S. Inflammatory bowel disease in children: current trends. *J Gastroenterol.* 2010;45(7):673–682.

Strouse PJ. Pediatric appendicitis: an argument for US. *Radiology.* 2010;255(1):8–13.

References

Full references for this chapter can be found on www.expertconsult.com.

Chapter 108

Intussusception

KIMBERLY E. APPLEGATE

Intussusception is an acquired invagination of the bowel into itself, usually involving both small and large bowel (Fig. 108-1). The more proximal bowel that invaginates into more distal bowel is termed the intussusceptum, whereas the recipient bowel that contains the intussusceptum is termed the intussuscipiens. Invagination of the bowel leads to edema, and ischemic changes eventually supervene; thus intussusception is an urgent condition, but prolonged delay in diagnosis is not uncommon, resulting in increased risk for patients to present with obstruction, necrosis, and bowel perforation.

Intussusception occurs with an incidence of at least 56 per 100,000 children per year in the United States, and it is the most common cause of small bowel obstruction in children.[1] In frequency, it is second only to pyloric stenosis as a cause of gastrointestinal tract obstruction in children, occurring in boys more often than girls at a ratio of 3:2. Classic pediatric intussusception involves invagination of the distal ileum into the colon, as ileocolic or ileoileocolic intussusception; however, intestinal intussusception may occur along the entire length of the bowel from the duodenum to the colon. Cases of intussusception range from the classic, symptomatic, and urgent presentation, to short-segment, transient, and asymptomatic events, typically isolated to the small bowel, and seen increasingly on ultrasound or on computed tomography (CT) of the abdomen performed for other indications (e-Fig 108-2).[2] This chapter will focus on ileocolic and ileo-ileocolic intussusception.

Etiology

Most cases of ileocolic intussusception occurring in children are idiopathic. It is hypothesized that the typical childhood ileocolic intussusception results from hypertrophied lymphoid tissue in the terminal ileum (Peyer patches). Some reports suggest a viral etiology, most commonly adenovirus, but enterovirus, echovirus, and human herpes virus 6 also have been implicated.[1,3] An accompanying pathologic lead-point mass lesion may be present in 5% to 6% of all children,[4,5] particularly when intussusception occurs outside of the typical idiopathic age range or when symptomatic intussusception is confined to the small bowel or the colon.

ROTAVIRUS VACCINE

Shortly after the first rotavirus vaccine was introduced in the United States in 1998 for routine vaccination of infants at ages 2, 4, and 6 months, several reports to the Centers for Disease Control and Prevention suggested an association between the vaccine and intussusception. The vaccine was removed from the world market in 1999. Subsequent investigations have demonstrated clear benefits in reducing morbidity and mortality, although some authors report a very small risk of intussusception after rotavirus vaccination.[6,7] Two new vaccines are now available.

PATHOLOGIC LEAD POINTS

Approximately 5% to 6% of intussusceptions in children are caused by pathologic lead points, either focal masses or a diffuse bowel wall abnormality.[4,5,8] The traditional view is that focal lead points are more common in older children. Although the absolute numbers of lead points are approximately equal in infants and in older children, the percentage of lead points in infants is lower because of the greater number of intussusceptions occurring in this age group.[4] The most common focal lead points are (in decreasing order of incidence) Meckel diverticulum, duplication cyst, polyp, and lymphoma. In older children, lymphoma is the more likely lead point, typically Burkitt lymphoma. Diffuse lead points are most commonly associated with cystic fibrosis or Henoch-Schönlein purpura. Colonic polyps can result in colocolic intussusception.

Clinical Presentation

Idiopathic intussusception occurs most commonly in infants between 2 months and 3 years of age, with a peak at age 5 to 9 months; authors of studies with a large series report that 57% to 85% of cases present before the age of 1 year (average, 67%).[8,9]

The classic clinical presentation of the child with intussusception is colicky abdominal pain, vomiting, bloody stools, and a palpable abdominal mass.[9] Children with intussusception should be diagnosed as early as possible to avoid bowel ischemia, necrosis, and surgery; however, this goal remains elusive. The clinical signs and symptoms of intussusception are often nonspecific and may overlap with those of gastroenteritis, malrotation with volvulus, and in older children, Henoch-Schönlein purpura. The classic triad of colicky abdominal pain (58% to 100% of cases), vomiting (up to 85% of cases), and bloody stools (up to 75% of cases)[10,11] is present in less than 25% of children.[10,12] No reliable clinical

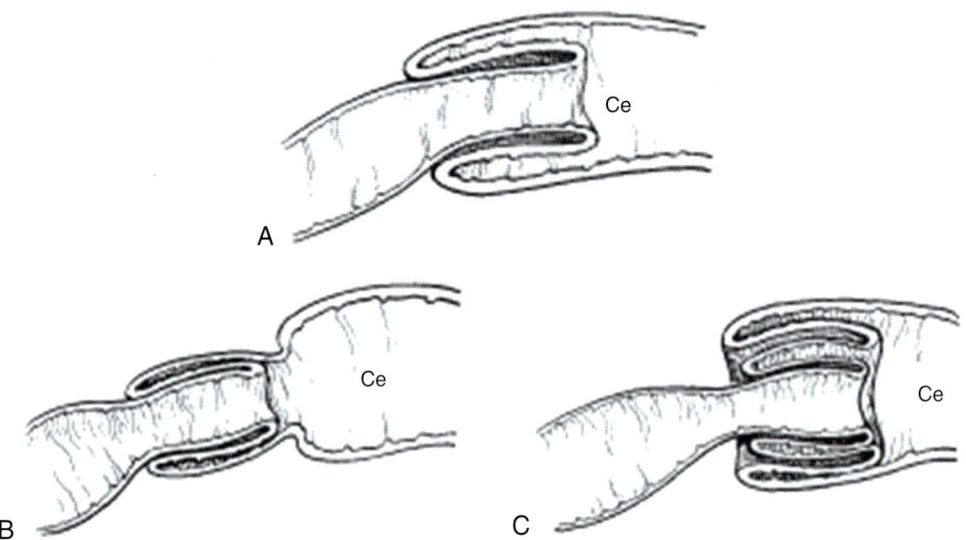

Figure 108-1 The common types of infantile intussusception, in longitudinal section. **A,** Ileocecal. **B,** Ileoileal. **C,** Ileoileocolic. *Ce,* Cecum.

prediction models exist that can identify all children with intussusception.[12-14] In one study, it was found that only 50% of children were correctly diagnosed at initial presentation to a health care provider.[15]

Vomiting or diarrhea may lead to dehydration, which exaggerates lethargy. Venous hypertension leads to hematochezia, with a typical mixture of stool, blood, and blood clots described as "currant jelly stools," a finding highly suggestive of intussusception. Intussuscepted bowel may prolapse through the rectum.

CLINICAL PREDICTORS OF INTUSSUSCEPTION AND NONSURGICAL REDUCTION

The most important factor, either alone or in combination with other factors, that predicts an unsuccessful enema reduction is a longer duration of symptoms; 48 to 72 hours typically is considered a significant delay.[8,9] Other factors associated with lower rates of successful reduction include age less than 3 months, dehydration, small bowel obstruction, and intussusception encountered in the rectum (resulting in a 25% reduction rate).[8,9,15-17] Additional findings that affect bowel edema, bowel viability, and success of nonsurgical reduction relate to imaging findings and are addressed in the next section. On the basis of sonographic or enema diagnosis before surgery, the rate of spontaneous reduction is estimated to be 10%.[4,18,19]

Diagnosis and Imaging

Box 108-1 summarizes the evidence regarding imaging management of intussusception.

ABDOMINAL RADIOGRAPHS

Abdominal radiographs have a limited sensitivity and specificity for the detection of intussusception, even when viewed by experienced pediatric radiologists.[9,20] Sargent and colleagues[16] reported a sensitivity of 45% in 60 children when

they were evaluated prospectively by pediatric radiologists, using an enema as the reference standard. Adding a left side down decubitus has been shown to improve sensitivity.[21] The presence of a curvilinear mass within the course of the colon (the crescent sign), particularly in the transverse colon just beyond the hepatic flexure, is a nearly pathognomonic sign of intussusception (Fig. 108-3). The absence of stool or recognizable colonic gas in the ascending colon is one of the more suggestive signs of intussusception on radiographs. However, fluid filling the ascending colon in a patient with gastroenteritis may falsely suggest intussusception, and small bowel gas located in the right abdomen on radiographs may mimic ascending colon or cecal gas.

Abdominal radiographs also may serve to screen for other diagnoses suggested by a patient's symptoms, such as constipation or gastroenteritis/colitis. Abdominal radiographs are important to assess for the presence of small bowel obstruction, which is one of the signs indicating greater bowel edema and diminished success of nonoperative reduction, as

---

Box 108-1 Management of Intussusception

Abdominal radiographs are useful for:
- Determining a differential diagnosis
- Showing bowel obstruction
- Identifying free air

Ultrasound is highly sensitive in detecting:
- Intussusception
- A lead point

The chance for nonoperative reduction is diminished if:
- Trapped fluid is present
- Doppler evaluation shows absence of flow

Enema is indicated for reduction in the absence of:
- Free air
- Peritoneal signs

  Air is the preferred contrast agent, but water-soluble positive-contrast media may be used.

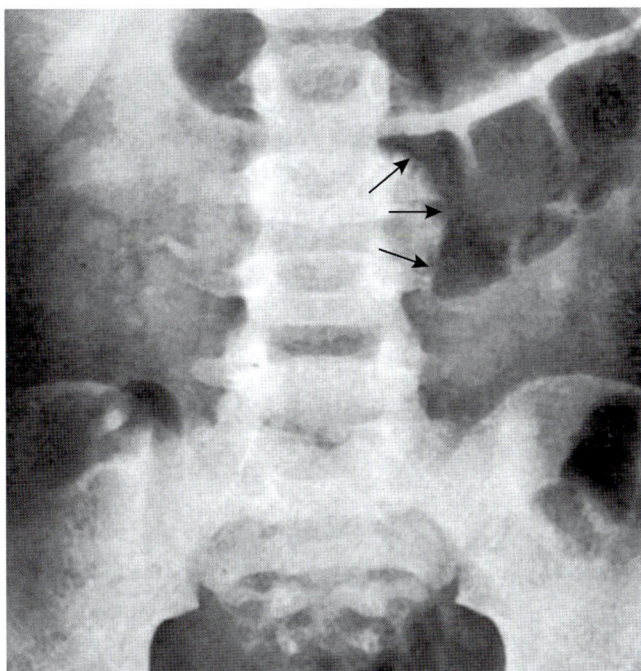

Figure 108-3 Ileocolic intussusception in a 4-year-old child. The leading edge of the intussusception (*arrows*) is seen on this radiograph outlined by gas within the transverse colon. No gas can be seen in the cecum or in the ascending colon.

Table 108-1

Sensitivity and Specificity of Diagnostic Imaging for Ileocolic Intussusception		
Test	**Sensitivity (%)**	**Specificity (%)**
Abdominal radiograph	45	Unknown
Ultrasound	98-100	88-100
Enema*	100	100

*Reference standard.

well as to evaluate for the potential finding of free intraperitoneal gas, although this finding is seldom seen before reduction occurs.

ULTRASONOGRAPHY

Ultrasound is highly sensitive in the detection of intussusception (see Table 108-1), even when it is performed by relatively inexperienced operators and with equipment that is no longer state of the art.[22,23] Although the diagnosis can be confirmed when the enema procedure is performed, ultrasound is the primary imaging modality for the initial diagnosis outside of the United States; it is used by 93% of European pediatric radiologists,[24] as well as by a growing number of

pediatric radiologists in the United States. Initial evaluation by ultrasound circumvents the more invasive enema in patients who do not have intussusception, and it allows diagnosis of other conditions, such as mesenteric adenitis or colitis, for which performance of an enema would not be the procedure of choice.[12,25,26]

Intussusception can be diagnosed by ultrasound when a donut, target, or "pseudokidney" sign is seen, most often in the right upper quadrant of the abdomen.[27] This appearance arises from intussuscepted bowel and mesentery within the intussuscipiens, producing the donut or target appearance on transverse images and a hypoechoic mass with hyperechoic center on longitudinal images; the hyperechoic center represents the intussuscepted mesentery. Using a linear transducer, the more specific bowel-within-bowel appearance can be seen, and the leading edge of the intussusception can be inspected to confirm that a pathologic lead point is not present (Fig. 108-4). Optimal sonographic techniques are well described,[26-28] and there are no known contraindications to, or complications resulting from, ultrasound used for this purpose.

After reduction enema, ultrasound also can be helpful in determining the presence of a residual intussusception, although this identification can be difficult until after some of the gas introduced during the air enema reduction has been evacuated.

Ultrasound evaluation in children suspected of intussusception has been suggested to reduce cost, radiation exposure, and anxiety in both patients and parents over the discomfort of the enema.[12] The accuracy of ultrasound evaluation

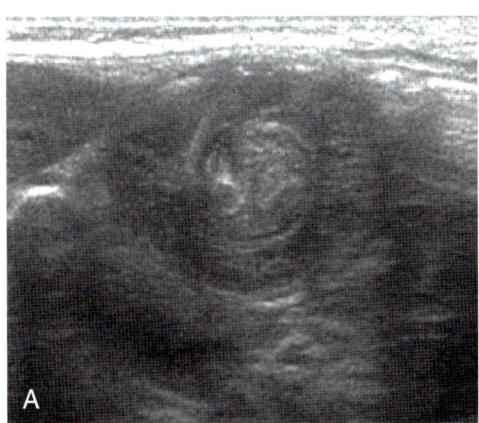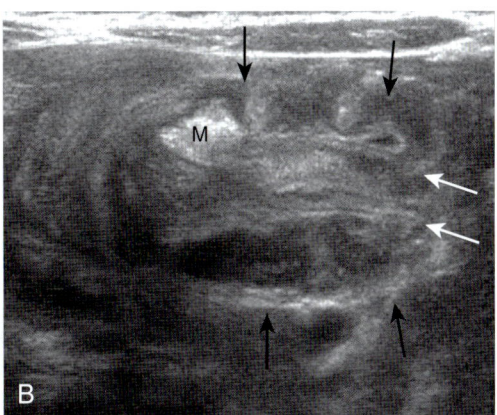

Figure 108-4 Intussusception. **A,** A 3-month-old boy with intussusception. A transverse ultrasound image through the intussusceptum complex shows the donut or target sign, with intussusceptum composed of small bowel, nodes, and mesentery surrounded by the intussuscipiens. **B,** A longitudinal section of intussusception in the same patient as depicted in part **A**. The image shows the terminal end of the intussusception, with the inner and outer sleeves of the intussusceptum (*white arrows*) containing the intussuscepted mesentery (*M*). Black arrows outline the outer edge of the intussuscipiens. Note that no lead point is present. (Courtesy Dr. Marta Hernanz-Schulman, Nashville, TN.)

approaches 100% with a sensitivity of 98% to 100% and a specificity reported at 88% to 100%.[12,22,23,29] Its cost effectiveness, of course, depends on the prevalence of intussusception, because very few positive diagnoses would be expected in a population in which the prevalence of intussusception is very low.

Ultrasound Predictors of Enema Reducibility and Bowel Necrosis

Anechoic fluid trapped between the intussusceptum and the intussuscipiens has been associated with lack of reducibility, whereas abundant flow on color Doppler interrogation is a predictor of reducibility (Fig. 108-5).[25,30] Free intraperitoneal fluid in small or moderate amounts is present in approximately half of children,[27] and reports are conflicting as to whether free peritoneal fluid is associated with fewer successful reductions.[18,28] Similarly, authors of some reports note that a thicker bowel wall is associated with fewer successful enema reductions, but others have not been able to verify this association. Other authors report that the presence of lymph nodes within the intussusceptum complex is associated with decreased success of reduction.[22,27,31] Although some of these findings are associated with fewer successful reductions, none represents a contraindication to enema reduction. Contraindications to enema reduction are signs of peritonitis or free intraperitoneal air.

Pathologic Lead Points

The detection of lead points by imaging is challenging. Ultrasound is the noninvasive standard of reference (Fig. 108-6). Ultrasound is reported to identify approximately 66% of lead points,[32] whereas approximately 40% are identified by positive-contrast liquid enema.[4,8,9,32] Air enema has a lower rate of detection (11%), leading some investigators to suggest that ultrasound be used afterward to search for lead points.[19] However, such an approach would be hindered by air introduced during the enema, and it seems to offer little

advantage over a pre-enema diagnostic ultrasound examination. Other cross-sectional imaging modalities, such as CT, can be used for further evaluation in selected patients (see Fig. 108-7).

CT and MRI are not part of the routine evaluation of suspected intussusception in children, although CT may be the initial modality in a child presenting with atypical abdominal pain. If the examination is done for other reasons, the intussusception should be recognized either in the cross-sectional or longitudinal plane, with the characteristic bowel-within-bowel appearance. As is the case with ultrasound, attention should be given to the potential existence of a lead point, such as an ileal duplication cyst in a young infant, or Burkitt lymphoma in an older child (Fig. 108-7).

Treatment

Enema reduction should be undertaken in children with intussusception after surgical consultation. As previously indicated, the only absolute contraindications to enema reduction are signs of peritonitis on clinical examination or free air on abdominal radiographs (Box 108-2). The rate of successful overall reduction is better with air enema than with liquid enema, but the outcome depends on the patient's risk factors and on the experience of the radiologist. Children with intussusception have fewer surgeries and a lower cost of care when they are treated at a children's hospital, where staff tend to have greater familiarity with the condition, along with greater expertise and experience with nonoperative reduction and expedient management of potential complications.[33] Between 1979 and 1997, 323 intussusception-associated deaths in U.S. infants were reported to the Centers for Disease Control and Prevention, with a higher rate of intussusception-related deaths among infants whose mothers were younger than 20 years old, unmarried, and nonwhite and who had less than a grade 12 education, suggesting that reduced access to specialized care or delay in seeking care contribute to the mortality risk.[1]

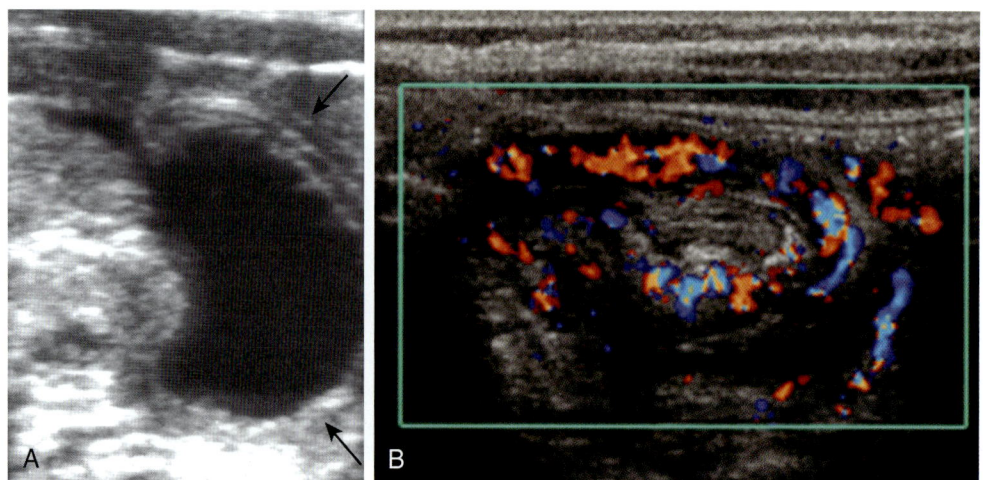

Figure 108-5 Intussusception. **A,** Trapped fluid in an infant with intussusception. Fluid is visible at the leading edge of the intussusceptum complex. Arrows point to the outer edge of the intussuscipiens. **B,** A color Doppler transverse image of the right flank in a different patient outlines abundant flow to intussusceptum and intussuscipiens. The intussusception was successfully and rapidly reduced with air enema. (**A,** Courtesy Dr. Marta Hernanz-Schulman, Nashville, TN.)

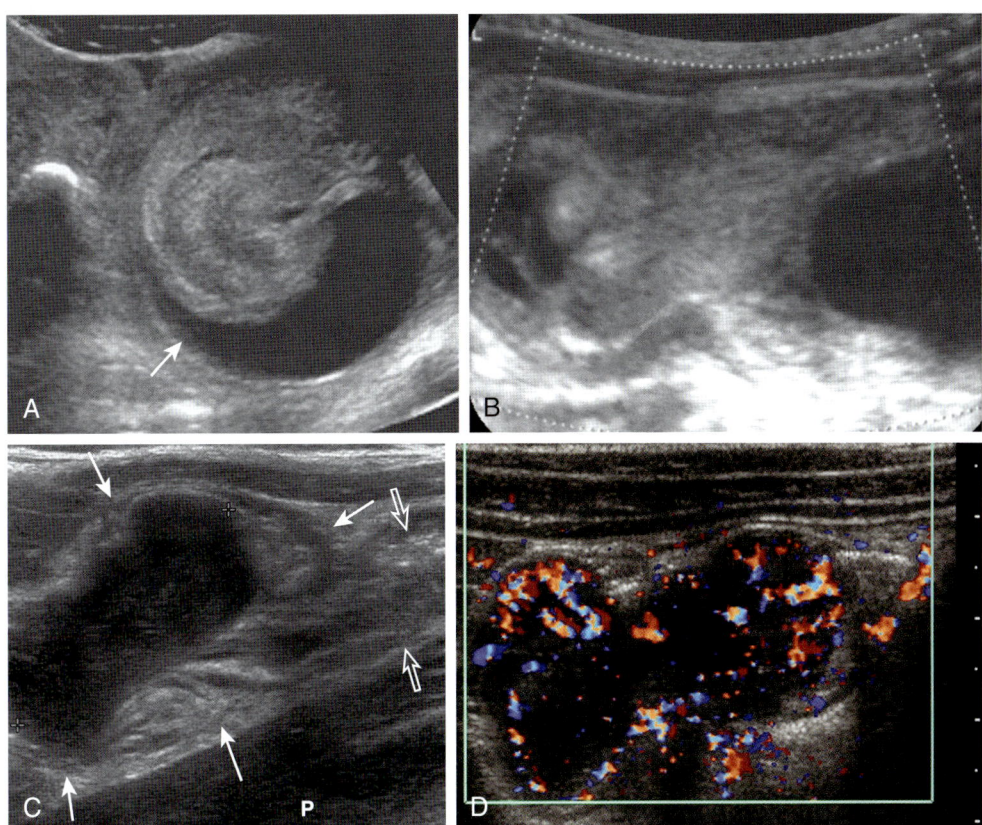

Figure 108-6   Lead points. **A,** An adolescent boy with Burkitt lymphoma presenting with intussusception. An ultrasound image shows the intussuscepted mass and bowel, with anechoic fluid (*arrow*) trapped within the lumen of the intussuscipiens adjacent to the intussusceptum. **B,** A 3 month-old infant with intussusception as a result of an ileal duplication cyst that is acting as a lead point. Note the difference in appearance from that of trapped fluid in a child without a lead point (Fig. 108-5, *A*). **C** and **D,** 8-year-old boy presenting with severe, intermittent abdominal pain. Examination of the right lower quadrant shows an anechoic, solid mass (between crosshairs) with abundant flow on color Doppler interrogation (**D**), intussuscepted into the cecum (*arrows*). Open arrows indicate the terminal ileum. *P,* Psoas muscle. The pathologic diagnosis was Burkitt lymphoma. (**B,** Courtesy Dr. Marta Hernanz-Schulman, Nashville, TN.)

ENEMA TECHNIQUES AND REDUCTION RATES

For reduction of intussusception, the air enema is considered superior to the positive-contrast liquid enema, and since its introduction, the air enema has had increasing acceptance among pediatric radiologists; in 2004, 65% of pediatric radiologists in the United States reported using air enema, a proportion that is likely higher today.[34] An air enema is considered superior for several reasons. It is cleaner, because no liquid or stool spillage occurs on the table, on the patient, or on the field of view. It is much easier to see the progress of the reduction through the distended sigmoid when it is filled with gas than when it is filled with dense positive-contrast media. An air enema is also considered safer than a liquid enema because if perforation does occur, it has been shown that there is less spillage of fecal material and

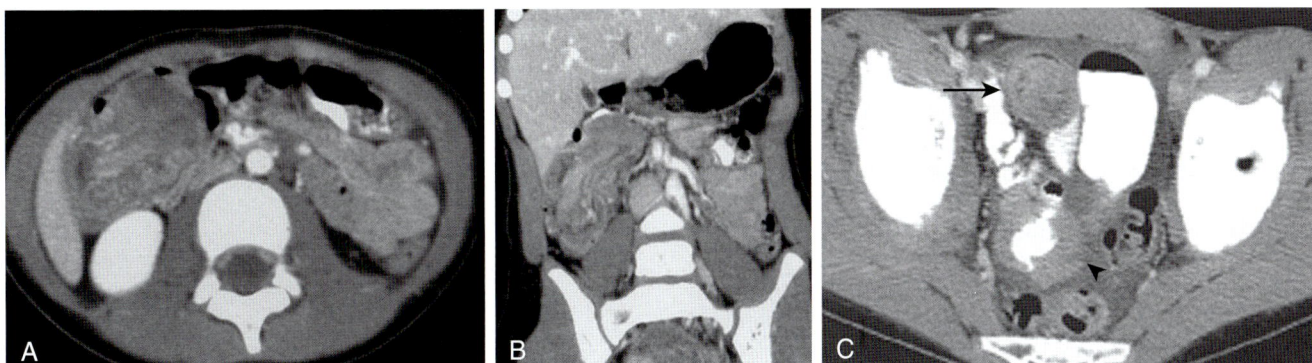

Figure 108-7   Intussusception on computed tomography (CT) images. **A** and **B,** Axial and coronal reformatting of a CT scan of a 6-year-old girl presenting with abdominal pain. The examination shows an intussusception with a solid mass at the leading end in the proximal transverse colon; the pathologic diagnosis was Burkitt lymphoma. **C,** CT in an adolescent with Burkitt lymphoma presenting with abdominal pain. The examination shows both the intussusception in the right lower quadrant anteriorly (*arrow*) and also ascites and tumor caking (*arrowhead*) on the outer wall of a loop of ileum dorsal to the intussusception.

Box 108-2 Image-Guided Reduction of Intussusception

Absolute Contraindications

- Peritonitis
- Free intraperitoneal air

Relative Contraindications

- High fever, leukocytosis, abdominal tenderness (especially rebound tenderness)
- Severe dehydration or profound lethargy

Pneumatic Reduction Technique

- Be certain the patient is well hydrated
- Be sure the buttocks are well sealed
- Use available measurement devices to control pressure
- Start at 80 mm Hg; do not exceed 120 mm Hg mean pressure
- Even after the small bowel is filled with air, evaluate the cecum for a residual mass

Hydrostatic Reduction Technique

- Be certain the patient is well hydrated
- Be sure the buttocks are well sealed
- Maintain a pressure head no greater than 1 meter H_2O
- Make three attempts of 3 minutes each
- Reduction is incomplete unless substantial amounts of small bowel are easily filled

liquid into the peritoneal cavity. Reduction usually is achieved more quickly, and air is less dense than positive-contrast media, translating into less radiation exposure. The rates of recurrence of intussusception after air or after liquid enema reductions do not differ; both are approximately 10%.[11,15,35-37]

In more than 70 published studies of enema reduction, investigators report an average reduction rate of 76% (Table 108-2).[8,38] When the reduction rates are weighted by the number of children in each study, the average reduction rate for air is significantly better than for liquid (82% for air and 73% for liquid). In the largest published series, Gu and colleagues[36] used air enema in 9028 children and reported reduction rates of 95%. However, although the air enema may be preferred in experienced hands, the liquid enema is also effective. In two randomized, controlled trials of reduction rate or air versus liquid enema, one trial concluded that air enema was superior to liquid enema,[39] and the other showed no difference,[40] although the sample size was small.

A surgical consultation should be obtained for all children before an enema is performed for the following reasons: (1) to assess for peritoneal signs precluding enema, (2) to identify children whose intussusception may not be reduced with enema or who are found to have perforation, (3) for urgent surgery in case of perforation, and (4) for management after reduction. Before enema reduction, dehydration should be treated with intravenous fluid resuscitation. Children with evidence of peritonitis, shock, sepsis, or free air on abdominal radiographs are not candidates for an enema.

Air Enema Technique

To perform the air enema technique, the enema tip should be placed in the child's rectum and taped in place. The tape can be shaped into a funnel along the tube to help form a seal. The buttocks are taped together tightly, and an assistant should hold the buttocks closed, whether the child is in a supine or a prone position. This technique is important because air leaking around the tube diminishes the pressure head. Air is rapidly insufflated into the colon under fluoroscopic observation, up to a constant mean pressure of 120 mm Hg, thus maximizing reduction and minimizing the risk for perforation. Once the intussusception is encountered, it is monitored fluoroscopically until it is completely reduced. The use of pulsed fluoroscopy at a low frame rate is an important factor for reducing the radiation dose, particularly when the reduction is lengthy. Fluoroscopy "grabs" (or "last image hold") can document the progress of the reduction, without additional exposures. Air should flow freely from the cecum into the distal small bowel loops to signify complete reduction (Fig. 108-8; Video 108-1).

The radiologist should be vigilant for the appearance of free intraperitoneal air, which can be inconspicuous at first. In case of perforation, it is very important to open the buttocks and the rectal tube to allow colonic air to escape outside the patient; in addition, it is also very important to have a large-gauge needle available to decompress the peritoneal cavity if respiratory distress develops, because air that escapes the colon and enters the cavity can result in a tension pneumoperitoneum, elevating the diaphragm and impeding adequate breathing. Images with the intussusception reduced to the cecum can be compared with later images to help determine the distension of small bowel loops with insufflated air, thus outlining a successful reduction, particularly in potentially confusing cases that involve small bowel loops that already are dilated because of preexistent small bowel obstruction. When using the air enema technique, many pediatric radiologists suggest limiting each attempt to 4 minutes.

A positive-contrast liquid enema tends to outline the small bowel loops to better advantage and may outline the

Table 108-2

Summary of Published Studies* of Enema Reduction and Perforation Rates[†]

		Studies (N)	Reduction Rate (%)	Studies (N)	Perforation Rate (%)
All	Simple	74	72.8 (1.8)	66	0.80 (0.16)
	Weighted	—	75.9 (0.4)	—	0.76 (0.10)
Hydrostatic	Simple	48	68.6 (2.4)	42	0.71 (0.19)
	Weighted	—	73.0 (0.5)	—	0.57 (0.10)
Pneumatic	Simple	26	81.3 (1.3)	24	0.98 (0.31)
	Weighted	—	81.5 (0.7)	—	1.02 (0.16)
P value[‡]	—	—	<.001	—	.02

*Excludes two very large studies by Guo et al. (1986) and Zhang et al. (1986).
[†]All values are mean (standard error) from unweighted (simple) and weighted estimates. Weighted estimates use the sample size to adjust the reported mean reduction and perforation rates.
[‡]p-values based on logistic regression. Compare hydrostatic with pneumatic rate and perforation rate.
Reprinted with permission from Applegate KE. Intussusception in children: diagnostic imaging and treatment. In: Medina LS, Applegate KE, Blackmore CC, eds. *Evidence-based imaging in pediatrics.* New York: Springer; 2010.

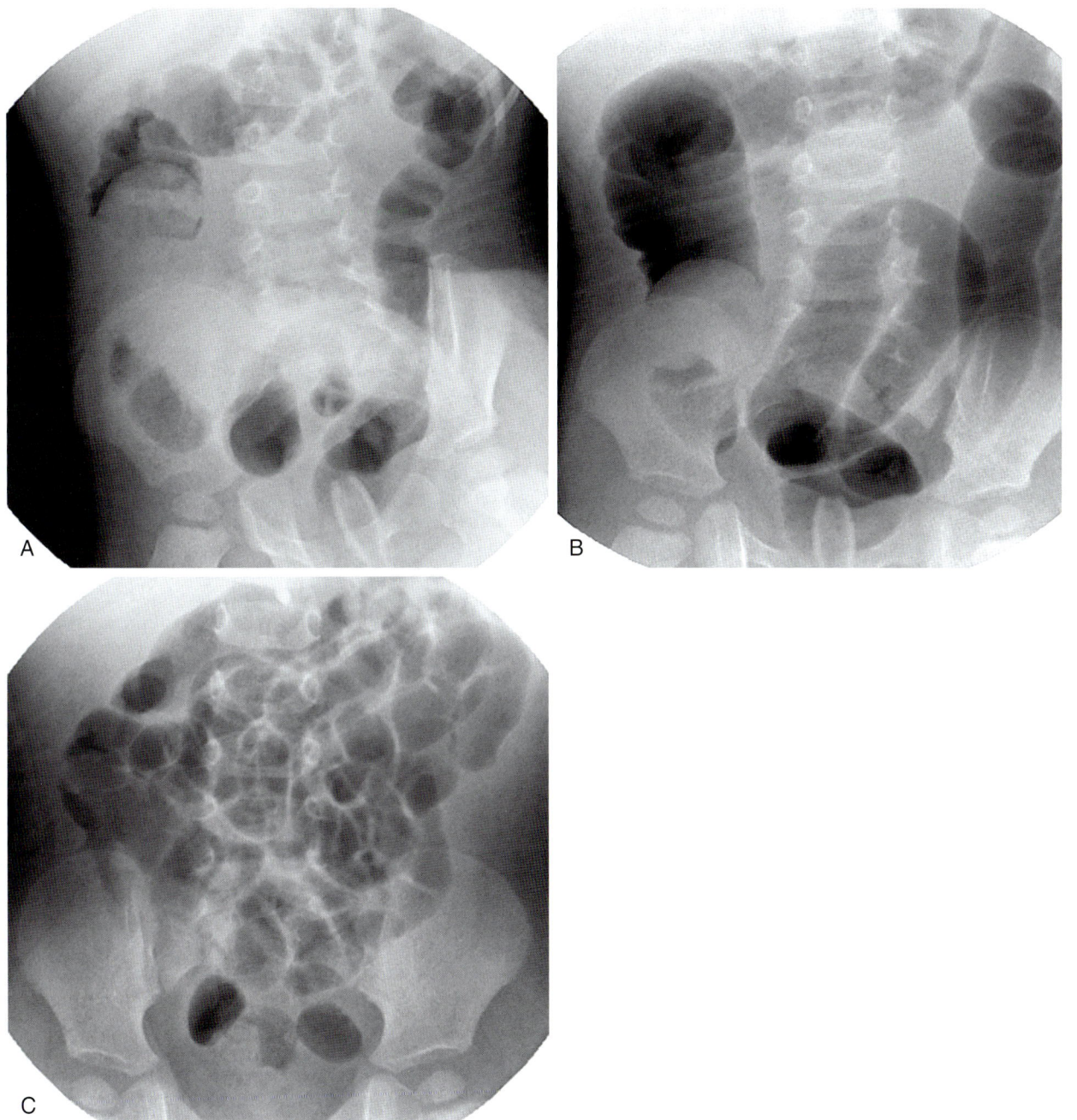

Figure 108-8 Pneumatic reduction of intussusception. **A,** An initial fluoroscopic image shows the tube tip in the rectum and the leading edge of the intussusception at the hepatic flexure. **B,** After continued insufflation and further distension of the colon, the leading edge has moved into the right lower quadrant. **C,** After successful reduction, gas fills multiple loops of small bowel. (Courtesy Dr. Marta Hernanz-Schulman, Nashville, TN.)

appendix at the cecal tip (e-Fig. 108-9). Ileoileal components may be more conspicuously identified. Rarely, the appendix intussuscepts into the cecum, causing abdominal pain (e-Fig. 108-10). A general guideline to the liquid enema technique is the "rule of 3s": three attempts of 3 minutes' duration, with the liquid enema bag at 3 feet above the fluoroscopy table (see Box 108-2). Although little evidence exists to support this rule, particularly regarding the height of the enema bag,[8,41] it serves well as a general guideline. A study by Kuta and Benator[42] of the pressures generated by a column of liquid media indicates that media differ in the height at which a pressure of 120 mm Hg is generated. This differs

from the air enema technique, which allows control and documentation of the pressure used. The examination is tailored to the patient and performed in collaboration with the surgeon.

Radiation Exposure

The radiation exposure a child receives depends on a number of factors, including the type of fluoroscopy equipment, the use of pulsed fluoroscopy, the ease or rapidity of reduction, the fluoroscopy time, and the contrast medium used. Experienced pediatric radiologists performing an air enema average approximately 95 seconds of fluoroscopy time to reduce an intussusception.[36] Air enema radiation exposures have been calculated to be less than one third those given during a barium enema.[43] In 2003, Henrikson and coworkers[26] estimated that the mean radiation exposure was 25 mSv for enema reductions in a group of patients receiving both air and positive-contrast media reductions.

Perforation

The potential complication of enema reduction that causes the most concern is bowel perforation.[11,44,45] The risk for perforation depends on each radiologist's patient population and technique. Although determination of clinical predictors of perforation is complicated by a lack of prospective studies, a key factor is symptoms that last longer than 48 hours. Several reports of studies in porcine models and in children suggest that a preexisting focal perforation in the necrotic intussuscipiens or less commonly the intussusceptum, may exist that is rarely radiographically apparent as free air before reduction but is uncovered during the reduction process.[8,11,15,44-46] The most common site is at or just proximal to the intussusception in the transverse colon.

In a summary of more than 60 studies, the mean perforation rate is less than 1%[39] (see Table 108-2). In 1989, Campbell[47] surveyed enema techniques and complications of North American pediatric radiologists. Respondents' combined experience was 14,000 intussusception enemas. Although they did not report enema reduction rates, the combined perforation rate was 0.39% (55 per 14,000, or 1 per 250 to 300 patients), with only one death. This study remains the basis for the perforation risk when it is explained to parents prior to enema reduction.[47]

Barium is no longer the liquid contrast medium of choice for reduction of intussusception among most pediatric radiologists because of the risks for barium peritonitis, infection, and adhesions when perforation occurs during the enema. If liquid media are to be used, iodinated contrast material is now preferred and is considered a safer agent than barium; nevertheless, such media are hypertonic and may produce fluid and electrolyte shifts if perforation occurs.[11,46,48-50]

One complication unique to air enema is tension pneumoperitoneum. In an early report, two deaths occurred as a result of this complication, leading the proponents of air enema to advise having an 18-gauge needle readily available in the fluoroscopy room for emergent decompression. Although development of an air embolism is theoretically possible, no reports of an air embolism have been published.

Alternative Enema Approaches

A number of different approaches have been described to try to improve intussusception reduction via enema. These approaches include sedation, anesthesia, use of glucagon, manual palpation, and a delayed repeat enema. Except for the delayed repeat enema, none of these approaches has been proved to increase the rate of successful reduction. Sedation may reduce the intraabdominal pressure children create by the Valsalva maneuver, a factor that increases success of reduction and decreases the perforation rate.[8,35]

Fluoroscopy Versus Sonography

In North American and most European centers, fluoroscopy is almost always used during enema reduction. In Asian and some European centers, sonographic guidance is used, thus avoiding any radiation exposure. Reports on the use of sonography with water or other liquid media such as normal saline solution show rates of successful reduction to be as high or higher than with fluoroscopic techniques.[51,52] However, the experience level required for these techniques has not been evaluated.

Delayed Repeat Enema

When an initial enema reduction attempt fails to completely reduce the intussusception, a delayed repeat enema may be successful and thus avoid the need for surgical reduction. The use of such an additional, delayed attempt between 30 minutes and 19 hours after the initial procedure has shown promise in increasing the success of enema reductions. Four studies report further reduction in 50% to 82% of cases in which reduction fails at the initial enema.[53-55] Further research to understand optimal timing and technique for delayed repeat enemas is needed. The largest reported experience to date suggests a delay of 2 to 4 hours, until further research yields more rigorous guidelines.[8] The child must remain clinically stable and be appropriately monitored during this time interval. A delayed enema is useful when movement of the intussusception occurred at the initial attempt, but the final reduction could not be accomplished; a delayed enema should not be attempted if the intussusception is not partially reduced during the initial attempt.

SURGICAL MANAGEMENT AND COMPLICATIONS

The costs of surgical care are four to five times the costs of nonsurgical management.[33,56] Depending on the patient population, approximately 20% to 40% of children for whom nonsurgical treatment fails and who undergo surgical reduction of their intussusception will require bowel resection.[57]

MANAGEMENT OF RECURRENT CASES

In patients with recurrent intussusception, including multiple recurrences, enema remains the preferred method of reduction. Intussusception recurrence rates average up to 10% in large series (range, 5% to 15%), regardless of whether the reduction technique involved an air or liquid enema. The recurrence rates are less than or equal to 5% when surgical reduction is performed, presumably because of the development of adhesions.[58] Enema reduction is both safe and effective in cases of recurrent intussusception, as long as the child remains clinically stable. Approximately 50% of children in whom recurrent intussusception develops present within 48 hours, although recurrences have been reported up to 18 months later. No clear risk factors have been discovered to explain why some children have recurrences, although some children have focal pathologic lead points. Nevertheless, the risk for lead points in children with recurrent intussusception remains low. In a large series of 763 children reported by Daneman and colleagues,[46] lead points were present in only

8% of recurrent intussusceptions, only slightly higher than the 5% to 6% incidence of lead points at first presentation of intussusceptions.

No predictive clinical factors have been identified for the presence of lead points in children with recurrent intussusception. In children with a diffuse bowel abnormality such as cystic fibrosis, Henoch-Schönlein purpura, or celiac disease, enema reduction may be used more aggressively than in children with focal lead points who require surgery.

When the presence of pathologic lead points is a concern, ultrasound may play an important role, detecting as many as 60% of the lead points (see Fig. 108-6).[4,5] Although ultrasound does not detect all lead points, the risk of missing a lead point without other signs or symptoms to guide management is thought to be unlikely.[5,58] To test the hypothesis that recurrent intussusception in some patients might be related to lymphoid hyperplasia at the terminal ileum, Lin and colleagues[3] conducted a randomized, double-blind trial comparing 144 children who received intramuscular corticosteroid drugs with 137 children who received placebo before air enema reduction. No recurrences occurred in the children who received dexamethasone, compared with a 5% recurrence rate in the placebo group. These investigators hypothesized that steroids decreased the volume of mesenteric adenopathy and lymphoid hyperplasia in the terminal ileum and thus decreased the risk for recurrence.[3] However, further investigation is needed for confirmation and to evaluate the risks and benefits of this intervention.

Key Points

Intussusception is the most common cause of small bowel obstruction in children.

Most cases of ileocolic intussusception occurring in children are idiopathic. An accompanying pathologic lead-point mass lesion may be found in 5% to 6% of all children.

The most common focal lead points are (in decreasing order of incidence) Meckel diverticulum, duplication cyst, polyp, and lymphoma.

The classic clinical presentation of the child with intussusception is colicky abdominal pain, vomiting, and bloody stools; a palpable abdominal mass is found in fewer than 25% of patients.

The most important factor that predicts an unsuccessful enema reduction is a longer duration of symptoms.

Abdominal radiographs have a limited sensitivity and specificity for the detection of intussusception.

Ultrasound is the primary imaging modality for the initial diagnosis of intussusception.

The only absolute contraindications to enema reduction are signs of peritonitis on clinical examination or free air on abdominal radiographs.

For reduction of an intussusception, an air enema is considered superior to a positive-contrast liquid enema.

The perforation rate during intussusception enema reduction is <1%.

Intussusception recurrence rates average up to 10%.

Suggested Readings

Applegate KE. Clinically suspected intussusception in children: evidence-based review and self-assessment module. *AJR Am J Roentgenol.* 2005; 185(suppl 3):S175-S183.
Daneman A, Navarro O. Intussusception. Part 1: A review of diagnostic approaches. *Pediatr Radiol.* 2003;33:79-85.
Daneman A, Navarro O. Intussusception. Part 2: An update on the evolution of management. *Pediatr Radiol.* 2004;34:97-108.
Navarro O, Daneman A. Intussusception. Part 3: Diagnosis and management of those with an identifiable or predisposing cause and those that reduce spontaneously. *Pediatr Radiol.* 2004;34:305-312.

References

Full references for this chapter can be found on www.expertconsult.com.

Chapter 109

Tumors and Tumorlike Conditions

JEFFREY TRAUBICI and ALAN DANEMAN

Tumors and tumorlike conditions affecting the colon in children can be divided into several categories. For the purpose of this chapter, we will discuss benign lymphoid hyperplasia, vascular lesions of the colon, and neoplasms. Several neoplasms arise in patients with genetic disorders, and in those cases, we have attempted to provide a brief description of the disorder. Although these colonic lesions, particularly the neoplastic ones, tend to be rare in children, it is incumbent on the radiologist to be familiar with them to be able to provide a thoughtful and thorough consultation with respect to the imaging findings.

Nonneoplastic Lesions

BENIGN LYMPHOID HYPERPLASIA

Overview Benign lymphoid hyperplasia is believed to represent a benign condition of the bowel and is most frequently found in the distal ileum and in the colon. These lesions represent patches of lymphoid tissue and can be seen in both adults and children. The precise prevalence in children is unknown, but the entity has been found in up to 30% of symptomatic patients undergoing colonoscopy.[1]

Etiology A number of possible causes have been postulated. The observation of benign lymphoid hyperplasia in families suggests that genetic or environmental factors could be pertinent.[2] A recent study by Krauss et al.[3] found that the prevalence of lymphoid hyperplasia at colonoscopy also is high in adults, and they postulated that it may relate to an enhanced immune response. In children, a number of theories have been proposed, including a local response to infection, immunodeficiency states, and local hypersensitivity reaction. Controversy also exists regarding the association of benign lymphoid hyperplasia and the autism spectrum disorder.[4]

Clinical Presentation Benign lymphoid hyperplasia is usually discovered incidentally either on imaging or at endoscopy. As such, it is almost certainly underrecognized, and its true prevalence is unknown. Visual inspection at colonoscopy will demonstrate multiple raised, closely spaced areas along the bowel wall.

Imaging The appearance on imaging studies is that of innumerable small filling defects, mostly uniform in size, at times umbilicated, and most commonly seen on double-contrast imaging of the colon (Fig. 109-1). These lesions are often too small to be detected on a single-contrast examination. One of the earliest imaging descriptions stressed their benign nature and the need to distinguish the lesion from true polyps,[5] citing instances in which colectomies were performed because the benign nature of these lesions was not recognized. This pattern of innumerable small lesions (often in the range of 2 to 3 mm) also should be distinguished from benign lymphoid polyps, which are more common in adults and can become fairly large and pedunculated.[6]

Treatment Lymphoid hyperplasia itself requires no specific treatment. If it is associated with another condition, then that condition would be treated accordingly.

VASCULAR LESIONS

Overview A number of vascular lesions and vascular tumors can arise within the colon. They are rare in children but can have specific clinical settings and imaging findings, which can allow for a specific diagnosis. Some vascular lesions will be found incidentally. Others can present as lower gastrointestinal (GI) tract bleeding.

Etiology Vascular lesions of the colon represent a wide array of conditions. The etiology is known for some lesions and remains unknown for others. Colonic varices (particularly in the rectal region) can be seen as mural lesions and typically are seen with portal hypertension, providing a collateral pathway between the portomesenteric and the systemic venous systems. This collateral pathway has been reported to occur in nearly one third of children with portal hypertension. In that group of patients, significant rectal bleeding was seen in 7%.[7]

Other vascular lesions also can result in lower GI bleeding. Venous malformations, arteriovenous malformations, angiodysplasia, telangiectasias, and hemangiomas all have been described in the colon in children but are rare.[8] Their etiology is not well understood.

Clinical Presentation Because vascular lesions of the colon tend to come to light when they are symptomatic, the true incidence is unknown, but they are believed to be rare in children. The presentation can be that of lower GI bleeding or anemia. It should be noted that hemangiomas, which fall under the category of vascular tumors of the GI tract, can be associated with cutaneous hemangiomas in up to 50% of cases.

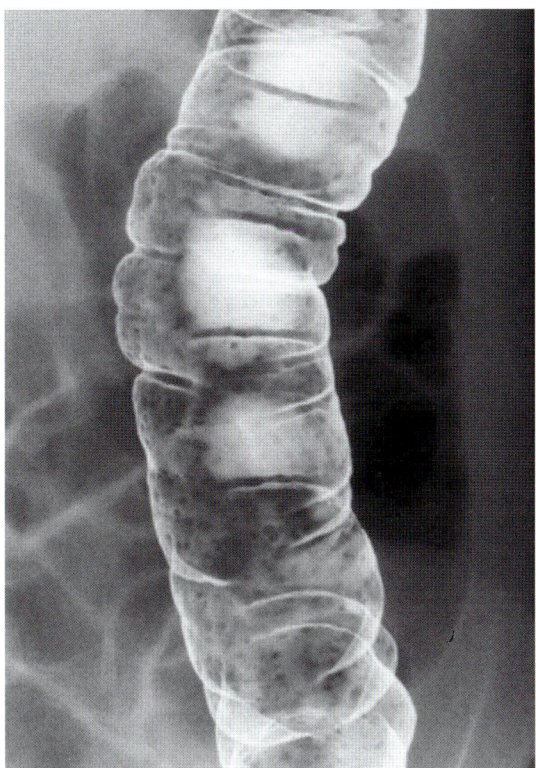

Figure 109-1 Benign lymphoid hyperplasia. An 11-year-old girl had a double-contrast barium enema as part of the workup for rectal bleeding. A spot image of the descending colon from that examination demonstrates numerous filling defects that are uniform in size. The findings are consistent with benign lymphoid hyperplasia. Similar findings were seen throughout the colon.

Imaging The lesions are difficult to resolve with most imaging modalities. Multidetector computed tomography (CT) with imaging in the early arterial phase after contrast injection can demonstrate these lesions. Involved bowel will show intense enhancement (Fig. 109-2). Some patients will

have abnormal supplying arteries or draining veins visible on CT. In a minority of cases with bleeding, active extravasation can be visualized.[9]

Treatment Much like vascular lesions elsewhere in the GI tract and indeed elsewhere in the body, the treatment of the lesion depends on the specific lesion, its location, the degree and extent of involvement, and the clinical status of the patient. These lesions can be treated medically or surgically, embolized via a catheter, or sclerosed endoscopically.

Although treatment very much depends on the type of lesion, some controversy exists with regard to the classification of intestinal vascular anomalies in children. Many persons advocate applying a classification system used for other vascular anomalies, such as the system proposed by Fishman and Mulliken,[10] although other persons advocate use of a broader system.[11]

Neoplastic Lesions

Neoplasms of the colon are rare in children. Most are benign juvenile polyps. Polyps associated with the hereditary polyposis syndromes are quite rare, and there is often a known family history. Primary malignancies arising from the colon and metastatic disease to the colon are rarer still. These three groups will constitute the remainder of this chapter.

In the past, the double-contrast barium enema has been the study of choice in the investigation of colonic neoplasms. However, more recently, ultrasound, CT, and magnetic resonance imaging (MRI) increasingly have been used. Often these modalities are used in the initial stages of the investigation, but the final diagnosis is established after endoscopy, snare resection, and/or surgical intervention.

JUVENILE POLYPS

Overview Juvenile or hamartomatous polyps are the most common intestinal tumors in childhood, with a prevalence

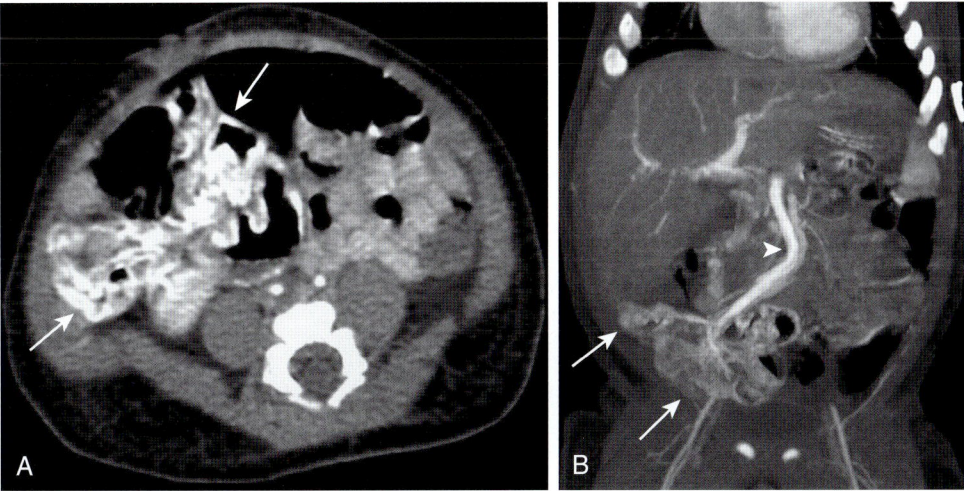

Figure 109-2 Colonic infantile hemangioma. An infant presented at 4 weeks of age with gastrointestinal bleeding requiring multiple transfusions. An enhanced computed tomography scan of the abdomen and pelvis was done in the arterial phase. Axial (**A**) and coronal reconstruction (**B**) demonstrates intense enhancement of the wall of the distal ileum and cecum (*arrows*). Venous drainage is through a markedly dilated mesenteric vein (*arrowhead* in **B**). The affected segment was resected, and pathology confirmed that it was an infantile hemangioma.

of 1% to 3%. They may be single or multiple, and most are found in the sigmoid colon and rectum, but they can arise anywhere along the GI tract.

Etiology Histologically these lesions appear as mucus-filled glands, and they might be related to blocked, hyperplastic mucus glands. A dense infiltrate of inflammatory cells suggests an inflammatory inciting event, and thus the synonymous term "inflammatory polyp." However, the underlying etiology of these isolated polyps remains to be determined.

Clinical Presentation Although presentation is rare in the first year of life, most patients present in the first decade, typically between 2 and 5 years of age. The most common presenting symptom is painless bright red rectal bleeding. Pain is associated with the rare complication of colocolic intussusception. Some children present with iron deficiency anemia. Others can present with a prolapsing mass, which can be mistaken for rectal prolapse.[12]

Imaging In the past, investigation for colonic neoplasms such as the juvenile polyp in a child with rectal bleeding often included a double-contrast enema. On such an examination, these lesions are typically smooth and can be sessile or pedunculated; most measure 3 cm or less. Currently the diagnosis is more frequently made endoscopically or on cross-sectional imaging, in which the lesions appear as nonspecific intraluminal masses (Fig. 109-3).

Treatment Because these solitary lesions carry no increased risk of malignancy, the treatment is polypectomy alone. Most commonly, a polypectomy is performed with snare resection during a colonoscopy. The anemia is treated with iron supplementation or transfusion if necessary. With resection of the polyp, the blood loss should cease. If multiple polyps are present or a family history of juvenile polyps is uncovered, then the patient should be evaluated for the juvenile polyposis syndrome (JPS), discussed later in this chapter.

Polyposis Syndromes

Although the inherited polyposis syndromes are rare, they have the potential to cause serious morbidity and mortality within affected families. A proper understanding of the various conditions is important for the primary clinician and consultant. Genetic screening and initiation of a surveillance plan is mandatory. Surveillance should include the GI tract as well as extraintestinal sites of potential disease.[13]

SYNDROMES ASSOCIATED WITH JUVENILE OR HAMARTOMATOUS POLYPS

Juvenile Polyposis Syndrome

Overview First described in the literature in 1964,[14] JPS is an autosomal-dominant condition that is characterized by a multiplicity of GI hamartomatous polyps. It is the most common of the hamartomatous syndromes.

Etiology In approximately 75% of cases, a family history of the disease will be present. The condition also can occur sporadically as a result of new mutations. Mutations have been identified in the *SMAD4* gene on chromosome 18 and the *BMPR1A* gene on chromosome 10.[15]

Clinical Presentation From a clinical standpoint, the disease should be considered in any patient with five or more juvenile polyps in the colon, extracolonic juvenile polyps, or with any number of polyps when associated with a positive family history.[16] The clinical presentation can be more variable than in the patient with nonsyndromic juvenile polyps. In addition to rectal bleeding, anemia, and intussusception, patients with JPS in whom there is involvement of a large segment of the GI tract can present with failure to thrive, malabsorption, or hypoalbuminemia. Associated congenital anomalies include hydrocephalus and hypertelorism. Small series have described JPS in association with other conditions, including hereditary hemorrhagic telangiectasia.[17]

Imaging The imaging appearance of polyps in JPS differs in the number of polyps identified, but otherwise it is similar to that of isolated lesions.

Treatment Patients with JPS have an increased risk of colonic malignancy that is reported to be as high as 50% on the basis of family studies.[18] Screening of these children can

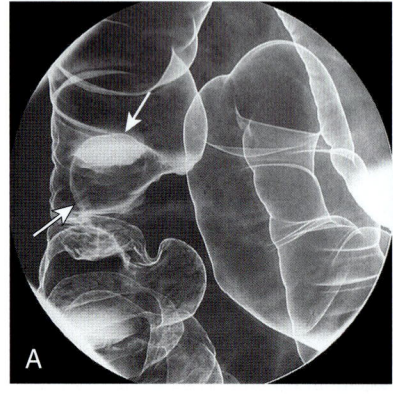
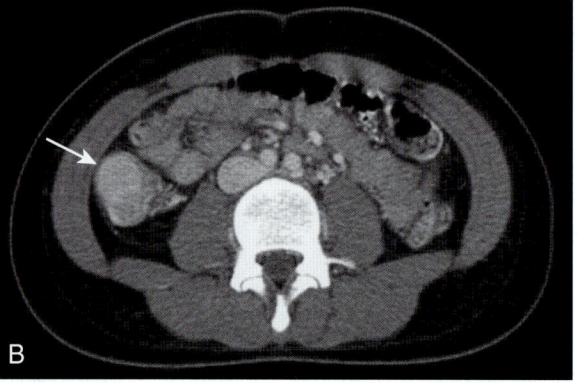

Figure 109-3 Juvenile polyp. A 15-year-old girl presented with a 2-month history of abdominal pain. **A,** A double-contrast enema demonstrates a sessile mass consistent with a polyp arising from the wall of the ascending colon (*arrows*). **B,** A computed tomography scan in the same patient demonstrated an enhancing mass (*arrow*) within the lumen of the ascending colon.

be done with a combination of endoscopy, various imaging modalities, and capsule endoscopy. Polyps typically are removed via snare polypectomy.

Cowden Syndrome

Overview   Cowden syndrome is a rare autosomal-dominant syndrome with an estimated prevalence of 1:200,000 individuals.[19] Features include hamartomatous polyps of the GI tract, hamartomatous lesions of the skin, hamartomas of other solid organs, and neoplasms of the breast, thyroid, and endometrium.[19] GI tract polyps arising in these patients include inflammatory, hyperplastic, lipomatous, and even adenomatous lesions.

Etiology   Cowden syndrome is one of several disorders that fall under the category of the protein tyrosine phosphatase and tensin (PTEN) hamartoma tumor syndromes. Mutations in the tumor suppressor gene *PTEN* are present in up to 80% of patients with Cowden syndrome.[19,20]

Clinical Presentation   The presentation of patients with Cowden syndrome can be similar to the other conditions in which colonic polyps occur. Patients with Cowden syndrome also have an increased risk of neoplasms of the thyroid, endometrium, and breast. The lifetime risk of breast cancer in women with Cowden syndrome is between 25% and 50%. In these women, the onset of breast cancer is earlier than in sporadic cases. At present, the risk of GI malignancy in these patients is unknown.[19]

Imaging   The imaging appearance of polyps in Cowden syndrome is similar to that of polyps described earlier in the chapter.

Treatment   Polyps in patients with Cowden syndrome are treated with snare polypectomy; screening can include endoscopy, fluoroscopic and cross-sectional imaging

modalities, and capsule endoscopy. Anemia is treated with iron supplementation and transfusion if necessary. Appropriate screening for the associated neoplasms also must be initiated. This screening consists of early breast self-examination and perhaps early initiation of mammography. Thyroid and uterine surveillance with screening ultrasound also is recommended.

Peutz-Jeghers Syndrome

Overview   Peutz-Jeghers syndrome is an autosomal-dominant syndrome with an incidence of approximately 1:120,000 people.[21] It was described separately, in 1921 and 1949, by the authors after whom the syndrome was named. In this condition, hamartomatous polyps develop in the GI tract, in association with skin and mucosal hyperpigmented lesions.

Etiology   Peutz-Jeghers syndrome can be divided into two types. In the familial type, evidence indicates that the syndrome relates to mutations in the *STK11* (serine threonine kinase) gene. In up to 50% of cases, no family history of the disease is present, which suggests a fairly high rate of new mutation.[22]

Clinical Presentation   The condition is characterized by pigmented lesions of the lips and buccal mucosa, as well as by hamartomatous polyps of the GI tract. The polyps can occur anywhere in the GI tract, although they are most commonly found in the small bowel, particularly in the jejunum. Polyps in the large and small bowel tend to be pedunculated. Those in the stomach tend to be more sessile (Fig. 109-4, *A*). Polyps also can arise in the gall bladder, bronchi, urinary bladder, and ureter.

The most common GI-related clinical presentation is one of abdominal pain as a result of intussusception, with a polyp as a pathological lead point. Patients also can present with clinical findings related to GI hemorrhage.

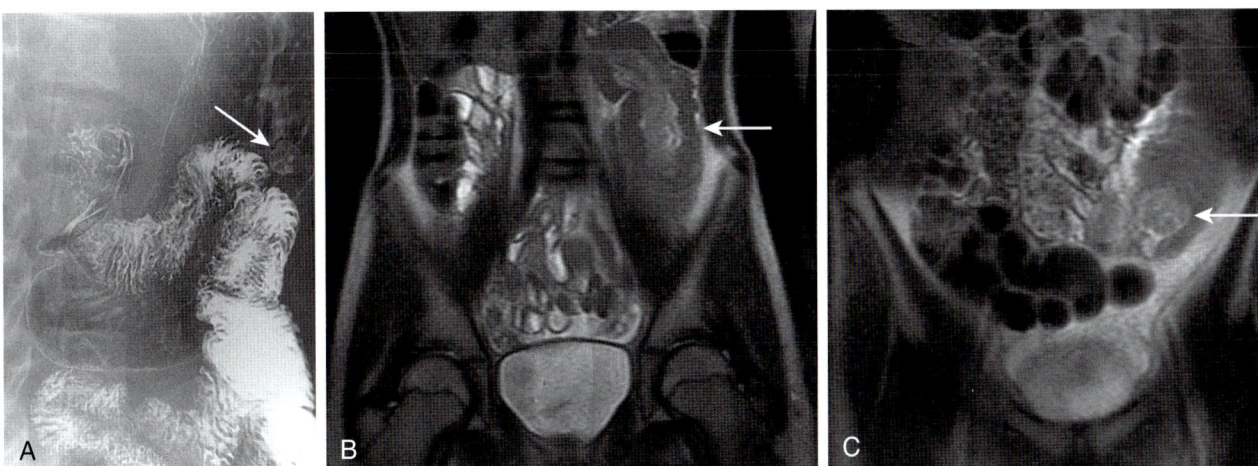

Figure 109-4   Peutz-Jeghers syndrome in a 14-year-old girl. **A,** A double-contrast upper gastrointestinal series demonstrates a small polyp (*arrow*) arising in the proximal body of the stomach. **B** and **C,** Several years later, the patient presented with abdominal pain and was found to have a small bowel intussusception (*arrow*). **B,** A coronal magnetic resonance imaging single shot fast spin echo sequence demonstrates the intussusception along the left flank (*arrow*). **C,** What was believed to be a polyp functioning as a lead point (*arrow*) was seen lower in the pelvis on a more anterior image of the same sequence.

Imaging   The appearance of the polyps in Peutz-Jeghers syndrome does not differ significantly from that seen in other hamartomatous polyposes. It is not unusual for patients to present with intussusception. In that situation, the appearance is typical of an intussusception (see Chapter 108), with the polyp acting as a pathological lead point (Fig. 109-4, *B* and *C*).

Treatment   The treatment of the polyps is removal, either surgically or endoscopically, when necessary. Anemia is treated with iron supplementation and transfusion if necessary. Although it is not clear whether the polyps themselves have malignant potential, it is now accepted that there is an overall increased risk of neoplasms in patients with Peutz-Jeghers syndrome, typically in adulthood. Colorectal, breast, and ovarian tumors predominate.[21]

POLYPOSIS SYNDROMES ASSOCIATED WITH ADENOMATOUS POLYPS

Several conditions fall under the category of polyposis syndromes associated with adenomatous polyps. These conditions include familial adenomatous polyposis (FAP), attenuated FAP, Gardner syndrome, and Turcot syndrome. In all these conditions, a germline mutation occurs in the adenomatous polyposis coli (*APC*) gene, located on the long arm of chromosome 5.

Familial Adenomatous Polyposis and Variants

Overview   The prevalence of FAP is believed to be between 1:5000 and 1:17,000, depending on the series.[23] Although the condition is defined by the presence of more than five adenomatous polyps, affected persons often will have hundreds, if not thousands, of polyps.

Extraintestinal lesions also are well described. In nearly 1 in 5 patients, a desmoid tumor will develop (e-Fig. 109-5), which will be discussed further later in this chapter. Congenital hypertrophy of the retinal pigment epithelial cells is seen in 60% to 90% of patients and is present at birth and can be assessed with fundoscopy. Lesions that can develop later in life include osteomas (often in the skull and mandible), lipomas, fibromas, and epidermoid cysts. An increased risk exists of developing hepatoblastoma (e-Fig. 109-6), thyroid and pancreatic cancers, cholangiocarcinoma, and central nervous system (CNS) tumors, particularly medulloblastoma.[24] It is believed that with better management of the intestinal manifestations of FAP and subsequent longer life spans of affected patients, the incidence of these extraintestinal manifestations will likely increase.

In patients with attenuated FAP, fewer polyps are present and the inevitable development of malignancy occurs nearly a decade later than in the classic form. Patients with attenuated FAP manifest similar extraintestinal lesions and also exhibit a propensity for extracolonic polyps.

Gardner syndrome is believed to represent a variant of FAP, rather than a separate syndrome; some clinicians include these patients within the FAP group and agree that the term Gardner syndrome is now obsolete, although others continue to use the term in cases where the extraintestinal disease is particularly prominent. In Gardner syndrome, one sees the typical GI manifestations of FAP, including the plethora of polyps and the associated malignancies. Desmoid tumors often are cited as a classic extracolonic lesion in persons with Gardner syndrome; these tumors are a local aggressive form of fibromatosis and arise from the fascial tissue associated with muscle or from the mesentery. The tumors typically appear in the abdomen or in the abdominal wall.[25] They may develop after trauma, such as after a prophylactic colectomy, and are a major cause of morbidity and mortality in these patients.[25]

In addition to desmoid tumors, patients with Gardner syndrome develop osteomas (particularly of the mandible), periampullary duodenal polyps, lipomas, fibromas, nasopharyngeal angiofibromas, and epidermoid cysts.

Etiology   FAP is an autosomal-dominant condition in which a mutation is present in the adenomatous polyposis coli (*APC*) gene; approximately 30% of cases result from spontaneous mutations.[26] This mutation results in a failure of apoptosis, and in uncontrolled cell growth, with the ultimate development of polyps—in this case, adenomatous ones.

Clinical Presentation   Polyps tend to develop in the second and late in the first decades of life, and often it is not until the third decade that symptoms arise. Therefore, unless screened, patients may not present with symptoms until adulthood. The most common presentation in childhood is rectal bleeding.[23]

Imaging   In classic FAP, the colon is carpeted with lesions (Fig. 109-7). The polyps tend to vary in size and lack the central umbilication often seen in benign lymphoid hyperplasia.

A desmoid tumor is most often hypoechoic and at times nearly anechoic on ultrasound. On CT, the lesion often will

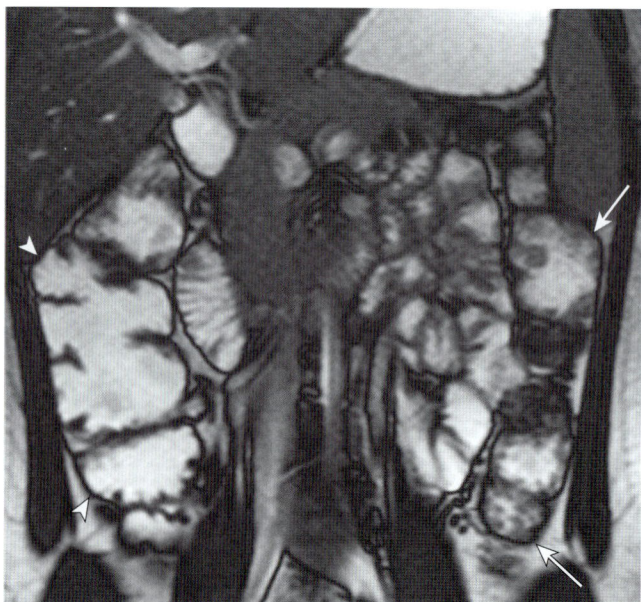

Figure 109-7   Familial adenomatous polyposis (FAP). A 17-year-old girl with FAP. A coronal true fast imaging with steady state precession magnetic resonance series through the abdomen demonstrates multiple nodular lesions consistent with small polyps along the descending colon (*arrows*). The ascending colon (*arrowheads*) also was involved to a lesser degree.

be low attenuation, exhibit little enhancement in the portal venous phase, and may show increased enhancement in a delayed phase. Signal characteristics vary on MR. The lesion is usually of low signal intensity on T1-weighted sequences and of high signal on T2-weighted sequences (see e-Fig. 109-5).

Treatment Colorectal carcinoma will develop in nearly all patients with FAP if it is left untreated. The accepted standard of care, therefore, is prophylactic colectomy. Polyps also can develop in other parts of the GI tract in patients with FAP. Periampullary polyps of the duodenum are well described; however, the development of duodenal carcinoma is rare overall, particularly in children.[27] Nevertheless, surveillance of the upper GI tract is recommended after prophylactic colectomy. Any polyps that are found are removed endoscopically.

Turcot Syndrome

Overview Turcot syndrome originally was described in 1959 in siblings found to have adenomatous polyps of the colon and malignancies of the CNS.[28] It is now understood that the condition is one of adenomatous polyposis, with an increased risk of colorectal carcinoma and an increased risk of CNS tumors. Within the past decade, the syndrome has been reclassified to include two separate conditions with distinct genetic and molecular abnormalities and phenotype. One of these is termed the brain tumor-polyposis syndrome-1; the second group is termed brain tumor-polyposis syndrome-2. Myriad colonic polyps characteristically develop in patients, with carcinoma typically developing by 40 years of age. Medulloblastoma is the more common CNS tumor that develops in these patients.[29]

Etiology Brain tumor-polyposis syndrome-1 is inherited as an autosomal-recessive condition and is the result of a defect in mismatch repair (*MMR*) genes, which correct deoxyribonucleic acid replication errors. This genetic abnormality is unusual in that, when heterozygous, the gene expresses a different phenotype, termed Lynch syndrome, also known as hereditary nonpolyposis colorectal cancer syndrome. Brain tumor-polyposis syndrome-2 is inherited as an autosomal-dominant condition, with mutations in the *APC* (adenomatous polyposis coli) gene.[29,30]

Clinical Presentation The clinical presentation is similar to that seen in FAP. Patients also can exhibit café au lait–type lesions and multiple lipomas. Patients with brain tumor-polyposis syndrome-1 are characterized by development of primarily astrocytomas and glioblastomas, as well as hematologic malignancies. Colorectal carcinomas arise at a mean age of 16 years; colon adenomas and carcinomas of the small bowel also develop in persons with this syndrome. Myriad colonic polyps characteristically develop in patients with brain tumor-polyposis syndrome-2, with carcinoma typically developing by 40 years of age; medulloblastoma is the more common CNS tumor that develops in these patients.[29]

Imaging The imaging of colonic polyps has been described earlier. The appearance of the polyps in patients with Turcot syndrome does not differ from that seen in other polyposes.

The CNS malignancies typically are investigated initially and followed up with MRI.

Treatment The treatment in patients with Turcot syndrome depends on the individual clinical presentation and concerns. Polyps can be removed by snare polypectomy; however, given the risk of colorectal carcinoma, the patient may undergo a prophylactic colectomy. The CNS malignancies or other tumors are treated accordingly.

Other Colonic Neoplasms

BENIGN NEOPLASMS

Rarely, other benign neoplasms can arise in the pediatric colon; they are largely sporadic and are not associated with other conditions. Lipomas (e-Fig. 109-8), leiomyomas, and neurofibromas have all been described. Hemangiomas and vascular malformations were discussed earlier in this chapter.

MALIGNANT NEOPLASMS

Isolated malignant colorectal neoplasms are quite rare in pediatric patients. Because of this rarity, larger series are limited and tend to represent years and decades of collected cases, during which time diagnostic methods and treatment protocols change. In addition, such reports tend to represent the experience of referral centers where more complicated patients with more advanced disease might be treated.

ADENOCARCINOMA

Overview Adenocarcinoma of the colon is exceedingly rare in children, with a prevalence of 1 in 1,000,000 persons younger than 19 years of age.[31] Mucinous carcinoma is the most common subtype described in sporadic cases of pediatric colon cancer. The tumor is more often associated with underlying predisposing conditions, such as FAP and its variants, hereditary nonpolyposis colorectal cancer syndrome, Peutz-Jeghers syndrome, and JPS, as well as Crohn disease and ulcerative colitis.[31]

Etiology The etiology of colorectal adenocarcinoma is not completely understood. What is known is that a number of risk factors relate to age, ethnicity, diet, other medical conditions, smoking, and alcohol consumption.

Clinical Presentation Presenting symptoms include abdominal pain, an abdominal mass, "constipation," weight loss, and GI bleeding. Whereas these symptoms might lead to immediate consideration of a GI malignancy in adults, that might not be an early consideration in a child. As a consequence, diagnosis may be delayed.[32]

Imaging Radiographs may be normal or suggest a bowel obstruction. Rarely one might see a mass or mass effect. Calcifications can be seen in the mucinous forms, both in the primary tumor and in the metastatic lesions (Fig. 109-9). Contrast enema may show irregularity of the bowel wall, a mural lesion, or circumferential narrowing (Fig. 109-10). CT and MRI are the modalities used to evaluate for local and

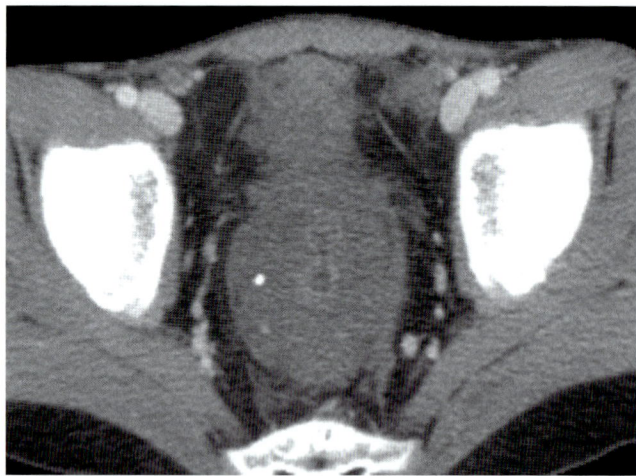

Figure 109-9 Rectal mucinous adenocarcinoma. A 12-year-old boy presented with several weeks of rectal bleeding and an 11-lb weight loss. Computed tomography with intravenous contrast material shows marked thickening of the rectal wall with internal calcifications. At surgery, diffuse carcinomatosis with peritoneal implants was also found. (Figure courtesy Marta Hernanz-Schulman, MD, Nashville, TN.)

distant spread. The most common sites of metastases are lymph nodes, liver, lung, and adrenal glands.

Treatment The treatment is primarily surgical, followed by chemotherapy and, at times, radiation therapy. In some cases of metastatic disease, particularly to the liver, locally directed therapy is used.

CARCINOID

Overview Carcinoid tumors are neoplasms of epithelial origin, which are most commonly periappendiceal (Fig. 109-11). Attempts have been made to establish a staging system that would help predict prognosis.[33] The most important prognostic criteria appear to be patient age, tumor size,

histology, and the presence or absence of lymph node involvement or distant metastases. In larger series, approximately 40% of lesions are well differentiated. The remainder are almost equally split between moderately and poorly differentiated lesions.[33]

Etiology The inciting event for the development of carcinoid tumor is not yet clear. These tumors may be seen in patients who have other malignant neoplasms.

Clinical Presentation When a carcinoid tumor involves the GI tract, it most commonly arises in the appendix. Patients can present with abdominal pain. Commonly the lesion is discovered only at appendectomy in a patient thought to have acute appendicitis. In some cases the lesion may act as a lead point for an intussusception. Patients with liver metastases can manifest the carcinoid syndrome, although it is extremely rare in the pediatric age group.

Imaging The imaging findings depend on the size of the mass, its location, and the extent of disease. If it is sufficiently small, the lesion can present by occluding the appendiceal lumen, resulting in a distended/obstructed appendix (see Fig. 109-11). In such a case it may mimic acute appendicitis. Otherwise a nonspecific mass is seen with or without metastatic spread. As in cases of adenocarcinoma, CT and MRI can be used to assess for extent of disease. The tumor can metastasize to the liver, lungs, and bone.

Treatment If the lesion is small (less than 2 cm) and no evidence is found of metastatic spread, the treatment is surgery alone. If evidence of metastatic spread is found, chemotherapy is administered.

LYMPHOMA

Overview The colon can be a site of involvement in patients with lymphoma, although the small bowel is more commonly involved. Primary colorectal lymphoma accounts for less than

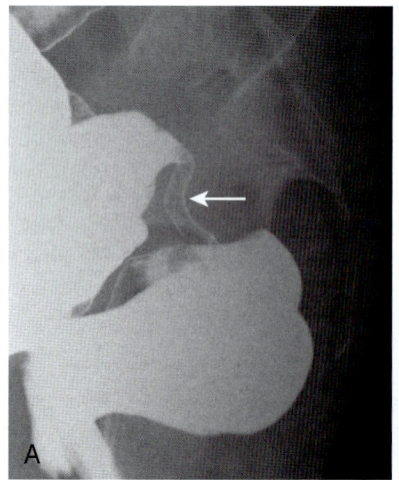
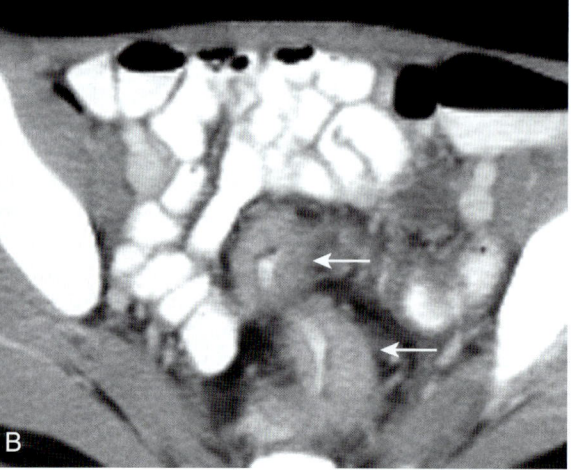

Figure 109-10 Rectosigmoid adenocarcinoma. A 14-year-old boy presented with rectal bleeding. **A,** Lateral projection from a double-contrast barium enema demonstrates an area of circumferential narrowing (*arrow*) near the junction of the sigmoid colon and rectum. **B,** A contrast-enhanced computed tomography scan also demonstrates circumferential soft tissue narrowing the lumen (*arrows*). The lesion was resected and found to be an adenocarcinoma.

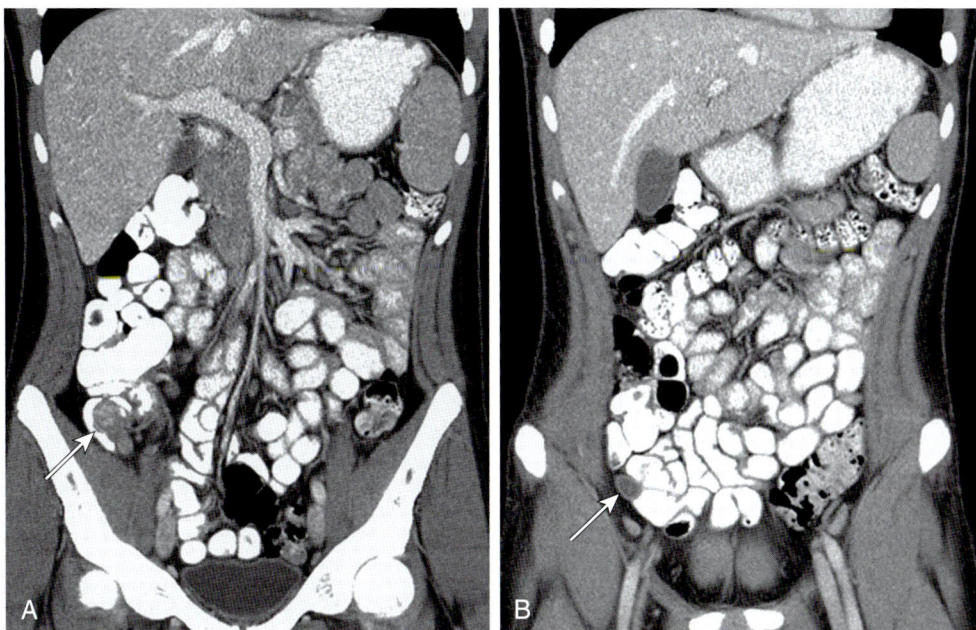

Figure 109-11   An appendiceal carcinoid tumor. A 16-year-old boy presented with intermittent right lower quadrant pain. **A,** A contrast-enhanced computed tomography coronal reformat demonstrates a mass at the base of the appendix invaginating into the cecum (arrow). **B,** The obstructed appendix is distended to its tip with fluid (arrow).

1% of all colorectal malignancies and occurs most often in the cecum.[34] Disorders predisposing developing bowel lymphoma include ataxia-telangiectasia, Wiskott–Aldrich syndrome, agammaglobulinemia, severe combined immunodeficiency, and solid organ or bone marrow transplantation. It is becoming understood that patients with inflammatory bowel disease (IBD) also can have an increased risk of developing lymphoma. IBD per se may result in chronic antigenic stimulation,[34] but data suggest that patients with IBD undergoing treatment with immunosuppressive and biologic agents are at greater risk of developing lymphoma.[35] The risk of developing a neoplasm must be weighed against the risks associated with not adequately treating the primary disease.

Etiology Lymphoma in the colon may arise as a result of conditions such as immunosuppression after transplantation, as noted above. Some investigators have postulated a genetic component, because in some cases a family history can be elicited. Others have postulated a role for infectious agents,

particularly the Epstein-Barr virus in patients with underlying IBD.[36]

Clinical Presentation The presenting symptoms in patients with GI lymphoma are often nonspecific and include abdominal pain and weight loss. Bleeding and a change in bowel habits occur less frequently. If the lesion is large enough, it can present as a palpable mass. In some cases the presentation is one of a colocolic intussusception (Fig. 109-12).[37]

Imaging If contrast enema is performed, the appearance can be one of irregularity of the bowel wall, a smooth or lobulated mural mass, or circumferential narrowing. A long segment of the bowel can be affected. On ultrasound the lesion is typically, although not always, hypoechoic, but is proved to be a solid mass by demonstration of flow on Doppler imaging. On CT or MRI an enhancing soft tissue mass is seen (e-Fig. 109-13), which can be associated with adenopathy and/or solid visceral involvement.

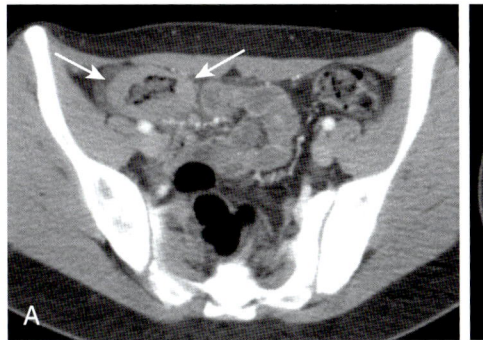
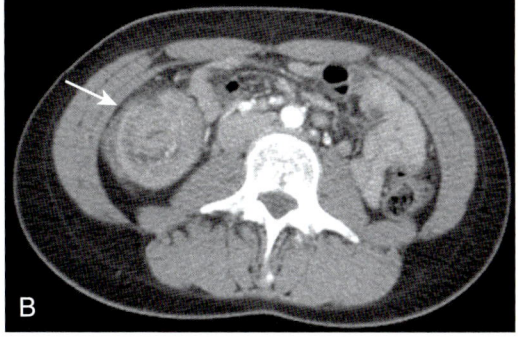

Figure 109-12   B-cell lymphoma of the ileum and ascending colon. **A** and **B**, Axial images from a contrast-enhanced computed tomography scan of the abdomen in a 17-year-old girl demonstrate a mass of the ascending colon (arrows in **A**) with an associated colo-colic intussusception (arrow in **B**).

Key Points

Benign lymphoid hyperplasia most frequently involves the terminal ileum and colon. On double-contrast enema, the lesions are uniform in size (usually 2 to 3 mm) and can be umbilicated.

Vascular lesions of the colon are rare but can present as lower GI bleeding. They can be difficult to demonstrate with imaging, although cross-sectional imaging may be useful, particularly arterial phase CT.

The isolated juvenile polyp is the most common intestinal tumor in childhood. It has no known malignant potential and is treated with polypectomy alone.

The hamartomatous syndromes include juvenile polyposis syndrome, Peutz-Jeghers syndrome, and Cowden syndrome.

The adenomatous syndromes include classic FAP, attenuated FAP, Gardner syndrome, and Turcot syndrome. Most persons believe that the term Gardner syndrome is obsolete and include the condition in FAP.

Benign tumors of the colon tend to be sporadic and include lipomas, leiomyomas, and neurofibromas.

Malignancies are rare but include adenocarcinoma, carcinoid tumor, and lymphoma.

Treatment Treatment consists of chemotherapy and radiation therapy. In cases of relapse, high-dose chemotherapy followed by stem cell transplantation has been used.

Suggested Readings

Alkhouri N, Franciosi JP, Mamula P. Familial adenomatous polyposis in children and adolescents. *J Pediatr Gastroenterol Nutr.* 2010;51:727-732.

Barnard J. Screening and surveillance recommendations for pediatric gastrointestinal polyposis syndromes. *J Pediatr Gastroenterol Nutr.* 2009;48(suppl 2):S75-S78.

Hill DA, Furman WL, Billups CA, et al. Colorectal carcinoma in childhood and adolescence: a clinicopathologic review. *J Clin Oncol.* 2007;25: 5808-5814.

Krauss E, Konturek P, Maiss J, et al. Clinical significance of lymphoid hyperplasia of the lower gastrointestinal tract. *Endoscopy.* 2010;42: 334-337.

Landry CS, Woodall C, Scoggins CR, et al. Analysis of 900 appendiceal carcinoid tumors for a proposed predictive staging system. *Arch Surg.* 2008;143:664-670.

Pickhardt PJ, Kim DH, Menias CO, et al. Evaluation of submucosal lesions of the large intestine: part 2. Nonneoplastic causes. *Radiographics.* 2007;27:1693-1703.

Shih SL, Liu YP, Tsai YS, et al. Evaluation of arterial phase MDCT for the characterization of lower gastrointestinal bleeding in infants and children: preliminary results. *AJR Am J Roentgenol.* 2010;194:496-499.

Wong MT, Eu KW. Primary colorectal lymphomas. *Colorectal Dis.* 2006;8:586-591.

References

Full references for this chapter can be found on www.expertconsult.com.

Chapter 110

Abdominal Trauma

GEORGE A. TAYLOR and CARLOS J. SIVIT

Overview

Trauma in children accounts for more than 500,000 hospital admissions and 20,000 deaths per year. After cranial trauma, the abdomen is the second most common site of injury, and approximately 80% of abdominal injuries are due to blunt force trauma. The most common reported mechanism is motor vehicle crashes, followed by automobile–pedestrian injuries. Other common causes of injury include bicycle trauma and falls from a height. In young children, injuries also may result from intentional or nonaccidental trauma.[1]

Clinical Presentation

Clinical variables that have been associated with a high risk of injury include gross hematuria, abdominal tenderness, seat belt ecchymoses, and a low trauma score. Seat belt ecchymoses across the lower abdomen or flank represent an important high-risk marker for injury.[2,3] Such ecchymoses are associated with a complex of injury to the lumbar spine, bowel, and bladder that accounts for most injuries to belted motor vehicle passengers.

Several points to be noted regarding hematuria and abdominal injury include the following: (1) most children with hematuria do not have a urinary tract injury; (2) a non–urinary tract injury is observed more frequently than a urinary tract injury in children with hematuria; and (3) asymptomatic hematuria is a low-risk indicator for abdominal injury.

Imaging

Computed tomography (CT) is the imaging method of choice in the evaluation of abdominal and pelvic injury after blunt trauma in hemodynamically stable children. Evaluation with CT allows for accurate detection and characterization of injury to solid and hollow viscera. CT also identifies and quantifies intraperitoneal and extraperitoneal fluid and blood and can detect active bleeding. Additionally, CT reveals associated bony injury to the ribs, spine, and pelvis. The role of CT in the assessment of injured children includes establishing

the presence or absence of visceral and bony injury, identifying injury that requires close monitoring and operative or endovascular intervention, and estimating associated blood loss. Normal CT findings also serve an important function in management of the injured child and in exclusion of an intraabdominal or pelvic source of blood loss.

The rapid and accurate evaluation of injured children with CT has resulted in improved triage, has contributed to reduced morbidity and mortality, and along with improvements in supportive care, has played a critical role in the success of nonoperative management of solid organ injuries. CT findings have been shown to change the initial management plan in nearly half of children assessed after blunt abdominal trauma.[4-6]

COMPUTED TOMOGRAPHY TECHNIQUE

Children should be hemodynamically stable before undergoing a CT scan. An unstable patient must be stabilized or should proceed directly to surgery for evaluation and treatment.

A precise protocol is important in minimizing the length of the examination and radiation dose exposure and in maximizing the information obtained. Sedation is rarely required before performing a CT scan in an injured child. However, because excessive patient motion results in image degradation, in select instances, a short-acting sedative may be necessary if diagnostic images are to be obtained.

The use of intravenous (IV) contrast material by rapid bolus injection is essential for maximizing the opacification of solid viscera and ensuring adequate injury detection. We administer 2 mL/kg to a maximum amount of 120 mL. Without appropriate IV administration of contrast material, solid organ laceration or hematoma may be relatively inconspicuous or missed. Additionally, the use of IV contrast material permits the detection of active hemorrhage. Multiphase imaging is not necessary for the detection of abdominal injury and adds an unnecessary radiation burden.

We do not routinely use oral contrast material in CT scanning after blunt abdominal trauma. In our experience, the potential advantages of enhanced detection of small intramural or mesenteric hematomas and the detection of oral contrast extravasation as a sign of bowel rupture are small and outweighed by its potential disadvantages, including delay in performance of the examination and possibility of aspiration. If oral contrast material is used, dilute (2%) water-soluble contrast material should be administered at least 30 minutes before the scan is performed.

SONOGRAPHY IN THE ASSESSMENT OF ABDOMINAL TRAUMA

Sonography remains widely used in the screening of injured children and adults and has been shown to have high sensitivity and specificity in the detection of hemoperitoneum; however, its utility is limited in comparison with CT. Solely identifying fluid does not necessarily reveal the cause or the site of injury, and the presence of hemoperitoneum in a hemodynamically stable child typically does not affect clinical management decisions. Furthermore, sonography provides no diagnostic information regarding injury to the bony pelvis or lumbar spine, it cannot be used in the diagnosis of hollow viscus injury, and it has been shown to miss approximately one fourth to one third of solid organ injuries.[7] Thus if one relies on identification of peritoneal fluid as a marker for hepatic and splenic injury, one will miss a significant number of injuries. Nevertheless, sonography has a potential role in diagnosing hemodynamically unstable patients because it can be performed rapidly at the bedside before the patient is taken to the operating room. In this role, it serves as a fast, non-invasive replacement for diagnostic peritoneal lavage. Recent studies suggest that contrast-enhanced sonography may have improved accuracy in delineating solid organ injuries.[8]

Computed Tomography Findings

HEPATIC INJURY

The liver is the most frequently injured viscus after blunt trauma in children, in whom this organ is poorly protected from injury by overlying ribs because the immature chest wall is easily deformed by external forces. A hepatic laceration appears as a nonenhancing region of varying configuration (Fig. 110-1) that may be linear or branching. Lacerations may be associated with a parenchymal or a subcapsular hematoma.

The liver is surrounded by a thin capsule that in turn is covered by a peritoneal reflection of thin connective tissue. The presence of hemoperitoneum associated with hepatic injury principally relates to violation of the liver capsule at the site of injury. In several large series, hepatic injury was associated with hemoperitoneum in approximately two thirds of cases. Associated hemoperitoneum may be seen throughout the greater peritoneal cavity. Often the largest fluid pockets are located in the pelvis. Hepatic injury may not be associated with intraperitoneal hemorrhage if the injury does not extend to the surface of the liver, if the hepatic capsule is not disrupted, or if the injury extends to the liver surface in the bare area of the liver, which is devoid of peritoneal reflection (Fig. 110-2). Injury that extends to the bare area may lead to associated retroperitoneal hemorrhage, with blood often surrounding the right adrenal gland or extending into the anterior pararenal space.

Circumferential zones of periportal low attenuation may be seen in the liver after trauma. The presence of these low attenuation zones does not indicate hepatic injury. They most likely represent distended periportal lymphatics as a result of intravascular third-space fluid losses that occur after fluid resuscitation.[9,10]

Treatment A number of grading scales have been proposed to quantify the severity of hepatic injury. These scales emphasize the anatomic extent of the injury, including capsular integrity, extent of subcapsular collection, extent of parenchymal disruption, and involvement of the vascular pedicle. The most widely used grading scale was developed by the American Association for the Surgery of Trauma. It was devised initially to reflect surgical findings but often is used to report severity of organ injury upon CT scanning. In children, these scales are not predictive of the need for operative management because in the vast majority of hepatic injuries, bleeding typically stops spontaneously and the injuries can be managed successfully without surgery regardless of the severity.[11] This response likely is a result of

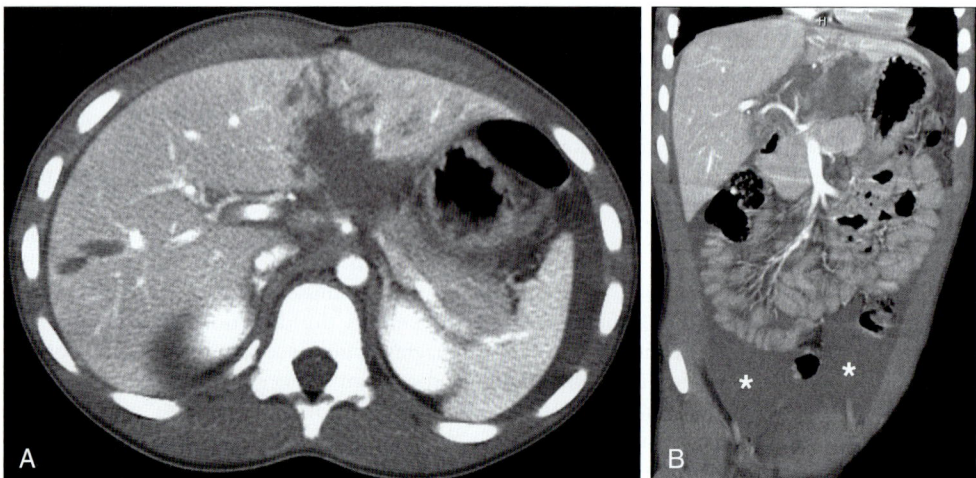

Figure 110-1 Hepatic laceration and hemoperitoneum. Contrast-enhanced axial computed tomography scan through the upper abdomen (**A**) reveals a complex hepatic laceration involving segment four and a simple laceration of segment 5. A coronal reformat image (**B**) shows a large associated hemoperitoneum in the pelvis (*asterisk*).

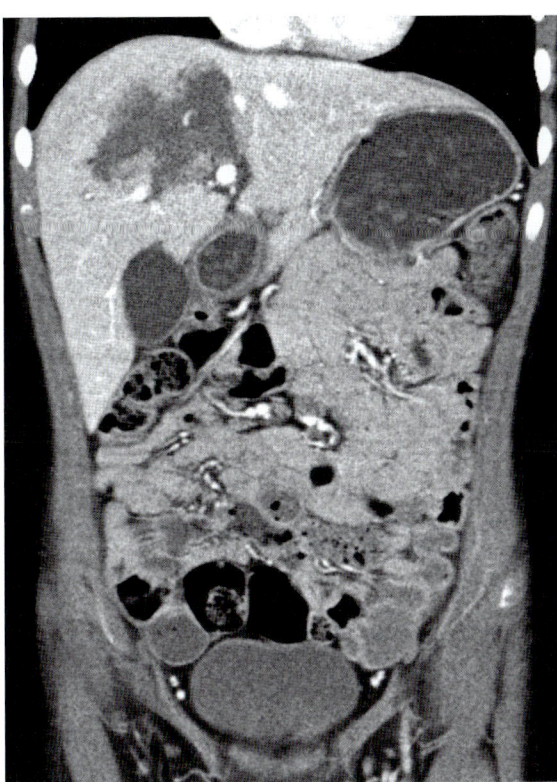

Figure 110-2 Hepatic laceration without hemoperitoneum. Coronal reformat of a contrast-enhanced computed tomography scan reveals a laceration of segment 8. No associated hemoperitoneum is present.

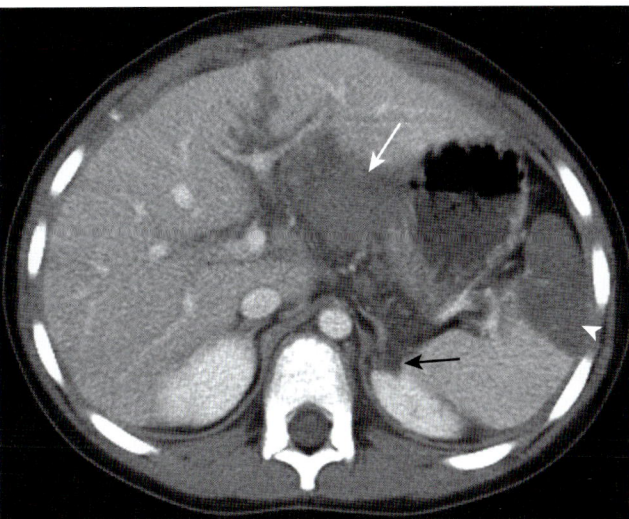

Figure 110-3 Hepatic, splenic, and renal injury. A contrast-enhanced axial computed tomography scan through the upper abdomen reveals a laceration to segment 3 of the left hepatic lobe (*white arrow*), a splenic hematoma (*arrowhead*), and a small laceration to the left kidney (*black arrow*).

the relatively smaller size of blood vessels and the enhanced vasoconstrictive response in children relative to adults. Between 1% and 3% of children with hepatic injury require surgical or endovascular hemostasis. However, injury grading scales often are used in the decision algorithm of patient management regarding intensity and length of hospitalization and activity restriction.

SPLENIC INJURY

Splenic injury also is common after blunt trauma and frequently is associated with other organ injuries (Fig. 110-3). Because the spleen is much smaller than the liver, complex injury results in shattering or fragmentation of the organ (Fig 110-4). Associated intraparenchymal or subcapsular hematoma may be present. As with hepatic injury, associated intraperitoneal hemorrhage is not always present, especially when the splenic capsule remains intact. Absence of hemoperitoneum is observed in approximately 25% of splenic injuries. After injury involving the splenic hilum, blood also can track along the splenorenal ligament into the anterior pararenal space surrounding the pancreas.

Pitfalls that may result in false-positive diagnosis of splenic injury include heterogeneous early splenic enhancement and splenic lobulations or clefts that mimic a laceration. The heterogeneous splenic enhancement is due to differences in enhancement between red and white pulp in the spleen. This artifact can be avoided by instituting a delay of at least 70 seconds prior to scanning after IV administration of contrast material. Splenic clefts and lobulations typically have smooth

contours and thus can be differentiated from lacerations, which typically have irregular contours.

Treatment Various injury grading scales have been described to objectively quantify injury to the spleen. As is true for hepatic injury, these scales are not predictive of surgical treatment in children because bleeding typically stops spontaneously and nonoperative management is successful in most splenic injuries.[11,12] Grade of injury often is used for nonoperative clinical decision making, similar to the use of grading in hepatic injury.[12-14]

PANCREATIC INJURY

Pancreatic injury is relatively uncommon in children. Injury to the body of the pancreas typically results from direct

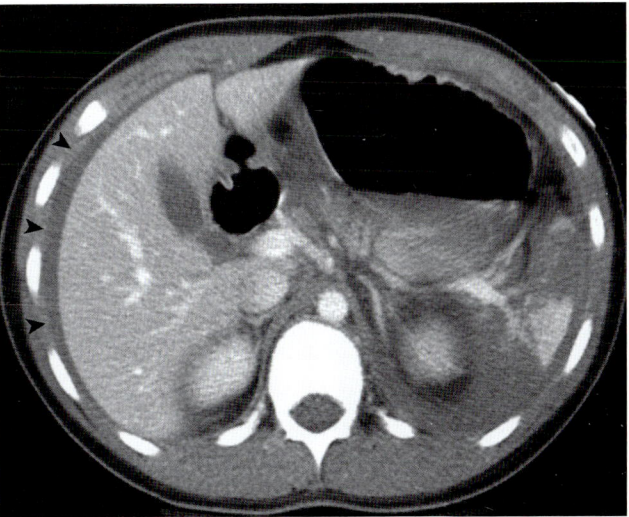

Figure 110-4 A shattered spleen. A contrast-enhanced axial computed tomography scan through the upper abdomen shows a shattered spleen with only a small amount of central contrast enhancement. Note right perihepatic hemoperitoneum (*arrowheads*).

compression of the gland against the vertebral column, whereas injury to the head or tail of the pancreas results from a blow to the flank. Impact by bicycle handlebars is a common mechanism of injury to the pancreas. Direct signs of injury may be difficult to identify because of the small size of the gland, the paucity of surrounding fat, and the minimal separation of fracture fragments.

The best indicator of pancreatic injury at CT is unexplained peripancreatic fluid (i.e., fluid in the anterior pararenal space or lesser sac) (Fig. 110-5). This finding may be seen more often than the actual laceration. When fluid collects in the anterior pararenal space, it also may dissect between the pancreas and the splenic vein. However, pancreatic injury is only one cause of fluid in the anterior pararenal space.[1] Other causes include third-space intravascular fluid loss, blood that extends from injury to the spleen or to the bare area of the liver, blood or bowel contents from a duodenal injury, and blood or urine that exudes from a renal injury after disruption of the renal fascia.

Additional CT signs of posttraumatic pancreatitis include focal or diffuse gland enlargement, stranding of peripancreatic and/or mesenteric fat, thickening of the anterior renal fascia, and free peritoneal fluid.

A false-positive diagnosis of pancreatic injury may result from the partial volume effect caused by the gland's small size and undulating nature. This pitfall may be avoided by obtaining thin-section axial reconstructions through the pancreas either routinely or in equivocal cases and by creating coronal reformatted images using unfolded and overlapped data.

Pancreatic injury may be complicated by peripancreatic fluid collections, which may evolve into pancreatic pseudocysts. Approximately half of focal fluid collections that develop after pancreatic injury spontaneously resolve, and half evolve into pseudocysts that may require percutaneous or surgical drainage. The most common location for pseudocyst formation is the intrapancreatic or peripancreatic anterior pararenal space, or lesser sac (Fig. 110-6). However, pseudocysts may develop anywhere in the abdomen or pelvis.

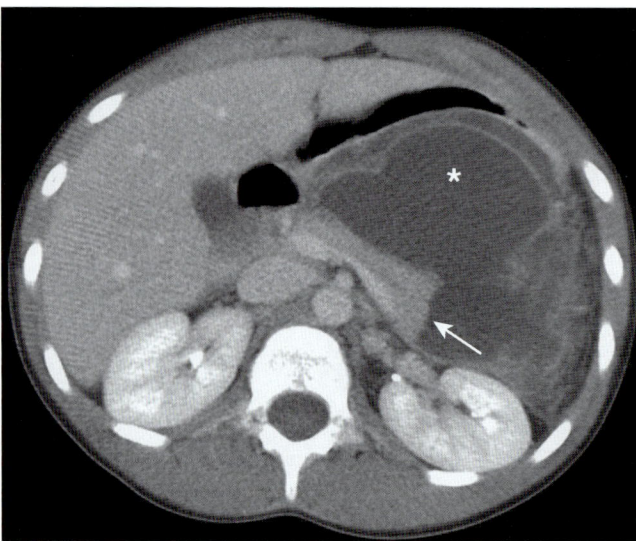

Figure 110-6 A pancreatic pseudocyst. A contrast-enhanced axial computed tomography scan through the upper abdomen shows a laceration of the pancreatic tail (*arrow*) with a large, thick-walled focal fluid collection (*asterisk*) representing a pancreatic pseudocyst in the anterior pararenal space.

MR cholangiopancreatography can be very useful in subsequent imaging evaluation of pancreatic injury, especially in patients with transection of the pancreatic duct (Fig. 110-7).

Treatment   Currently, divergent opinions have been expressed regarding the management of pancreatic injury. Some practitioners have shown that nonoperative management of most pancreatic injury is successful, even when the pancreatic duct is involved. Others believe that distal pancreatectomy for transections occurring to the left of the spine is the treatment of choice because it is definitive and is accompanied by an acceptable level of morbidity.[15-17]

PERITONEAL FLUID AND HEMORRHAGE

Attenuation values of blood in the peritoneal cavity vary widely, depending on whether it is unclotted blood (hemoperitoneum), clotted blood, or active hemorrhage. Furthermore, several factors affect measured attenuation values for peritoneal fluid on CT, including measurement technique, fluid location within the field, artifacts, and delayed fluid enhancement after IV administration of contrast material. Unclotted hemoperitoneum has attenuation values that range from 20 to 60 Hounsfield units (HU). Approximately one third of fluid pockets exhibit attenuation values lower than 30 HU. Low attenuation fluid (<60 HU) in an acutely injured child also may represent bile, urine, bowel contents, third-space fluid losses, or preexisting ascites.

Clotted blood has higher attenuation values (60 to 90 HU) than does free-flowing blood because of its greater density and hemoglobin content. Because clotted blood typically is seen adjacent to the site of injury, the presence of focal, higher attenuation clotted blood has been described as the "sentinel clot" sign; it is a marker for the principal site of hemorrhage and occasionally may be useful in localizing the site of injury.

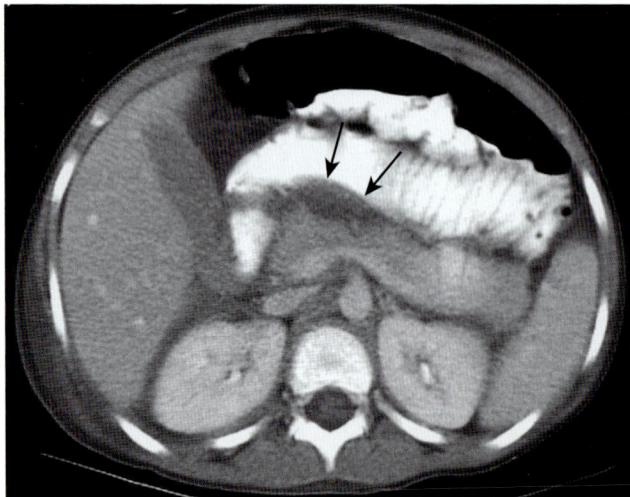

Figure 110-5 Pancreatic injury with associated peripancreatic fluid. A contrast-enhanced axial computed tomography scan through the upper abdomen shows fluid in the anterior pararenal space surrounding the pancreas (*arrows*).

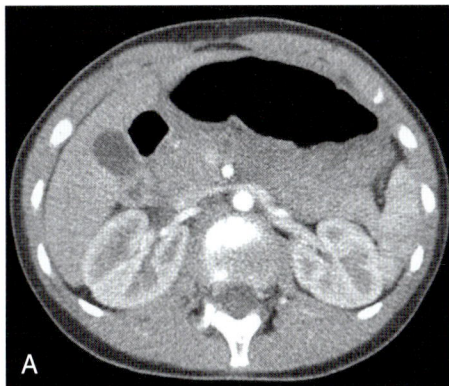
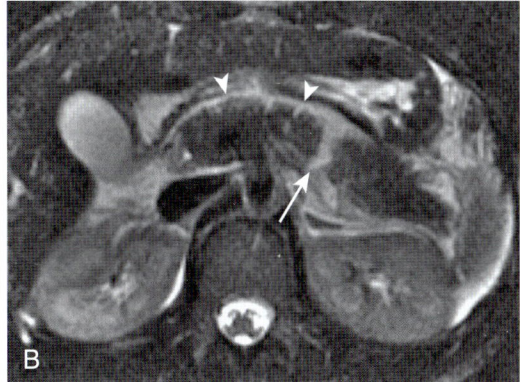

Figure 110-7 Pancreatic injury missed on an initial computed tomography (CT) scan. A contrast-enhanced CT through the upper abdomen (**A**) shows a heterogeneous ill-defined pancreas but no focal laceration. An axial T2-weighted fast spin echo magnetic resonance image with fat saturation obtained the same day (**B**) shows peripancreatic fluid (*arrowheads*) and a laceration of the pancreatic body (*arrow*).

Occasionally, CT may reveal active hemorrhage in children who appear hemodynamically stable. The amount of hemoperitoneum noted on CT is not a measure of ongoing hemorrhage; rather, it reflects the cumulative amount of bleeding that occurred between the time of injury and the time the CT scan was obtained. The only sign of active hemorrhage on CT is the presence of focal or high attenuation areas (>90 HU) (Fig. 110-8). This finding also has been referred to in the literature as a contrast blush.[13] The rate of active bleeding required for detection on CT is unclear. CT is useful in identifying active bleeding but may have difficulty in localizing the site of the hemorrhage. The torn blood vessel may be difficult to see because of diminished contrast enhancement caused by vasoconstriction and loss of blood containing contrast material. Occasionally, this finding may be observed only on delayed scanning.

The absence of peritoneal fluid or blood does not exclude the presence of hepatic or splenic injury. More than one third of hepatic injuries and one fourth of splenic injuries in children have no associated peritoneal fluid. The relatively high prevalence of hepatic and splenic injury without associated peritoneal fluid has significant implications for imaging strategies in the assessment of injured children.

Treatment Most children with active hemorrhage detected on CT do not require operative intervention. It has been reported that 20% or fewer children with hepatic or splenic injury and active hemorrhage have required operative hemostasis.[14,18,19]

BOWEL AND MESENTERIC INJURY

Bowel and mesenteric injuries are uncommon after blunt trauma, occurring in 6% to 16% of injured children. The most common mechanisms of injury associated with bowel and mesenteric injury are motor vehicle crashes, handlebar injuries, nonaccidental trauma, and falls. Intestinal injury is the result of direct force on the gastrointestinal tract and mesentery leading to a crush injury, rapid deceleration producing a shearing force between fixed and mobile portions of bowel or mesenteric attachments, and a sharp increase in intraluminal pressure resulting in rupture of the gut.[20] Bowel rupture most commonly occurs in the mid to distal small intestine. The presence of seat belt ecchymosis and an acute hyperflexion (Chance) fracture of the lumbar spine are the only physical findings found to have a strong and significant association with bowel and mesenteric injury.[3] Nonaccidental injury always must be considered in a child with a history of minor blunt trauma who has a bowel perforation.[21,21a]

Clinical signs and symptoms may be absent, minimal, or delayed, and CT plays an important role in early and accurate diagnosis. Delayed diagnosis can result in bowel ischemia, peritonitis, and, in rare cases, death as a result of sepsis. The main challenge for the radiologist is to distinguish between injuries that do and do not require surgical intervention. CT findings that are specific to bowel injury include the presence of extraluminal gas, extravasation of oral contrast material, and bowel discontinuity (Fig. 110-9).[22,23] The latter two findings are very uncommon in pediatric practice. Extraluminal gas, however, is present in 20% to 30% of children with bowel injury and is a highly specific finding, with, unfortunately, low sensitivity. In a supine patient, extraluminal gas tends to accumulate at the convexity of the abdominal wall and in the porta hepatis (Fig. 110-10). Blunt abdominal

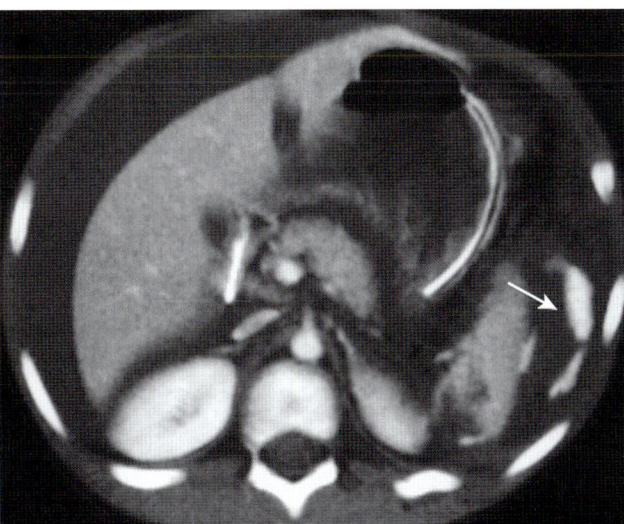

Figure 110-8 Active hemorrhage. A contrast-enhanced axial computed tomography scan through the upper abdomen shows a focal high attenuation collection representing intravenous contrast extravasation from a splenic arterial tear (*arrow*).

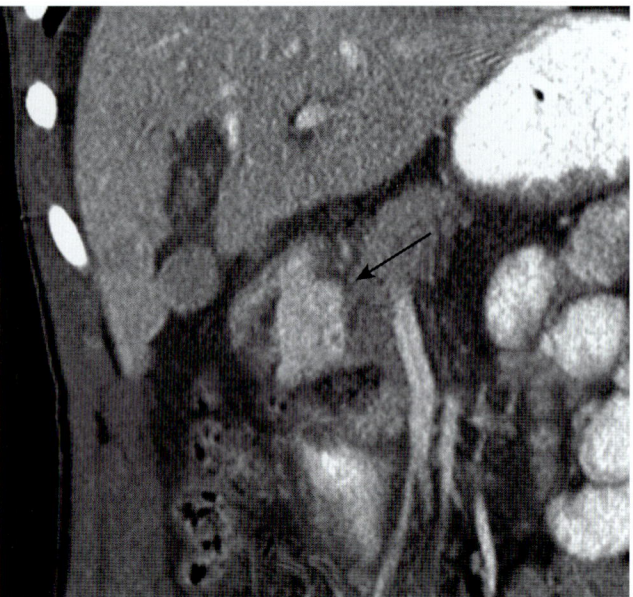

Figure 110-9 Duodenal perforation with extravasation of oral contrast material. Coronal reformat of a contrast-enhanced computed tomography scan shows extravasation of oral contrast in the retroperitoneum (*arrow*) medial to the duodenal sweep.

injury also can lead to intravasation of gas into the mesenteric and portal venous system, presumably through mucosal disruption, or because of ischemic changes resulting from mesenteric tears.[24] Injury to the retroperitoneal duodenum often results in localized bubbles of gas immediately adjacent to a

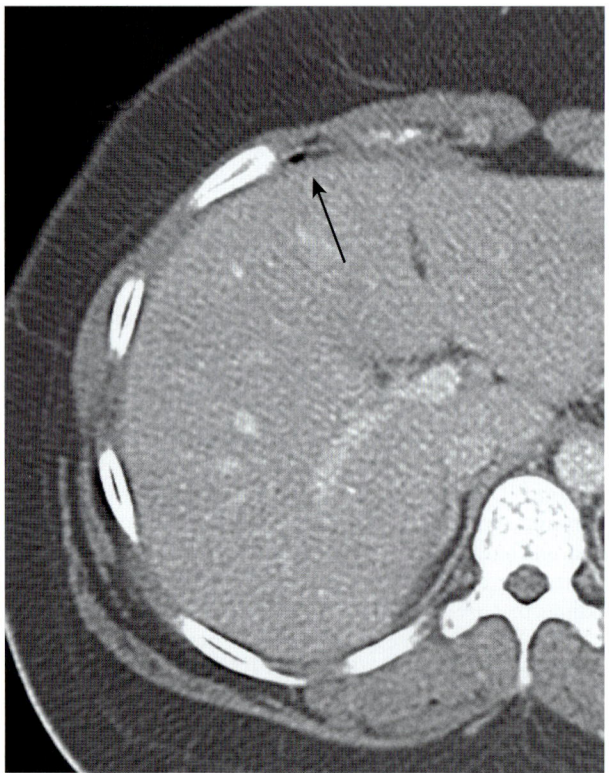

Figure 110-10 Ileal perforation and extraluminal gas. A contrast-enhanced computed tomography image through the liver shows a small collection of extraluminal gas anterior to the right hepatic lobe (*arrow*).

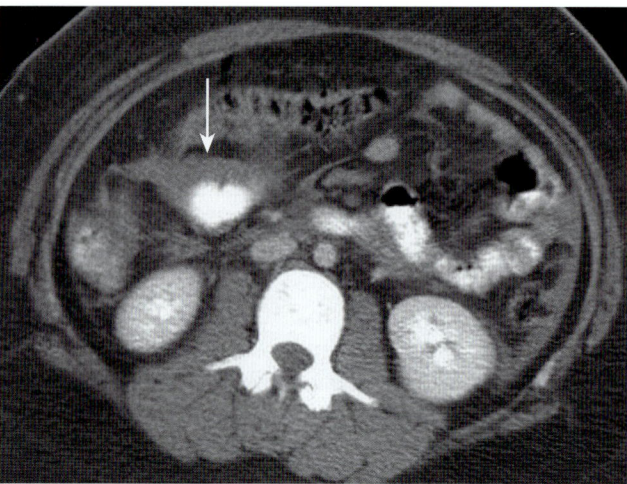

Figure 110-11 Mesenteric tear and ischemic bowel. A contrast-enhanced axial computed tomography image through the mid abdomen shows a focal area of eccentric bowel wall thickening (*arrow*) due to a mesenteric tear. Ischemic bowel was confirmed at surgery.

thickened and distorted duodenum and pancreas. Review of the examination at a wide window setting is helpful in the detection of small amounts of extraluminal gas. Several other CT findings are common in injured patients but are less specific for significant bowel injury; these findings include focal bowel wall thickening and mesenteric fluid or stranding.

Intramural hematoma results from hemorrhage into the bowel wall after a partial-thickness tear has occurred; these injuries usually can be managed nonoperatively. The most common location is the duodenum. The CT appearance is that of focal bowel wall thickening that often is eccentric (Fig. 110-11). Large duodenal hematomas may appear dumbbell shaped. Because the injury is intramural, no extraluminal air or extravasated contrast material should be present. Large hematomas can result in obstruction of the bowel proximal to the injury.

CT signs that are highly specific for significant mesenteric injury are related to vascular injury and include mesenteric vascular beading, abrupt termination of mesenteric vessels, and mesenteric vascular extravasation (Fig. 110-12 and Box 110-1).[22] These findings are rare in children, and their sensitivity and specificity are not known. Abnormalities that are less specific for the need for surgical intervention in mesenteric injury are mesenteric stranding and hematoma; these findings may represent a range of injuries from minor mesenteric bruising to underlying vascular disruption.

The most frequent CT finding associated with bowel rupture and mesenteric injury is "unexplained" peritoneal

---

Box 110-1 High-Specificity Computed Tomography Findings in Bowel and Mesenteric Injury

Extraluminal gas

Extraluminal oral contrast material

Bowel discontinuity

Mesenteric vascular beading

Abrupt termination of mesenteric vessels

Mesenteric vascular extravasation

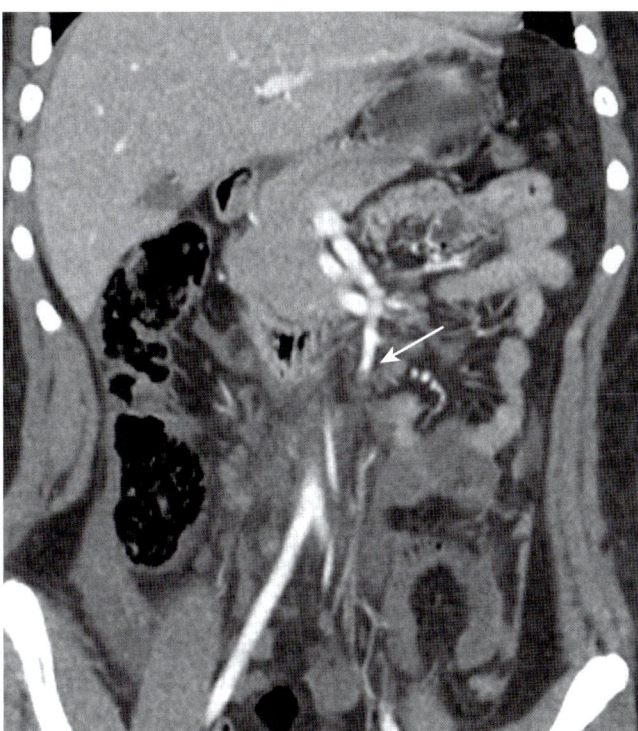

Figure 110-12 Superior mesenteric artery occlusion. Coronal reformat of a contrast-enhanced computed tomography scan shows abrupt termination of the superior mesenteric artery (*arrow*). The patient had subsequent mesenteric ischemia and bowel perforation.

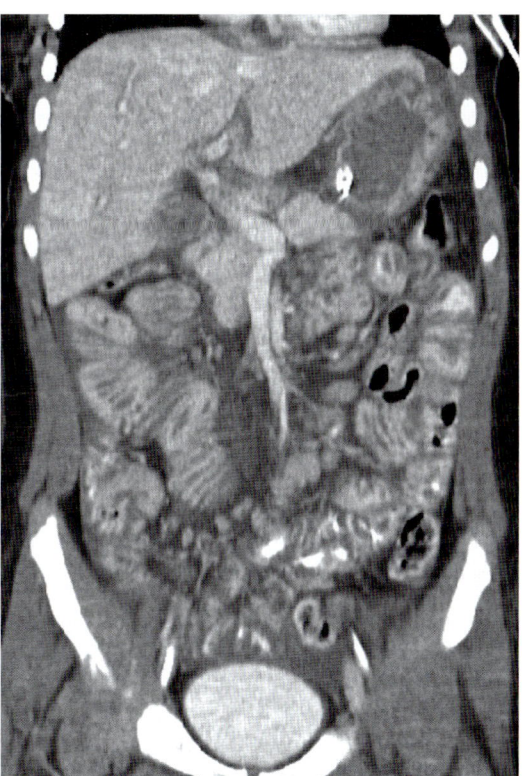

Figure 110-14 Hypoperfusion complex. Coronal reformat of a contrast-enhanced computed tomography image shows diffuse intestinal thickening, dilation with fluid, intense contrast enhancement of the bowel wall, low periportal attenuation, and ascites indicative of partially compensated shock.

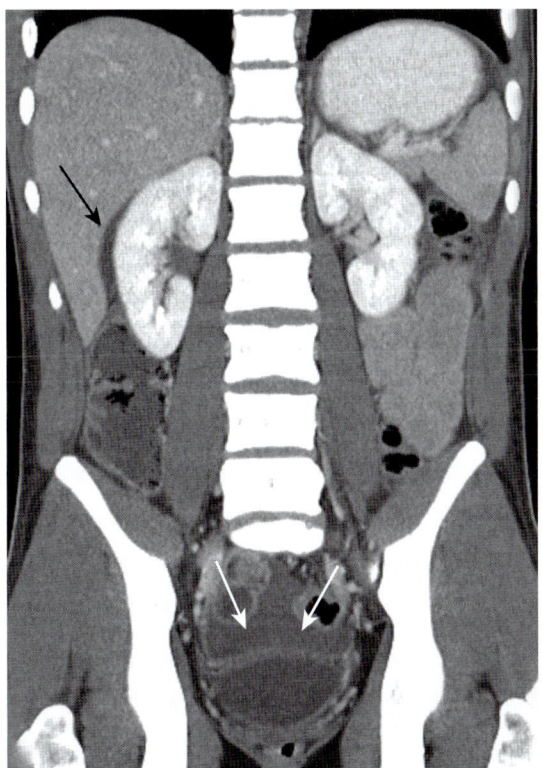

Figure 110-13 Bowel rupture with a moderate amount of "unexplained" peritoneal fluid. Coronal reformat of a contrast-enhanced computed tomography (CT) image shows a moderate amount of peritoneal fluid in the cul-de-sac (*white arrows*), and in the subhepatic space (*black arrow*). No other abnormalities were noted on CT. A jejunal rupture was identified at surgery.

fluid (i.e., moderate to large amounts of fluid in the absence of solid viscus injury or bony pelvic fracture) (Fig. 110-13). Although nonspecific, unexplained peritoneal fluid is an important marker of potentially serious bowel or mesenteric injury. Approximately half the children with a moderate to large quantity of peritoneal fluid as the only finding on CT after blunt trauma have intestinal injury.[25] Follow-up CT imaging in patients with initially equivocal findings and persistent abdominal symptoms has been reported to improve the detectability of intestinal injuries.[23]

Multidetector scanners have improved the accuracy of CT for the diagnosis of bowel and mesenteric injuries. However, the reported sensitivity values (80%-95%) and specificity values (48%-84%) vary widely among studies.[22,23]

HYPOPERFUSION COMPLEX

A characteristic complex of findings on CT associated with partially compensated hypovolemic shock in severely injured children has been characterized as the "hypoperfusion complex." Most of these children have required extensive resuscitation for arterial hypotension on admission.[26]

CT findings in all children with the hypoperfusion complex include diffuse intestinal dilation with fluid. Abnormally intense contrast enhancement of bowel wall, mesentery, kidneys, aorta, and inferior vena cava is present, as well as diminished caliber of the aorta and inferior vena cava (Fig. 110-14). Variable findings include periportal low attenuation zones, intense adrenal, pancreatic and mesenteric enhancement, decreased pancreatic and splenic enhancement, peritoneal and retroperitoneal fluid, and bowel wall thickening.[26,27]

The hypoperfusion complex is a marker for a tenuous hemodynamic state and a predictor of a poor outcome. The mortality rate in children with this constellation of findings on CT approaches 80%.[26]

Key Points

Clinical variables associated with a high risk of injury include gross hematuria, abdominal tenderness, and seat belt ecchymoses.
Multiphase CT scanning is not necessary in children who have sustained blunt trauma.
Hepatic injury extending to the bare area of the liver may be associated with retroperitoneal hemorrhage.
Heterogeneous early splenic enhancement, splenic lobulations, or clefts may mimic a splenic laceration.
Most hepatic and splenic injuries in children can be treated safely without operative intervention.
Pancreatic injury may be difficult to identify in children because of a paucity of surrounding fat and the minimal separation of fracture fragments. The best indicator of pancreatic injury at CT is unexplained peripancreatic fluid.

The size of hemoperitoneum on CT reflects the cumulative amount of bleeding; it is not a measure of ongoing hemorrhage.
The absence of peritoneal fluid or blood does not exclude the presence of hepatic or splenic injury.
A sentinel clot can indicate the site of injury.
The most frequent CT finding associated with bowel rupture and mesenteric injury is "unexplained" peritoneal fluid.

Suggested Readings

Brofman N, Atri M, Epid D, et al. Evaluation of bowel and mesenteric trauma with multi-detector CT. *Radiographics*. 2006;26:1119-1131.

Lynn KN, Werder GM, Callaghan RM, et al. Pediatric blunt splenic trauma: a comprehensive review. *Pediatr Radiol*. 2009;39:904-916.

Mattix KD, Tataria M, Holes J, et al. Pediatric pancreatic trauma: predictors of nonoperative management failure and associated outcomes. *J Pediatr Surg*. 2007;42:340-344.

Sokolove PE, Kupperman N, Holmes JF. Association between the "seat belt sign" and intra-abdominal injury in children with blunt torso trauma. *Acad Emerg Med*. 2005;12:808-813.

Van der Vlies CH, Saltzherr TP, Wilde JCH, et al. The failure rate of nonoperative management in children with splenic or liver injury with contrast blush on computed tomography: a systematic review. *J Pediatr Surg*. 2010;45:1044-1051.

References

Full references for this chapter can be found on www.expertconsult.com.

SECTION 7

Genitourinary System

Chapter 111

Embryology, Anatomy, and Variants of the Genitourinary Tract

MARY P. BEDARD, SALLY WILDMAN, and JONATHAN R. DILLMAN

The urinary system and the genital system are closely associated embryologically and begin to develop during the fourth week of gestation.[1,2] Both develop from the intermediate mesoderm along the posterior wall of the abdominal cavity. A longitudinal elevation of the mesoderm, the urogenital ridge, forms on both sides of the abdominal aorta. Part of the urogenital ridge gives rise to the nephrogenic cord, which will form the urinary system, and another part gives rise to the gonadal ridge, which will form the genital system (see Chapter 125).[1]

The nephrogenic cord gives rise to the mesonephros, which consists of glomeruli and mesonephric tubules. The mesonephric tubules open into the mesonephric duct, which soon opens into the cloaca.[1,3] The mesonephros degenerates toward the end of the first trimester, although their tubules persist in males and participate in the formation of the genital system.[2] During the fifth week of gestation, the metanephros begins to develop. The definitive kidneys develop from the ureteric bud (metanephric diverticulum), an outgrowth of the mesonephric duct, and the metanephric blastema, which is derived from the nephrogenic cord.

The ureteric bud is responsible for the development of the collecting system (ureter, renal pelvis, and calyces).[1,2,4] The stalk of the ureteric bud forms the ureter. The ureteric bud grows into the metanephric blastema, where branching leads to the formation of the renal pelvis, major and minor calyces, and the collecting tubules (Figs. 111-1 and 111-2). Nephrons form in the metanephric blastema as the result of induction by the collecting tubules. The embryonic kidneys initially lie in the pelvis. As the abdomen grows, the kidneys "ascend" and rotate 90 degrees. By the ninth week of gestation, the kidneys come in contact with the adrenal glands as they attain their final position. The fetal kidney has a lobulated external contour that will disappear as the nephrons continue to grow. The full complement of glomeruli is present by 36 weeks' gestation.

Congenital anomalies of the urinary tract are common.[1,4] Early degeneration of a ureteric bud or involution of the metanephros leads to regression of the metanephric blastema and renal agenesis. If the ureteric bud and metanephric blastema do not join normally, abnormal induction of the blastemal elements is likely to result in a multicystic dysplastic kidney. Bifurcation of the ureteric buds results in partial duplication of the collecting system. When the location of the origin of the ureteric bud is abnormal or if the origin itself is maldeveloped, the potential for vesicoureteral reflux (VUR) or ureteral ectopia exists (Fig. 111-3).

The bladder arises from the most superior portion of the urogenital sinus.[1,2,5] It is initially continuous with the allantois. With constriction of the allantois, the lumen is obliterated, and a thick, fibrous cord, the urachus, remains. The urachus connects the apex of the bladder with the umbilicus. Persistence of the allantoic lumen may result in urachal fistulas, sinuses, or cysts. The ureterovesical junction (UVJ) develops as the distal parts of the mesonephric duct are incorporated into the enlarging bladder. As the mesonephric ducts are absorbed, the ureters come to open separately into the urinary bladder with the orifice moving superolaterally and the distal ureteral segments entering obliquely through the base of the bladder. The middle portion of the urogenital sinus develops into the prostatic urethra in males and the entire urethra in females. The distal portion of the male urethra is derived from a cord of ectoderm that grows from the tip of the glans penis to meet the spongy portion of the urethra derived from the caudal (phallic) portion of the urogenital sinus. Development of the ureters and bladder is complete by the fourth gestational month.

The fetus begins to make urine by the ninth week of gestation, and the urine contributes the largest component of the amniotic fluid.[6] Oligohydramnios is often a marker of urinary tract abnormalities, and severe oligohydramnios may lead to pulmonary hypoplasia.

During the first few days after birth, the neonate has a low glomerular filtration rate (GFR) and low urine output.[7] This is especially true of premature infants. The newborn kidney also has a limited ability to concentrate urine and decreased tubular reabsorption of sodium. GFR and urine output increase significantly over the first week of life. This immaturity of renal function is an important factor to keep in mind in the ordering and interpretation of renal imaging studies. For example, the low urine output present on day one of life may mask the presence of hydronephrosis on renal ultrasonography.

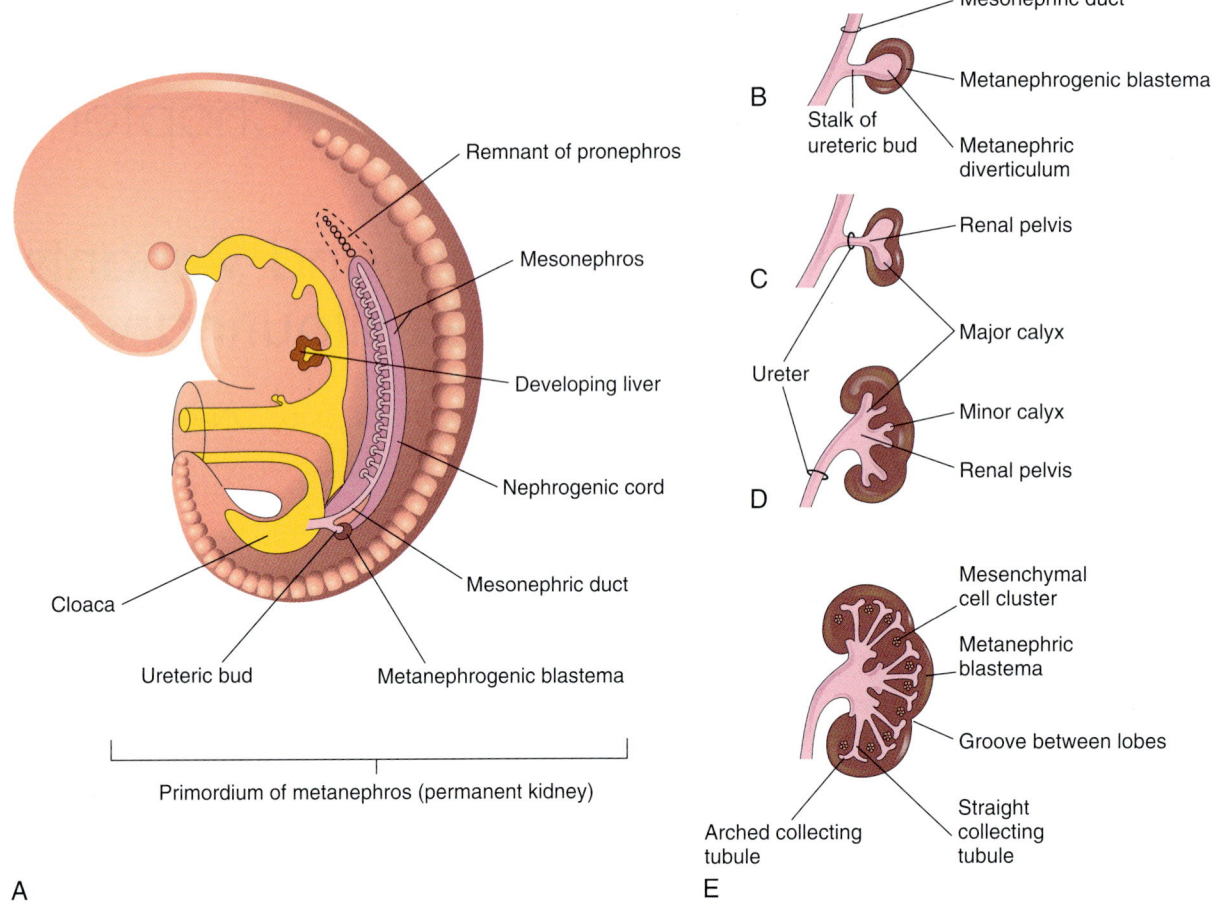

Figure 111-1 Development of the metanephros, the primordium of the permanent kidney. **A,** Lateral view of a 5-week embryo, showing the primordium of the metanephros. **B** to **E,** Successive stages in the development of the metanephric diverticulum or ureteric bud (fifth to eighth weeks). Observe the development of the ureter, renal pelvis, the calices, and the collecting tubules. (From Moore KL, Persaud TVN. The urogenital system. In: *Before we are born: essentials of embryology and birth defects.* 7th ed. Philadelphia: Saunders Elsevier; 2003.)

Normal Anatomy

KIDNEY

The renal parenchyma is composed of two distinct regions: (1) the outer cortex, and (2) the inner medulla (Fig. 111-4). Within the cortex are the nephrons. The medulla is composed of 8 to 13 pyramids, which terminate in the renal papillae at the level of the calyces. Two or more pyramids may drain into the same papilla (confluent papilla), and two or more papillae may drain into a single calyx (compound calyx). A column of Bertin represents the renal cortex extending centrally between the pyramids (e-Fig. 111-5), most often occurring at the junction of the middle and upper groups of calyces or between the two central renal hypoechoic complexes of a duplex kidney.[8,9]

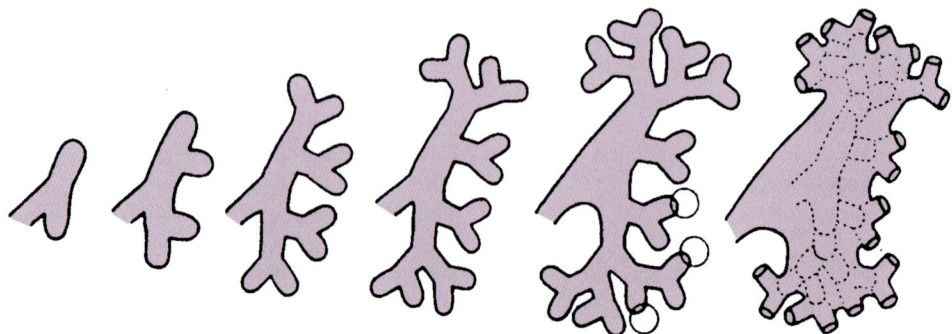

Figure 111-2 Ureteric bud with multiple divisions leading to development of the calyceal system. (Adapted from Parrott TS, Skandalakis JE, Gray SW. The kidney and ureter. In: Skandalakis JE, Gray SW, eds. *Embryology for surgeons: the embryological basis for the treatment of congenital anomalies.* 2nd ed. Baltimore: Williams & Wilkins; 1994.)

URETER DUPLICATION

Reflux and ectopy

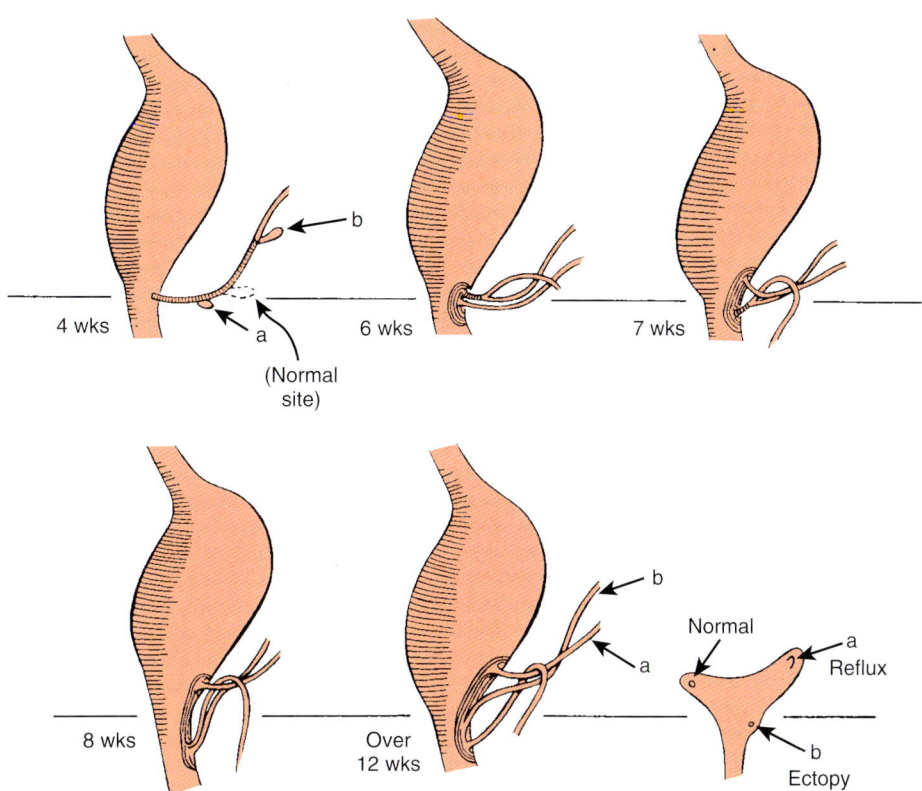

Figure 111-3   The ureteric bud and its relationship to the bladder. The drawing shows how ectopia may occur.

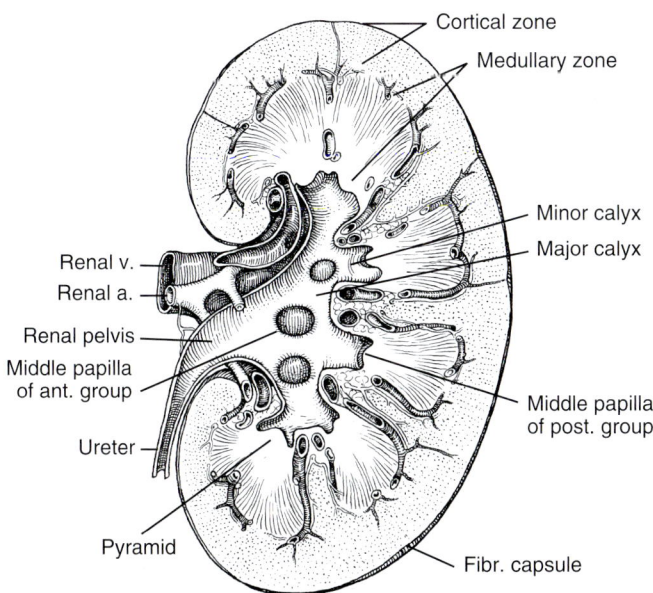

Figure 111-4 Macroscopic anatomy of the kidney in longitudinal section. The right kidney is seen from the back; the renal artery is posterior to the renal vein. (Redrawn from Kelly HA, Burnam CF. *Diseases of the kidneys, ureters and bladder.* 2nd ed. New York: Appleton; 1922.)

Multiple renal lobules fuse to form the kidney. The junction of these lobules sometimes persists and may be seen as a scalloping of the cortical border (Fig. 111-6). The junctional parenchymal defect is similarly derived from a variation in the fusion of the fetal renunculi or lobules. It appears as a thick, triangular, echogenic notch in the anterosuperior or posteroinferior aspect of the kidney (more often on the right) and mimics a cortical scar. The junctional parenchymal defect may be connected to the renal hilum by an echogenic line called the *inter-renuncular septum* (Fig. 111-7). The left kidney is apt to be more triangular in shape, with a distinct bulge along its lateral aspect, the so-called *dromedary kidney* (Fig. 111-8).[10-13]

In newborns and infants, the kidneys have a larger medullary and a smaller cortical volume than in later life. On ultrasonography, the neonatal renal cortex is moderately hyperechoic, close to the echogenicity of adjacent liver and spleen. In newborn and premature infants, the cortical echogenicity may actually be greater than that of the liver (see Fig. 111-8). The pyramids are relatively hypoechoic. Between ages 6 months and 2 years, the echogenicity of the medulla and cortex resembles that of adult kidneys.[14-17]

The kidney is usually supplied by a single artery arising from the aorta. After the renal artery enters the renal hilum, posterior and slightly superior to the renal vein, it divides into anterior and posterior branches, which, in turn, generally divide into superior and inferior branches (e-Fig. 111-9).

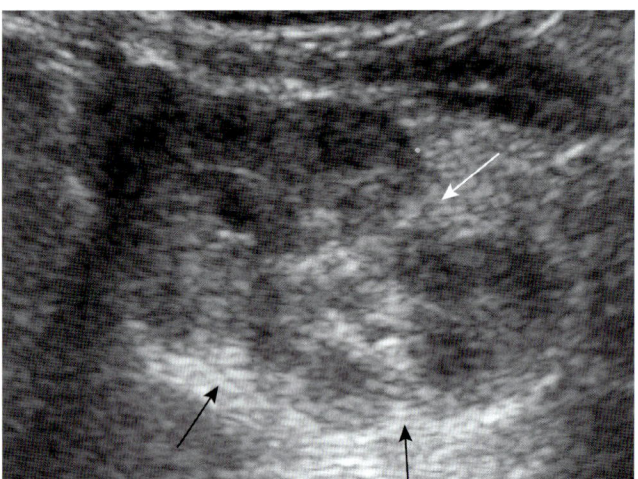

Figure 111-6 Fetal lobulations. Residual fetal lobulations are responsible for the scalloped border of the kidney (*black arrows*) on this sagittal sonogram. A prominent junctional cortical defect is also present (*white arrow*).

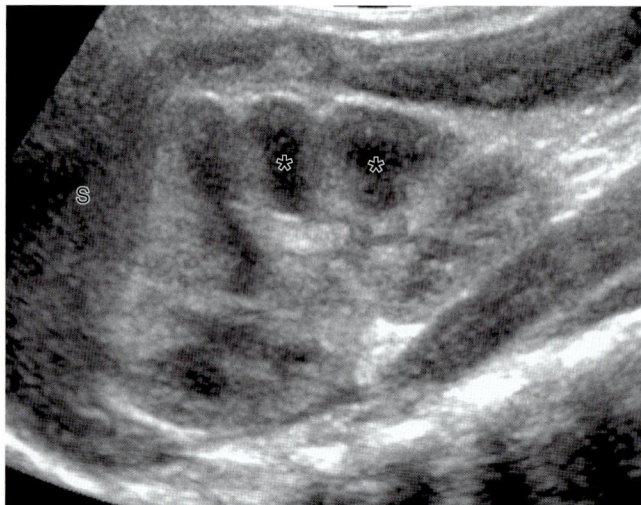

Figure 111-8 Normal neonatal kidney. Supine longitudinal sonogram of the left kidney shows the sharp corticomedullary differentiation common in infancy and early childhood. The hypoechoic triangular renal pyramids (*asterisks*) are surrounded by cortex that is more echogenic than the adjacent spleen (*S*). The spleen has flattened the upper renal contour and produces the appearance of a dromedary kidney. (Courtesy Brian D. Coley, MD, Cincinnati, OH.)

Variations exist at all levels. About 20% to 30% of kidneys have a second or accessory renal artery, which also arises from the aorta. The normal renal vein lies anterior and slightly inferior to the renal artery. The left renal vein is longer than the right, courses anterior to the aorta, and receives the ipsilateral suprarenal and gonadal veins before entering the inferior vena cava.[8,9,18]

Renal length is the most commonly measured parameter and has been correlated to age, body height and weight, and height of the first three or four lumbar vertebral bodies. Standards for renal size have been developed for ultrasonography (e-Fig. 111-10). The left kidney may be slightly longer than the right. Kidneys with complete or partial collecting system duplication are longer than normal kidneys. The width of the kidney is approximately 50% of its length and is relatively thicker in neonates than in older children. Cortical thickness of the upper renal pole is normally slightly thicker than the lower pole, and the renal cortex is slightly thinner in the center of the kidney. Extra cortical tissue may be noted about the renal hilum and may impinge from above or below on the renal pelvis (suprahilar or infrahilar bulge, or hilar lips).[19-25]

PELVOCALYCEAL SYSTEM

The renal pelvis varies in size from a small, poorly defined sac to a large, boxlike structure. The pelvis may lie entirely within (intrarenal) or almost beyond (extrarenal) the renal sinus. The configuration of the pelvocalyceal system is quite variable. In most kidneys, the pelvis branches into two major infundibula (or major calyces). The inferior infundibulum is commonly broad and short and is connected with a larger number of calyces compared with the upper infundibulum.

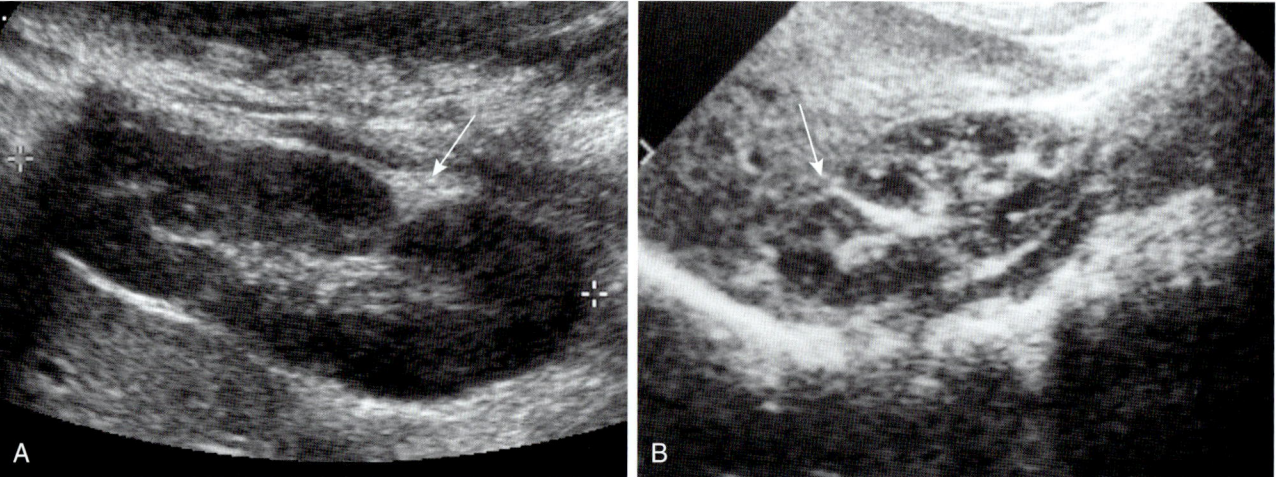

Figure 111-7 Junctional parenchymal defects. **A,** Longitudinal prone sonogram shows a fat-filled cleft (*arrow*) in the posterior kidney. **B,** Longitudinal supine sonogram in another patient shows a renicular septum (*arrow*). Both are normal findings, probably related to a demarcation of embryonic reniculi.

Each kidney has about 8 to 13 calyces. These have a cup-shaped appearance that results from the protrusion of the renal papilla into the calyx. Two or more papillae may enter one calyx (compound calyx). Most calyces are directed laterally and either slightly anteriorly or posteriorly within the kidney.[4,6,18,24,26]

URETER

The ureter is a tubular structure that courses retroperitoneally from the kidney to the bladder and has three major components: (1) the ureteropelvic junction (UPJ) and upper ureter, (2) the midureter, and (3) the lower ureter and the UVJ (including the transmural ureter and the ureteral orifice). The abdominal or upper ureter starts at the UPJ with a smooth tapering from the renal pelvis. The abdominal ureter lies adjacent to the psoas muscle, being crossed by the gonadal vessels before passing behind the iliac vessels. The lower ureter lies along the lateral pelvic wall, coursing downward behind the bladder. As the ureter enters the bladder wall, it takes an oblique course from a superolateral entry point to an inferomedial ostium and eventually opens into the bladder. Its course through the bladder wall may be seen (called the *plica ureterica* at cystoscopy) and constitutes the lateral border of the bladder trigone. Three muscular layers constitute the ureteral wall, with a thick outer adventitial covering that contains a rich vascular layer and lymphatic plexus.[4,6,27-29]

The vascular supply of the ureter is from bladder vessels (inferior vesical artery), gonadal arteries (testicular artery), and the renal artery superiorly. Nerves supplying the ureter follow the same course as that of arteries. Rhythmic peristaltic ureteral contractions transport urine from the renal pelvis into the urinary bladder and occur two to seven times per minute.[4,6]

The anatomic relationship of the distal ureter to the bladder wall at the UVJ is important in preventing VUR. Normally, the distal ureter inserts into the bladder, courses through the bladder musculature at an oblique angle, and then continues inferomedially and submucosally to its ostia in the lateral corner of the trigone (Fig. 111-11). The UVJ acts as a passive flap valve. Continence is ensured by apposition of the roof and floor of the submucosal tunnel when intravesical pressure increases and is enhanced by the action of the intrinsic local musculature. A normal ureteral tunnel length to ureteral diameter ratio in children is 5:1. A ratio of at least 3:1 is necessary for UVJ competence.[30-34]

BLADDER

In the neonate and young child, the dome and body of the bladder are located primarily in the abdomen and anterior, whereas its base is intrapelvic and posterior. Bowel impressions are common and may impress on the intraabdominal bladder when it is filled. This normal appearance should not be confused with an intravesical mass or extrinsic compression by a pelvic mass. A urachal remnant may also be seen at the bladder dome. Normal bladder capacity may be predicted on the basis of weight in infancy and by age for the older child. For infants under 1 year of age, bladder capacity in milliliters is predicted by multiplying the weight in kilograms by 7. The predicted bladder capacity in milliliters of children more than 1 year old is the age in years plus 2

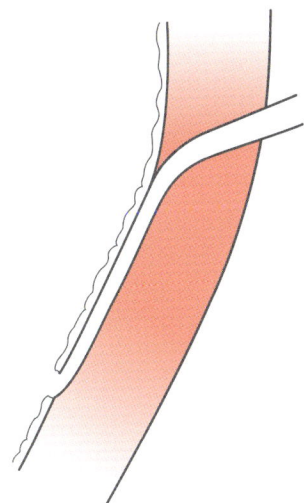

Figure 111-11 Course of the distal segment of ureter within the bladder wall. The ureter at first traverses the bladder musculature almost perpendicularly and then descends submucosally for a much longer segment (submucosal tunnel).

multiplied by 30. Ultrasonography best demonstrates normal bladder wall thickness, which should be no more than 3 mm when distended and 6 mm when collapsed.[5,35-43]

URETHRA

The female urethra corresponds anatomically to the posterior urethra of the male. Anatomic features of the female urethra include the internal sphincter at the bladder neck, intermuscular incisura, membranous urethra at the level of the urogenital diaphragm or external urethral sphincter, and the fossa navicularis.[5,44,45]

The components of the normal male urethra include the prostatic or posterior urethra, the membranous urethra, the bulbous urethra, and the penile urethra. Normal anatomic features of the male prostatic urethra include the internal sphincter, the intermuscular incisura, and the verumontanum. The membranous urethra runs through the urogenital diaphragm or the external urethral sphincter, after which come the bulbous urethra, the penile urethra, and the fossa navicularis (e-Fig. 111-12). The intermuscular incisura produces an indentation in the midportion of the posterior urethra at the level of the verumontanum and is caused by an abundance of collagenous tissue at this location (more prominent anteriorly). The verumontanum is a focal elevation in the posterior wall of the prostatic urethra where the paired ejaculatory ducts enter, seen as a small ovoid filling defect in the posterior portion of the prostatic urethra. The plicae colliculae are normal folds that extend from the distal verumontanum to the posterior urethra and may produce circumferential impressions on urethral images.[5,44,46-50]

The muscles related to bladder continence and micturition are the detrusor muscle of the bladder, the musculature of the bladder neck and proximal urethra at the internal urethral sphincter, and the external urethral sphincter. The urethra is also affected indirectly, at the level of the urogenital diaphragm, by the striated voluntary muscles of the pelvic floor.

Congenital Anatomic Variants and Anomalies

KIDNEY

Renal Agenesis (Unilateral and Bilateral)

True renal agenesis is thought to be caused by failure of the ureteric bud to contact the ipsilateral metanephric blastema. Unilateral renal agenesis is present in about 1 : 1000 live births. Children with true unilateral renal agenesis lack the ipsilateral ureter and hemitrigone of the urinary bladder. Those children with an absent kidney but a normally developed bladder and a distal ureter of varying length probably represent the involution of a multicystic dysplastic kidney.[36] Associated anomalies include VACTERL association (e-Fig. 111-13), unicornuate uterus, uterus didelphys, and Mayer-Rokitansky-Küster-Hauser syndrome in females, and seminal vesicle cysts, absence of the vas deferens, and cystic dysplasia of the rete testis in males (Box 111-1).[36,51-58]

Bilateral renal agenesis is uniformly lethal with an incidence of 1 : 10,000 to 3 : 10,000 live births. Boys are affected more commonly compared with girls. Pulmonary hypoplasia is generally the cause of death and may be associated with neonatal pneumothorax and pneumomediastinum. The Potter sequence is manifest at birth: small chest, abnormal facial features (micrognathia, beaked nose, epicanthic folds, low-set ears), and limb deformities (tightly apposed fingers, dislocated hips, clubfeet).[36]

Imaging Ultrasonography demonstrates the absence of the kidney and the presence of an abnormally configured (elongated or elliptical) adrenal gland, rather than its normal triangular or Y-configuration (Fig. 111-14).[36,59-61] Because the embryology of the adrenal gland is independent of that of the kidney, it is usually located in its expected position, even when the kidney does not reach the renal fossa. Ultrasonography and magnetic resonance imaging (MRI) are most commonly used to evaluate associated uterine and vaginal anomalies in girls and seminal vesicle cysts in boys (Fig.

111-15).[50-54] Because of the increased incidence of VUR into the remaining solitary kidney and the need to protect its parenchyma, a study to exclude reflux is recommended early in life.

Renal Ectopia (Pelvic Kidney and Ectopic Intrathoracic Kidney)

Renal ectopia is diagnosed when a kidney fails to migrate to its appropriate renal fossa, occurring with an incidence of 1 : 800 to 1 : 1000.[62] The pelvic kidney is the most common type of renal ectopia (accounting for about 60% of cases). Pelvic kidneys are prone to VUR and in about 10% of children may be the only kidney. In some children, both kidneys are in the pelvis and may be fused into a single unit, the so-called *cake kidney* or *lump kidney*. Ectopic intrathoracic kidney is the least common form of renal ectopia,

---

Box 111-1 Genital Anomalies Associated with Unilateral Renal Agenesis

Female
- Absence or hypoplasia of vagina
- Absence of uterus
- Failure of fusion of midline structures (Müllerian derivatives)
  - Bicornuate uterus, uterus didelphys
  - Obstructed hemivagina and hemiuterus and hydrocolpos, hematocolpos, hematosalpinx
- Gartner duct cyst
- Ipsilateral absence of uterine horn and fallopian tube (unicornuate uterus)

Male
- Ipsilateral anomalies
  - Absence of epididymis
  - Absence of seminal vesicle
  - Absence of vas deferens
  - Absence or hypoplasia of testis
  - Seminal vesicle cyst

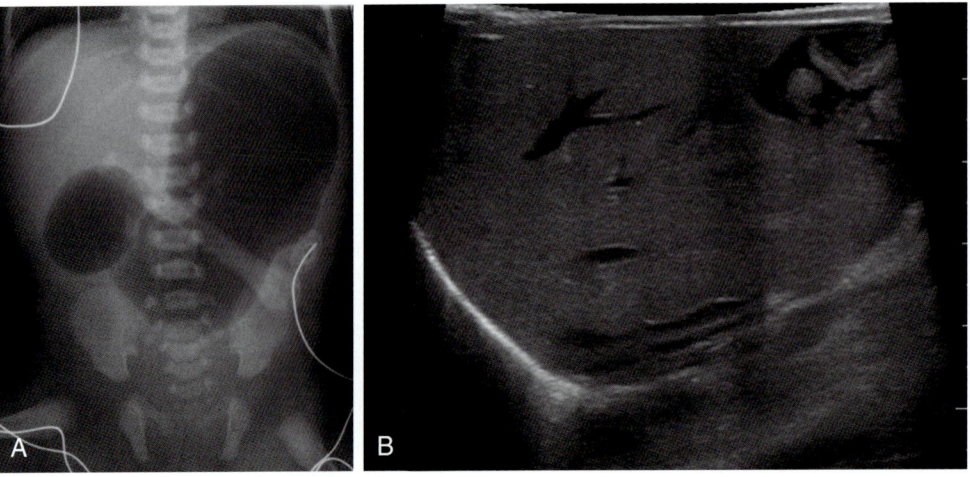

Figure 111-14 A female newborn with unilateral renal agenesis and VACTERL association. **A,** A supine abdominal radiograph shows marked gastric and proximal duodenal gaseous distention, the so-called "double bubble sign." No identifiable distal bowel gas exists. Both esophageal atresia (with distal fistula) and duodenal atresia were confirmed at surgery. **B,** Longitudinal ultrasonographic image through the right renal fossa confirms congenital absence of the right kidney. The right adrenal gland is abnormally elongated.

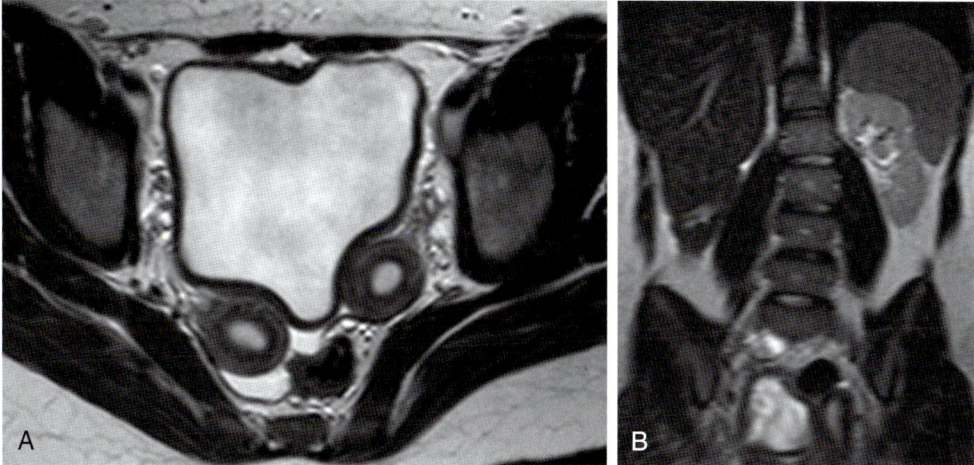

Figure 111-15 A 14-year-old girl with unilateral renal agenesis and Mullerian anomaly. **A,** Anaxial T2-weighted magnetic resonance image through the pelvis shows two separate uterine horns, proven to be uterus didelphys. **B,** A coronal single-shot fast spin-echo image through the retroperitoneum confirms congenital absence of the right kidney.

representing less than 5% of cases.[63,64] This condition may occur as an isolated lesion with an intact diaphragm but is more often part of a larger intrathoracic herniation through the foramen of Bochdalek.[63] Anomalies of rotation and blood supply are to be expected with renal ectopia.[36]

Imaging On ultrasonography, the pelvicalyceal system of the pelvic kidney may be predominantly extrarenal, resulting in images in which the kidney lacks the usual central renal echo complex.[62] Corticomedullary differentiation may be indistinct (Fig. 111-16). UPJ obstruction is common in pelvic kidneys because the abnormal orientation of the ureter relative to the renal pelvis impedes drainage. Renal scintigraphy is often used to both locate and define the morphology of ectopic kidneys, but computed tomography (CT), MRI, and excretory urography are also effective (e-Fig. 111-17).[65] The thoracic kidney is located in the posterior mediastinum and on chest radiographs may be mistaken for the usual neurogenic tumors that develop in this region (e-Fig. 111-18).

ANOMALIES OF FUSION: HORSESHOE KIDNEY AND CROSSED RENAL ECTOPIA

Horseshoe Kidney

Horseshoe kidney is the most common renal fusion anomaly, noted in 1 : 400 to 1 : 1000 autopsies.[36,66-68] It derives its name from the U-shape configuration of the kidneys, produced by the fusion of the lower pole moieties, which are more medially located than the upper poles (Fig. 111-19).[66-68] The bridging tissue, known as the *isthmus*, is more commonly composed of functioning renal parenchyma than fibrous tissue.[36,66,69] The isthmus is located just below the origin of the inferior mesenteric artery.[36,68] This condition is caused by in utero fusion of the metanephric blastemas in the pelvis during the sixth or seventh week of gestation.[67] The vascular supply of horseshoe kidneys is quite variable, arising from the abdominal aorta, iliac arteries, and inferior mesenteric artery.[66,68,69]

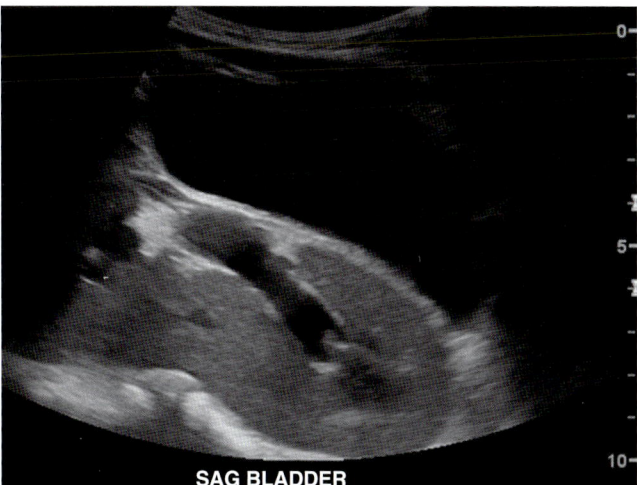

Figure 111-16 A 5-year-old boy with pelvic kidney. Longitudinal ultrasonographic image through the pelvis reveals an ectopic kidney located posterior to urinary bladder. The kidney is nonrotated with its hilum and extrarenal pelvis oriented anteriorly.

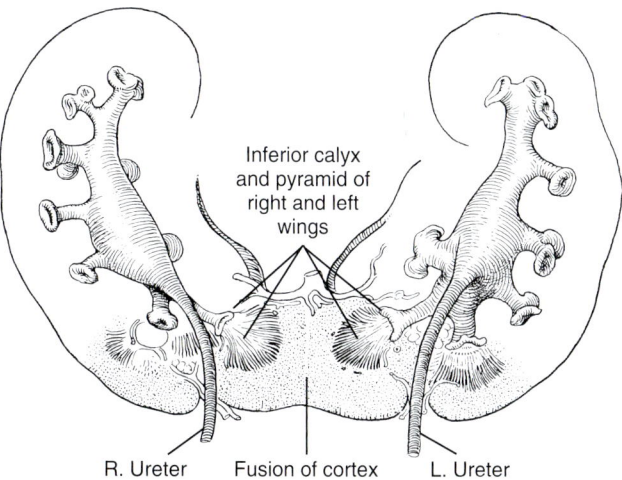

Figure 111-19 Horseshoe kidney with fusion of the inferior poles, spreading apart of the superior poles, and failure of rotation. The renal pelves enter the kidneys on their anterior aspect. (Redrawn from Kelly HA, Burnam CF. *Diseases of the kidneys, ureters and bladder.* 2nd ed. New York: Appleton; 1922.)

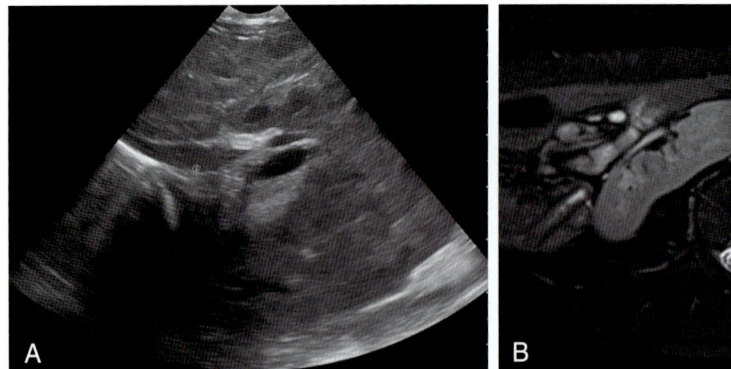

Figure 111-20 Horseshoe kidney. **A,** Coronal oblique ultrasonographic image through the retroperitoneum shows a horseshoe kidney with a parenchymal isthmus overlying the abdominal aorta. Abnormal longitudinal axis of the kidneys is seen. **B,** An axial T2-weighted magnetic resonance image with fat-saturation shows fusion of the kidneys in the midline just below the level of the inferior mesenteric artery. The kidneys are malrotated with the collecting systems oriented anteriorly (Courtesy Damien Grattan-Smith, MD.)

Clinical Presentation Horseshoe kidneys may be an asymptomatic; however, an increased incidence of UPJ obstruction, VUR, and ureteral duplication predispose affected individuals to both urolithiasis and infection.[36,68-70] Because horseshoe kidneys overly the spine and lack protective surrounding ribs, they are prone to injury from direct trauma.[68] A slight increased risk of Wilms tumor in horseshoe kidneys compared with normal kidneys has been reported.[36,67,68,71,72]

Imaging Ultrasonography demonstrates the upper portion of each kidney in a low paraspinal location. The isthmus may be identified in many cases anterior to the lumbar spine, especially when mild compression is used to displace interposed bowel loops. The renal long axis is abnormal and may be curved (Fig. 111-20).[73] Anterior orientation of the renal pelvis from malrotation is common as are extrarenal pelves.[69,73] CT and magnetic resonance angiography may be used to establish renal artery anatomy. CT also excellently depicts renal parenchymal and collecting system injuries in the setting of abdominal trauma (e-Fig. 111-21). Magnetic resonance urography or renal scintigraphy may be performed to assess for suspected UPJ obstruction (e-Fig. 111-22).[68] Voiding cystourethrogram (VCUG) may help assess for VUR.

Crossed Renal Ectopia

Clinical Presentation Crossed renal ectopia occurs when both kidneys are located on one side of the spine; a portion of the lower kidney, usually the one that has moved from its normal position (most commonly the left kidney), may extend over the spine.[36,74] This anomaly is seen in 1 : 7500 children, affects boys more often than girls, and is the second most common renal fusion anomaly after horseshoe kidney.[36,66,74,75] The ureter from the lower kidney crosses the midline to insert into the bladder in its normal position.[74] Although most are oriented in a relatively vertical axis, the lower kidney may be obliquely or horizontally related to the superior kidney (Fig. 111-23). The position of the upper (uncrossed) kidney may also be ectopically low. Approximately 85% of crossed kidneys are fused and encompassed by a common renal fascia—hence the term *crossed fused renal ectopia*.[36] As expected in any type of ectopia, the arterial vascularity may be

anomalous, and the renal pelvis, especially of the lower kidney, may be malrotated.[64,74,76]

Imaging Imaging demonstrates an empty renal fossa on one side and both kidneys located on the opposite side of the spine (Fig. 111-24).[77] MRI and CT show two separate ureters, each entering its appropriate trigone.[36] Doppler ultrasonography may be used to demonstrate jets of urine emanating from the normally positioned UVJs. Ultrasonography, MRI, and CT may allow visualization of a small indentation at the site of fusion (e-Fig. 111-25).[77,78]

Ureter

URETEROPELVIC JUNCTION

The transition between the renal pelvis and the ureter, or the UPJ, may be sharply or poorly defined. Both extrinsic filling defects and local narrowing are commonly observed at the UPJ without resultant hydronephrosis. An inferior polar artery may produce a small extrinsic defect or notch in the ureter near the UPJ (e-Fig. 111-26). A sharp kink without obstruction is occasionally seen in the proximal portion of the ureter as a transient or constant finding. Retained fetal folds in the upper ureter (e-Fig. 111-27), mild elongation and tortuosity of the ureter, and mild widening of the midureter may all be seen normally in the urogram in the infant. They are believed to represent a persistence of fetal characteristics, and disappear in early childhood.[17,79-83]

DUPLICATION

Ureteral duplication (duplication of the renal pelvis and ureter) is one of the most common anomalies of the urinary tract (Fig. 111-28). Incomplete duplication ranges from a bifid renal pelvis to two ureters joining anywhere along their course and continuing inferiorly as a single structure. In completely duplicated systems, the two ureters are separate throughout their entire course. The ureter draining the upper pole of the kidney normally inserts into the bladder more caudad and more medially than the lower pole ureter (Weigert-Meyer rule) and has a longer submucosal tunnel

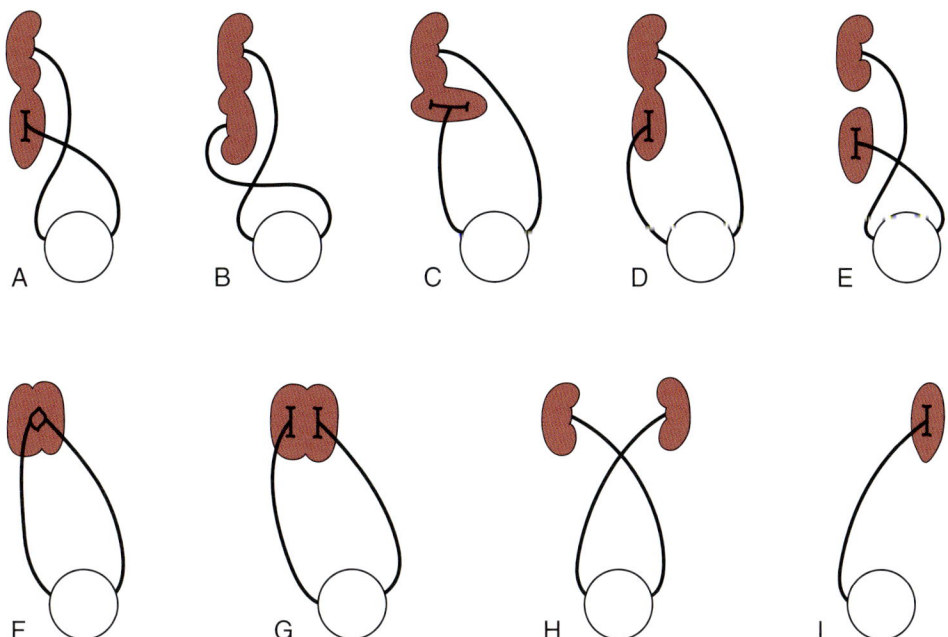

Figure 111-23 **Various types of crossed renal ectopia. A,** Unilateral fused kidney (inferior renal ectopia), the most common form. **B,** Sigmoid or S-shaped kidney. **C,** L-shaped kidney. **D,** Unilateral fused kidney (superior renal ectopia). **E,** Crossed ectopia without fusion. **F,** Unilateral disk kidney. **G,** Unilateral lump kidney. **H,** Bilateral crossed ectopia. **I,** Crossed ectopia of a solitary kidney (solitary crossed renal ectopia).

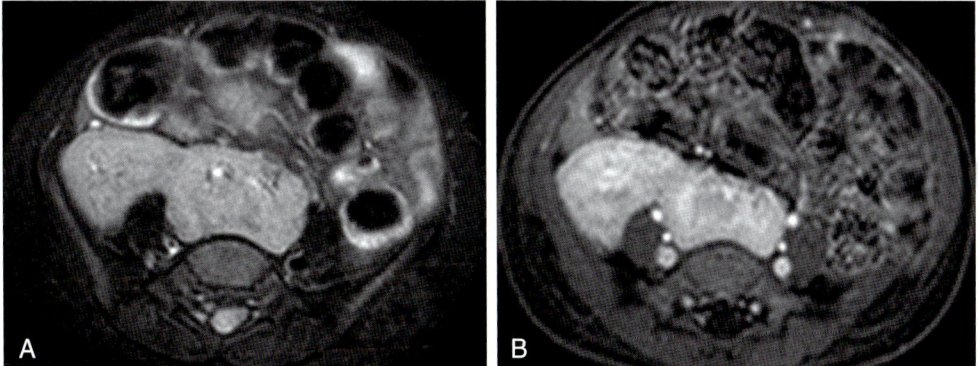

Figure 111-24 A 2 year-old girl with crossed fused renal ectopia and magnetic resonance imaging. **A** and **B,** Axial T2-weighted and T1-weighted postcontrast images with fat-saturation show renal fusion, with both kidneys located to the right of the midline. The left (lower) moiety partly overlies the spine.

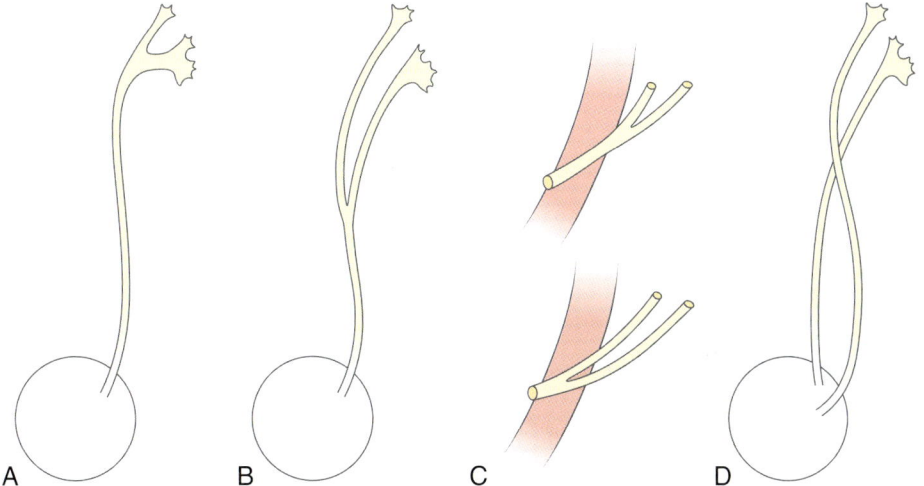

Figure 111-28 **Various forms of ureteral duplication. A,** Bifid pelvis. **B,** Partial ureteral duplication (Y-ureter). **C,** Incomplete ureteral duplication with the ureters joining near the bladder or within the bladder wall (V-ureter). **D,** Complete ureteral duplication with separate ureteral orifices. The upper pole ureter inserts distally and medially to the lower pole ureter (Weigert-Meyer rule).

than the lower pole ureter. Ureteral duplication is more commonly unilateral, although it may be bilateral. Ureteral duplication is of no clinical importance unless complicated by another congenital lesion or an acquired process. These conditions such as ureteral ectopia, VUR, urinary tract infection, and congenital UPJ obstruction are addressed in later chapters.[84-91]

Other variants of ureteral duplication probably related to ureteral duplication include the accessory ureter or a ureteral stump. The accessory ureter is a tubular structure originating from a distal normal ureter at the bladder, and extending cephalad along the normal ureter to end blindly proximally, without connection to a pelvocalyceal system or renal parenchyma. The ureteral stump varies in length from a few centimeters to a narrow but patent cord that extends almost to the kidney (e-Fig. 111-29).[92-96]

Ureteral triplication (e-Fig. 111-30) is another rare anomaly in which three ureters arise from the kidney, one from the upper pole, the second from the midzone of the kidney, and the third from the lower pole The three ureters may drain separately into the bladder, or one may end ectopically; the parenchyma drained by the ectopic ureter is usually small and poorly functioning. In a second type, two of the three ureters may join in the lumbar area to form a single Y-shaped ureter that drains usually into the bladder, together with a normal third ureter. In a third type, the three ureters join in the lumbar area to form a common distal ureter that drains into the bladder. More than half the cases of ureteral triplication defy the Weigert-Meyer rule. Four ureters emanating from a single kidney have been described.[97-100]

Bladder

Bladder ears are normal lateral protrusions of the urinary bladder (Fig. 111-31). They are most frequently seen in infants less than 6 months of age as transient protrusions that are most apparent when the bladder is partially full. Bladder ears represent extraperitoneal herniations of the bladder through the internal inguinal ring into the inguinal canal. An association of bladder ears with inguinal hernia may reflect the presence of a patent or partially patent processus vaginalis. Rarely, lateral protrusions of the rectum occur in this same location, producing a normal anatomic variant termed *rectal ears*.[101-103]

Urethra

Several normal findings exist and should not be confused with pathologic processes, including normal anatomic folds of the posterior urethra of the male, and urinal and foreskin artifact. Normal anatomic folds are frequently visualized in the posterior urethra of the male and should not be confused with congenital obstructing membranes. Unlike congenital obstructing membranes, these folds do not produce dilatation of the proximal posterior urethra or decrease the urinary stream.[104-108]

Urinal artifact may be produced in the male during voiding. The urethral stream is compressed at the level of the penoscrotal junction by the plastic urinal and should not be confused with a stricture of the penile urethra. A film during voiding without urethral compression by the urinal confirms normal urethral caliber.[109]

Foreskin artifact is caused by retraction of a tight foreskin and consequent narrowing of the distal urethra. This appearance may also mimic a urethral stricture. Reduction of the foreskin while voiding makes the appearance normal.

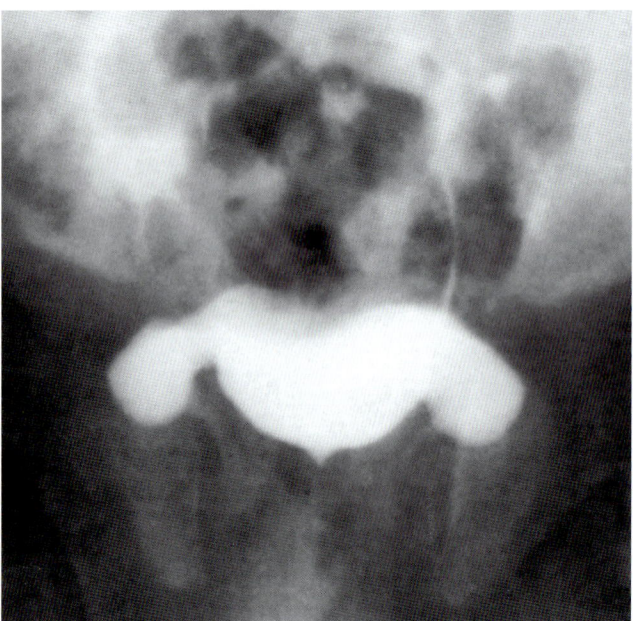

Figure 111-31 **Bladder ears.** A voiding cystourethrogram shows transient lateral herniation of the bladder ("bladder ears") in a normal infant. (Courtesy Sandra K. Fernbach, MD, and Kate A. Feinstein, MD.)

✓ WHAT THE CLINICIAN NEEDS TO KNOW

- Renal number, location, size, echogenicity, and presence of duplication
- Expected bladder capacity is achieved on VCUG based on weight in infancy and by age for the older child
- Associated genital anomalies with unilateral renal agenesis
- Presence of an abnormally configured (elongated or elliptical) adrenal gland
- UPJ obstruction, VUR, ureteral duplication, urolithiasis, infection with renal fusion anomalies, or all of these conditions

Key Points

The urinary and genital systems are closely associated embryologically.

The neonatal kidney has immature function during the first days after birth with decreased GFR and urine output, and limited concentrating ability.

Variants in imaging of the childhood kidney include the column of Bertin, junctional parenchymal defect, scalloping of the cortical border, interrenuncular septum, dromedary hump, hilar lips, and hypoechoic pyramids.

Renal length is correlated to age, height, and weight.

Horseshoe kidneys have an increased incidence of UPJ obstruction, VUR, and ureteral duplication, and injury from direct trauma. A slight increased risk of Wilms tumor has been reported.

The ureter from the lower kidney of crossed, fused kidneys crosses midline to insert into the bladder in its normal position.

Ureteral duplication may be partial or complete. Incomplete duplication ranges from a bifid renal pelvis to two ureters joining anywhere along their course and continuing inferiorly as a single structure. In completely duplicated systems, the two ureters are separate throughout their entire course.

Suggested Readings

Fernbach SK, Feinstein KA, Schmidt MB. Pediatric voiding cystourethrography: a pictorial guide. *Radiographics*. 2000;20(1):155-168.

Glodny B, Petersen J, Hofmann KJ, et al. Kidney fusion anomalies revisited: clinical and radiological analysis of 209 cases of crossed fused ectopia and horseshoe kidney. *BJU Int*. 2009;103:224-235.

Moore KL, Persaud TVN. The urogenital system. In: *Before we are born: essentials of embryology and birth defects*. 7th ed. Philadelphia, PA: WB Saunders, 2003

Patel U. *Congenital anomalies of the bladder imaging and urodynamics of the lower urinary tract*. London, U.K.: Springer; 2010:23-27.

Shapiro E. Clinical implications of genitourinary embryology. *Curr Opin Urol*. 2009;19(4):427-433.

References

Full references for this chapter can be found on www.expertconsult.com.

Chapter 112

Imaging Techniques

AMY B. KOLBE, LARRY A. BINKOVITZ, M. BETH MCCARVILLE,
J. DAMIEN GRATTAN-SMITH, and BRIAN D. COLEY

Radiographic Procedures

INTRAVENOUS UROGRAPHY

In the past, intravenous (IV) urography was the imaging method of choice for the kidneys and collecting system, but it has been supplanted by magnetic resonance imaging (MRI) and computed tomography (CT) and is rarely the preferred imaging method in current pediatric practice. IV urography uses the physiologic excretion of injected iodinated contrast media for visualization of the renal cortex, medulla, and collecting system. Anatomic details of the renal parenchyma and collecting system and general information concerning renal function are obtained.

Imaging begins with a frontal radiograph of the abdomen to identify any calcifications or masses. After this preliminary radiograph is obtained, low osmolar contrast media with a high iodine content is administered intravenously at a dose of 2 mL/kg (maximum, 150 mL) to obtain adequate iodine concentration in the renal tubules and collecting system. The filming sequence is tailored to the individual examination. An initial frontal radiograph within 1 to 2 minutes of injection images the nephrographic phase. Assessment of this radiograph determines subsequent filming. Upon routine examination, a radiograph at approximately 5 to 10 minutes allows visualization of the kidneys and their collecting systems, including the bladder (e-Fig. 112-1). In the prone position, the higher specific gravity of the contrast material allows better visualization of the anteriorly positioned renal pelves and proximal ureters.

The nephrographic phase provides a gross estimate of renal function, as well as information on renal size and parenchymal contour. A poorly visible nephrogram may indicate a technical problem in achieving optimal plasma concentration of contrast material or some degree of renal failure or diminished renal function. A dense and prolonged nephrogram indicates obstruction of the renal collecting system or renal tubules, hypotension, hypovolemia, or acute tubular necrosis.

RETROGRADE URETHROGRAPHY

Retrograde urethrograms are obtained infrequently in children but sometimes are performed in boys to evaluate possible urethral injury or rupture after a straddle injury or pelvic trauma. A small catheter is introduced into the anterior urethra to or slightly past the fossa navicularis, and the meatus is occluded. With the patient in a steep oblique position, a small amount of contrast material is injected through a syringe to allow evaluation of the urethra to the level of the external sphincter. Spasm of the external sphincter sometimes prevents filling of the most proximal portion of the posterior urethra. Although urethrograms are rarely performed in girls, the tip of a small Foley catheter with the balloon distended can be placed into the urethra and then taped to the perineum to allow retrograde evaluation of the urethra.

VOIDING CYSTOURETHROGRAPHY

Antegrade voiding cystourethrography (VCUG) is the traditional examination of choice for detailed anatomic evaluation of the bladder, study of the anatomy of the male urethra, and identification of vesicoureteral reflux (VUR). The bladder is filled by gravity pressure, using dilute sterile contrast media with an iodine concentration of 80 to 100 mg/mL. The predicted bladder capacity (in milliliters) for children younger than 1 year is the child's weight in kilograms multiplied by 7. In children older than 1 year, the predicted capacity is the child's age in years plus 2, multiplied by 30.[1,2]

An early bladder filling image is obtained to evaluate for ureteroceles or masses. Images with a full urinary bladder are obtained in the lateral oblique projections to look for VUR. Voiding films are useful to evaluate the bladder and urethra (particularly the male urethra) and for the diagnosis of VUR, which may occur only during voiding. After voiding, an image of the bladder documents any postvoid residual, and an image of the kidneys documents any reflux that occurred during the examination. Neonates should undergo at least two filling and voiding cycles to increase the chance of detecting VUR.[3-6] Pulsed fluoroscopy, last image hold recording, and videotaping are important imaging strategies for reducing radiation exposure.[7-10]

Ultrasound

CONTRAST-ENHANCED VOIDING ULTRASONOGRAPHY

The intravesical instillation of ultrasound contrast agents in the urinary bladder allows the sonographic evaluation of VUR without the use of ionizing radiation.[11-14] These microbubble contrast agents are composed of an outer shell of lipid,

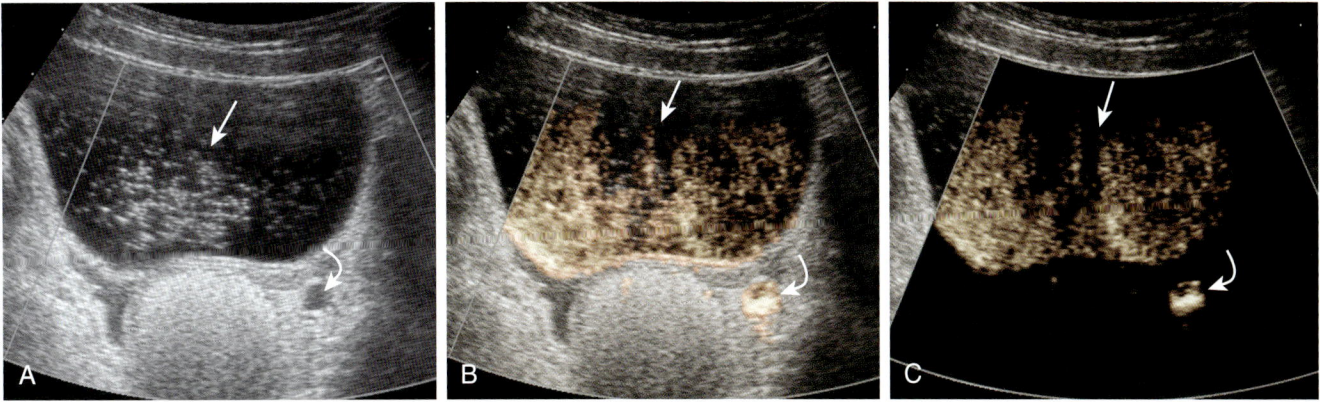

Figure 112-2 Contrast-enhanced cystosonography. Transverse ultrasound images after instillation of an ultrasound contrast agent into the urinary bladder. **A,** On gray-scale imaging, the contrast agent appears as hyperechoic material in the bladder (*straight arrow*) surrounded by anechoic urine. Reflux into the distal left ureter (*curved arrow*) is present but somewhat difficult to appreciate. **B,** Color overlay technology shows the contrast agent to better advantage as bright orange material in the bladder (*straight arrow*) and distal ureter (*curved arrow*). **C,** Subtraction technology further accentuates the presence of contrast material by eliminating non–contrast-enhanced background tissue. Contrast material in the bladder (*straight arrow*) and ureter (*curved arrow*) are readily apparent. (Images courtesy Dr. Kassa Darge.)

protein, or polymer that encases a gas, most commonly a perfluorocarbon.[15] The gas is highly reflective on ultrasound imaging (Fig. 112-2) and can be detected even when administered in very small volumes. The ultrasound transducer is positioned intermittently over the bladder, ureters, and kidneys while the bladder is filled. On grayscale imaging, the microbubbles appear echogenic. Refluxed contrast material is easily detected in the ureters and kidneys (Fig. 112-3). Although this technique does not avoid catheterization, it does eliminate radiation exposure. Results indicate that the sensitivity for VUR detection is comparable with that of standard techniques. A reflux grading system for contrast-enhanced voiding ultrasonography has been developed and is similar to the international grading system for VCUG.[12] Urethral visualization is possible with contrast–enhanced voiding ultrasonography but remains challenging.

RENAL ULTRASONOGRAPHY

Ultrasonography is an ideal method for examining the kidneys and bladder in infants and children because of their small physical habitus and lack of abdominal fat and because ultrasonography does not utilize ionizing radiation. Variable transducer frequencies and transducer design (e.g., sector, phased, curvilinear, and linear array) allow for individualized approaches. Doppler ultrasound is valuable for the detection of blood flow, to confirm arterial perfusion, or to exclude venous thrombosis. Measurable blood flow parameters from spectral Doppler analysis include peak systolic velocity, end-diastolic velocity, and acceleration times. The normal renal artery has a prompt systolic upstroke with an acceleration time of 70 msec or less and a visible early systolic peak (e-Fig. 112-4). The normal resistive index depends on the patient's age; it may be as high as 0.9 in a preterm infant and falls to around the adult value of 0.7 in the first few months of life.[16-19]

In young children, it is advisable to initiate the urogenital ultrasound examination with an examination of the bladder. The full bladder of an infant usually empties when the transducer is placed in the suprapubic region. Kidneys are imaged in the longitudinal and transverse planes. The kidneys are ovoid solid organs with fine, medium-level echoes arising from the cortex, a well-delineated corticomedullary junction with brightly echoic arcuate arteries, and pyramid-shaped, relatively large medullary rays that are hypoechoic. Cortical echogenicity in neonates and young infants is higher and the medullary pyramids are more hypoechoic than in older children (Fig. 112-5). The cortical echogenicity is increased

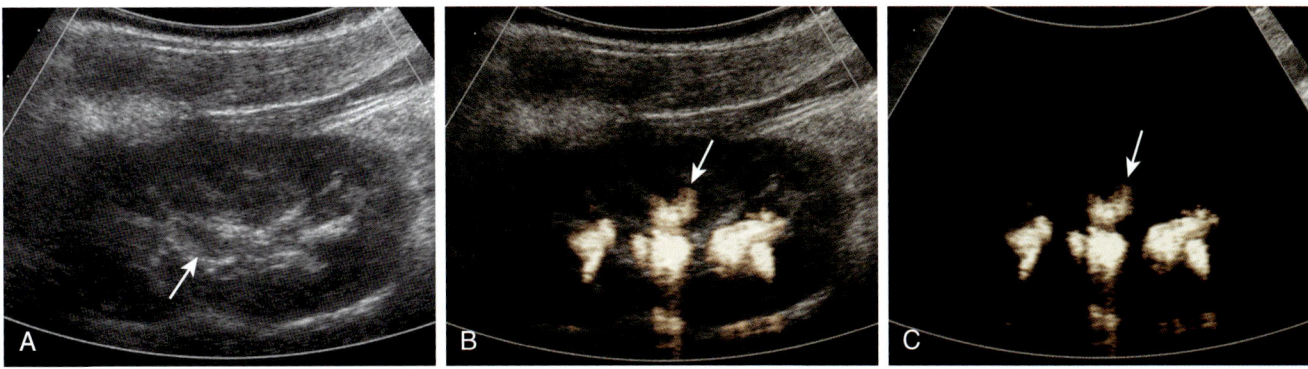

Figure 112-3 Contrast-enhanced cystosonography. Longitudinal ultrasound images of the kidney, obtained during contrast-enhanced voiding ultrasonography, demonstrate reflux into the renal collecting system (*arrows*) on gray-scale (**A**), color-overlay (**B**), and subtraction (**C**) images. (Images courtesy Dr. Kassa Darge.)

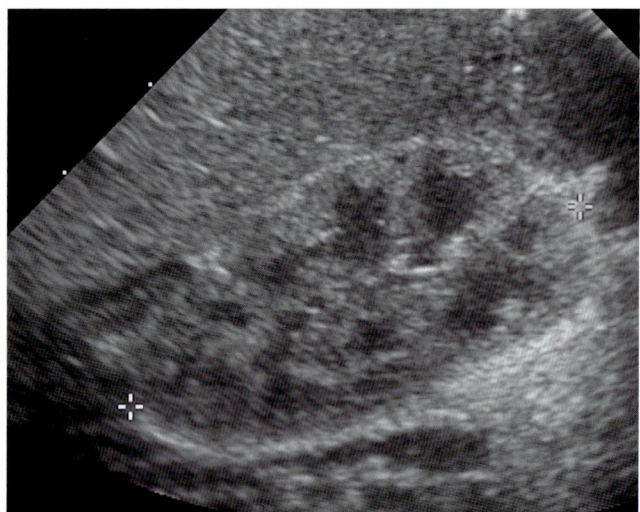

Figure 112-5   **A normal newborn kidney.** A longitudinal sonogram shows that the right renal cortex is slightly more echogenic than the adjacent liver. The hypoechoic medullary pyramids are quite distinct.

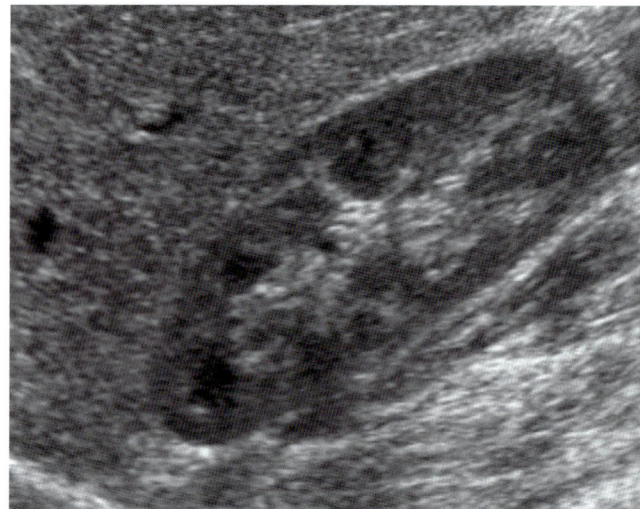

Figure 112-6   **A normal pediatric kidney.** A longitudinal sonogram in a 5-year-old child shows that the renal cortex is hypoechoic relative to the adjacent liver. The medullary pyramids are still distinct. Note the minimal echogenicity of the renal sinus as a result of a paucity of renal sinus fat.

compared with the liver and spleen in preterm infants, isoechoic in neonates and young infants, and diminishes progressively in older children. The transition from the infant renal echo pattern to that of the child typically occurs between 6 and 9 months (Fig. 112-6). Normal pediatric sonographic measurements of right and left kidney length, based on height and age, are provided in Table 112-1.[20-25]

Nuclear Medicine

NUCLEAR CYSTOGRAPHY

Nuclear cystography is performed for the assessment of VUR and is an alternative to fluoroscopic VCUG. The examination is performed by direct instillation of radiotracer (technetium-99m–sulfur colloid) and sterile saline solution into the bladder after sterile catheterization[26] or indirectly after nuclear renography with planar images obtained during voiding.[27] Dynamic imaging of the bladder and kidney regions is acquired with use of a posterior gamma camera throughout the filling and voiding cycle. The data can be grouped (in 10- or 60-second intervals) and viewed dynamically. VUR is documented when tracer is shown to ascend into a tubular structure corresponding to the ureter or when the renal collecting system is visualized. The dose of tracer is dependent on bladder volume: 300 mCi for bladder volumes up to 300 mL, and 600 mCi for larger bladder volumes. A cyclic cystogram is recommended for children younger than 2 years, for children with previously documented VUR or a high suspicion for VUR, and for children

Table 112-1

Normal Sonographic Renal Lengths in Children Based on Height and Age													
Subjects			**Left Kidney Length (mm)**					**Right Kidney Length (mm)**					
				Percentile		**Suggested Limits of Normal**			**Percentile**		**Suggested Limits of Normal**		
Body Height (cm)	**No.**	**Age Range**	**Mean (SD)**	**5th**	**95th**	**Lower**	**Upper**	**Mean (SD)**	**5th**	**95th**	**Lower**	**Upper**	
48-64	50	1-3 mo	50 (5.5)	42	59	35	65	50 (5.8)	40	58	35	65	
54-73	39	4-6 mo	56 (5.5)	47	64	40	70	53 (5.3)	50	64	40	70	
65-78	17	7-9 mo	61 (4.6)	54	68	45	75	59 (5.2)	52	66	45	70	
71-92	18	1-2.5 y	66 (5.3)	57	72	50	80	61 (3.4)	55	65	50	75	
85-109	22	3-4.9 y	71 (4.5)	61	76	55	85	67 (5.1)	59	75	55	80	
100-130	26	5-6.9 y	79 (5.9)	70	87	60	95	74 (5.5)	65	83	60	85	
110-131	32	7-8.9 y	84 (6.6)	73	93	65	100	80 (6.6)	70	91	65	95	
124-149	27	9-10.9 y	84 (7.4)	75	97	65	105	80 (7.0)	69	89	65	100	
137-153	15	11-12.9 y	91 (8.4)	77	102	70	110	89 (6.2)	82	100	70	105	
143-168	22	13-14.9 y	96 (8.9)	84	110	75	115	94 (5.9)	85	102	75	110	
152-175	11	15-16.7 y	99 (7.5)	90	110	80	120	92 (7.0)	83	102	75	110	

From Konus OL, Ozdemir A, Akkaya A, et al. Normal liver, spleen, and kidney dimensions in neonates, infants, and children: evaluation with sonography. *AJR.* 1998;171:1693-1698.

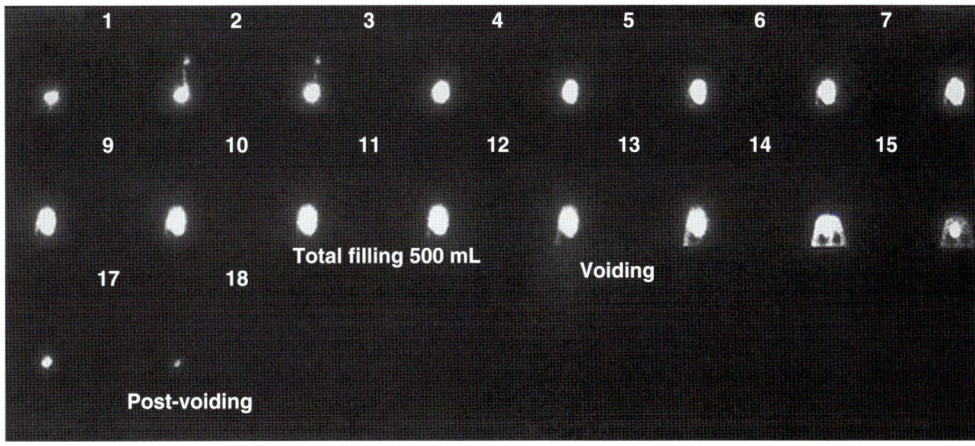

Figure 112-8   Vesicoureteral reflux. Early in the study, this nuclear cystogram shows intermediate-grade vesicoureteral reflux that later fully drains and does not recur through voiding. Continuous acquisition of the nuclear cystogram allowed the demonstration of this transient reflux, which likely would have been missed with fluoroscopic voiding cystourethrography.

who void well before the expected bladder capacity is reached. The procedure is identical to the standard cystogram; however, the catheter is left in the bladder after the first voiding cycle and is used to refill the bladder for a repeat void. As with VCUG, cyclic studies increase the diagnostic yield (e-Fig. 112-7), identifying an additional 10% to 15% of children with VUR compared with noncyclic voiding studies.[28]

Nuclear cystography offers three main advantages over fluoroscopic VCUG: increased detection of VUR (up to an additional 20%) (Fig. 112-8), frequent detection of a higher grade of VUR,[29,30] and reduced radiation dose (tenfold) (Table 112-2). Disadvantages of nuclear cystography include a lack of detailed anatomic visualization of the urethra and collecting systems and limited identification of bladder abnormalities (such as periureteric diverticula); in addition, the classification of VUR with nuclear cystography is less refined than that with VCUG. The nuclear cystography VUR grades of low, intermediate, and high roughly correspond to the fluoroscopic grades of 1 (low), 2 or 3 (intermediate), and 4 or 5 (high).[26]

Table 112-2

Effective Radiation Doses (mSv) for Boys and Girls			
Age (y)	VCUG[30]	RNC[31]	VCUG/RNC
Boys			
0	0.104	0.024	
1	0.121	0.024	5.4
5	0.162	0.024	
10	0.233	0.048	4.9
Girls			
0	0.137	0.024	
1	0.164	0.024	7.6
5	0.246	0.024	
10	0.522	0.048	10.9

RNC, Radionuclide cystogram; *VCUG,* voiding cystourethrogram.

DIURETIC RENOGRAPHY

Diuretic renography is used to distinguish obstructive from nonobstructive hydronephrosis.[31] It attempts to quantify urinary obstruction based on the relative function of the hydronephrotic kidney compared with the normal kidney and the rate of urinary excretion of radiotracer (technetium-99m mertiatide or technetium-99m diethylene triamine pentaacetic acid) from the renal pelvis (and, in the presence of hydroureter, from the ureter) after a diuretic challenge (1 mg/kg IV furosemide). The graphic presentation of renal excretion using a time versus intensity curve is termed a *renogram* (e-Fig. 112-9); normal, equivocal, and obstructed patterns of excretion after a diuretic challenge, termed *washout,* have been described[31] (Fig. 112-10). Additionally, the time required for half the tracer in the collecting system to pass across the ureteropelvic junction after the administration of furosemide, termed *diuretic T½,* is stratified to indicate a normal (0 to 10 minutes), equivocal (10 to 20 minutes), or obstructed (>20 minutes) pattern.[32,33] These values are useful in distinguishing obstructive from nonobstructive hydronephrosis in older children and adults. However, application of these guidelines can lead to the misdiagnosis of obstruction in a large number of young infants with hydronephrosis demonstrated on routine prenatal sonography (e-Fig. 112-11).[34] The high capacitance of the dilated renal pelvis and relatively low renal urine output in young infants limit the accuracy of this test in the setting of hydronephrosis in children younger than 2 years.[33] Increasing hydronephrosis, decreasing split renal function of the hydronephrotic kidney, and a worsening washout curve all suggest the possibility of significant obstruction (Fig. 112-12).

CORTICAL SCINTIGRAPHY

A renal cortical scan is performed for the assessment of acute pyelonephritis or its sequela, atrophic pyelonephritic scarring, or for the identification and characterization of functioning renal tissue. A cortical scan also can be used to identify renal anomalies of fusion or location, although sonography is the examination of choice because of its lack of ionizing radiation, increased availability, better anatomic detail, and lower cost.

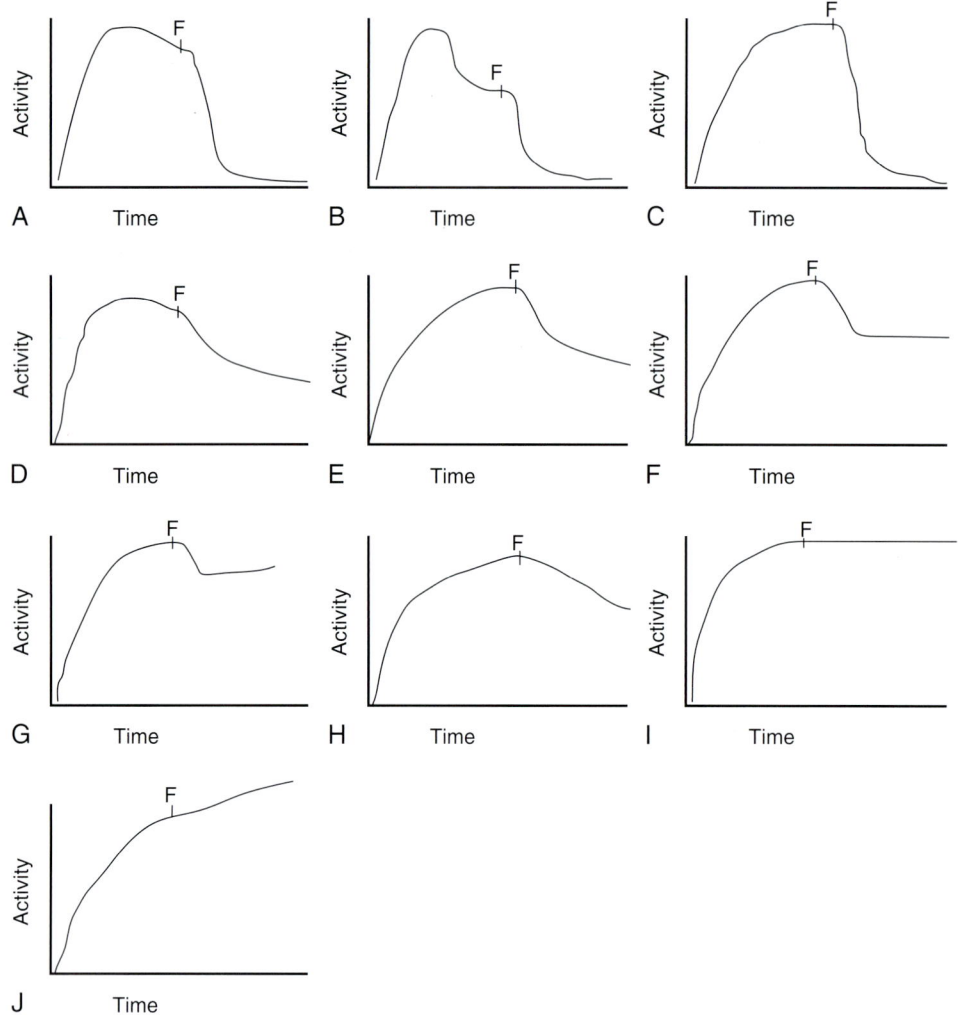

Figure 112-10 Diuretic renogram patterns. Patterns **A, B,** and **C** are typically indicative of nonobstructed systems. Patterns **D** and **E** are equivocal in older children but usually indicate no obstruction in neonates and young infants with hydronephrosis. Patterns **F** and **G** often indicate flow-related obstruction. Patterns **H, I,** and **J** typically indicate obstruction in older children but are seen frequently in neonates and infants with nonobstructive hydronephrosis. *F,* Furosemide injection.

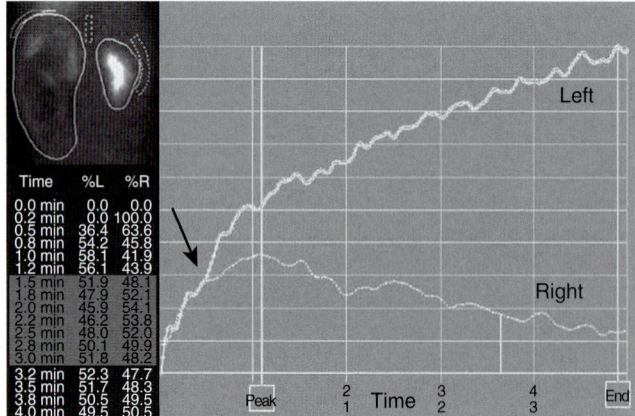

Figure 112-12 Hydronephrosis. A markedly enlarged left kidney with central photopenic regions consistent with marked hydronephrosis. The renogram shows tracer accumulation and retention throughout, with no discernible washout after administration of a diuretic. Note that the renogram tracings of the two kidneys are superimposed during the first few minutes after injection of the tracer (*arrow*), which indicates nearly equal split renal function, as shown on the function table between 1.5 and 3 minutes.

The renal cortical scan typically is performed with technetium-99m–labeled dimercaptosuccinic acid. This agent is extracted by and then binds to cells of the proximal convoluted tubule. It does not accumulate in the medulla or collecting system, thus accounting for the scan appearance of cortical uptake with relative central photopenia of the medulla and renal sinus (Fig. 112-13). Imaging typically occurs 2 to 3 hours after injection and should be performed with pinhole collimation or single photon emission CT acquisition with a dual-headed camera.[35,36] The accuracy in demonstrating acute pyelonephritis exceeds 95%.[37] A defect that appears as a vague area of photopenia not associated with volume loss is more consistent with acute pyelonephritis, whereas a triangular, well-demarcated photopenic focus with volume loss typically is considered an atrophic scar (Fig. 112-14), although it also may be related to focal renal dysplasia. Most areas of infection resolve without residual scarring, especially in older children, but resolution may not occur until 6 months or longer after the acute event. Therefore a definitive diagnosis of a scar requires a follow-up study at least 6 months after the acute infection.[38] Rounded defects

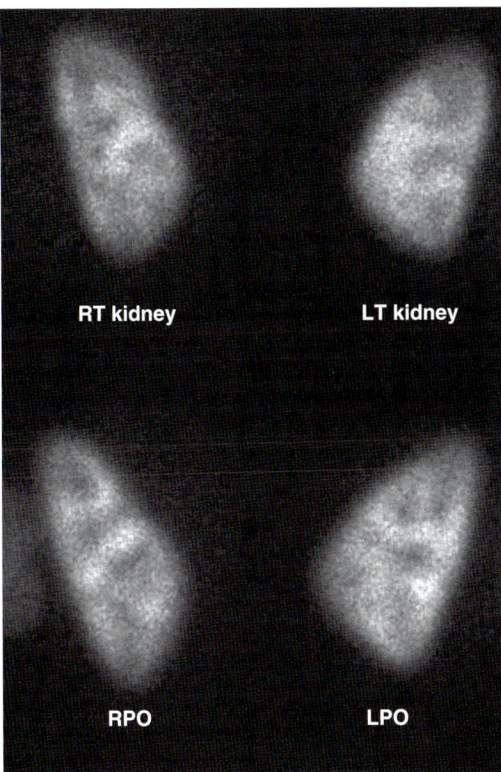

Figure 112-13 A normal dimercaptosuccinic acid cortical scan. Note the relative photopenia of the medulla due to a lack of uptake by the deeper portions of the loop of Henle. Also note the decreased intensity of the polar regions as a result of the relatively thinner polar cortex when compared with the midpolar region. *LPO,* Left posterior oblique; *LT,* left; *RPO,* right posterior oblique; *RT,* right.

identified with cortical scintigraphy should be further characterized with ultrasound to assess for a cyst or mass (e-Fig. 112-15).

MISCELLANEOUS RENAL NUCLEAR STUDIES

Quantitation of renal function is possible with nuclear imaging techniques.[39] The relative function of each kidney can be assessed during the renogram before tracer exits the renal pelvis or with cortical scintigraphy. Regions of interest for each kidney are drawn from a posterior image, and relative function is given in terms of a percentage of total renal counts. The normal value is 50% ± 5%. Absolute renal function quantitation in terms of glomerular filtration rate or effective renal plasma flow can be performed with technetium-labeled mertiatide and dimercaptosuccinic acid, respectively, but these techniques require one to four blood samples.[39] Renal function increases rapidly in the first 2 years of life and reaches adult values, when normalized to body surface area, by age 2 years (normal values range from 80 to 140 mL/min/1.73 m²).[39]

Computed Tomography

CT is one of our most powerful imaging tools. High-quality CT can be performed in patients of all ages and sizes and is not limited by bone or bowel gas. Relative immobility is required, and in children, reassurance, explanation of the procedure, the presence of a parent, sedation, and immobilization all contribute to a successful diagnostic study. Multidetector scanners that operate quickly obviate the need for sedation in most patients. Multiplanar reformatting, especially in the coronal plane, can depict the entire course of the urinary collecting system.[40-42]

Noncontrast imaging is performed for calcifications or nephrolithiasis, but most CT imaging of the genitourinary

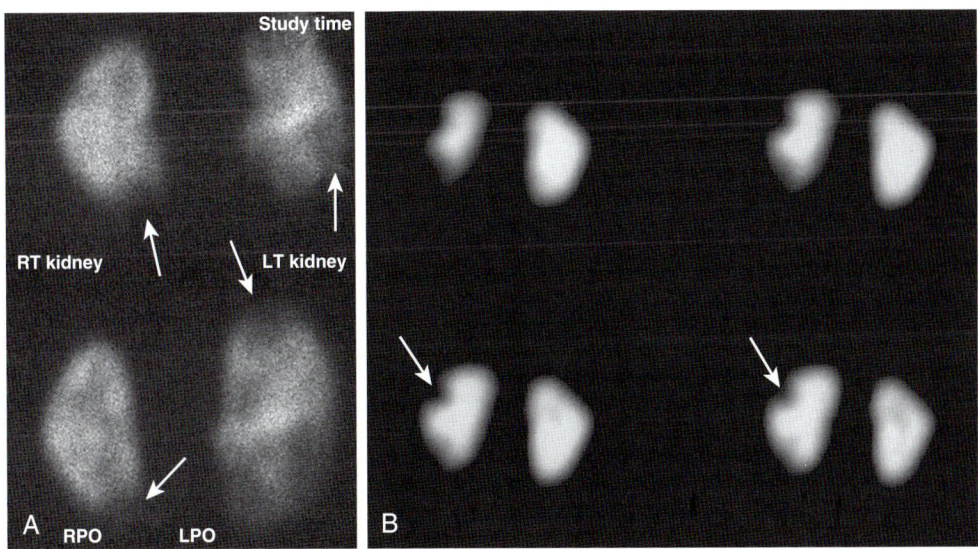

Figure 112-14 Pyelonephritis versus scarring. **A,** Pinhole dimercaptosuccinic acid (DMSA) images obtained for split uptake assessment show bilateral photopenic defects that are rather poorly defined and not associated with renal parenchymal volume loss (*arrows*) indicating pyelonephritis. **B,** Coronal single photon emission computed tomography glucoheptonate images show sharply defined wedge-shaped defects (*arrows*) indicative of renal scars. Glucoheptonate has been largely replaced by DMSA for cortical scintigraphy because of better binding characteristics. *LPO,* Left posterior oblique; *LT,* left; *RPO,* right posterior oblique; *RT,* right.

system is performed with IV contrast. Contrast enhancement is required for the evaluation of renal lesions and the vessels of the abdomen. Delayed imaging is useful for assessing the integrity of the collecting system (such as after trauma), assessing the course of the ureter, and evaluating renal masses and cysts. CT radiation doses should be reduced and optimized based on patient size and the purpose of the study. Scanning begins based on the speed of the particular CT scanner and the information being sought. By showing the progression of contrast enhancement of the cortex, medulla, and collecting system of the kidney, CT provides some assessment of renal function and anatomy.[43-48]

Magnetic Resonance Imaging

MRI has superior tissue characterization, multiplanar capabilities, and the ability to gather functional and anatomic information. Meticulous attention to patient preparation and scanning technique is essential to reliably obtain high-quality images. The typical imaging parameters are described in Table 112-3.

Urine in the collecting system and ureter has low signal intensity on T1-weighted images and higher signal intensity on T2-weighted scans. The kidney is easily visualized with an intermediate signal on T1-weighted sequences. The renal cortex has an intermediate signal close to that of the spleen, and the medullary pyramids show a lower intensity signal on T1-weighted images. The kidney has a uniformly high signal on T2-weighted scans (Fig. 112-16).[49-56]

MAGNETIC RESONANCE UROGRAPHY

MR urography (MRU) represents the next stage in the evolution of uroradiology, fusing superb anatomic and functional imaging into a single test that does not use ionizing radiation (Fig. 112-17).[57-63] In addition to spin echo T1- and T2-weighted images, dynamic imaging is performed in conjunction with the injection of a gadolinium-based contrast agent to assess the concentrating and excretory functions of the kidney (e-Fig. 112-18). The evaluation of the contrast dynamics is similar to renal scintigraphy but with the important distinction that the signals originating from the renal parenchyma can be separated from those originating from the collecting system. The primary indication for MRU is in the evaluation of hydronephrosis (e-Fig. 112-19). Other evolving indications for MRU include evaluation of renal scarring and dysplasia, identification of ectopic ureters in children with urinary incontinence, and characterization of renal masses.

Hydronephrosis and Obstructive Uropathy

Hydronephrosis is the most common indication for MRU in infants and children.[64] Ureteropelvic junction obstruction is the most common cause of neonatal hydronephrosis. Obstructive uropathy occurs in a subset of children with hydronephrosis and refers to obstruction that results in an injury to the kidney.[65] The kidney damage is not simply a result of mechanical impairment of urine flow but rather occurs as a result of a complex syndrome caused by the interaction of a variety of vasoactive factors and cytokines, leading to alterations of both glomerular hemodynamics and tubular function.[66] It is necessary to try to determine if the degree of obstruction present will lead to either a loss of renal function in the future or, in the case of children, will limit the future development of the kidney.

In children, obstruction is usually both chronic and partial. The partial obstruction results in equilibrium between urine production, impaired urine outflow, and pelvic reservoir capacity.[67] A steady state is reached between the amount of urine produced and the volume of the renal pelvis so that the pressure in the renal pelvis is in the normal range. This dynamic balance may be upset during diuresis or when the

Table 112-3

Standard Image Acquisition Parameters for Magnetic Resonance Urography						
	2D T1 Weighted	**2D T2 Weighted**	**3D Urogram**	**3D Dynamic**	**Post IR**	**Post 3D HR**
Sequence	TSE (ETL = 23)	TSE (ETL = 29)	TSE (ETL = 122)	3D GRE	TSE (ETL = 9)	3D GRE
Orientation	Axial	Coronal	Coronal	Coronal	Coronal	Sagittal
TR (ms)	6000	6000	Resp triggered	3.30	2000	3.5
TE (ms)	144	200	360	1.15	7.5	1.27
BW	137 Hz/pixel	200 Hz/pixel	326 Hz/pixel	590 Hz/pixel	241 Hz/pixel	530 Hz/pixel
Slice thickness (mm)	3.0	3.0	1.1	2.0	3.0	1.0
No. slices	20	19	60	32	13	160
FOV (mm)	160 × 120	220 × 172	230 × 220	240 × 195	192 × 192	240 × 165
Phase o/s	100%	100%	0	0	100%	0
NEX	3	2	2	1	2	1
Matrix	320 × 216	256 × 160	256 × 220	256 × 220	256 × 243	256 × 256
Options	Fat sat	Fat sat	Fat sat I-PAT = 2	Fat sat I-PAT = 2	TI = 165	Fat sat
Scan time (min)	6:03	2:36	~5 min	8 sec (per vol)	3:42	2:12

BW, Bandwidth; *ETL,* echo train length; *FOV,* field of view; *GRE,* gradient recalled echo; *I-PAT,* acceleration factor for parallel imaging; *IR,* inversion recovery; *HR,* high resolution; *NEX,* number of excitations; *o/s,* oversampling; *resp,* respiratory; *sat,* saturation; *TE,* echo time; *TI,* inversion time; *TR,* repetition time; *TSE,* turbo spin echo; *2D,* two dimensional; *3D,* three dimensional.

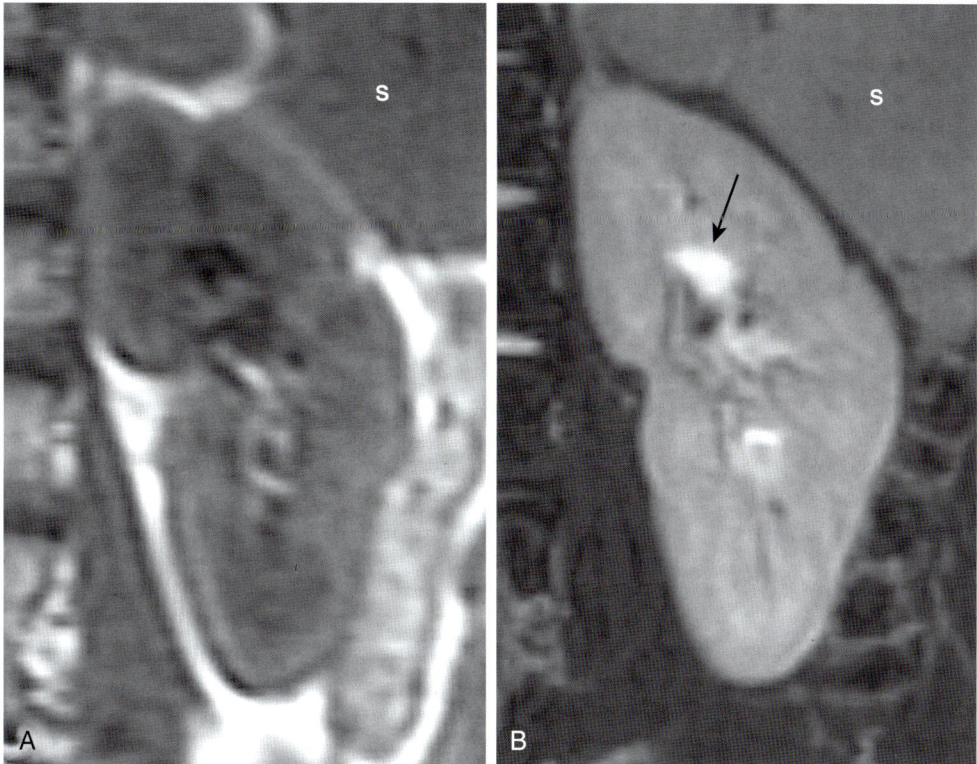

Figure 112-16   A normal renal magnetic resonance image. **A,** A coronal T1-weighted image shows that the renal cortex is isointense to the adjacent spleen (*S*) and the medulla is hypointense relative to the cortex. **B,** A coronal T2-weighted fat-saturated image shows diffuse hyperintensity of the renal parenchyma relative to the spleen (*S*), with the urine in the central pelvis appearing quite hyperintense (*arrow*).

obstruction is exacerbated. The loss of balance results in a transient increase in pelvic pressure. It is unclear whether it is the frequency, duration, or severity of these transitory elevations in renal pelvic pressure that are responsible for renal damage and progressive loss of renal function.

One of the key strengths of MRU is its ability to dynamically assess signal intensity changes occurring within the renal parenchyma after administration of contrast material and in response to a fluid and diuretic challenge. Changes in renal physiology can be evaluated rapidly by examining how the perfusion, filtration, and concentration affect the handling of the contrast agent by the kidney.

With MRU, the hydronephrotic kidney is subjected to both a fluid challenge (IV hydration) and a diuretic challenge (IV furosemide administered 15 minutes before the administration of contrast material). The response of the kidney to this challenge determines the appearance of the MR nephrogram. If symmetric changes in the signal intensity of the nephrogram occur, the hydronephrosis is classified as a compensated hydronephrotic system—that is, the fluid challenge has been accommodated without increasing the pressure in the pelvicalyceal system. However, when the signal intensity changes are asymmetric, they most often indicate acute or chronic obstruction—that is, the fluid challenge has exceeded the capacity for renal drainage, and the pressure in the collecting system rises. This hydronephrosis is classified as a decompensated hydronephrotic system. Signs associated with decompensation include parenchymal edema on the T2-weighted images, delayed calyceal transit time, and a delayed and increasingly dense nephrogram (Fig. 112-20).

These two patterns have different prognostic implications; little improvement in renal function can be expected after pyeloplasty in compensated kidneys, but significant improvement is seen in decompensated systems.[68]

The quality of the renal parenchyma is assessed both on the high-resolution T2-weighted images and during the parenchymal phase of the nephrogram. Signs that suggest underlying uropathy and permanent damage include architectural disorganization with loss of the corticomedullary differentiation, small subcortical cysts, and low cortical T2 signal intensity (e-Fig. 112-21). The nephrogram in these cases usually shows dim and patchy contrast enhancement reflecting damage to the microvasculature, as well as to the glomeruli and tubules. These imaging findings probably reflect the histologic changes of renal damage based on reduced glomerular number, glomerular hyalinization, cortical cysts, and interstitial inflammation and fibrosis.[69] In contrast to uropathic kidneys, edematous kidneys typically show increased signal intensity on the T2-weighted images, as well as a delayed dense nephrogram. The edematous pattern typically is seen either with decompensated hydronephrosis or acute pyelonephritis.

Anatomic information includes grading the hydronephrosis, identification of transition in the caliber of the ureter, and evaluation of underlying causes such as kinks, strictures, or crossing vessels. Both the T2-weighted and delayed postcontrast images are used to define the pelvicalyceal and ureteric anatomy. The T2-weighted images are particularly helpful in children with severe hydronephrosis and/or poorly functioning systems. Volumetric T2 and postcontrast images can be

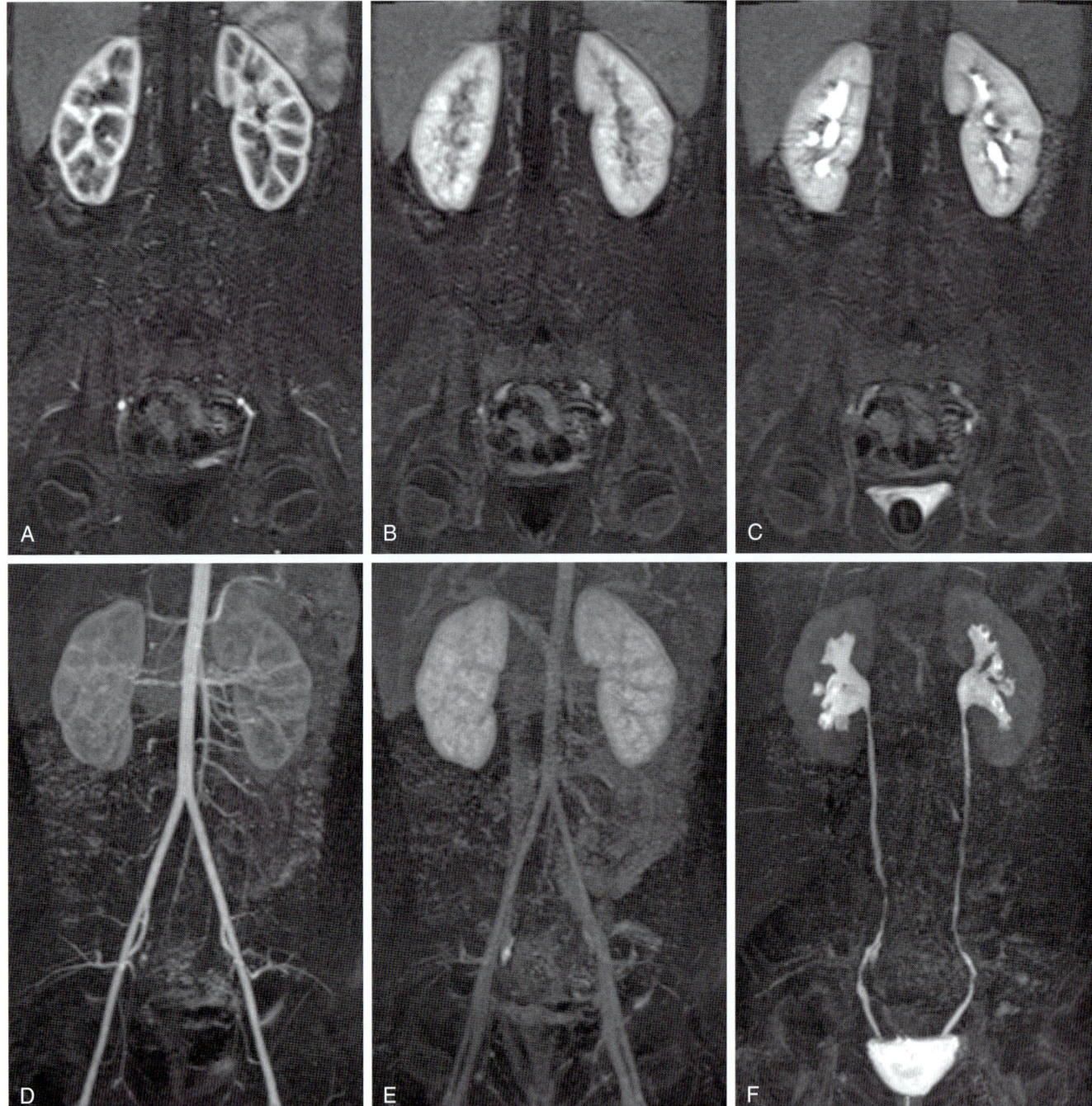

Figure 112-17 A normal magnetic resonance urogram in an 8-year-old girl. Images **A, B,** and **C** show the same slice from three volume acquisitions acquired at time points corresponding to the cortical (arterial), parenchymal, and excretory phases of renal function, respectively. Images **D, E,** and **F** are maximum intensity projections derived from the total volume for the three same time points.

used to generate exquisite volume-rendered images of the pelvicalyceal systems and ureters.

Congenital Malformations, Renal Scarring, and Dysplasia

Anomalies of renal fusion, position, and rotation are clearly demonstrated with MRU. Horseshoe and ectopic kidneys easily can be separated from the background and overlying tissues. Pelvic kidneys in particular are clearly demonstrated with MRU. Hypoplastic kidneys associated with ureteric ectopia and supernumerary kidneys usually can be demonstrated even if minimal renal function exists. MRU is the method of choice in the evaluation of incontinence associated with ectopic insertion of the ureter (Fig. 112-22).[70]

MRU enables identification of the acquired segmental scars most often associated with pyelonephritis and differentiation of areas of acute pyelonephritis from developed scars

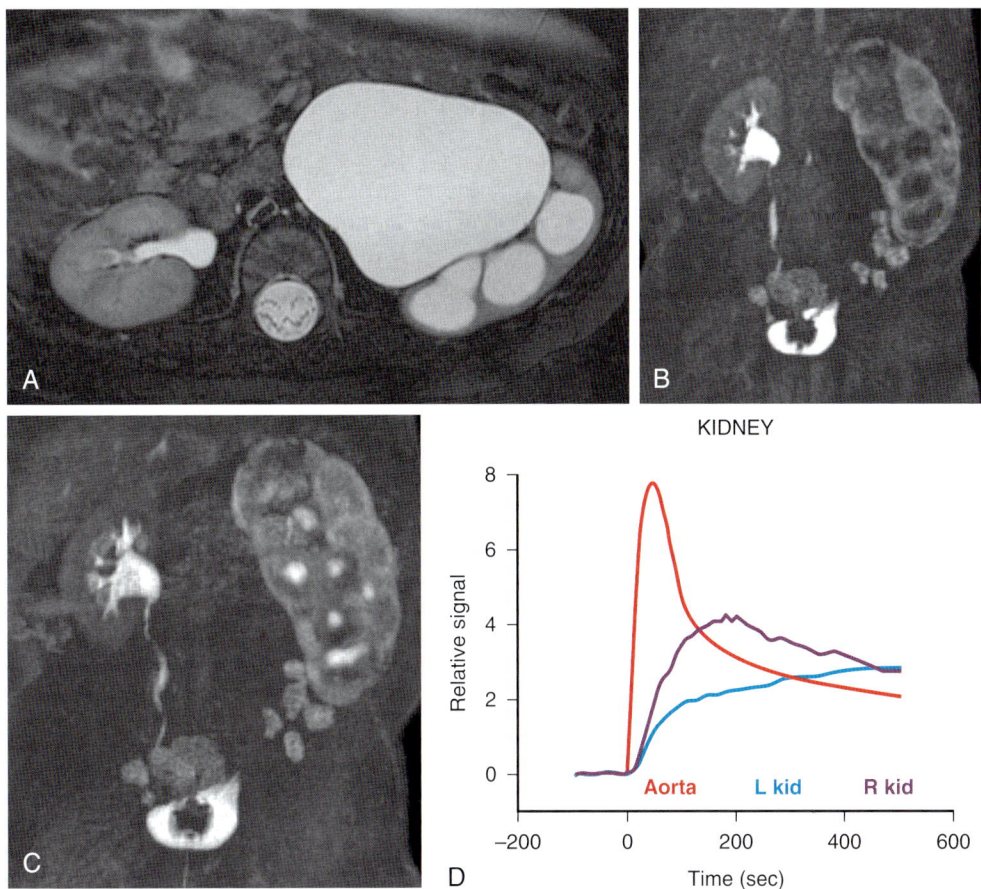

Figure 112-20 Decompensated ureteropelvic junction obstruction in a 3-month old-girl. **A,** The axial T2-weighted image demonstrates marked hydronephrosis of the left kidney with ballooning of the calyces and thinning of the renal parenchyma. After administration of contrast material, calyceal excretion of contrast material is delayed on the left side (**B**), and an increasingly dense nephrogram is seen (**C**). The signal intensity versus time curve (**D**) shows delayed peak enhancement with gradual accumulation of signal within the parenchyma of the left kidney. *L,* Left; *R,* right.

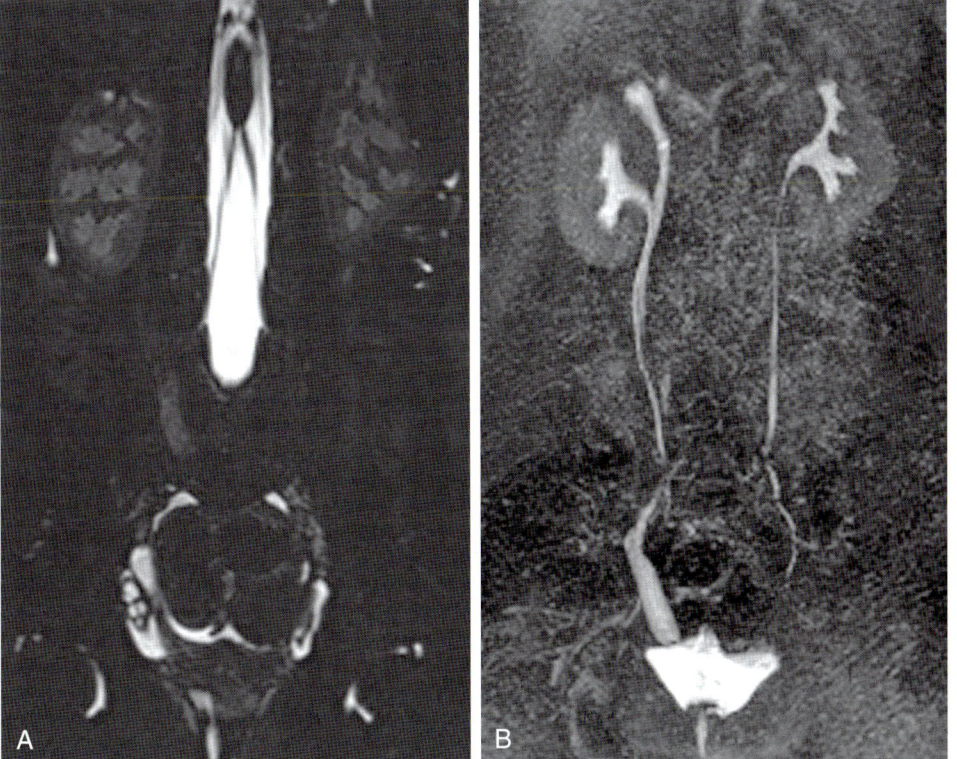

Figure 112-22 Ectopic ureteric insertion in a 9-year-old girl with incontinence. The T2-weighted image (**A**) shows a small cystic and dysplastic right upper pole moiety with a dilated ureter seen extending below the bladder base. On the delayed postcontrast maximum intensity projection image (**B**), the dilated ectopic ureter is seen inserting distally into the vagina.

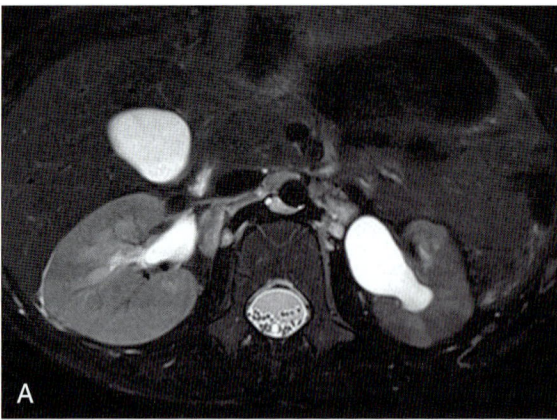
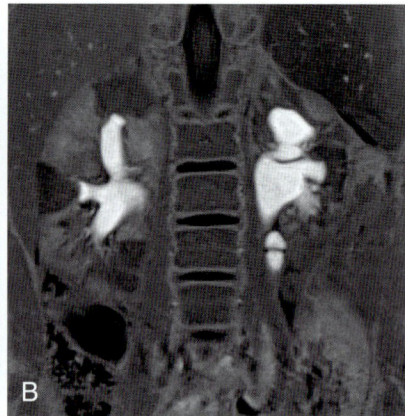

Figure 112-23 Renal scarring in a 5-year-old girl with a history of a recurrent urinary tract infection. An axial T2-weighted image (**A**) shows a smaller left kidney with disorganization of the renal parenchyma and focal areas of low signal intensity. Minimal abnormality is seen on the right. The inversion recovery image after administration of contrast material (**B**) shows triangular areas of decreased intensity with associated deformity of the renal contour. The scars are seen adjacent to the calyces.

on the basis of mass effect and inflammatory changes. Acute pyelonephritis is associated with edema, mass effect, and swelling of the kidney. Mature scars are characterized by volume loss and contour defects of the kidney on T2-weighted images and perfusion defects on the dynamic contrast-enhanced images, and they exhibit dilatation of the adjacent calyx, indicating transmural parenchymal loss. Affected regions demonstrate no appreciable contrast enhancement, reflecting fibrosis and microvascular damage (Fig. 112-23).

The typical imaging features associated with dysplastic kidneys include small size, disorganized architecture with loss of normal corticomedullary differentiation, small subcortical cysts, decrease in signal intensity on T2-weighted images, poor perfusion, a dim and patchy nephrogram, and dysmorphic calyces.

Acknowledgments

We wish to recognize the contributions of Dr. Jack O. Haller, Dr. Beverly P. Wood, Dr. Guido Currarino, and Dr. Douglas F. Eggli from previous editions of this book.

WHAT THE CLINICIAN NEEDS TO KNOW

- Renal size, echogenicity, number and location, and/or the presence of congenital malformations, obstruction, scarring, or mass lesions
- Ureteral dilation and the presence of a ureterocele or extravesical ectopia
- Strengths and weakness of VCUG versus nuclear cystography
- Strengths and imaging indications for MRU
- Imaging guidelines for detection and follow-up of childhood urologic disease

---

Key Points

Antegrade VCUG is the examination of choice for detailed anatomic evaluation of the bladder, study of the anatomy of the male urethra, and identification of VUR.

Nuclear cystography is performed as an alternative to VCUG for the assessment of VUR. Advantages include continuous imaging, which increases detection of VUR, reduced radiation dose, and detection of higher grade VUR. Disadvantages include lack of detailed anatomic information and decreased information about the grade of VUR.

Contrast-enhanced voiding ultrasonography sensitivity for VUR detection is comparable with that of standard techniques.

Cyclic voiding studies increase the detection of VUR in infants.

Diuretic nuclear renography distinguishes obstructive from nonobstructive hydronephrosis based on the characteristics of the renogram generated, including differential renal function, renal extraction of radiotracer, and washout of radiotracer from the urinary collecting system. The examination is less accurate in young infants because of a high capacitance renal pelvis and relatively low urine output.

The ability of MRU to provide a more complete characterization of renal anatomy and physiology has provided insights into the pathophysiology of hydronephrosis and the complex interaction of renal development, dysplasia, and scarring. MRU has the potential to revolutionize the imaging approach to renal disease in children.

MRU is the method of choice in the evaluation of incontinence associated with ectopic insertion of the ureter.

Suggested Readings

Darge K, Grattan-Smith JD, Riccabona M. Pediatric uroradiology: state of the art. *Pediatr Radiol.* 2011;41(1):82-91.

Jones RA, Grattan-Smith JD, Little S. Pediatric magnetic resonance urography. *J Magn Reson Imaging.* 2011;33:510 526.

Jones RA, Votaw JR, Salman K, et al. Magnetic resonance imaging evaluation of renal structure and function related to disease: technical review of image acquisition, postprocessing, and mathematical modeling steps. *J Magn Reson Imaging.* 2011;33:1270-1283.

Riccabona M, Lindbichler F, Sinzig M. Conventional imaging in pediatric uroradiology. *Eur J Radiol.* 2002;43:100-109.

Riccabona M, Mache CJ, Lindbichler F. Echo-enhanced color Doppler cystosonography of vesicoureteral reflux in children: improvement by stimulated acoustic emission. *Acta Radiol.* 2003;44:18-23.

Sukan A, Bayazit AK, Kibar M, et al. Comparison of direct radionuclide cystography and voiding direct cystography in the detection of vesicoureteral reflux. *Ann Nucl Med.* 2003;17:549-553.

References

Full references for this chapter can be found on www.expertconsult.com.

Chapter 113

Prenatal Imaging and Intervention

TERESA CHAPMAN

Overview

Fetal genitourinary system abnormalities encompass a wide spectrum of disorders varying in degrees of severity and include developmental anomalies, obstructive lesions in the urinary tract, and renal parenchymal diseases. The prenatal evaluation of the genitourinary system includes assessment of the amniotic fluid, the kidneys, the bladder, and associated anomalies. Amniotic fluid is important for normal fetal development, particularly the fetal lungs. In the first trimester, amniotic fluid forms as a dialysate of maternal serum. Fetal urine production begins by 12 weeks of gestation and becomes the major source of amniotic fluid by 16 weeks. Fetal urine production is typically 120 mL/day at 20 weeks and increases gradually to 1200 mL/day by term. The fetus voids every 30 to 60 minutes. The bladder should be visualized at least once during an examination.[1,2]

Identification of the fetal urinary bladder is attempted in the first trimester ultrasound, and more detailed evaluation of the kidneys and bladder is a fundamental part of the second trimester fetal anatomic assessment. Complex cases such as exstrophy, confusing duplex collecting systems, and obstructive masses may be further evaluated by fetal magnetic resonance imaging (MRI).[3-5] Sonographic fetal anatomic assessment may be limited in the setting of oligohydramnios, and MRI may be particularly useful. Prenatal findings may influence the further pursuit of genetic and laboratory testing or surgical intervention and may guide the delivery plan.

Normal Fetal Genitourinary Tract

Overview and Imaging Fetal kidneys can be identified at 13 weeks of gestation. Normal renal sizes at various gestations (mean kidney length in millimeters is slightly longer than weeks of gestation) are shown in Table 113-1.[6,7] Corticomedullary differentiation is apparent by 20 weeks of gestation (Fig. 113-1). Renal calyces and ureters typically are not seen on ultrasound unless they are pathologically dilated,[8] and the renal pelvis is only readily visualized once the anterior-posterior diameter exceeds 2 mm.[9] The fetal bladder can be visualized at 10 weeks of gestation. The bladder wall should not measure more than 3 mm. Bladder wall thickening may be a sign of outlet obstruction.[10,11]

As mentioned earlier, the amniotic fluid volume is a reflection of renal health. Oligohydramnios (defined by an amniotic fluid index less than 8 cm)[12] may be seen in the setting of placental insufficiency, intrauterine growth retardation, chromosomal abnormality, premature rupture of membranes, post-dates gestation, or urologic pathology (Box 113-1).[13]

Renal Parenchymal Disorders

Overview Fetal renal echogenicity may be abnormally increased as a normal variant but more often reflects an underlying abnormality. The fetal kidney is considered echogenic if sonographically it is brighter than the fetal liver. Echogenic kidneys are observed in approximately 1 to 2 per 1000 fetal ultrasounds, and approximately 10% of cases of renal malformations include echogenic kidneys.[14,15] Etiologic considerations for the echogenic kidney are summarized in Box 113-2.[16-24] If echogenic kidneys are identified and the amniotic fluid volume is normal, the findings suggest nonlethal renal disease. Echogenic kidneys with oligohydramnios portend a very poor prognosis.[25]

Cystic Renal Disease

Overview Congenital cystic renal diseases occur in about 2 to 4 in 1000 live births and include autosomal-dominant and autosomal-recessive polycystic kidney disease (Fig. 113-2 and Video 113-1), multicystic dysplastic kidney (Fig. 113-3), cystic glomerulopathies, and other cystic renal dysplasias. The complex pathogenesis of these disorders involves an abnormal orchestration of transcription and growth factor expression (Table 113-2), as well as ciliopathies affecting the renal tubule primary cilium (Table 113-3).[26-29] Structural and functional abnormalities in primary cilia contribute to various cystic phenotypes that involve not only the kidney but the liver and pancreas as well.[27]

Imaging These types of cystic renal dysplasias may be demonstrated in the fetus either by ultrasound or MRI.[27,30-37] Fetal sonographic evaluation of the kidneys should include renal length, overall echogenicity, preservation of corticomedullary differentiation, and presence of macroscopic cysts. Renal size may be considered abnormally increased if it is ≥2 standard deviations (moderately enlarged) or ≥4 standard deviations (markedly enlarged) greater than expected for gestational age.[6] Renal echogenicity greater than that of the liver or

Table 113-1

Normal Fetal Renal Lengths		
Gestational Age (wk)	Mean Kidney Length (cm)	95% Confidence Interval (cm)
18	2.2	1.6-2.8
19	2.3	1.5-3.1
20	2.6	1.8-3.4
21	2.7	2.1-3.2
22	2.7	2-3.4
23	3	2.2-3.7
24	3.1	1.9-4.4
25	3.3	2.5-4.2
26	3.4	2.4-4.4
27	3.5	2.7-4.4
28	3.4	2.6-4.2
29	3.6	2.3-4.8
30	3.8	3.9-4.6
31	3.7	2.8-4.6
32	4.1	3.1-5.1
33	4	3.3-4.7
34	4.2	3.3-5
35	4.2	3.2-5.2
36	4.2	3.3-5
37	4.2	3.3-5.1
38	4.4	3.2-5.6
39	4.2	3.5-4.8
40	4.3	3.2-5.3
41	4.5	3.9-5.1

Modified from Cohen HL, Cooper J, Eisenberg P, et al. Normal length of fetal kidneys. *AJR Am J Roentgenol.* 1991;157:545-548.

spleen is abnormal (Fig. 113-4), and corticomedullary differentiation may be lost or reversed if renal parenchymal disease is present.[27] MRI also readily shows abnormalities in renal size and detects renal cysts. Dysplastic parenchyma typically increases the T2-weighted signal (e-Fig. 113-5).

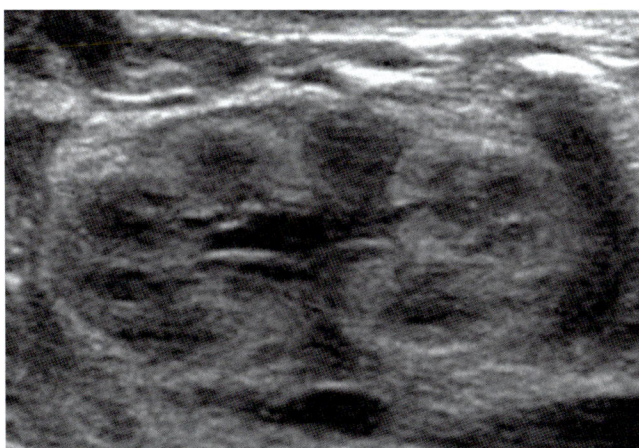

Figure 113-1 **A normal fetal kidney at 32 weeks of gestation.** A longitudinal sonogram of the fetal kidney shows a thin layer of perinephric fat with normal corticomedullary differentiation. Fetal lobulation is present. A small amount of fluid is present in the central renal pelvis.

Box 113-1 Renal Etiologies for Oligohydramnios

1. Bilateral renal agenesis
2. Bilateral multicystic dysplastic kidney
3. Bilateral severe ureteropelvic junction obstruction
4. Bilateral renal disease with one kidney each involved with items 1, 2, or 3 above
5. Severe prune-belly syndrome
6. Severe autosomal recessive polycystic kidney disease
7. Severe renal dysplasia as a result of posterior urethral valves or urethral atresia

Approach to Diagnosis A differential diagnostic approach to fetal echogenic renal cystic diseases is summarized in Table 113-4. If macroscopic cysts are observed without abnormal renal echogenicity, possible etiologies will depend on the number of cysts observed. Visualization of a single renal cyst should prompt consideration of a cystic tumor, a duplex collecting system with cystic dysplasia of the upper pole, urinoma, asymmetric presentation of autosomal-dominant polycystic kidney disease (ADPKD), or an isolated cyst in an otherwise normal kidney. Multiple cysts may be seen with multicystic dysplastic kidney, ADPKD, tuberous sclerosis complex, and TCF2 gene mutation–associated nephropathy.

Renal Tumors

Overview and Imaging A solid, rounded echogenic mass in the fetal kidney (Fig. 113-6) is most likely to be a congenital mesoblastic nephroma (CMN), also known as a leiomyomatous hamartoma or a fetal renal hamartoma, although a Wilms tumor may present in the fetus as well.[38] Both tumor types can replace the kidney or be localized. Tumors may be vascular with cystic areas as a result of hemorrhage and cystic degeneration. Polyhydramnios may occur (it is seen in 40% of renal tumor cases) and may lead to premature labor. Although the CMN is benign, a low-grade malignancy cannot be excluded, and resection is recommended. In one review of 28 prenatally diagnosed renal masses, 26 were CMNs and two were Wilms tumors (stage 1). The two children with Wilms tumors were followed up and remained disease free at ages 4 and 5 years.[39]

Antenatal Hydronephrosis

Overview A commonly seen fetal renal abnormality is pyelectasis (dilatation of the fetal renal collecting system), which is seen in 1% to 5% of screened fetuses.[40-46] Numerous factors influence renal pelvis dilation, including maternal hydration, fetal bladder filling, or the presence of an extrarenal pelvis

Box 113-2 Causes of Fetal Echogenic Kidney

- Idiopathic
- Cystic renal disease
- Infection
- Chromosomal abnormalities
- Toxic and ischemic insults

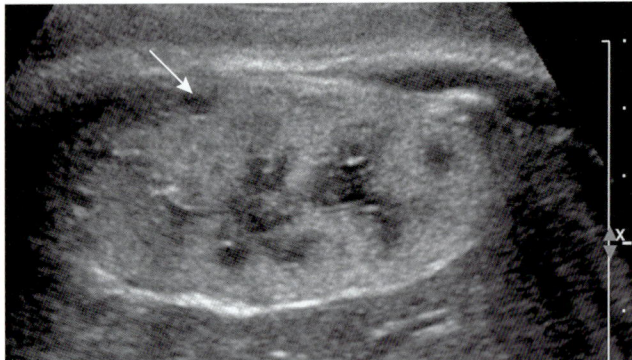

Figure 113-2 Autosomal-dominant polycystic kidney disease (ADPKD). A longitudinal sonogram of a fetus at 36 weeks' gestational age shows an enlarged echogenic kidney measuring more than 6 cm in length with small peripheral cysts (arrow). The contralateral kidney also was large and echogenic. Amniotic fluid remained normal throughout the pregnancy. The father also has ADPKD. See also Video 113-1 for fetal autosomal-recessive polycystic kidney disease on fetal ultrasound (a cine loop).

Box 113-3 Bilateral Hydronephrosis: Etiologies in a Fetus

Ureteral Lesions
- Ureteropelvic junction obstruction
- Ureterovesicular junction obstruction

Bladder Outlet Lesions
- Ureterocele with obstruction
- Posterior urethral valves
- Urethral atresia
- Vesicoureteral reflux
- Prune-belly syndrome
- Megacystis-microcolon-hypoperistalsis syndrome

(Fig. 113-7). Fetuses with trisomy 21 have an increased incidence of mild pyelectasis (>4 mm in the second trimester).[47] Other anomalies or risk factors should be present before recommending an amniocentesis if mild pyelectasis is observed, because the specificity of aneuploidy with isolated pyelectasis is low.[48-50] Most fetuses with mild pyelectasis are normal (approximately 90% or more).[43,46,51,52] Regardless of the risk for chromosomal abnormalities, pyelectasis in the fetus may signify either obstruction (Fig. 113-8 and e-Fig.113-9) or vesicoureteral reflux, and therefore follow-up later in gestation and postnatally must be considered. Causes of bilateral hydronephrosis are presented in Box 113-3.

Imaging The degree of collecting system dilatation is based on the anterior to posterior diameter (APD) of the renal pelvis as imaged in transverse plane (Fig. 113-10). Other imaging characteristics that may be pertinent include the morphology of the collecting system (for instance, disproportionately dilated renal pelvis in a configuration suggesting a ureteropelvic junction obstruction), visualization of the ureter, and features of the renal parenchyma, such as cortical echogenicity and the presence of cortical thinning.

The thresholds used to declare abnormal dilatation of the collecting system vary at different centers and range from 4 to 10 mm in the second trimester and 7 to 10 m in the third trimester. Sensitivity and specificity rates will be influenced by the APD threshold that is chosen. Odibo et al.[45] showed that in scans after 32 weeks' gestation, the highest accuracy for predicting normal postnatal renal function relied on an APD threshold of 7 mm. A separate analysis performed on scans obtained between 18 to 32 weeks' gestational age

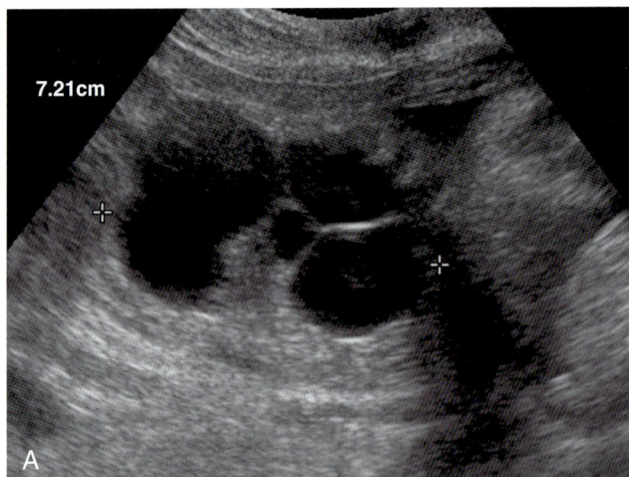

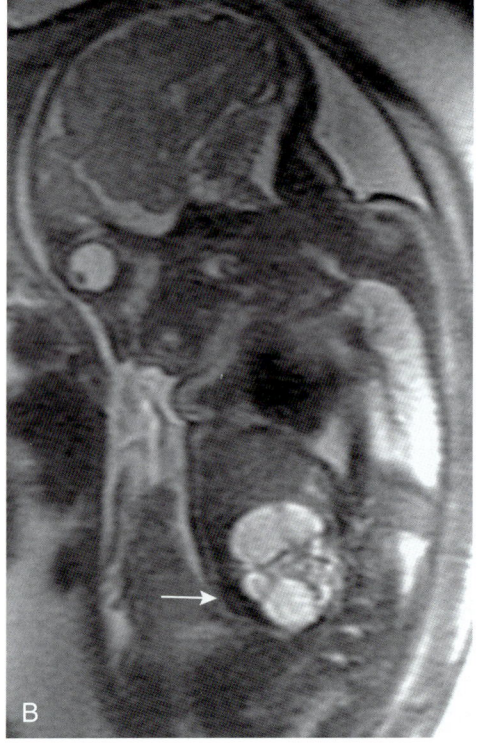

Figure 113-3 A multicystic dysplastic kidney. **A,** A sagittal ultrasound view of the right kidney in this 31-week gestational age fetus shows an enlarged kidney with macroscopic cysts not communicating with the collecting system. The minimal amount of discernible renal parenchyma is echogenic and disorganized. **B,** A sagittal single-shot fast-spin echo T2-weighted magnetic resonance image of a 32-week gestational age fetus shows a multicystic mass (arrow) in the renal fossa with no normal renal tissue.

Table 113-2

Selected Examples of Gene Mutations Resulting in Congenital Urinary Tract Abnormalities						
Renal Abnormality	**PAX2**	**TCF2**	**EYA1**	**SIX1**	**SALL1**	**GATA3**
Dysplasia	√	√	√	√	√	√
Renal agenesis			√	√		√
Renal hypoplasia	√	√			√	
Ureteropelvic junction obstruction	√	√			√	
Vesicoureteral reflux					√	√
Glomerulocystic kidney disease		√				
Syndrome	Renal-coloboma	MODY5	BOR	BOR	Townes-Brock	HDR

BOR, Brachio-oto-renal; *HDR*, hypoparathyroidism, deafness, and renal dysplasia; *MODY5*, maturity-onset diabetes, type 5.
Modified from Bonsib SM. The classification of renal cystic diseases and other congenital malformations of the kidney and urinary tract. *Arch Pathol Lab Med*. 2010;134(4):554-568.

Table 113-3

Ciliopathies: Molecular, Genetic, and Pathologic Features			
Ciliopathy	**Protein**	**Inheritance**	**Lesions**
Autosomal-dominant PKD	Polycystin 1, Polycystin 2	AD	Cysts within the entire nephron
Autosomal-recessive PKD	Fibrocystin	AR	Collecting duct cysts
Meckel-Gruber syndrome	MKS proteins 1, 3	AR	Cystic dysplasia
Oral-facial-digital syndrome	OFD protein	X-linked	Glomerular kidney disease
Bardet-Beidl syndrome	BBS proteins 1-8	Digenic	Tubulointerstitial nephritis
Von Hippel-Lindau	VHL protein	AR	Clear cell cysts and cancer

AD, Autosomal dominant; *AR*, autosomal recessive; *PKD*, polycystic kidney disease.
Modified from Bonsib SM. The classification of renal cystic diseases and other congenital malformations of the kidney and urinary tract. *Arch Pathol Lab Med*. 2010;134(4):554-568.

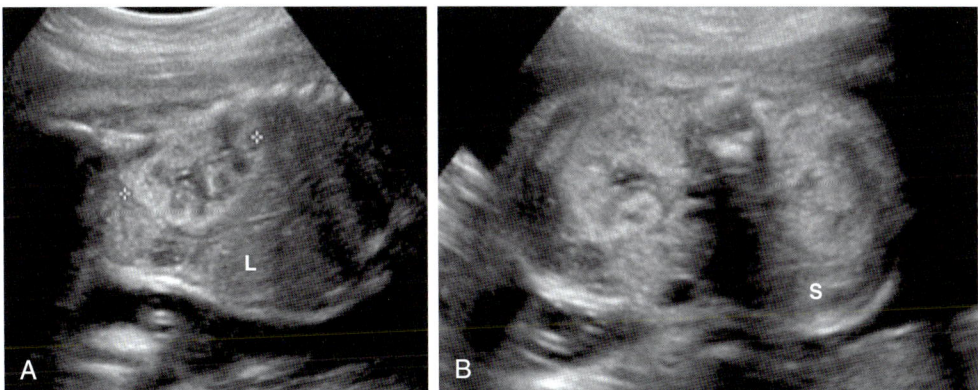

Figure 113-4   Echogenic kidneys in a fetus at 29 weeks' gestational age by ultrasound. **A,** The sagittal plane through the right kidney. **B,** The transverse plane through both kidneys. The renal cortices are brighter than the liver (*L*) and spleen (*S*). Renal length is normal for this gestational age, and the amniotic fluid volume is normal.

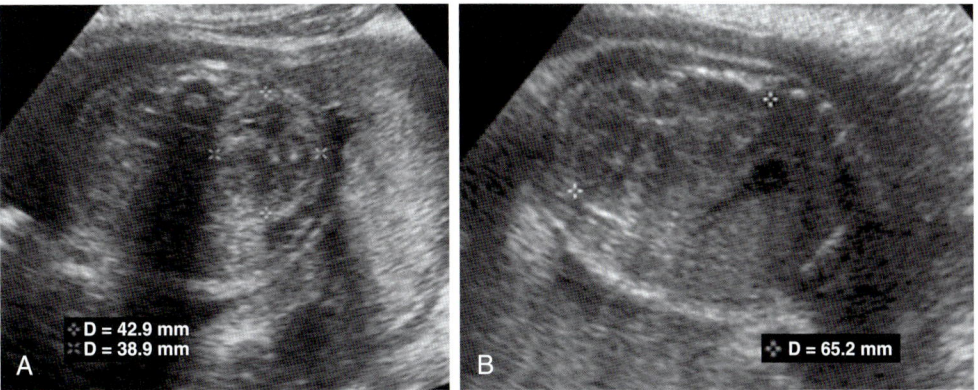

Figure 113-6   Fetal mesoblastic nephroma. Transverse (**A**) and sagittal (**B**) sonograms of a fetus at 30 weeks' gestational age show a well-circumscribed heterogeneously echogenic left renal mass. The other differential consideration would be a Wilms tumor.

Table 113-4

Differential Diagnosis: Fetal Renal Cystic Disease with Echogenic Kidneys by Ultrasound[78,211]			
Diagnosis	**Gestational Age at Diagnosis**	**Degree of Renal Enlargement**	**Additional Findings**
Meckel-Gruber Syndrome	Late first trimester, early second trimester	Markedly enlarged	Hypoechoic renal medulla; polydactyly; cerebral anomalies
ARPKD	Mid to late second trimester, third trimester	Moderately to markedly enlarged	Reversal of corticomedullary differentiation; possible oligohydramnios; few visible cysts are rare but possible
Bardet-Biedl syndrome	Second trimester, third trimester	Markedly enlarged	Postaxial polydactyly; cysts may be observed
ADPKD	Second trimester, third trimester	Moderately enlarged	
TCF2 gene mutation– associated nephropathy	Second trimester, third trimester	Moderately enlarged	Family history of diabetes is frequent; spectrum of expression includes glomerulocystic change, renal dysplasia, and renal agenesis; cysts may be observed

From Avni FE, Hall M. Renal cystic diseases in children: new concepts. *Pediatr Radiol.* 2010;40:9399-946; and Cassart M, Eruin D, Didier F, et al. Antenatal renal sonographic anomalies and postnatal follow-up of renal involvement in Bardet-Biedl syndrome. *Ultrasound Obstet Gynecol.* 2004;24:51-54. *ADPKD,* Autosomal-dominant polycystic kidney disease; *ARPKD,* autosomal-recessive polycystic kidney disease.

showed an optimal threshold of 6 mm APD, although the accuracy of predicting normal renal function was lower than in the post–32-week analysis. The authors point out that using the 6-mm threshold in the second trimester increases the false-positive rate to 20% and does not improve the sensitivity; therefore the assessment after 32 weeks is best for counseling parents. They propose an alternative approach of only following pregnancies with APDs greater than 6.0 mm after 32 weeks' gestation, and if on follow-up at 32 weeks the APD remains less than 7.0 mm, then parents can be counseled regarding the association with a good postnatal outcome. A commonly used system for characterizing antenatal pyelectasis is presented in Table 113-5.

When pyelectasis is encountered, an overlap exists between obstructive and nonobstructive causes, and follow-up examinations are useful. Third-trimester sonograms are the best predictor of significant postnatal uropathy, with a cutoff of 11 mm as an effective prognostic indicator, specifically of neonatal nephrouropathy requiring surgery.[45] Additional findings that predict a poorer postnatal outcome include bilateral involvement, hydroureter, renal cortical echogenicity, renal cysts, oligohydramnios, and associated anomalies. The main goals of follow-up imaging are to identify fetal kidneys at risk for renal failure and at higher risk for infection and to identify fetuses that may benefit from fetal surgical intervention (discussed later in this chapter).

Counseling patients about the significance of antenatally detected pyelectasis can be based on a large number of studies reviewing outcomes of otherwise normal fetuses found to have varying degrees of pyelectasis.[41-44,46,53] A meta-analysis[46] combining the findings 1678 cases of antenatal hydronephrosis gathered from 17 independent studies found that even mild degrees of prenatally diagnosed hydronephrosis may indicate pathology requiring postnatal management (11.9%) (Table 113-6).

Grading of Hydronephrotic Abnormalities

Overview Postnatal ultrasound usually is performed at least 3 to 5 days after birth to avoid underestimating collecting

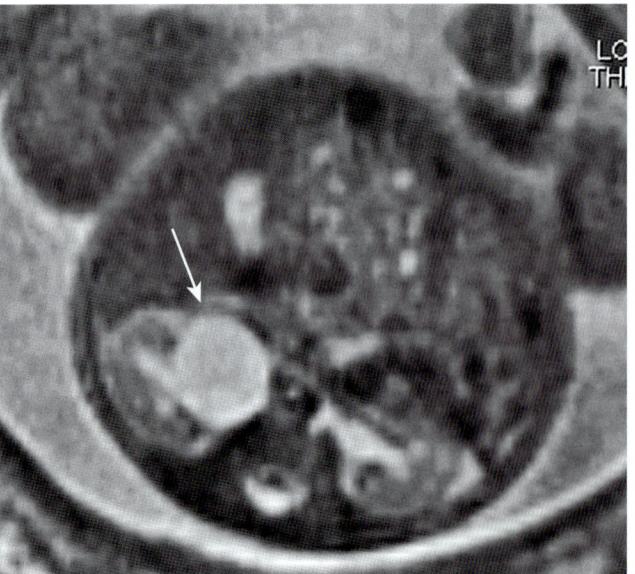

Figure 113-7 Extrarenal pelvis. An axial single-shot fast-spin echo T2-weighted magnetic resonance image of both fetal kidneys shows a large extrarenal pelvis on the right (*arrow*). The renal cortex remains thick.

Table 113-5

Defining Degree of Hydronephrosis in the Fetus*	
Trimester	**Degree of Hydronephrosis**
Second Trimester	
Mild pyelectasis	4-7 mm
Moderate pyelectasis	8-10 mm
Severe pyelectasis	>10 mm
Third Trimester	
Mild pyelectasis	7-10 mm
Moderate pyelectasis	10-15 mm
Severe pyelectasis	>15 mm

* Chosen thresholds vary across fetal imaging centers. Thresholds presented here are commonly adopted measures and are provided as guidelines.[46]

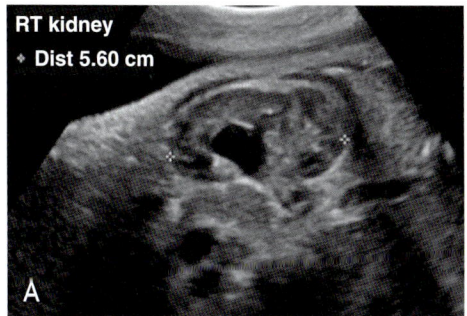
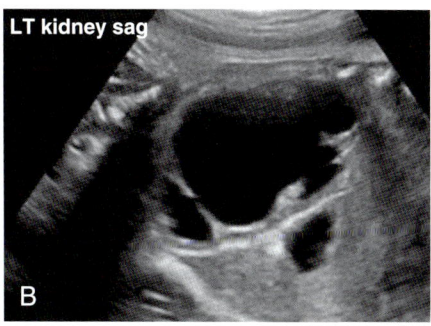
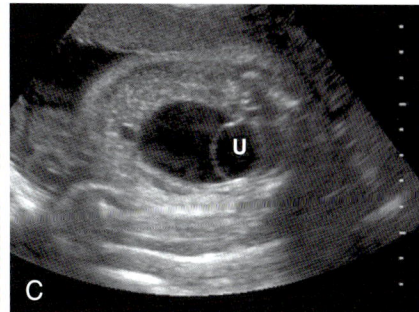

Figure 113-8   A unilateral duplex collecting system with a ureterocele. Sagittal ultrasound images of the right (**A**) and left (**B**) kidneys of a 28-week gestational age fetus show abnormal kidneys bilaterally. A right duplex right collecting system is present with pelvocaliectasis. The left kidney shows massive, disproportionate dilatation of the upper collecting system suggestive of a duplex system. A sagittal view of the left aspect of the fetal bladder (**C**) shows a thin-walled anechoic structure within the bladder lumen consistent with a ureterocele (*u*).

system dilatation as a result of physiologic oliguria in the first 48 hours of life.[54,55] Most centers evaluate postnatal hydronephrosis using the grading system of the Society of Fetal Urology (Box 113-4).[56] This system offers prognostic information; long-term follow-up of children with antenatally diagnosed hydronephrosis indicates that higher grades of hydronephrosis are more likely to require surgery.

Megacystis

Overview and Imaging   An abnormally large bladder, or megacystis, manifests in the first trimester in approximately 1 in 1800 pregnancies. A longitudinal bladder diameter greater than 15 mm during weeks 10 to 14 may indicate obstruction and portends a poor prognosis.[57] Lesser bladder diameters of 8 to 12 mm may resolve by 20 weeks.[11,58,59] In the second trimester, megacystis is defined as simply an abnormally large-appearing bladder, with or without the failure of the bladder to empty over 45 minutes.[60] An enlarged fetal bladder observed by ultrasound or MRI usually simply reflects normal variation in bladder filling, although if bilateral hydroureteronephrosis also is observed, then pathologies such as a serious

obstruction or functional emptying abnormalities must be considered. These abnormalities include posterior urethral valves (Fig. 113-11 and e-Fig. 113-12), prune-belly syndrome (Eagle-Barrett syndrome), and megacystis-microcolon-intestinal hypoperistalsis syndrome. An enlarged fetal bladder also merits close evaluation of the spine, given that caudal regression and neural tube defects may present with a neurogenic bladder.

Fetal Bladder Outlet Obstruction: Surgical Interventions

Overview   At a minimum, management of urinary tract outlet obstruction in the fetus involves serial ultrasounds through the second and third trimester and may merit delivery of the fetus at a tertiary care center. The role for procedural intervention in the fetus with bladder outlet obstruction has been well investigated during the past few decades; much of the research is directed toward identifying the appropriate fetal population that would benefit from intervention. Although the fetus with a high-grade bladder outlet obstruction may progress during pregnancy and be accompanied by development of renal dysplasia, cases of high-grade obstruction with oligohydramnios in the second trimester have been reported that spontaneously improve and later manifest only a low-grade obstruction with normal amniotic fluid volume.[61] Further, animal studies have shown that the severity of renal damage from obstruction depends on numerous factors, including the timing, duration, and severity of the obstruction.[62-64] The primary challenge is to identify the fetuses for intervention that have severe enough obstruction that renal function and pulmonary development would be compromised by progression of disease but who maintain the potential for improved renal development after the obstruction is relieved.

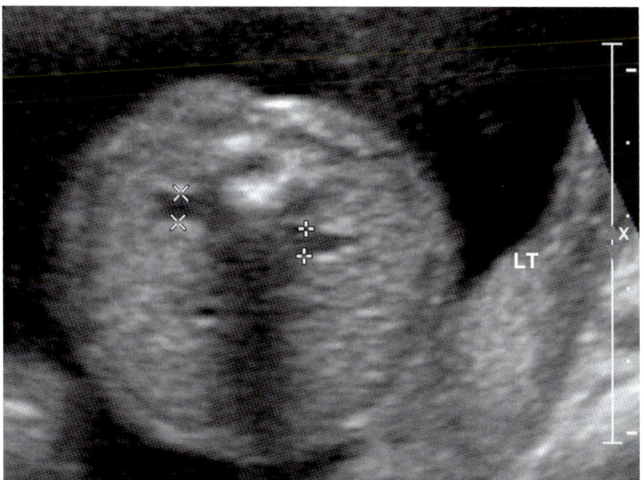

Figure 113-10   Measurement of renal pelvic diameter in the fetus. A transverse image through this fetus at 23 weeks' gestational age shows calipers marking the anterior-posterior diameter of the bilateral renal pelves. *LT,* Left.

Box 113-4	Society for Fetal Urography Grading System for Hydronephrosis
Grade 1	Dilation of renal pelvis only
Grade 2	Dilation of renal pelvis and not all of the calyces
Grade 3	Dilation of renal pelvis and all of the calyces
Grade 4	Grade 3 plus parenchymal thinning

Table 113-6

Summary of Postnatal Pathology Found in Different Categories of Antenatal Hydronephrosis					
Degree of pyelectation	Mild (n = 587)	Mild to moderate (n = 213)	Moderate (n = 235)	Moderate to severe (n = 179)	Severe (n = 94)
Second trimester AP renal diameter	≤7 mm	<10 mm	7-10 mm	≥7 mm	≥10 mm
Third trimester AP renal diameter	≤9 mm	<15 mm	9-15 mm	≥9 mm	≥15 mm
Postnatal pathology, % (95% CI)					
Any pathology	11.9 (4.5-28.0)	39.0 (32.6-45.7)	45.1 (25.3-66.6)	72.1 (47.6-88.0)	88.3 (53.7-98.0)
UPJ	4.9 (2.0-11.9)	13.6 (9.6-18.9)	17.0 (7.6-33.9)	36.9 (17.9-61.0)	54.3 (21.7-83.6)
VUR	4.4 (1.5-12.1)	10.8 (7.3-15.7)	14.0 (7.1-25.9)	12.3 (8.4-17.7)	8.5 (4.7-15.0)
PUV	0.2 (0.0-1.4)	0.9 (0.2-3.7)	0.9 (0.2-2.9)	6.7 (2.5-16.6)	5.3 (1.2-21.0)
Ureteral obstruction	1.2 (0.2-8.0)	11.7 (8.1-16.8)	9.8 (6.3-14.9)	10.6 (7.4-15.0)	5.3 (1.4-18.2)
Other	1.2 (0.3-4.0)	1.9 (0.7-4.9)	3.4 (0.5-19.4)	5.6 (3.0-10.2)	14.9 (3.6-44.9)

The percentage of total number of cases in each degree of antenatal hydronephrosis is indicated, along with a 95% CI.
AP, Anteroposterior; CI, Confidence interval; PUV, posterior urethral valve; UPJ, ureteropelvic junction; VUR, vesicoureteral reflex.
Modified from Lee RS, Cendron M, Kinnamon DD, et al. Antenatal hydronephrosis as a predictor of postnatal outcome: a meta-analysis. *Pediatrics.* 2006;118:586-593.

Monitoring the function of fetal kidneys primarily requires assessing amniotic fluid volume and the sonographic appearance of the kidneys; more eloquent measurements that add to this assessment include sampling various fetal urine electrolytes and proteins after 20 weeks' gestational age. Many investigators have evaluated the potential of fetal urine electrolyte concentrations in identifying renal functional prognosis.[65-68] Fetuses with obstructive uropathy and a subsequent poor outcome are "salt wasters," and fetuses with a decent outcome have hypotonic urine.[69] Nicolini et al[67] found that elevated fetal urinary calcium levels was the most sensitive (100%) predictor of renal dysplasia (specificity 60%), and elevated urinary sodium levels were the most specific (80%) predictor of renal dysplasia. Urinary phosphate, creatine, and urea were not useful in predicting the likelihood of renal dysplasia. Elevated levels of the protein β2-microglobulin within fetal urine also has been shown to be useful in the prediction of postnatal renal function,[68] particularly in identifying fetuses at risk for renal damage by obstruction even when amniotic fluid volume remains normal.

Treatment and Complications Surgical intervention for bladder outlet obstruction and decreasing amniotic fluid volume or oligohydramnios is considered in the fetus with a good prognostic electrolyte panel (i.e., Na <100 mEq per liter, Cl <90 mEq per liter, and osmolarity <210 mEq per liter) and no evidence of renal dysplasia by ultrasound.[66,70] Surgical interventions to treat bladder outlet obstruction include vesicoamniotic shunt, fetoscopic valve ablation, fetoscopic urethral stent placement, and open fetal surgery for vesicostomy. The vesicoamniotic shunt is placed percutaneously under ultrasound guidance to allow for emptying of the obstructed bladder directly into the amniotic cavity. Clinical experience remains somewhat limited, and no randomized-controlled trial has been performed to evaluate the effective outcomes of this procedure. Seven clinical series in the literature[66,71-76] offer the combined experience of 195 fetuses. A meta-analysis[77] incorporating studies of both these controlled series and additional case studies pooled the odds ratios to summarize measures of effect of this procedure. This analysis found that bladder drainage markedly improved perinatal survival, specifically in the subgroup of fetuses with a poor predicted prognosis (based on urine electrolytes and amniotic fluid volume). The procedure, when successful, restores amniotic fluid volume and allows for improved development of the fetal lungs. Although the vesicoamniotic

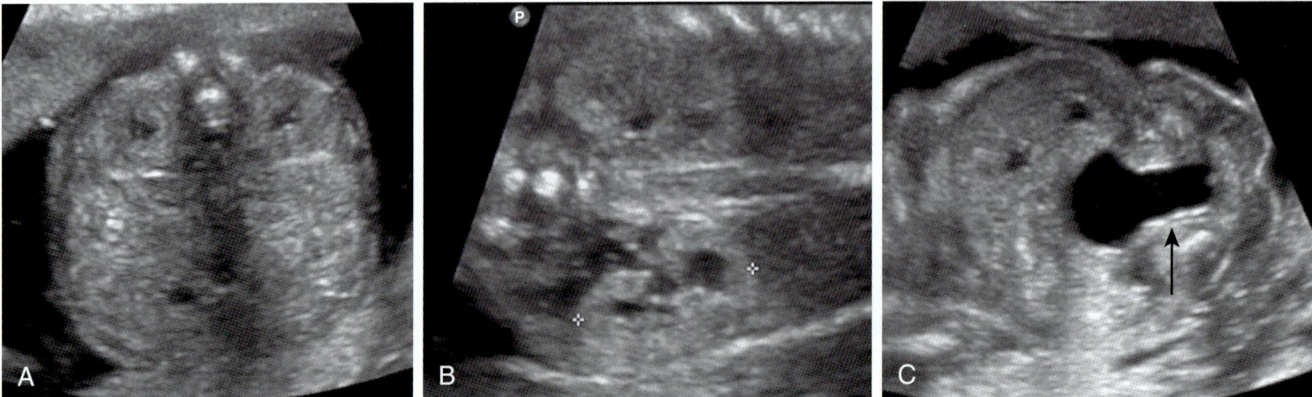

Figure 113-11   Posterior urethral valves and oligohydramnios. Fetal ultrasound at 20 weeks' gestational age shows bilateral echogenic kidneys in transverse (**A**) and coronal (**B**) projections. The fetal bladder (**C**) is abnormally large with distention of the posterior urethra (*arrow*) in a configuration called the "keyhole" sign.

shunt has the potential to improve pulmonary development, the shunt does not necessarily benefit the kidneys. Further, shunt placement does not address the severe bladder dysfunction seen with outlet obstruction, and animal studies have shown that decompressing a normal fetal bladder by shunting leads to a fibrotic and noncompliant bladder wall.[78] The bladder dysfunction is a potential obstacle to renal transplantation. Complication rates from vesicoamniotic shunt placement are as high as 50% to 60%[74,79,80] and include inadequate shunt drainage, shunt migration, premature labor, urinary fetal ascites, chorioamnionitis, and iatrogenic gastroschisis. However, with evolving technology and experience, outcomes appear more promising. A disc-shaped shunt may eliminate the risk of shunt migration,[81] and one study reviewing clinical outcomes in 20 pregnancies with a singleton male fetus treated by vesicoamniotic shunting for lower urinary tract obstruction reported acceptable renal and bladder function, although one third of the survivors required dialysis and transplantation.[82]

Fetoscopic surgery may be performed to introduce urethral stents or to ablate posterior urethral valves.[83] A small number of cases in the literature[84-89] show gradually improving outcomes as the technology advances. Earlier survival rates were less than 50%, and more recent experience shows that laser fulguration and hydroablation are the best option for urethra disruption, with neonatal survival rates of approximately 70% to 75%.[90] Little published evidence exists regarding the effectiveness of therapeutic fetal cystoscopy as an intervention for congenital lower urinary tract obstruction, and it is still considered an experimental intervention.[91]

Open fetal surgery for vesicostomy (bladder marsupialization) is the only approach that completely decompresses the entire urinary tract and eliminates the transmission of pressure to the kidney. Candidates for this procedure are male fetuses with posterior urethral valves less than 24 weeks' gestational age presenting with oligohydramnios, normal fetal urine electrolytes, and no evidence of renal cystic dysplasia or abnormally increased renal echogenicity, and who have normal karyotypes. Only a small amount of clinical experience exists in this advanced arena of fetal surgical intervention, and vesicostomy currently carries a 50% neonatal mortality.[92-94] Animal studies evaluating use of robot-assisted laparoscopy to perform vesicostomy show promise for improving survival.[95]

WHAT THE CLINICIAN NEEDS TO KNOW

- Renal length correlated to expected for gestational age
- Presence of developmental renal anomalies, obstructive lesions, or parenchymal diseases
- APD of a dilated renal pelvis
- Unilateral or bilateral antenatal hydronephrosis
- Bladder visualized and longitudinal bladder diameter
- Amniotic fluid index
- Fetal lung development

Key Points

The prenatal evaluation of the genitourinary system includes assessment of the amniotic fluid, the kidneys, the bladder, and associated anomalies.

Fetal urine production begins by 12 weeks of gestation.

The fetal kidney is considered echogenic if sonographically it is brighter than the fetal liver. Echogenic kidneys with oligohydramnios portend a very poor prognosis.

Visualization of a single renal cyst should prompt consideration of a cystic tumor, duplex collecting system with cystic dysplasia of the upper pole, urinoma, asymmetric presentation of ADPKD, or an isolated cyst in an otherwise normal kidney. Multiple cysts may be seen with multicystic dysplastic kidney, ADPKD, tuberous sclerosis complex, and TCF2 gene mutation–associated nephropathy.

A solid, rounded echogenic mass in the fetal kidney is most likely to be a CMN.

If at 32 weeks, the APD of the renal pelvis remains less than 7.0 mm, then parents can be counseled regarding the association with a good postnatal outcome.

If an enlarged fetal bladder is associated with bilateral hydroureteronephrosis, a serious obstruction or functional emptying abnormality must be considered. These abnormalities include posterior urethral valves, prune-belly syndrome (Eagle-Barrett syndrome) and megacystis-microcolon-intestinal hypoperistalsis syndrome.

Complex cases such as exstrophy, confusing duplex collecting systems, and obstructive masses may be evaluated further by fetal MRI.

Surgical intervention for bladder outlet obstruction and decreasing amniotic fluid volume or oligohydramnios is considered in the fetus with a good prognostic electrolyte panel (Na <100 mEq per liter, Cl <90 mEq per liter, and osmolarity <210 mEq per liter) and no evidence of renal dysplasia by ultrasound.

Surgical interventions to treat bladder outlet obstruction include a vesicoamniotic shunt, fetoscopic valve ablation, fetoscopic urethral stent placement, and open fetal surgery for vesicostomy.

Suggested Readings

Aksu N, Yavascan O, Kangin M, et al. Postnatal management of infants with antenatally detected hydronephrosis. *Pediatr Nephrol.* 2005; 20:1253-1259.

Bonsib SM. The classification of renal cystic diseases and other congenital malformations of the kidney and urinary tract. *Arch Pathol Lab Med.* 2010;134:554-568.

Deshpande C, Hennekam RCM. Genetic syndromes and prenatally detected renal anomalies. *Semin Fetal Neonatal Med.* 2008;13:171-180.

Gunay-Aygun M. Liver and kidney disease in ciliopathies. *Am J Med Genet Part C Semin Med Genet.* 2009;151C:296-306.

Hormann M, Brugger PC, Balassy C, et al. Fetal MRI of the urinary system. *Eur J Radiol.* 2006;57:303-311.

Kemper MJ, Mueller-Wiefel DE. Prognosis of antenatally diagnosed oligo-hydramnios of renal origin. *Eur J Pediatr.* 2007;166:393-398.

Kohl T. Minimally invasive fetoscopic interventions: an overview in 2010. *Surg Endosc.* 2010;24:2056-2067.

Kumari N, Pradhan M, Shankar VH, et al. Post-mortem examination of prenatally diagnosed fatal renal malformation. *J Perinatol.* 2008; 28:736-742.

Leclair MD, El-Ghoneimi A, Audry G, et al. French Pediatric Urology Study Group. The outcome of prenatally diagnosed renal tumors. *J Urol.* 2005;173:186-189.

Morris RK, Ruano R, Kilby MD. Effectiveness of fetal cystoscopy as a diagnostic and therapeutic intervention for lower urinary tract obstruction: a systematic review. *Ultrasound Obstet Gynecol.* 2011;37(6):629-637.

Mure PY, Pierre Mouriquand P. Upper urinary tract dilatation: prenatal diagnosis, management and outcome. *Semin Fetal Neonatal Med.* 2008;13:152-163.

Quintero RA, Gomez Castro LA, Bermudez C, et al. In utero management of fetal lower urinary tract obstruction with a novel shunt: a landmark development in fetal therapy. *J Matern Fetal Neonatal Med.* 2010;23:806-812.

Rosenblum ND. Developmental biology of the human kidney. *Semin Fetal Neonatal Med.* 2008;13:125-132.

Witzani L, Brugger PC, Hormann M, et al. Normal renal development investigated with fetal MRI. *Eur J Radiol.* 2006;57:294-302.

Wood AS, Price KL, Scambler PJ, et al. Evolving concepts in human renal dysplasia. *J Am Soc Nephrol.* 2004;15:998-1007.

Yiee J, Wilcox D. Abnormalities of the fetal bladder. *Semin Fetal Neonat Med.* 2008;13:164-170.

References

Full references for this chapter can be found on www.expertconsult.com.

Chapter 114

Congenital and Neonatal Abnormalities

JONATHAN R. DILLMAN and D. GREGORY BATES

Kidney and Ureter

MULTICYSTIC DYSPLASTIC KIDNEY

Overview, Etiology, and Clinical Presentation A multicystic dysplastic kidney (MCDK) is the most common form of cystic renal dysplasia. With high-grade obstruction or atresia of the upper urinary tract (renal pelvis and/or ureter) during early renogenesis, disordered parenchymal development results in an MCDK.[1] Two types of MCDK exist: the pelvoinfundibular type (common) and the hydronephrotic type (uncommon).[2,3] MCDK can occur in half of a duplex kidney (usually the upper moiety) or in renal fusion anomalies, such as a horseshoe kidney and crossed fused renal ectopia. MCDK is sporadic in most cases, although familial cases have been described.[1,4] Vesicoureteral reflux (VUR) (both ipsilateral and contralateral) and contralateral ureteropelvic junction obstruction are common.[1,5] Long-term sequelae (e.g., infection and hypertension) are rare, because most affected kidneys either partially or completely involute on their own over time.[6-9]

Imaging On ultrasound, computed tomography (CT), and magnetic resonance imaging (MRI), a classic MCDK is characterized by multiple cysts of various sizes (ranging from 1 mm to several cm) that do not communicate, with no normal intervening renal parenchyma (Fig. 114-1). The affected kidney may be small, normal, or enlarged.[1] Compensatory hypertrophy of the contralateral kidney often is present.[10] The hydronephrotic form has cysts that communicate, mimicking pelvocaliectasis, but no normal functioning renal tissue.[2] The diagnosis of both classic and hydronephrotic MCDK can be confirmed by diuretic renal scintigraphy (e-Fig. 114-2) or MR urography (MRU) (e-Fig. 114-3). A voiding cystourethrogram (VCUG) may reveal VUR into a blind-ending ureter on the side of the MCDK.[11,12]

Treatment Follow-up ultrasound typically demonstrates involution of the cysts over time, eventually resulting in remnant dysplastic renal tissue that may be impossible to visualize.[13,14] Immediate resection of an MCDK is rarely indicated[15] and is reserved for cases in which the size of the kidney is a problem. In the past, routine nephrectomies were performed because of a fear of malignant degeneration. Current belief discounts this possibility, and as long as no other complication exists, surgery is not indicated.

AUTOSOMAL-DOMINANT POLYCYSTIC KIDNEY DISEASE

Overview and Etiology Autosomal-dominant polycystic kidney disease (ADPKD), the most common form of inherited renal cystic disease, is seen in 1 in 800 live births.[16,17] Two types of ADPKD exist, each with clearly defined chromosomal mutations. The more severe form (PKD1) accounts for about 85% to 90% of cases, whereas the milder phenotype (PKD2) presents later in life, results in less morbidity, and is less common.[16,18] Cysts arise from both the renal cortex and the medulla.[16,19]

Clinical Presentation Systemic hypertension, hematuria, and slowly progressive renal insufficiency are the typical clinical manifestations.[1,20] ADPKD is very rarely detected prenatally because fewer than 5% of nephrons are cystic before birth.[1] Diagnosis of ADPKD early in life portends a poor prognosis; 43% of affected persons die in the first year of life, hypertension develops in 67%, and some affected children progress rapidly to end-stage renal disease.[20] Because it can be difficult to delineate between autosomal-recessive and autosomal-dominant forms of polycystic kidney disease in a neonate, screening of siblings and parents may be helpful.

Imaging The diagnosis of ADPKD usually is made on the basis of ultrasound (Fig. 114-4), although CT or MRI also can suggest it. Although the kidneys may be normal during the first decade of life, they also may contain one or more simple cysts (Fig. 114-5).[16,21] The kidneys may be abnormally enlarged and echogenic, mimicking autosomal-recessive polycystic kidney disease (ARPKD) in early life (e-Fig. 114-6).[16,22] Although it is typically a bilateral process, imaging findings may be asymmetric, and in young children they can manifest as a unilateral abnormality.[16,21,23] Microscopic cysts, as well as larger cysts that can be detected by cross-sectional imaging techniques, are common in the liver and less frequent in the pancreas, spleen, lungs, thyroid, ovaries, and testes.[19] The remainder of the urinary tract is usually normal.

Treatment Although renal function is generally maintained during childhood, ADPKD is responsible for the need for chronic dialysis in 10% to 12% of adult patients.[1] Hypertension should be managed medically to prevent long-term complications. About 12% to 15% of patients with ADPKD have

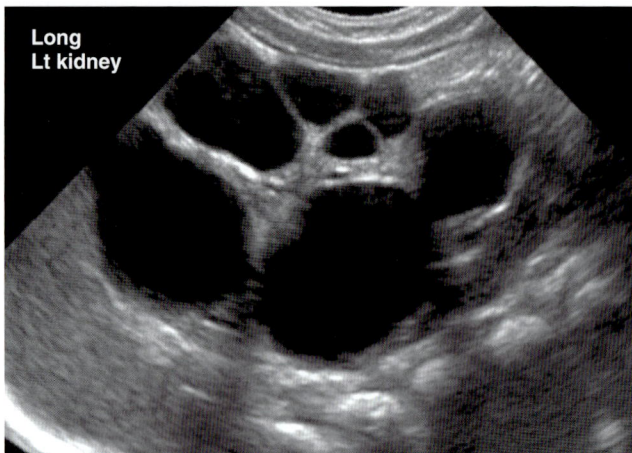

Figure 114-1 A multicystic dysplastic kidney in a 3-month-old boy. A longitudinal ultrasound image of an enlarged left kidney shows multiple noncommunicating simple cysts of variable size, mimicking hydronephrosis. The very small amount of remaining renal parenchyma is abnormally echogenic.

an intracranial aneurysm, most often arising from the circle of Willis.[19,23-25] Screening MR angiography usually is not performed in childhood, however, because aneurysm rupture is rare in this period.

AUTOSOMAL-RECESSIVE POLYCYSTIC KIDNEY DISEASE

Overview   ARPKD is a rare disorder (occurring in 1:20,000 live births) that affects both kidneys.[26,27] Genetic studies have localized the inheritance of ARPKD to chromosome 6p.[27,28] The *PKHD1* gene is expressed in fetal and adult kidneys and livers, the two major sites affected by the disease.[28] Approximately 1 in 70 persons are a carrier for this condition.[26,27]

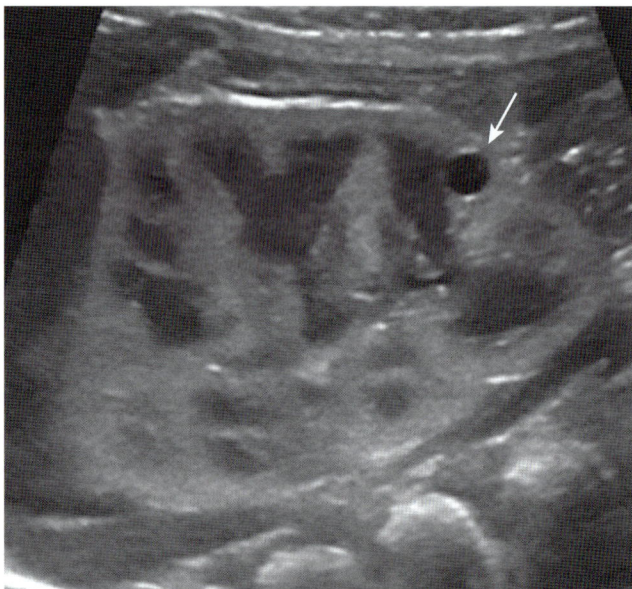

Figure 114-4 Autosomal-dominant polycystic kidney disease in a newborn. A longitudinal ultrasound image shows a small lower pole simple renal cyst (*arrow*). The renal cortex appears echogenic as well. Three additional simple renal cysts were identified in this neonate with a maternal history of autosomal-dominant polycystic kidney disease.

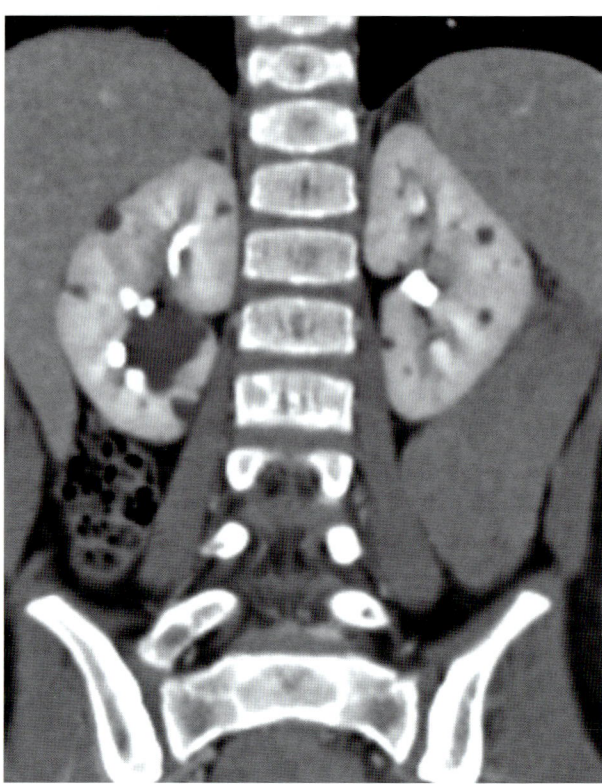

Figure 114-5 Autosomal-dominant polycystic kidney disease in an 8-year-old girl. A coronal reformatted contrast-enhanced computed tomography image shows multiple low attenuation lesions in both kidneys due to the presence of cysts.

Clinical Presentation   ARPKD has been subdivided into categories based on clinical presentation. The perinatal and neonatal forms, which have the poorest prognosis, are associated with severe renal dysfunction and minimal hepatic portal tract fibrosis. Affected children often die of the disease early in life.[27,29] Infantile and juvenile forms are associated with less severe renal dysfunction and more significant hepatic fibrosis.[27] The degrees of renal and hepatic abnormalities tend to be inversely proportional.[17,27] A number of children with ARPKD also have Caroli disease (see Chapter 88).[27]

Pathology   Histologically, the kidneys have a spongelike appearance, replaced by myriad minute 1- to 2-mm cysts of relatively uniform size, representing markedly dilated and elongated collecting ducts.[1,27] These cysts radiate from the hilum to the surface of the kidney without a clear demarcation between the medulla and cortex. Fibrosis is present in the renal interstitium. Children with significant hepatic involvement are at increased risk for complications related to portal hypertension, and ascending cholangitis can lead to sepsis and death.[27]

Imaging   Abdominal radiography in the neonatal period commonly reveals bilateral abdominal or flank masses with centralized gas-filled bowel loops. The lungs may appear small because of a combination of pulmonary hypoplasia and mass effect from marked nephromegaly (e-Fig. 114-7).[27]

   On ultrasound, affected neonatal kidneys tend to be smoothly enlarged (frequently more than four standard deviations above the mean expected length for age), are

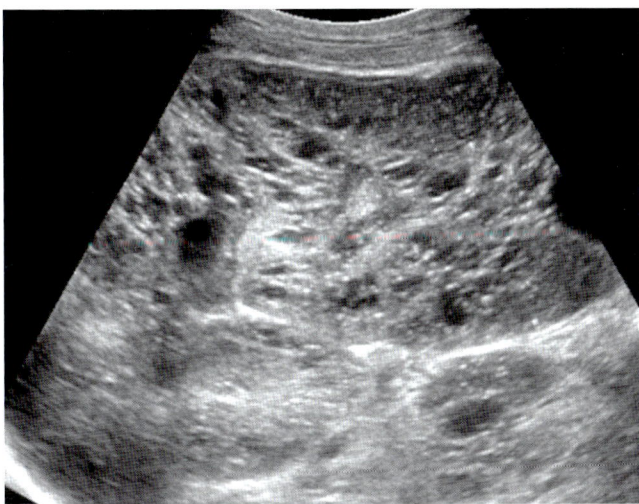

Figure 114-9 Autosomal-recessive polycystic kidney disease in a 6-month-old boy presenting with acute renal failure and bilateral renal masses. A longitudinal ultrasound image of the right kidney shows nephromegaly, loss of normal corticomedullary differentiation, and innumerable tiny cystic structures replacing the renal parenchyma.

hyperechoic as a result of the multiple acoustic interfaces at the walls of the dilated ducts, and have poor corticomedullary differentiation (e-Fig. 114-8).[1,27,29,30] On occasion, discrete cysts (solitary or multiple) of variable size (most commonly <1 cm) may be seen (Fig. 114-9).[26,30] A sonolucent rim may be seen at the periphery of the kidney, especially in older infants, as a result of cortical compression and relative sparing.[26,27] Contrast-enhanced CT (Fig. 114-10) or MRI show delayed opacification of the renal parenchyma with a prolonged and striated nephrogram. When studied with MRI, the dilated tubules in affected kidneys appear linear and hyperintense on T2-weighted imaging, radiating from the medulla toward the cortex (Fig. 114-11).[31]

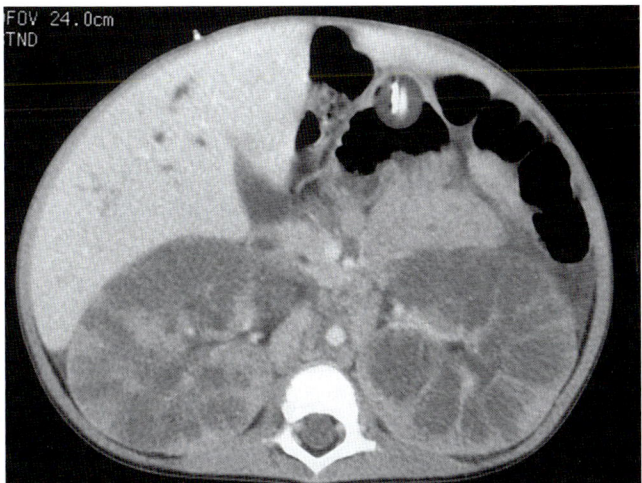

Figure 114-10 Autosomal-recessive polycystic kidney disease. A computed tomography image shows that the pathologic process is primarily medullary. The dilated tubules have produced a linear pattern that can be seen clearly in a few regions. Marked cortical thinning present along the anterior aspect of each kidney is not a typical finding, because the cortex is usually spared.

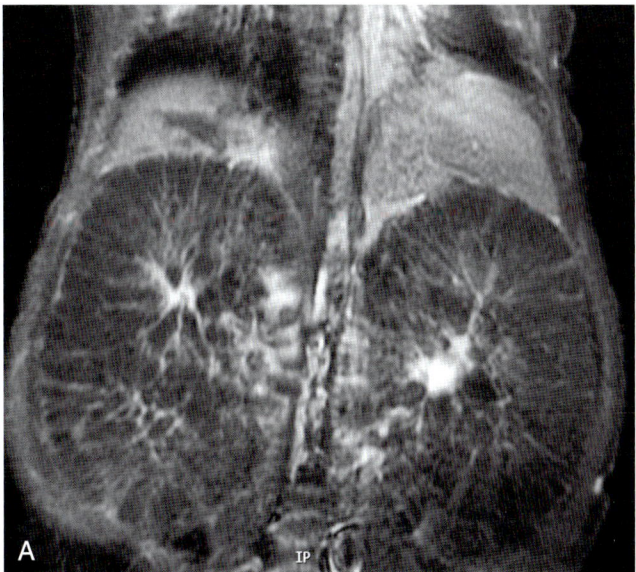

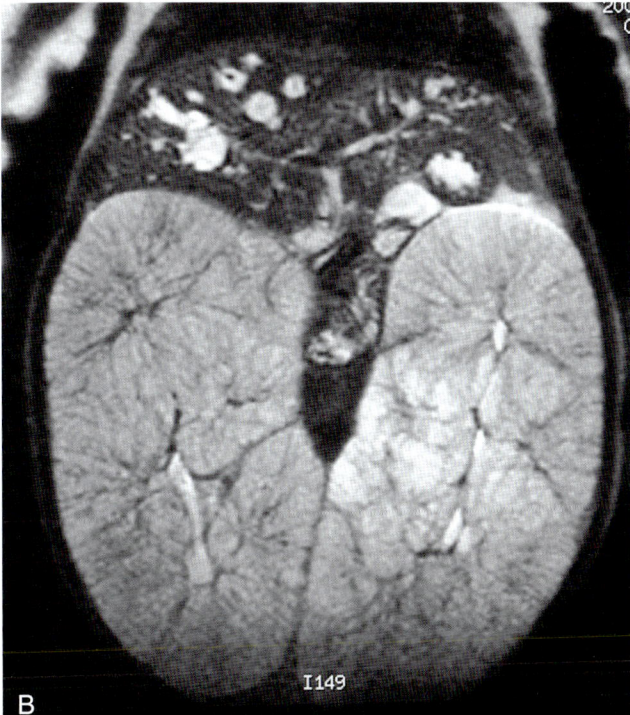

Figure 114-11 Autosomal-recessive polycystic disease. T1-weighted (**A**) and T2-weighted (**B**) magnetic resonance images of an infant with autosomal-recessive polycystic disease. The kidneys are enormously enlarged, and on the T1-weighted image, the spoke wheel is appreciated. The patient also has Caroli disease as seen by the dilated biliary system on the T2-weighted image.

Treatment Eighty-six percent of patients who survive beyond 1 month of age are alive at 1 year, and 67% are alive at 15 years.[32] In infants who have initially adequate (although not normal) renal function, the disease may not be detected until later in the first decade, when ultrasound is being performed for unrelated purposes. Systemic renovascular hypertension may occur and require medical management.[17,27] Persons with ARPKD who have severely impaired renal function eventually will require renal replacement therapy, either dialysis or renal transplantation.

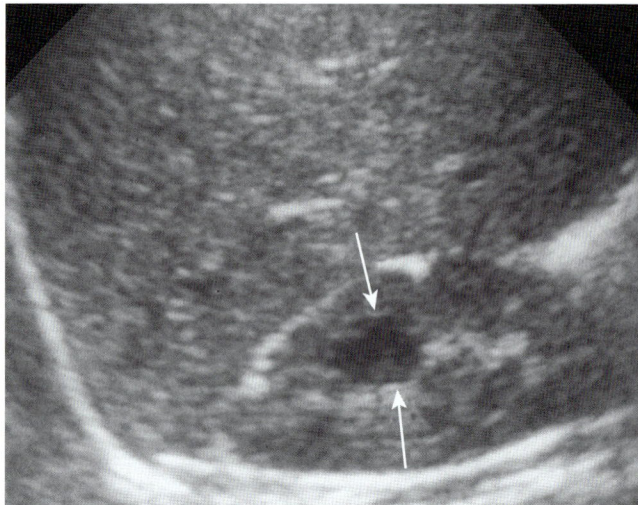

Figure 114-12 Calyceal diverticulum. A longitudinal ultrasound image reveals a medullary cyst (*arrows*). On a subsequent intravenous urography procedure, the cyst filled with contrast material.

OTHER RENAL CYSTIC DISEASES IN CHILDREN

Many rare inherited syndromes and genetic disorders are associated with renal cystic disease (Box 114-1).

CALYCEAL DIVERTICULUM

Overview, Etiology, and Clinical Presentation A calyceal diverticulum represents a focal outpouching of the renal collecting system that is located within the renal parenchyma and that contains urine.[33] This condition has an incidence of 3.3-4.5:1000 in children, based on excretory urography.[34-36] Calyceal diverticula are likely developmental in origin; they are lined with urothelium and surrounded by muscularis mucosa.[33,35] Although these structures most commonly are an incidental finding, they can be associated with both infection and calculus formation as a result of urinary stasis.[33,35,37]

Imaging Abdominal radiographs may be normal or may demonstrate one or more calculi (or milk of calcium) within a calyceal diverticulum.[35] Upon ultrasound, such diverticula may mimic a solitary renal cyst, appearing as a round, thin-walled anechoic structure (Fig. 114-12).[34] They can vary in size ranging from a few millimeters to several centimeters (with a mean size around 11 mm).[35,37] They most commonly occur within the upper pole of the kidney.[33] Upon excretory phase imaging (including excretory urography, MRI, and

CT), calyceal diverticula typically fill with contrast material (Fig. 114-13). A thin connection, or neck, to an adjacent calyceal fornix may or may not be identified.[35]

Treatment A symptomatic calyceal diverticulum may require surgical ablation. Although both lithotripsy of calculi within the diverticulum and percutaneous ablation of the cavity have decreased the invasive treatment in adults,[37,38] such techniques have not yet been applied widely to children.

CONGENITAL INFUNDIBULOPELVIC STENOSIS

Overview, Etiology, and Clinical Presentation Congenital infundibulopelvic stenosis is a very rare congenital anomaly of the renal collecting system that presents as unilateral or bilateral caliectasis. Although the exact etiology of this condition is uncertain, Lucaya et al.[39] hypothesized that this abnormality is a milder manifestation of the process that results in multicystic dysplastic kidney. Affected children may be predisposed to urinary tract infections, and this condition may be associated with other renal and urinary tract anomalies.[39]

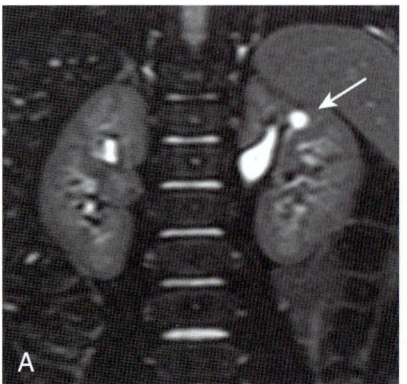
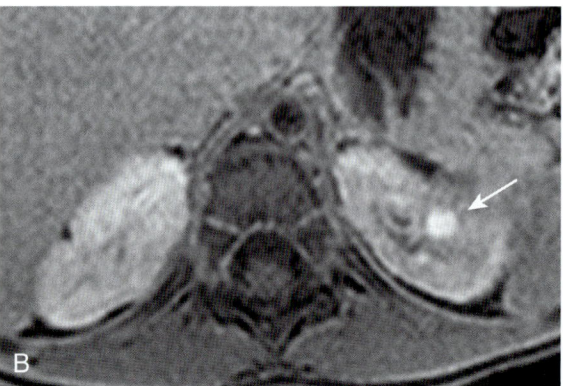

Figure 114-13 Calyceal diverticulum in a 4-year-old girl. **A,** A coronal three-dimensional T2-weighted fast spin echo magnetic resonance (MR) image with fat saturation shows a round structure within the upper pole of the left kidney demonstrating signal intensity identical to urine. **B,** An axial delayed postcontrast T1-weighted MR image with fat saturation reveals excreted contrast material filling this abnormality.

Imaging Upon contrast-enhanced excretory phase imaging studies (including excretory urography, MRU, and CT), this condition has a specific appearance: the renal collecting system infundibula are abnormally narrowed but not entirely obliterated, and the calyces appear abnormally rounded and dilated (Fig. 114-14). The renal pelvis also appears narrowed as a result of stenosis or hypoplasia. This condition may be unilateral or bilateral. Despite the cystlike appearance of the calyces on such contrast-enhanced studies, the ultrasound appearance of the kidneys can be normal. Renal function may be normal to severely impaired.[39]

Treatment Most affected individuals demonstrate normal or stable renal function and do not require treatment. Surgical approaches to manage this condition have been described, including ureterocalicostomy and renal transplantation.[39]

Congenital Megacalyces (Megacalycosis)

Overview, Etiology, and Clinical Presentation Congenital megacalyces is a very rare anomaly of the renal collecting system that may be easily confused for hydronephrosis.[40] Calyceal involvement may be unilateral or bilateral. This abnormal calyceal dilatation is not due to urinary tract obstruction but instead is likely a result of underdevelopment/hypoplasia of the renal medullary pyramids.[41,42] Boys are more commonly affected than are girls. Associated urinary stasis may predispose affected children to urinary tract infection and urolithiasis.[41]

Imaging Congenital megacalyces may be misidentified as obstructive caliectasis by ultrasound. With excretory urography, however, this condition is easily identifiable because of the presence of abnormally dilated calyces that lack normal papillary impressions, have a polygonal or faceted shape, and appear to be increased in number (20 or more calyces may be seen) (Fig. 114-15).[42] The renal parenchyma overlying affected calyces may appear thin. The renal pelvis can be normal in caliber or mildly dilated,[41] and classically, no related urinary tract obstruction should be present. This appearance of the calyces on MRU and excretory-phase CT (CT urography) also should suggest the diagnosis.

Treatment Congenital megacalyces usually are an incidental finding that requires no specific treatment.

URETEROPELVIC JUNCTION OBSTRUCTION

Overview Ureteropelvic junction (UPJ) obstruction is the most common type of congenital urinary tract obstruction, occurring in 3 per 1000 live births. Boys are more frequently affected than are girls, and the left kidney is more commonly involved than the right kidney. About 30% of cases are bilateral, although severity of obstruction and pelvocaliectasis may be asymmetric.[1]

Pathophysiology An intrinsic narrowing (e.g., smooth muscle deficiency, increased fibrosis and collagen, stricture, valve, kinking, and altered peristalsis) occurs at the level of the UPJ,

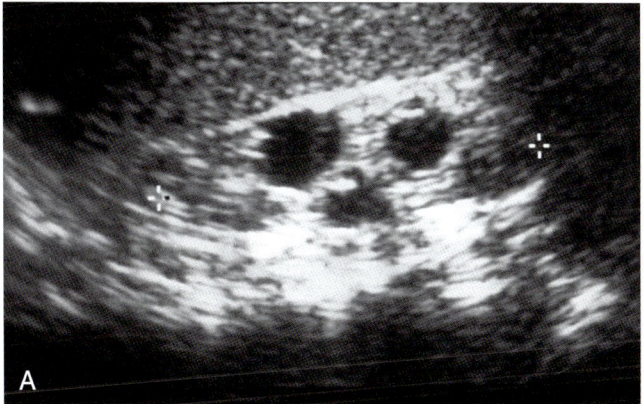
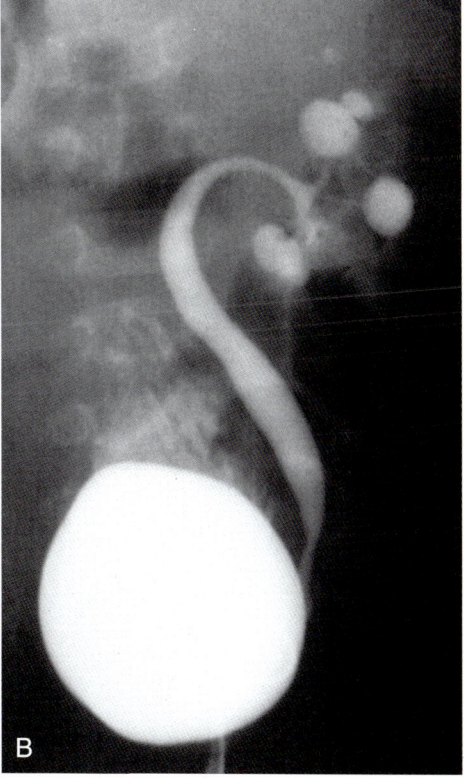

Figure 114-14 Infundibulopelvic stenosis simulating cystic kidney disease. **A,** A longitudinal ultrasound image shows multiple "cysts" scattered throughout the kidney in this child with VACTERL association. **B,** A voiding cystourethrogram shows vesicoureteral reflux into the abnormal pelvocalyceal system. The ureter has a greater caliber than the renal pelvis, infundibula, and calyces. The most peripheral portion of each calyx is rounded, producing the cystic spaces seen with ultrasound.

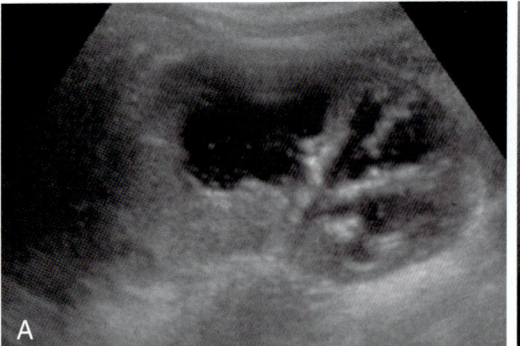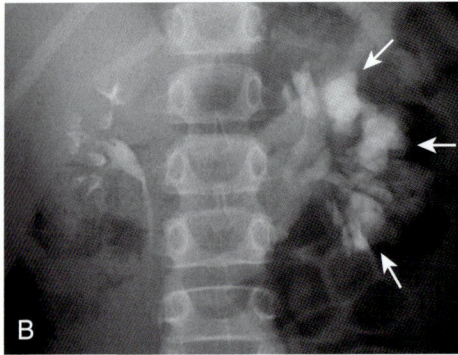

Figure 114-15 Congenital megacalyces in a 6-year-old boy. **A,** A longitudinal ultrasound image shows multiple dilated calyces with overlying parenchymal thinning. Debris within the renal collecting system was due to infection. **B,** A subsequent excretory urography image demonstrates contrast material filling an increased number of left kidney polygon-shaped calyces (*arrows*), confirming the diagnosis of congenital megacalyces.

leading to dilatation of the pelvicalyceal system.[1,43] On occasion, extrinsic narrowing can be seen from a crossing renal vessel in older children and adults.[44] UPJ obstruction often is seen in association with other urinary tract anomalies, such as contralateral multicystic dysplastic kidney, upper urinary tract duplication,[45,46] VUR,[47] and ureterovesical junction obstruction.[48]

Clinical Presentation When UPJ obstruction is not detected prenatally, affected children commonly present with a palpable abdominal mass in the neonatal period. Older children may present with intermittent hydronephrosis and flank pain, often associated with crossing vessels. UPJ obstruction can be complicated by calculi, infection (pyonephrosis), and hemorrhage, especially when diagnosis is delayed.[29]

Imaging On ultrasound, abnormal dilatation of the pelvicalyceal system of varying degrees is seen, whereas the ureter is normal in caliber.[1,29] Ultrasound findings suggestive of renal dysplasia may be present in cases of severe obstruction (described later). Debris within the collecting system can represent infection or hemorrhage (Fig. 114-16). Careful

interrogation of the UPJ region with Doppler ultrasound may identify a crossing vessel, when present.[49] Frequently, separating dilated nonobstructed from dilated obstructed renal collecting systems is difficult by ultrasound alone.

Abdominal radiographs may show soft tissue fullness, bulging of the flank, and displacement of bowel loops from the affected side (e-Fig. 114-17). On contrast-enhanced excretory phase CT, the obstructed kidney demonstrates delayed opacification and excretion of contrast material.[43] CT angiography with multiplanar reformatted and three-dimensional images may be used to depict suspected crossing vessels as a cause of UPJ obstruction in older children and adults.[50]

Diuretic renal scintigraphy is commonly used to evaluate UPJ obstruction; both renal function (including perfusion and differential function) and drainage are evaluated (e-Fig. 114-18).[51,52] MRU is an increasingly important tool in the evaluation of untreated and treated UPJ obstructions.[53] This imaging technique currently allows for the detailed assessment of urinary tract anatomy, while also providing information regarding renal function, including differential renal function, and the presence or absence of obstructive uropathy (Fig. 114-19).[53-55] Both a retrograde pyelogram and a antegrade nephrostogram also can be performed to establish the level of upper urinary tract obstruction, if clinically necessary.

Treatment Recent literature has emphasized the conservative management of neonates with UPJ obstruction, especially with preserved renal function shown by biochemical parameters and renal scintigraphy.[1,56-58] A substantial number of cases that are identified prenatally resolve spontaneously without requiring surgery.[56-58] Indications for surgery include reduced renal function, sustained increase in pelvicalyceal dilation, breakthrough infections, a solitary kidney, and severe bilateral hydronephrosis.[58,59] Treatment, if deemed necessary, usually is accomplished with a dismembered pyeloplasty.[1]

UPPER URINARY TRACT DUPLICATION

Overview and Etiology A duplex kidney consists of a single renal unit that is drained by two collecting systems. If two ureteric buds are present or the ureteric bud bifurcates before meeting the metanephric blastema, duplication of the renal collecting system and ureter occur.[60] Possibilities include a simple bifid renal pelvis, a bifid ureter (i.e., incomplete ureteral duplication), complete ureteral duplication, an ectopic

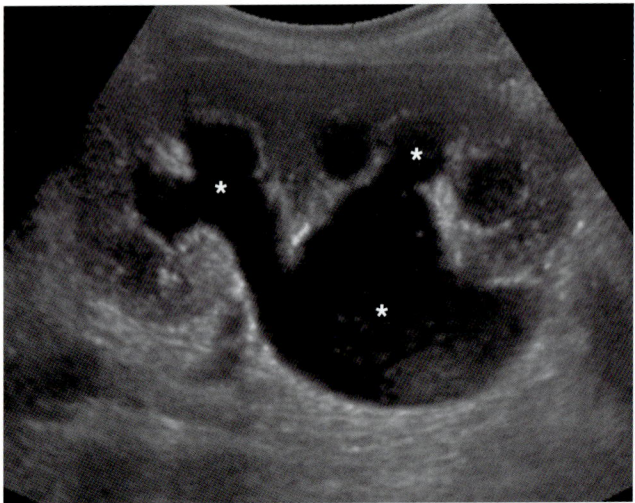

Figure 114-16 Ureteropelvic junction obstruction in a newborn boy with a typical ultrasound appearance. A longitudinal image of the left kidney shows moderate to severe dilatation of the pelvicalyceal system (*asterisks*), with the renal pelvis being more dilated that the calyces. The proximal ureter could not be seen. Debris is present in the renal pelvis.

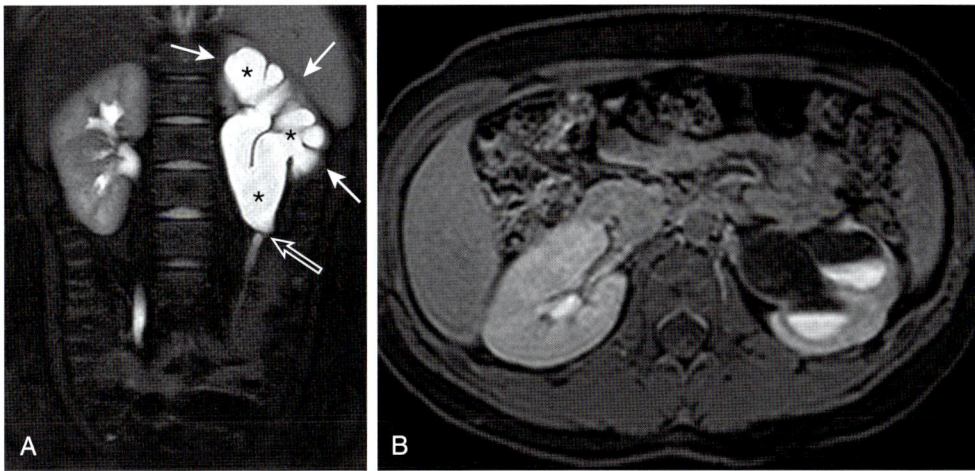

Figure 114-19   Ureteropelvic junction obstruction in a 9-year-old girl. **A,** A coronal T2-weighted magnetic resonance (MR) image with fat saturation shows moderate to severe left pelvocaliectasis (*asterisks*) with overlying parenchymal thinning (*white arrows*). The left ureter is normal in caliber, and there is apparent kinking of the left ureteropelvic junction (*open arrow*). **B,** A postfurosemide axial T1-weighted MR image with fat saturation obtained 20 minutes after intravenous contrast material injection confirms left obstructive uropathy. Only a small amount of contrast material is present in the left collecting system, and multiple urine-contrast levels are present as a result of stasis. Because a substantial amount of enhancing left renal parenchyma was seen, the patient was treated with surgical pyeloplasty to preserve renal function.

ureter, and an ectopic ureterocele. Incomplete duplication of the upper urinary tract is more common than is complete duplication. Even when two ureters are present distally, they frequently enter the bladder via a common sheath.

In cases of complete ureteral duplication, one ureter takes up a near-normal position within the urinary bladder, and the other moves inferiorly with the mesonephric (Wolffian) duct into an abnormal location (e.g., the bladder neck, urethra, vagina, or perineum in girls or the ejaculatory system in boys).[60] The Weigert-Meyer rule, which is applied only to complete duplications, states that the ureter that drains the upper moiety inserts inferior and medial to the lower moiety ureter (Fig. 114-20). In addition, the ectopic ureter is more

likely to be obstructed, whereas the lower moiety ureter is more likely to reflux. Extravesical ureter insertion is far more common in girls than in boys. Extravesical ureter insertions in boys are almost always above the sphincter mechanism; they can be below the sphincter mechanism in girls and present with urinary dribbling and daytime and nighttime wetness. On occasion, ectopic ureteroceles may be detected in the setting of a diminutive pelvicalyceal system, the so-called "ureterocele disproportion."[60,61]

Clinical Presentation   Clinically, incomplete duplication of the upper urinary tract may be asymptomatic or may present with urinary tract infections as a result of ureteroureteral reflux and stasis (so-called "yo-yo" reflux).[60] Children with complete duplication may present in a variety of manners, including hydronephrosis, urinary tract infection, and bladder outlet obstruction due to a large ureterocele.[60,62] Complete duplications in girls also may present with enuresis (both daytime and nocturnal wetness) as a result of insertion of the ectopic ureter into the urethra below the level of the sphincter mechanism or vagina.[60]

Imaging   Ultrasound may identify a prominent renal parenchymal column that appears to separate the sinus fat, providing indirect evidence of collecting system duplication (Fig. 114-21). More commonly, complete duplications present with upper moiety hydronephrosis. Dilatation of the lower moiety can be due to VUR or, less often, concomitant UPJ obstruction (e-Fig. 114-22).[45,60] Ultrasound of the urinary bladder may show a thin-walled intraluminal cystic structure, consistent with a ureterocele (Fig. 114-23).[1] Ureteroceles can vary in size and may appear septated or multiloculated, and when they are located in the midline, it may be difficult to establish the exact side from which they arise.[62]

In the early bladder filling phase of a VCUG examination, a smooth round filling defect is observed, consistent with a ureterocele (Fig. 114-24). Ureteroceles become more difficult to visualize as the urinary bladder distends with contrast material because of obscuration, flattening, or even

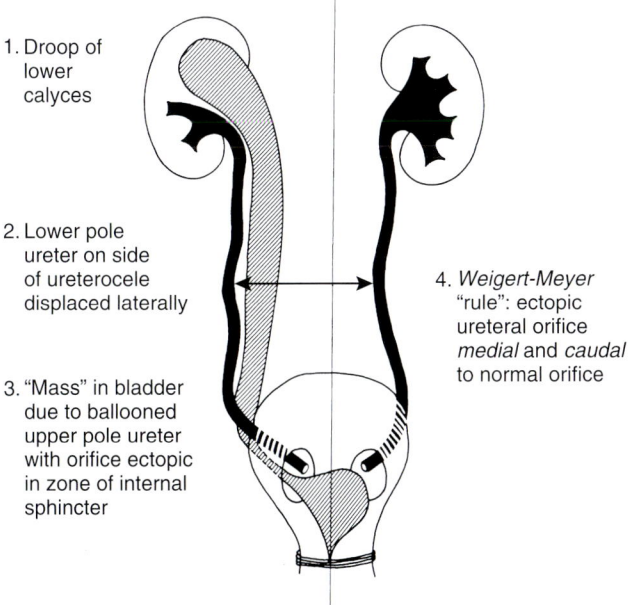

1. Droop of lower calyces

2. Lower pole ureter on side of ureterocele displaced laterally

3. "Mass" in bladder due to ballooned upper pole ureter with orifice ectopic in zone of internal sphincter

4. *Weigert-Meyer "rule"*: ectopic ureteral orifice *medial* and *caudal* to normal orifice

Figure 114-20   Diagram of the Weigert-Meyer rule. (From Berdon WE, Baker DH, Becker JA, et al. Ectopic ureterocele. *Radiol Clin North Am.* 1968;6:205-214).

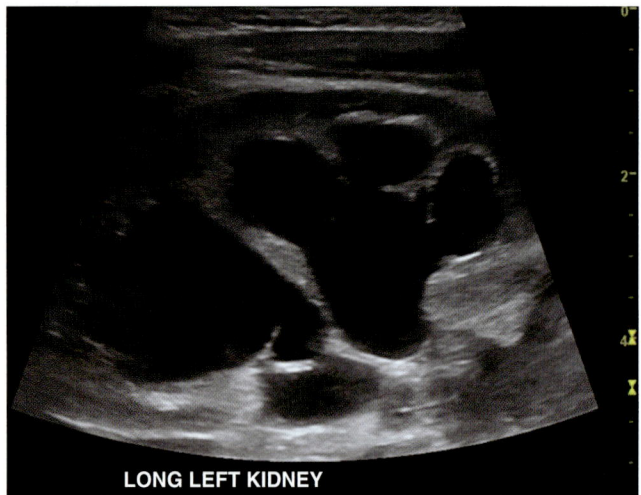

LONG LEFT KIDNEY

Figure 114-21 Upper urinary tract duplication in a 6-week-old girl. A longitudinal ultrasound image through the left kidney shows separate abnormally dilated upper and lower moiety collecting systems. Thinning of overlying renal parenchyma is seen.

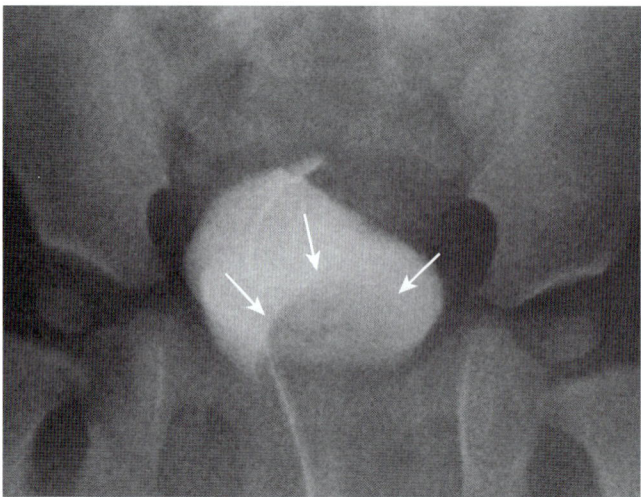

Figure 114-24 Left upper urinary tract duplication in a 1-year-old girl. A voiding cystourethrogram image demonstrates a large urinary bladder-filling defect (*arrows*), consistent with a ureterocele. No vesicoureteral reflux was visualized.

eversion.[60,62] VUR into the lower moiety collecting system of a duplex kidney commonly reveals too few calyces and has a "drooping lily" appearance as a result of abnormal long-axis orientation (Fig. 114-25).[60] The normal long axis of the renal collecting system should parallel that of the ipsilateral psoas muscle. On occasion, VUR may be noted involving the upper moiety of a duplicated system (in about 11% of children), sometimes only after ureterocele incision.[60,63] VUR also can be used to discriminate incomplete from complete ureteral duplications (Fig. 114-26).

MRI (particularly MRU) provides a precise assessment of duplicated upper urinary tract anatomy (e-Fig. 114-27). A variety of T2-weighted imaging techniques can be used to image urine-filled structures, even in the setting of obstruction. MRU also allows for the assessment of renal function and the presence of obstructive uropathy and is optimal

for the assessment of the extravesical ureteric insertions (e-Fig. 114-28).[60,64]

Treatment Incomplete duplications of the upper urinary tract are frequently asymptomatic and require no specific treatment. Specific treatments for upper moiety obstruction

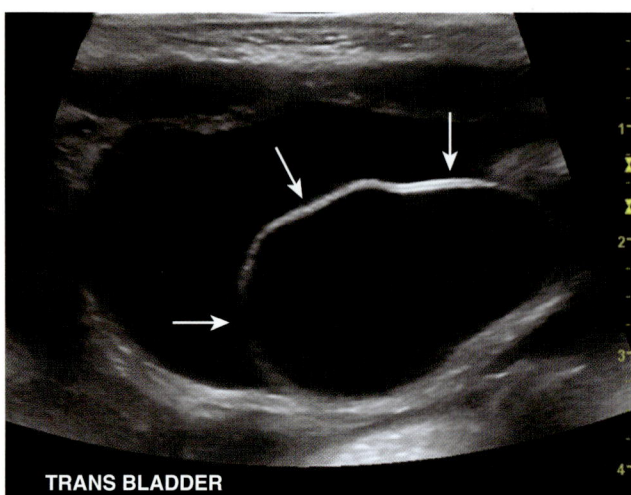

TRANS BLADDER

Figure 114-23 Upper urinary tract duplication in a 6-week-old girl. A transverse ultrasound image through the bladder confirms the presence of a large left ureterocele (*arrows*).

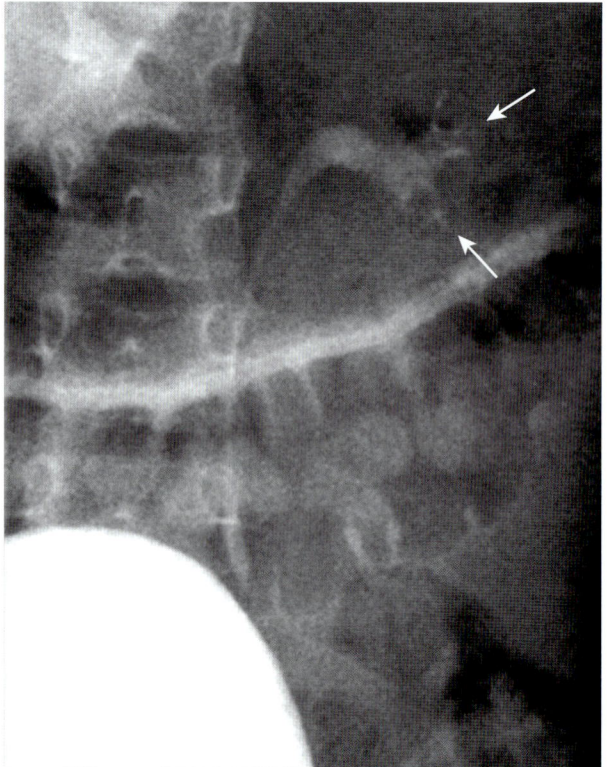

Figure 114-25 Left upper urinary tract duplication in a 6-year-old girl. A voiding cystourethrogram image shows left grade 2 vesicoureteral reflux. The left renal collecting system has too few calyces and its axis is abnormally oriented, giving rise to the "drooping lily" appearance (*arrows*).

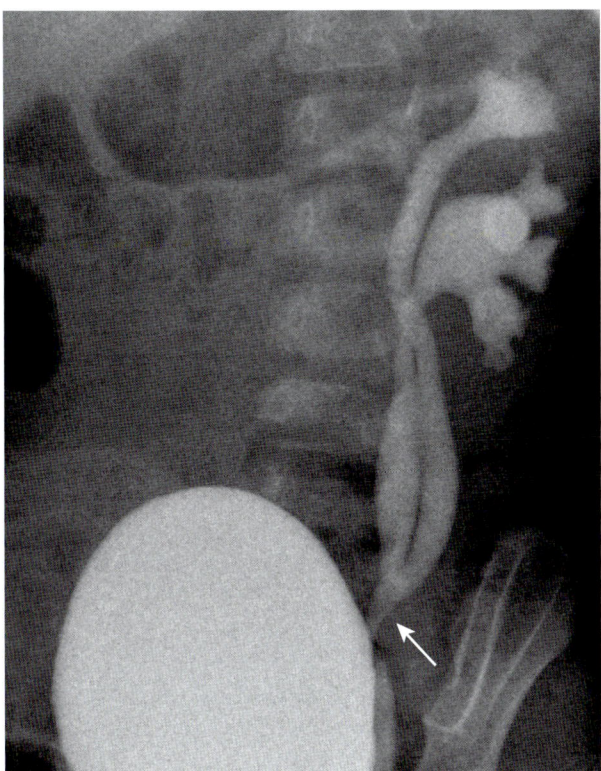

Figure 114-26 Incomplete duplication of the left upper urinary tract in a 1-year-old girl. A voiding cystourethrogram image shows reflux of contrast material into two separate left renal collecting systems and proximal/mid ureters. The ureters join distally (*arrow*), above the left ureterovesical junction.

include endoscopic puncture or excision of an obstructing ureterocele, ureteroureterostomy, and upper moiety heminephrectomy in the setting of poor or absent function.[60,65,66] Lower moiety dilatation due to VUR may require ureteral reimplantation, whereas dilatation due to UPJ obstruction may require surgical pyeloplasty. Multicystic dysplastic upper moieties commonly involute over time without the need for surgical intervention.[67]

Urinary Bladder

PRUNE-BELLY SYNDROME (EAGLE-BARRETT SYNDROME)

Overview, Etiology, and Clinical Presentation Prune-belly syndrome, also known as Eagle-Barrett or triad syndrome, includes the constellation of bilateral cryptorchidism, anterior abdominal wall muscular deficiency, and a variety of urinary tract anomalies, including megacystis and hydroureteronephrosis.[68,69] The appearance of the abdominal wall on physical examination and radiographs has a characteristic appearance. Although the pathogenesis of prune-belly syndrome is controversial, two main theories are currently suggested: (1) bladder outlet obstruction early in utero and (2) a primary mesodermal defect.[68-70] This condition is usually nonhereditary (although familial cases have been reported), almost always affects boys (3% to 5% of cases occur in girls), and is present in 1:29,000 to 1:50,000 live births.[68,69] Associated anomalies of the cardiovascular, musculoskeletal, and gastrointestinal systems also may be present.

Imaging On physical examination and radiographs, the abdominal wall of affected neonates has a characteristic wrinkled appearance with bulging of the flanks resulting from muscular deficiency (e-Fig. 114-29). VCUG allows depiction of the urinary bladder and urethral anatomy, identifies VUR, and determines whether a urachal anomaly is present. Markedly dilated, tortuous ureters are common because of a combination of muscular deficiency and VUR, which is present in approximately 75% of patients with prune-belly syndrome (Fig. 114-30).[69] Upper urinary tract obstruction typically is not present. The urinary bladder usually has a smooth wall, increased capacity (megacystis), and may contain multiple diverticula. Urethral findings include dilatation and elongation of the prostatic urethra (e-Fig. 114-31), an enlarged utricle, megalourethra (e-Fig. 114-32), and rarely urethral atresia.[68] A minority of patients with prune-belly syndrome have urethral obstruction due to an obstructing membrane or valve.[68] The primary role of ultrasound in the neonatal period is to establish the status of the kidneys. The kidneys commonly show

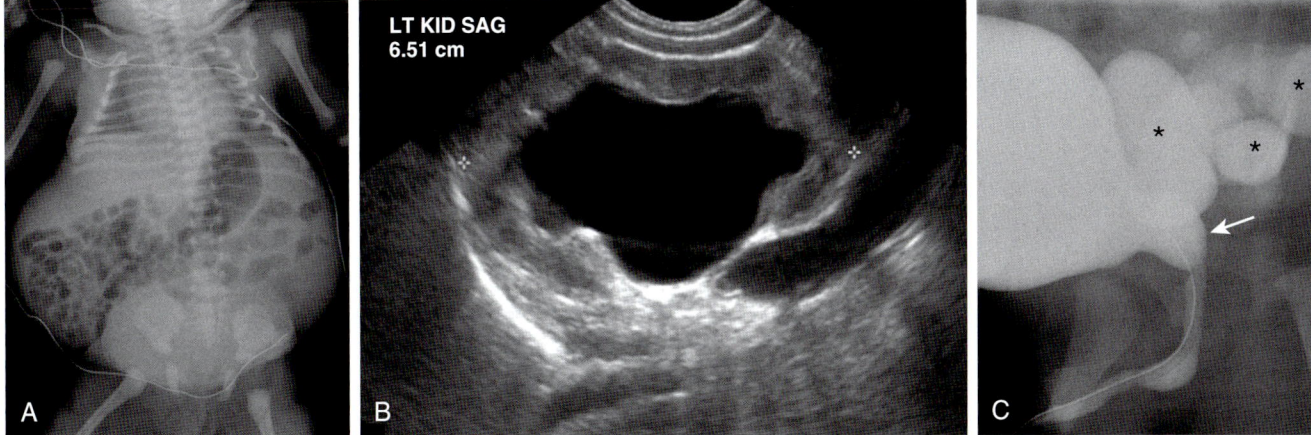

Figure 114-30 A neonatal boy with prune-belly syndrome. **A,** An abdominal radiograph shows laxity of the anterior abdominal wall and bulging flanks. **B,** A longitudinal ultrasound image of the left kidney shows dilatation of the collecting system and proximal ureter. The kidney demonstrates abnormally increased parenchymal echogenicity and contains a few subcortical cysts (not shown), suggestive of renal dysplasia. **C,** A voiding cystourethrogram demonstrates dilatation of the posterior urethra (*arrow*) and high-grade vesicoureteric reflux (*asterisks*).

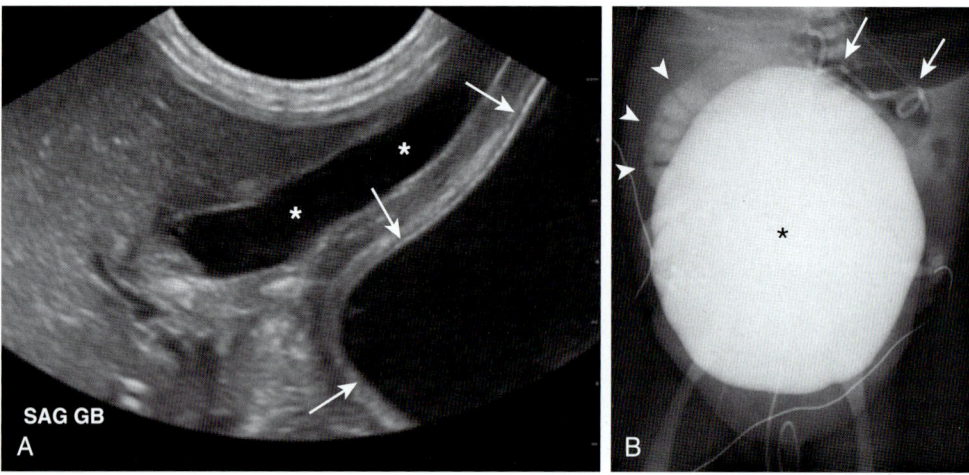

Figure 114-33 A 1-day-old boy with megacystis-microcolon-intestinal hypoperistalsis-malrotation syndrome (Berdon syndrome). **A,** A longitudinal ultrasound image demonstrates a markedly dilated urinary bladder (*arrows*), which extends into the upper abdomen and abuts the gallbladder (*asterisks*). **B,** A voiding cystourethrogram image shows the urinary bladder (*asterisk*) occupying most of the abdomen and pelvis. High-grade right vesicoureteral reflux is present (*arrowheads*), and a retained peritoneoamniotic shunt (*arrows*) projects over the left upper quadrant of the abdomen.

findings compatible with renal dysplasia, including small size, abnormally increased parenchymal echogenicity, loss of corticomedullary differentiation, and cortical cysts.

Treatment Children with prune-belly syndrome may require multiple surgical procedures. The testes should be relocated from the abdomen to the scrotum (orchiopexy) to minimize the risk of future testicular torsion and neoplasm.[68] Urethral obstruction, if present, should be surgically addressed. VUR and poor upper urinary tract drainage may be managed with chronic antibiotic prophylaxis (which is currently preferred) or surgical reimplantation of the ureters to attempt to preserve renal function. Megacystis and poor urinary bladder emptying may be treated with reduction cystoplasty or vesicostomy.[71] In more severe cases, anterior abdominal wall surgical reconstruction (abdominoplasty) is performed and may improve urinary bladder emptying.[68,71] Because of chronic kidney disease and frequent underlying renal dysplasia, affected children eventually may require renal transplantation or dialysis therapy.

MEGACYSTIS-MICROCOLON-INTESTINAL HYPOPERISTALSIS-MALROTATION SYNDROME

Overview, Etiology, and Clinical Presentation The name "megacystis-microcolon-intestinal hypoperistalsis-malrotation syndrome" actually describes the pertinent clinical and radiologic findings. Features of this syndrome may overlap with prune-belly syndrome. This syndrome is an autosomal-recessive disorder seen mostly in girls. It presents clinically with severe abdominal distention during the neonatal period because of functional bowel obstruction and severe urinary bladder distention.[72,73]

Imaging Abdominal radiography may demonstrate a large, round mass emanating from the pelvis because of megacystis. Ultrasound and VCUG show an abnormally distended urinary bladder (Fig. 114-33) and, in most cases, hydroureteronephrosis.[73] Urinary bladder emptying is abnormal, although no

anatomic obstruction is found. Contrast enema examination reveals a severe microcolon and diminished or absent colonic peristalsis (Fig. 114-34).[72,73]

Treatment This syndrome is commonly fatal in the first year of life because of malnutrition or sepsis, unless the patient receives parenteral nutrition.[72-75] Bowel transplantation has been attempted as a treatment option.[76] A cutaneous vesicostomy or suprapubic cystostomy may assist with urinary bladder drainage.[73]

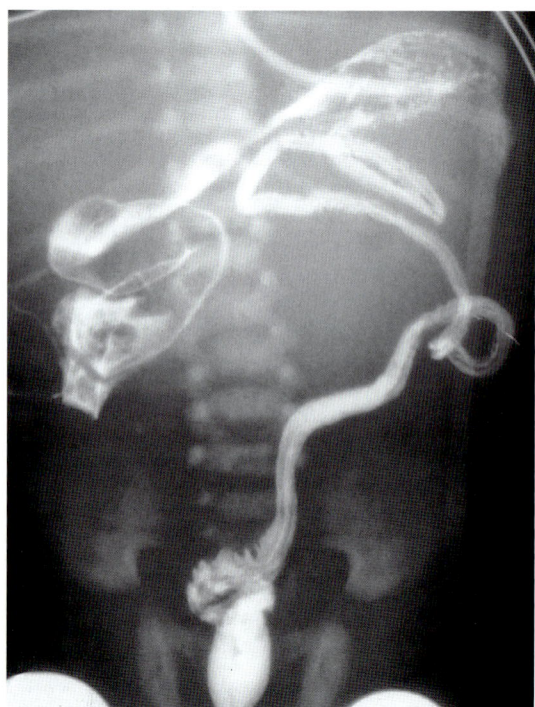

Figure 114-34 Megacystis-microcolon. The anterior view from a contrast enema reveals a severe microcolon.

BLADDER EXSTROPHY

Overview Deficiency of the anterior abdominal wall with an open, everted, incompletely formed urinary bladder is referred to as *bladder exstrophy*. The anterior wall of the urinary bladder and overlying skin are absent, and the rectus abdominis muscles are separated inferiorly.[1,77] The remaining posterior urinary bladder wall is continuous with the skin.[77]

Etiology and Clinical Presentation Failure of migration of mesenchymal cells between ectoderm and cloaca during the fourth week of fetal life leads to incomplete closure of the midline lower anterior abdominal wall in utero, resulting in bladder exstrophy.[1,77,78] This rare, unpredictable, congenital defect occurs in 1:10,000 to 1:40,000 live births and is more common in boys.[1] Upon physical examination, the ureteral orifices may be visualized draining into the posterior urinary bladder wall. Epispadias in boys and bifid clitoris in girls often are noted as well.[77] Other skeletal, scrotal, renal, spinal, and anorectal anomalies also may be present.[1,77]

Imaging Radiographs show abnormal pubic symphyseal widening (Fig. 114-35).[77,79] The hips may be dislocated. Renal imaging is most commonly normal at birth.[77] Recently, MRI has been used to assess pelvic anatomy after bladder exstrophy repair.[80]

Treatment The prognosis for bladder exstrophy is generally good. Although certain patients may be amenable to complete primary closure,[81] others may require multiple surgeries

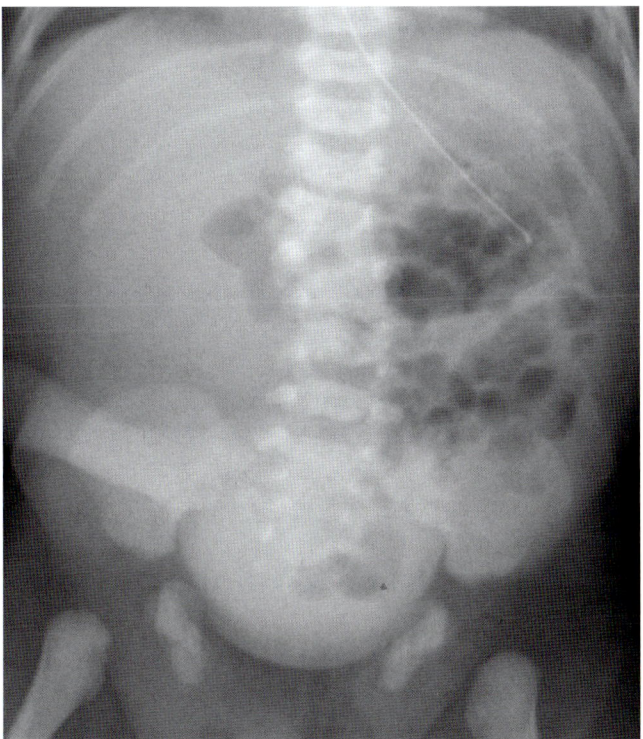

Figure 114-35 A neonate with bladder exstrophy and a bifid scrotum. An abdominal radiograph shows symphyseal diastasis, consistent with bladder exstrophy. A round, masslike opacity projecting over the pelvis is due to a large umbilical hernia. Incidental note is made of multiple lumbar vertebral anomalies.

involving the genitourinary and skeletal systems early in life. An increased incidence of adenocarcinoma of the bladder later in life is found compared with age-matched control subjects.[1,82]

Cloacal Exstrophy

Overview, Etiology, and Clinical Presentation Cloacal exstrophy is a nonhereditary constellation of congenital anomalies that involves the anterior abdominal wall and multiple organ systems. This condition is a result of maldevelopment of the cloacal membrane during organogenesis. The infraumbilical cloacal membrane persists, which interferes with normal infraumbilical anterior abdominal wall closure and leads to failure of urogenital septum separation from the rectum. Two hemibladders are separated by ileocecal bowel mucosa.[83] The terminal ileum prolapses through the exposed cecum (sometimes called an "elephant trunk" deformity).[83] Associated anomalies include omphalocele, abnormal genitalia, a two-vessel umbilical cord, closed spinal defects, and renal abnormalities.

Imaging Radiographs may demonstrate a variety of abnormalities, including abnormal widening of the pubic symphysis, lumbosacral spine anomalies, developmental dysplasia of the hip, and clubfoot. Imaging of the kidneys may reveal agenesis or ectopia, and various Müllerian anomalies may be detected in the pelvis (Fig. 114-36 and Box 114-2). Ultrasound and MRI imaging of the spine commonly reveal spinal dysraphism and spinal cord tethering (e-Fig. 114-37). At some point, upper gastrointestinal series evaluation should be performed because midgut malrotation may be present in up to 30% of affected children.[83]

Treatment This condition commonly requires a multistage approach to surgical reconstruction.[84] Advances in surgical technique and supportive care have improved survival and functional outcomes.

Box 114-2 Genital Anomalies Associated with Unilateral Renal Agenesis

Female
- Absence or hypoplasia of vagina
- Absence of uterus
- Failure of fusion of midline structures (Müllerian derivatives)
  - Bicornuate uterus, uterus didelphys
  - Obstructed hemivagina and hemiuterus and hydrocolpos, hematocolpos, hematosalpinx
- Gartner duct cyst
- Ipsilateral absence of uterine horn and fallopian tube (unicornuate uterus)

Male
- Ipsilateral anomalies
  - Absence of epididymis
  - Absence of seminal vesicle
  - Absence of vas deferens
  - Absence or hypoplasia of testis
  - Seminal vesicle cyst

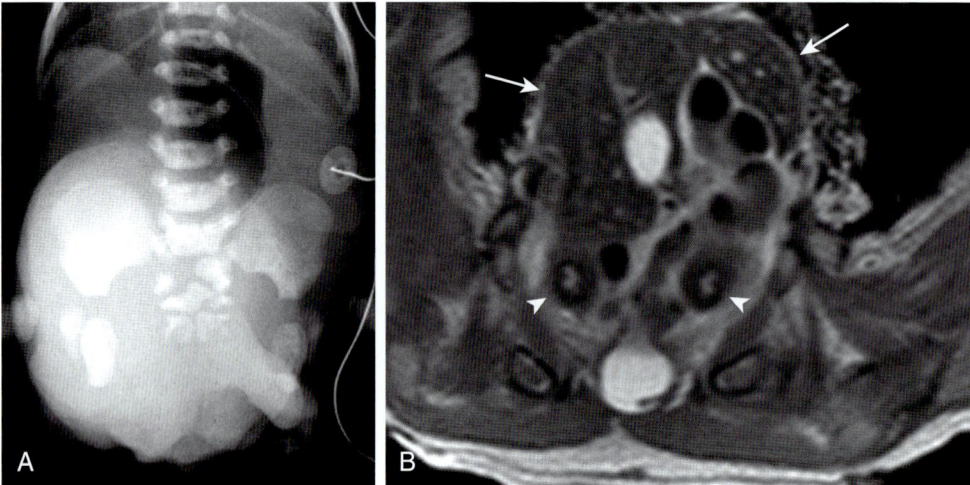

Figure 114-36 A neonate with cloacal exstrophy. **A,** An abdominal radiograph shows multiple sacral anomalies and abnormal widening of the pubic symphysis. A masslike opacity projecting over the lower abdomen and pelvis was due to a large omphalocele. **B,** An axial T2-weighted magnetic resonance image shows a large liver-containing omphalocele at the level of the pelvis (*arrows*). Two separate uterine horns (*arrowheads*) can be seen, consistent with uterus didelphys. The ileum had prolapsed through the exposed cecum on physical examination (the so-called "elephant trunk" deformity).

Cloacal Malformation

Overview, Etiology, and Clinical Presentation Cloacal malformation is diagnosed when the urinary, genital, and gastrointestinal tracts all come together to form a single outflow channel of variable length.[62,85] On physical examination, the perineum has a single opening that eliminates urine, feces, and genital tract secretions.[85] Unlike with cloacal exstrophy, the anterior abdominal wall is intact.[62] Although the etiology of this congenital anomaly is not entirely understood, it is thought to be the result of failure of urorectal septum to join the cloacal membrane in utero.[62] This condition only affects 1:40,000 to 1:50,000 phenotypic newborn girls.[85]

Imaging Contrast injection through a catheter placed within the single perineal orifice under fluoroscopic observation can be used to confirm the diagnosis and definitely characterize perineal anatomy.[62,85] Jaramillo et al.[85] divided these malformations into urethral and vaginal subtypes based on the appearance of the common channel. Numerous genitourinary tract abnormalities may be seen in the setting of cloacal malformation, including VUR, ureteral ectopia, urinary bladder diverticula, urinary bladder duplication, urachal anomalies, urethral duplication, and a variety of uterine and vaginal anomalies.[85] Renal abnormalities may include agenesis, obstruction, and horseshoe kidney, whereas osseous abnormalities may include widening of the pubic symphysis and partial sacral agenesis. Abnormalities of the spinal cord may be present and are best characterized by ultrasound or MRI (Fig. 114-38). Contrast material injection through the distal limb of a diverting colostomy also may be performed to further assess perineal anatomy.[62,85]

Treatment The goals of surgery are to achieve urinary and fecal continence and to preserve future sexual function. The surgical approach depends, at least in part, on the length of the common channel. A diverting colostomy may be performed soon after birth as a temporizing measure. Hematocolpos/hydrocolpos due to vaginal obstruction should be drained when present. Posterior sagittal anorectovaginourethroplasty often is performed to definitely repair the entire malformation with good results, although laparotomy also may be required.[86]

WHAT THE CLINICIAN NEEDS TO KNOW

- Renal size, position, number, corticomedullary differentiation, and the presence of hydronephrosis and/or hydroureter
- The presence of noncommunicating cysts and dysplastic renal parenchyma of MCDK
- The presence of renal cysts in a child with a family history of ADPKD
- The imaging appearance of both the kidneys and the liver in persons with ARPKD
- Renal cystic disease suggesting an inherited syndrome or genetic disorder
- Severity of hydronephrosis, current and follow-up renal functional imaging status, the presence of VUR, and any associated complications in persons with UPJ obstruction
- Complete versus incomplete renal duplication and associated ectopic ureteral position
- The presence of severe urinary bladder distention in combination with microcolon
- The status of the spinal cord in patients with cloacal exstrophy or cloacal malformation

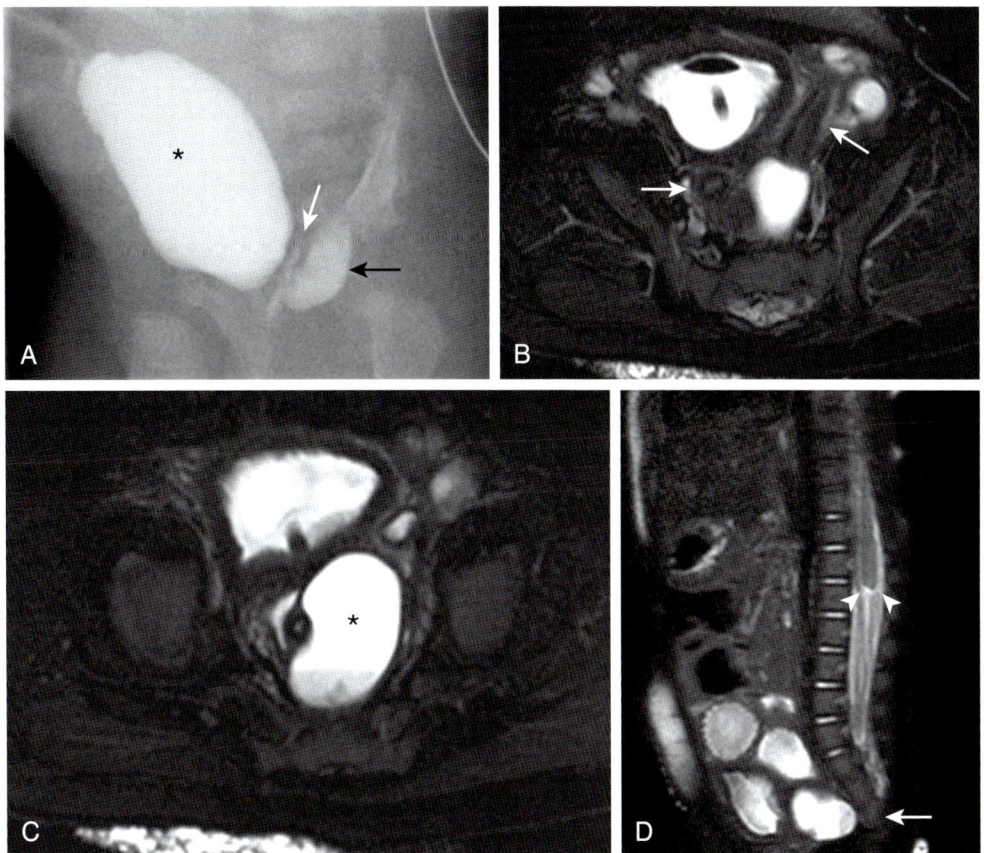

Figure 114-38 Cloacal malformation in a 2-month-old girl. **A,** Fluoroscopic contrast material injection through the common channel fills the urinary bladder (*asterisk*), vagina (*white arrow*), and rectum (*black arrow*). **B,** An axial heavily T2-weighted magnetic resonance (MR) image with fat saturation shows two separate uterine horns (*arrows*), consistent with uterus didelphys. A balloon catheter is present in the urinary bladder. **C,** Another axial MR image at a slightly lower level reveals two vaginas. The left hemivagina is obstructed (*asterisk*) and contains a fluid-fluid level due to hematocolpos. **D,** A sagittal single shot fast spin echo MR image with fat saturation demonstrates partial sacral agenesis (*arrow*) and truncation of the lower spinal cord with blunting of the conus medullaris (*arrowheads*). (From Jarboe MD, Teitelbaum DH, Dillman JR. Combined 3D rotational fluoroscopic MRI cloacagram procedure defines luminal and extraluminal pelvic anatomy prior to surgical reconstruction of cloacal and other complex pelvic malformations. *Pediatr Surg Int.* 2012;28:757-763.)

Key Points

MCDK typically involutes over time, eventually resulting in remnant dysplastic renal tissue that may be impossible to visualize.

Two types of ADPKD exist, each with clearly defined chromosomal mutations.

ARPKD has been subdivided into categories based on clinical presentation. The degrees of renal and hepatic abnormalities tend to be inversely proportional.

About 30% of UPJ cases are bilateral, although the severity of obstruction and pelvocaliectasis may be asymmetric.

The Weigert-Meyer rule, which applies only to complete duplications, states that the ureter that drains the upper moiety inserts inferior and medial to the lower moiety ureter. The upper moiety ectopic ureter is more likely to be obstructed, whereas the lower moiety ureter is more likely to reflux.

Calyceal diverticula most commonly occur within the upper pole.

Congenital megacalyces is a very rare anomaly of the renal collecting system that may be confused easily with hydronephrosis.

Prune-belly syndrome, also known as Eagle-Barrett or triad syndrome, includes the constellation of bilateral cryptorchidism, anterior abdominal wall muscular deficiency, and a variety of urinary tract anomalies, including megacystis and hydroureteronephrosis.

Megacystis-microcolon-intestinal hypoperistalsis-malrotation syndrome presents clinically with severe abdominal distention during the neonatal period as a result of functional bowel obstruction and severe urinary bladder distention.

Cloacal malformation has a single perineal opening that eliminates urine, feces, and genital tract secretions. Unlike with cloacal exstrophy, the anterior abdominal wall is intact.

Suggested Readings

Avni FE, Guissard G, Hall M, et al. Hereditary polycystic kidney diseases in children: changing sonographic patterns through childhood. *Pediatr Radiol.* 2002;32:169-174.

Avni FE, Nicaise N, Hall M, et al. The role of MR imaging for the assessment of complicated duplex kidneys in children: preliminary report. *Pediatr Radiol.* 2001;31:215-223.

Berrocal T, Lopez-Pereira P, Arjonilla A, et al. Anomalies of the distal ureter, bladder, and urethra in children: embryologic, radiologic, and pathologic features. *Radiographics.* 2002;22:1139-1164.

Jain M, LeQuesne GW, Bourne AJ, et al. High-resolution ultrasonography in the differential diagnosis of cystic diseases of the kidney in infancy and childhood: preliminary experience. *J Ultrasound Med.* 1997;16:235-240.

Jaramillo D, Lebowitz RL, Hendren WH. The cloacal malformation: radiologic findings and imaging recommendations. *Radiology.* 1990; 177:441-448.

McDaniel BB, Jones RA, Scherz H, et al. Dynamic contrast-enhanced MR urography in the evaluation of pediatric hydronephrosis: Part 2, anatomic and functional assessment of uteropelvic junction obstruction. *AJR Am J Roentgenol.* 2005;185:1608-1614.

Rabelo EA, Oliveira EA, Diniz JS, et al. Natural history of multicystic kidney conservatively managed: a prospective study. *Pediatr Nephrol.* 2004;19:1102-1107.

Traubici J, Daneman A. High-resolution renal sonography in children with autosomal recessive polycystic kidney disease. *AJR Am J Roentgenol.* 2005;184(5):1630-1633.

References

Full references for this chapter can be found on www.expertconsult.com.

Chapter 115

Acquired Abnormalities
(Stone Disease and Infection)

ROBERT G. WELLS

Renal Infection

ACUTE BACTERIAL PYELONEPHRITIS

Overview   The term *pyelonephritis* encompasses infections of the renal parenchyma and pelvocaliceal system. Bacterial infections of the kidneys are further categorized as acute or chronic, unilateral or bilateral, and focal, multifocal, or diffuse. Potential complications of pyelonephritis include renal or perinephric abscess. A bacterial infection in which purulent material fills a dilated collecting system is termed *pyonephrosis.*[1]

Pathophysiology and Clinical Presentation   The most common cause of acute bacterial pyelonephritis is ascending infection from the lower urinary tract. Parenchymal renal infection occasionally occurs as a result of hematogenous inoculation; this mechanism is more common in infants than in older children. Although children with vesicoureteral reflux are at elevated risk for pyelonephritis, reflux is not a prerequisite for renal infection. Potential clinical manifestations of acute bacterial pyelonephritis include flank pain, abdominal pain, fever, pyuria, nausea, and vomiting. Young infants with pyelonephritis often have nonspecific findings such as irritability and poor feeding; fever is sometimes lacking.[2-4]

Imaging   Renal cortical scintigraphy with technetium-99m dimercaptosuccinic acid (DMSA) or technetium-99m glucoheptonate is highly sensitive (at least 90%) for the detection of acute bacterial pyelonephritis. Infected regions of the kidneys have diminished or absent accumulation of the radiopharmaceutical agent, often with a spherical or flarelike pattern (Fig. 115-1). A renal abscess produces a scintigraphic defect that usually is indistinguishable from that of uncomplicated parenchymal infection.[5,6]

Contrast-enhanced computed tomography (CT) provides sensitivity that is similar to renal cortical scintigraphy for the diagnosis of acute bacterial pyelonephritis. Infected renal parenchyma has diminished contrast enhancement on images obtained immediately after injection of contrast material (Fig. 115-2). Potential patterns of infected parenchyma include radially oriented linear streaks of diminished attenuation, round or irregular hypoattenuating foci, wedge-shaped defects, and heterogeneous diminished enhancement throughout an enlarged kidney. The nephrogram intensity usually is diminished relative to the contralateral normal kidney. Delayed CT images of the infected kidney show retention of contrast in obstructed tubules. A parenchymal abscess appears as a hypoattenuating focus, sometimes with a prominently enhancing rim. A perinephric abscess also is hypoattenuating.[7]

Renal parenchymal edema resulting from infection leads to diminished signal intensity on T1-weighted magnetic resonance imaging (MRI) and increased signal intensity on T2-weighted images (Fig. 115-3). Nephromegaly or localized parenchymal expansion may be present. Corticomedullary differentiation is sometimes deficient. The parenchyma may have a striated appearance. Edema in the perinephric space is a common MRI finding. As with CT, contrast enhancement is deficient in the involved portions of parenchyma. Urothelial thickening is sometimes appreciable.[8,9]

Reported sensitivities of sonography for the detection of acute bacterial pyelonephritis range from 25% to 50%. The findings include nephromegaly, abnormal parenchymal echogenicity, loss of corticomedullary differentiation, renal sinus hyperechogenicity, and urothelial thickening. Color Doppler or power Doppler imaging demonstrates diminished perfusion of the infected regions of parenchyma, sometimes with a wedge shape (Fig. 115-4). A parenchymal abscess usually appears as a spherical hypoechoic focus with acoustic enhancement. Occasionally, pus within the cavity results in an isoechoic or hypoechoic appearance. A perinephric abscess appears as a hypoechoic fluid collection immediately peripheral to the capsule.[10-13]

Treatment and Follow-up   Longer and more intensive antibiotic therapy is required for upper urinary tract infections than for those confined to the bladder. Antibiotic prophylaxis against reinfection is indicated for selected patients, particularly for those with predisposing factors. The utility of follow-up diagnostic imaging studies for children with acute bacterial pyelonephritis is a topic of ongoing investigation and debate.[14,15]

PYONEPHROSIS

Overview   Pyonephrosis is a bacterial infection of the kidney in which purulent material fills a dilated collecting system. Most often, a preexisting chronic obstruction is present, such as congenital ureteropelvic junction obstruction. Acute obstruction because of a calculus is an occasional cause in children. The clinical presentation of pyonephrosis is similar to that of other bacterial urinary tract infections. Fever, flank pain, pyuria, and hematuria are common.[16]

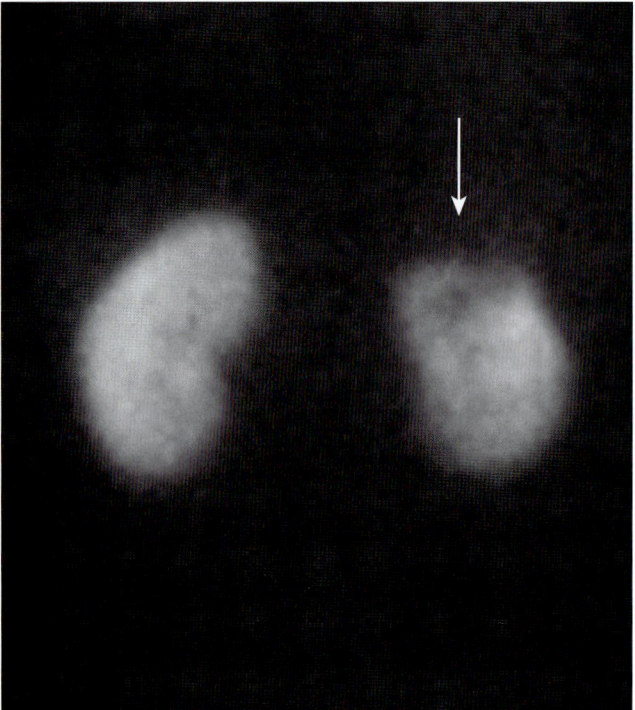

Figure 115-1 Acute bacterial pyelonephritis. A posterior technetium-99m dimercaptosuccinic acid image of a febrile 16-year-old shows absent uptake in the upper pole of the left kidney (*arrow*).

Imaging Sonography shows echogenic material within a dilated pelvocaliceal system (Fig. 115-5). The purulent material often layers in the dependent portions of the collecting system and may shift with changes in patient position. Thickening of the wall of the dilated renal pelvis usually is present.

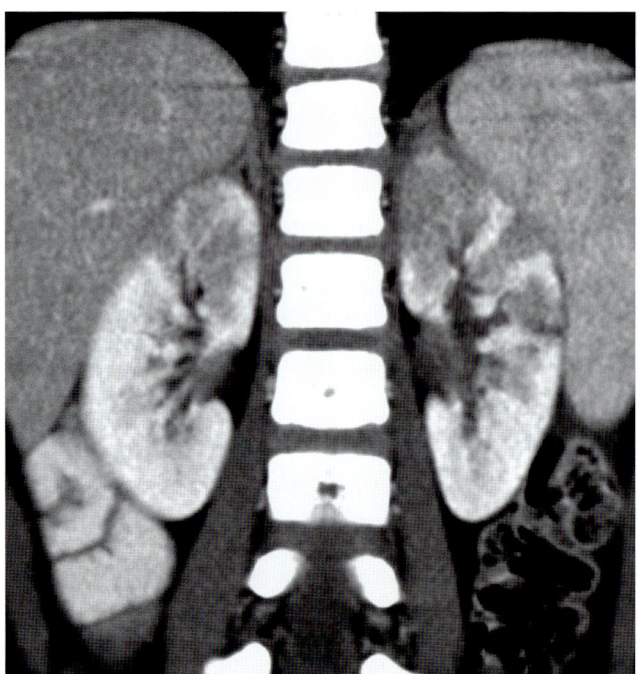

Figure 115-2 Multifocal bacterial pyelonephritis. Multiple areas of deficient contrast enhancement of the kidneys are present on this coronal computed tomography image of a 6-year-old girl.

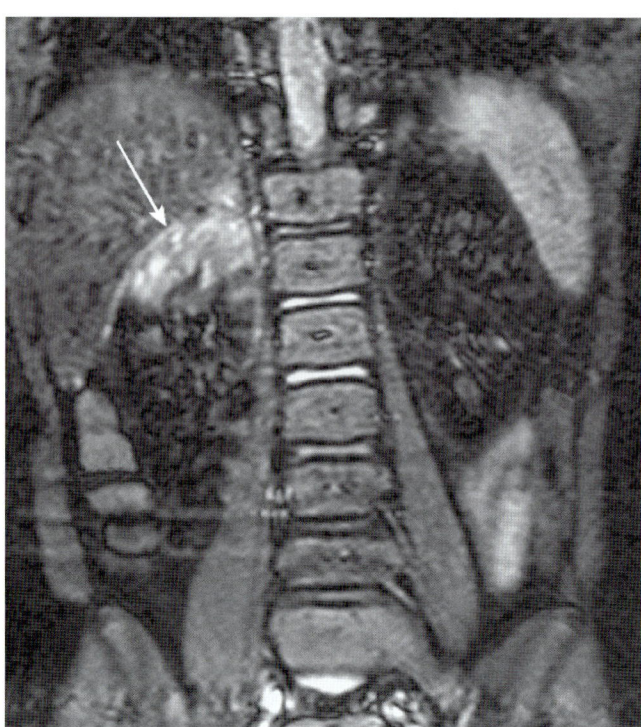

Figure 115-3 Acute bacterial pyelonephritis. A coronal contrast-enhanced short tau inversion recovery magnetic resonance image shows abnormal increased signal in the upper pole of the right kidney (*arrow*). Normal renal parenchyma is hypointense. (Courtesy Damien Grattan-Smith, MD, Atlanta, GA.)

Uncommon additional potential findings include a fluid-debris level in the collecting system, echogenic foci due to gas-forming organisms, and complete filling of the dilated collecting system with echogenic material.[17,18]

Imaging of pyonephrosis with CT, MRI, or scintigraphy shows diminished function of the involved kidney. Deficient excretion of intravenously administered contrast or radiopharmaceutical material is noted. Contrast enhancement of the renal parenchyma of the infected kidney is heterogeneous and delayed on CT. Excreted contrast may outline filling defects in the dilated collecting system on delayed images. Debris usually is visible in the dilated renal collecting system on MRI. The renal parenchyma has abnormal heterogeneous signal intensity. The pus-filled collecting system is markedly hyperintense on diffusion-weighted images. Contrast-enhanced MRI confirms reduced function of the kidney.[19]

Treatment and Follow-up The treatment of pyonephrosis includes prompt initiation of aggressive antimicrobial therapy. Drainage of the obstructed collecting system often is required, usually by percutaneous nephrostomy. Surgical correction of the underlying obstruction typically is performed after resolution of the acute infection.

XANTHOGRANULOMATOUS PYELONEPHRITIS

Overview Xanthogranulomatous pyelonephritis (XGP) is an uncommon form of severe chronic renal parenchymal infection. The pathogenesis typically involves chronic infection of an obstructed kidney. Histologic examination demonstrates inflammatory cells interspersed within fibrogranulomatous

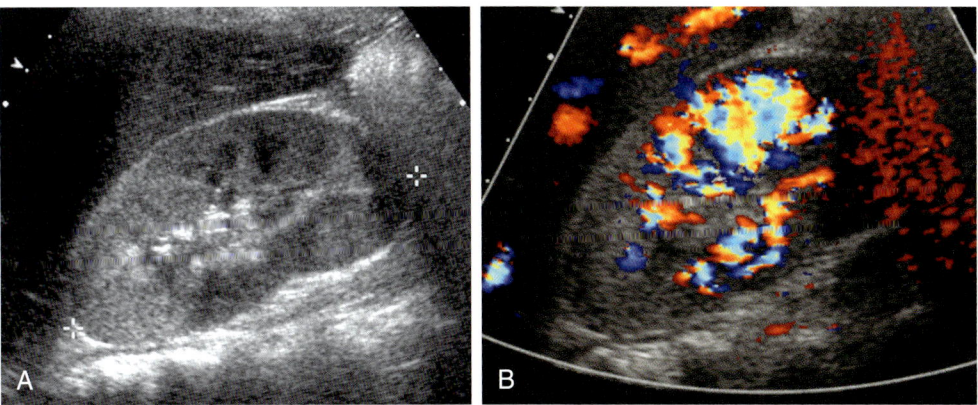

Figure 115-4 Acute bacterial pyelonephritis. **A,** Sonography shows increased echogenicity and deficient corticomedullary differentiation in the upper pole. **B,** Diminished perfusion is present in the edematous infected upper pole.

tissue, nodules of lipid laden macrophages, and areas of necrotic parenchyma. Diffuse involvement of the kidney is most common; segmental or focal forms also can occur, sometimes in association with obstruction of a duplicated system or infundibulum. Common clinical findings include fever, flank pain, malaise, pyuria, weight loss, and anemia.[20-22]

Imaging In the early stages of XGP, the involved portion of the kidney typically has an irregular hyperechoic character on sonography. With the diffuse form, the kidney may be massively enlarged but usually maintains a reniform shape. Echogenic foci with shadowing indicate the presence of calcifications. With progression, necrotic tissue and fluid are usually hypoechoic. Echogenic debris is sometimes visible within abscesses or the dilated collecting system.[23]

CT of diffuse XGP typically demonstrates an enlarged nonfunctioning kidney that has multiple low-attenuation parenchymal foci (Fig. 115-6). A staghorn calculus often is present in a contracted renal pelvis. Irregular contrast enhancement of the inflamed renal parenchyma occurs, often accompanied by inflammatory enhancement of the perinephric fat. Abscesses are moderately hypoattenuating and do not enhance

with contrast. The pus-filled collecting system also is hypoattenuating. Little or no contrast excretion occurs. Regional retroperitoneal lymphadenopathy is common. With the focal form of XGP, CT typically demonstrates an expansile renal mass. Peripheral granulation tissue or compressed renal parenchyma may result in an enhancing peripheral rim. The involved renal parenchyma typically has low or intermediate signal intensity on T1-weighted MRI and high intensity on T2-weighted images.[24]

Treatment and Follow-up The usual treatment for XGP is antibiotic therapy followed by nephrectomy or heminephrectomy. A percutaneous biopsy occasionally is useful to allow differentiation from a neoplasm and to provide material for

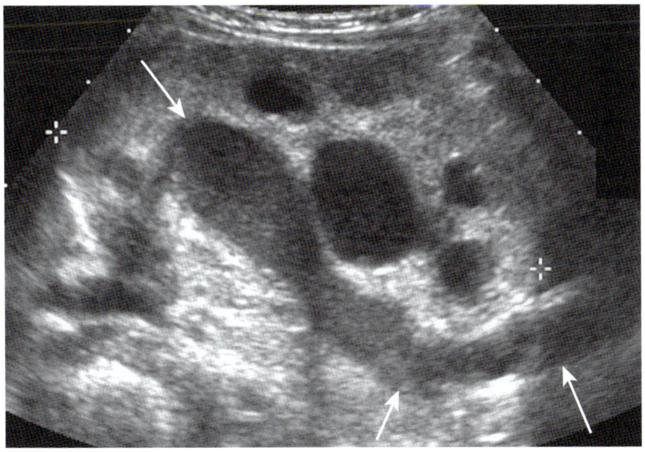

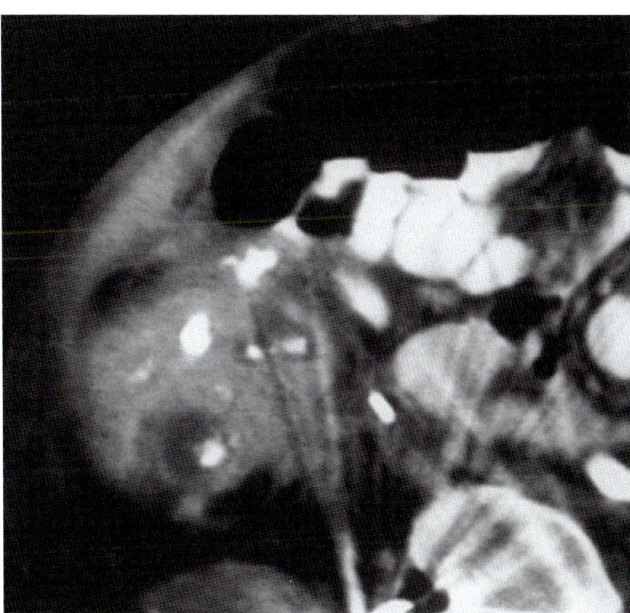

Figure 115-6 Xanthogranulomatous pyelonephritis. Contrast-enhanced computed tomography shows a right kidney that contains multiple stones surrounded by low-attenuation regions of abscess or necrosis. The process extends into the perirenal tissues, which are edematous and poorly defined, and into the soft tissues beneath the right abdominal wall, which are thickened. Metal-induced artifacts are produced by spinal fixation hardware in this child with dysraphism.

Figure 115-5 Pyonephrosis. A longitudinal sonogram shows a hydronephrotic duplex collecting system. Echogenic debris is present within the upper pole collecting system and ureter (*arrows*). Lesser debris is present within the lower pole collecting system.

culture. With acute disease, percutaneous abscess drainage can serve as a temporizing measure.

CANDIDIASIS

Overview Candidiasis, typically due to *Candida albicans*, accounts for about 80% of renal fungal infections. Premature neonates are particularly susceptible. The clinical presentation in neonates usually is nonspecific: hypertension, oliguria, or anuria. Older children with renal candidiasis usually have immunocompromise. The clinical findings typically are indistinguishable from those of a bacterial infection: fever, chills, dysuria, and flank pain.[25]

Imaging Potential sonographic findings of renal candidiasis include parenchymal hyperechogenicity, nephromegaly, one or more small abscesses, and debris within the collecting system. A fungus ball (mycetoma) in the pelvocaliceal system appears as an echogenic object, with or without acoustic shadowing (Fig. 115-7). Dilation of the collecting system proximal to a fungus ball is common. Findings on contrast-enhanced CT include nephromegaly, diffuse or multifocal edema, renal abscess, and hydronephrosis. Infected parenchyma lacks normal contrast enhancement. Disseminated candidiasis sometimes results in tiny bilateral renal lesions, which often are associated with splenic and hepatic disease. CT may demonstrate organ enlargement and a heterogeneous (salt and pepper) pattern of contrast enhancement.[26,27]

Treatment and Follow-up The typical treatment for renal candidiasis is systemic antifungal medication. Percutaneous nephrostomy is an option for children with an obstructing fungus ball. This treatment allows decompression of the collecting system and provides a pathway for installation of antifungal medication.

TUBERCULOSIS

Overview The urinary system is the most common site of extrapulmonary tuberculosis. Initial infection of the kidney

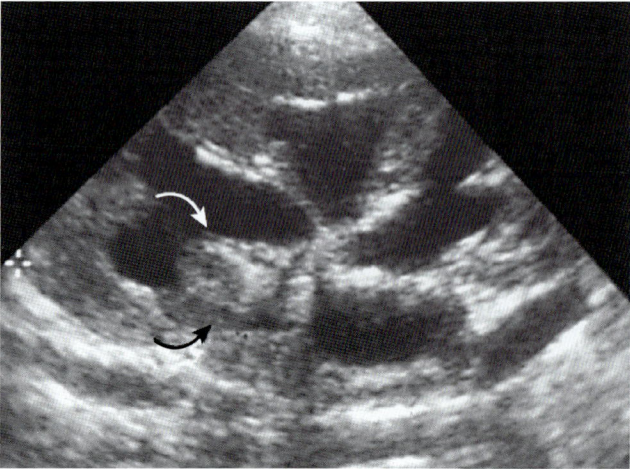

Figure 115-7 Candidiasis. A longitudinal renal sonogram of a premature infant with urinary candidiasis shows hydronephrosis and a small fungus ball in the collecting system (*arrows*). (Courtesy Dr. Beverly Wood, Los Angeles, CA.)

consists of small caseous foci in the renal parenchyma that release the organism into the collecting tubules. Eventually, a larger mass may develop in the renal cortex, resulting in additional discharge of bacteria. Antegrade seeding frequently allows spread of infection to the ureters, prostate, or epididymis. Involvement of the collecting system can progress to fibrosis and calcification, sometimes leading to obstruction. Potential symptoms of urinary tuberculosis include dysuria, flank pain, and gross hematuria.[28]

Imaging In the acute phase of tuberculous infection, imaging of the renal parenchyma may be normal or show manifestations of edema and vasoconstriction. Involved areas lack normal contrast enhancement on CT and MRI and sometimes have altered echogenicity on sonography. Inflamed urothelium may appear thickened on cross-sectional imaging studies and undergo prominent contrast enhancement. Parenchymal edema and large tubercles may cause distortion of the calyceal system. Later in the course of the disease, compromised renal function results in diminished contrast excretion. Contrast sometimes pools within parenchymal cavitations. Multiple small filling defects may be present in the collecting system or ureter. Fibrotic strictures of the collecting system that are common late in the course of the disease result in focal dilation or hydronephrosis. Dystrophic calcifications develop in persons with necrotic parenchyma.[29,30]

Treatment and Follow-up The mainstay treatment of urinary system tuberculosis is systemic antituberculous medication. Imaging studies serve to monitor treatment effectiveness and to detect complications. Apparent obstructive strictures of the ureter sometimes are due to edema that can regress during treatment. A persistent stricture may require surgical intervention.

Stone Disease

OVERVIEW

Urinary system calcifications can occur within the kidneys, ureters, bladder, or urethra. *Urolithiasis* refers to intraluminal stones. The term *nephrolithiasis* indicates calculi within the pelvicalyceal system. *Nephrocalcinosis* refers to intraparenchymal renal calcifications, either medullary or cortical. *Dystrophic* calcification of abnormal tissue, such as the wall of a renal cyst, inflammatory tissue, or a neoplasm, is a potential source of calcifications throughout the urinary system.

NEPHROCALCINOSIS

Medullary Nephrocalcinosis

Overview In more than 90% of children with nephrocalcinosis, the calcification predominantly is in the medullary region. The most common causes of medullary renal calcification in children are metabolic conditions such as renal tubular acidosis, diuretic use, and metabolic conditions that produce hypercalcemia and hypercalciuria (Box 115-1).[31-33]

Etiologies, Pathophysiology, and Clinical Presentation Type 1 renal tubular acidosis (RTA) is the most common metabolic condition associated with nephrocalcinosis in children.

Box 115-1 Causes of Medullary Nephrocalcinosis

Hypercalciuria

Endocrine
- Hyperparathyroidism
- Cushing syndrome
- Diabetes Insipidus
- Hyperthyroidism

Renal
- Renal tubular acidosis

Alimentary
- Milk alkali syndrome
- Hypervitaminosis D

Skeletal
- Immobilization
- Metastatic disease

Drugs
- Furosemide
- Steroids

Miscellaneous
- Idiopathic hypercalciuria
- Idiopathic hypercalcemia
- Nephropathic cystinosis

Urinary Stasis

Obstructive uropathy
Medullary sponge kidney

Hyperoxaluria

Primary

Hyperuricosuria

Secondary

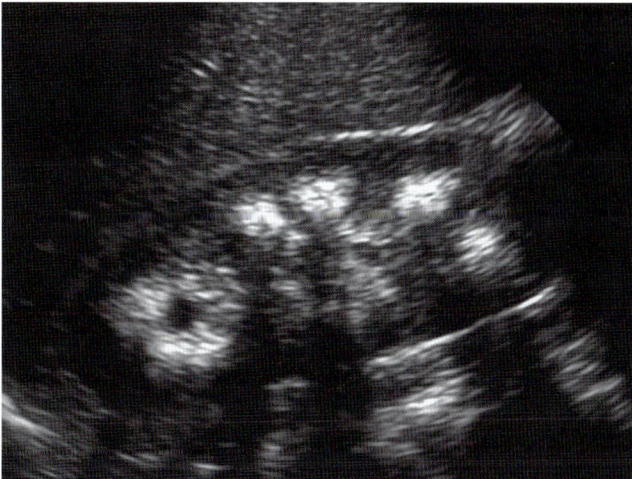

Figure 115-8 Medullary nephrocalcinosis. A longitudinal sonographic image of a child with type 1 renal tubular acidosis and medullary nephrocalcinosis shows markedly echogenic renal pyramids, some of which produce acoustic shadowing.

Nephrocalcinosis occurs in about three quarters of patients with type 1 RTA. Progression to urolithiasis can occur.

The long-term administration of loop diuretics, such as furosemide, is an important cause of nephrocalcinosis in neonates. The typical time course to the earliest manifestations of stone formation is approximately 30 days after the start of diuretic therapy. Spontaneous resolution occurs in most, but not all, of these infants within several months.

Medullary sponge kidney is an idiopathic developmental abnormality in which collecting tubule dilation occurs in one or more renal pyramids. Calcifications can form within the dilated collecting tubules, with the potential for migration into the pelvicalyceal system. Macroscopic renal calcifications are present in about 15% of patients with medullary sponge kidney.

Imaging The major sonographic feature of medullary nephrocalcinosis is hyperechogenicity of one or more renal pyramids (Fig. 115-8). With macroscopic calcification, acoustic shadowing is present. The earliest sonographic sign of medullary nephrocalcinosis is loss of normal papillary hypoechogenicity. In some instances, hyperechogenicity occurs only at the tips of the pyramids.[34,35]

With extensive nephrocalcinosis, medullary calcifications are visible on standard radiographs. Most common are diffuse or uniform calcifications within the medullary pyramids,

resulting in a triangular pattern. Renal calcification in patients with type 1 RTA typically is quite dense and involves all the medullary pyramids in a uniform fashion. Calcifications associated with medullary sponge kidney tend to be asymmetric.[36]

CT allows definitive localization of calcifications to the medullary or cortical regions (Fig. 115-9). With medullary sponge kidney, medullary calculi typically occur in clusters within the renal pyramids. Stagnation of contrast material is evident within the dilated collecting tubules on enhanced CT. With mild disease, stagnation of contrast material appears as linear papillary opacities; small cystic components may be visible with more advanced disease. With medullary sponge kidney, contrast material within the collecting tubules surrounds calculi. In patients with type 1 RTA, the contrast does not uniformly surround calcific deposits because the calcifications are within the medullary interstitium and tubular lumina.[37]

The Anderson-Carr-Randall progression theory of urolithiasis suggests that microscopic calcifications within a renal

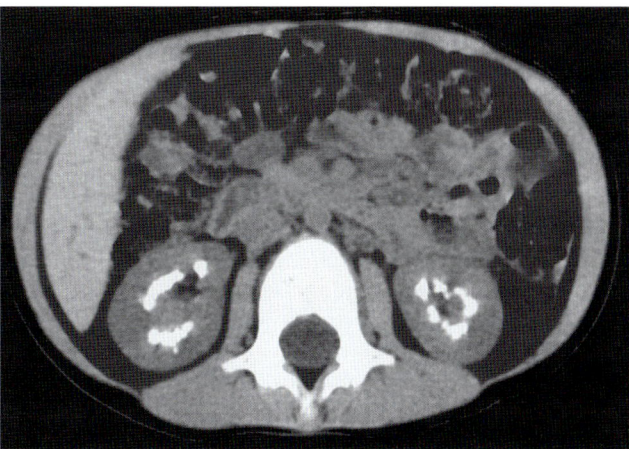

Figure 115-9 Medullary nephrocalcinosis. Unenhanced computed tomography shows dense renal pyramid calcifications in a child with type 1 renal tubular acidosis.

Box 115-2   Causes of Cortical Nephrocalcinosis

- Renal cortical necrosis
- Chronic glomerulonephritis
- Renal transplant rejection
- Alport syndrome
- Ethylene glycol poisoning
- Hyperoxaluria
- Acquired immunodeficiency syndrome–associated infections

pyramid can coalesce to form a plaque that migrates toward the calyx and thereby form a stone nidus. High-resolution ultrasonography of young children may reveal papillary hyperechogenicity caused by these microscopic calcifications, despite normal findings on other imaging studies. Hyperechoic pyramids are present in about 50% of children with diseases that predispose to nephrocalcinosis. Subepithelial calcium phosphate plaques sometimes are visible on radiographs or CT as slivers of calcification adjacent to the papillary tip.[38]

Treatment and Follow-up   Adequate hydration is an important preventive measure in patients with known nephrocalcinosis or a metabolic condition that can cause nephrocalcinosis. Various medical therapies are designed to reduce renal calcium excretion and increase the solubility of urinary calcium. These techniques occasionally serve to lessen the severity of nephrocalcinosis over time. However, nephrocalcinosis is irreversible for most patients. Imaging studies provide early detection of renal calcifications, monitor response to therapy, and detect complications such as obstructive urolithiasis.

Cortical Nephrocalcinosis

Overview and Imaging   Cortical nephrocalcinosis involves the periphery of the kidney and the central septa of Bertin. In the pure forms of cortical nephrocalcinosis, the medullary pyramids are spared. The most common causes of cortical nephrocalcinosis are chronic glomerulonephritis, acute cortical necrosis, and oxalosis (Box 115-2). Standard abdominal radiographs may show thin linear peripheral calcifications, diffuse homogeneous renal calcification, or diffuse punctate calcifications. On sonography, the involved cortex is echogenic, but acoustic shadowing does not occur unless conglomerate calcifications are present. CT accurately demonstrates the cortical location of calcification.[33,39]

Hyperoxaluria can cause nephrocalcinosis or nephrolithiasis. Renal calcifications in these patients often are predominantly cortical and can have a patchy or homogeneous character. Occasionally, calcification occurs throughout the cortical and medullary regions. During infancy, sonography may reveal enlarged hyperechoic kidneys without acoustic shadowing or other manifestation of macroscopic calcification. Eventually, parenchymal thickness decreases.

Cortical hyperechogenicity in patients with acute renal cortical necrosis may be visible on sonography within a few weeks of the injury. Calcifications become more obvious sonographically and radiographically over time. Progressive renal atrophy also occurs. Various patterns of nephrocalcinosis can occur in these patients: (1) punctate, (2) bandlike peripheral calcification with perpendicular extensions into the columns of Bertin, and (3) thin, parallel curvilinear calcifications at the interface between the necrotic cortex and the viable subcapsular cortex (i.e., the "tram-track" pattern).

UROLITHIASIS

Overview   The prevalence of urolithiasis varies according to geographic area, age, sex, and race. In the United States, urolithiasis affects approximately 1 in 1000 children. Urolithiasis is slightly more common in Europe than in North America and is considerably more common in Asia. In American children, the prevalence of urolithiasis is greatest in southern California and in the southeastern states. Urolithiasis is more common in white persons than in African Americans.[31,40-42]

Pathophysiology   About 70% of patients with urolithiasis have a known predisposing condition such as hypercalciuria, urinary stasis, or chronic infection (Table 115-1). A genitourinary anomaly is present in at least one third of children with nephrocalcinosis and in nearly all patients with renal calculi related to infection. Urolithiasis is common in patients

Table 115-1

Causes of Urolithiasis and the Most Commonly Associated Types of Stones	
Underlying Condition	**Associated Stones**
Idiopathic	Calcium
Urinary stasis 　Congenital obstruction 　Neurogenic bladder 　Pyelocalyceal diverticulum 　Surgical urinary diversions	Calcium
Urinary tract infection	Struvite, triple phosphate
Hypercalciuria 　Idiopathic hypercalciuria 　Idiopathic infantile hypercalcemia 　Hyperparathyroidism 　Sarcoidosis 　Type 1 renal tubular acidosis 　Immobilization 　Long-term diuretic use 　Hypervitaminosis D 　Hyperthyroidism 　Bone metastasis 　Prolonged corticosteroid therapy 　Fanconi syndrome	Calcium
Hyperoxaluria 　Primary oxaluria 　Small-bowel disease	Calcium oxalate
Hyperuricosuria 　Lymphoproliferative and myeloproliferative disorders 　Tumor lysis 　Lesch-Nyhan syndrome	Uric acid
Cystinuria 　Hereditary cystinuria	Cystine
Xanthinuria 　Hereditary xanthinuria 　Allopurinol therapy	Xanthine

with a urinary tract infection because of a urea-splitting gram-negative enteric organism. These "infection stones" usually are a mixture of magnesium ammonium phosphate (struvite) and calcium phosphate (apatite), that is, a "triple phosphate stone." Struvite is the predominant composition of most staghorn calculi. Nonstruvite stones that occur in association with urinary tract infections are termed "infection-associated stones." Patients with a neurogenic bladder, a congenital urinary tract obstruction, and other forms of urinary stasis have a propensity for calcium stones and infection stones.[43-45]

Hypercalciuria is a common cause of calcium stones. Hyperoxaluria is an additional potential cause of urinary stones that contain calcium. Uric acid stones due to hyperuricosuria account for only 5% of stones in North American children, but they are common in some areas of the world (e.g., Israel). Cystinuria and xanthinuria are rare causes of urolithiasis. Matrix stones are rare stones that consist of nonradiopaque inspissated mucoproteins, usually in conjunction with laminated or scattered calcific components. About 30% of pediatric urolithiasis is idiopathic. The typical composition of idiopathic stones is calcium phosphate or calcium oxalate. Idiopathic calcium stones sometimes have a nucleus of urate.[46]

Bladder stones can either originate from the upper urinary tract or develop within the bladder (Fig. 115-10). Bladder stones often are laminated and sometimes reach a very large size. Bladder stones also can form in a bladder diverticulum, surgical pouch, or urachal remnant.

Urethral calculi are rare and only occur in males (Fig. 115-11). They can originate from a more proximal portion of the urinary tract or arise locally. Primary urethral calculi

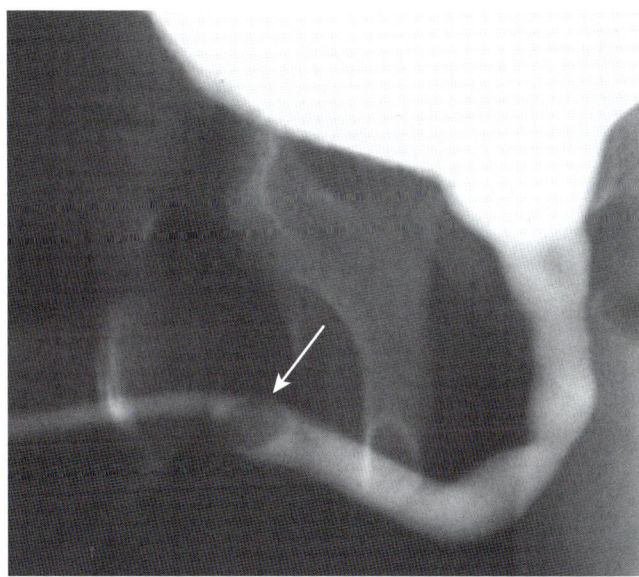

Figure 115-11 **Urethral calculus.** A urethrogram shows a partially obstructing urethral calculus as a filling defect (*arrow*) in the contrast column.

sometimes develop in association with prolonged obstruction or within a urethral diverticulum or the prostatic utricle.

Clinical Presentation   Pain is present in 50% to 75% of children with urolithiasis at the time of diagnosis. Pain can localize to the abdomen or flank and may or may not radiate. Additional potential clinical manifestations include hematuria (which is common), urgency, dysuria, frequency, fever, pyuria, and bacteriuria. Urinary retention can occur in patients with stones of the bladder or urethra.

Imaging   About 90% of urinary tract calculi are sufficiently radiopaque for visualization on standard radiographs (Table 115-2). Classification of a stone as radiopaque versus nonopaque (or radiolucent) is according to its appearance on standard radiographs (Fig. 115-12); most nonopaque stones are hyperattenuating on CT. In general, calcium stones are radiopaque. Stones composed of pure uric acid, xanthine, or struvite usually are nonopaque. Cystine stones are moderately radiopaque.[47,48]

Both radiopaque and nonopaque urinary tract stones appear echogenic on sonography and produce acoustic shadowing (Fig. 115-13). Sonography is sensitive for the

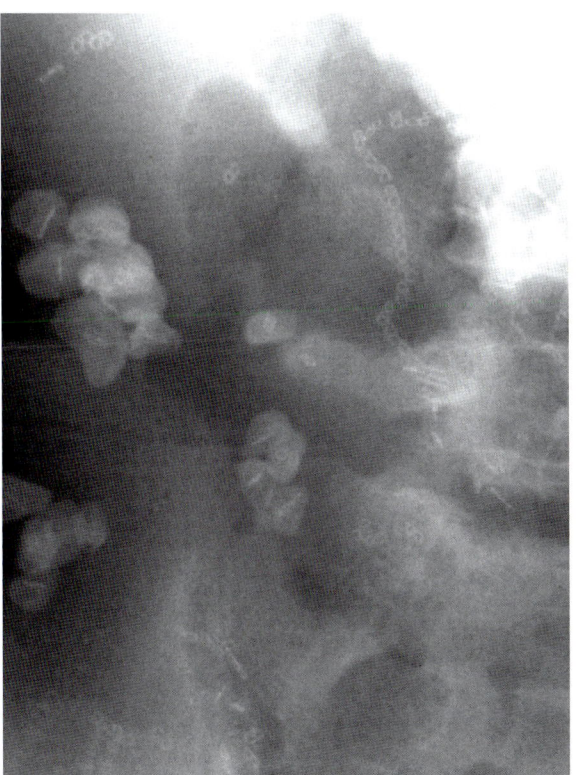

Figure 115-10 **Bladder calculi.** A radiograph of the right lower quadrant shows multiple calculi within a bladder augmentation. A surgical clip serves as the nidus for each of the stones.

Table 115-2

Radiopacity of Urinary Stones and Relative Frequency in North American Children		
Stone	**Opacity**	**% of Stones**
Calcium stones	+++	75-80
Struvite	−	10-15
Triple phosphate	++	
Cystine	+	Rare
Uric acid	−	5
Xanthine	−	Rare
Matrix	−	Rare

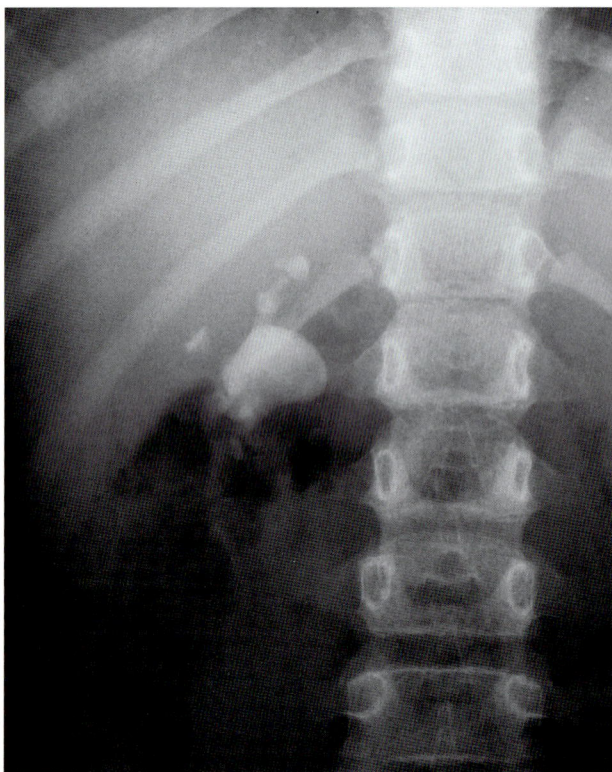

Figure 115-12 **Staghorn calculus.** This triple phosphate infection stone is radiopaque.

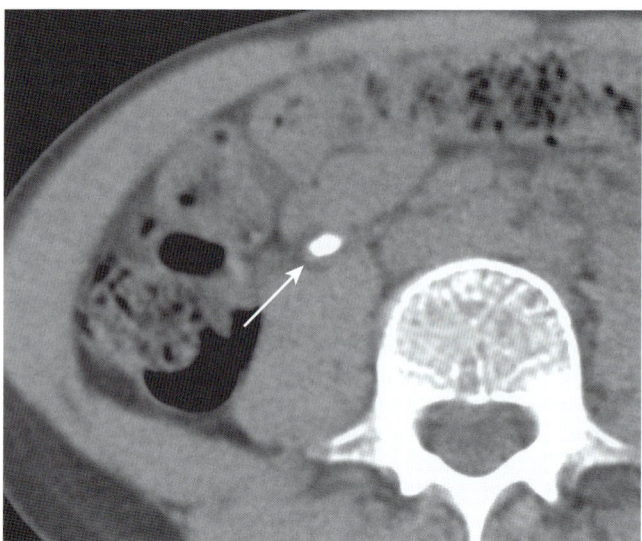

Figure 115-14 **Ureteral calculus.** Unenhanced computed tomography shows a right ureteral calculus with a surrounding thickened ureteral rim (*arrow*).

detection of nephrolithiasis but is of limited utility for visualizing calculi in the ureters. An obstructing ureteral calculus usually is associated with some degree of ureteropelvocalyectasis, however. The sonographic appearance of acoustic shadowing aids in the differentiation of a bladder calculus from blood clot, debris, or tumor.

Multi-detector CT is the most sensitive imaging technique for the detection of urolithiasis (Fig. 115-14). Regardless of composition, nearly all urinary tract stones are hyperattenuating on CT. Calcium oxalate stones generally have attenuation values in the 800 to 1000 HU range, infection stones are in

the 300 to 900 HU range, and uric acid stones usually measure between 150 to 500 HU. Secondary CT signs of an obstructing urinary tract stone include hydronephrosis, hydroureter, nephromegaly, delayed nephrogram, periureteral edema, and perinephric stranding or fluid. Usually, the portion of the ureteral wall that surrounds a calculus thickens (the "rim sign"); this sign typically is lacking with a phlebolith or other mimicking calcification. A linear soft tissue density (the involved pelvic vein) often extends from a phlebolith; this feature is the "comet tail sign."[47,49,50]

WHAT THE CLINICIAN NEEDS TO KNOW

- Echogenicity/attenuation/signal intensity of parenchyma
- Scintigraphic or enhancement defects
- Renal or perirenal abscess
- Caliber of collecting system
- Locations and radiopacity of stones
- Parenchymal calcifications

Key Points

Renal cortical scintigraphy and contrast-enhanced CT are highly sensitive for the detection of parenchymal renal infections.

Renal candidiasis usually occurs in premature infants and immunocompromised persons.

Pyelonephritis in children can occur without pyuria or vesicoureteral reflux.

Most children with nephrocalcinosis have hypercalcemia and/or hypercalciuria.

Most children with urolithiasis have a known predisposing condition such as hypercalciuria, urinary stasis, or chronic infection.

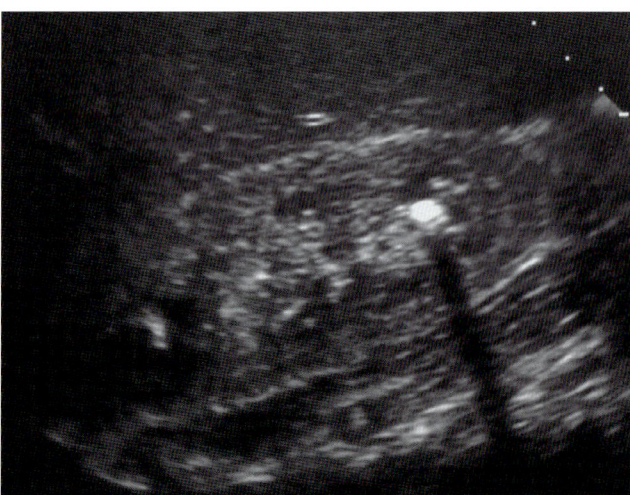

Figure 115-13 **Nephrolithiasis.** A longitudinal sonographic image of an infant with hypercalcemia and Williams syndrome reveals an echogenic calculus in a right lower pole calyx.

Suggested Readings

Craig WD, Wagner BJ, Travis MD. Pyelonephritis: radiologic-pathologic review. *Radiographics*. 2008;28(1):255-277; quiz 327-328.

Lavocat MP, Granjon D, Allard D, et al. Imaging of pyelonephritis. *Pediatr Radiol*. 1997;27(2):159-165.

Hoppe B, Kemper MJ. Diagnostic examination of the child with urolithiasis or nephrocalcinosis. *Pediatr Nephrol*. 2010;25(3):403-413.

Kraus SJ, Lebowitz RL, Royal SA. Renal calculi in children: imaging eatures that lead to diagnoses: a pictorial essay. *Pediatr Radiol*. 1999; 29(8):624-630.

References

Full references for this chapter can be found on www.expertconsult.com.

Chapter 116

Renal Neoplasms

D. GREGORY BATES and KATE A. FEINSTEIN

Nephroblastomatosis Complex

Overview and Pathophysiology Nephrogenesis is completed by the 36th gestational week. A focus of fetal metanephric blastema or embryonal renal tissue that persists beyond 36 weeks gestation is called a nephrogenic rest. Multiple foci or diffuse nephrogenic rests are termed *nephroblastomatosis*. Nephrogenic rests are identified in about 1% of neonatal autopsies but usually are no longer found after 4 months of age. Malignant transformation of the fetal metanephric blastema may occur, along with development of a Wilms tumor (nephroblastoma), or nephroblastomatosis may resolve spontaneously.[1-3]

Nephrogenic rests can occur anywhere in the kidney, depending on when nephrogenesis is interrupted. These rests may be located in the renal lobe (intralobar) or in the cortex that envelops the renal lobe (perilobar). The two types of nephrogenic rests have different appearances, malignant potential, and associated genetic abnormalities. Nephrogenic rests also are classified according to histologic features of development; hyperplastic and neoplastic rests are thought to be active and to have malignant potential, whereas dormant or sclerosing nephrogenic rests are considered inactive.[1-4]

Intralobar nephrogenic rests are less common than perilobar nephrogenic rests and are more likely to degenerate into a Wilms tumor. Intralobar nephrogenic rests tend to be few and are located randomly in the renal lobe; they are seen in patients with sporadic aniridia, Drash syndrome (i.e., male pseudohermaphrodism and nephritis), and WAGR syndrome (i.e., Wilms tumor, aniridia, genital anomalies, and mental retardation). Patients with sporadic aniridia have a 30% to 40% risk of having a Wilms tumor develop, which represents the greatest likelihood of all of the genetic and syndromic abnormalities associated with nephroblastomatosis.[1-4]

Perilobar nephrogenic rests are multiple and are located at the corticomedullary junction or in the cortex. Also called diffuse perilobar nephrogenic rests or diffuse perilobar nephroblastomatosis, they are found in persons with hemihypertrophy and in persons with Beckwith-Wiedemann syndrome (i.e., macroglossia, macrosomia, and omphalocele), Perlman syndrome (i.e., fetal gigantism and multiple congenital anomalies), and trisomy 18 syndrome. Patients with hemihypertrophy and Beckwith-Wiedemann syndrome have about a 5% risk of having a Wilms tumor develop.[1,3-5]

Imaging Microscopic nephrogenic rests cannot be identified radiologically. Diffuse perilobar nephroblastomatosis and multifocal nephroblastomatosis can be evaluated through ultrasonography, computed tomography (CT), and magnetic resonance imaging (MRI). In diffuse perilobar nephroblastomatosis, the affected kidney may be enlarged. On sonography, corticomedullary differentiation is absent. Regions of nephroblastomatosis may be hypoechoic or isoechoic with respect to normal renal cortex (Fig. 116-1). Multifocal nephroblastomatosis is more difficult to identify on sonography.[2,3,6]

CT is more sensitive than ultrasound for the evaluation of nephroblastomatosis. On contrast-enhanced CT, areas of nephroblastomatosis are well defined because they enhance to a lesser extent than does normal renal cortex (Fig. 116-2). Bulky masses of nephroblastomatosis may distort the pelvicalyceal system. Involvement may be symmetric or asymmetric (e-Fig. 116-3). In diffuse perilobar nephroblastomatosis, a thick rind of lower attenuation tissue encases normally enhancing but architecturally distorted parenchyma. In persons with multifocal nephroblastomatosis, multiple round masses of low attenuation are present. Flat or plaquelike areas of involvement may be difficult to identify on CT.[2,3,6]

On MRI, nephroblastomatosis cannot be distinguished from normal renal parenchyma on T1-weighted sequences and is isointense or hyperintense on T2-weighted sequences. Nephroblastomatosis appears hypointense relative to normal renal parenchyma after administration of contrast material on T1-weighted sequences, which are the most sensitive for detection. Active areas of nephroblastomatosis typically are hyperintense on T2-weighted sequences, and inactive areas are hypointense. The signal intensity of nephroblastomatosis is homogeneous, whereas foci of Wilms tumor tend to be heterogeneous.[2,3,6-8]

Treatment and Follow-up Although the subject is somewhat controversial, presently no specific treatment is advocated for nephrogenic rests/nephroblastomatosis. Close radiologic follow-up is recommended for children with genetic abnormalities or syndromes associated with nephroblastomatosis. Patients should be monitored to detect Wilms tumor development, because the prognosis for Wilms tumor is best with small lesions. Children with hemihypertrophy or Beckwith-Wiedemann syndrome are at risk for the development of other embryonal tumors, such as hepatoblastoma and adrenal

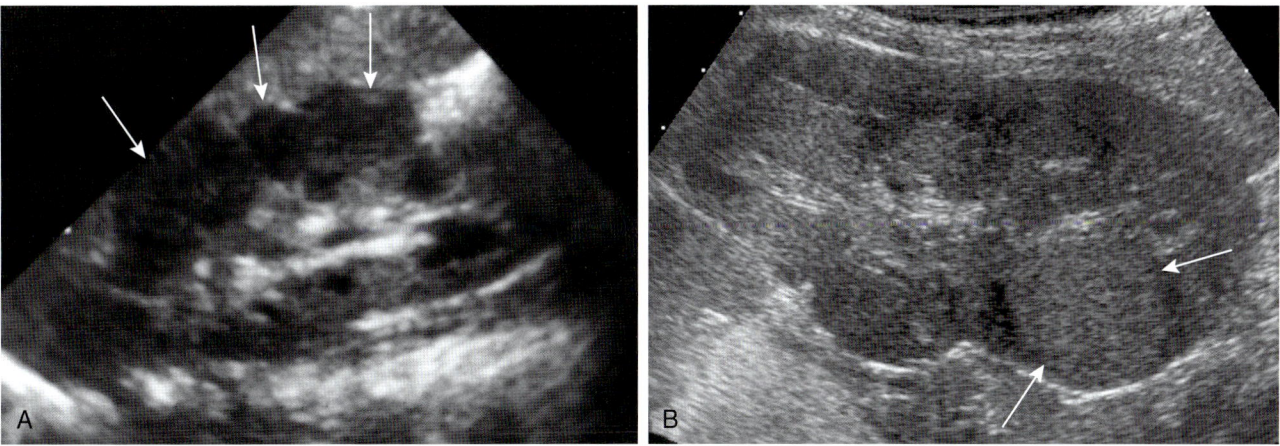

Figure 116-1 Nephroblastomatosis. **A,** Diffuse perilobar form. A longitudinal sonogram shows an enlarged right kidney with lobulated contour and hypoechoic cortical masses (*arrows*). **B,** Focal intralobar form. A longitudinal sonogram shows a lower pole mass (*arrows*) that is isoechoic with renal cortex.

cell carcinoma. No large studies have been performed to establish the optimal screening interval for Wilms tumor surveillance; however, large tumors with metastases that develop within a 6-month period are reported. A baseline CT of nephroblastomatosis-related genetic abnormalities or syndromes at 6 months of age (or at diagnosis if the patient is older than 6 months), followed by ultrasound examinations every 3 to 4 months until the child is 8 years of age, is recommended on the basis of results from the National Wilms Tumor Studies. An area of nephroblastomatosis that grows larger and rounder is suspicious for malignant degeneration.[2,3,9-13]

Wilms Tumor

Overview, Pathophysiology, and Staging Wilms tumor is the most common abdominal malignancy of childhood and

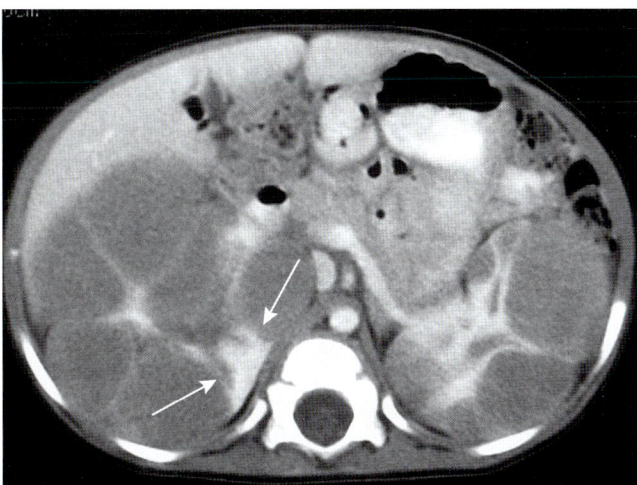

Figure 116-2 Diffuse perilobar nephroblastomatosis with symmetric involvement. On a contrast-enhanced computed tomography scan, the kidneys are enlarged and multiple, round, peripheral masses of low attenuation are present. Architectural distortion at this level is pronounced; in the medial portion of the right kidney, only a peripheral area of normally enhancing kidney (*arrows*) is present.

accounts for 87% of renal masses. Its peak incidence is at 3 to 4 years of age (80% occur in children <5 years), but it has been described in the fetus, neonate, teenager, and adult. Clinical presentation includes a palpable mass, abdominal pain, hematuria, and occasional hypertension (from tumor renin production). As discussed in the Nephroblastomatosis Complex section of this chapter, certain syndromes and genetic abnormalities predispose to development of a Wilms tumor (e-Fig. 116-4). Two loci on chromosome 11 have been implicated in the genesis of Wilms tumors: 11p13 (*WT1* gene—WAGR or Drash syndrome) and 11p15 (*WT2* gene—Beckwith-Wiedemann syndrome or hemihypertrophy). Bilateral Wilms tumors occur almost exclusively in patients with nephroblastomatosis. Most Wilms tumors arise from the renal parenchyma; however, extrarenal Wilms tumors rarely may develop in the abdomen or at distant sites.[1,14-17]

In the United States, tumor stage (Box 116-1) is determined operatively, and the grade is established on pathologic examination. The classic triphasic Wilms tumor arises from mesodermal precursors of the renal parenchyma (metanephros) and contains blastemal, stromal, and epithelial elements. The "teratoid Wilms tumor" contains tissue not normally found in the kidney (e.g., bone, cartilage, and muscle). Tumors with a favorable histology do not contain any anaplastic changes. The prognosis for tumors with a favorable histology is excellent, even for those at higher stages. In Europe, the staging system is based completely on radiologic findings. Tumors are classified on the basis of their imaging appearance, and chemotherapy is given before definitive surgery is performed. Tumors with extension into the inferior vena cava or invasion through the renal capsule are easier to resect after tumor shrinkage produced by chemotherapy.[1,2,18]

Imaging Radiologic evaluation of Wilms tumor is focused on identifying the site(s) of involvement, extension, and metastases to assist in surgical planning. Preoperative imaging may include conventional chest radiography, abdominal and pelvic sonography, and thoracic, abdominal, and pelvic CT, MRI, and potentially fluorine deoxyglucose positron emission tomography (FDG-PET) fused with CT (PET-CT).[1,2,19,20]

Box 116-1   Children's Oncology Group Staging of Wilms Tumor

Stage I

- A completely resected tumor limited to the kidney with an intact capsule
- No biopsy or rupture of tumor prior to removal
- No involvement of vessels or renal sinuses
- No tumor at or beyond the margins of resection
- Regional lymph nodes are negative for tumor

Stage II

- A completely resected tumor
- No tumor at or beyond the margins of resection
- Regional lymph nodes are negative for tumor
- One or more of the following findings:
  - Penetration of the renal capsule
  - Invasion of vasculature extending beyond the renal parenchyma

Stage III

- Residual tumor is present after surgery, confined to the abdomen, with one or more of the following attributes present:
  - One or more regional lymph nodes are positive for tumor
  - The tumor is implanted on or penetrating through the peritoneum
  - The presence of gross unresected tumor or tumor at the margin of resection
  - Any tumor spillage occurring before or during surgery, including biopsy
  - The tumor was removed in more than one piece

Stage IV

- The presence of hematogenous metastasis (e.g., lung, liver, bone, or brain)
- The presence of lymph node metastasis outside the abdomen and pelvis

Stage V

- Wilms tumor in both kidneys

From Gratias EJ, Dome JS. Current and emerging chemotherapy treatment strategies for Wilms tumor in North America. *Paediatr Drugs.* 2008;10(2):115-124.

On sonography, a Wilms tumor is an intrarenal mass of heterogeneous echogenicity. Some Wilms tumors may contain cystic components, portions of obstructed and entrapped pelvicalyceal systems, or hemorrhagic and necrotic tumor. Extension into the inferior vena cava and the right atrium are characteristic routes of tumor growth and can be well visualized on ultrasound (e-Fig. 116-5), CT (Fig. 116-6), and MRI. The tumor typically forms a pseudocapsule but may invade the renal capsule, seed the peritoneal space, or grow directly into the mesentery and omentum. Hepatic metastases also are possible. The contralateral kidney may contain a smaller Wilms tumor or nephroblastomatosis. Synchronous or metachronous bilateral Wilms tumor may occur in up to 10% of patients.[1,2,6]

On CT, Wilms tumor is generally spherical and intrarenal. It may contain small amounts of fat or fine calcification (Fig. 116-7 and e-Fig. 116-8) because the metanephric blastema cell is a pluripotential embryonal cell. Dystrophic calcifications are seen in about 9% of Wilms tumors. The tumor enhances to a lesser extent than does renal parenchyma. In patients who have been screened ultrasonographically because of genetic or syndromic conditions, the tumor is usually smaller than 4 cm in diameter. Children who are evaluated because of physical examination abnormalities generally have tumors larger than 10 cm in diameter. CT and conventional radiographs of the chest are used to identify pulmonary metastases.[1,2,6,21,22]

On MRI, a Wilms tumor is isointense with respect to normal renal parenchyma on T1-weighted sequences and hyperintense with respect to normal renal parenchyma on T2-weighted sequences. After administration of contrast material, a Wilms tumor is hypointense relative to normal renal parenchyma and has inhomogeneous signal intensity (Fig. 116-9). An effectively treated Wilms tumor may be hypointense on T2-weighted sequences.[1,2,7,8,23]

FDG-PET fused with CT is a rapidly developing modality for imaging accelerated metabolism in malignant tissue. FDG-PET has better accuracy than MRI and bone scanning for staging. Wilms tumors are presumed to be FDG-avid, but the role of FDG in Wilms evaluation is as yet unclear. FDG-PET can help with a targeted biopsy of a viable Wilms tumor and biologically aggressive elements (e.g., anaplastic Wilms). Sensitivity for lung metastases is dependent on nodule size and respiratory motion. Treatment response of the primary tumor can be monitored. Potential benefits of FDG-PET will require ongoing investigation.[2]

Treatment   Surgery for a Wilms tumor typically begins with a complete abdominal exploration before attention is given to the kidneys. The unaffected kidney initially is visualized and palpated to assess for masses or areas of superficial nephroblastomatosis before en bloc resection of the affected kidney is performed. An excisional biopsy of lung nodules is performed to ensure that the stage of the tumor is correctly assigned. Patients with bilateral disease undergo staging surgery as well. Results of the surgical staging and the histologic examination determine the selection of therapy. In patients with bilateral disease, treatment is provided according to the tumor histology of the higher stage side, along with later nephron-sparing surgery. When the tumor is very large or when the tumor extends into the right atrium via the inferior vena cava, the surgeon may defer surgery until several courses of chemotherapy have reduced the tumor size or extension. Substantial progress in therapy for persons with a Wilms tumor over recent decades has resulted in a greater than 90% long-term survival for localized disease and greater than 70% survival for metastatic disease.[1,2,24-30]

Clear Cell Sarcoma of the Kidney

Overview   Clear cell sarcoma of the kidney accounts for approximately 5% of primary renal tumors in childhood and was considered a sarcomatous subtype of Wilms tumor before 1978. It was reclassified as a separate entity from Wilms tumor because of the tumor's histologically and biologically unique features. No familial or syndrome association has been identified. Clear cell sarcoma occurs in an age group similar to that affected by Wilms tumor (1 to 4 years of age), and has a male predominance. Immunohistochemical staining has

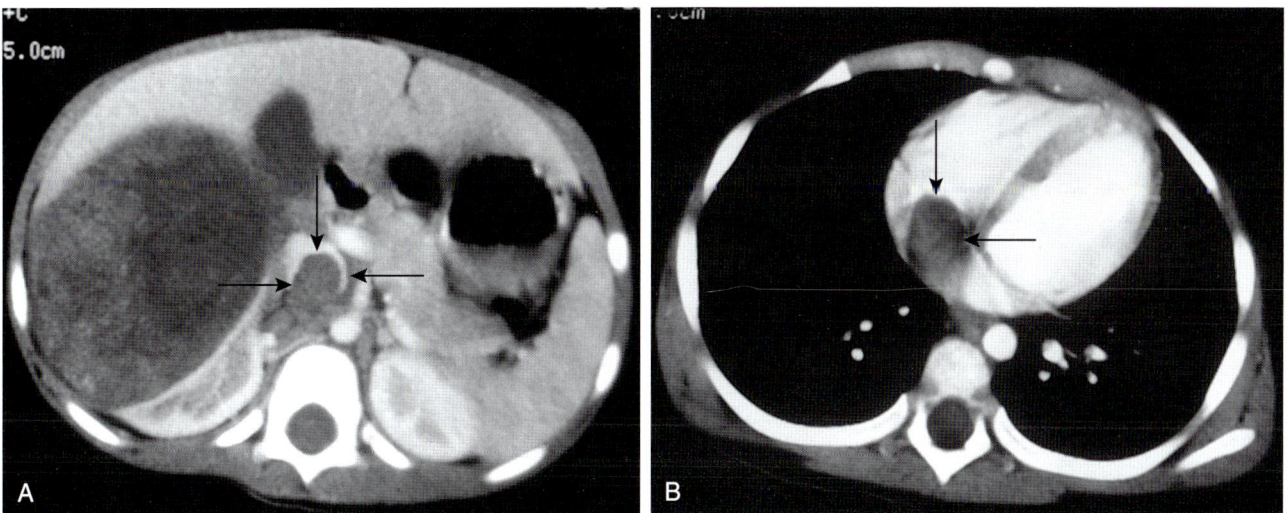

Figure 116-6   A Wilms tumor extending into the inferior vena cava and right atrium. **A,** A contrast-enhanced computed tomography scan reveals a large, round, heterogeneous mass in the right kidney that enhances to a lesser extent than normal renal parenchyma. Contrast material opacifies the lateral and anterior margins of the inferior vena cava that contain hypoattenuating tumor (*arrows*). **B,** The tumor (*arrows*) extends into the right atrium.

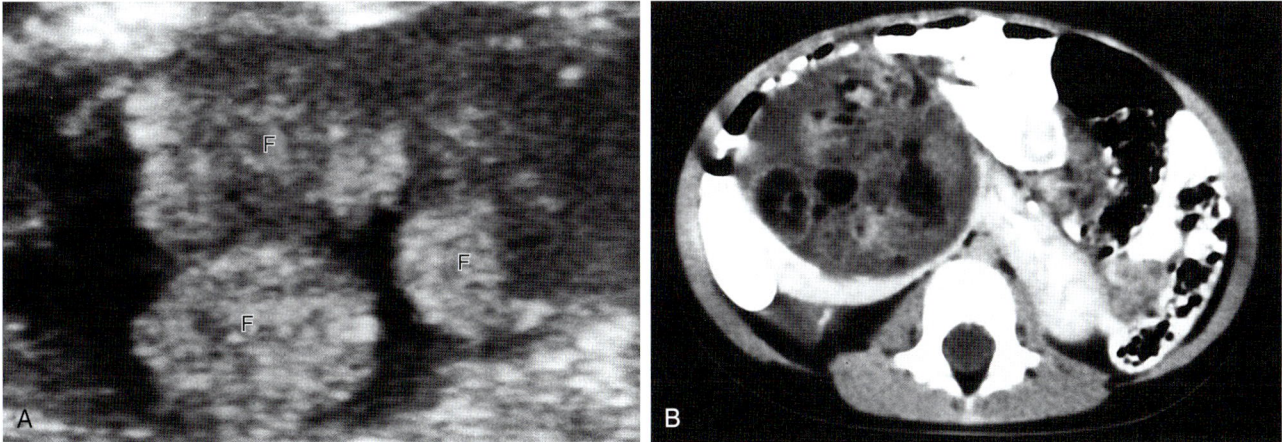

Figure 116-7   A Wilms tumor containing fat in a horseshoe kidney. **A,** An axial sonogram of part of the Wilms tumor reveals hyperechoic lobules containing fat (*F*). **B,** A contrast-enhanced computed tomography scan shows areas of fat within the mass. The isthmus of the renal parenchyma extends across the midline.

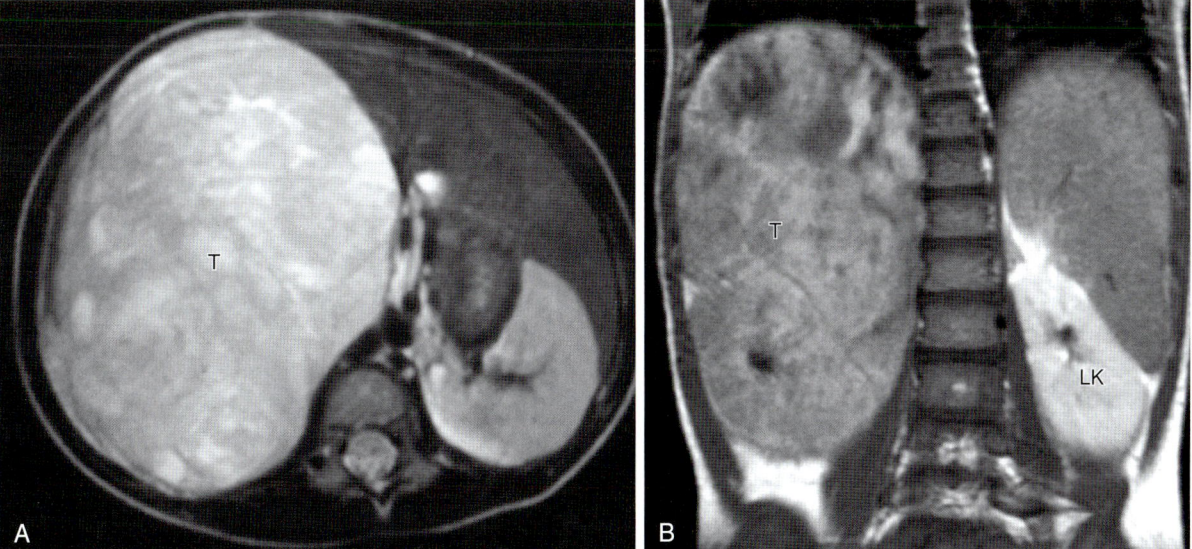

Figure 116-9   A Wilms tumor. **A,** Axial T2-weighted magnetic resonance imaging (MRI) shows a large tumor (*T*) replacing the right kidney, which is hyperintense to other soft tissue structures. **B,** Coronal T1-weighted MRI after gadolinium in the same patient shows that the large tumor (*T*) is hypointense relative to the normally enhancing left kidney (*LK*).

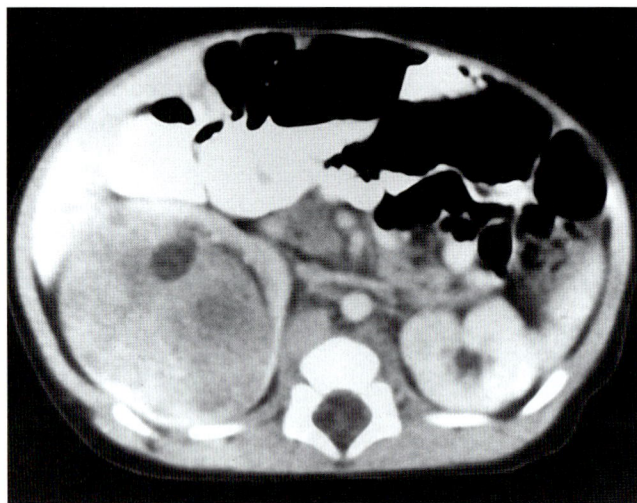

Figure 116-10 **A clear cell sarcoma of the kidney.** A contrast-enhanced computed tomography (CT) scan shows a large, round heterogeneous right renal mass. The mass was identified on antenatal sonography, and CT was performed on the second day of life.

shown no characteristic marker pattern, but negativity to the *WT1* gene is important.

Imaging and Treatment   Clear cell sarcoma imaging features are not distinct from those of the Wilms tumor (Fig. 116-10). Clear cell sarcoma has a predilection for bone metastases (formerly known as the bone metastasizing renal tumor of childhood) that may occur at presentation or upon relapse. A pathologic diagnosis of clear cell sarcoma necessitates an evaluation of the skeletal system. Bone scintigraphy or a conventional radiographic skeletal survey may be used. However, metastases to lymph nodes, lung, and liver still are seen more frequently than bone metastases. Because of the aggressive behavior of clear cell sarcoma, it is associated with a higher rate or relapse and mortality than is Wilms tumor, with a reported long-term survival of 60% to 70%. Treatment consists of nephrectomy and aggressive chemotherapy.[1,31-38]

Rhabdoid Tumor of the Kidney

Overview   Rhabdoid tumor of the kidney accounts for 2% of pediatric renal malignancies and was considered a sarcomatous variant of Wilms tumor before 1978, when it was reclassified as a separate entity. The name is derived from its monomorphous histologic appearance resembling that of skeletal muscle, although a myogenic origin has not been proved. Rhabdoid tumors occur in a younger age group than do Wilms tumors (80% occur in children younger than 2 years of age). The most common clinical presentation is hematuria secondary invasion of the renal pelvis. Fever, hypertension, hypercalcemia (elevated parathormone levels), and cutaneous nodules ("blueberry muffin baby") also are reported.

Imaging   As is seen with clear cell sarcoma of the kidney, rhabdoid tumors of the kidney have imaging features similar to those of Wilms tumors. Imaging features that may suggest the diagnosis include subcapsular fluid collections, medial location within the kidney, and tumor lobules separated by

low-density hemorrhage or necrosis and outlined by calcifications. Rhabdoid tumor of the kidney is highly aggressive, metastasizes early, and presents with advanced disease. A distinct association with synchronous or metachronous primary or metastatic central nervous system lesions is seen, often in the posterior fossa. Primitive neuroectodermal tumors, medulloblastomas, ependymomas, and cerebellar and brainstem astrocytomas all have been reported. After tissue diagnosis, MRI of the brain is recommended.

Treatment   Rhabdoid tumors have the worst prognosis of all of the childhood renal tumors, with an 18-month survival rate of only 20%. Treatment includes nephrectomy, radiation therapy to the tumor bed, and aggressive chemotherapy.[1,39-46]

Congenital Mesoblastic Nephroma

Overview   Congenital mesoblastic nephroma (CMN) is the most common solid renal tumor of infancy. Originally thought to represent a congenital Wilms tumor, it is recognized as a distinct neoplasm and also is referred to as a fetal renal hamartoma. It usually is identified in the first 3 months of life. Clinical presentation is that of a palpable abdominal mass and, less frequently, hematuria. Histologically, the tumor is composed of monomorphic infiltrating spindle-shaped mesenchymal cells and embryonal metaplasia of entrapped renal tissue. CMN is subtyped into classic, cellular, and mixed forms. On gross sectioning, the tumor resembles a uterine leiomyoma.

Imaging   A mesoblastic nephroma tends to be a large infiltrative mass; it has poorly defined margins and lacks a capsule. Ultrasound should be the initial imaging study performed. A mesoblastic nephroma is predominantly solid but may contain cystic components (Fig. 116-11). A concentric hyperechoic and hypoechoic ring pattern may be seen reflecting dilated vasculature and entrapped nephrons. The mass may distort and displace the pelvicalyceal system. On CT, CMN may be homogeneous or heterogeneous, is unilateral and unifocal,

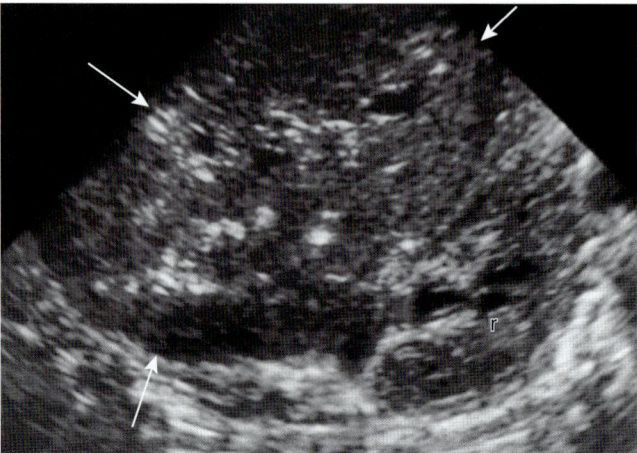

Figure 116-11 **A congenital mesoblastic nephroma.** On coronal sonography, the large, round mass (*arrows*) is predominantly solid, with foci of hyperechogenicity. A portion of the normal kidney (*r*) is present inferomedially.

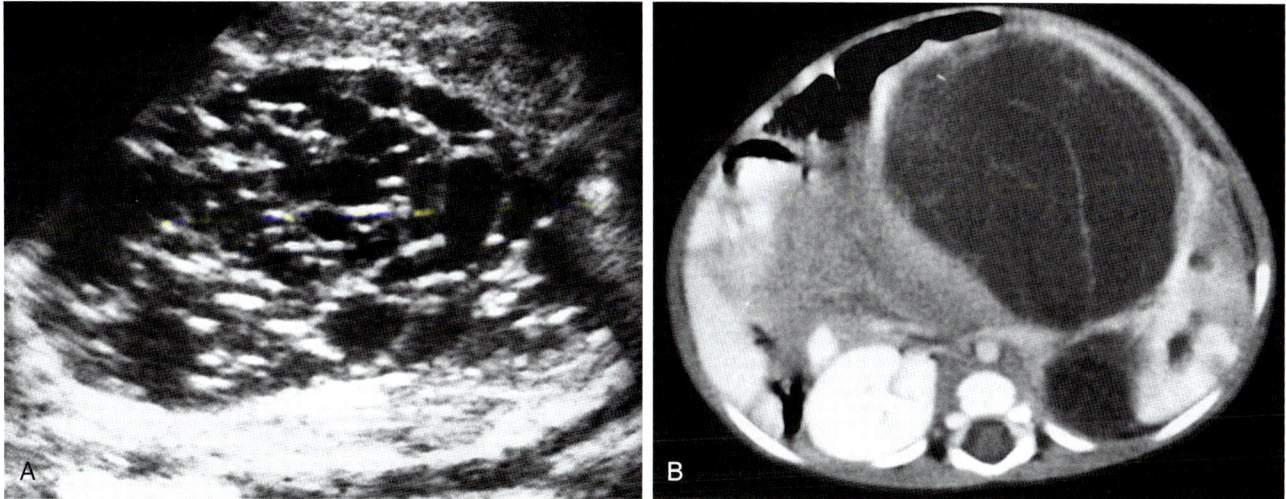

Figure 116-12 A partially differentiated cystic nephroblastoma. **A,** A sagittal sonogram of the left kidney reveals a cystic mass that contains many septa and locules of varying sizes. **B,** A contrast-enhanced CT scan reveals the hypoattenuating mass with very delicate-appearing septa.

displaces adjacent vasculature without invasion, and shows no calcification. Low-density foci representing necrosis, seroma, fluid-filled cysts, or hemorrhage may be seen. Enhancement patterns are variable and can be related to entrapped functioning nephrons. On MRI, the tumor typically has a low signal on T1-weighted images both before and after administration of contrast material and has a variable signal on T2-weighted sequences. T1 shortening is associated with hemorrhage.

Treatment CMN usually is associated with a favorable outcome after complete surgical excision. However, the cellular variant (resembling congenital infantile fibrosarcoma) is associated with local recurrences (10%) and metastases. Adjuvant chemotherapy is not recommended if complete resection is feasible in either classic or cellular variants of CMN.[1,47-53]

Multilocular Cystic Renal Tumor

Overview and Pathophysiology Multilocular cystic renal tumor occurs predominantly in boys during infancy and toddler stages (3 months to 4 years) and in women during their seventh and eighth decades. Multilocular cystic tumors with fibrous septa that contain mature tubules are called cystic nephromas. When the cystic mass has blastemal elements within its septa, it is called a cystic partially differentiated nephroblastoma. A cystic Wilms tumor is present if solid masses of nephroblastomatous tissue are present. A potential theory suggests that cystic nephromas, cystic partially differentiated nephroblastomas, and Wilms tumors represent benign and malignant ends of a spectrum, analogous to the continuum of ganglioneuromas, ganglioneuroblastomas, and neuroblastomas. Partially differentiated cystic nephroblastomas present in childhood, whereas cystic nephromas are more commonly identified in adult women. Lesions are nonfamilial, are sporadically associated with congenital anomalies, and present clinically as painless abdominal masses.

Imaging Partially differentiated cystic nephroblastomas and cystic nephromas cannot be distinguished on the basis of

imaging features. The multilocular cystic renal tumor may involve the entire kidney or only a small portion of it. Ultrasound is more sensitive than CT for identification of septa (Fig. 116-12). The lesions are well-circumscribed, encapsulated masses of multiple anechoic cysts varying in size from a few millimeters to 4 cm. When the cystic spaces are small, the lesion may appear solid. The septa may be thin or thick. The pelvicalyceal system may be distorted and displaced. On CT, the septa enhance but the locules do not enhance, and contrast material does not accumulate within individual locules (Fig. 116-13). Small curvilinear calcifications occasionally are identified. Herniated tumoral cysts may project within the renal pelvis. MRI demonstrates a low T1 and variable T2 signal, depending on the cyst's contents (hemorrhage or protein). After administration of gadolinium, the cyst septa enhance.

Treatment Surgical excision generally is curative, and the prognosis is excellent. Imaging on a regular interval is recommended for follow-up. Local recurrence may occur if the tumor is incompletely excised. Recurrence is treated with

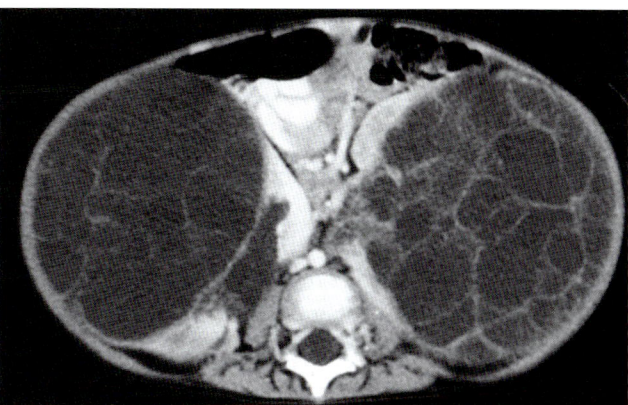

Figure 116-13 A bilateral, partially differentiated cystic nephroblastoma. A contrast-enhanced computed tomography scan shows the septa, with similar attenuation to renal parenchyma, coursing through low-density masses.

radiation therapy and chemotherapy. Metastases have not been reported.[1,54-66]

Renal Cell Carcinoma

Overview Renal cell carcinoma (RCC) is rare in the first two decades of life and accounts for approximately 5% of all renal tumors (median age at diagnosis is 9 to 12 years). Increasing evidence indicates that RCC in children differs from adult RCC in biology and behavior. Translocation RCC accounts for most instances of childhood RCC and generally involves the *TFE3* gene on chromosome Xp11.2 and less commonly the *TEFB* gene on chromosome 6p21. Prior chemotherapy currently is the only known risk factor for the development of Xp11 translocation RCC. Children with tuberous sclerosis complex, von Hippel–Lindau syndrome, and neuroblastoma appear to be at increased risk for the development of RCC. Histologically, nearly 80% of RCCs are predominately papillary in architecture. Wilms tumors outnumber RCCs in the first decade of life by a ratio of 30:1. During the second decade of life, a solid renal mass is equally likely to be an RCC or a Wilms tumor. Clinical presentation includes gross hematuria, flank pain, and a palpable abdominal mass. Fever, hypercalcemia, polycythemia, and hypertension are uncommon.

Imaging Although an RCC tends to be smaller than a Wilms tumor, its gross morphology is similar, and the two can be indistinguishable preoperatively. The tumor forms an infiltrative mass with variable necrosis, hemorrhage, calcification, and cystic degeneration. The tumor invades locally and spreads to retroperitoneal nodes. Metastases to the lungs, bones, liver, or brain are found in 20% of patients at diagnosis. Compared with Wilms tumors, RCCs are more likely to be bilateral and have bone metastases. Well-defined intrarenal lesions have been described on ultrasound (Fig. 116-14). On CT and MRI, an RCC appears as a nonspecific solid intrarenal mass with little enhancement. Regions of hemorrhage and necrosis may be present. In some case reports, the tumor has been of increased attenuation relative to renal parenchyma. About 25% of renal cell carcinomas contain calcifications. RCC enhances to a lesser extent than does normal renal parenchyma.

Treatment Staging uses the Tumor, Node, Metastasis system. The standard therapy for RCC in children and adolescents remains radical nephrectomy; RCC is among the tumors most resistant to systemic chemotherapy or radiotherapy. Nephron-sparing surgery currently is recommended only in adults. Retroperitoneal lymph node dissection remains controversial in children. Overall survival rates are approximately 50% to 60%, with the best prognosis for localized disease confined to the kidney. Xp11 translocation RCC has the potential to metastasize late, as many as 20 or 30 years after diagnosis.[1,67-78]

Medullary Carcinoma of the Kidney

Overview Medullary carcinoma of the kidney was described as a distinct entity in 1995. It is a highly aggressive malignant tumor of epithelial origin that appears almost exclusively in patients of African descent with the sickle cell (SC) trait or hemoglobin SC disease. The tissue of origin appears to be within the caliceal epithelium, a common region of papillary necrosis in the SC population. The age at presentation is 20 years (range, 10 to 39 years). A male-to-female ratio of 3:1 is seen in patients younger than 25 years. Presenting symptoms include gross hematuria, abdominal or flank pain, a palpable mass, and weight loss. A medullary carcinoma metastasizes rapidly to regional lymph nodes and the lungs.

Imaging Medullary carcinomas develop in the renal medulla, infiltrate the cortex, encase the renal pelvis, invade the lymphatics and vasculature, and have a predilection for the right kidney. Ultrasound (Fig. 116-15) and CT show a centrally located, infiltrative lesion with peripheral calyectasis, reniform enlargement, and peripheral satellite nodules. The tumor has a heterogeneous echotexture on ultrasound and shows heterogeneous enhancement on CT, which is related to hemorrhage and extensive necrosis. MRI is superior for revealing the extent of parenchymal and nodal invasion, as well as intratumoral hemorrhage and liver metastases.

Treatment The tumor generally responds poorly to chemotherapy or radiation therapy, with a mean survival of 15 weeks from diagnosis.[1,79-82]

Renal Angiomyolipoma

Overview Angiomyolipomas are lesions consisting of a disordered arrangement of vascular, smooth muscle, and fatty elements. Histologic composition suggests a hamartoma, but currently angiomyolipomas are thought to represent a true neoplasm. In children, angiomyolipomas are rare in the absence of tuberous sclerosis. In most children with tuberous sclerosis, angiomyolipomas develop by 10 years of age. Angiomyolipomas also are associated with neurofibromatosis and

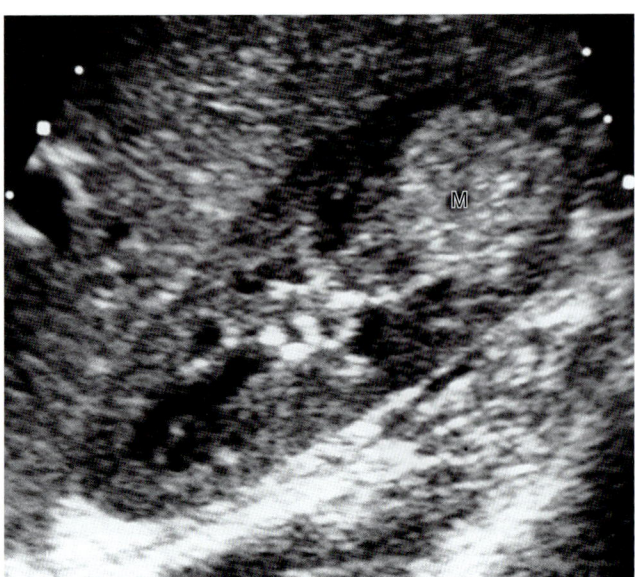

Figure 116-14 **A renal cell carcinoma.** A sagittal sonogram of the right kidney shows a round, hyperechoic mass (*M*) in the lower pole.

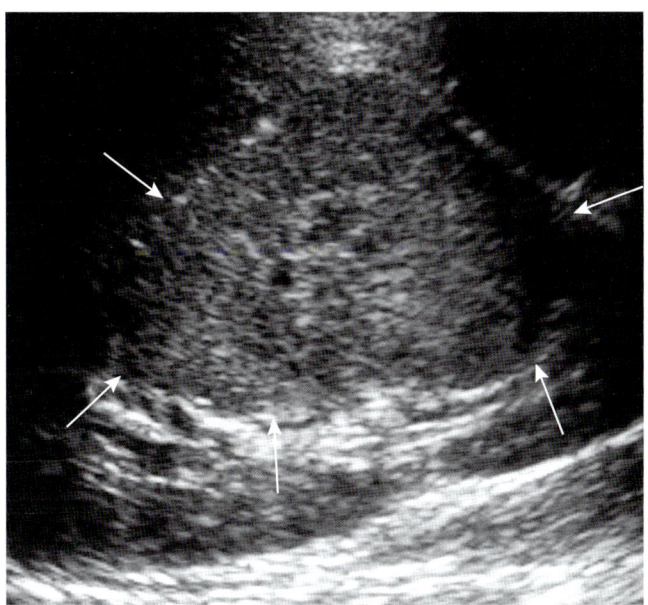

Figure 116-15 A medullary carcinoma of the kidney. A sagittal sono-gram of the right kidney shows a mass (*arrows*) that is isoechoic to parenchyma effacing and abutting the renal pelvis.

von Hippel–Lindau syndrome. Lesions that are smaller than 4 cm typically are asymptomatic. Larger lesions are susceptible to spontaneous hemorrhage, resulting in flank or abdominal pain, hematuria, and severe retroperitoneal hemorrhage (Wunderlich syndrome).

Imaging The imaging appearance of angiomyolipomas is variable depending on the histologic contents. CT (Fig. 116-16) and MRI generally are diagnostic when fat density or signal is identified within the lesion, remembering that fat may be seen in Wilms tumors and RCCs. Ultrasound will identify highly echogenic nonshadowing lesions. Bilateral lesions often are seen in persons with tuberous sclerosis. On angiography, angiomyolipomas demonstrate characteristic tortuous, dilated vessels with aneurysm formation. Rarely are lesions hypovascular.

Treatment Lesions larger than 4 cm may be selectively embolized or surgically removed to prevent a life-threatening hemorrhage. Ultrasound screening to monitor angiomyolipoma size is recommended every 2 to 3 years before puberty and then annually after puberty.[1,83-92]

Renal Lymphoma

Overview Lymphoma of the kidney is due to hematogenous spread or extension from retroperitoneal sites; the kidney normally does not contain lymphoid tissue, and for this reason, primary renal lymphoma is rare. In children, non-Hodgkin lymphoma (especially Burkitt lymphoma) is most common. Lymphomatous involvement of the kidney typically does not produce symptoms until late in its course. Flank pain, abdominal pain, hematuria, anemia, weight loss, and a palpable mass are most common.

Imaging The most common radiographic pattern is multiple parenchymal masses distorting the collecting system; less common findings are a solitary renal mass, diffuse infiltration, and isolated perinephric disease. Both CT and MRI are better than sonography for locating renal lesions and identifying extension into adjacent structures. On CT, multiple round homogeneous and hypoattenuating masses are seen on precontrast and postcontrast images (Fig. 116-17). The CT findings of perinephric disease include thickening of Gerota fascia, soft tissue attenuating nodules, or a hypoechoic plaque that is hyperattenuating on nonenhanced images and hypoattenuating on contrast-enhanced images. MRI demonstrates that lymphomatous masses are isointense or slightly hypointense on T1-weighted images and hypointense on T2-weighted images relative to the renal cortex. Enhancement of the lesions after administration of gadolinium usually is less intense than surrounding renal parenchyma, particularly on postcontrast images. On sonography, the mass(es) typically are hypoechoic, with frequent through transmission. Hypoechoic, isoechoic, and hyperechoic subcortical masses all have been described (e-Fig. 116-18). Lymphomatous lesions, however, may be occult or may present as nephromegaly because of diffuse tumor infiltration as the only finding.[1,93-99]

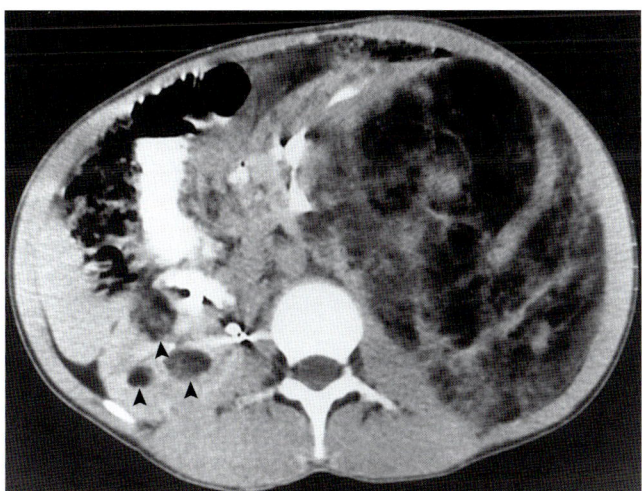

Figure 116-16 Angiomyolipomas of the kidneys. A contrast-enhanced computed tomography scan depicts a huge angiomyolipoma in the left kidney and three smaller ones (*arrowheads*) in the right kidney.

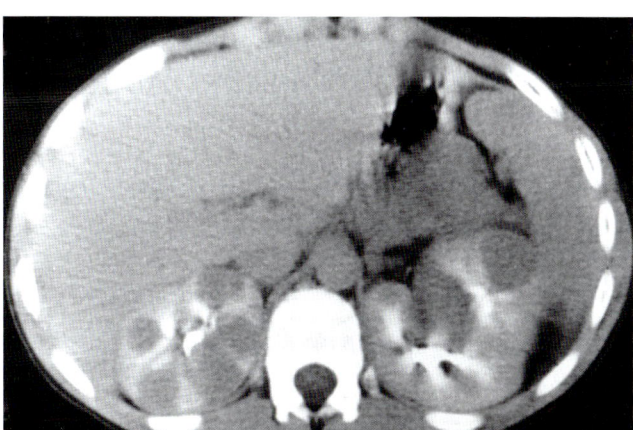

Figure 116-17 Non-Hodgkin lymphoma of the kidneys. A delayed contrast-enhanced computed tomography image reveals multiple, round hypoattenuating cortical masses.

Ossifying Renal Tumor of Infancy

Overview An ossifying renal tumor of infancy is an exceedingly rare benign renal mass presenting in children; only 13 cases have been reported in the literature. The age at presentation ranges from 6 days to 14 months. Boys are affected more commonly, with a lesion predilection for the left kidney and upper pole calices. Hematuria is the presenting symptom. Histologically, the lesion consists of an osteoid core, osteoblasts, and spindle cells.

Imaging The mass arises from the urothelium at the papillary region of the renal pyramids, is polypoid in configuration, and is 2 to 3 cm in size. At imaging, filling defects are seen in the collecting system with partial obstruction. On ultrasound, the mass is echogenic with acoustic shadowing. On CT, a well-defined calcified mass is seen with poor contrast enhancement.

Treatment The treatment is resection—either complete or partial nephrectomy was performed in the reported cases. The biologic behavior appears to be benign, with no case of malignant spread or postsurgical disease at follow-up.[1,100-102]

WHAT THE CLINICIAN NEEDS TO KNOW

- Renal involvement (unilateral or bilateral)
- Size and imaging characteristics (a solid, cystic, or mixed lesion and the presence of fat)
- Extent (confined to the kidney or extrarenal extension)
- Vascular invasion (inferior vena cava) and extent and distribution of metastatic disease
- Imaging recommendations for further diagnostic evaluation and follow-up

Key Points

Nephroblastomatosis commonly regresses and resolves spontaneously; however, it may degenerate into a Wilms tumor.

Children with genetic and syndromic abnormalities associated with nephroblastomatosis should be screened for Wilms tumor by ultrasound at 3- to 4-month intervals.

Wilms tumors may contain soft tissue, fluid, fat, and calcific elements.

The imaging features of clear cell sarcoma of the kidney are similar to those of Wilms tumor. Clear cell carcinoma has a predilection for bone metastases.

Rhabdoid tumor of the kidney has the worst prognosis of all of the childhood renal tumors and is associated with primary or metastatic central nervous system lesions.

CMN is a solid neoplasm in the neonatal period; the enhancement pattern is variable and is related to entrapped functioning nephrons within the tumor.

Multilocular cystic renal tumors occur in two distinct groups: young boys and elderly women.

RCC in children differs from adult RCC in biology and behavior.

Life-threatening retroperitoneal hemorrhage is a complication of angiomyolipomas that are larger than 4 cm.

Medullary carcinoma of the kidney is a highly aggressive malignant tumor of epithelial origin that occurs almost exclusively in patients of African descent who have the SC trait or hemoglobin SC disease.

Suggested Readings

Argani P, Ladanyi M. Recent advances in pediatric renal neoplasia. *Adv Anat Pathol.* 2003;10(5):243-260.

Broecker B. Non-Wilms' renal tumors in children. *Urol Clin North Am.* 2000;27(3):463-469, ix.

Cohen MM Jr. Beckwith-Wiedemann syndrome: historical, clinicopathological, and etiopathogenetic perspectives. *Pediatr Dev Pathol.* 2005;8(3):287-304.

Geller E, Kochan PS. Renal neoplasms of childhood. *Radiol Clin North Am.* 2011;49(4):689-709, vi.

Glick RD, Hicks MJ, Nuchtern JG, et al. Renal tumors in infants less than 6 months of age. *J Pediatr Surg.* 2004;39(4):522-525.

Lowe LH, Isuani BH, Heller RM, et al. Pediatric renal masses: Wilms tumor and beyond. *Radiographics.* 2000;20(6):1585-1603.

Miniati D, Gay AN, Parks KV, et al. Imaging accuracy and incidence of Wilms' and non-Wilms' renal tumors in children. *J Pediatr Surg.* 2008;43(7):1301-1307.

Powis M. Neonatal renal tumours. *Early Hum Dev.* 2010;86(10):607-612.

Sarhan OM, El-Baz M, Sarhan MM, et al. Bilateral Wilms' tumors: single-center experience with 22 cases and literature review. *Urology.* 2010;76(4):946-951.

Sebire NJ, Vujanic GM. Paediatric renal tumours: recent developments, new entities and pathological features. *Histopathology.* 2009;54(5):516-528.

Shet T, Viswanathan S. The cytological diagnosis of paediatric renal tumours. *J Clin Pathol.* 2009;62(11):961-969.

Zhang J, Israel GM, Krinsky GA, et al. Masses and pseudomasses of the kidney: imaging spectrum on MR. *J Comput Assist Tomogr.* 2004;28(5):588-595.

References

Full references for this chapter can be found on www.expertconsult.com.

Chapter 117

Vascular Conditions

ROBERT G. WELLS

Renovascular Hypertension

Overview Approximately 5% to 10% of children and adolescents with severe hypertension have an underlying renal vascular lesion. In infants, up to 70% of clinically significant hypertension is due to renovascular disease. Myriad developmental and acquired causes of renovascular hypertension exist (Box 117-1). A complication related to umbilical artery catheterization is the most common cause of renovascular hypertension in neonates. In older children, renal arterial fibromuscular dysplasia is the most common cause.[1-4]

Imaging Asymmetry of the kidneys on sonography is an important sign of possible renovascular hypertension. The affected kidney often is small and may have manifestations of scarring. Direct visualization of a stenotic renal arterial lesion is uncommon with sonography, however. Evaluation of the aorta also is an important component of the examination. With Doppler evaluation, a renal artery-to-aorta peak systolic velocity ratio of greater than 3.5 carries a strong association with renal arterial stenosis. A peak velocity in the renal artery of greater than 180 cm/s also is suggestive of renal artery stenosis. Distal to the stenotic lesion, the systolic peak of the renal arterial waveform often appears flattened (Fig. 117-1). With severe stenosis, Doppler evaluation of distal arteries shows a tardus-parvus pattern, with slow systolic acceleration and diminished peak systolic velocity. Diastolic flow in the main renal artery sometimes is elevated.[5]

The most useful scintigraphic technique for detection of renovascular hypertension involves the evaluation of renal function without and with the use of an angiotensin-converting enzyme inhibitor, usually captopril or enalaprilat. MAG3 is the optimal imaging agent for this study. In the presence of renovascular disease, imaging in conjunction with angiotensin-converting enzyme inhibitor therapy typically shows diminished perfusion, diminished initial uptake, and poor parenchyma clearance of the affected kidney. Comparative imaging in the absence of antihypertensive therapy shows improved function (Fig. 117-2). The sensitivity of this technique for the detection of renovascular hypertension is approximately 85% to 90%. Bilateral renal artery stenosis or markedly compromised renal function can lead to false-negative examinations.[6]

Transcatheter angiography is the most sensitive and specific technique for the detection and identification of small-vessel renal artery disease. Computed tomographic angiography (CTA) and magnetic resonance angiography (MRA) are important noninvasive techniques for visualization of renal vascular anatomy. Upon administration of contrast material, global and regional alterations in kidney perfusion and function also can be assessed with computed tomography (CT) and magnetic resonance imaging (MRI). In general, >50% narrowing of the renal arterial diameter is hemodynamically significant. The presence of enlarged collateral pathways is an additional indicator of significant renal artery stenosis. Transcatheter renal vein renin sampling is useful in selected cases of suspected renal hypertension (Fig. 117-3).[7,8]

Renal Fibromuscular Dysplasia

Overview Renal fibromuscular dysplasia (FMD; arterial fibrous dysplasia) is the most common cause of renal artery stenosis in children. Subcategorization of FMD is based on the layer of the arterial wall that is involved. This classification is important because each type of FMD has distinct histologic and angiographic features and occurs in a different clinical setting.[9-11]

PRIMARY INTIMAL FIBROPLASIA

Primary intimal fibroplasia is characterized by circumferential accumulation of collagen subintimally and within the internal elastic membrane. This form of FMD is the most common cause of renal artery stenosis in children. Imaging shows a smooth, bandlike, tubular, or funnel-shaped stenosis that usually involves the distal two thirds of the renal artery or a branch vessel (Fig. 117-4).

PERIMEDIAL OR SUBADVENTITIAL FIBRODYSPLASIA

Perimedial or subadventitial fibrodysplasia involves collagen deposition in the outer border of the media over a variable length of the renal artery. Angiography typically shows severe long-segment beaded narrowing of the renal artery. This disease occurs almost exclusively in girls older than 10 years of age, and it involves only the renal arteries or branches. About 15% of cases are bilateral.

FIBROMUSCULAR HYPERPLASIA

Fibromuscular hyperplasia is an extremely rare vasculopathy that can occur in childhood. Concentric thickening of the

Box 117-1 Causes of Renovascular Hypertension

Fibromuscular Dysplasia

Inflammatory Disease

- Takayasu arteritis
- Kawasaki disease
- Moyamoya disease
- Irradiation

Genetic Disorders

- Williams syndrome
- Neurofibromatosis
- Klippel-Trenaunay-Weber syndrome
- Feuerstein-Mims syndrome
- Rett syndrome
- Degos-Köhlmeier disease
- Marfan syndrome

Atherosclerosis

- Hyperlipidemias

Vascular Anomaly

- Renal arteriovenous malformation
- Renal artery aneurysm
- Renal artery hypoplasia

Thromboembolism

- Umbilical artery catheterization
- Neonate of diabetic mother
- Sepsis/dehydration

Renal Transplantation

- Rejection
- Arterial narrowing

Other

- Congenital rubella
- Compression by mass
- Congenital fibrous band
- Posttraumatic cause
- Retroperitoneal fibrosis

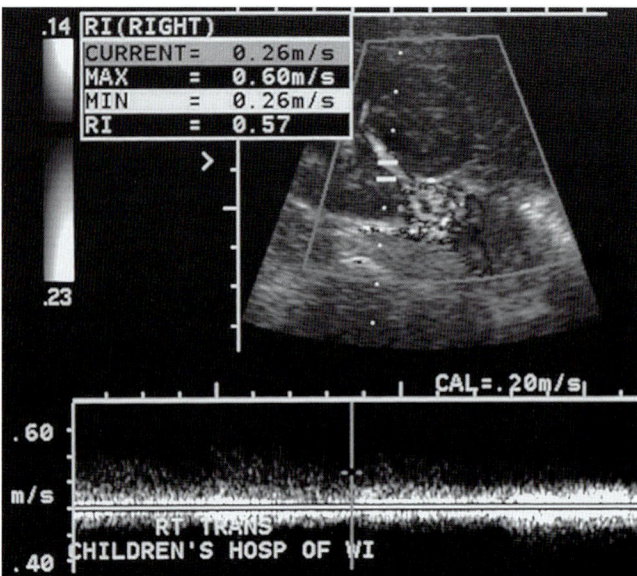

Figure 117-1 Renal artery stenosis. Doppler evaluation of the renal artery distal to a severe stenosis in a child with renal fibromuscular dysplasia shows a low-velocity monophasic arterial waveform.

renal arterial wall is due to proliferating smooth muscle and fibrous tissue. Angiographically, this lesion appears as a smooth stenosis of the renal artery or its branches. The appearance often is indistinguishable from that of intimal fibroplasia.

MEDIAL FIBROPLASIA

Medial fibroplasia is the most common cause of nonarteriosclerotic renovascular disease in adults, but it is rare in children. Alternating areas of focal thinning of the internal elastic membrane and focal collagenous thickening of the medial

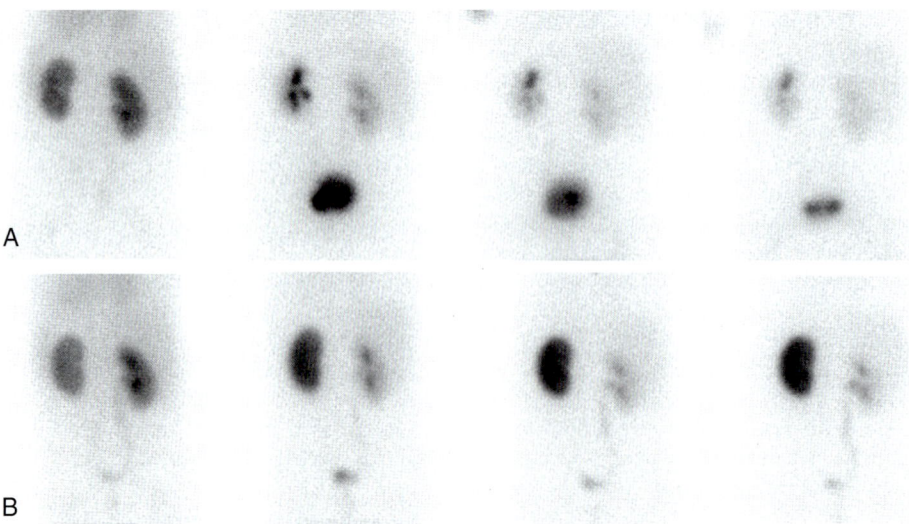

Figure 117-2 Renovascular hypertension and angiotensin-converting enzyme (ACE) inhibition scintigraphy. **A,** A renogram shows normal uptake and excretion from both kidneys. **B,** A renogram after administration of an ACE inhibitor shows marked radiopharmaceutical retention in the left kidney, indicating renal artery stenosis. (Courtesy Douglas F. Eggli, MD, Hershey, PA.)

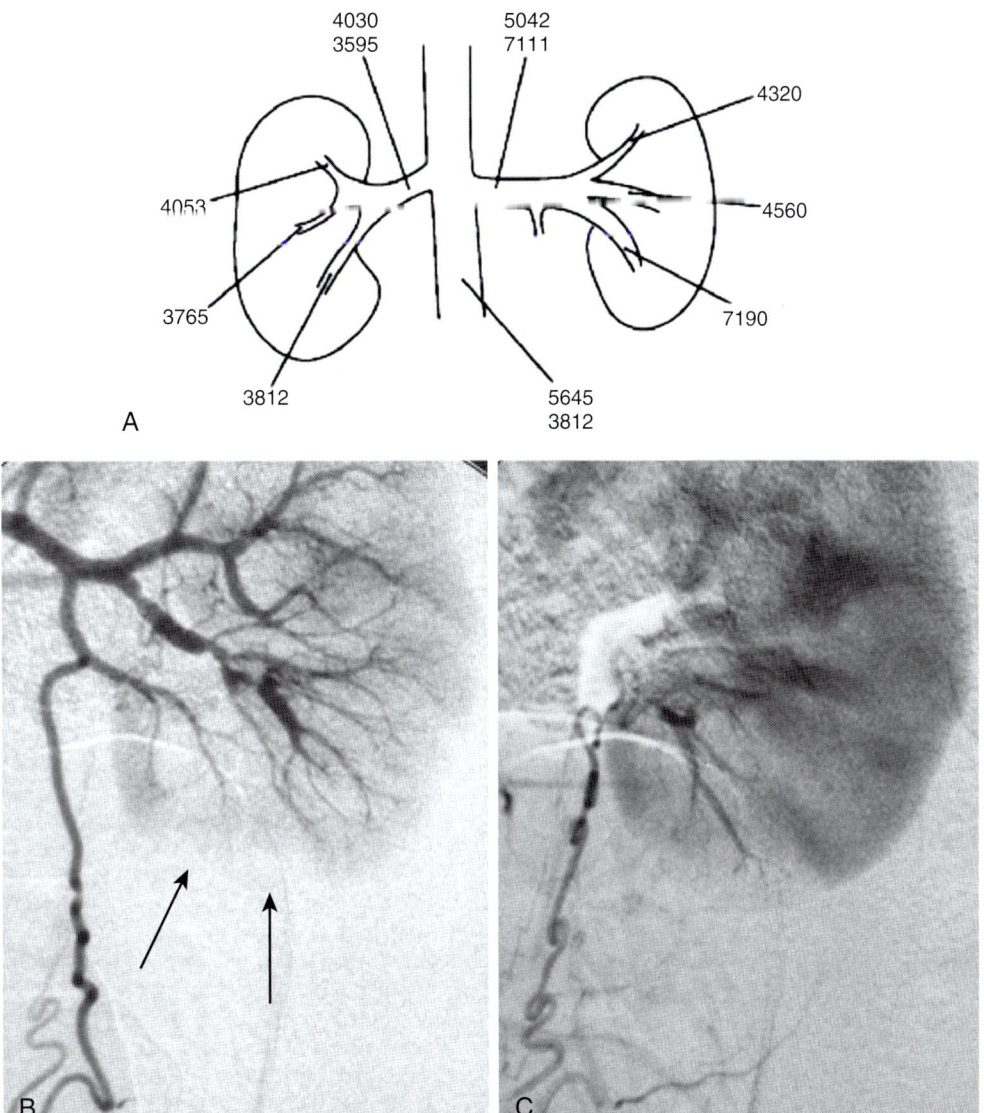

Figure 117-3 An 11-year-old girl with hypertension. **A,** A map of renal vein renin activity shows that the hypertension is driven by a focus in the left lower pole. **B,** Arterial phase angiography shows complex segmental stenoses, an area of delayed perfusion owing to a "missing vessel" (*arrows*), and a prominent collateral ureteric artery. **C,** Capillary phase angiography shows that the ureteric artery collateral reconstitutes the "missing vessel," completing the nephrogram. (From Roebuck DJ. Paediatric interventional radiology. *Imaging.* 2001;13:302-320.)

muscular layer are present. Angiographically, medial fibrodysplasia produces a string-of-beads appearance, typically involving the distal two thirds of the main renal artery and its branches. Areas of dilation between stenoses are usually greater in caliber than the normal renal artery.

Neurofibromatosis

Overview The most common vascular pathology in patients with neurofibromatosis type 1 involves stenosis of the aorta or a large branch vessel as a result of proliferation of neural tissue in the arterial wall and perivascular space. Occasionally, an aneurysm occurs. In the kidney, a small-vessel mesodermal dysplasia also can occur. Arterial stenosis usually occurs at the vessel origin or in the proximal third of the main renal artery. Concomitant aortic stenosis is common.[12]

Takayasu Arteritis

Overview Takayasu arteritis is a rare idiopathic chronic inflammatory arteritis. Hypertension as a result of renal arterial stenosis or abdominal aortic narrowing is common. CT and MRI features of Takayasu arteritis include narrowing, mural thickening, adherent thrombus, and mural calcification of the aorta, pulmonary arteries, and major aortic branch vessels (Fig. 117-5). With active disease, the thickened vascular wall has prominent contrast enhancement.[13-15]

Middle Aortic Syndrome

Overview Middle aortic syndrome (midaortic dysplastic syndrome) is an acquired, progressive vascular disorder that

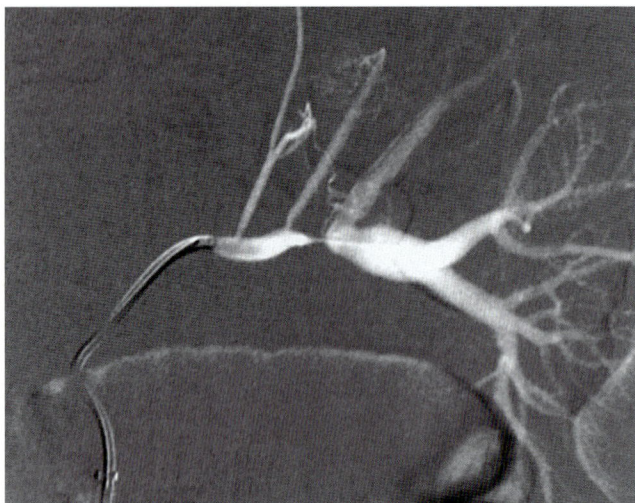

Figure 117-4 **Renal artery stenosis.** A selective renal arteriogram of a 12-year-old girl with hypertension due to primary intimal fibroplasia shows severe stenosis of the main renal artery. Poststenotic dilation is present.

involves the midthoracic through abdominal segments of the aorta and usually is accompanied by narrowing of major visceral branches, including the renal arteries. Imaging studies show diffuse narrowing of the thoracoabdominal segment of the aorta and the major branch vessels (Figs. 117-6 and 117-7). If renal artery narrowing is severe, collateral flow to the kidneys usually occurs via ureteral, adrenal, and gonadal arteries that fill from lower intercostal vessels.[16,17]

Renovascular Trauma

Overview Potential renal arterial injuries include intimal disruption, main renal artery avulsion, branch vessel transection, false aneurysm, and arteriovenous fistula. Most renal injuries in children result from blunt trauma; penetrating injuries are uncommon. The intima is most susceptible to a stretching injury because it is less elastic than the media and the adventitia. An intimal tear can precipitate dissection, luminal occlusion, or thrombosis. Stretching injury also can cause spasm of the renal artery without a tear. With severe, rapid motion of the kidney, vascular avulsion can occur. Penetrating injuries and iatrogenic mechanisms such as a needle biopsy can lead to an intrarenal arteriovenous fistula.[18]

Imaging Globally deficient parenchymal contrast enhancement is an important CT indicator of possible disruption, thrombosis, or spasm of the main renal artery. Contrast enhancement in the periphery of an ischemic kidney (the "cortical rim sign") is a radiographic indicator of acute renal arterial occlusion. The cortical rim sign does not develop until at least 8 hours after the onset of ischemia; in many patients, it is not present until a few days after the injury. This sign generally indicates that renal salvage is not possible because of the prolonged nature of the ischemia.

With complete traumatic disruption of the main renal artery, CT shows a large adjacent hematoma. A localized renal infarction due to traumatic occlusion of an intrarenal vessel results in a wedge-shaped or rounded area of absent enhancement, often with sharp margins. With partial main renal artery occlusion, the nephrogram intensity is diminished.

Aneurysm

Overview Renal artery aneurysms are rare in childhood. Classifying features include location (extraparenchymal and intraparenchymal) and morphology (saccular, fusiform, dissecting, and false). Some pediatric renal artery aneurysms are idiopathic; others are due to infection (i.e., mycotic aneurysms), renal artery stenosis (often related to neurofibromatosis type 1 or fibromuscular dysplasia), or autoimmune vasculitis (e.g., polyarteritis nodosa). Aneurysms of the renal artery can occur in patients with Kawasaki disease and Ehlers-Danlos syndrome. The most common clinical manifestations of a renal artery aneurysm are hematuria and flank pain.[19]

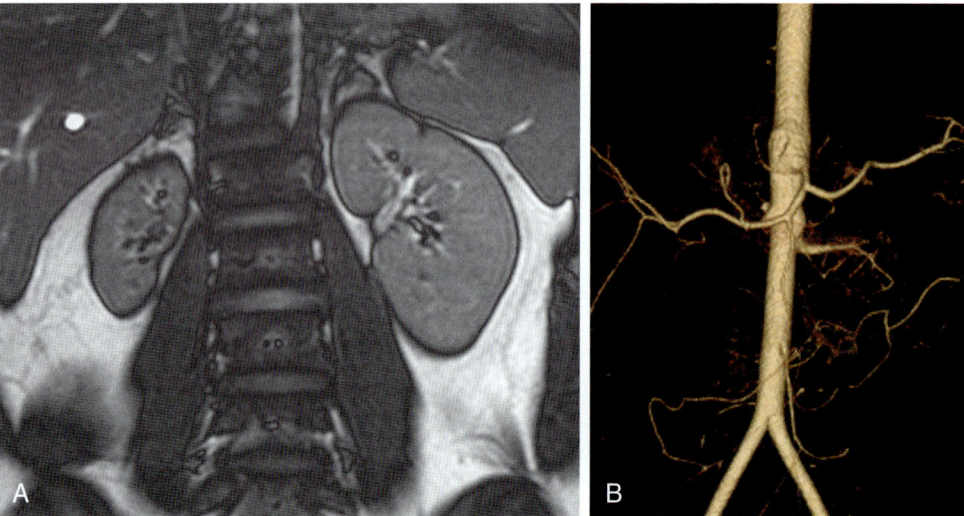

Figure 117-5 **Takayasu arteritis. A,** A coronal magnetic resonance image of a teenager with hypertension shows a markedly small right kidney. **B,** No flow in the right renal artery is visible on this magnetic resonance angiography image.

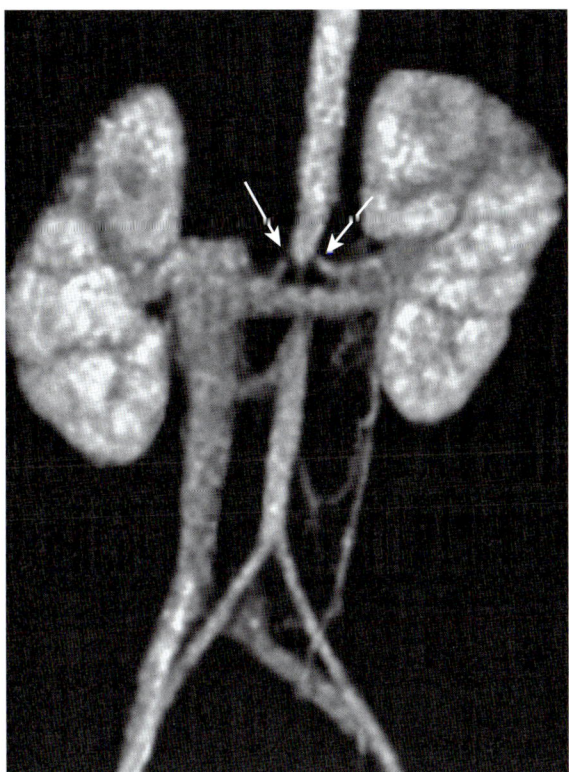

Figure 117-6 **Middle aortic syndrome**. Computed tomographic angiography of a child with middle aortic syndrome reveals severe narrowing of the renal arteries (*arrows*) and infrarenal portion of the abdominal aorta.

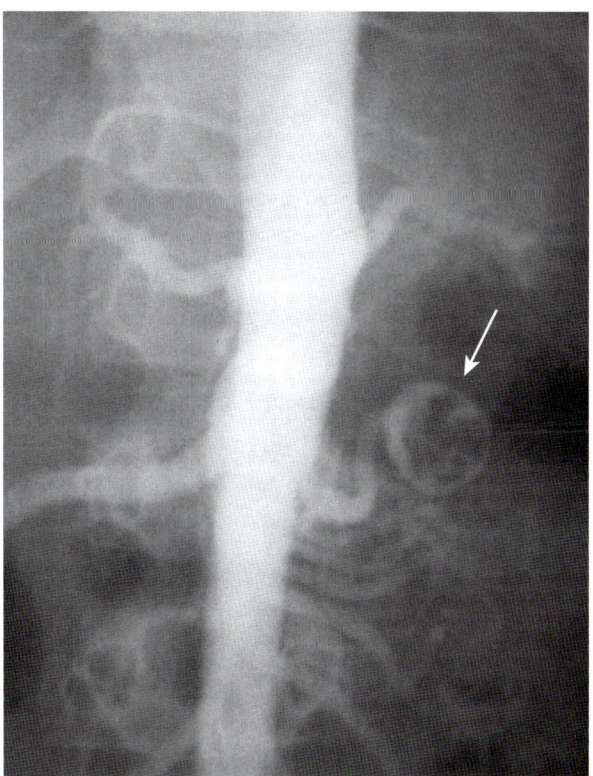

Figure 117-8 **Renal artery aneurysm**. An abdominal aortogram shows a partially thrombosed saccular aneurysm (*arrow*) of the left renal artery.

Imaging Renal artery aneurysms can be single or multiple; most are saccular. A clot or calcification occasionally is present within the aneurysm (Fig. 117-8). Aneurysms that occur in patients with polyarteritis nodosa tend to be small, multiple, and intraparenchymal. Most are detectable with sonography, CTA, or MRA. Conventional angiography sometimes is required for the detection and characterization of small lesions.[20]

Arteriovenous Malformation and Fistula

Overview and Imaging About three quarters of renal arteriovenous fistulas are iatrogenic or related to trauma. Congenital arteriovenous malformations of the kidney are rare. Hematuria and a bruit are common clinical findings. A large lesion can cause congestive heart failure. Imaging studies of a renal arteriovenous fistula show a focal abnormal direct communication between an artery and a vein, whereas shunting in an arteriovenous malformation occurs through a nidus of abnormal vessels. Supplying and draining vessels are enlarged. Doppler analysis shows turbulent flow and arterial velocity in the draining veins. Conventional angiography shows rapid flow through the lesion.[21,22]

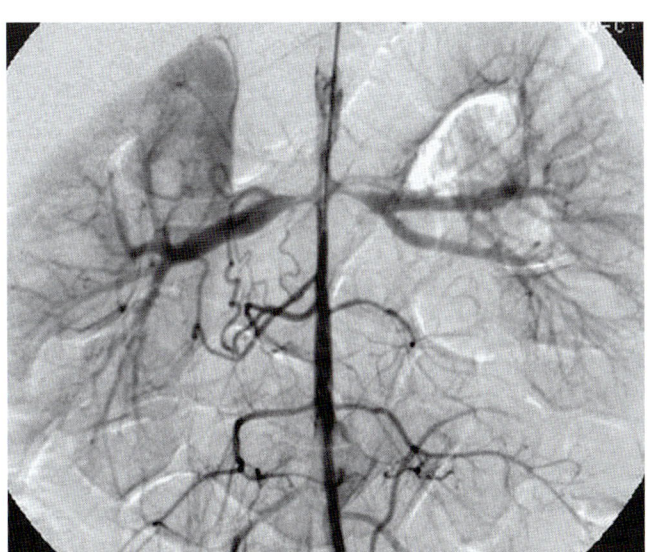

Figure 117-7 **Middle aortic syndrome**. An aortogram of a 3-month-old boy with severe hypertension reveals a hypoplastic abdominal aorta and bilateral renal artery stenoses.

Thrombosis, Embolism, and Infarction

Overview Thromboembolic disease of the renal arteries is uncommon in children. Predisposing conditions include sepsis, prolonged hypotension, severe dehydration, congenital heart disease, trauma, and hypercoagulable disorders. In

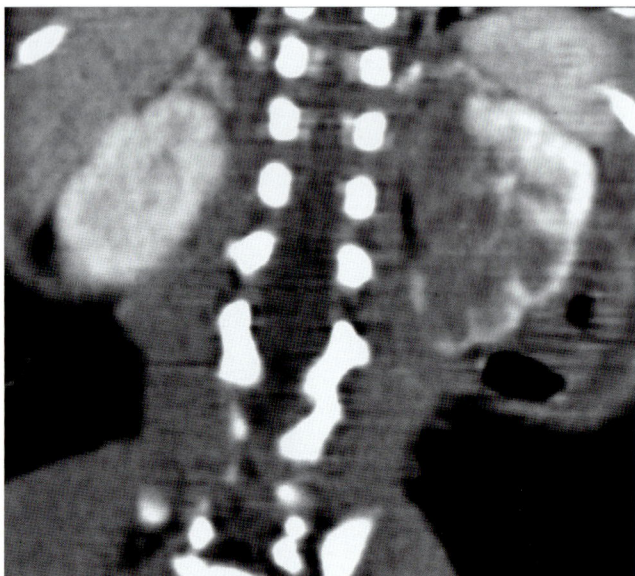

Figure 117-9 Acute renal artery thrombosis in a neonate. Contrast enhancement is deficient in most of the left kidney on this coronal reformatted computed tomography image. Note preserved enhancement of a thin peripheral rim of cortex.

neonates, the most common cause is an umbilical arterial catheter, particularly when the catheter tip is near the origins of the renal arteries. Infants of diabetic mothers are at increased risk for renal arterial thrombosis. In older children, acute occlusion of a major renal artery causes flank pain, nausea, vomiting, fever, and hematuria. Small emboli or minor thrombosis may be asymptomatic, although hypertension is a common complication.[23]

Imaging In the acute phase of renal artery thromboembolism, sonography is normal or shows nonspecific renal enlargement and cortical hyperechogenicity. Doppler evaluation sometimes reveals global, focal, or multifocal perfusion deficits. Flow within the capsule may be increased. Careful evaluation of the main renal artery sometimes demonstrates an echogenic clot, as well as abnormal arterial waveforms. If the main renal artery is patent in a patient with renal infarction, the resistive index often is elevated.

CTA and MRA of patients with renal arterial thromboembolic disease may reveal filling defects or narrowing of the renal artery. With global renal infarction, renal parenchymal enhancement and normal contrast media excretion are lacking. One or more wedge-shaped enhancement defects may occur in the presence of segmental renal infarction. In about 50% of patients with renal infarction, a thin, prominently enhancing rim is visible at the peripheral margin of an infarction (Fig. 117-9).

Diseases of the Intrarenal Arteries

RENAL VASCULITIS

Overview The kidney is a relatively common site of involvement in various forms of vasculitis. The most widely used classification of vasculitis is based on the size of the predominantly involved vessels. Takayasu arteritis is an example of large-vessel vasculitis. Polyarteritis nodosa and Kawasaki disease predominantly involve medium-sized vessels. The presence or absence of antineutrophil cytoplasmic antibodies (ANCAs) allows subcategorization of the small-vessel vasculitides. Henoch-Schönlein purpura (HSP) is ANCA negative; ANCA-positive vasculitides that can affect the kidney include Wegener granulomatosis and microscopic polyarteritis. Small-vessel vasculitis also can occur in association with various infectious diseases, such as Rocky Mountain spotted fever, human immunodeficiency virus, hepatitis B, and tuberculosis.[24]

POLYARTERITIS NODOSA

Overview Polyarteritis nodosa is a rare idiopathic focal segmental necrotizing vasculitis. Renal involvement occurs in slightly more than half of affected children. Clinical manifestations of kidney involvement include hematuria, proteinuria, and hypertension. Imaging studies of the kidneys may show manifestations of focal or multifocal renal ischemia. Intraparenchymal or perirenal hemorrhage can occur as the result of aneurysm rupture. Arteriography reveals small aneurysms, typically located at the bifurcations of interlobular or arcuate arteries. Small intrarenal vessels are irregular and tortuous because of vascular and perivascular inflammation (Fig. 117-10).[25]

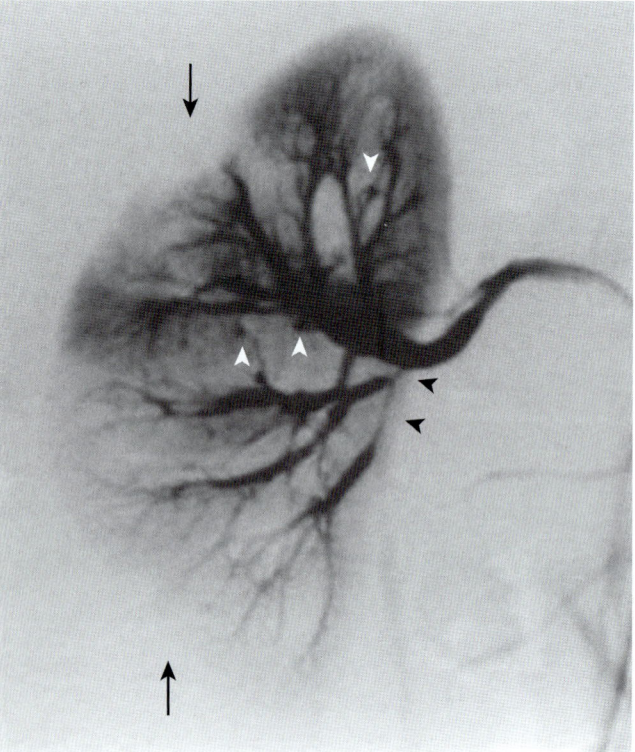

Figure 117-10 This patient had an established diagnosis of polyarteritis nodosa for 1 year and new onset of hypertension. A right renal angiogram shows segmental narrowing of the intrarenal branch to the lower pole (*black arrowheads*), small saccular aneurysms at vessel branch points (*white arrowheads*), and patchy perfusion deficits in the upper and lower poles (*arrows*).

WEGENER GRANULOMATOSIS AND MICROSCOPIC POLYARTERITIS

Overview Wegener granulomatosis is a rare necrotizing vasculitis that predominantly affects the respiratory tract. Up to 80% of patients have evidence of renal involvement, as manifested by hematuria, proteinuria, and (in many patients) diminished glomerular filtration rate. Similar clinical findings occur in patients with microscopic polyarteritis, although respiratory system involvement is lacking with this disorder. Diagnostic imaging findings of kidney involvement with these two vasculitides are nonspecific. Foci of parenchymal scarring may occur as the result of ischemia. Parenchymal or perirenal hemorrhage can occur as a result of rupture of a small-vessel aneurysm. The imaging findings are similar to those of polyarteritis nodosa.[26,27]

SYSTEMIC LUPUS ERYTHEMATOSUS

Overview Systemic lupus erythematosus is a systemic autoimmune disease. Up to 75% of children with this disorder have clinical manifestations of renal involvement. A clinical spectrum ranges from mild asymptomatic disease to severe forms that lead to end-stage renal disease or death. The major pathologic manifestation is thickening of the basement membrane as a result of focal glomerulonephritis; inflammatory narrowing of interlobular arteries also may be evident. In the absence of renal failure, the kidneys often appear normal on imaging studies. Mild nephromegaly is common. Diffuse or multifocal hyperechogenicity of the renal parenchyma may be present on sonography. Elevation of the resistive index on Doppler ultrasonography may be predictive of worsening renal function.[28,29]

HEMOLYTIC-UREMIC SYNDROME

Overview Hemolytic-uremic syndrome is the most common cause of acute renal failure in early childhood. The pathogenesis involves endothelial cell damage within glomeruli and renal arterioles. The kidney is the main target of this microangiopathy, although the intestines, lung, and brain variably are affected. In most cases of hemolytic-uremic syndrome, fever, vomiting, bloody diarrhea, and abdominal discomfort develop in an otherwise healthy infant. Affected children beyond infancy are usually around 3 years of age. The child may become critically ill, with signs and symptoms that include pallor, irritability, seizures, heart failure, hypertension, gastrointestinal bleeding, and oliguria. Acute renal failure usually lasts for 1 to 4 weeks, with subsequent slow improvement. Clinical recovery is complete in most patients, but some children have permanent neurologic or renal damage.[30]

Imaging Early in the disease, sonography is normal or shows minimal nephromegaly. Subsequent abnormally increased parenchymal echogenicity usually is most prominent in the glomerular and subcortical regions. The degree of cortical echogenicity correlates with the severity of the illness. In most patients, the kidney returns to a normal size as the disease resolves, but more severe injury is associated with eventual kidney atrophy; nephrocalcinosis can occur.[31,32]

HENOCH-SCHÖNLEIN PURPURA

Overview HSP is a hypersensitivity vasculitis that affects small vessels and is an important cause of nephritis in children. The clinical tetrad includes a purpuric rash, arthralgias, abdominal pain, and glomerulonephritis. Between 20% to 30% of patients with HSP have hematuria, and 50% to 70% have proteinuria. In patients with profound proteinuria, nephrotic syndrome and renal insufficiency can occur. Clinical signs of renal involvement may follow or coincide with the appearance of purpura, but they rarely antedate the skin findings. HSP usually is a self-limited disorder, but it can be complicated by hypertension or chronic renal failure.[33,34]

Imaging Sonography of patients with HSP may show normal or bilaterally enlarged kidneys. Hyperechogenicity of the renal cortex is usually diffuse, and the medullary pyramids remain hypoechoic. Renal cortical hyperechogenicity diminishes as the acute disease regresses. Occasionally, cross-sectional imaging studies show an intramural hematoma of the bladder wall or ureter. Ureteral fibrosis is a rare complication.

SICKLE CELL DISEASE

Overview Sludging of red blood cells within the medulla is common in patients with sickle cell disease. Recurrent episodes of medullary ischemia lead to alterations in papillary morphology. Papillary necrosis develops when medullary ischemia is severe. Cortical hypertrophy may occur. Nephropathy of sickle cell disease involves the entire renal parenchyma. Histologic features include dilation and engorgement of cortical capillary tufts, glomerulosclerosis, increased mesangial matrix, and iron deposition in the glomerular epithelium and glomerular basement membrane. Occasionally, glomerular sclerosis progresses to complete obliteration of glomerular tufts.[35]

Imaging Intravenous urography and CT may show calyceal blunting and prominent papillae with broad, deep calyces. The collecting system often is distorted because of cortical hypertrophy (Fig. 117-11). In some patients, papillary necrosis is evident. Nephromegaly, usually bilateral, is common. Recurrent infarction and subsequent fibrosis eventually may lead to scarring and atrophy.[36]

Renal sonography of patients with sickle cell disease typically shows mild diffuse enlargement, hyperechogenicity, and loss of corticomedullary differentiation (Fig. 117-12). A perirenal hematoma can occur as a complication of renal infarction. Doppler sonography serves to detect renovascular disease. MRI shows decreased cortical signal relative to the medulla on T1-weighted and T2-weighted images as a result of iron deposition in the renal cortex.[37,38]

Renal Vein Thrombosis

Overview Renal vein thrombosis (RVT) is the most common renal vascular abnormality of neonates. Most affected infants have a predisposing systemic abnormality such as dehydration, sepsis, polycythemia, or maternal diabetes mellitus. Small intrarenal vessels are the initial or only site of thrombosis in

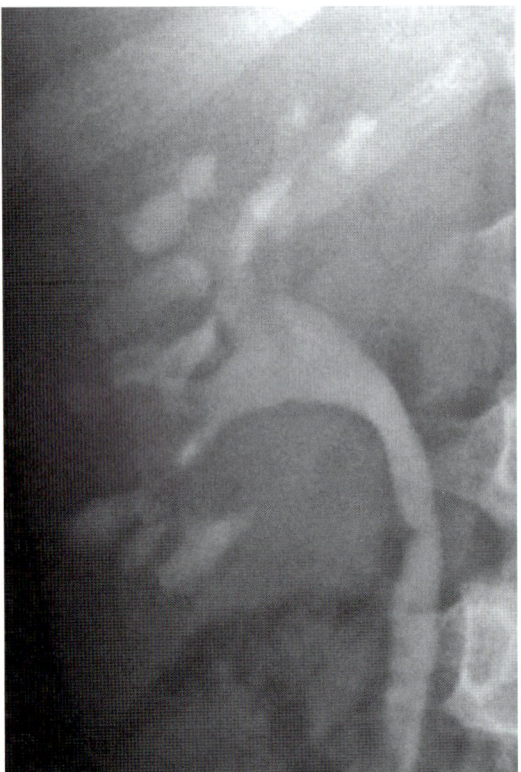

Figure 117-11 **Sickle cell disease.** An intravenous urogram of a 13-year-old child with sickle cell disease shows calyceal dilation and collecting system distortion.

many cases of RVT. Propagation of a central venous catheter–related inferior vena cava clot is an additional potential mechanism. Renal vein thrombosis in older patients can occur as the result of nephrotic syndrome, glomerulonephritis, a hypercoagulable state, trauma, or a retroperitoneal tumor. Typical clinical manifestations of RVT include nephromegaly, signs of renal insufficiency, hematuria, and hypertension.[39]

Imaging The typical sonographic features of RVT are abnormal parenchymal echogenicity and loss of

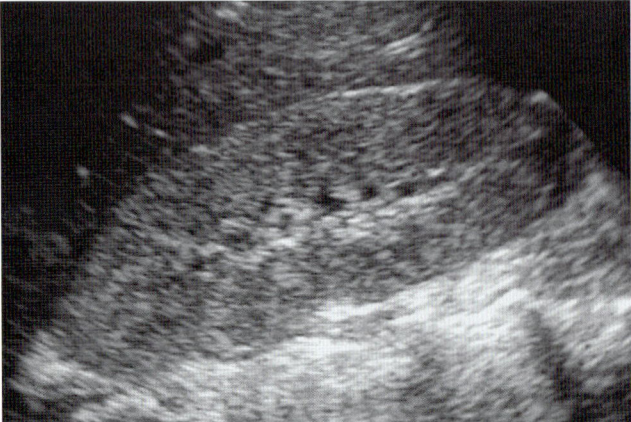

Figure 117-12 **Sickle cell disease.** A longitudinal sonographic image of a 15-year-old boy with sickle cell disease shows hyperechogenicity of the kidney and absent corticomedullary differentiation.

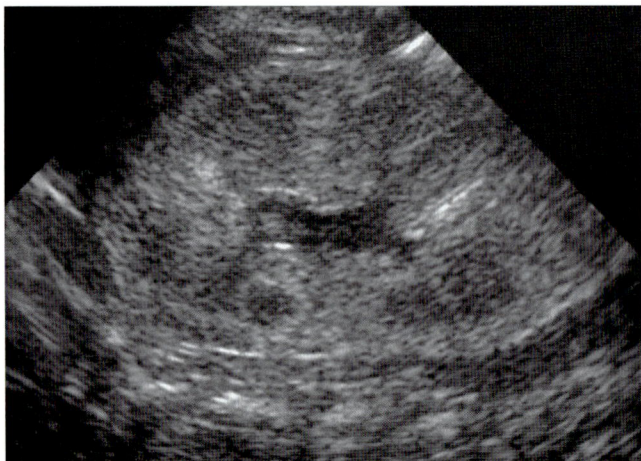

Figure 117-13 **Renal vein thrombosis.** Sonography of an infant with renal vein thrombosis shows an enlarged, echogenic kidney with loss of corticomedullary differentiation.

corticomedullary differentiation; in some cases, interlobular echogenic streaks are present (Fig. 117-13). Interstitial hemorrhage occasionally leads to parenchymal hyperechogenicity. Elevation of the arterial resistive index occurs as a result of venous outflow obstruction (Fig. 117-14). Narrowing of the systolic peak also is common. Careful sonographic evaluation of the renal veins sometimes reveals an echogenic clot; however, the absence of a clot within the major renal veins does not exclude the diagnosis of small vessel renal vein thrombosis. With severe involvement, Doppler evaluation

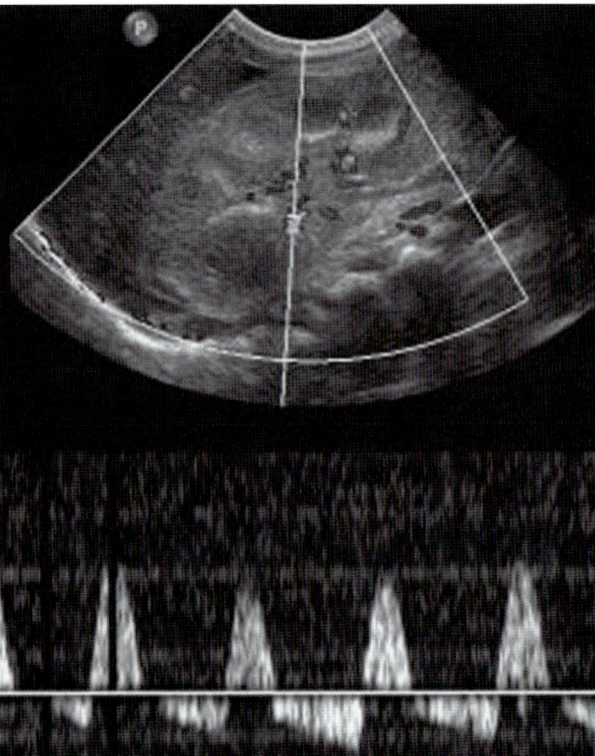

Figure 117-14 **Renal vein thrombosis.** The kidney of this 2-day-old infant is enlarged and echogenic. A highly resistive pattern of intrarenal arterial flow is present.

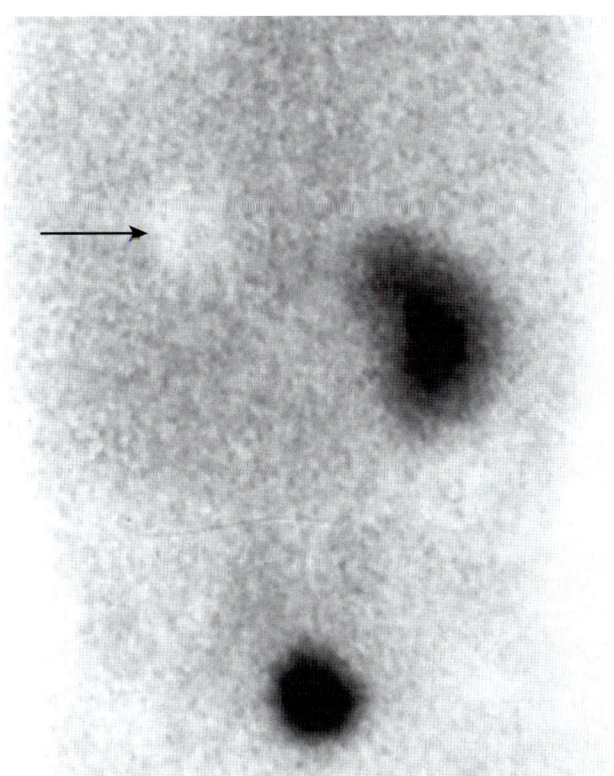

Figure 117-15 Renal vein thrombosis. A posterior technetium-99m diethylenetriaminepentaacetic acid scintigraphic image of an infant with left renal vein thrombosis shows absent left renal function. An oval suprarenal photopenic focus (*arrow*) is a result of concomitant adrenal hemorrhage.

imaging occasionally demonstrates a reticular pattern of calcification within the intrarenal veins; this finding is essentially pathognomonic of previous renal vein thrombosis.

WHAT THE CLINICIAN NEEDS TO KNOW

- Kidney sizes
- Parenchymal echogenicity
- Doppler flow characteristics of main renal arteries and veins
- Resistive indices of main renal arteries and intrarenal arteries
- Narrowing or thrombosis of renal arteries or veins

Key Points

Renal fibromuscular dysplasia is the most common cause of renal arterial stenosis in children.

Most renal arteriovenous fistulas are iatrogenic.

Renal artery thromboembolism in infants often is related to an umbilical artery catheter.

Hemolytic-uremic syndrome is the most common cause of acute renal failure in childhood.

Renal vein thrombosis is the most common neonatal renovascular abnormality.

may show an absence of flow within the main renal vein. In other patients, renal vein flow is monophasic.[40-42]

Treatment and Follow-up Therapy of RVT is supportive and directed toward treatment of the underlying cause. Renal scintigraphy during the acute phase provides prognostic information; mild compromise of uptake and excretion indicates a good prognosis (Fig. 117-15). Within a few weeks of onset of RVT, the affected kidney decreases in size. In some patients, progression to global atrophy occurs. Follow-up

Suggested Readings

Cakar N, Ozcakar ZB, Soy D, et al. Renal involvement in childhood vasculitis. *Nephron Clin Pract*. 2008;108(3):c202-c206.

Lau KK, Stoffman JM, Williams S, et al. Neonatal renal vein thrombosis: review of the English-language literature between 1992 and 2006. *Pediatrics*. 2007;120(5):e1278-e1284.

Olin JW, Sealove BA. Diagnosis, management, and future developments of fibromuscular dysplasia. *J Vasc Surg*. 2011;53(3):826-836, e821.

Tullus K, Brennan E, Hamilton G, et al. Renovascular hypertension in children. *Lancet*. 2008;371(9622):1453-1463.

References

Full references for this chapter can be found on www.expertconsult.com.

Chapter 118

Renal Failure and Transplantation

HARRIET J. PALTIEL

Acute Renal Failure

Overview Acute renal failure is defined as a sudden loss of renal function that may be due to inadequate renal perfusion, renal cell injury, or obstruction to urine flow. Recently, the term "acute kidney injury" (AKI) has been proposed to replace the term acute renal failure and is gaining wide acceptance.[1] AKI usually develops in hospitalized children as a result of systemic illness or its treatment and not from primary renal disease. The most common causes of AKI in children are renal ischemia, nephrotoxic drugs, and sepsis.[2] Other important causes are listed in Box 118-1. AKI from any cause can lead to chronic kidney disease.[3-7] Recovery of renal function depends on the underlying events leading to injury.

Imaging In general, sonography should be the first diagnostic imaging study performed in the workup of persons with AKI, and in most cases, it is the only imaging required. The role of sonography is to determine renal size and exclude anatomic abnormalities as the cause of AKI. The renal cortex, medulla, and collecting system have different acoustic properties, and pathologic changes are readily detected and correlate well with histologic findings. Doppler techniques provide information about renal perfusion and vascular abnormalities. Sonography also is used to localize the kidneys for percutaneous biopsy. More precise functional information may be obtained with nuclear medicine studies that can aid in differentiating between prerenal, renal, and postrenal causes of AKI.

Prerenal Injury In persons with prerenal injury, the kidney is intrinsically normal, and renal function is diminished as a result of decreased renal perfusion. Sonographic examination of the kidneys is normal. Restoration of renal perfusion results in a prompt return of renal function.

Intrinsic Renal Disease Renal ischemia due to a prolonged prerenal injury or a severe hypoxic/ischemic insult can lead to acute tubular necrosis. Imaging findings depend on the severity of parenchymal injury. A generalized increase in renal cortical echogenicity indicates intrinsic renal disease (Fig. 118-1). In mild cases, the kidneys may appear normal or may demonstrate slightly increased renal cortical echogenicity. Decreased corticomedullary differentiation may be noted. Doppler flow may be normal in mild disease, whereas poor peripheral perfusion and diminished arterial diastolic flow due to increased peripheral vascular resistance occur in more severe cases.

Nephrotoxic drugs commonly associated with AKI include antibiotics, chemotherapeutic agents, and nonsteroidal antiinflammatory medications.[8] Some agents such as aminoglycoside antibiotics cause tubular injury. Methicillin and other penicillin analogues, cimetidine, sulfonamides, rifampin, and nonsteroidal antiinflammatory drugs may cause acute interstitial nephritis, which is thought to be related to a hypersensitivity reaction with development of antitubular basement membrane antibodies in some cases. Children with acute lymphocytic leukemia and B-cell lymphoma are at risk for the development of uric acid nephropathy and tumor lysis syndrome. One mechanism of injury believed to be of importance in uric acid nephropathy is precipitation of uric acid crystals in the renal microvasculature leading to obstruction of renal blood flow, or precipitation in the renal tubules leading to obstruction of urine flow. Tumor lysis syndrome is a constellation of metabolic abnormalities resulting from spontaneous or treatment-related tumor necrosis. As tumor cells are lysed, rapid increases in serum potassium, uric acid, and phosphorus occur, with a decrease in serum calcium. Patients who are treated with allopurinol, a purine analog used to diminish the excretion of uric acid, instead excrete large quantities of the uric acid precursors xanthine and hypoxanthine. Precipitation of these compounds is thought to play a role in the development of AKI. In patients who are in septic shock, AKI can develop from hypotension, leading to renal ischemia and acute tubular necrosis, or AKI can develop as a result of the use of nephrotoxic medications.

Obstructive Uropathy and Lower Tract Lesions A urinary tract obstruction can develop in persons with AKI if the obstruction affects a solitary kidney, both ureters, or the urethra. Congenital causes include ureteropelvic junction obstruction, ureterovesical junction obstruction, and posterior urethral valves. Acquired urinary tract obstruction can be caused by urinary tract stones or, rarely, tumors. Bladder rupture is another rare cause of AKI associated with ascites. Bladder rupture in children usually is due to trauma; it also can occur as a complication of infection, chemotherapy, and radiotherapy.[9,10]

Box 118-1 Common Causes of Acute Kidney Injury

Prerenal Failure
- Decreased true intravascular volume
- Decreased effective intravascular volume

Intrinsic Renal Disease
- Acute tubular necrosis (vasomotor neuropathy)
  - Hypoxic/ischemic insults
  - Drug induced
  - Toxin mediated
    Endogenous toxins—hemoglobin, myoglobin
    Exogenous toxins—ethylene glycol, methanol

Uric Acid Nephropathy and Tumor Lysis Syndrome

Interstitial Nephritis
- Drug induced
- Idiopathic

Glomerulonephritis

Vascular Lesions
- Renal artery thrombosis
- Renal vein thrombosis
- Cortical necrosis
- Hemolytic uremic syndrome

Hypoplasia/Dysplasia with or Without Obstructive Uropathy
- Idiopathic
- Exposure to nephrotoxic drugs in utero

Hereditary Renal Disease
- Autosomal-dominant polycystic kidney disease
- Autosomal-recessive polycystic kidney disease
- Alport syndrome
- Sickle cell nephropathy
- Juvenile nephronophthisis

Obstructive Uropathy/Lower Tract Lesions
- Obstruction in a solitary kidney
- Bilateral ureteral obstruction
- Urethral obstruction
- Bladder rupture

From Andreoli SP. Clinical evaluation of acute kidney injury in children. In: Avner ED, ed. *Pediatric Nephrology*. 6th ed. Berlin: Springer-Verlag; 2009.

Chronic Renal Failure

Overview The terms "chronic renal failure" and "chronic renal insufficiency" have been used historically to describe varying degrees of renal dysfunction. Currently, the term *chronic kidney disease* (CKD) is used by both adult and pediatric nephrology communities throughout the world.[11] The classification of CKD published by the National Kidney Foundation's Kidney Disease Outcomes Quality Initiative is based on the estimated glomerular filtration rate and is applicable to children older than 2 years and to adults.[12] The classification categorizes CKD into five different stages and is widely used in clinical practice (Table 118-1). Recently it has been recognized that most patients with CKD (estimated to be one in eight adults) never reach end-stage renal disease and the need for renal replacement therapy because they are

at risk for accelerated cardiovascular disease and are more likely to die prematurely from cerebrovascular or cardiovascular disease.[13] Therefore clinical management requires measures to diminish cardiovascular risk factors in both adult and pediatric patients. According to the North American Pediatric Renal Trials and Collaborative Studies 2007 report,[14] the most common causes of pediatric CKD in North America are congenital disorders such as obstructive uropathy, renal dysplasia, and reflux nephropathy (Fig. 118-2; Table 118-2). In contrast, in Japan, 34% of pediatric CKD is due to glomerulonephritis, primary focal segmental glomerulosclerosis, and immunoglobulin A nephropathy.[15] In Jordan[16] and Iran,[17] where consanguinity is more common, heritable disorders such as cystic kidney disease, primary hyperoxaluria, cystinosis, Alport syndrome, and congenital nephrotic syndrome represent a greater proportion of cases of CKD. In the developing world, acquired causes of CKD predominate, particularly infection-related glomerulopathies.[18,19] The worldwide incidence and prevalence of CKD is greater for boys than for girls because of the higher incidence of congenital causes of CKD in boys.[14-21]

Imaging Imaging plays an essential role in diagnosis, assessment of function, and monitoring of the effects of treatment at all stages of CKD, from the antenatal period to pretransplantation evaluation. Many urinary tract abnormalities are discovered by prenatal sonography. Postnatal imaging usually focuses on growth, function, and assessment of complications. A multimodality approach often is required, including radiography, sonography, fluoroscopy, nuclear medicine, and magnetic resonance imaging.

As with AKI, sonography is the primary imaging modality used to investigate CKD and guide performance of a biopsy. Assessment of renal and bladder morphology permits detection of congenital anomalies such as ureteropelvic junction obstruction, posterior urethral valves, duplex collecting systems and ureters, and ectopic ureteral insertion. Determination of kidney size is critical for long-term follow-up. Enlarged kidneys may occur in the setting of obstruction, cystic disease, and glomerulonephritis. Hypoplastic and scarred kidneys usually are small. A gradual reduction in kidney size usually occurs in persons with CKD. With progressive CKD, a concomitant loss of corticomedullary differentiation usually occurs, and most patients will have echogenic renal

Table 118-1

Kidney Disease Outcomes Quality Initiative Stages of Chronic Kidney Disease		
Stage	**Description**	**GFR (mL/ min/1.73 m²)**
1	Kidney damage with normal or increased GFR	≥90
2	Kidney damage with mild decrease in GFR	60-89
3	Moderate decrease in GFR	30-59
4	Severe decrease in GFR	15-29
5	Kidney failure	<15 (or dialysis)

GFR, Glomerular filtration rate.
From VanDeVoorde RG, Warady BA. Management of chronic kidney disease. In: Avner ED, ed. *Pediatric nephrology*. 6th ed. Berlin: Springer-Verlag; 2009.

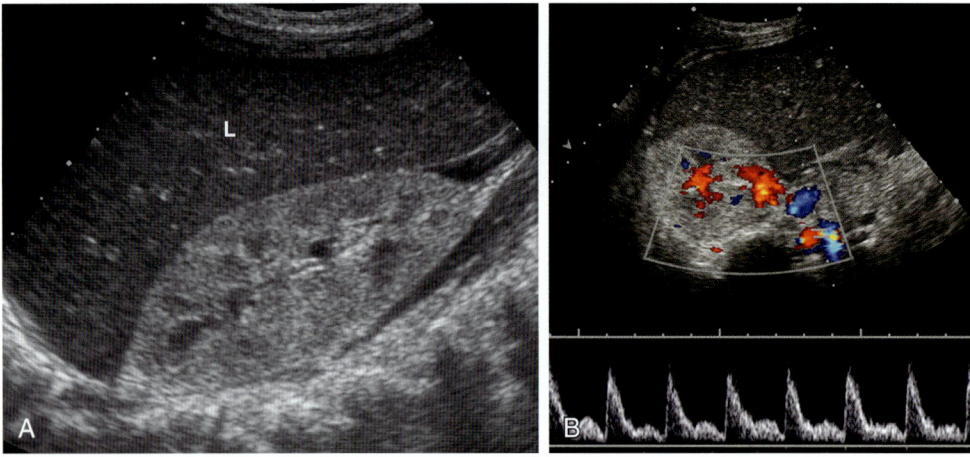

Figure 118-1   Hemolytic-uremic syndrome. **A,** A sonogram of an 18-month-old boy with impaired renal function shows an enlarged right kidney with parenchymal echogenicity greater than that of the adjacent liver (*L*) and decreased corticomedullary differentiation. **B,** A pulsed Doppler waveform from the main renal artery shows diminished diastolic flow.

parenchyma. However, increased renal parenchymal echogenicity is nonspecific and is not linked to the severity of disease.[22] Dysplastic kidneys have disordered development that generally is manifested as a combination of echogenic parenchyma and cysts (Fig. 118-3). Dysplasia may be focal or diffuse and generally appears sonographically as echogenic tissue without recognizable corticomedullary differentiation. Total bilateral renal dysplasia is incompatible with life. Multicystic dysplastic kidney is the most common form of unilateral dysplasia and consists of multiple large, noncommunicating cysts of varying size and minimal intervening echogenic parenchyma. Most of these kidneys eventually will involute.[23] Monitoring of the contralateral functioning kidney is critical in these patients, because associated abnormalities

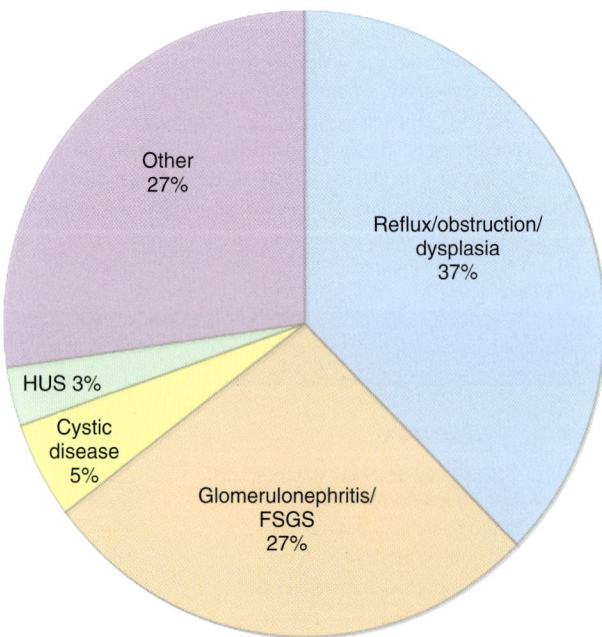

Figure 118-2   Primary causes of end-stage renal disease in pediatric patients. *HUS,* Hemolytic uremic syndrome; *FSGS,* focal segmental glomerulosclerosis. (Modified from Eddy A, Pathophysiology of progressive renal disease. In: Avner ED, ed. *Pediatric nephrology.* 6th ed. Berlin: Springer-Verlag; 2009.)

Table 118-2

2007 North American Pediatric Renal Trials and Collaborative Studies Report, Primary Diagnosis of Chronic Renal Insufficiency

Primary Diagnosis	No. of Patients (N = 6794)	%
Obstructive uropathy	1436	21.1
Aplastic/hypoplastic/dysplastic kidney	1187	17.5
Focal segmental glomerulosclerosis	589	8.7
Reflux nephropathy	568	8.4
Polycystic disease	271	4.0
Prune belly	192	2.8
Renal infarct	157	2.3
Hemolytic uremic syndrome	138	2.0
Systemic lupus erythematosus nephritis	108	1.6
Familial nephritis	108	1.6
Membranoproliferative glomerulonephritis, types I and II	102	1.5
Cystinosis	100	1.5
Pyelonephritis/interstitial nephritis	95	1.4
Medullary cystic disease	86	1.3
Chronic glomerulonephritis	81	1.2
Congenital nephritic syndrome	74	1.1
Immunoglobulin A (Berger) nephropathy	66	1.0
Idiopathic crescentic glomerulonephritis	46	0.7
Henoch-Schönlein nephritis	42	0.6
Membranous nephropathy	35	0.5
Wilms tumor	31	0.5
Other systemic immunologic disorders	25	0.4
Wegener granulomatosis	21	0.3
Sickle cell nephropathy	14	0.2
Diabetic glomerulopathy	11	0.2
Oxalosis	7	0.1
Drash syndrome	6	0.1
Other	1020	15.0

From VanDeVoorde RG, Warady BA. Management of chronic kidney disease. In: Avner ED, ed. *Pediatric nephrology.* 6th ed. Berlin: Springer-Verlag; 2009.

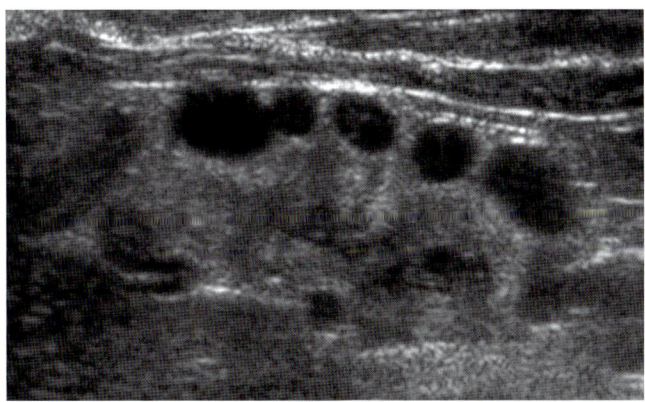

Figure 118-3 **Renal dysplasia.** A sagittal sonogram of the right kidney in a 7-week-old boy with renal failure shows that the kidney is small, with echogenic parenchyma and multiple peripheral cysts. The left kidney had a similar appearance (not shown).

are common.[24] Renal scarring may occur as a sequela of infection or vesicoureteral reflux. Sonography is relatively insensitive in the detection of scarring, and nuclear scintigraphy with dimercaptosuccinic acid may be required for more precise assessment of renal parenchymal integrity.[25] Patients with autosomal-recessive polycystic kidney disease have large, echogenic kidneys with poor corticomedullary differentiation due to the presence of microscopic cysts. Visible cysts less than 1 cm in diameter are detected in about 50% of children (Fig. 118-4). Evaluation of the liver is necessary because of the high association of parenchymal cysts and fibrosis. Autosomal-dominant polycystic kidney disease may manifest in childhood, although associated CKD is rare. The kidneys usually appear normal initially, with cystic changes developing later in life. Occasionally, cysts may be present at birth.[26-29] Renal vascularity reflects functional status and will decrease in persons with CKD. Several recent publications suggest that the renal arterial resistive index may correlate with creatinine levels and may be an independent risk factor for the progression of CKD.[30,31]

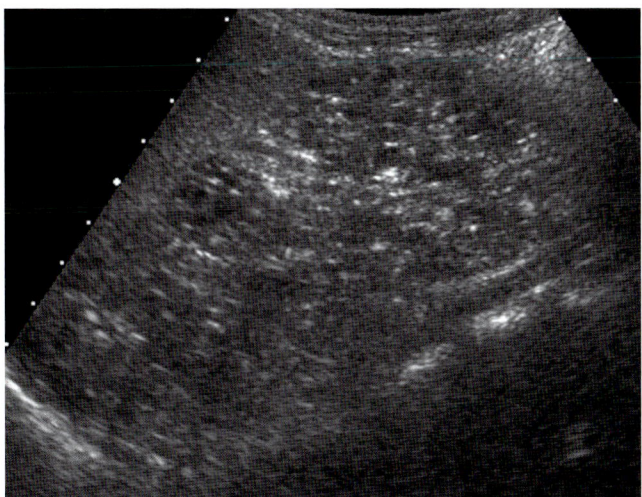

Figure 118-4 **Autosomal-recessive polycystic kidney disease.** A sagittal sonogram in a 6-year-old girl reveals an enlarged, echogenic right kidney containing innumerable tiny cysts. The left kidney had a similar appearance (not shown).

Transplantation

Overview Renal transplantation is the treatment of choice in children with end-stage renal disease, with improved patient survival and quality of life compared with dialysis. However, renal transplantation in children is associated with a number of specific problems, including a higher incidence of graft failure and posttransplant malignancy than in adults, as well as growth retardation. Furthermore, it may be challenging technically to transplant a relatively large adult kidney into a small pediatric abdomen. Transplantation of kidneys from donors younger than 5 years usually is avoided because the risk of early graft failure is increased, mainly as a result of graft thrombosis.[32] Adult kidneys almost always are used. An allograft may be from a living, related donor, from a living, unrelated donor, or it may be cadaveric in origin. In the United States, more than 50% of transplanted kidneys in children are from living, adult donors.[33]

Imaging Assessment of the transplant kidney is similar to that of a native kidney, with an emphasis on graft perfusion and vascular anastomoses; sonography is the primary imaging technique. Familiarity with the surgical anatomy is essential to a complete evaluation of the vasculature. In small children, the kidney is placed intraperitoneally with anastomosis of the donor renal artery and vein to the recipient distal aorta and inferior vena cava, respectively. In older children, the graft is placed in a retroperitoneal location within an iliac fossa. The donor renal artery is anastomosed either to the recipient external (more commonly) or to the internal iliac artery, and the donor vein is anastomosed to the recipient external iliac vein. The donor ureter is anastomosed to the recipient urinary bladder (ureteroneocystostomy).

A normal kidney transplant has a sonographic appearance similar to that of a normal native kidney. The close proximity of the graft to the body surface accentuates the distinction between the renal cortex, medullary pyramids, and central sinus. Doppler evaluation reveals continuous antegrade flow within the main renal artery throughout the cardiac cycle, with low-impedance arterial waveforms in the intrarenal vessels. The intrarenal arterial resistive indices range from 0.4 to 0.8, with a mean value of 0.6.[34] Flow within the main renal vein and intrarenal veins is opposite in direction to that in the arteries and usually is mildly pulsatile, reflecting normal cardiac and respiratory motion.

In the immediate postoperative period, the most common complications are acute tubular necrosis, vascular thrombosis, and rejection. These entities may be difficult to distinguish with imaging techniques. In all three entities, the graft will appear swollen, with loss of normal corticomedullary differentiation and elevated arterial resistive indices. Renal vein thrombosis usually occurs in the first postoperative week and manifests as decreased or absent flow within the main renal vein associated with elevated arterial resistive indices (Fig. 118-5). Additional acute complications include urine leaks, other fluid collections (e.g., hematoma or abscess), urinary obstruction, and vesicoureteral reflux, all of which are readily demonstrated by imaging.[35-37] Lymphoceles are the most common fluid collections and are caused by lymphatic disruption. They usually develop weeks to months after transplantation (Fig. 118-6).[38]

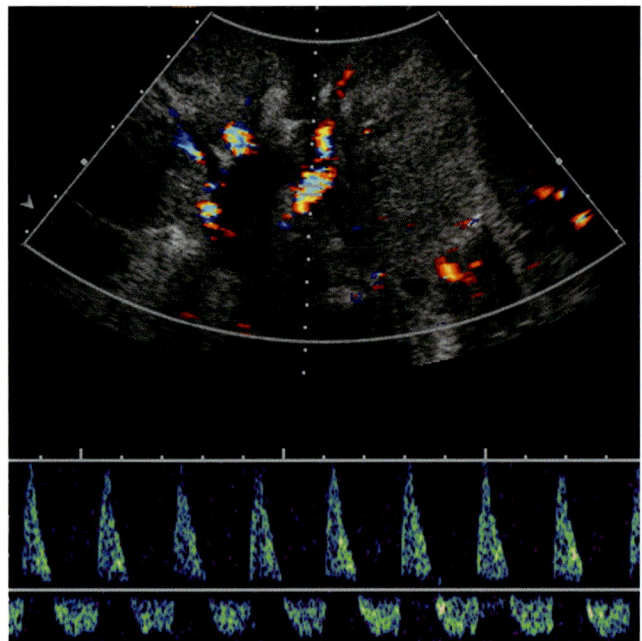

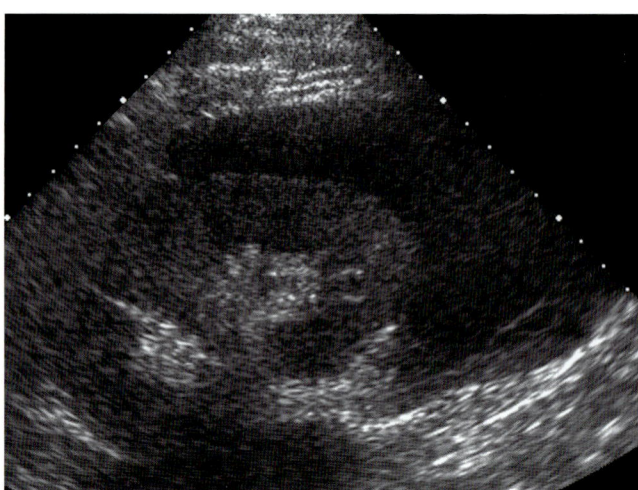

Figure 118-6 **Lymphocele.** A sagittal sonogram of a 16-year-old boy obtained 5 weeks after living-related donor transplantation depicts a large fluid collection surrounding the lower pole of the left-sided kidney.

Figure 118-5 Transplant renal vein thrombosis. A longitudinal sonogram of a 20-month-old boy 1 day after living-related donor transplantation shows a swollen, echogenic kidney with diminished corticomedullary differentiation. Marked pulsatility of the main renal arterial waveform is noted with reversed diastolic flow, reflecting increased peripheral resistance.

Renal artery stenosis usually occurs within the first 3 years after transplantation.[39,40] Doppler sonography may demonstrate an elevated velocity within the main renal artery of greater than 200 cm/sec (Fig. 118-7), as well as a *pulsus parvus et tardus* waveform in the arteries distal to the stenotic site. Although Doppler sonography is the screening modality of choice, significant stenotic lesions can be missed.

Computed tomographic angiography and magnetic resonance angiography are useful problem-solving techniques when sonography is inconclusive. However, catheter angiography remains the "gold" standard imaging technique for renal artery imaging.[40-42]

Important late complications include chronic rejection and posttransplant lymphoproliferative disorder (PTLD). Chronic rejection is manifested sonographically by a gradual reduction in graft size, increased parenchymal echogenicity, and decreased perfusion.[37] In the pediatric renal transplant population, two large series have reported an incidence of 1.2%[43] and 4.5%.[44] PTLD is the most common neoplastic disorder in pediatric transplant recipients, accounting for 52% of all malignancies in this patient population,[45] and is associated

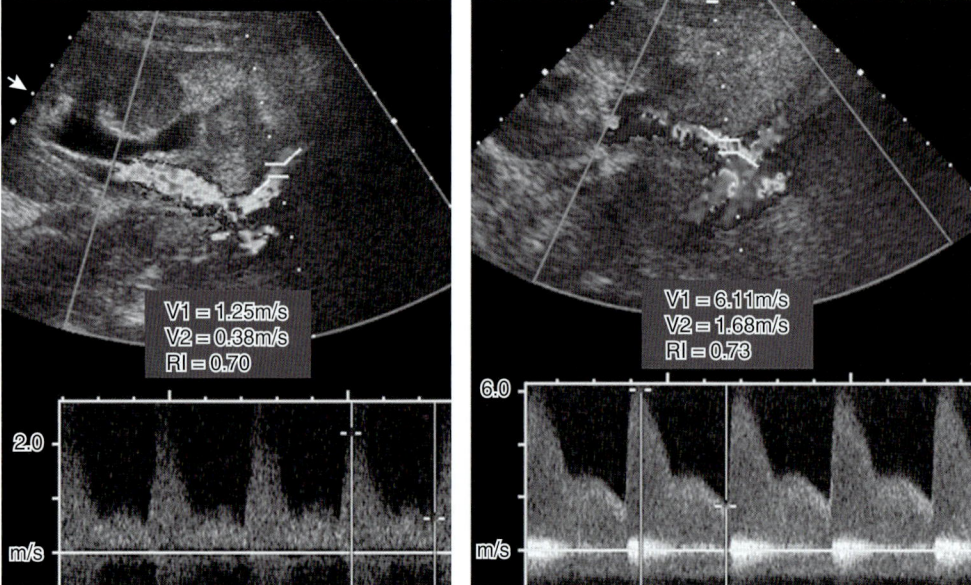

Figure 118-7 Transplant renal arterial stenosis. A Doppler sonogram of a patient with a rising creatinine level shows a nearly fivefold increase in renal arterial peak systolic velocity (right image) compared with the supplying external iliac artery (left image), indicating hemodynamically significant stenosis.

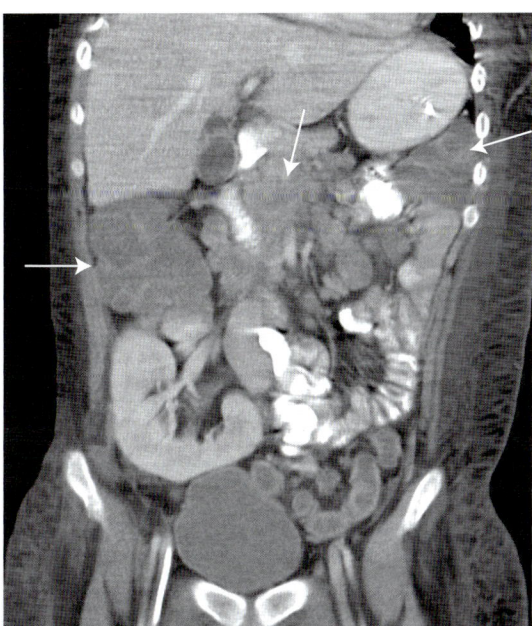

Figure 118-8 Posttransplant lymphoproliferative disorder. A coronal reformatted image from contrast-enhanced computed tomography in a 17-year-old boy shows a right lower quadrant renal transplant. Multiple low-density conglomerate masses within the abdomen represent lymphoproliferative tissue (arrows).

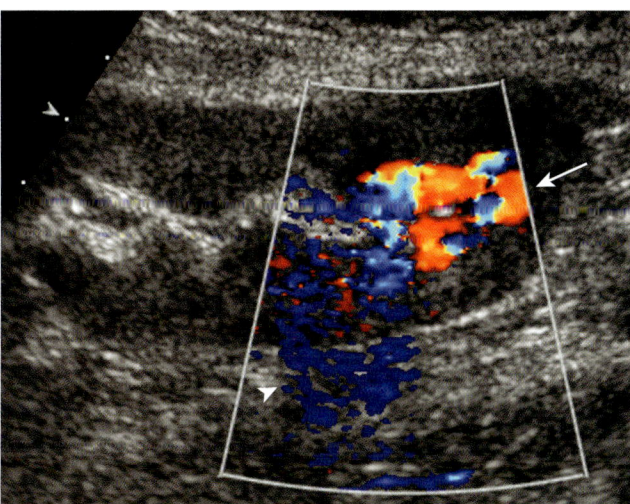

Figure 118-9 **A postbiopsy arteriovenous fistula.** A color Doppler sonogram shows enlarged vessels in the lower pole of a renal homograft (*arrow*) associated with soft tissue vibration artifact (*arrowhead*).

with Epstein-Barr virus (EBV) infection. In immune-suppressed persons with impaired T-cell immune surveillance, EBV infection can cause abnormal B-cell proliferation, especially in persons who were seronegative at the time of transplantation.[45,46] Patients at risk will have elevated EBV titers, and sonographic follow-up must include a search for lymph node enlargement and solid masses of the abdominal and pelvic viscera (Fig. 118-8).

Renal biopsy may be indicated at any stage after transplantation and often is performed under sonographic guidance. Iatrogenic complications of biopsy include hemorrhage and arteriovenous fistula formation (Fig. 118-9). Sonographic monitoring of the native kidneys always should be performed because of an increased risk of malignancy.[47,48]

WHAT THE CLINICIAN NEEDS TO KNOW

- Dilated or nondilated renal collecting system
- Parenchymal echogenicity, corticomedullary differentiation, and renal size
- Congenital versus acquired malformations
- Presence of posttransplant urinomas, lymphoceles, hematomas, urinary obstruction, and/or masses
- Renal vein patency and renal artery spectral wave form, peak systolic velocity, and resistive index

Key Points

Sonography is the first imaging study performed for evaluation for AKI and CKD and often is the only imaging required.

Nuclear medicine studies provide functional information that helps distinguish prerenal, renal, and postrenal causes of AKI and CKD.

Sonography is the technique of choice for detecting complications of renal transplantation.

PTLD is the most common neoplastic disorder in pediatric transplant recipients.

Sonographic monitoring of native kidneys in transplant recipients is necessary because of an increased risk of malignancy.

Suggested Readings

Akbar SA, Jafri SZ, Amendola MA, et al. Complications of renal transplantation. *Radiographics.* 2005;25:1335-1356.

Borhani AA, Hosseinzadeh K, Almusa O, et al. Imaging of posttransplantation lymphoproliferative disorder after solid organ transplantation. *Radiographics.* 2009;29:981-1000.

Irshad A, Ackerman SJ, Campbell AS, et al. An overview of renal transplantation: current practice and use of ultrasound. *Semin Ultrasound CT MRI.* 2009;30:298-314.

Kalantarinia K. Novel imaging techniques in acute kidney injury. *Curr Drug Targets.* 2009;10:1184-1189.

Khati NJ, Hill MC, Kimmel PL. The role of ultrasound in renal insufficiency: the essentials. *Ultrasound Q.* 2005;21:227-244.

References

Full references for this chapter can be found on www.expertconsult.com.

Chapter 119

The Ureter

D. GREGORY BATES and MICHAEL RICCABONA

Embryology

The ureter develops from a branch of the mesonephric duct called the ureteric bud. It arises during the fourth to fifth week of pregnancy and grows dorsally and upward until it contacts the nephrogenic cord. This contact of the ureteric bud with the metanephric blastema induces normal kidney development. The ureterovesical junction (UVJ) develops as the distal parts of the mesonephric duct are incorporated into the enlarging bladder originating from the urogenital sinus. As the mesonephric ducts are absorbed, the ureters come to open separately into the urinary bladder, with the orifice moving superolaterally and the distal ureteral segments entering obliquely through the base of the bladder. During this complex course of development, numerous variations concerning the position of the kidney, the course of the ureter, and the anatomy of the UVJ, as well as the ureteropelvic junction (UPJ), may arise.[1-11]

Imaging On ultrasonography, the ureter can only be visualized when it is sufficiently filled with urine. The UPJ usually can be sonographically visualized in well-hydrated patients with a tapering of the pelvis toward the proximal ureter, using the kidney as an acoustic window from a dorsal or lateral approach. For visualizing the distal ureter, a sufficiently distended urinary bladder is mandatory, because it serves as a window to the retrovesical space. With sufficient bladder filling, the normal ureter can be detected and followed superiorly for several centimeters. Further visualization up to the iliac vessels or higher is only possible in cases with a significantly dilated ureter and sufficient sonographic access.[1]

The patency of the ureteral orifice can be sonographically assessed by observing the urine inflow jet into the urinary bladder. This ureteral jet sometimes can be seen on gray scale as a rush of pseudoechoes from the ureteral ostium into the bladder lumen, but it is more easily seen with color Doppler ultrasonography. Color Doppler imaging allows not only visualization of ureteral patency and osteal position but also evaluation of the frequency of the inflow jet, indicating ureteric peristaltic activity. Thus asymmetric jets, atypical direction of the ureteral jet, lateralized orifice position, and unusual ostial shape and impaired ureteral peristalsis may be used as indirect signs for ureteral pathology or dysfunction such as obstruction or vesicoureteral reflux (VUR).[1,12-14]

Modern multislice computed tomography (CT) is a powerful imaging tool that provides high spatial and anatomic resolution, but it may impose a significant radiation burden even using low-dose pediatric protocols. Thus in pediatric uroradiology, CT should be restricted to uncommon and complicated cases. Contrast-enhanced CT allows for excellent delineation of the entire ureter. By using three-dimensional reformatting and viewing techniques, an intravenous urography–like comprehensive overview over the entire ureter can be achieved. This technique usually is applied in rare or difficult cases, such as for assessment of a retrocaval ureter, ureteral tumors, and paraureteral pathology compressing or displacing the ureter.[1,15-17]

Magnetic resonance urography (MRU) is a powerful new tool for imaging the ureter and urinary tract. By applying heavily T2-weighted sequences, a sufficiently distended or dilated ureter can be visualized in its entire course without administration of a contrast agent. However, diuretic stimulation before the investigation is helpful and even mandatory in many cases. Diuretic contrast-enhanced MRU additionally allows for functional assessment by using fast T1-weighted sequences (usually three-dimensional gradient-echo or turbo-flash). The spatial resolution of MRU is less than on CT, and thus small folds or tiny stones can be overlooked or only inferred from indirect signs. In the lower parts of the ureter, where motion from breathing is less likely, high-resolution magnetic resonance (MR) sequences can improve spatial resolution for depiction of small structures, such as an unusual course or insertion site of an ectopic ureter.[1,18-22]

The current best method for assessment of ureteral function and drainage is dynamic nuclear scintigraphy. Serial image acquisitions are obtained after intravenous injection of technetium-99m–labeled mercaptoacetyltriglycine and diuretic stimulation. Ureteral drainage can be visualized and quantified in a standardized fashion. However, the normal ureter usually is difficult to assess by this method and, despite its excellent functional information, anatomic resolution is poor.[1,23-25]

Obstruction of the Ureter

Overview Obstruction may be severe, threatening renal function and urine drainage, or it may be partial and minor without any clinical consequence. Most ureteral obstructions occur at the UPJ or UVJ. Obstructive lesions between these two points are uncommon and include retrocaval ureter, retroiliac ureter, ureteral obstruction caused by other vessels, ureteral valves, acquired ureteral strictures, ureteral urolithiasis, ureteral neoplasms, and extrinsic lesions affecting the ureter.[1]

Ureteral Valves and Striations

Overview Ureteral valves are said to consist of a cusplike fold or an iris diaphragm composed of ureteral mucosa and smooth muscle fibers (Fig. 119-1). They are more commonly found in the lower third of the ureter. In neonates and infants, ureteral valves may be difficult to differentiate from physiologic ureteral folds, which are immature remnants that disappear during the first years of life. Ureteral striations are longitudinal mucosal folds that may be seen in normal ureters but often are a sign of inflammatory disease, VUR, or previous obstruction. They must be distinguished from submucosal hemorrhage and collateral circulation resulting from renal vein or inferior vena cava thrombosis.[1,26-32]

Vascular Obstruction

Overview A retrocaval or circumcaval ureter (Fig. 119-2) is an uncommon anomaly in which the right ureter passes behind the inferior vena cava, emerges between the cava and

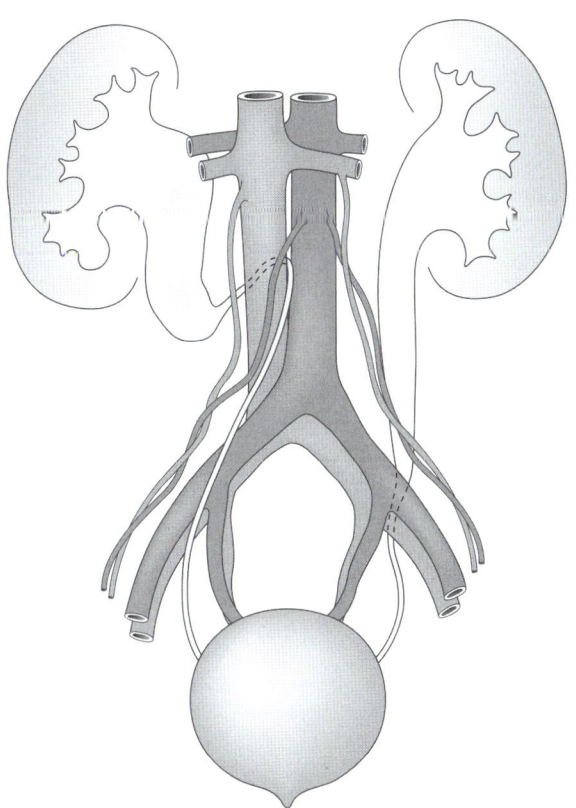

Figure 119-2 **Abnormal ureteral course.** An anatomic diagram shows a right retrocaval ureter and a left retroiliac ureter.

the aorta, and then curves around and in front of the cava to return to its normal position in the pelvis. This anomaly results from abnormal persistence of the subcardinal vein in the definitive inferior vena cava. The ureter descends from the renal pelvis and crosses behind the inferior vena cava near its bifurcation. It then curves medially and upward, forming a reversed-J appearance (Fig. 119-3). Ureteral obstruction at this level is common. The retrocaval ureter is more common in males than in females and usually manifests in adult life, perhaps because the hydronephrosis is slow to develop. The anomaly may be demonstrated with contrast-enhanced multidetector CT, but MRU (with or without contrast) provides a less invasive and nonionizing imaging option.[1,33-35] Ureteral obstructions caused by accessory renal arteries, iliac vessels, ovarian arteries, and hypogastric arteries (e-Fig. 119-4) are rare. Normal vascular impressions occasionally are seen on imaging (e-Fig. 119-5).[36-37]

Ureteral Ectopia: Intravesical Versus Extravesical

Overview An ectopic ureter is one that drains in an abnormal location (outside the posterolateral angle of the trigone) either within the bladder or extravesically. Extravesical ureteral ectopia is more common and clinically more important than the intravesical type. It also is more common in girls than in boys, with some anatomic and functional differences between the two sexes (Table 119-1). It is more common in ureteral duplication anomalies (up to 80%).[1,11,38-41]

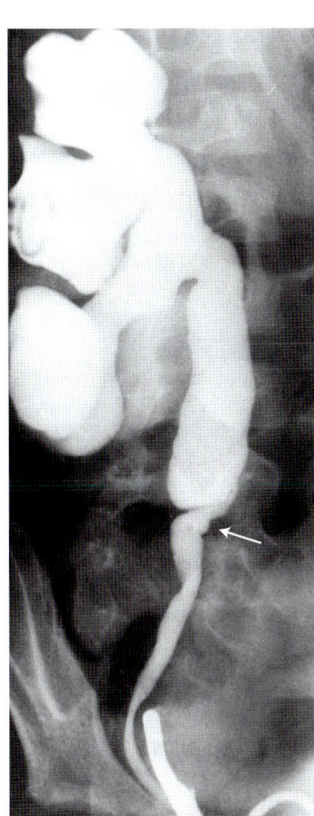

Figure 119-1 **Ureteral mucosal fold.** Retrograde study shows midureteral obstruction and hydronephrosis caused by a congenital valve-like mucosal fold (*arrow*).

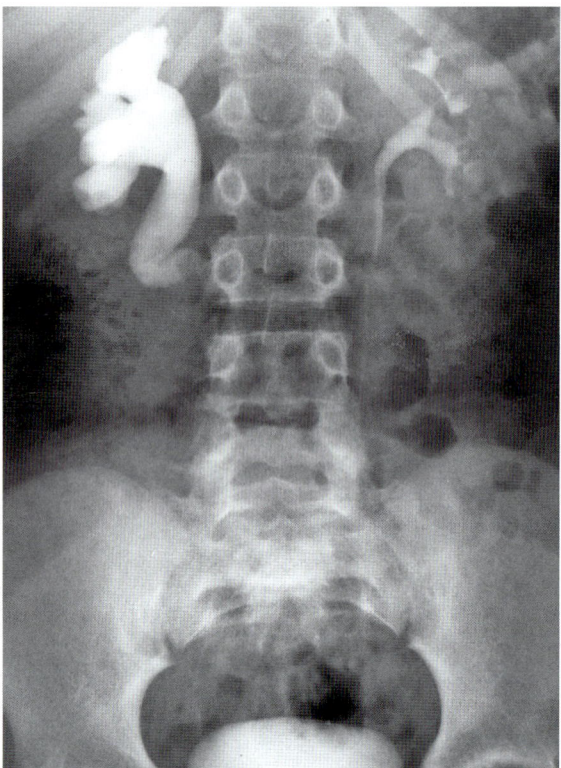

Figure 119-3 **Retrocaval ureter.** Intravenous urography image shows right hydronephrosis. The dilated right ureter passes behind the inferior vena cava in front of the L3 pedicle.

Table 119-1

Extravesical Ureteral Ectopia		
	Girls	**Boys**
Duplicated system	More common	Less common
	Inserts into the urethra, vestibule, vagina	Inserts into the prostatic urethra, bladder neck, genital ducts
	Urethral-ending ureter refluxes	Same
	Ectopic ureter normal	Same
	Drains atrophic nubbin	Same
	Lower pole refluxes	Same
	Chief complaint: continuous urine leakage	Chief complaint: infection
Single system	Uncommon	Uncommon
	Associated with a small, often ectopic kidney	Associated with a dysplastic kidney
	May insert in the urethra, vestibule, vagina	May insert in the seminal vesicle
	Gartner duct cyst	Ejaculatory duct wolffian tissue posterior to bladder

Intravesical Ureteral Ectopia Two types of intravesical ureteral ectopia are recognized: lateral and caudal. In lateral ectopia, the more common of the two, one or both ureters (the lower pole ureter in a duplicated system) drain into the bladder more superior and laterally than normal. The intramural submucosal tunnel of the affected ureter tends to be short or otherwise defective, leading to VUR in many cases.

In the second type, one or both ureters (the upper pole ureter in a duplicated system) drain inferior and medial to the usual site along a line extending from the normal lateral corner of the trigone to the bladder neck. These ureters are less prone to VUR than the lateral type.[1,38,41]

Extravesical Ureteral Ectopia Extravesical ureteral ectopia in girls (Fig. 119-6) is associated with a duplicated system in at least 85% of cases and affects the upper pole ureter in practically all cases. The ectopic ureter may end in the urethra or in the vestibule or, less commonly, in the vagina (Fig. 119-7).

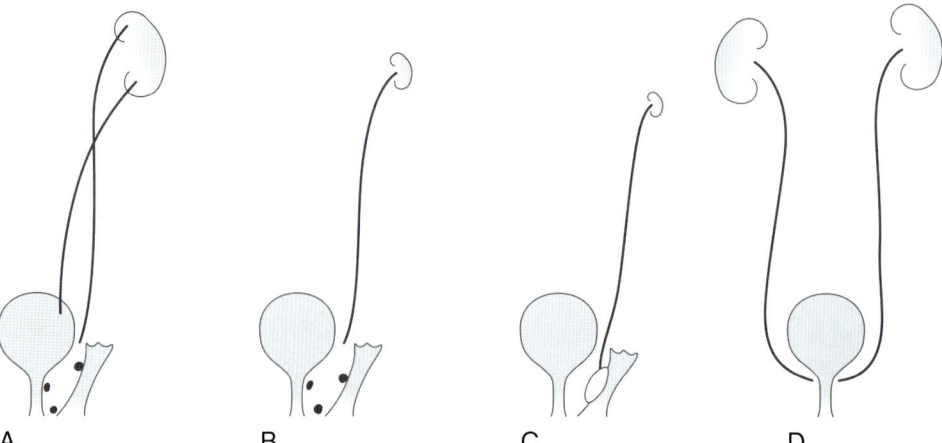

A   B   C   D

Figure 119-6 **Types of ureteral ectopia in females. A,** In the most common variant, ureteral duplication is present, with the upper pole ureter draining into the urethra, into the perineum near the urethral meatus, or into the vagina. **B,** Ectopic ureteral drainage as in **A,** but from a single collecting system. The kidney may be small and dysplastic. **C,** Ectopic drainage from a single system into a Gartner duct cyst in the wall of the vagina. The ipsilateral kidney may not be identifiable. **D,** Bilateral single-system ectopic drainage into the bladder neck or proximal urethra. This uncommon form is found almost exclusively in females and usually is associated with a wide bladder neck, a defective internal sphincter, sometimes a malformed urethra, and urinary incontinence.

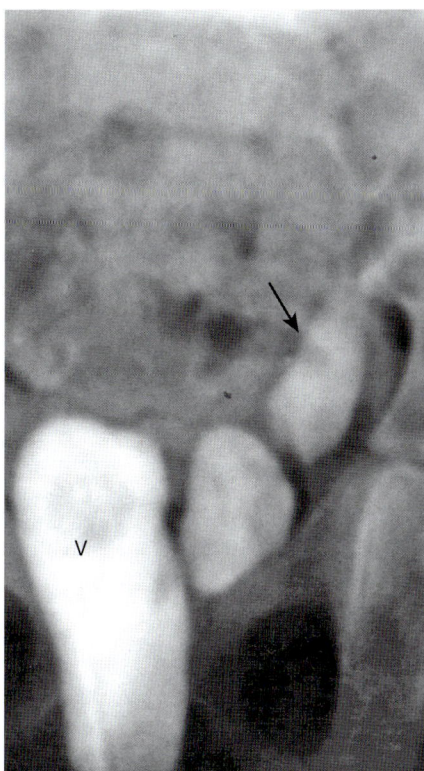

Figure 119-7 Ureteral ectopia. Contrast medium injected into the vagina (*V*) is seen filling the distal left ureter (*arrow*).

A common presenting complaint is continuous leakage of urine in the context of an otherwise normal voiding pattern. Leakage of urine is observed even if the anomalous ureter ends in the proximal urethra, as a result of the relative weakness of the external urethral sphincter in girls. The renal parenchyma drained by the ectopic ureter often is dysplastic with decreased or absent function. The ipsilateral lower pole ureter may be normal or dilated and frequently is the site of reflux.[1,42-46]

Single (unduplicated) ureteral ectopia in girls is uncommon and usually unilateral. The corresponding kidney frequently is small and dysplastic and may be ectopic. Sometimes the ectopic ureter is connected with a multicystic dysplastic kidney or ends blindly superiorly without renal tissue (renal agenesis). The anomalous ureter may terminate in the urethra, vestibule, or vagina. Occasionally, a single ectopic ureter ends in a blind cystic structure in the lateral wall of the vagina (a Gartner duct cyst) (Fig. 119-8). Developmental anomalies of the vagina, uterus, and ipsilateral ovary may be encountered.[1,42-46]

Extravesical ureteral ectopia in boys occurs much less commonly than in girls. The anomaly commonly involves the upper pole ureter in a duplex system but also may occur in a single, unduplicated ureter. The anomalous ureter may insert in the prostatic urethra, sometimes near the bladder neck, and much less often in the genital ducts (seminal vesicle, vas deferens, or ejaculatory duct) (Fig. 119-9). Ureteral ectopia to the posterior urethra usually ends slightly above or at the level of the verumontanum (Fig. 119-10). Ureteral ectopia to the genital ducts ends in a markedly dilated, cystic mass behind the trigone of the bladder. The renal parenchyma drained by the ectopic ureter is commonly small and dysplastic and often nonfunctioning. Urinary incontinence rarely is a problem in boys because the ectopic ureter drains above the strongly developed external urethral sphincter. Cryptorchidism or testicular hypoplasia on the side of the lesion is common.[1,11,38,47-49]

Imaging Ultrasound is the initial imaging method of choice and often is diagnostic, particularly when the anomalous

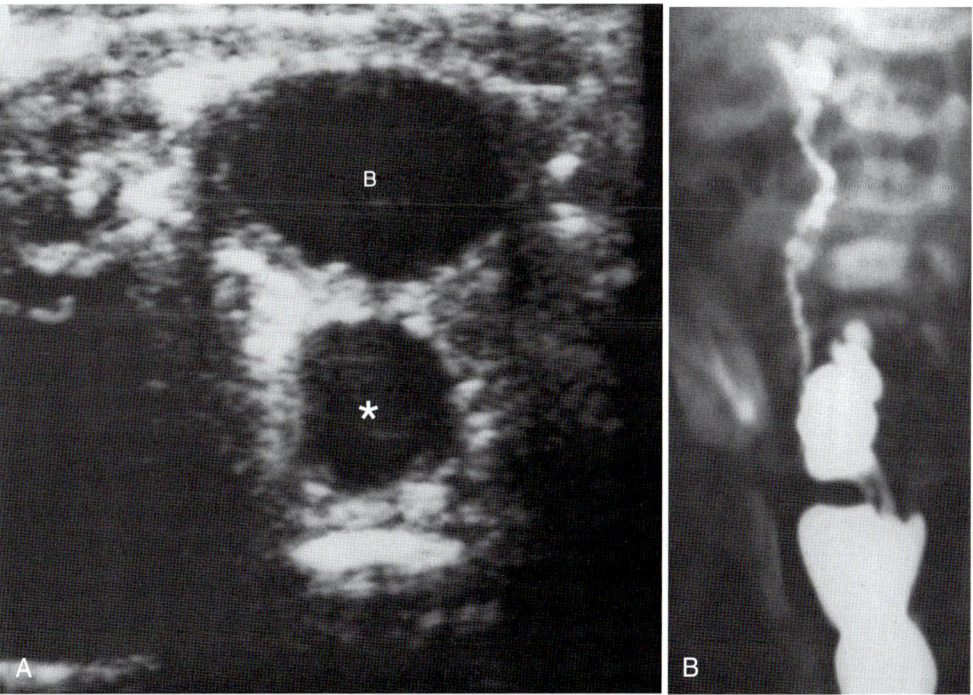

Figure 119-8 Ureteral ectopia into Gartner duct cyst. **A,** A transverse sonogram shows a cystic structure (*asterisk*) posterior to the bladder (*B*). **B,** A voiding cystourethrogram image shows filling of the bladder, through the Gartner duct cyst, and through the ureter to the upper pole.

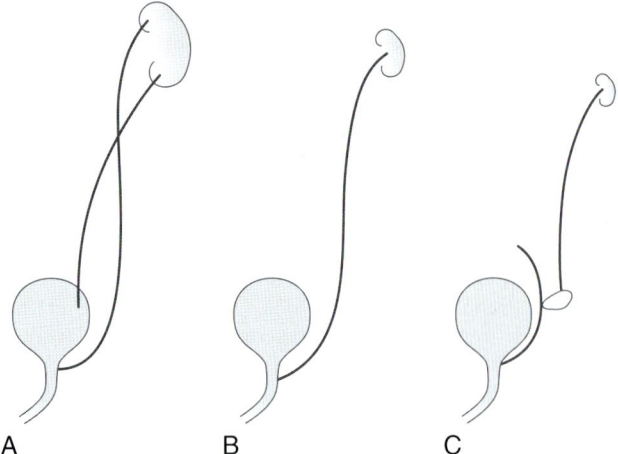

Figure 119-9 Types of ureteral ectopia in males. **A,** In the most common variant, ureteral duplication is present with the upper pole ureter draining into the posterior urethra. **B,** Ectopic ureteral drainage as in **A** but from a single collecting system. The kidney may be small and dysplastic. **C,** Ectopic drainage from a single system into a seminal vesicle, vas deferens, or ejaculatory duct. The ipsilateral kidney may not be identifiable.

ureter is dilated and sufficient renal parenchyma or even cysts of the corresponding renal moiety are present. The course of this ureter often may be followed down to and beyond the bladder. A vaginal ectopic ureter may be shown by ultrasound to be connected with a urine-filled vagina (e-Fig. 119-11). A nonfunctioning system is best visualized by MRU (Fig. 119-12). When the aberrant ureter empties in the urethra, VUR into the ectopic ureter occasionally is demonstrated by voiding cystourethrogram (VCUG) (Fig. 119-13 and e-Fig. 119-14). A vaginogram or genitogram may show reflux in the affected ureter if it terminates in the vagina (see Fig. 119-7). Note that many of these anomalies are accompanied by ipsilateral malformations of the genitalia. A thorough investigation of the vagina, the uterus, and the ovaries by ultrasound or magnetic resonance imaging (MRI) is recommended.[1,11,18,20-22,38,39,50-52]

Ureterocele

Overview A ureterocele is a cystlike expansion of the terminal segment of the ureter projecting into the lumen of the urinary bladder. The anomaly is relatively common and has two subtypes: (1) intravesical ureterocele, which is located entirely within the bladder, and (2) ectopic ureterocele, which usually is large and extends to the bladder neck area or proximal urethra. Both forms may be associated with a duplicated or an unduplicated system. More than 90% of the cases are discovered in children younger than 3 years of age, and most cases are diagnosed prenatally or in the newborn period. Urinary tract infection (UTI) is the most common presenting clinical manifestation. Failure to thrive, difficulty voiding, urinary retention, flank pain, and sometimes chronic

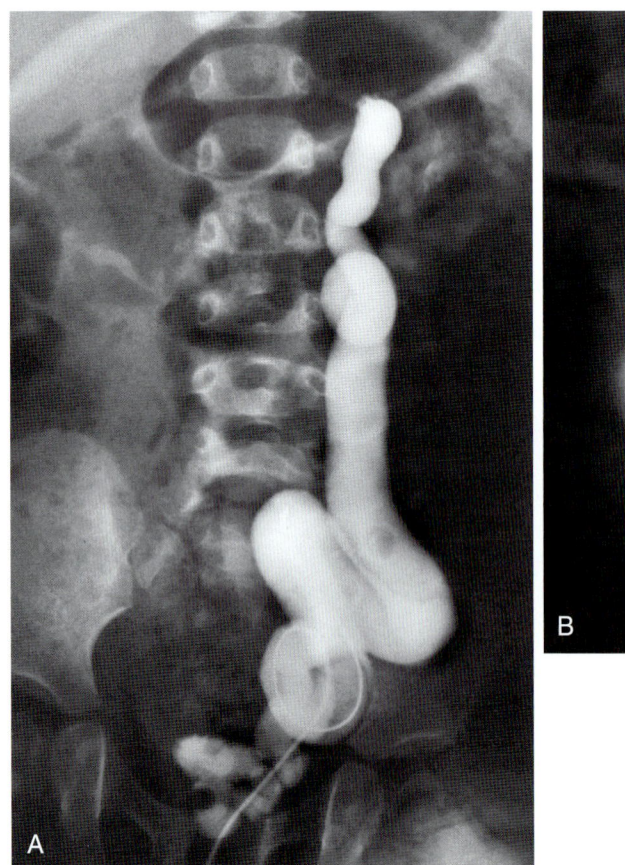

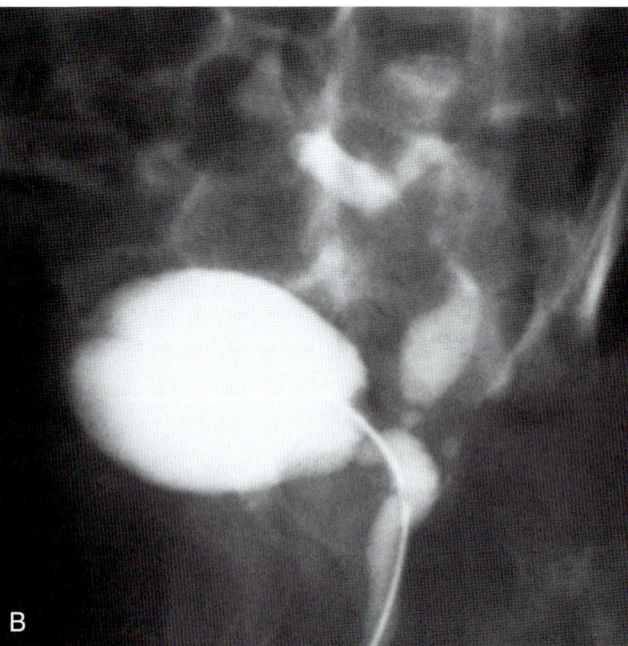

Figure 119-10 Ureteral ectopia into the urethra. **A,** A voiding cystourethrogram image shows that the catheter has passed from the urethra directly into the ureter, which drains an atrophic upper pole. **B,** A voiding cystourethrogram image during voiding shows vesicoureteral reflux into the ureter, which drains into the posterior urethra.

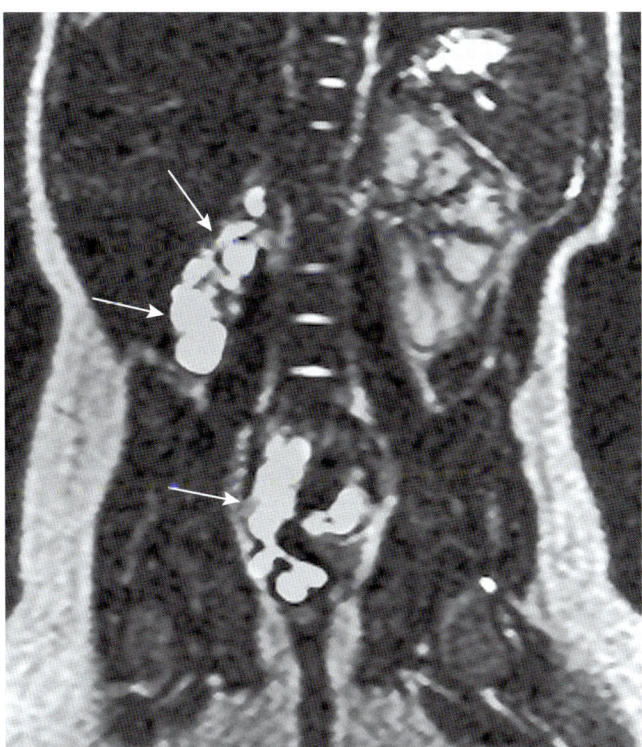

Figure 119-12 Ectopic ureteral insertion. Magnetic resonance urography demonstrating a cystic remnant of an ectopic renal bud (*top arrows*) with only minimal residual function and a dilated and tortuous dysplastic ureter (*bottom arrow*) ectopically inserting into the vagina.

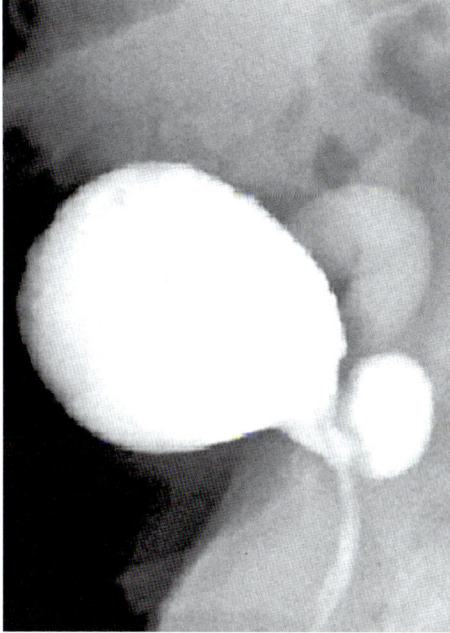

Figure 119-13 A voiding cystourethrogram image series in a girl with a refluxing ectopic ureterocele inserting into the urethra and filling of a diverticula-shaped ureterocele connected to the posterior urethra during voiding (see e-Fig. 119-14).

renal failure are prominent manifestations of the anomaly in older infants and in children.[1,53,54]

The intravesical ureterocele (also called stenotic, orthotopic, simple, or adult-type ureterocele) is more common in adults than in children, suggesting that it may be acquired in many cases. In children it is more frequently associated with significant hydroureteronephrosis. The ureterocele is located at the orthotopic ureteric ostium position (i.e., at the lateral angle of the trigone) and is entirely within the bladder (Fig. 119-15). The ureteral orifice of the ureterocele is variably stenotic. Intravesical ureteroceles may be bilateral and, although commonly seen in single (unduplicated) ureters, may involve the upper and sometimes the lower pole ureter of a duplicated system.[1,53,54]

The ectopic or infantile ureterocele is more common in children and is five to seven times more frequent in females than males. It is unilateral in 90% of cases and bilateral in 10% of cases. Ectopic ureteroceles most often occur in a duplicated system and almost always are connected with the upper pole ureter. The ureter connected with the ureterocele enters the bladder wall at the normal site, descends toward the bladder neck submucosally, passes through the internal urethral sphincter, and terminates ectopically in the proximal urethra. In contrast to a simple ureterocele, in which the "cyst" is formed by herniation of the distal end of the ureter, the ectopic ureterocele represents a dilatation and protrusion of the entire submucosal segment of the ureter into the lumen of the bladder and at the bladder neck. The ureterocele may obstruct the bladder neck or the opposite ureteral orifice, and in patients with ureteral duplication, it may deform the musculature or position and

course of the adjacent ureter so that VUR into the lower pole ureter occurs (in 40% to 50% of cases). Occasionally the ureterocele herniates into the urethra, causing urethral obstruction.[1,11,53-55]

Imaging Ultrasound imaging demonstrates an intravesical cystic lesion of variable size attached to the posterolateral wall of the bladder and protruding into the lumen of the bladder ("cyst within cyst"), which often is associated with a cystic structure in the upper pole moiety of the ipsilateral kidney (in duplicated systems) (Fig. 119-16 and e-Fig. 119-17). The dilated ureter connecting with the ureterocele may be demonstrated, as well as the corresponding renal unit. In duplex

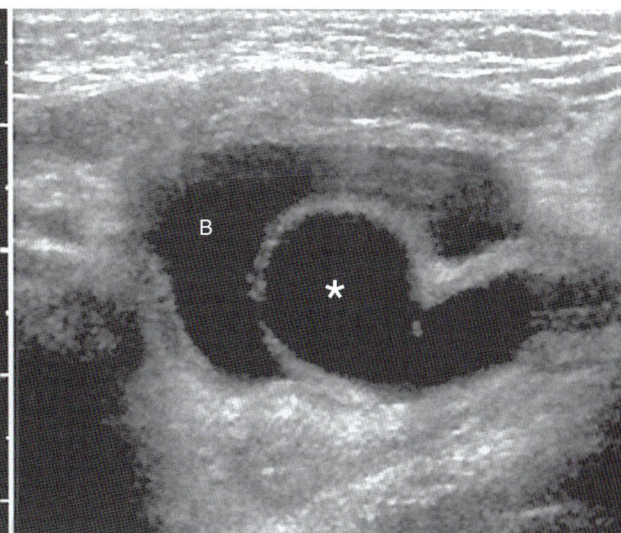

Figure 119-15 A ureterocele. A typical sonogram of a large ureterocele (*asterisk*) protruding into the bladder (*B*) lumen.

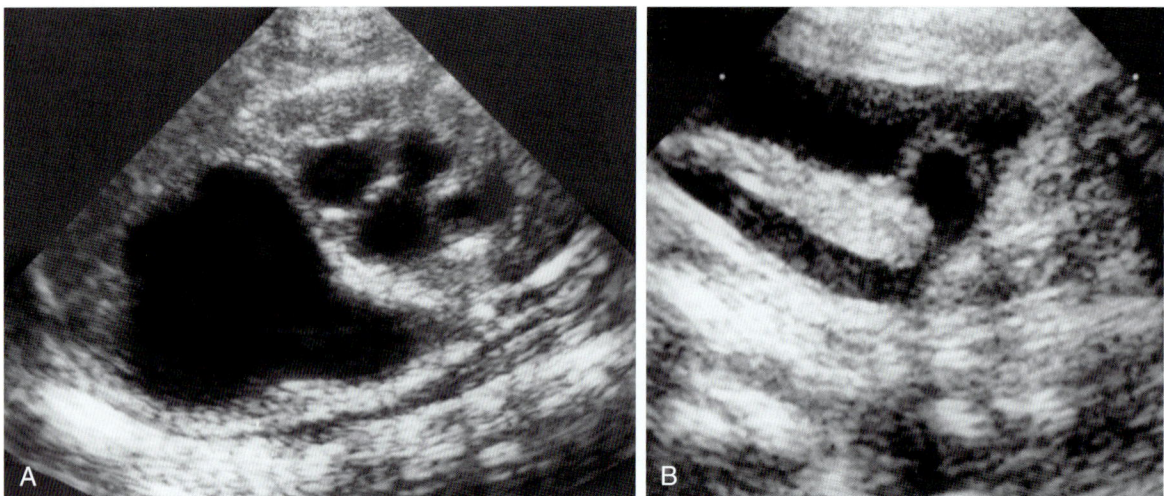

Figure 119-16   A ureterocele. **A,** A longitudinal sonogram of the right kidney shows marked upper pole hydronephrosis and parenchymal thinning along with mild lower pole hydronephrosis. **B,** A longitudinal sonogram of the right pelvis shows a dilated right ureter ending in a ureterocele that protrudes into the bladder.

systems, both ureters on the side of the ureterocele may be dilated.[1,10,11,55]

A radiolucent filling defect within the bladder is demonstrated on VCUG and is best imaged during the early filling. As bladder capacity is reached and luminal pressure rises, the ureterocele may be compressed and flattened against the bladder wall (Fig. 119-18 and e-Fig. 119-19) and can even evert (e-Fig. 119-20), simulating a paraureteral

diverticulum. During voiding the VCUG may show prolapse of the ureterocele into the urethra (Fig. 119-21), where it may produce bladder outlet obstruction. VUR into an ureterocele is rare initially, but common after endoscopic incision (e-Fig. 119-22).

Renal scintigraphy reveals decreased function at the superior pole of the kidney and often a photopenic area in the bladder corresponding to the ureterocele. Intravenous

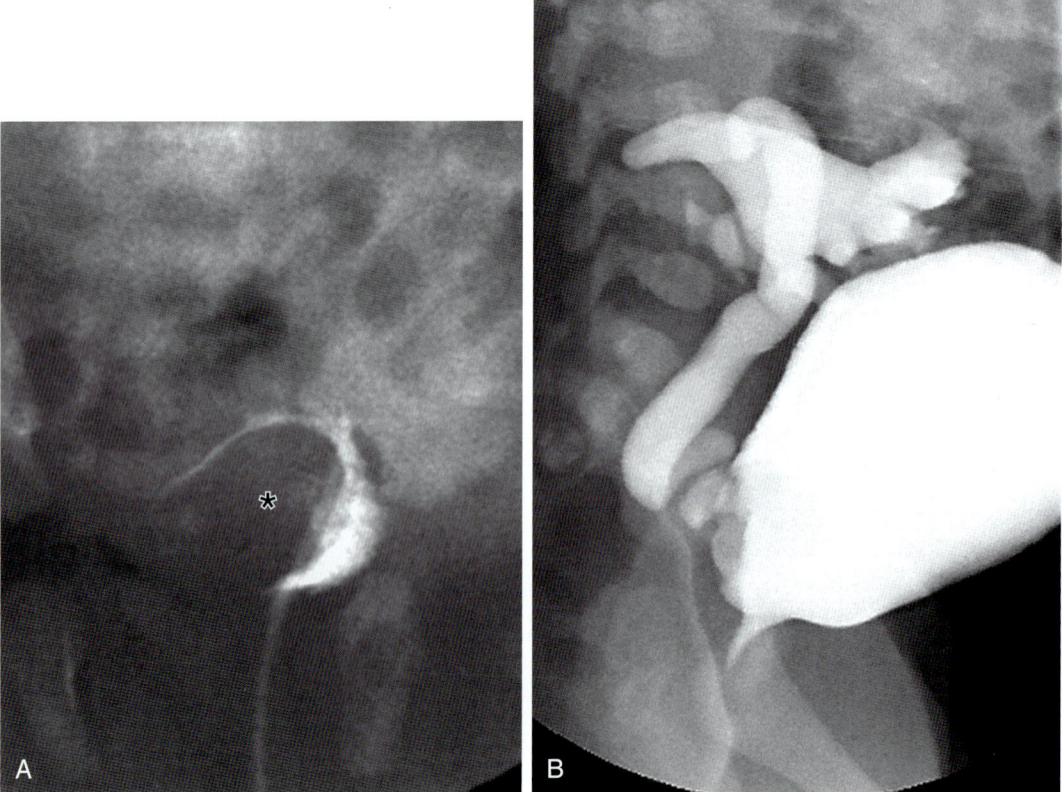

Figure 119-18   Ureterocele and vesicoureteral reflux. A voiding cystourethrogram series demonstrating the defect caused by the ureterocele (*asterisk*) during early bladder filling (**A**) and effacement of the ureterocele during late filling (**B**).

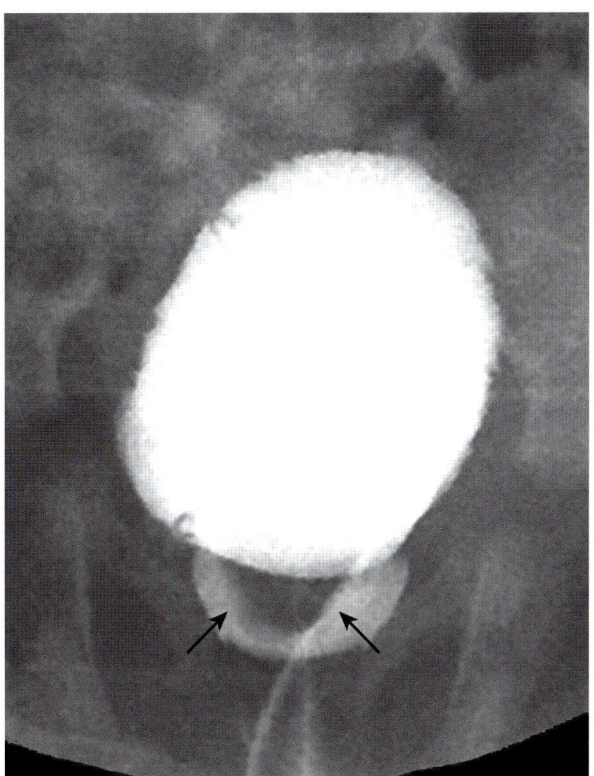

Figure 119-21 A ureterocele. A voiding cystourethrogram demonstrates inferior herniation of a ureterocele (*arrows*) into the bladder neck.

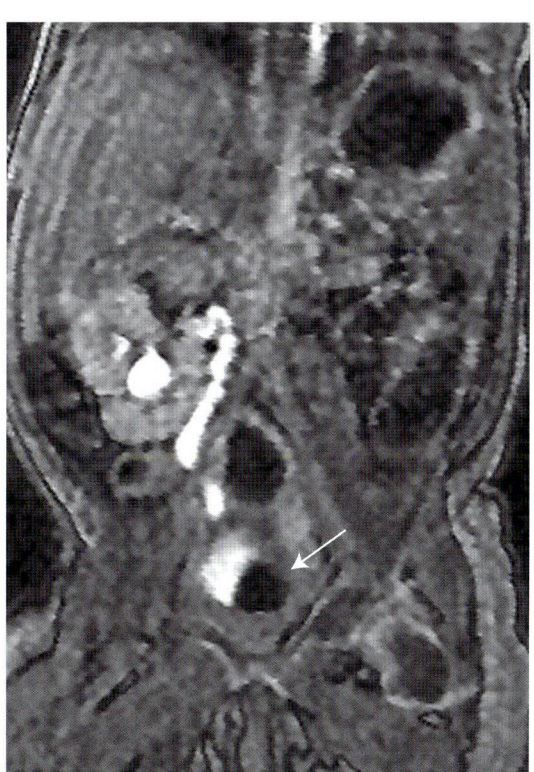

Figure 119-23 A typical magnetic resonance urography finding in ureteroceles. A contrast-enhanced T1-weighted gradient-recalled echo sequence delineating the non–contrast filled ureterocele in the urinary bladder (*arrow*).

urography has been replaced by methods such as dynamic MRU as the modality of choice for preoperative imaging because it provides all the functional information along with superior anatomic detail and can reveal associated renal abnormalities and genital malformations (Fig. 119-23 and e-Fig. 119-24) (Box 119-1).[1,10,11,18-25]

Treatment Treatment consists of cystoscopic fenestration of the ureterocele and/or resection and reimplantation of the ureter, especially if the ureterocele causes VUR or bladder outlet obstruction.[1,56,57]

Box 119-1 Imaging Findings in Ectopic Ureterocele

- Poor or nonfunctioning upper pole, with dysplasia, dilatation, and poor vascularization on ultrasound
- "Drooping lily" appearance on intravenous urography or voiding cystourethrogram (if refluxing lower moiety)
- Filling defect in bladder, often double filling defect (intravenous urography + voiding cystourethrogram on early filling of bladder)
- Cystic structure in or adjacent to the bladder on ultrasound
- Seldom refluxes, but may occur after injury by instrumentation or catheterization
- May evert, simulating diverticulum
- May show as urethral mass and may cause bladder outlet obstruction
- Nuclear medicine studies show decreased function in upper pole and a photon-deficient area in the bladder
- Magnetic resonance: "cyst in cyst" often poorly visualized on nonenhanced acquisitions but becomes obvious on contrast-enhanced diuretic T1-weighted magnetic resonance urography

---

Acquired Ureteral Obstruction

Overview Acquired strictures of the body of the ureter are uncommon. They may be due to a local surgical procedure, instrumentation, ureteral wall inflammation, or periureteral infection; they may be a complication of Henoch-Schönlein purpura, periarteritis nodosa, tuberculosis, or granulomatous disease of childhood (e.g., Crohn disease); they may be the result of trauma or submucosal hemorrhage in patients on anticoagulant medication; or they may follow local radiation. Other acquired intrinsic ureteral obstructions include sludge balls, blood clots, various calculi, and fungus balls. Note that acute obstructions may exhibit only minor collecting system dilatation, but patients will have severe pain and renal colic.

Imaging usually starts with ultrasound, with assessment of the distal ureter and the ureteral inflow jet through a sufficiently distended urinary bladder. The upper ureter and pelvocalyceal system then are evaluated before looking at the renal parenchyma and renal blood flow and Doppler changes. Ultrasound usually is supplemented with an abdominal radiograph. Although it is rarely used in Europe, CT (with or without contrast medium enhancement) often is used in North America. Advanced imaging such as MRU is rarely necessary.[1,58-64]

Primary Ureteral Neoplasms

Overview Primary neoplasms of the renal pelvis and ureters, such as rhabdomyosarcoma or urothelial cell carcinoma, are extremely rare in children. Secondary involvement of the pelvocalyceal system by Wilms tumor, as well as Wilms tumor implants in the ureter, may occur. The ureter may be infiltrated or secondarily involved by other retroperitoneal tumors of infancy and childhood, such as neuroblastoma, rhabdomyosarcoma, peripheral neuroectodermal tumor, or malignant teratoma. Instances of benign and usually pedunculated fibrous polyps in the upper third of the ureter (occasionally bilateral) have been reported (Fig. 119-25 and e-Fig. 119-26). They may cause hematuria, or rarely obstruction, and have no malignant potential. Fibrous polyps are more common in adults. Ultrasound is only useful to detect large tumors with a significant extraureteral component or to visualize indirect signs caused by the obstruction. Otherwise, imaging relies on CT, MRI, or even ureterography.[1,65-71]

Primary Megaureter

Overview Two forms of megaureter are described: (1) a megaureter resulting from an organic lesion (Box 119-2) and (2) a primary megaureter, which is mostly functional in origin. A primary megaureter is an uncommon, nonhereditary lesion that is probably congenital in origin. It is caused by an adynamic distal ureteral segment, usually 0.5 to 4 cm in length, which prevents normal caudal propagation of ureteral peristalsis. The disorder is discovered in patients of any age and is more common in males than in females. Three fourths of cases are unilateral, with the left ureter being involved more often than the right ureter. Bilateral cases are more common in children younger than 1 year. The affected

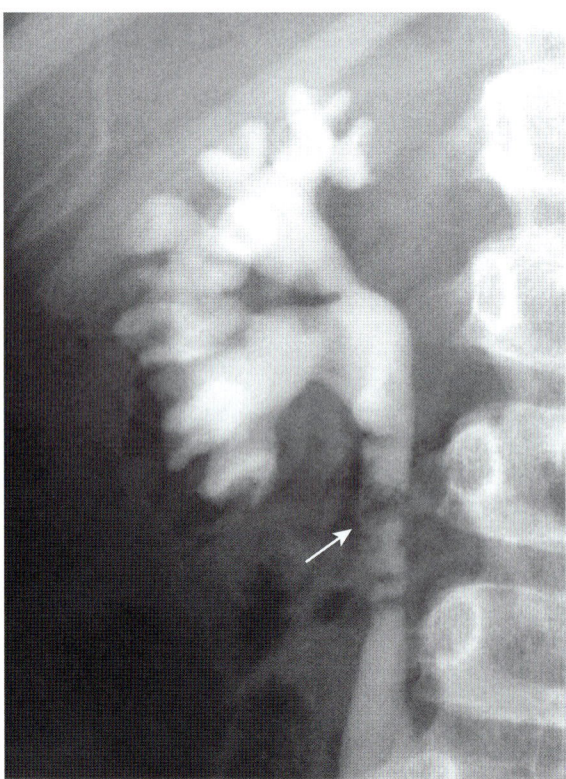

Figure 119-25 Ureteral obstruction from ureteral polyps. An intravenous urography image shows mild hydronephrosis and proximal ureteral filling defects (*arrow*) surgically proven to be polyps.

> **Box 119-2 Types of Megaureter**
>
> • Primary megaureter
> • Congenital ureterovesical junction obstruction
> • Retrocaval or retroiliac megaureter
> • Prunebelly syndrome
> • Refluxing megaureter
> • Megaureter caused by stone, fungus balls, polyps, valves and folds, or other intrinsic lesions
> • Bladder outlet obstruction
> • Megaureter caused by extrinsic compression (masses)
> • Postoperative megaureter, or as a result of other acquired strictures

ureter is variously dilated but tapers down rather abruptly to a curved, short distal segment that appears normal in caliber or slightly narrowed on imaging. The dilatation often is limited to (or is most marked in) the lower half of the ureter. The renal parenchyma usually is of normal thickness, but in more severe cases it is variously thinned or even dysplastic and atrophic. The symptoms of a primary megaureter include recurrent UTI, abdominal pain (and distention if the megaureter is severe and bilateral), and hematuria. Ureteral stone formation has been reported. However, a primary megaureter often is discovered as an incidental finding in asymptomatic patients.

At gross pathology, the distal segment of the ureter appears normal, without evidence of intrinsic narrowing upon probing with ureteral catheters. Histologically, however, the ureter shows normal ganglion cells (which may be reduced in number), hypoplasia and atrophy of muscle fibers, and an increase in collagen tissue. The remaining muscle fibers are predominantly circular, and in severe cases little or no muscle tissue is present. The proximal dilated segment of the ureter shows muscular hypertrophy that results from hyperperistalsis. Cytoscopically the ureteral orifices are normal.[1,72,73]

Imaging The findings on imaging reflect the pathologic changes in the ureter and kidney (Fig. 119-27 and e-Fig. 119-28). As seen fluoroscopically on ureterography, by ultrasound, and by dynamic MRU, the ureter shows normal or hyperactive peristalsis with waves starting in the proximal ureter and increasing in amplitude and fading distally into the dilated portion of the ureter. Antiperistaltic waves may be observed. A VCUG shows no organic or functional abnormalities of the bladder or urethra. VUR is not a typical feature of the disorder but does occur in some children. Renal agenesis and other contralateral abnormalities have been described, and ipsilateral megacalycosis and hydronephrosis may occur.[1,74-77]

Hypotonia, Hypomotility, and Dyskinesia

Overview and Imaging Hypotonia, hypomotility, and dyskinesia are disturbances of the ureter that primarily affect motility and function. An adynamic or dysplastic ureteral segment may cause functional impairment and cause segmental

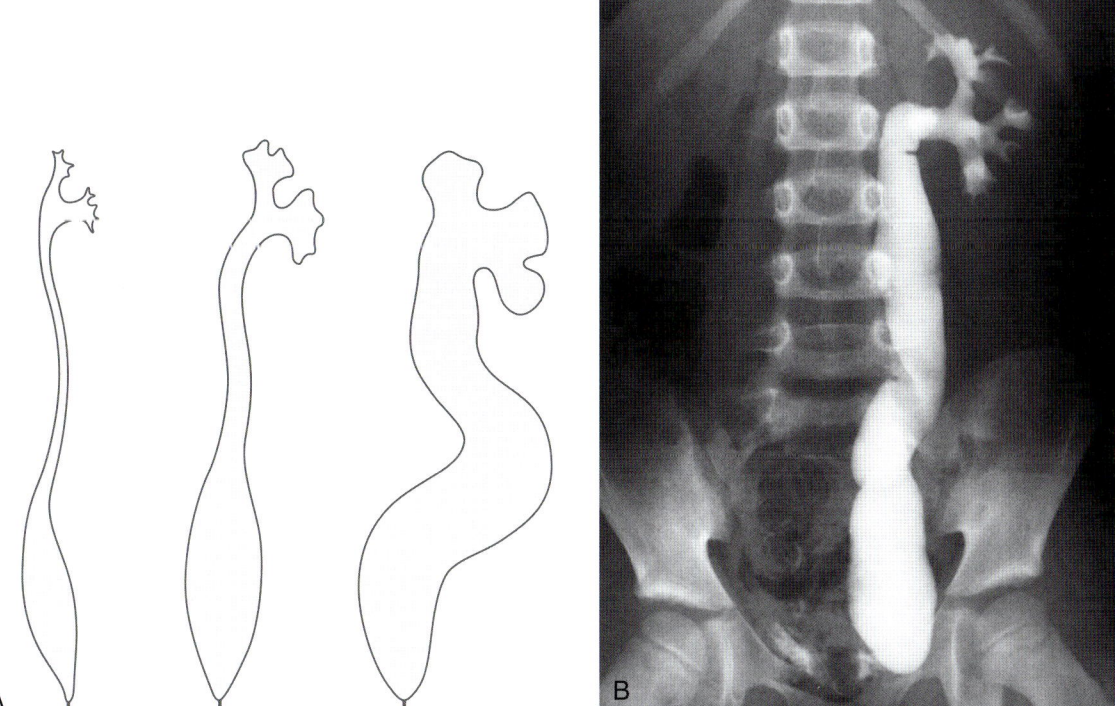

Figure 119-27 **Megaureter. A,** A diagram of the ureter and collecting system in primary megaureters of varying severity. **B,** A postvoid voiding cystourethrogram image shows left vesicoureteral reflux and ureterovesical junction obstruction, suggesting a primary megaureter. The ureteral dilatation is most pronounced in the lower ureter; the renal pelvis and calyces are little affected.

ureteral dilatation, with urine drainage relying on gravity. Furthermore, peristalsis and loss of muscular tone may be seen during and shortly after UTI, as well as after instrumentation, operations, or with in situ foreign bodies such as nephroureteral stents, causing reactive hypotonia with an adynamic or hypoperistaltic ureter. Finally, transient hypomotility of the ureter may be observed in postoperative settings and as a result of medications that affect the smooth muscles. Ureteral peristalsis may be assessed and documented using ultrasound cine-loop clips (e-Fig. 119-29); ureteral drainage and function is evaluated by mercaptoacetyltriglycine scintigraphy or dynamic MRU.[1,23-25,78,79]

Miscellaneous Conditions

Overview Preoperative imaging needs to reveal all relevant information the surgeon requires for either planning or performing the operation. Because a comprehensive overview and display may be crucial, ultrasound alone often is considered insufficient, particularly because of its limited potential to visualize the entire ureter. Therefore VCUG (in refluxing units) and MRU usually are integrated in a standard preoperative imaging workup; more invasive procedures such as ureterography may be performed at the beginning of or during surgery in the course of the same anesthesia.[1]

Postoperative imaging is heavily based on ultrasound. However, ultrasound is poor in assessment and grading of

urinary drainage; therefore a functional scintigraphic study, as well as MRU (or CT), sometimes may prove helpful. If postoperative complications occur (e.g., ureteral obstruction after antireflux procedures, ureteral obstruction due to blood clots, manifestation of UPJ obstruction after ureteral surgery, ureteral fibrosis, stenosis, and compression), imaging not only may detect them but also may offer treatment options. These image-guided interventions and treatment strategies consist of ureteral recanalization, balloon dilatation of fibrous stenoses and ureteral stenting for keeping a compressed or recanalized ureter patent, and percutaneous nephrostomy.[1,80-82]

> ### WHAT THE CLINICIAN NEEDS TO KNOW
> - The presence or absence of a dilated ureter
> - A proximal versus distal ureteral obstructive pattern
> - The presence of a single collecting system versus a duplex kidney
> - The presence of a ureterocele
> - The ectopic ureteral insertion site
> - The presence of vesicoureteral reflux; unilateral or bilateral
> - Ureteral function and drainage by dynamic nuclear scintigraphy
> - The need for functional MRU

Key Points

The ureter is much more difficult to image than other parts of the urinary system.

MRU is a powerful new tool for imaging the ureter.

Diuretic scintigraphy currently provides the best assessment of ureteral drainage.

Most ureteral obstructions occur at the UPJ or UVJ.

Distal ureteral obstruction and VUR may coexist.

Early filling VCUG images are essential in demonstrating ureteroceles.

A history of constant urine leakage in a girl with otherwise normal voiding should suggest extravesical ureteral ectopia.

A primary megaureter is caused by an adynamic distal ureteral segment that prevents normal caudal propagation of ureteral peristalsis.

Suggested Readings

Cerwinka WH, Damien Grattan-Smith J, Kirsch AJ. Magnetic resonance urography in pediatric urology. *J Pediatr Urol.* 2008;4(1):74-82, quiz 82-83.

Ehammer T, Riccabona M, Maier E. High resolution MR for evaluation of lower urogenital tract malformations in infants and children: Feasibility and preliminary experiences. *Eur J Radiol.* 2011;78(3):388-393.

Gordon I, Riccabona M. Investigating the newborn kidney—update on imaging techniques. *Semin Neonatol.* 2003;8:269-278.

Jones RA, Perez-Brayfield MR, Kirsch AJ, et al. Renal transit time with MR urography in children. *Radiology.* 2004;233(1):41-50.

Kim S, Jacob JS, Kim DC, et al. Time-resolved dynamic contrast-enhanced MR urography for the evaluation of ureteral peristalsis: initial experience. *J Magn Reson Imaging.* 2008;28(5):1293-1298.

Riccabona M, Fotter R. Radiographic studies in children with kidney disorders: what to do and when. In: Hogg R, ed. *Kidney disorders in children and adolescents.* Birmingham: Taylor & Francis; 2006.

Riccabona M, Fritz G, Ring E. Potential applications of three-dimensional ultrasound in the pediatric urinary tract: pictorial demonstration based on preliminary results. *Eur Radiol.* 2003;13:2680-2687.

Riccabona M, Lindbichler F, Sinzig M. Conventional imaging in paediatric uroradiology. *Eur J Radiol.* 2002;43:100.

Riccabona M, Simbrunner J, Ring E, et al. Feasibility of MR-urography in neonates and infants with anomalies of the upper urinary tract. *Eur Radiol.* 2002;12:1442.

Riccabona M, Sorantin E, Hausegger K. Imaging guided interventional procedures in paediatric uroradiology—a case-based overview. *Eur J Radiol.* 2002;43:167.

Riccabona M, Uggowitzer M, Klein E, et al. Contrast enhanced color Doppler sonography in children and adolescents. *J Ultrasound Med.* 2000;19:783.

Roy Choudhury S, Chadha R, Bagga D, et al. Spectrum of ectopic ureters in children. *Pediatr Surg Int.* 2008;24(7):819-823.

References

Full references for this chapter can be found on www.expertconsult.com.

Chapter 120

Vesicoureteral Reflux

D. GREGORY BATES and MICHAEL RICCABONA

Definition and Imaging Objectives

Overview Vesicoureteral reflux (VUR) refers to the retrograde passage of urine from the urinary bladder into the ureter and often to the calyces. It is a common and potentially important childhood problem that generally is regarded as abnormal at all ages. Because of recent insights into the natural history of fetal and neonatal urinary tract development, this judgment is increasingly under discussion and review. VUR itself causes neither urinary tract infection (UTI) nor renal damage, but it may be associated with bladder dysfunction. However, VUR is a risk factor for the development of upper UTI and pyelonephritis, with consequent renal scarring and potential long-term sequelae (Box 120-1).[1-15]

The major objective in the evaluation of children with documented UTI traditionally has been to diagnose or exclude VUR. Today, the focus of imaging in UTI has shifted to evaluation of renal inflammatory involvement or existing renal scarring and to assessment of structural or functional abnormalities of the urinary tract that may predispose to renal damage (i.e., prenatal "hydronephrosis"), complicated UTI, and VUR, particularly early depiction of anomalies that may require prompt interventional or surgical treatment to prevent renal damage.[1,16-34]

Etiology

Overview The most common cause of VUR is a developmental anomaly of the ureterovesicular junction (UVJ) in which the ureteral orifice may be lateralized or too large ("golf hole ostium") or the submucosal ureter is too short and/or deficient in longitudinal muscle fibers. VUR often is seen in patients with other urinary tract anomalies (Box 120-2). Additionally, some sort of immaturity of the UVJ may play a role in fetal and neonatal VUR, because a large percentage of congenital VUR decreases spontaneously within the first years of life. This type of VUR, often referred to as *primary* or *congenital* VUR, is seen more frequently in girls than in boys. High-grade congenital VUR in male infants, often with severe congenital renal dysplasia ("congenital reflux nephropathy"), constitutes a different entity with a far more serious prognosis.

Secondary VUR is seen in patients with bladder outlet obstruction (e.g., posterior urethral valves) or with neurogenic bladder disease (e.g., myelomeningocele). It is caused in part by thinning and weakening of the UVJ musculature precipitated by chronically increased intravesical pressure. However, the fact that VUR in these disorders may be absent and frequently is unilateral suggests the possibility of an associated congenital weakness of the UVJ or a protective measure of a potentially thickened bladder wall that otherwise may lead to ureteral obstruction. Although lesser degrees of lower urinary tract obstruction per se do not seem to cause VUR in patients with a completely normal UVJ, they may precipitate VUR (with ascending spread of infection to the kidneys) in people with ostia of borderline competence as the result of local edema and cellular infiltration, causing further weakening of the UVJ.[1,35-38]

Imaging Techniques

Overview The diagnostic imaging modalities available for the evaluation of VUR include ultrasound, voiding cystourethrogram (VCUG), and nuclear cystography (Box 120-3). A new method for VUR assessment is contrast-enhanced voiding urosonography (ce-VUS). This method uses ultrasound contrast material (e.g., shaken saline solution, air, or commercially available contrast agents) instilled into the urinary bladder via suprapubic or transurethral catheterization and bladder filling (Fig. 120-1 and e-Fig. 120-2). The reflux of contrast into the upper tracts can be appreciated readily by alternately scanning both kidneys as well as the retrovesical space during filling and before and after voiding. Ultrasound techniques such as harmonic imaging, stimulated acoustic emission, or other contrast-specific techniques have further enhanced ce-VUS potential for VUR depiction and grading, resulting in a reported sensitivity and specificity equal to VCUG (Fig. 120-3 and e-Fig. 120-4).[1,39-55]

VCUG is and remains the basic imaging technique for VUR assessment. It uses radiopaque contrast material instilled into the catheterized and emptied urinary bladder for detection of VUR into the upper urinary tract. For a reliable assessment, the bladder must be filled to near capacity. For infants younger than 1 year of age, bladder capacity in milliliters is determined by the patient's weight in kilograms × 7. For patients older than 1 year of age, bladder capacity in milliliters equals age in years plus 2, multiplied by 30. Fluoroscopic observation of the (early) filling phase, the distal ureters (in oblique projections), the renal collecting system, and the urethra during voiding (lateral projection in boys)

Box 120-1   Findings in Patients with Vesicoureteral Reflux

- African Americans have lower vesicoureteral reflux (VUR) incidence.
- VUR has a family history component: parent-child or sibling-sibling.
- Children with VUR have twice the incidence of pyelonephritis.
- Fifty percent of children with postinfectious nephropathy do not have VUR.
- Cyclic voiding studies increase the rate of VUR detection in infants.
- For VUR assessment, a voiding cystourethrogram, a radionuclide cystogram, and echo-enhanced urosonography can be used.
- Filling the initially empty bladder to capacity increases VUR detection; assessment also occurs during and after voiding, as well as in the early filling phase.
- The prevalence of VUR in children without a urinary tract infection (UTI) is almost equal to that in children with a UTI.
- Bladder infections do not cause VUR.
- UTI is independent of the presence of VUR.
- Sterile VUR does not produce renal scars or other damage.
- New scars rarely develop after puberty; the kidney is most vulnerable during the first years of life.
- Despite the initial severity or persistence of VUR, renal growth rates remain unaffected, except for associated congenital dysplasia.
- VUR and asymptomatic bacteriuria do not result in scars.
- In the treatment of VUR, no difference exists between continuous antibiotic prophylaxis or just treating episodes of UTI in terms of renal scar development.
- Most patients with VUR do not demonstrate defects upon dimercaptosuccinic acid scintigraphy, and children with defects often do not have VUR.
- Symptomatic and asymptomatic VUR have the same natural history and resolution.
- Bladder urodynamics are related to the presence and resolution of VUR.
- Breakthrough infections, changes in renal function or growth, and new or progressive scarring are seen with similar frequency in both medical and surgical treatment of VUR.

Box 120-2   Causes and Associations of Vesicoureteral Reflux

Primary

- Developmental, idiopathic, and immaturity
- Anomalous development at the ureterovesical junction
- Prunebelly syndrome
- Diverticula

Secondary

- Bladder outlet obstruction, particularly posterior urethral valves
- Neurogenic bladder/myelomeningocele
- Bladder dyssynergia and dysfunctional voiding
- Postoperative bladder
- Indwelling catheter
- Foreign body
- Bladder calculi
- Iatrogenic
- Ureterocele surgery

Box 120-3   Imaging Studies for Vesicoureteral Reflux

Voiding Cystourethrogram

- Defines anatomy (urethra in males)
- Accurate grading of vesicoureteral reflux (VUR) and good comparability upon follow-up
- Visualization of diverticula and (if refluxing) ureterovesical junction + ureteral anatomy

Nuclear Studies

- Decreased ability to see urethra in males
- Continuous imaging
- Less accurate VUR grading
- Don't need to see the urethra in females: can be used as an initial study in females
- Decreased gonadal radiation dose: good for screening familial VUR and for follow-up examinations

Echo-enhanced Urosonography

- No radiation, and thus it is ideal for screening, follow-up, and in females
- A longer observation period than with a voiding cystourethrogram (VCUG) and a similar or higher VUR incidence/detection rate
- Tends to grade low-degree VUR slightly higher than VCUG
- Provides fewer anatomic details (e.g., urethra, ureters, and diverticula) and a less panoramic display
- Provides information on renal parenchyma, prefilling anatomy, and nonrefluxing systems

enables focused imaging of critical areas and conditions such as intrarenal VUR and UVJ anatomy. Cyclic VCUG should be performed in infants to avoid missing significant VUR, because VUR may not occur during the first fill and void.[1,56-69]

For studying the renal parenchyma, ultrasound and dimercaptosuccinic acid (DMSA) scintigraphy commonly are used. Other methods for the evaluation of the upper tract are contrast-enhanced computed tomography (CT) and magnetic resonance imaging (MRI), which may become indicated for assessment of complicated disease. The choice of imaging method for VUR assessment depends in large part on individual preference, availability, and the experience of the examiner. Other variables include the age, sex, and race of the patient; whether an initial or a follow-up examination is being done; and the cost of and time required to perform the procedure. All male infants and all patients before surgery should have a conventional VCUG performed for detailed anatomic assessment.[1,20,21,23,24,28,30,31,70-85]

Grading

Overview   The international criteria for grading VUR is based on the VCUG (Fig. 120-5). Similar comparable grading scales exist for ce-VUS and nuclear cystography. Although simple and easy to use, this classification and other similar classifications reflect only the appearance of the upper tracts and do not take into consideration other important factors such as the age and sex of the patient, the presence of intrarenal reflux or urinary tract obstruction, renal function and scarring, high- or low-pressure VUR, early or late VUR,

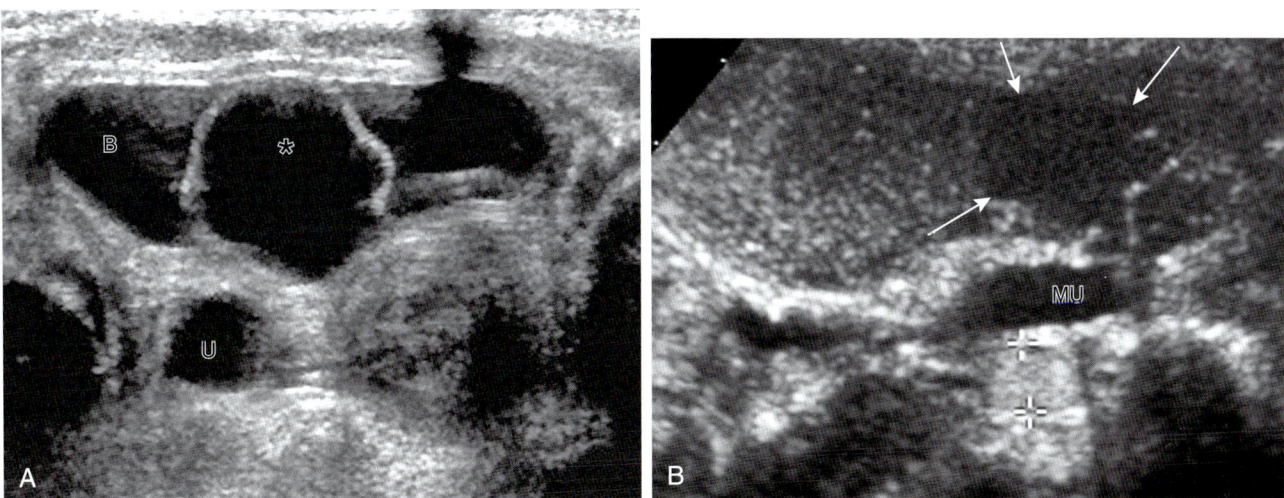

Figure 120-1 Vesicoureteral reflux demonstrated by echo-enhanced urosonography. **A,** A transverse unenhanced bladder sonogram reveals a ureterocele (*asterisk*) within and a dilated ureter (*U*) behind the urinary bladder (*B*). **B,** A longitudinal sonogram after instillation of contrast material (Levovist) into the urinary bladder shows the nonrefluxing ureterocele (*arrows*) and corresponding megaureter (*MU*) and echogenic contrast material within the refluxing lower pole ureter (*cursors*). See also e-Figure 120-2.

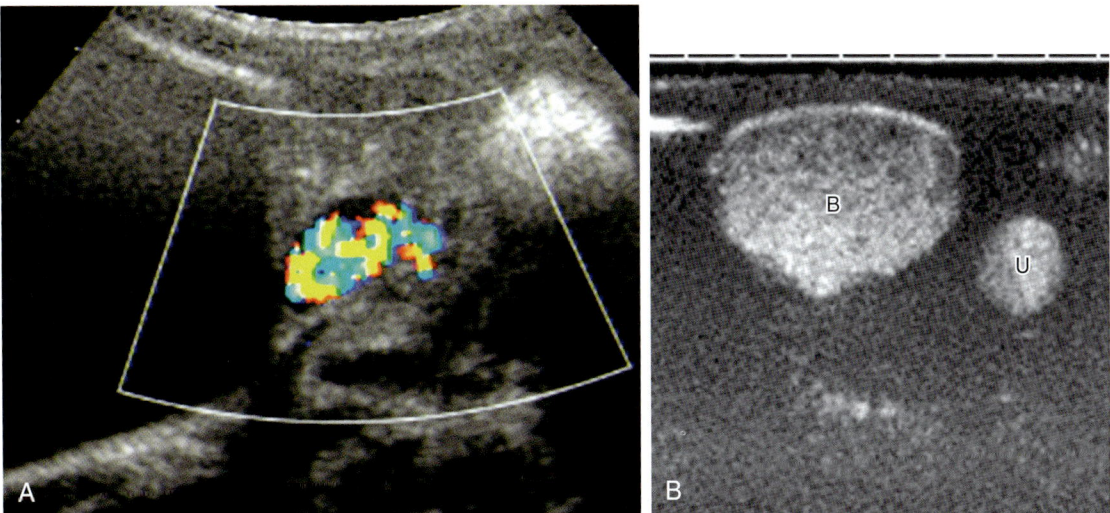

Figure 120-3 Improved detection of vesicoureteral reflux using contrast-specific techniques. **A,** The same patient as in Figure 120-1 and e-Figure 120-2, with reflux into the right lower moiety. Reflux is now depicted using stimulated acoustic emission with high ultrasound power (high mechanical index) to burst the contrast bubbles, thus creating strong color signals. **B,** Contrast-specific imaging techniques (CDI, Siemens, Mountain View, CA) provide exquisite contrast delineation in a patient with refluxing megaureter, using double-image technique for visualization contrast image (*B*, bladder; *U*, ureter). See e-Figure 120-4 for a generic image with simultaneous contrast and harmonic imaging gray-scale information.

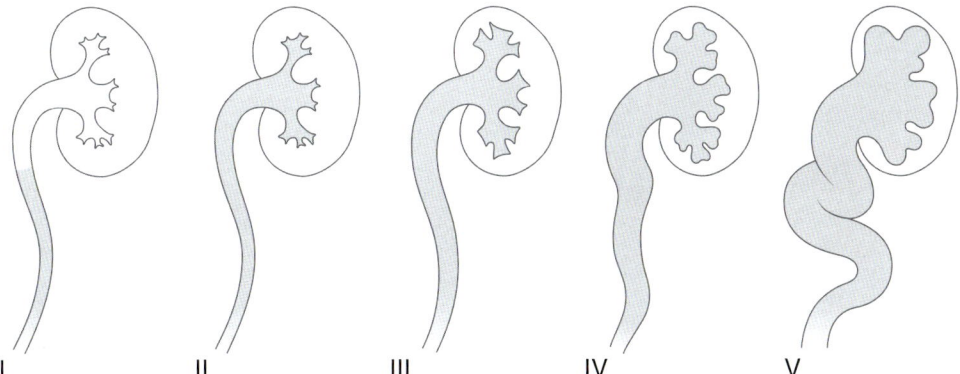

Figure 120-5 A schematic drawing demonstrating the vesicoureteral reflux grading system on a voiding cystourethrogram. (From Lebowitz RL, Olbing H, Parkkulainen KV, et al. International reflux study in children: international system of radiographic grading of vesico-ureteral reflux. International Reflux Study in Children. *Pediatr Radiol.* 1985;15:105.)

slow or quick clearance from the upper collecting system, cystoscopic findings, and the presence or absence of associated disorders (e.g., ureteral duplication, ureteral ectopia, ureterocele, bladder diverticula, prunebelly syndrome, urethral obstruction, megacystis-megaureter association, or neurogenic bladder). This additional information sometimes is essential for making decisions about therapy.[1,86-88]

VUR Imaging

ULTRASOUND

On ultrasound, the ureters and pelvocalyceal systems of patients with VUR often appear normal even if they appear dilated on VCUG (particularly when the bladder is empty or catheterized). Indirect sonographic signs for VUR are uroepithelial thickening of the ureter or renal pelvis, changing diameter of the pelvocalyceal system and ureter, quick refilling of the bladder after voiding, asymmetric ureteral inflow jets, and a lateralized position or unusual shape of the ureteral ostium (Fig. 120-6). In more severe cases, the refluxing upper tracts are grossly dilated, with clubbing of the calyces and elongated and tortuous ureters (e-Fig. 120-7). Ureteral peristalsis generally is poor, especially in the presence of urinary infection and high-grade VUR. Kinks in the proximal ureter or distal segment of the ureter are common. Direct sonographic evidence of VUR may be identified on ce-VUS as described previously.[1,89-103]

VOIDING CYSTOURETHROGRAM

The appearance of refluxing ureters and pelvocalyceal systems on VCUG is quite variable, ranging from normal-sized upper tracts to extreme upper tract dilatation and marked ureteral tortuosity (Fig. 120-8 and e-Fig. 120-9). These changes may reflect only an increased volume and decreased motility of the ureters, but in some cases a developmental defect of the

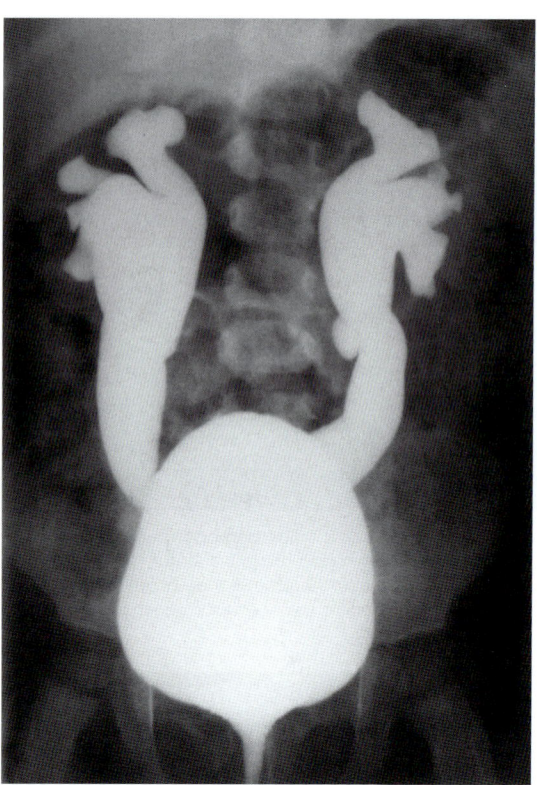

Figure 120-8   Vesicoureteral reflux. A voiding cystourethrogram image shows bilateral grade IV vesicoureteral reflux. Also see e-Figure 120-9.

ureter related either to inutero VUR or to an inadequate development of the ureteral musculature is suspected (e.g., prune-belly syndrome). In some patients, VUR is accompanied by marked ballooning of the pelvocalyceal system without evidence of UPJ obstruction (e-Fig. 120-10). The phenomenon may be transient and reflects an increased elasticity of unknown cause in the upper collecting system. Sometimes VUR may induce a kink at the UPJ, with a valvelike mechanism that may even deteriorate after antireflux procedures, producing a functional UPJ obstruction (Fig. 120-11). The obstruction may be related to local scarring from infection, anatomic kinks in the ureter, or overlying aberrant vessels or fibrous bands. Thus a primary congenital UPJ obstruction and primary VUR may coexist as associated anomalies.[1,104-107]

In patients with VUR to the calyces, one may observe transient pyelotubular and interstitial reflux of contrast material extending outward in a wedge-shaped pattern from one or more papillae to the renal cortical surface (Fig. 120-12). *Intrarenal reflux* is an important finding because of its association with renal scarring. It is believed that the morphology of the opening of the collecting ducts of Bellini on the renal papilla is partly responsible for intrarenal reflux. The opening of these ducts on compound, flat-topped papillae (more common at the poles) are round and therefore less resistant to retrograde flow than the slitlike openings of the ducts of simple or conical papillae. The fact that intrarenal reflux does not occur in all infants and that it is rarely seen after age 4 years suggests an additional local defect that improves with age.[1-3,6,8,9,12,15,19,56-59,62,63,66,69,88,105,107]

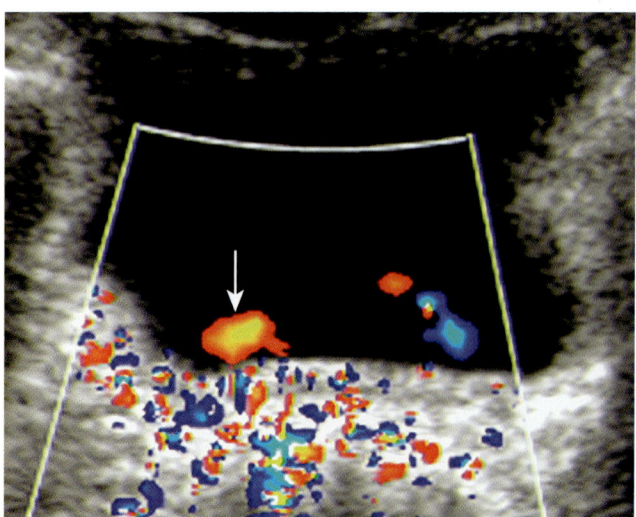

Figure 120-6   Lateralized ureteral orifice. A transverse color Doppler image shows a laterally positioned and abnormally oriented right ureteral jet (*arrow*). Such indirect signs may help ultrasound diagnosis of vesicoureteral reflux.

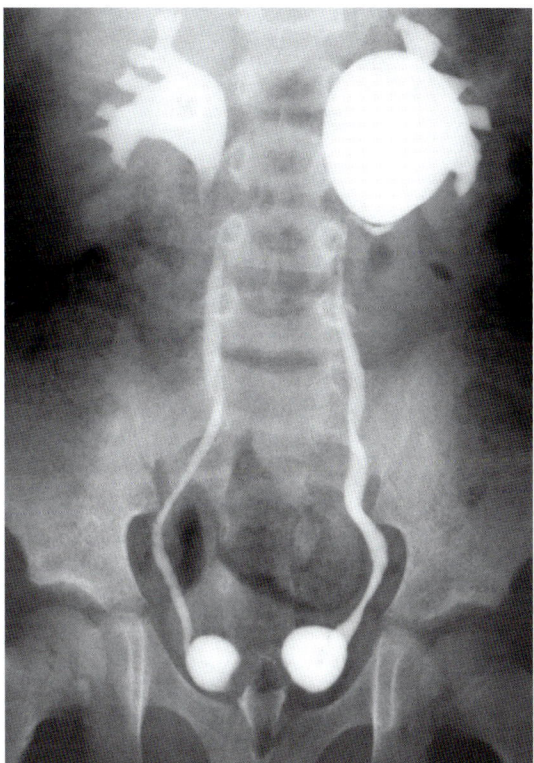

Figure 120-11   Vesicoureteral reflux and functional ureteropelvic junction obstruction. A voiding cystourethrogram image after voiding shows bilateral vesicoureteral reflux and ballooning of the left renal pelvis. The intravenous urogram image (not shown) was entirely normal. Bilateral paraureteral (Hutch) diverticula also are present.

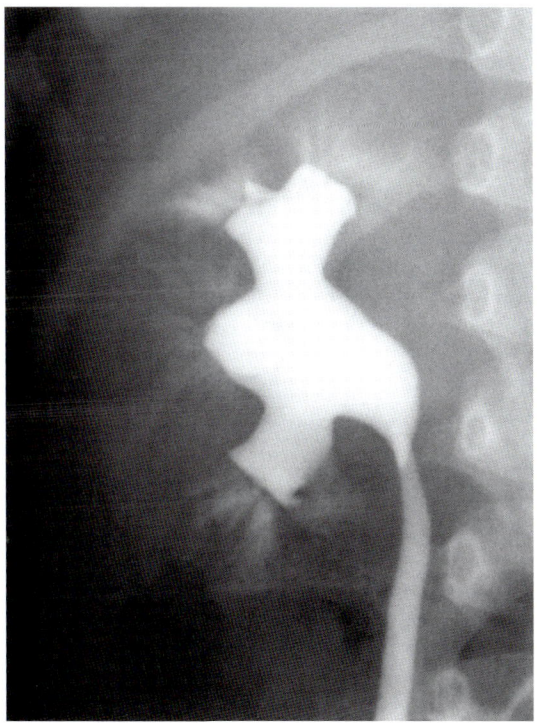

Figure 120-12   Intrarenal reflux. A voiding cystourethrogram image in a 2-year-old girl shows right vesicoureteral reflux and diffuse intrarenal reflux.

Natural History

Overview   VUR has a tendency to improve and to disappear spontaneously during the first decade of life, often during the preschool years. This tendency is attributed to a maturation process of the UVJ with age, with an increase in the length of the intramural ureter and strengthening of its musculature. Mild VUR (grades I and II) with normal-sized ureters and ureteral orifices has a favorable prognosis and disappears with time in more than 80% of cases, whereas more severe forms of VUR with dilated ureters have a lower incidence of spontaneous recovery (grade III, about 50%; grade IV, 30%; grade V, rarely). VUR that is associated with anatomic anomalies such as a large ureteral orifice and a short submucosal tunnel at cystoscopy is not likely to resolve. VUR occurring in an ectopically ending ureter (i.e., defective UVJ accompanying lateral ureteral ectopia of the lower pole moiety of a duplex kidney) or associated with a large paraureteral diverticulum also tends to persist, especially if the ureter ends in the diverticulum. VUR that occurs in patients with a lower urinary tract obstruction may disappear after correction of the lesion but is considered uncured if it is still present 1 year postoperatively. VUR that occurs in persons with neurogenic bladder disease or bladder dysfunction also tends to persist until the functional disturbance is treated successfully.[1,108-117]

Renal Scarring and VUR

Overview and Pathophysiology   Renal scarring is a common and potentially serious problem in patients with VUR and upper UTI (acute pyelonephritis). Renal scarring is characterized by one or more areas of renal cortical atrophy that is almost always associated with blunting or distortion of the underlying calyx or group of calyces, retraction of the papillae, and reduction of the medullary zone. Histologically, the affected kidneys show areas of cortical loss with tubular destruction and atrophy and interstitial fibrosis. Obliteration of glomeruli, arteriolar changes, and minor signs of interstitial inflammation also may be observed. The scarring characteristically has a focal or segmental pattern with a predisposition for the upper pole (38%) and less frequently for the lower pole. In some cases the process affects the entire kidney diffusely. The areas of scarring result in one or more clefts or depressions of various sizes in the outline of the kidney. The unaffected renal parenchyma may be hypertrophied, sometimes simulating a renal mass (pseudotumor). When the process is diffuse and severe, it results in global renal atrophy.

VUR is of paramount importance in the transport of bacteria from the bladder to the upper tract. However, because scarring may be seen in persons with and without reflux, VUR is not necessary to develop scars. The observation that scars are located preferentially in the renal poles, where compound papillae and intrarenal reflux predominate, has suggested the theory that intrarenal reflux may play an important role in the development of renal scars. Although sterile intrarenal reflux does not seem to cause parenchymal scarring (except perhaps prenatally in some severe cases), evidence both clinically and from animal experiments indicates that renal scars may result in part from the intrarenal reflux of infected urine.

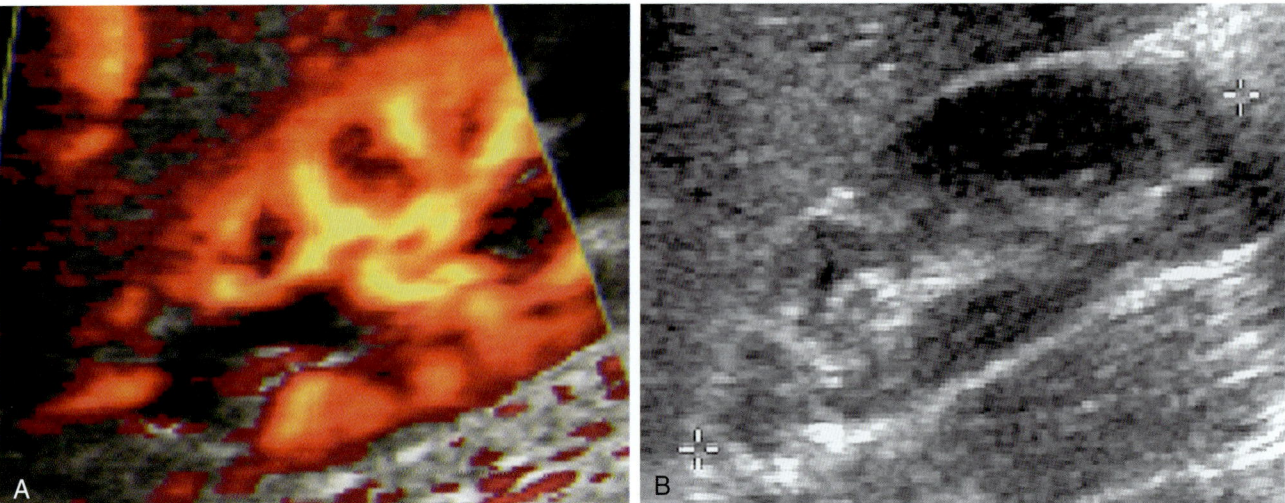

Figure 120-13   Acute pyelonephritis. **A,** A longitudinal color Doppler image shows a focal perfusion defect in the upper pole associated with a dilated calyx in an infant with acute febrile upper urinary tract infection. Evaluation found grade III vesicoureteral reflux. **B,** A follow-up longitudinal sonogram shows the development of upper pole scarring.

Imaging   The parenchymal changes may be directly depicted by ultrasound as areas of depression in the outline of the kidney with increased echogenicity of the nondifferentiated parenchyma at the dilated and distorted calyx; color Doppler imaging reveals focally reduced peripheral vascularity (Fig. 120-13). Nuclear scintigraphy, using a cortical agent such as DMSA, is especially sensitive in detecting renal cortical scars and is considered the gold standard. Magnetic resonance urography has been shown to hold great potential for diagnosis of renal involvement in persons with a UTI and renal scarring. Parenchymal changes also are visualized on contrast-enhanced CT, but this study is not indicated for the evaluation of renal scarring.

It may take a few weeks to several months for a scar to become apparent on imaging. Some apparently new renal scars that are seen in follow-up examinations may represent the end stage of an old insult to the kidney that was not apparent earlier or may be a result of intercurrent infections. In addition, what appears to be a progression of a previously demonstrated scar on follow-up may only reflect continuing growth and hypertrophy of adjacent normal renal tissue contrasting with a fixed atrophic area, creating an increasing mismatch during physiologic growth.[1,118-139]

End-Stage Renal Disease

Overview and Pathophysiology   Severe renal scarring is associated with decreased renal function of varying severity and is a relatively common cause of end-stage renal disease (ESRD), leading to dialysis and renal transplantation. Severe renal scarring is responsible for 8% of all cases of ESRD, but establishing how many children with scarred kidneys eventually experience this complication is difficult because VUR may not be demonstrated at the time of diagnosis (as a result of previous ureteral reimplantation or spontaneous resolution of the VUR). ESRD resulting from scarring is seen most commonly in older children, adolescents, and young adults, with an increased risk in patients with hypertension. The ESRD of these patients is probably the result of a decrease in the number of nephrons, a limited growth potential of the unaffected nephrons, plus an acquired glomerulosclerosis caused by an increased workload (hyperperfusion) of these unaffected glomeruli, similar to patients with a posterior urethral valve who also have congenital renal hypodysplasia.[1,140-144]

Treatment

Overview   Eradication or early treatment of UTI and the prevention of recurrences are the main therapeutic objectives in children with VUR, with an emphasis on infants and small children who are at particularly high risk of experiencing renal scars. These objectives may be attained by long-term suppressive medication with antibiotics until the patient is 4 to 5 years of age or until VUR ceases. This medical treatment is thought to be often sufficient in patients with low-grade VUR. However, with the new knowledge of the natural history of VUR and the increasing number of resistant bacteria causing breakthrough infections, this strategy is increasingly under discussion, particularly in persons with low-grade VUR. An antireflux procedure may become necessary in many patients with symptomatic and persisting high-grade VUR and usually is indicated in persons with grade V VUR, the latter sometimes after temporary urinary diversion via a ureterostomy. The success rate of ureteral reimplantation is high (up to 95%) in patients with grade I and II VUR, but the success rate decreases as the size of the affected ureter increases (a 60% success rate in persons with grade V VUR has been reported). Endoscopic intravesical injection of a small amount of some material (e.g., Silicon, Teflon paste, or dextranomer/hyaluronic acid [Deflux]) into the bladder wall behind the submucosal ureteral tunnel offers an alternative to the surgical procedures (Fig. 120-14). The injected material elevates and narrows the ureteral tunnel and causes a localized protrusion of the bladder wall at the lateral angle of the trigone containing the ureteral orifice. The injected material is well visualized by ultrasound as a rounded echogenic focus (Fig. 120-15 and e-Fig. 120-16).[1,145-171]

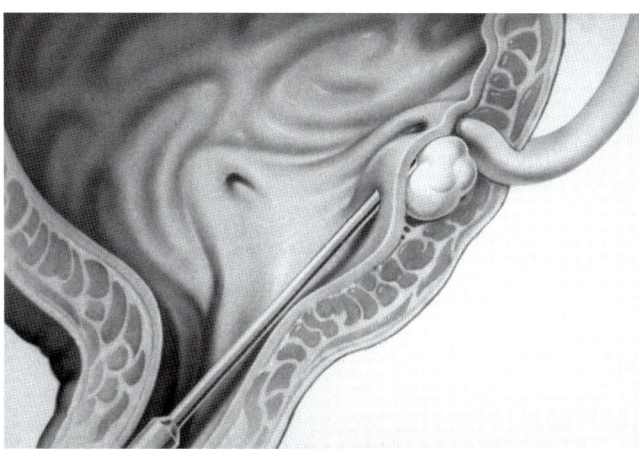

Figure 120-14 Subureteric injection. A diagrammatic representation of injection of material under the entrance of the ureter into the bladder to eliminate vesicoureteral reflux.

Imaging Algorithms for Evaluation and Follow-up

Overview Different recommendations exist for VUR imaging and imaging during or after UTI in different parts of the world. With the new knowledge and insight into the nature and pathophysiology of VUR and renal damage, many of these imaging algorithms are undergoing changes. Imaging is increasingly focused on phenomena that define prognosis and risk for long-term sequelae, such as the kidney with potential renal scars and bladder functional disturbances. We want to avoid diagnostic overimaging for economic reasons and patient concerns.

Imaging In large parts of Europe and North America, VUR assessment is considered to be indicated in all infants and children up to 2 years of age after the first UTI and in older children if a UTI has occurred with proven renal

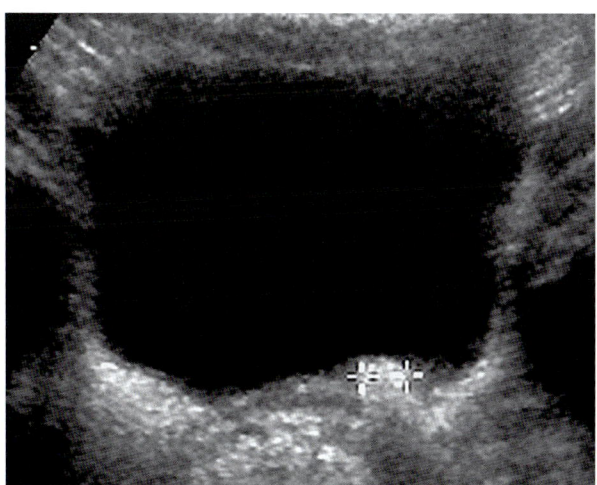

Figure 120-15 Postoperative imaging for vesicoureteral reflux. A transverse bladder sonogram after cystoscopic injection shows echogenic material at the left ureterovesical junction (*cursors*). See e-Figure 120-16 for the parasagittal view.

> **Box 120-4** Imaging Objectives and Imaging Algorithms in Urinary Tract Infections
>
> - Differentiate between lower and upper urinary tract infection (UTI) (renal involvement)
> - Assess for renal scarring and growth after a UTI
> - Find preexisting urinary tract malformations
> - Find signs of a complicated or atypical infection
> - Find complications in patients with a protracted clinical course and help with the differential diagnosis
> - Assess for vesicoureteral reflux, particularly in patients with upper UTI and renal scars

involvement, scars, or recurrent upper UTI. Furthermore, some sort of cystogram is considered indicated in all neonates with significant hydronephrosis and in all patients with significant urinary tract malformations, particularly preoperatively. School-age patients with a UTI should undergo an initial ultrasound, potentially a urodynamic assessment, and a late DMSA scan; VUR assessment is promoted only in persons with renal scarring, severe functional disorders, and recurrent infections. In teenage girls with a UTI who are afebrile, have no previous history of urinary tract disease, and have clinical signs of cystitis, ultrasound of the upper tracts may be the only procedure necessary. Patients with a family risk can undergo ultrasound and cystography, with ce-VUS and nuclear cystography being preferred in this patient group to minimize radiation exposure.

In persons with a UTI, imaging is increasingly being focused on the kidney; thus an early ultrasound or DMSA study is considered compulsory in any febrile patient with an upper UTI. To differentiate acute renal inflammatory changes from persisting scars, a DMSA study 6 to 12 months after the infection is recommended. In follow-up examinations and in studies after reimplantation, a nuclear cystogram (or ce-VUS) may replace VCUG for evaluation of VUR, and ultrasound and DMSA scans may be used to monitor the upper tracts (Box 120-4 and Fig. 120-17).[1,172-185]

> ✓ **WHAT THE CLINICIAN NEEDS TO KNOW**
>
> - Renal size, echogenicity, and corticomedullary differentiation
> - The presence of obstructive uropathy or congenital malformations
> - The presence of pyonephrosis, acute pyelonephritis, or renal abscess
> - Doppler ultrasound or a DMSA perfusion defect in the setting of upper UTI
> - The presence of renal scarring
> - The grade of VUR on a cystogram
> - Recommendation and guidance for the need and type of follow-up imaging

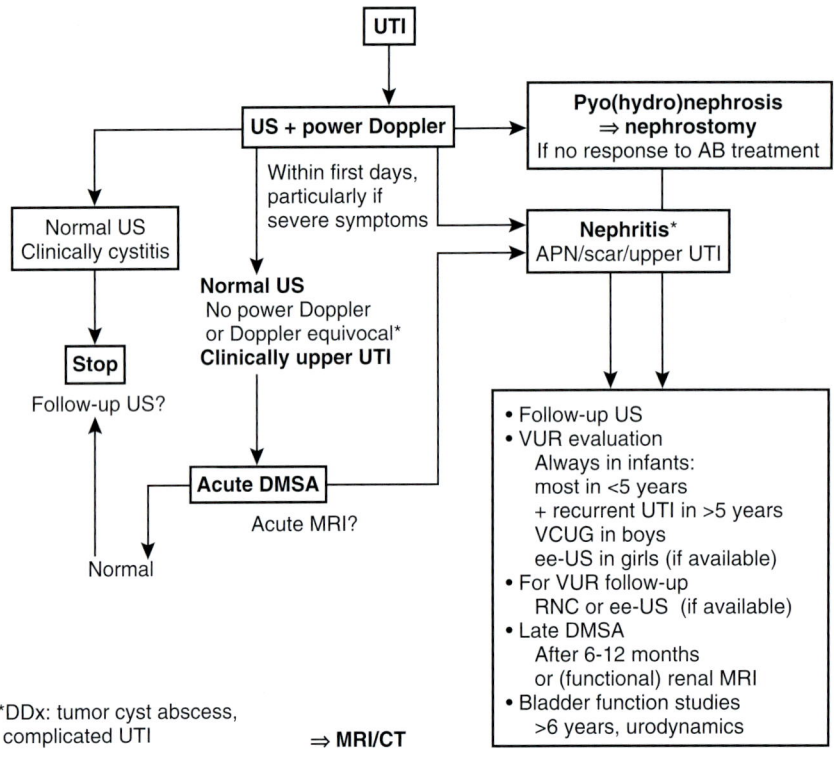

*DDx: tumor cyst abscess, complicated UTI   ⇒ **MRI/CT**

CT indications: complicated stone disease (unenhanced scan)

UTI criteria:
Urine sample and blood count, leukocyturia, positive nitrite, positive culture
(10^4 catheter sample, 10^6 normal voiding), leukocytosis, elevated C-reactive protein

Reliable clinical diagnosis is essential and the most important entry criteria for imaging!

Figure 120-17 Imaging algorithm. *AB*, Antibiotic; *APN*, acute pyelonephritis; *CT*, computed tomography; *DDx*, differential diagnosis; *DMSA*, dimercaptosuccinic acid; *ee-US*, echo-enhanced urosonography; *MRI*, magnetic resonance imaging; *RNC*, radionuclide cystogram; *US*, ultrasound; *UTI*, urinary tract infection; *VCUG*, voiding cystourethrogram; *VUR*, vesicoureteral reflux. (Modified from Riccabona M, Fotter R. Reorientation and future trends in paediatric uroradiology. Minutes of a symposium held in Graz, 5-6 September, 2002. *Pediatr Radiol*. 2004;34:295.)

Key Points

VUR itself causes neither UTI nor renal damage.

VUR is a risk factor for the development of upper UTI and pyelonephritis, with consequent renal scarring and potential long-term sequelae.

Mild VUR (grades I and II) in persons with normal-sized ureters and ureteral orifices has a favorable prognosis and disappears with time in more than 80% of cases, whereas more severe forms of VUR in persons with dilated ureters have a lower incidence of spontaneous recovery (grade III, about 50%; grade IV, 30%; grade V, rarely).

The importance of VUR presently is undergoing reestimation on the basis of new insights into natural history and new management strategies.

The focus of imaging in persons with a UTI has shifted to evaluation of renal inflammatory involvement or existing renal scarring and to assessment of structural or functional abnormalities of the urinary tract that may predispose a person to have renal damage.

Suggested Readings

Brandström P, Esbjörner E, Herthelius M, et al. The Swedish reflux trial in children: III. Urinary tract infection pattern. *J Urol*. 2010;184(1):286-291.

Brandström P, Nevéus T, Sixt R, et al. The Swedish reflux trial in children: IV. Renal damage. *J Urol*. 2010;184(1):292-297.

Fernbach SK, Feinstein KA, Schmidt MB. Pediatric voiding cystourethrography: a pictorial guide. *Radiographics*. 2000;20:155.

Fouzas S, Krikelli E, Vassilakos P, et al. DMSA scan for revealing vesicoureteral reflux in young children with urinary tract infection. *Pediatrics*. 2010;126(3):e513-e519.

Giordano M, Marzolla R, Puteo F, et al. Voiding urosonography as first step in diagnosis of vesicoureteral reflux in children: a clinical experience. *Pediatr Radiol*. 2007;37:674-677.

Hannula A, Venhola M, Renko M, et al. Vesicoureteral reflux in children with suspected and proven urinary tract infection. *Pediatr Nephrol*. 2010;25(8):1463-1469.

Hernandez RH, Goodsitt M. Reduction of radiation dose in pediatric patients using pulsed fluoroscopy. *AJR Am J Roentgenol*. 1996;167:1247.

Holmdahl G, Brandström P, Läckgren G, et al. The Swedish reflux trial in children: II. Vesicoureteral reflux outcome. *J Urol*. 2010;184(1):280-285.

Keren R, Carpenter MA, Hoberman A, et al. Rationale and design issues of the Randomized Intervention for Children with Vesicoureteral Reflux (RIVUR) study. *Pediatrics*. 2008;122(suppl 5):S240-S250.

Leslie B, Moore K, Salle JL, et al. Outcome of antibiotic prophylaxis discontinuation in patients with persistent vesicoureteral reflux initially presenting with febrile urinary tract infection: time to event analysis. *J Urol*. 2010;184(3):1093-1098.

Montini G, Tullus K, Hewitt I. Febrile urinary tract infections in children. *N Engl J Med.* 2011;365(3):239-250.

Peters CA, Skoog SJ, Arant Jr BS, et al. Summary of the AUA Guideline on Management of Primary Vesicoureteral Reflux in Children. *J Urol.* 2010;184(3):1134-1144.

Riccabona M, Fotter R. Reorientation and future trends in paediatric uro-radiology: minutes of a symposium. *Pediatr Radiol.* 2004;34:295.

Riccabona M. VUR. In: Carty H, Brunelle F, Shaw D, et al, eds. *Imaging children.* 2nd ed. Edinburgh: Churchill Livingstone; 2006.

Sillén U, Brandström P, Jodal U, et al. The Swedish reflux trial in children: v. Bladder dysfunction. *J Urol.* 2010;184(1):298-304.

Skoog SJ, Peters CA, Arant Jr BS, et al. Pediatric Vesicoureteral Reflux Guidelines Panel Summary Report: Clinical Practice Guidelines for Screening Siblings of Children With Vesicoureteral Reflux and Neonates/Infants With Prenatal Hydronephrosis. *J Urol.* 2010;184(3):1145-1151.

Subcommittee on Urinary Tract Infection, Steering Committee on Quality Improvement and Management. Roberts KB. Urinary tract infection: clinical practice guideline for the diagnosis and management of the initial UTI in febrile infants and children 2 to 24 months. *Pediatrics.* 2011;128(3):595-610.

Zier JL, Kvam KA, Kurachek SC, et al. Sedation with nitrous oxide compared with no sedation during catheterization for urologic imaging in children. *Pediatr Radiol.* 2007;37:678-684.

References

Full references for this chapter can be found on www.expertconsult.com.

Chapter 121

Bladder and Urethra

D. GREGORY BATES

Urachal Anomalies

Overview Fibrotic regression of the urachus typically extends from the umbilicus toward the bladder, resulting in the formation of the median umbilical ligament.[1,2] Failure of the urachus to normally regress results in one of four disorders: (1) patent urachus (50%), (2) urachal sinus (15%), (3) urachal diverticulum (3-5%), and (4) urachal cyst (30%) (Fig. 121-1).[3] Clinical symptoms include umbilical discharge, local infection, lower abdominal pain, and urinary tract infection.[4]

Imaging Abdominal ultrasound, voiding cystourethrography (VCUG), and fistulography are the primary imaging diagnostic tools for initial evaluation of suspected urachal anomalies.[5] In a patent urachus, the urachus fails to obliterate, resulting in a vesicoumbilical fistula (Fig. 121-2). The diagnosis may be confirmed by catheterization of the bladder through the umbilicus (Fig. 121-3) or by VCUG with films in the lateral projection. In urachal sinus, the urachus is closed at the level of the bladder but remains patent at the umbilicus (e-Fig. 121-4). The diagnosis of urachal sinus can be made only by catheterization and opacification of the umbilical fistula. In urachal diverticulum, the urachus is obliterated at the level of the umbilicus but communicates with the bladder. Ultrasound readily demonstrates this, but urachal diverticula are best shown on a cystogram in the lateral projection (Fig. 121-5). In urachal cyst, the urachus is obliterated at both ends but remains patent in its midportion. Multiple small urachal cysts may occur as a result of segmental urachal obliteration (e-Fig. 121-6).[1]

Treatment Urachal remnants in children younger than 6 months are likely to resolve with nonoperative management. However, if symptoms persist or the urachal remnant fails to resolve after 6 months of age, it should be excised to prevent recurrent infection.[1,2,6]

Bladder Diverticula

Overview Bladder diverticula, which may be primary (congenital), secondary, or iatrogenic (postoperative) (Box 121-1),[7] are the most common, are seen more often in males than in females, may be single or multiple, and occur most frequently in the trigonal area.[8,9] Secondary bladder diverticula are the result of chronically increased intravesical pressure and occur most commonly in the paraureteral area. Iatrogenic diverticula are seen most often in the anterior wall of the bladder at the site of a previous vesicostomy or suprapubic drainage catheter, and at the ureterovesical junction after ureteral reimplantation. Patients present with recurrent urinary tract infection, urinary retention, incontinence, stone formation, vesicoureteral reflux, and ureteral and bladder outlet obstruction.[10]

Imaging VCUG is the most efficient method of detection.[11] Bladder diverticula may become visible only during voiding when contractions of the bladder force urine into the diverticulum (Fig. 121-7). A paraureteral diverticulum or Hutch diverticulum[12] is located laterally and cephalad to the ureteral orifice (e-Fig. 121-8). If the diverticulum is large, it may engulf the ureteral meatus and the ureter may empty into the diverticulum. Associated vesicoureteral reflux is present in about half of the cases (e-Fig. 121-9).[13]

Treatment Surgical diverticulectomy may be performed by an intravesical, extravesical, or combined approach with satisfactory results.[14] The muscular defect in the bladder wall should be meticulously repaired. Surgical diverticulectomy often restores normal voiding dynamics.[10,15,16]

Neoplasms of the Bladder

RHABDOMYOSARCOMA

Overview Rhabdomyosarcoma (RMS) is the most common and important neoplasm of the lower genitourinary tract and accounts for about 20% of all RMS seen in children. RMS is the most frequent bladder neoplasm in children in the first two decades of life, presenting typically at ages 2 to 6 years or 15 to 19 years.[17,18] In males, more than 50% of the cases arise from the prostate. In females, RMS arises from the vagina and the uterine cervix. Histologically, the tumor is divided into three subtypes: (1) embryonal, (2) alveolar, and (3) polymorphic. Embryonal RMS is further subdivided into three categories: (1) classic embryonal, (2) botryoid, and (3) spindle cell. The embryonal form is, by far, the most common, accounting for approximately 90% of all RMS. The embryonal botryoid subtype accounts for one fourth of the cases and has a lobulated, polypoid appearance, resembling a bunch of grapes, hence the name *sarcoma botryoides*.[17,19-21]

RMS spreads by local extension from the bladder, prostate, and vagina into regional and retroperitoneal lymph

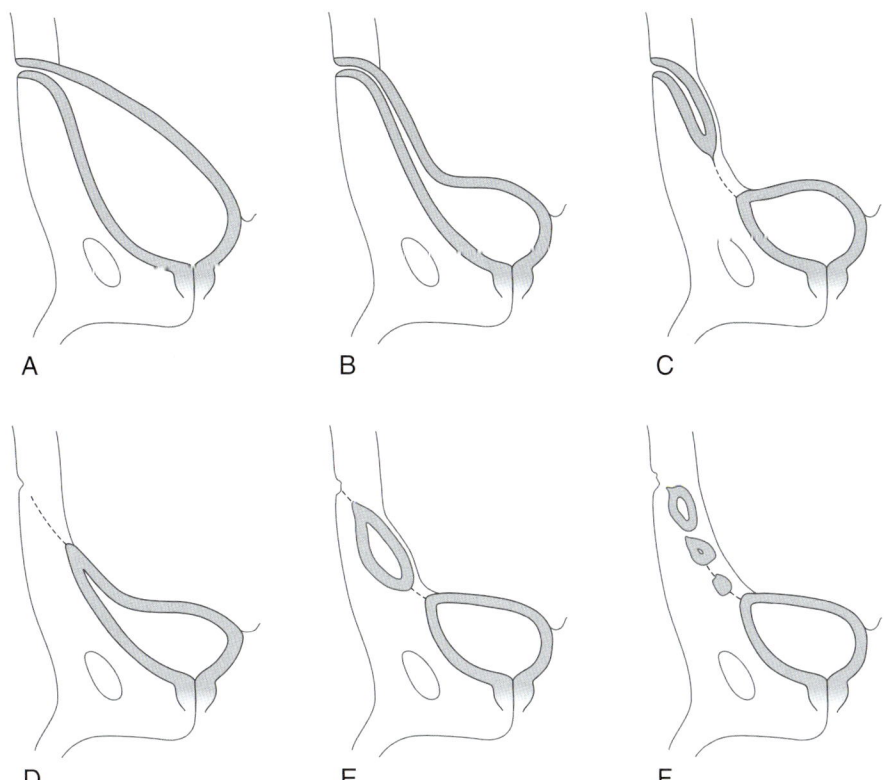

Figure 121-1 Development of the urachus and types of urachal anomalies. **A,** Appearance of the bladder in early fetal life, before development of the urachus. **B,** Patent urachus (vesicoumbilical fistula). **C,** Urachal sinus. **D,** Urachal (vesicourachal) diverticulum. **E** and **F,** Urachal cyst(s).

nodes and muscle. Lymph node involvement or distant tumor spread is found at initial diagnosis in 10% to 20% of patients.[22] Although RMS can metastasize to almost any site, it does so most commonly to the lungs, cortical bone, and lymph nodes, and less frequently to the bone marrow and liver. Hematuria, dysuria, frequency, urinary retention, and obstruction are the most frequent clinical manifestations. An abdominal mass may be palpated in some cases. In females, a vaginal tumor may manifest as a prolapsing mass in the introitus.[19]

Imaging On ultrasound, RMS is hyperechoic or hypoechoic, compared with surrounding healthy tissue, with or without focal anechoic regions representing necrosis and hemorrhage. Color and duplex Doppler evaluation show hypervascularity.[22] VCUG shows a filling defect in the posteroinferior aspect of the bladder (e-Fig. 121-10). When originating in the prostate (Fig. 121-11 and e-Fig. 121-12), the cystogram shows an upward displacement of the bladder floor or a smooth, lobulated mass at the base of the bladder.[19,22]

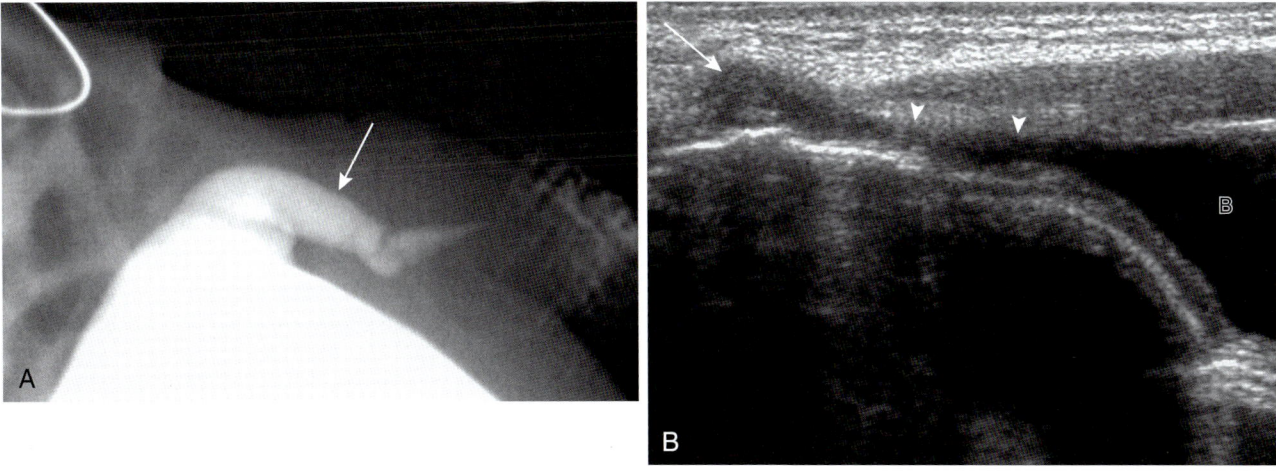

Figure 121-2 Patent urachus. **A,** Lateral view during a voiding cystourethrogram shows a fistulous tract (*arrow*) leading from the dome of the bladder to the umbilicus. **B,** Longitudinal sonogram shows a urine-filled patent urachus (*arrowheads*) extending from the dome of bladder (*B*) to the umbilicus (*arrow*).

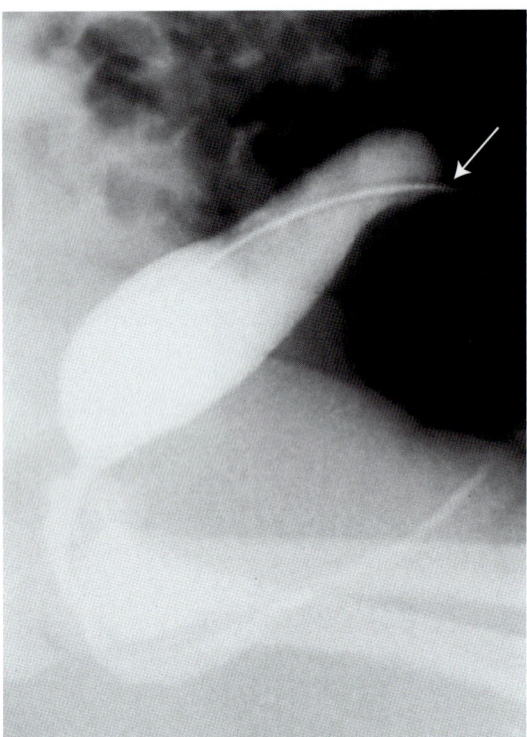

Figure 121-3 *Patent urachus.* Lateral view during voiding cystourethrography performed after catheterization of the bladder through the umbilicus (arrow).

Contrast-enhanced CT identifies RMS of the prostate or bladder base as a bulky pelvic mass of heterogeneous attenuation that may invade periurethral and perivesical tissues or may extend into the ischiorectal fossa. Calcification is rare. Vaginal tumors often arise high in the anterior vaginal vault and may be indistinguishable from a primary bladder tumor.[19] On magnetic resonance imaging (MRI) scans, RMS demonstrates nonspecific, low signal intensity on T1-weighted

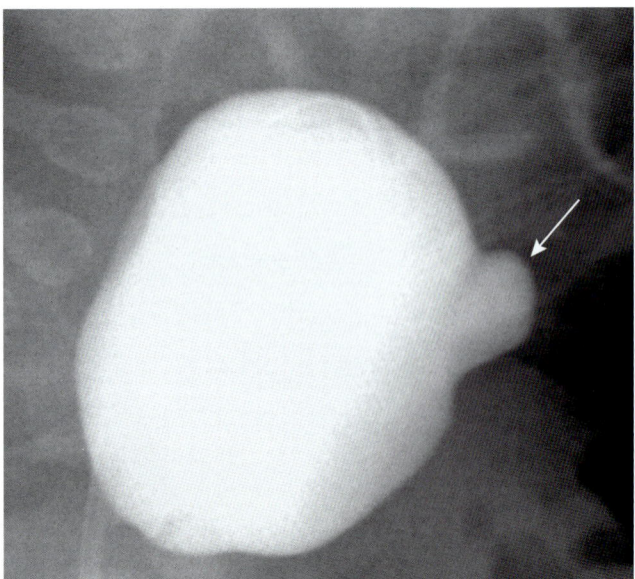

Figure 121-5 *Urachal diverticulum.* Lateral view during a voiding cystourethrography shows a urachal diverticulum extending from the bladder dome (*arrow*).

Box 121-1 Types and Causes of Bladder Diverticula

Primary (Congenital, Idiopathic)

Multiple syndromes: cutis laxa, Ehlers-Danlos, fetal alcohol, Menkes, Williams

Secondary

Posterior urethral valves

Urethral obstruction

Neurogenic bladder

Iatrogenic

Vesicostomy site

Suprapubic drainage site

Urethral reimplantation site

---

sequences and high signal intensity on T2-weighted sequences. After the administration of MRI contrast, RMS typically enhances heterogeneously.

Treatment The Children's Oncology Group and Intergroup Rhabdomyosarcoma Study staging and clinical system for neoplasms of the genitourinary system is given in Box 121-2.[18] Treatment combines surgical removal of as much of the tumor as possible, chemotherapy, and radiation therapy. Tumors of the urinary bladder and prostate have an overall 5-year survival rate of approximately 70%. Tumors originating in nonbladder or prostatic sites (paratesticular, vagina, and cervix) have better 5-year survival rates, between 84% and 89%.[23] Botryoid histology has the most favorable prognosis compared with all other histologies.[24]

Benign Neoplasms

Overview and Imaging Hemangioma of the bladder is probably the most common benign neoplasm (0.6% of all bladder tumors). Hemangioma presents as a discrete solitary mass of variable size (<1 cm to more than 10 cm), usually projecting from the posterior or lateral walls of the bladder.[25] Hematuria is the most common clinical presentation. Ultrasound will demonstrate bladder wall thickening, intramural anechoic spaces, and occasional calcification. CT and MRI may be required to fully define the extent of the lesion and for preoperative planning, since cystoscopy may only reveal a small portion of the mass.[26]

Box 121-2 Intergroup Rhabdomyosarcoma Study Staging System for Neoplasms of the Bladder

Stage I: Localized tumor, completely resected

Stage IIA: Localized tumor, grossly resected with microscopic residual

Stage IIB: Tumor with regional disease or lymph node involvement, completely resected

Stage IIC: Tumor with regional disease or involved lymph nodes, grossly resected with microscopic residual

Stage IIIA: Gross residual tumor after biopsy only

Stage IIIB: Distant metastases present at diagnosis

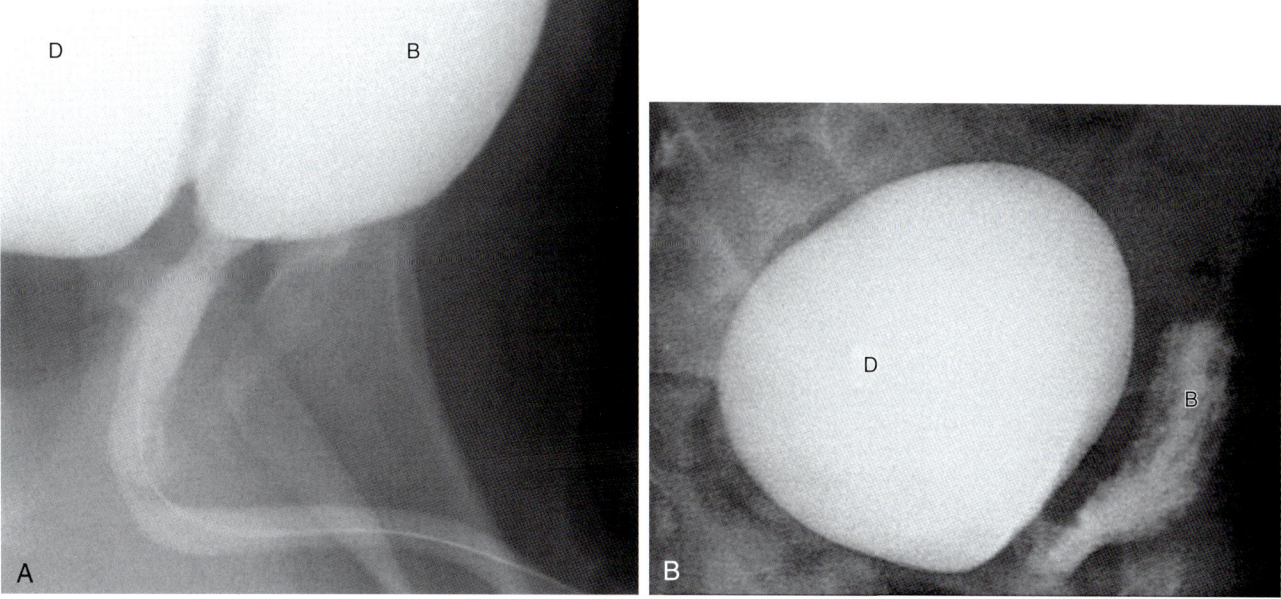

Figure 121-7 **Expanding diverticulum. A,** Oblique view during voiding cystourethrography showing an expanding right bladder diverticulum (*D*) during voiding. *B,* bladder. **B,** At the end of voiding, a large contrast medium–filled diverticulum (*D*) remains with an empty bladder (*B*).

Nephrogenic adenoma is a rare benign papillary lesion of the bladder. In most cases. a history of upper urinary tract infection, inflammation, trauma or recent surgery (ureteral re-implantation), calculi, or catheterization is present. The bladder is the most common site in children.[27] The female to male ratio in children is 3:1. Clinical presentation includes hematuria, frequency or urgency, and nocturia. Ultrasound demonstrates a nonspecific, echogenic papillary mass projecting from the bladder wall (Fig. 121-13).[28] Most nephrogenic adenomas are less than 1 cm in size; however, they may be

as large as 7 cm.[29] Treatment consists of transurethral resection and fulguration. The recurrence rate in children is 80%, with peak recurrence at approximately 4 years after treatment.[28,30]

Posterior Urethral Valves

Overview Posterior urethral valves (PUVs), more recently considered congenital obstructive posterior urethral

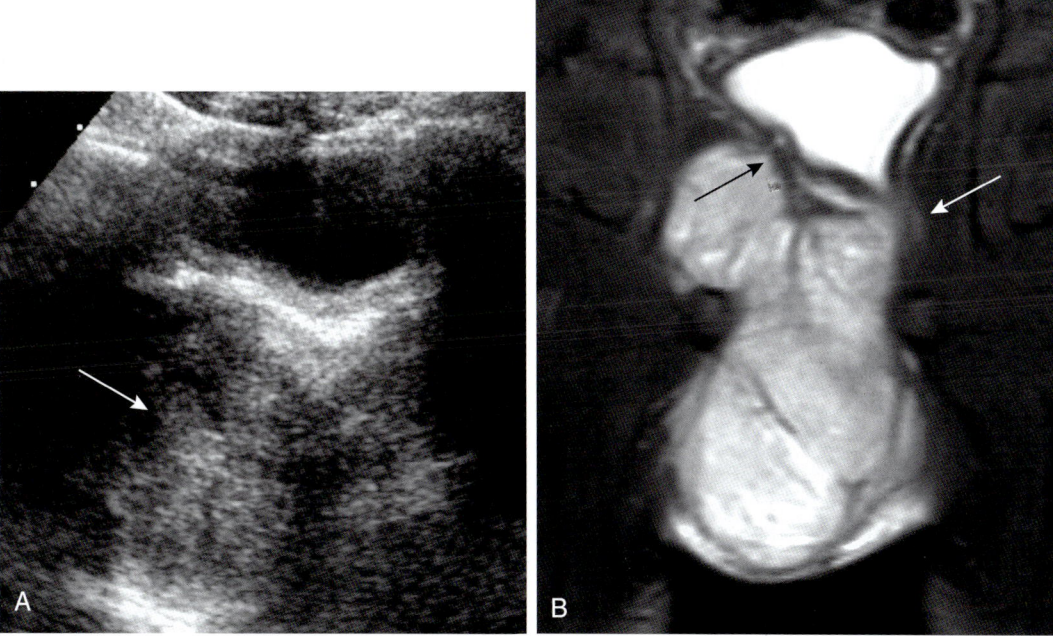

Figure 121-11 **Prostatic rhabdomyosarcoma. A,** A transverse sonogram of the pelvis in a 5-year-old boy shows a large predominately isoechoic mass below the bladder base (*arrow*). **B,** A coronal T2-weighted magnetic resonance imaging scan shows the bladder base displaced to the left (*black arrow*) and the rectum displaced to the left and partially encased (*white arrow*). See e-Figure 121-12.

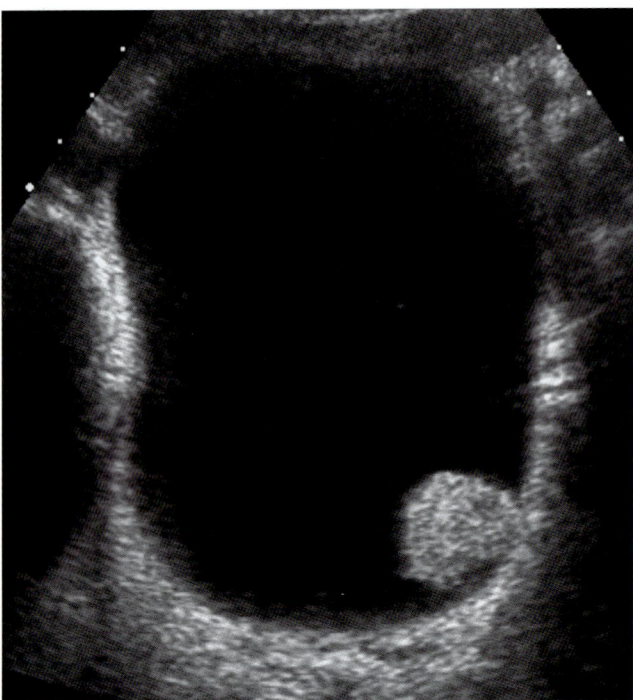

Figure 121-13 **Nephrogenic adenoma.** A transverse sonogram through the bladder shows an echogenic polypoid mass arising from the left side of the bladder floor.

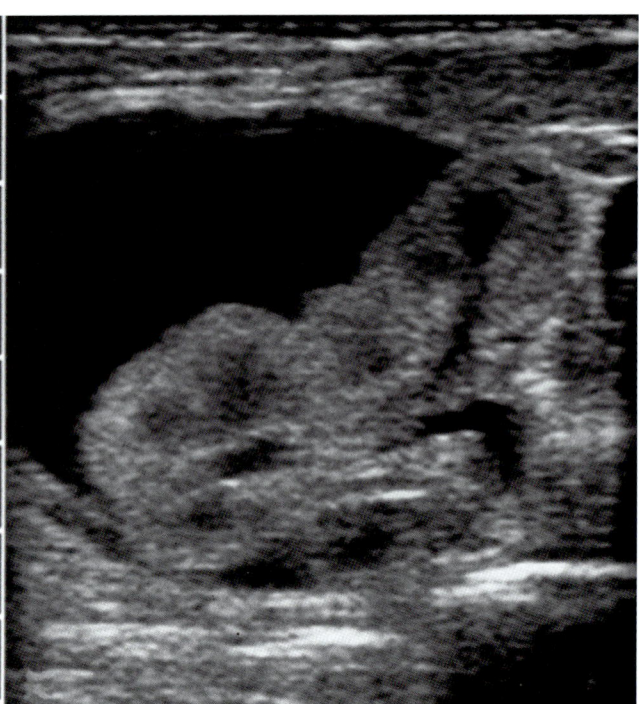

Figure 121-15 **Perinephric fluid collection.** A transverse prone image of a subcapsular urinoma with mass effect on the left kidney. See e-Figure 121-16.

membranes, are the most common cause of congenital bladder outlet obstruction.[31-34] The valves are identified at the base of the verumontanum, and the obstruction leads to posterior urethral dilation and chronic bladder outlet obstruction. The degree of urethral obstruction, however, is variable.[32,35-37] When detected prenatally, varying degrees of renal dysplasia result from pressure damage to the developing renal pelvis, collecting ducts, and parenchyma. If the fetus survives, up to 45% will develop renal insufficiency or end-stage renal disease requiring renal dialysis or transplantation before 5 years of age.[38-41] Those children who escape antenatal detection may present in the first months or years of life with urinary tract infections, sepsis, voiding disorders, hematuria, vomiting, failure to thrive, urinary retention, hydronephrosis, ascites, and congestive heart failure. At the other end of the spectrum are patients with late presentation of PUVs. These patients have a mild form of disease, and detection may be delayed as late as adolescence. These children may present with functional voiding disorders or urinary tract infections.[42,43]

Imaging Ultrasound shows varying degrees of hydroureteronephrosis and bladder wall thickening (e-Fig. 121-14). Dysplastic kidneys with increased echogenicity, decreased corticomedullary differentiation, and cortical cyst formation may be seen. Perinephric fluid collections (urinomas) are usually related to forniceal rupture (Fig. 121-15 and e-Fig. 121-16). When unexplained ascites is discovered in a male newborn, the diagnosis of urinary tract obstruction caused by PUVs should be strongly considered. Associated hydroureteronephrosis may not be present because the forniceal rupture and communication to the peritoneal cavity act as a "pop off" mechanism, allowing one or both kidneys to decompress. Transperineal ultrasound can show the dilated

posterior urethra, especially if the child is voiding at the time of the examination (e-Fig. 121-17).[44-50]

VCUG is the diagnostic study of choice for PUVs (Fig. 121-18 and e-Fig. 121-19). VCUG directly shows the PUVs and their effect on the urinary bladder; wall thickening, trabeculation with cellulae and sacculi, diverticula, and hypertrophy of the interureteric ridge (e-Fig. 121-20). Vesicoureteral reflux occurs in about one half to two thirds of male children with PUV, of whom approximately two thirds have unilateral reflux (e-Fig. 121-21) (Box 121-3).[34,35,51,52]

Treatment Transurethral resection or fulguration of the obstructing valvular structures is the recommended treatment for PUVs. Residual valve tissue with obstruction is not

---

Box 121-3 Imaging Findings in Patients with Posterior Urethral Valves

Ultrasonography
Renal cysts
Bilateral (unilateral) hydronephrosis
Thick-walled bladder
Actual valves

Voiding Cystourethrography
Dilated posterior urethra
Actual valves
Reflux into prostatic ducts, ejaculatory ducts, or both
Thick bladder neck
Trabeculated bladder
Reflux (50% of cases)

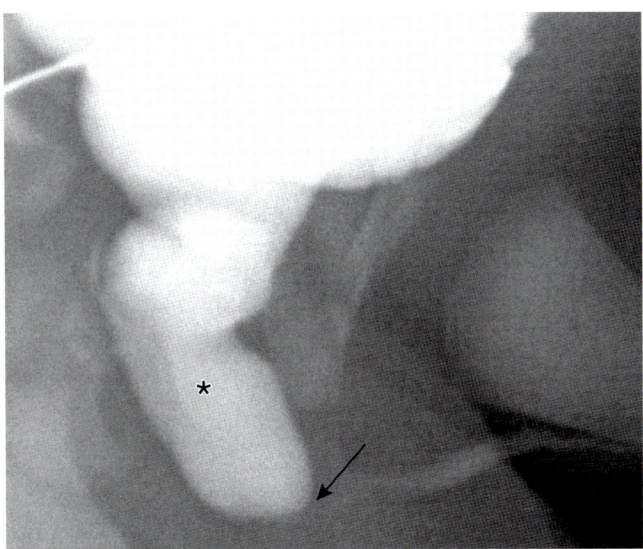

Figure 121-18 Posterior urethral valves. Oblique image during voiding cystourethrography shows a dilated posterior urethra (*asterisk*) with abrupt transition at level of valves to a narrow anterior urethra (*arrow*). See e-Figure 121-19.

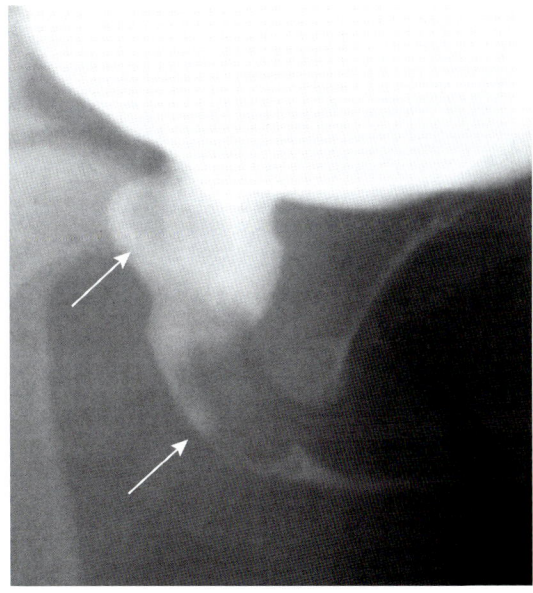

Figure 121-22 Urethral polyp. Oblique image during voiding cystourethrography shows a lobular filling defect in the posterior urethra representing a polyp on a stalk (*arrows*). See Figure 121-22.

uncommon, and stricture formation at the site of previous urethral valves or in the membranous urethra as a complication of surgery may occur. Urethroscopy is usually more reliable than the urethrogram in the diagnosis of these lesions.[53-63]

Posterior Urethral Polyps

Overview Urethral polyps typically arises from the posterior urethra and consist of an elongated, freely movable mass on a long stalk originating from the region of the verumontanum (Box 121-4).[64] The lesion is typically diagnosed in the first decade of life at a mean age of 8 to 10 years The classic symptoms are those of intermittent urethral obstruction with straining on voiding, abnormal voiding pattern, and urinary

---

Box 121-4

Characteristics of Posterior Urethral Polyps

Originate at verumontanum

Usually found at 3 to 6 years of age

Hamartoma with muscle, neural, and vascular tissues

Stalk present

Signs/Symptoms

Intermittent urethral obstruction

Urinary retention

Hematuria

Infections

Bladder tics

Imaging Findings

Filling defect at bladder neck–midurethra

Vesicoureteral reflux

Dilatation of upper tracts

---

retention.[65,66] Hematuria (30%–60%) and urinary tract infections may also be observed.[64-67]

Imaging VCUG remains the imaging gold standard. Before voiding, the tip of the polyp is frequently located at the level of the bladder neck, causing a small rounded filling (Fig. 121-22 and e-Fig. 121-23). In the voiding phase, the polyp moves downward into the distal posterior urethra and occasionally into the bulbar urethra. At the end of voiding, the polyp is displaced backward to the level of the bladder outlet by the contraction of the external urethral sphincter. Ultrasound may demonstrate a mobile pedunculated mass at the bladder base and indirect signs of bladder outlet obstruction (hydronephrosis and large bladder with or without bladder wall hypertrophy.[65-69]

Treatment Therapy of urethral polyps includes surgical resection (either by the transurethral endoscopic approach or through the suprapubic open cystostomy), transurethral fulguration, or laser (Nd:YAG, or neodymium-doped yttrium aluminum garnet).[65]

Prostatic Utricle

Overview The prostatic utricle is an epithelium–lined diverticulum of the prostatic urethra, the remnant of the fused caudal ends of the müllerian ducts. It is located in the verumontanum between the openings of the two ejaculatory ducts. When secretion or resistance to müllerian inhibitory factor is deficient, regression of the müllerian ducts is incomplete, resulting in an enlarged prostatic utricle and varying degrees of hypospadias (secondary to incomplete androgen-mediated closure of the urogenital sinus). The increasing severity of the hypospadias correlates with the increasing size of the utricle.[70] Poor emptying leads to urine retention and stasis. Clinically, this presents as lower urinary

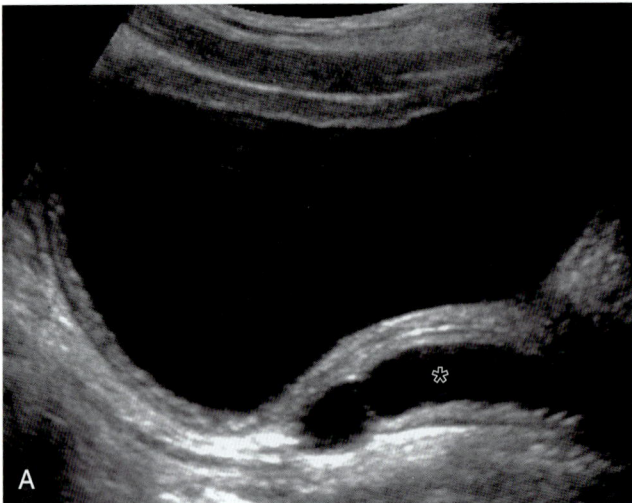
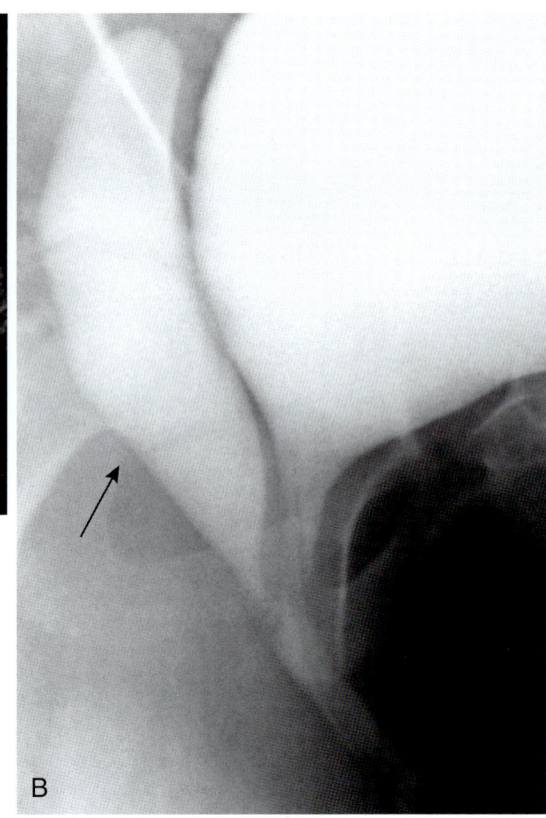

Figure 121-24 Utricle. **A,** A longitudinal ultrasound image of the bladder in patient with hypospadias shows a blind-ending anechoic tubular structure (*asterisk*) posterior to the bladder. **B,** Corresponding oblique view from a voiding cystourethrogram shows a large utricle (*arrow*) extending posterior to the bladder.

tract voiding symptoms, urinary retention, epididymitis, urethral discharge caused by urinary infection or stone formation, or postvoid dribbling caused by delayed utricle drainage.[71]

Imaging VCUG and retrograde urethrography (RUG) define the utricular size and its origin from the prostatic urethra, and associated hypospadias (Fig. 121-24). Direct catheterization of the bladder during VCUG may be difficult secondary to preferential passage into the utricle (e-Fig. 121-25). Transabdominal ultrasound may demonstrate a retrovesical cystic mass, with or without internal debris, tapering to the expected location of the posterior urethra. CT and MRI imaging will demonstrate a thin-walled cystic lesion originating from the prostatic urethral region, with or without associated mass effect on the bladder and ureters.[72,73]

Treatment Surgical excision is the definitive treatment of symptomatic müllerian duct remnants. Surgical management remains challenging because of the intimate association of these lesions to the ejaculatory ducts, pelvic nerves, rectum, vas deferens, and ureters.[74]

Abnormalities of Cowper's Glands

Overview Bulbourethral (Cowper's) glands are two pea–sized bodies on either side of the membranous urethra between the two layers of the urogenital diaphragm (Fig. 121-26). Their ducts are 2 to 3 cm in length and are directed forward through the bulb of the corpus spongiosum to end in the ventral aspect of the bulbar urethra. These accessory sexual organs secrete a clear mucous substance that acts as a lubricant for spermatozoa.[75-78]

Imaging Both the ducts and glands may opacify during VCUG when the distal orifice is patulous. A contrast medium–filled tubular structure is seen paralleling the undersurface of the bulbous urethra (e-Fig. 121-27). This finding, as a rule, is of no clinical significance. When the ductal orifice becomes stenotic, a dilated Cowper's gland (syringocele) and duct are formed. The diagnosis can be made at VCUG by demonstrating a smooth extrinsic mass effect along the ventral surface of the bulbous urethra (Fig. 121-28).[75,76,79,80]

Treatment At urethroscopy, these lesions appear cystic. Transurethral marsupialization or incision demonstrates these lesions to be filled with clear or blood–tinged fluid.[81,82]

Anterior Urethral Diverticula, Anterior Urethral Valve, and Megalourethra

Overview These uncommon anomalies of the male urethra are considered together because of common features and transitional forms suggesting a spectrum of related deformities.[83] The difference resides in their relationship to the corpus spongiosum. The urethral arch accompanying valves may

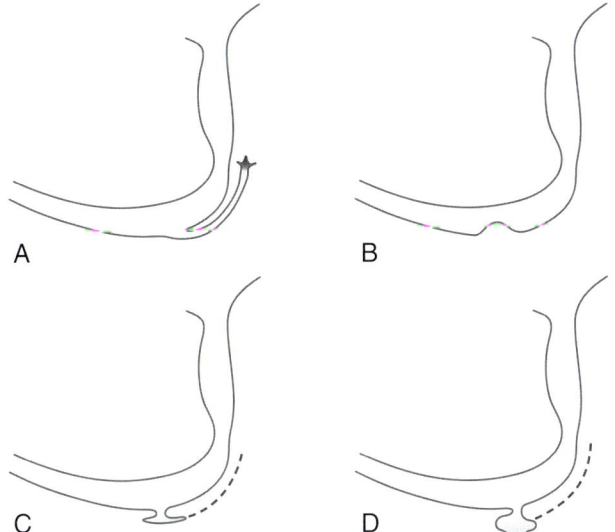

Figure 121-26 Various Configurations of Cowper's ducts and Cowper's glands on urethrography. **A,** Filling of the duct up to the gland. **B,** Opening of the duct is obliterated, causing a small mass on the floor of the bulbar urethra. **C** and **D,** Diverticula originating from the floor of the bulbar urethra; the duct is not usually opacified in these cases.

take on a "pseudodiverticular" appearance but remains bordered by the corpus spongiosum. In contrast, a true diverticulum develops outside the corpus spongiosum, which is completely absent from the margin of the diverticular pouch. The urethral diverticulum may be more anatomically linked to the megalourethra, in which the corpus spongiosum (scaphoid megalourethra), corpora cavernosa (fusiform megalourethra), or both are deficient.[84]

Anterior Urethral Diverticulum

Overview Anterior urethral diverticulum is a saccular outpouching of the ventral aspect of the anterior urethra into

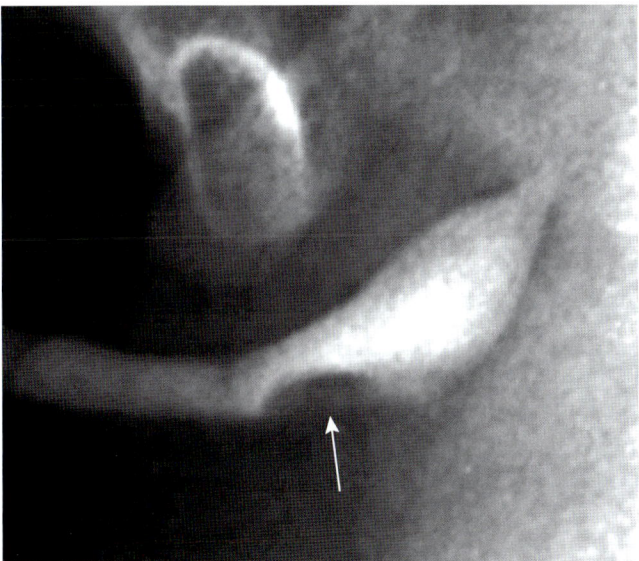

Figure 121-28 Cowper's duct cyst (syringocele). An oblique image from a retrograde urethrogram shows a lobular filling defect (*arrow*) along the ventral surface of the bulbous urethra.

the corpus spongiosum, usually near the penoscrotal junction.[83,85,86] The corpora cavernosa are intact. During voiding, urine distends the diverticulum and displaces the anterior lip of the diverticulum forward and against the dorsal wall of the urethra, obstructing the flow of urine. A tense bulge on the ventral aspect of the penis at the level of the diverticulum may be observed during voiding. The clinical symptoms depend on the degree of obstruction and include urinary retention, poor urinary stream, dribbling of urine, enuresis, and urinary tract infection.[87,88]

Imaging VCUG is the diagnostic tool of choice. Imaging of the urethra in an anterior oblique position will demonstrate a wide-mouthed, focal outpouching of the ventral urethra of variable size (up to 3 to 5 cm in diameter).[84] The urethra proximal to the diverticulum is dilated, with a sharp demarcation with the unobstructed distal urethra (Fig. 121-29). The proximal margin of the urethral diverticulum forms an acute angle with the floor of the ventral urethra.[83] The lesion is not clearly visualized on a retrograde urethrogram.[89]

Treatment Transurethral resection of the distal margin of the diverticulum with a hooked, single-wire or electrocautery knife is often successful. Open primary reconstruction, with diverticulectomy and urethroplasty, provides a more homogeneous caliber to the urethra. In the presence of infection, marsupialization of the diverticulum and urinary diversion followed by secondary repair is recommended.[83,85,87]

Anterior Urethral Valve

Overview Anterior urethral valves (AUVs) are congenital mucosal folds located distal to the membranous urethra.[90] The valvular tissue is directed backward and is anchored laterally such that it is raised up against the dorsal aspect of the urethra during voiding, obstructing the flow of urine. It differs from a urethral diverticulum in that it lacks a posterior lip and usually causes a lesser degree of localized swelling of the ventral aspect of the penis during micturition.[84] No abnormalities of the corpus spongiosum or corpora cavernosa are

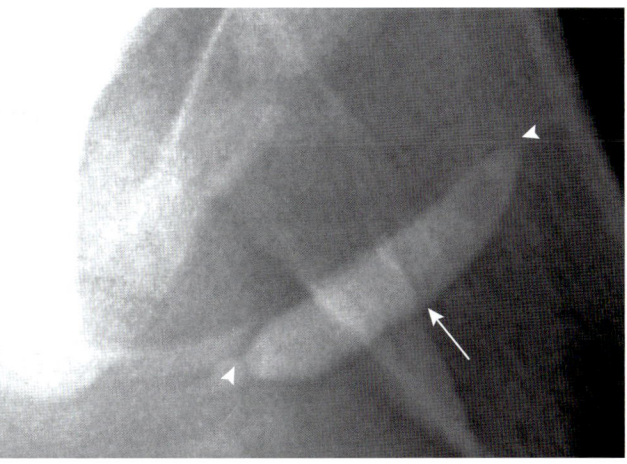

Figure 121-29 Urethral diverticulum. Oblique image during voiding cystourethrography shows saccular outpouching (*arrow*) along the ventral urethra. Acute angles are formed at the junction of the anterior and posterior lips with the urethra (*arrowheads*).

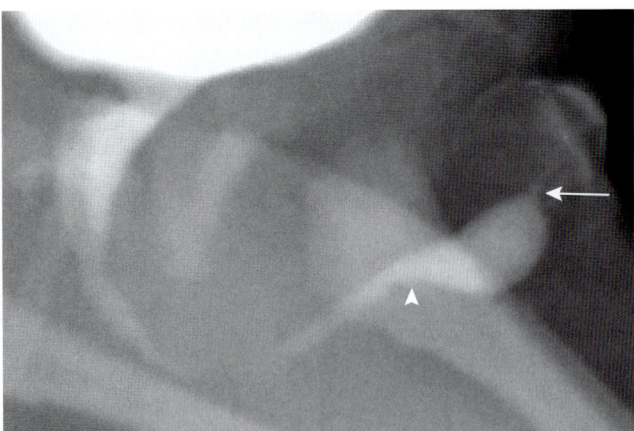

Figure 121-30 Anterior urethral valve. An oblique image during voiding cystourethrography shows a focal saccular dilation of the distal anterior urethra. Distally, an acute angle is formed at the junction with the narrowed urethra (*arrow*). Proximally, an obtuse angle is present (*arrowhead*). (From Bates DG, Coley BD. Ultrasound diagnosis of the anterior urethral valve. *Pediatr Radiol.* 2001;31:634-636.) See e-Figure 121-31.

present. The clinical manifestations and complications are the same as those described for anterior urethral diverticula but are often milder.

Imaging VCUG is the diagnostic tool of choice. The urethra has a more fusiform dilation proximal to the valve and is narrow distally. A thickened band of valvular tissue is seen at the transition, assuming an iris-like, semi-lunar, or cusp-like configuration (Fig. 121-30 and e-Fig. 121-31).[87,91] AUVs may produce a proximal dilation of the urethra that mimics a diverticulum. However, in "pseudodiverticula" formation caused by AUVs, the proximal end of the urethral dilation forms an obtuse angle with the ventral floor of the urethra, unlike the acute angle seen in a true urethral diverticulum.[83,91]

Treatment Transurethral valve ablation with the help of a pediatric resectoscope is the treatment of choice. Open urethrotomy and excision of the valve or segmental urethrectomy of the valve-bearing area along with a primary end-to-end anastomosis are alternative options.[91]

Scaphoid and Fusiform Megalourethra

Overview The scaphoid megalourethra is much more common than the fusiform type. It consists of a saccular dilatation of the penile urethra, caused by the absence or underdevelopment of the corpus spongiosum. Ventrally, the penis is soft and baggy with redundant skin. During voiding, the affected part of the urethra balloons markedly, causing a large, smooth bulge in the ventral surface of the penis. The penis and pendulous urethra assume a scaphoid (boat-shaped) configuration. The patient voids with a poor stream.[35,92]

Fusiform megalourethra, less common and more severe than the scaphoid form, is characterized by a diffuse ectasia of the penile urethra secondary to the absence or partial deficiency of the corpus spongiosum and corpora cavernosa. The penis is large, misshapen, and flabby, with redundant and wrinkled skin.[35] During voiding, the urethra and penis become markedly distended. The patient voids with a poor urinary stream. Clinical symptoms and the prognosis vary with the severity of the associated anomalies (e.g., "prune belly syndrome").

Imaging On VCUG or RUG, the dilated ventral segment of the scaphoid urethra dilates and blends gradually with a normal urethra distally and proximally. The fusiform megalourethra is markedly dilated, tapering both distally and proximally into a relatively normal urethra (Fig. 121-32). The proximal urethra may be dilated. Sometimes, the anomaly affects only a small portion of the urethra (e-Fig. 121-33).[93,94]

Urethral Duplication

Overview A single unifying theory does not exist to explain all the various forms of duplication, and more than one classification scheme exists in the literature. These developmental anomalies are characterized by the presence of a complete or partial accessory urethral channel arising from the bladder to the distal urethra. Incomplete duplications arise from the penile surface or from the urethral channel but end blindly in the periurethral tissue.[95-98] Sagittal plane duplication is most common with a ventral and dorsal urethra (one urethra atop the other). It is important to remember that in almost all cases, the ventral urethra is the functioning channel and contains the urethral sphincter and verumontanum. According to the location of the accessory urethral opening on the dorsal or ventral aspect of the penis, urethral duplications are divided into epispadic (the most common type) and hypospadic types, respectively.[99-101]

In the epispadic type, an incomplete accessory channel has a dorsal opening in the penis and ends blindly. The complete or partial forms originate from the bladder or proximal urethra and course through the dorsal aspect of the penis to end in an epispadic position anywhere between the glans and the root of the penis, or rarely they originate from a minute cavity (nonfunctional sagittal plane duplicated bladder) located behind the pubic symphysis and in front of the normal bladder. The ventral urethra is normally posi-

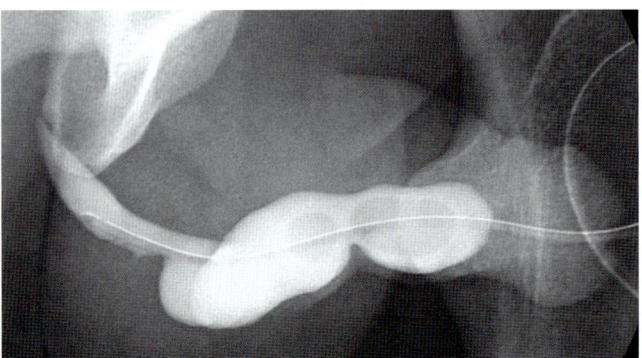

Figure 121-32 Megalourethra. An oblique image from a retrograde urethrogram shows fusiform dilation of the penile urethra.

tioned and ends in the glandular meatus (although rarely is hypospadic).[96,98-101]

In the hypospadic type, an incomplete accessory channel has a ventral opening in the penis and ends blindly or originates from the normal proximal urethra and ends blindly in the periurethral tissue, similar in appearance to a urethral diverticulum or Cowper's duct. Complete or partial duplications arise from the bladder or proximal urethra and course through the ventral aspect of the penis to end in a hypospadic position along the shaft.[96-98,102]

An important form of urethral duplication of the hypospadic type is referred to as *Y-type duplication*. The ventral urethra originates from the midprostatic urethra and terminates in the anal canal or in the perineum along the anterior anal margin. Urine flows preferentially through this ventral channel and is considered the normal urethra as it traverses the sphincter mechanism. A normally positioned dorsal urethra is usually stenotic or partially atretic.[103-106]

The congenital urethroperineal fistula has a similar location to the Y-type duplication, but is a distinctly different developmental anomaly (Fig. 121-34 and e-Fig. 121-35). The normally positioned dorsal channel is the functioning urethra in this case, and micturition is normal. Clinically, only a few drops of urine are present at the perineal opening.[107-109]

Accessory urethras may be asymptomatic or may cause a double urinary stream, urinary incontinence, urinary tract infections, and urinary retention.

Imaging Appropriate evaluation or urethral duplication includes anatomic evaluation of all channels, recognition of the functional urethra and identification of associated anomalies.[95,96,98] VCUG is adequate if both urethral channels can be clearly identified (Fig. 121-36 and e-Fig. 121-37). RUG may be necessary for hypoplastic channels not visualized on VCUG. Cystoscopy may be performed to confirm the radiographic findings and to precisely identify which

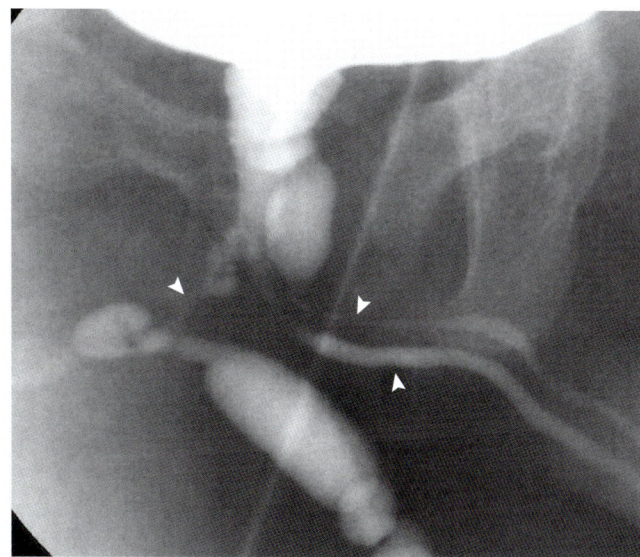

Figure 121-36 Urethral duplications. An oblique image during voiding cystourethrography shows triplication of the urethra (*arrowheads*) originating from the prostatic urethra. See e-Figure 121-37.

urethra contains the sphincteric mechanism and normal verumontanum.[97,102]

Treatment Preservation and reconstruction of the functional urethral channel is the primary goal of treatment. Ventral channel excision in congenital urethroperineal fistula is curative.[96,97,102,103,110]

Urethral Strictures

Overview Iatrogenic strictures, which account for about two thirds of the cases, are located predominantly near the penoscrotal junction, an area that is particularly vulnerable to internal trauma. Pelvic fractures, penetrating injuries, direct blows to the perineum, and straddle injuries are the most common forms of external trauma. Urethral infections are uncommon causes of urethral strictures in children as opposed to young adults, in whom urethral strictures are often due to *Neisseria gonorrhoeae* infection.[111-115] Urethral strictures of unknown cause in symptomatic boys are not rare. They may be the result of unrecognized external trauma or urethritis, Cowper's duct infection, or rupture of a Cowper's duct cyst, or they may be secondary to incomplete dissolution of the urogenital membrane at the junction of the cloaca and genital groove (Cobb's collar).[116,117] The clinical manifestations of urethral strictures include poor urinary stream, straining to void, urinary retention, painful urination, hematuria, urinary infections, and recurrent epididymitis.

Imaging The diagnosis is readily established by VCUG when the bladder can be catheterized. Compression of the distal penis during voiding (choke urethrogram) or RUG results in distention of the normal urethra and a better delineation of the true extent of the stricture. The membranous urethra is the area most often injured, owing to its fixation by the urogenital diaphragm. Strictures from straddle injuries

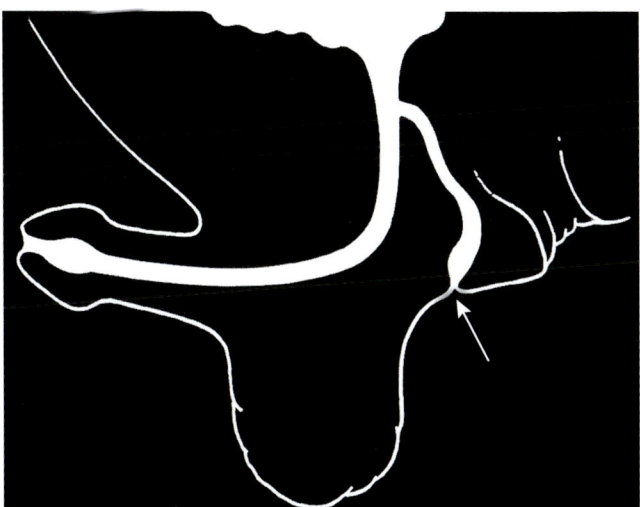

Figure 121-34 Urethroperineal fistula. Schematic diagram showing the perineal fistula (*arrow*) originating from the normal dorsal urethra. This is the exception to the rule that the ventral urethra is the normal urethra in duplications. (From Bates DG, Lebowitz RL. Congenital urethroperineal fistula. *Radiology.* 1995;194:501-504.) See e-Figure 121-35.

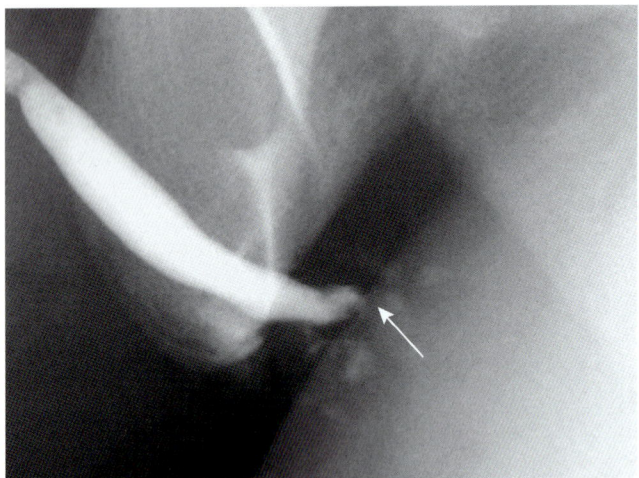

Figure 121-38 Straddle injury. A retrograde urethrogram shows bulbar urethral disruption (*arrow*) and contrast extravasation. See e-Figure 121-39.

are usually located in the bulbar urethra (Fig. 121-38 and e-Fig. 121-39). Congenital strictures are located most often in the bulbar urethra and are usually very short and diaphragm-like (Fig. 121-40). An alternative to fluoroscopic evaluation is ultrasound of the urethra, which provides information about the urethra as well as periurethral tissues. In the interpretation of the urethrogram, it is important to keep in mind those normal areas of narrowing at the level of the urogenital diaphragm or narrowing caused by spasm of the bulbocavernosus or external sphincter muscles that may simulate a stricture.[111,115,118-121]

Treatment Three major forms of treatment exist for urethral stricture: (1) *urethral dilation*, which is the oldest and simplest treatment; (2) *open reconstruction with urethroplasty*, which is regarded as the gold standard; and (3) *internal urethrotomy* by incising or ablating the stricture transurethrally.[122,123]

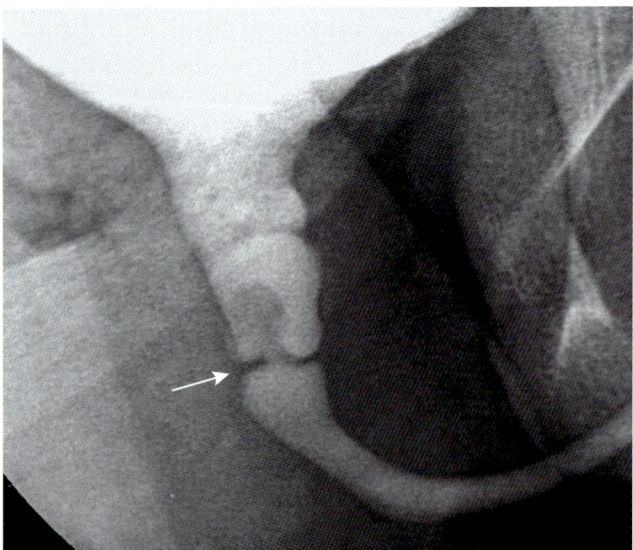

Figure 121-40 Congenital urethral diaphragm. An oblique image during voiding cystourethrography shows a linear filling defect in the posterior urethra at the base of the verumontanum (*arrow*). Mild posterior urethra dilation is present.

WHAT THE CLINICIAN NEEDS TO KNOW

- Type of urachal remnant
- Number, size, and location of bladder diverticuli
- Local spread and/or distant metastasis of bladder RMS, or both
- Identification of PUVs, associated bladder morphology, and presence of VUR
- Presence and size of prostatic utricle
- Presence of anterior urethral lesions—valve, diverticulum, or syringocele
- Classification of urethral duplication—particularly differentiation of congenital urethroperineal fistula versus Y-type duplication
- Urethral injury, stricture, or both

Key Points

Failure of the urachus to normally regress results in one of four disorders: patent urachus (50%), urachal sinus (15%), urachal diverticulum (3%–5%), and urachal cyst (30%).

Bladder diverticula may be primary (congenital), secondary, or iatrogenic (postoperative).

RMSs are the most common and important neoplasms of the lower genitourinary tract. The embryonal form of RMS is, by far, the most common, accounting for approximately 90% of all cases.

Late renal insufficiency or failure may develop in 25% to 40% of patients with PUV throughout adolescence and into adulthood.

Large prostatic utricles are typically associated with male hypospadias.

In Y-type urethral duplication, the ventral channel and is considered the normal urethra. In congenital urethroperineal fistula, the normally positioned dorsal channel is the functioning urethra.

Iatrogenic urethral strictures account for about two thirds of the cases in children.

Suggested Readings

Agrons GA, Wagner BJ, Lonergan GJ, et al. From the archives of the AFIP. Genitourinary rhabdomyosarcoma in children: radiologic-pathologic correlation. *Radiographics.* 1997;17(4):919-937.

Berrocal T, Lopez-Pereira P, Arjonilla A, et al. Anomalies of the distal ureter, bladder, and urethra in children: embryologic, radiologic, and pathologic features. *Radiographics.* 2002;22:1139-1164.

Evangelidis A, Castle EP, Ostlie DJ, et al. Surgical management of primary bladder diverticula in children. *J Pediatr Surg.* 2005;40:701-703.

Jones EA, Freedman AL, Ehrlich RM. Megalourethra and urethral diverticula. *Urol Clin North Am.* 2002;29:341-348.

Kawashima A, Sandler CM, Wasserman NF, et al. Imaging of urethral disease: a pictorial review. *Radiographics.* 2004;24(suppl 1):S195-S216.

Koff SA, Mutabagani KH, Jayanthi VR. The valve bladder syndrome: pathophysiology and treatment with nocturnal bladder emptying. *J Urol.* 2002;167(1):291-297.

Krishnan A, deSouza A, Konijeti R, et al. The anatomy and embryology of posterior urethral valves. *J Urol.* 2006;175:1214-1220.

Levin TL, Han B, Little BP. Congenital anomalies of the male urethra. *Pediatr Radiol.* 2007;37(9):851–862; quiz 945.

Little DC, Shah SR, St Peter SD, et al. Urachal anomalies in children: the vanishing relevance of the preoperative voiding cystourethrogram. *J Pediatr Surg.* 2005;40:1874-1876.

Pavlica P, Barozzi L, Menchi I. Imaging of the male urethra. *Eur Radiol.* 2003;13:1583-1596.

Poggiani C, Teani M, Auriemma A, et al. Sonographic detection of rhabdomyosarcoma of the urinary bladder. *Eur J Ultrasound.* 2001;13:35.

Schneider G, Ahlhelm F, Altmeyer K, et al. Rare pseudotumors of the urinary bladder in childhood. *Eur Radiol.* 2001;11:1024-1029.

Troiano RN, McCarthy SM. Müllerian duct anomalies: imaging and clinical issues. *Radiology.* 2004;233:19-34.

Wu HY, Snyder HM 3rd, Womer RB. Genitourinary rhabdomyosarcoma: which treatment, how much, and when? *J Pediatr Urol.* 2009; 5(6):501-506.

Yapo BR, Gerges B, Holland AJ. Investigation and management of suspected urachal anomalies in children. *Pediatr Surg Int.* 2008;24(5):589-592.

References

Full references for this chapter can be found on www.expertconsult.com.

Chapter 122

Congenital and Neonatal Conditions

OSCAR M. NAVARRO and ALAN DANEMAN

Normal Adrenal

At birth, the adrenal glands are relatively large because of the presence of the fetal adrenal cortex, which accounts for about 80% of the gland.[1] Because of this, both adrenals are easily visualized by using ultrasonography in the neonate (Fig. 122-1).

On ultrasonography, the normal adrenal gland has a central hyperechoic stripe surrounded by a hypoechoic rim. The hypoechoic rim represents the fetal and the peripheral definitive cortex (see Fig. 122-1). The central hyperechoic stripe includes the medulla, the central veins of the adrenal, connective tissue, and probably also part of the fetal cortex.[2] The surface of the adrenals is smooth or only slightly undulating (see Fig. 122-1). The easiest and most useful measurement of the adrenal is the limb width, which should normally be less than 4 mm.[3]

Computed tomography (CT) and magnetic resonance imaging (MRI) are rarely required to visualize the adrenals in a neonate unless a mass is present.

Abnormalities of Shape and Size

STRAIGHT OR DISCOID ADRENAL

Overview and Imaging A straight or discoid shape of the adrenal gland is seen on ultrasonography in association with certain congenital anomalies of the ipsilateral kidney, in which the kidney either is absent from its normal position in the renal fossa or is extremely small as a result of antenatal damage and dysplasia.[4] The adrenal gland otherwise develops normally but assumes a flattened, discoid shape (Fig. 122-2). On ultrasonography, the adrenal retains its normal pattern of echogenicity. Straight adrenals are longer than otherwise normal glands, and they tend to be slightly thicker.

HORSESHOE ADRENAL

Overview and Imaging Horseshoe adrenal is a rare congenital anomaly, in which the right and left adrenal glands are fused. It is often associated with other anomalies of the kidneys and the central nervous system, asplenia with visceral heterotaxy, and other anomalies.[5]

A horseshoe adrenal appears on ultrasonography as a band of normal adrenal tissue crossing the midline in the upper abdomen above the kidneys (e-Fig. 122-3). The adrenal maintains normal echogenicity. The isthmus of the horseshoe adrenal usually passes behind the aorta, but in asplenia, it usually passes in front of the aorta.[5]

Adrenal Congestion

Overview and Imaging Adrenal congestion may occur in perinatal asphyxia or stress, but the mechanism for this is not clearly understood. On ultrasonography, the glands appear markedly enlarged but maintain their general overall shape and smooth surface (Fig. 122-4). This usually occurs bilaterally but may be seen unilaterally or focally within one gland.[2] Loss of the normal central echogenic stripe occurs, and the fetal cortex may become a broad band of slightly increased echogenicity. A very thin peripheral anechoic rim that represents the definitive cortex may be present. Follow-up ultrasonography may show development of focal hypoechoic areas that represent focal hemorrhages or infarction.[2] The changes may be reversible and the sonographic pattern may return to that of normal adrenal glands in patients who survive.

Congenital Adrenal Hyperplasia

Overview *Congenital adrenal hyperplasia (CAH)* refers to a group of autosomal recessive disorders, in which an enzymatic defect occurs in the pathway for cortisol biosynthesis in the adrenal cortex. The most common defect is a deficiency of the enzyme 21-hydroxylase, which affects females much more commonly than males.[3] This leads to ambiguous sexual development in newborn girls or salt-losing crisis in newborns of either sex.

The diagnosis of CAH is confirmed by the presence of elevated serum 17-hydroxyprogesterone (17-OHP). In addition, in female neonates with genital ambiguity, normal internal genitalia are seen on pelvic ultrasonography, and a normal (46, XX) karyotype. The 17-OHP level is diagnostic only when measured after the third day of life because a relatively

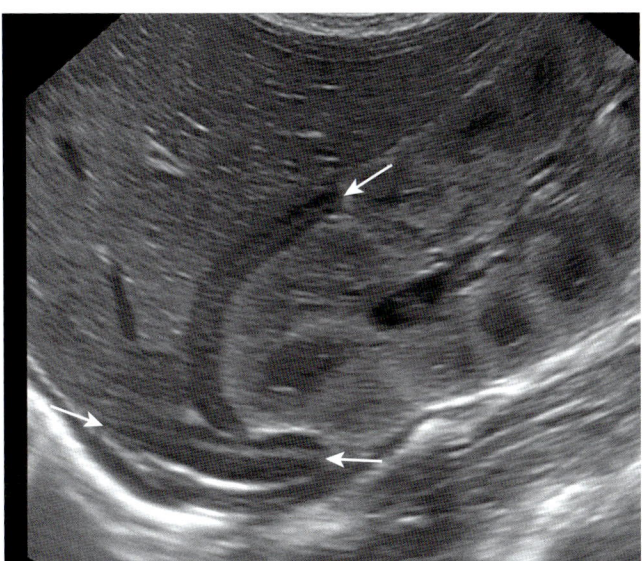

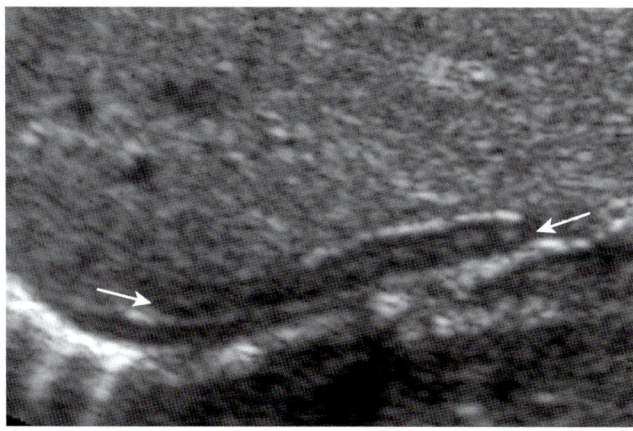

Figure 122-2 A longitudinal sonogram of the right adrenal gland shows a straight adrenal (*arrows*) in a patient with right renal agenesis. The adrenal gland is straight and lacks the angulation and shapes illustrated in Figure 122-1. The central hyperechoic stripe, surrounding hypoechoic zone, and smooth surface are preserved.

Figure 122-1 A longitudinal sonogram of a normal adrenal (*arrows*) in a 1-day-old newborn. The central hyperechoic stripe represents the central veins, connective tissue, medullary tissue, and congested sinusoids of the inner part of the fetal cortex. The surrounding hypoechoic zone represents the less congested outer part of the fetal cortex and the thin peripheral definitive cortex. The surface of the gland is smooth.

high level is present in the immediate neonatal period in a normal newborn. Furthermore, 17-OHP assays may not be easily available. These delays, although relatively short, may contribute to the diagnostic dilemma and heighten parental anxiety. Therefore, ultrasonography in the immediate neonatal period may play a role as some specific signs of CAH are seen on ultrasonography.[3]

Imaging Ultrasonography has shown to have a sensitivity of 92% and a specificity of 100% for the diagnosis of CAH with the use of the composite sonographic signs of adrenal gland size (limb width >4 mm), surface characteristics (cerebriform or crenated appearance), and internal echo pattern (diffusely stippled pattern of echogenicity or less commonly diffuse

thickened band of echogenicity) (Fig. 122-5) to make the diagnosis.[3] The presence of two or more of the three signs is diagnostic of CAH. These changes may also be present focally within the glands or may be markedly asymmetric between both adrenals.[3] Rarely, the adrenals may appear normal, emphasizing the fact that the absence of the signs does not exclude the diagnosis of CAH.

The sonographic changes in the adrenals with CAH are reversible with the introduction of therapy. Administration of steroids to the mother of the affected fetus seems to result in a normal sonographic appearance of the adrenals at birth.

Wolman Disease

Overview Wolman disease is a rare disorder of lipid metabolism (familial xanthomatosis). This inherited deficiency of lysosomal acid lipase leads to an accumulation of cholesterol esters and triglycerides in many organs, particularly the

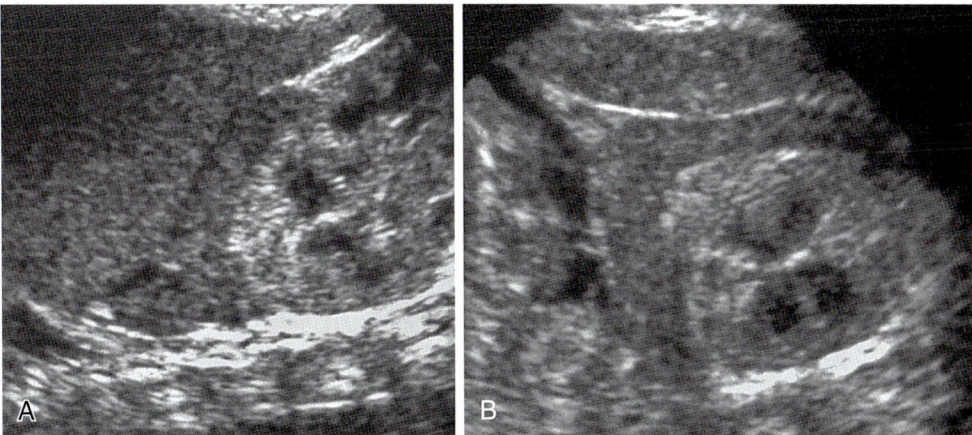

Figure 122-4 Adrenal congestion in an 8-day-old full-term boy who developed necrotizing enterocolitis, cardiovascular collapse, and multiorgan failure. Longitudinal (**A**) and transverse (**B**) sonograms reveal marked enlargement of the left adrenal, which, although has retained its normal shape and smooth surface, shows loss of the normal central echogenic stripe. The gland has a more homogeneous low-level echogenicity, and in parts, a peripheral anechoic thin rim is seen. A postmortem histologic examination revealed congestion of the fetal cortex. The peripheral thin rim represents the peripheral definitive cortex.

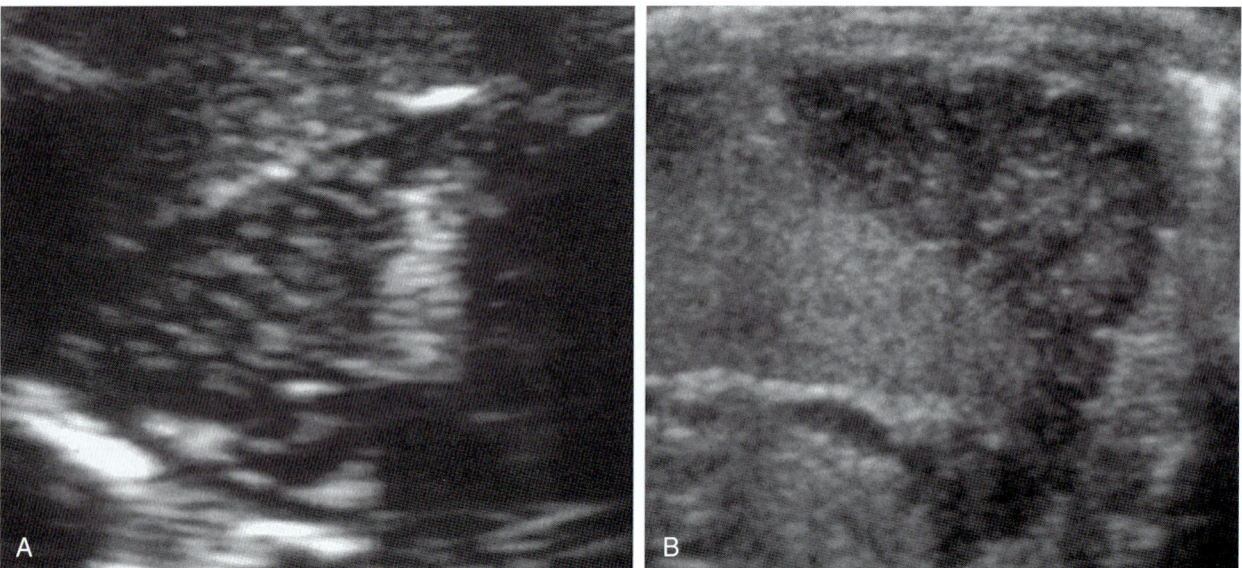

Figure 122-5 Congenital adrenal hyperplasia in a 26-day-old boy. Longitudinal (**A**) and transverse (**B**) sonograms of the left adrenal show marked enlargement of the gland, with a limb width greater than 4 mm in thickness. A clearly lobulated surface to the adrenal is seen better on transverse scan. The central echogenic stripe has been replaced by diffuse stippled echogenicity.

adrenals.[6] The disorder manifests in the early weeks of life, and hepatosplenomegaly, jaundice, vomiting, steatorrhea, abdominal distention, and growth failure may exist. The disease is rapidly progressive, and death occurs within the first year.

Imaging A marked enlargement of both adrenals, which retain their overall shape, is seen on imaging. This is associated with marked, diffuse, punctate calcification (e-Fig. 122-6).[6] This can be recognized on plain radiographs of the abdomen and cross-sectional imaging. On ultrasonography, the calcification in Wolman disease appears as dense punctate or granular calcification with marked posterior acoustic shadowing, the latter seldom seen with adrenal hemorrhage. On CT, the large size of both glands and the diffuse pattern of calcification differentiate this condition from resolving adrenal hemorrhage, in which the glands are smaller with more globular calcification.

Suprarenal Masses

Overview Adrenal masses in the neonate are mainly caused by hemorrhage or neoplasm, particularly neuroblastoma. Extra-adrenal masses are rare with the most common being intra-abdominal pulmonary sequestration. An accurate diagnosis is of the utmost importance because of the different management for these entities. However, the diagnosis may be difficult because of overlapping imaging features and, therefore, may not be established on the initial imaging findings alone, often requiring follow-up imaging (mainly with ultrasonography), correlation with clinical history, and measurement of urine catecholamines. Because of the relatively good prognosis of perinatal neuroblastoma, an initial conservative management is warranted. CT and MRI have little role in the diagnosis of these lesions and are mainly indicated to assess extent and for staging of a suspected neuroblastoma.

ADRENAL HEMORRHAGE

Overview Adrenal hemorrhage is the most common adrenal mass in neonates. It often occurs within the first few days of life but can occur prenatally and be seen on antenatal ultrasonography. It is more commonly right sided (70%) but may also be bilateral (10%).[7] It usually occurs in situations of perinatal stress, including difficult or traumatic delivery, hypoxia, and sepsis. It may also occur in bleeding diatheses. Large infants and infants of mothers with diabetes are particularly susceptible. Adrenal hemorrhages in neonates may not infrequently be an incidental finding.

Imaging Ultrasonography is the modality of choice for documentation of the presence of an adrenal hemorrhage and for follow-up. Ultrasonography shows a suprarenal mass of variable echogenicity (Fig. 122-7) without flow on color Doppler ultrasonography. These findings may overlap with those of neuroblastoma, and therefore, further confirmation of the diagnosis may be obtained from follow-up ultrasonography.[7] The adrenal hemorrhage decreases in size and changes echogenicity within the first week (see Fig. 122-7), followed by development of peripheral increased echogenicity due to calcification. The calcification becomes more compacted as the mass becomes smaller, and the adrenal eventually resumes its more normal shape and size.

NEUROBLASTOMA

Overview and Imaging Neuroblastoma is the most common adrenal neoplasm found in the fetus on ultrasonography and in neonates.[8] When detected antenatally, it is generally diagnosed in the third trimester. It is frequently right sided, may vary significantly in size (Fig. 122-8), and often has a more cystic appearance than in older infants and children (Fig. 122-9).[8,9] However, the echogenicity on ultrasonography varies; some may be evenly echogenic (Fig. 122-10), whereas others are highly heterogeneous. Flow is often

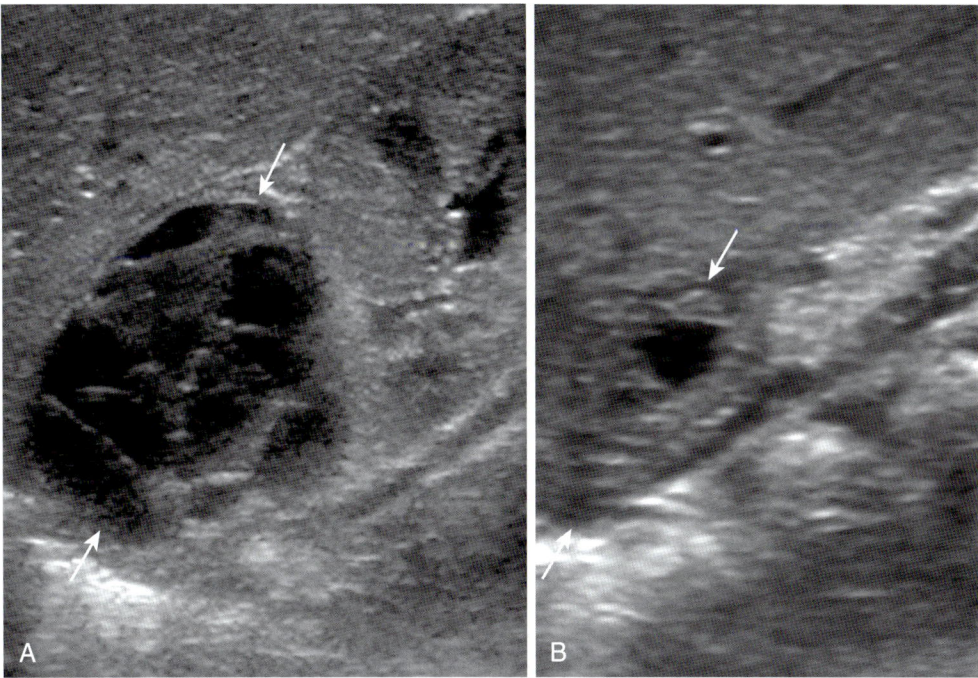

Figure 122-7 Adrenal hemorrhage detected in the third trimester of pregnancy in a neonate. **A,** A longitudinal sonogram of the right upper quadrant at 17 days of age shows a multiseptated predominantly cystic mass (*arrows*) superior to the right kidney. No flow in the septa was evident on color Doppler interrogation (*not shown*). **B,** The follow-up sonogram at 38 days of age shows significant decrease in size of the mass (*arrows*) as well as a change in its echogenicity. The pattern of evolution of this lesion is compatible with an adrenal hemorrhage. In addition, urine catecholamines and metaiodobenzylguanidine scan were negative in this patient.

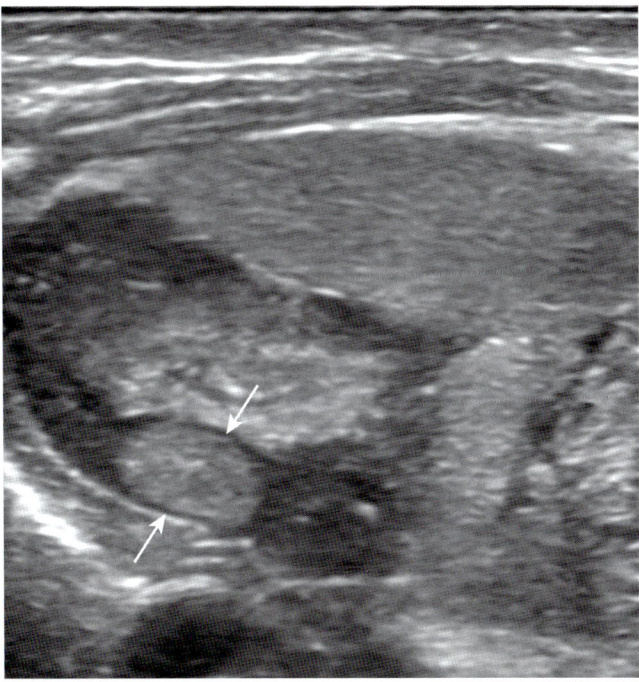

Figure 122-8 Left adrenal neuroblastoma found incidentally in a 13-day-old boy who had bladder perforation. A longitudinal sonogram of the left upper quadrant shows a very small hyperechoic mass (*arrows*) within one of the limbs of the left adrenal.

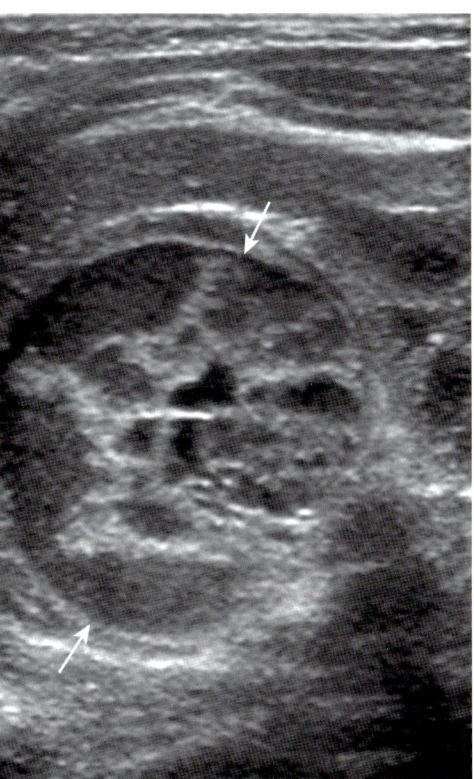

Figure 122-9 Right adrenal neuroblastoma detected in the third trimester of pregnancy in an 8-day-old girl. A longitudinal sonogram shows a complex, multiseptated, predominantly cystic mass (*arrows*) involving the right adrenal. No flow in the septa was evident on color Doppler interrogation (*not shown*). The mass has similar features to the adrenal hemorrhage illustrated in Figure 122-7, although in this case, urine catecholamines were elevated and the mass was metaiodobenzylguanidine avid.

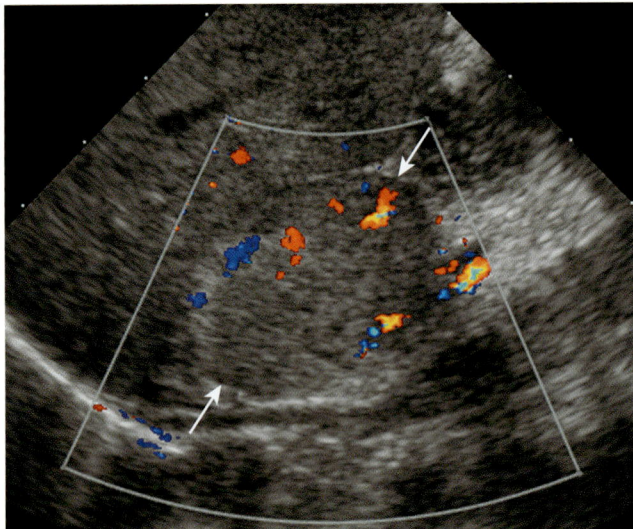

Figure 122-10 Right adrenal neuroblastoma detected in the third trimester of pregnancy in a 10-day-old boy. A longitudinal sonogram shows a relatively homogenous hyperechoic mass (*arrows*) arising in a somewhat exophytic fashion from the inferior and anterior aspect of the right adrenal. Intralesional flow is shown on color Doppler interrogation.

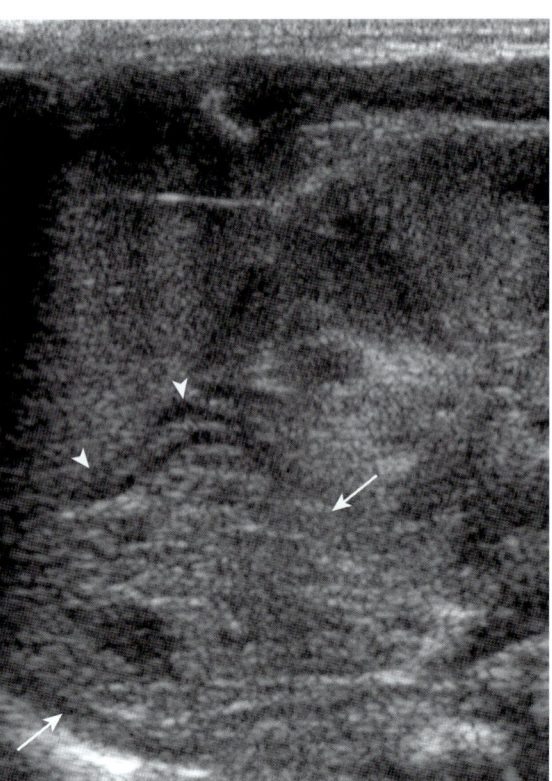

Figure 122-12 Left-sided intra-abdominal pulmonary sequestration detected in the second trimester of pregnancy in a 2-day-old girl. A relatively echogenic left suprarenal mass (*arrows*) displaces the normal left adrenal anteriorly (*arrowheads*), characteristic of sequestration. Within the mass, rounded hypoechoic areas represent cysts secondary to component of congenital pulmonary airway malformation.

detected on color Doppler ultrasonography aiding in the differentiation from hemorrhage (see Fig. 122-10). However, the absence of flow does not exclude the diagnosis of neuroblastoma.

Perinatal neuroblastoma also may present with metastatic disease, typically in the liver, skin, and bone marrow, corresponding to stage MS (equivalent to stage 4S of the formerly used International Neuroblastoma Staging System) (see Chapter 123). Diffuse infiltration of the liver may result in massive hepatomegaly (e-Fig. 122-11).

In contrast to neuroblastoma in older children, in perinatal neuroblastoma urinary catecholamine metabolites are elevated in only 40% of cases, and metaiodobenzylguanidine avidity exists in only 70% of cases.[8]

INTRA-ABDOMINAL PULMONARY SEQUESTRATION

Overview and Imaging Intra-abdominal pulmonary sequestration is a mass of pulmonary tissue, separate from the lung, with systemic arterial supply, more commonly found in the suprarenal region, usually left sided. In contrast to adrenal neuroblastoma and hemorrhage, these are commonly diagnosed in the second trimester of pregnancy.[10] In fact, a suprarenal mass diagnosed in the third trimester of pregnancy but with a normal second trimester sonogram militates against a sequestration. On ultrasonography, sequestrations appear homogeneously hyperechoic, although in more than half the cases, small (<5 mm), well-defined intralesional cysts exist because of the presence of associated congenital pulmonary airway malformation (Fig. 122-12).[10,11] The normal adrenal gland is often identified, displaced anteriorly by the sequestration. These sequestrations may significantly decrease in size and even disappear on follow-up ultrasonography.[11]

✓ WHAT THE CLINICIAN NEEDS TO KNOW

- Adrenal limb width
- Adrenal contours
- Adrenal echogenicity
- Presence of adrenal mass
- Flow present in adrenal mass
- Changes on follow-up examination

Key Points

A straight or discoid adrenal is a marker for an ipsilateral renal anomaly.

A horseshoe adrenal is associated with nongenitourinary anomalies, including asplenia.

Ultrasonography can be helpful in the expedient diagnosis of CAH.

Follow-up ultrasonography is helpful in the differentiation of adrenal neuroblastoma from adrenal hemorrhage.

Time of antenatal diagnosis is extremely helpful in the differentiation of adrenal neuroblastoma from intra-abdominal pulmonary sequestration.

Suggested Readings

Balassy C, Navarro OM, Daneman A. Adrenal masses in children. *Radiol Clin North Am.* 2011;49(4):711-727.

Paterson A. Adrenal pathology in childhood: a spectrum of disease. *Eur Radiol.* 2002;12:2491-2508.

Rosado-de-Christenson ML, Frazier AA, Stocker JT, et al. Extralobar sequestration: radiologic-pathologic correlation. *RadioGraphics.* 1993;13:425-441.

References

Full references for this chapter can be found on www.expertconsult.com.

Chapter 123

Acquired Conditions

OSCAR M. NAVARRO and ALAN DANEMAN

Neuroblastoma

Overview Neuroblastoma is the most common extracranial solid neoplasm in children and accounts for almost 10% of all childhood neoplasms.[1] Neuroblastoma arises in the abdomen in two thirds of cases; of these, about two thirds of lesions occur in the adrenal, whereas the remainder may arise anywhere along the sympathetic nerve chains.[1]

Neuroblastoma, ganglioneuroblastoma, and ganglioneuroma belong to a group of related neoplasms arising from neural crest tissue that are distinguished by their degree of cellular maturation and differentiation. Neuroblastoma accounts for the vast majority of these lesions and has the most primitive and malignant cells.[2] Ganglioneuroma represents the more differentiated end of the spectrum and is benign. Ganglioneuroblastomas represent an intermediate group with mixed histology.

Most children with neuroblastoma present between 1 and 5 years of age, with a median age of almost 2 years.[2] Neuroblastoma is more common in patients with neurofibromatosis type 1, Beckwith-Wiedemann syndrome, Hirschsprung disease, central hypoventilation syndrome, and DiGeorge syndrome.[2]

Neuroblastomas typically present as palpable masses or with symptoms and signs related to local tumor invasion, metastatic disease, and the effects of hormone production or autoimmune response (opsoclonus–myoclonus syndrome). Metastatic disease is seen in up to 70% of patients at presentation.[3] The most common sites include local and distant lymph nodes, bone, bone marrow, liver, and skin.

The diagnosis of neuroblastoma can be made by tissue biopsy, but a combination of positive bone marrow aspirate and increased urinary catecholamine metabolites (vanillylmandelic acid and homovanillic acid) is sufficient to confirm the diagnosis. The urinary level of catecholamine metabolites is increased in almost 90% of cases of neuroblastoma.[4] The International Neuroblastoma Staging System has been the most commonly used worldwide for staging neuroblastoma.[1,2,4] However, its application has encountered many difficulties, as it relies on the extent of tumor resected at surgery. For this reason, a new staging system, the International Neuroblastoma Risk Group Staging System, was developed in 2009, and this system relies on preoperative imaging findings (imaging risk factors) and detection of metastatic disease (Box 123-1).[5]

The prognosis of neuroblastoma depends on stage at presentation, patient's age (children younger than 12 to 18 months have better prognosis), histologic category, grade of tumor differentiation, status of the *MYCN* oncogene, chromosome 11q status, and deoxyribonucleic acid ploidy.[6]

Imaging Adrenal neuroblastomas and those arising from the adjacent retroperitoneal area are usually easily identified with ultrasonography, computed tomography (CT), or magnetic resonance imaging (MRI) because the mass is generally quite large by the time of presentation (Fig. 123-1). Very small masses are uncommon, and in those cases seen beyond the neonatal age, CT and MRI play a more important role than ultrasonography (Fig. 123-2). On ultrasonography, the masses have a variety of appearances with the most characteristic being that of a solid, heterogeneous, hyperechoic mass, often with small hyperechoic foci with or without acoustic shadowing caused by calcification (e-Fig. 123-3).[1,2,4] Anechoic areas resulting from cystic, hemorrhagic, or necrotic changes may be present (e-Fig. 123-4).

The new International Neuroblastoma Risk Group Staging System requires the use of CT, MRI, or both for staging.[5] On CT, neuroblastomas usually show heterogeneous enhancement, depicting solid areas along with areas of necrosis, hemorrhage, and cystic change (see Fig. 123-1). Calcification is present in more than 90% of cases (see Figs. 123-1, 123-2, and e-Figs 123-3 and 123-4).[4] On MRI, the lesions are usually heterogeneous, with predominantly low signal on T1-weighted images and high signal on T2-weighted images, and with variable degrees of enhancement (Fig. 123-5).[2,4]

A characteristic imaging feature of neuroblastoma is the displacement of adjacent organs and the displacement or encasement of adjacent major vessels (see Figs. 123-1 and 123-5).[4] Local spread may be to lymph nodes. Less frequently, direct invasion into the kidneys (Fig. 123-6) or liver may occur, and even less commonly, the tumor may extend into the spinal canal.

Neuroblastoma may also cause liver metastases. These may be single or multiple nodules or masses or may present with an infiltrative pattern, particularly in neonates (see Chapter 122). Metastases to bone are best identified with metaiodobenzylguanidine scan or with radionuclide bone scan.

If the lesion responds to chemotherapy, the mass regresses and shrinks to a very small amount of soft tissue that often becomes calcified.

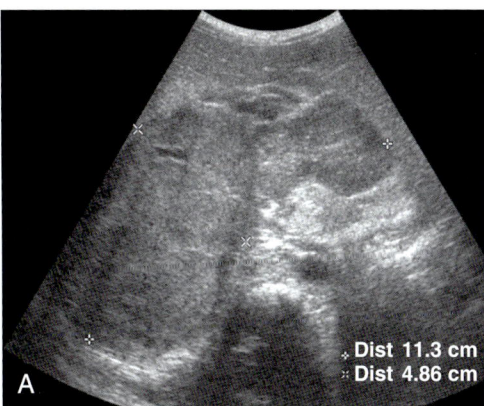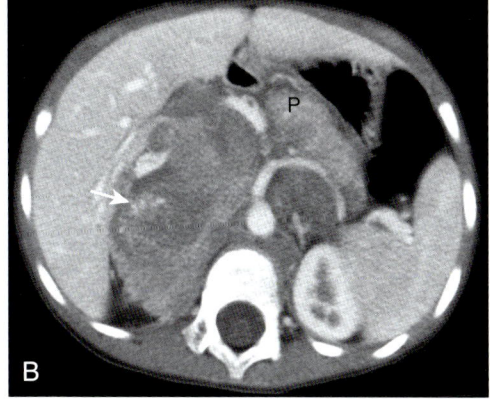

Figure 123-1 Large retroperitoneal neuroblastoma in a 4-year-old boy. **A,** A transverse sonogram. **B,** An axial contrast-enhanced computed tomography image of the abdomen show a large lobulated, solid mass centered in the right upper quadrant but with a significant component crossing the midline and extending into the left hemiabdomen. In **A,** the mass (between cursors) is relatively hypoechoic compared with the liver. In **B,** the mass is heterogeneous with hypodense and hyperdense areas as well as foci of calcification (*arrow*). Note the characteristic encasement of the major vessels by the mass, in this case the aorta, the celiac axis, and its major branches. The pancreas (*P*) is displaced anteriorly and to the left by the mass.

Ganglioneuroma

Overview Ganglioneuroma represents the mature, benign form of neural crest neoplasm. This type of tumor is far less frequent compared with neuroblastoma; it may develop from the maturation of a known malignant neuroblastoma, or it may be found de novo.[2]

Ganglioneuromas most frequently occur in the posterior mediastinum followed by the extra-adrenal retroperitoneum and the adrenal.[2] These tumors usually occur in older children, are frequently asymptomatic, and are often found incidentally on imaging. Occasionally, symptoms may result from tumor growth into the intervertebral foramina, causing cord compression. Urinary catecholamine levels are usually normal.

Imaging The imaging appearance of ganglioneuroma is most often indistinguishable from that of neuroblastoma (Figs. 123-7 and 123-8).[2] Therefore, definitive diagnosis depends on the histologic examination of tumor tissue.

Pheochromocytoma

Overview Pheochromocytoma is an uncommon neuroendocrine tumor of the adrenal arising from chromaffin cells. If the tumor is extra-adrenal, it is known as a paraganglioma,

with most common abdominal locations being in the vicinity of the renal vessels and at the organ of Zuckerkandl, near the origin of the inferior mesenteric artery. In children, 70% of pheochromocytomas occur in the adrenal gland, and 20% to 70% have bilateral adrenal involvement.[7] Malignancy is present in 12% of lesions in children.[8] The diagnosis of malignancy is often made on the basis of metastases rather than histology.[8]

Pheochromocytoma usually presents in older children (mean age 11 years). It is often sporadic but may be part of cancer predisposition syndromes, mainly von Hippel-Lindau disease and multiple endocrine neoplasias 2A and 2B, and less commonly neurofibromatosis type 1, multiple endocrine neoplasia 1, and tuberous sclerosis complex.[8]

The clinical presentation is usually related to the secretion of catecholamines. Patients present with hypertension, headache, tachycardia, diaphoresis, nervousness, and weight loss.[7]

Imaging CT and MRI are better imaging modalities than ultrasonography for accurate localization of these tumors.

Box 123-1 International Neuroblastoma Risk Group Staging System

Stage L1: Localized tumor confined to one body compartment without involvement of vital structures

Stage L2: Locoregional tumor with at least one image-defined risk factor

Stage M: Distant metastasis (excluding stage MS)

Stage MS: Child <18 months of age with metastasis confined to skin, liver, and/or bone marrow

Modified from Monclair T, Brodeur GM, Ambros PF, et al. The international neuroblastoma risk group (INRG) staging system: an INRG task force report. *J Clin Oncol.* 2009;27:298-303.

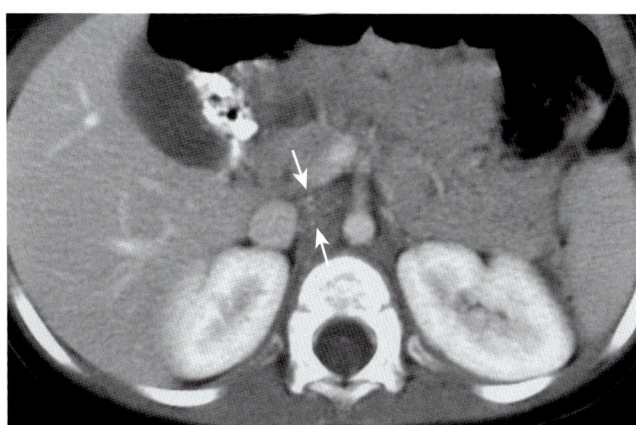

Figure 123-2 Small retroperitoneal neuroblastoma in a 19-month-old boy who presented with ataxia and nystagmus. Axial contrast-enhanced computed tomography image shows a small hypodense mass with punctate calcifications in the interaortocaval region (*arrows*). Because of its location and small size, this mass was difficult to appreciate on ultrasonography.

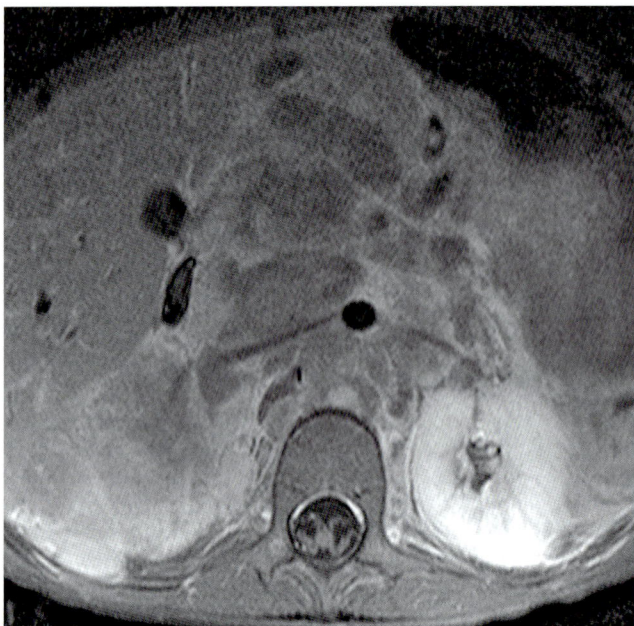

Figure 123-5 Retroperitoneal neuroblastoma in a 4-year-old girl. An axial gadolinium-enhanced T1 fat-suppressed magnetic resonance image shows a large retroperitoneal mass encasing the aorta and renal arteries and displacing the inferior vena cava to the right. The mass shows heterogeneous enhancement.

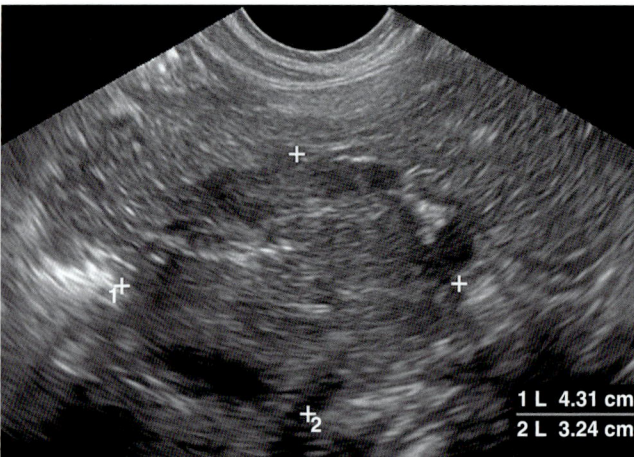

Figure 123-7 Retroperitoneal ganglioneuroma in a 7-year-old girl. A transverse sonogram shows a large rounded mass (between cursors) of intermediate echogenicity with scattered punctate calcifications in the midline retroperitoneum. The sonographic appearance of ganglioneuroma is indistinguishable from neuroblastoma.

Functional imaging with metaiodobenzylguanidine is more specific and has been reported to be more sensitive in detecting multifocal disease.[7,8]

On ultrasonography, pheochromocytoma may have a solid homogeneous or heterogeneous appearance (Fig. 123-9 and e-Fig 123-10). Heterogeneity is more commonly seen with larger lesions because of hemorrhage, necrosis, and less commonly calcification.[9] On CT, the lesions show avid enhancement except for areas of necrosis or hemorrhage.[1] The use of non–ionic low–osmolar intravenous contrast material for CT is safe in patients with pheochromocytoma. On MRI, pheochromocytoma is hypointense to isointense compared with the liver on T1-weighted images and hyperintense on

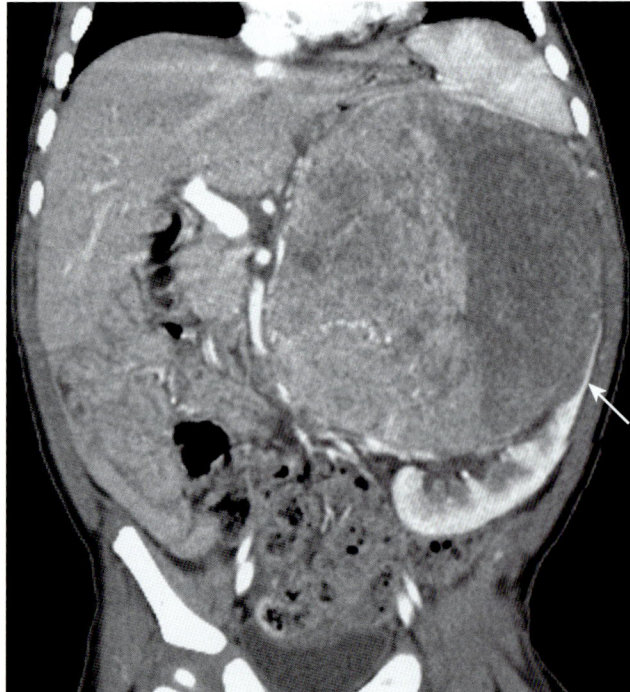

Figure 123-6 Left adrenal neuroblastoma in a 9-month-old girl. A reformatted coronal computed tomography image shows a large heterogeneous mass invading the left kidney. The left kidney is displaced caudally and laterally with suggestion of a partial "claw sign" (arrow), which may lead to the erroneous interpretation that the mass is arising from the left kidney.

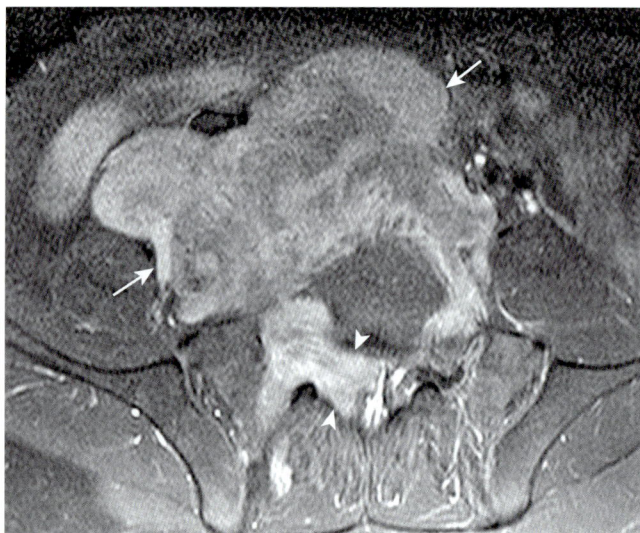

Figure 123-8 Retroperitoneal ganglioneuroma in a 10-year-old girl. An axial gadolinium-enhanced T1 fat-suppressed magnetic resonance image shows a large, heterogeneous, retroperitoneal mass (arrows), which extends into the sacral intervertebral foramina and into the distal spinal canal (arrowheads). The imaging features are similar to those seen in neuroblastoma.

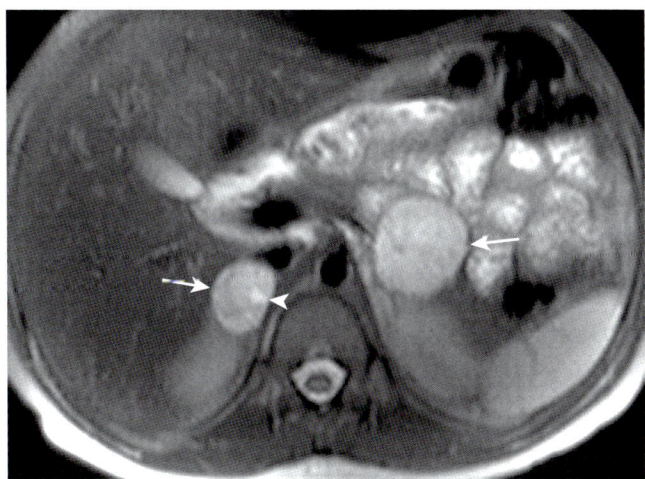

Figure 123-9 Bilateral pheochromocytoma in an 11-year-old boy with von Hippel–Lindau disease and arterial hypertension. An axial fat-suppressed T2-weighted magnetic resonance image shows bilateral adrenal masses (*arrows*), larger on the left. The masses are hyperintense with small cystic change on the right medially (*arrowhead*). See e-Figure 123-10.

T2-weighted images (see Fig. 123-9 and e-Fig. 123-10), with a pattern of intense enhancement after the administration of gadolinium.[1]

Treatment Surgical removal of all known lesions is usually curative. However, clinical follow-up is essential, along with urinary catecholamine measurement to detect recurrence or the development of new lesions.

Adrenocortical Neoplasms

Overview Adrenocortical neoplasms comprise two types of tumor: adenomas and carcinomas. Both are uncommon in children. A higher incidence is seen in children under the age of 4 years.[10] Girls are affected more commonly compared with boys, and carcinomas are much more common than are adenomas.[10] The vast majority of these tumors are functioning tumors, and the most common endocrine abnormality is overproduction of androgens. Girls present with virilization, and boys present with pseudoprecocious puberty. Often, mixed endocrine dysfunction is caused by the overproduction of both glucocorticoids and mineralocorticoids. Two cancer predisposition syndromes, Li-Fraumeni syndrome and Beckwith-Wiedemann syndrome, are strongly associated with adrenocortical neoplasms.[10]

Imaging At presentation, adrenocortical neoplasms in children are usually larger than 5 cm.[9] Most lesions can be documented with ultrasonography, but CT and MRI are particularly important for assessing large lesions and local invasion and spread. On all three modalities, smaller lesions tend to have a fairly homogeneous appearance. Areas of hemorrhage, necrosis, and calcification are seen more commonly in larger lesions, usually carcinomas (Fig. 123-11 and e-Fig 123-12).[9] In larger lesions, the characteristic appearance of a central scar, with radiating linear bands that represent

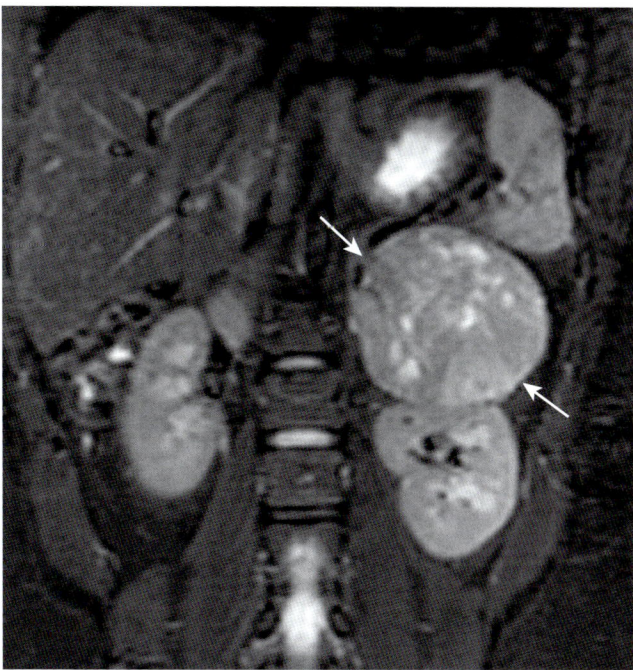

Figure 123-11 Adrenocortical carcinoma in a 14-year-old girl who presented with virilization signs and elevated testosterone levels. A coronal short inversion time inversion recovery magnetic resonance image shows a large heterogeneous left suprarenal mass (*arrows*) causing inferior displacement and flattening of the upper pole of the adjacent left kidney. The mass contains multiple hyperintense foci due to areas of necrosis. See e-Figure 123-12.

areas of necrosis and calcification (Fig. 123-13), may be seen.[1] It is not always possible to predict accurately which masses are malignant, unless local spread and invasion have occurred or metastatic disease is present. Metastatic disease most commonly occurs to the lungs, liver, and bone.

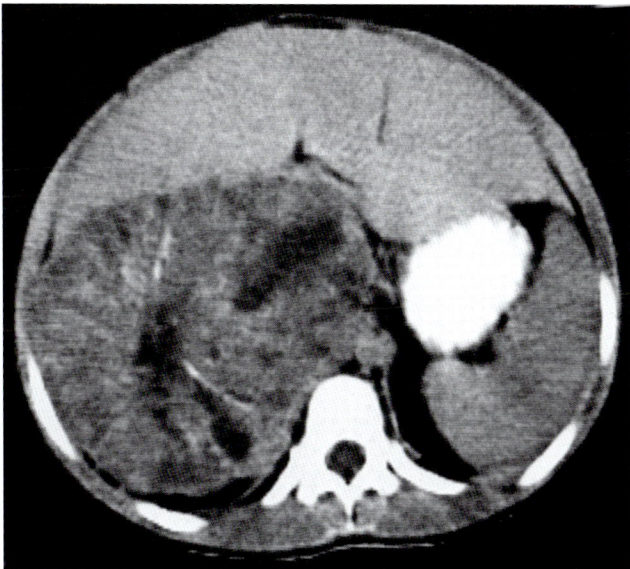

Figure 123-13 Adrenocortical carcinoma in an 8-year-old girl with precocious puberty. A contrast-enhanced axial computed tomography image shows a large, relatively well-defined right adrenal mass with heterogeneous attenuation. A radial pattern of calcification in the mass is seen, with adjacent areas of decreased attenuation caused by necrosis, which is characteristic of adrenocortical carcinoma.

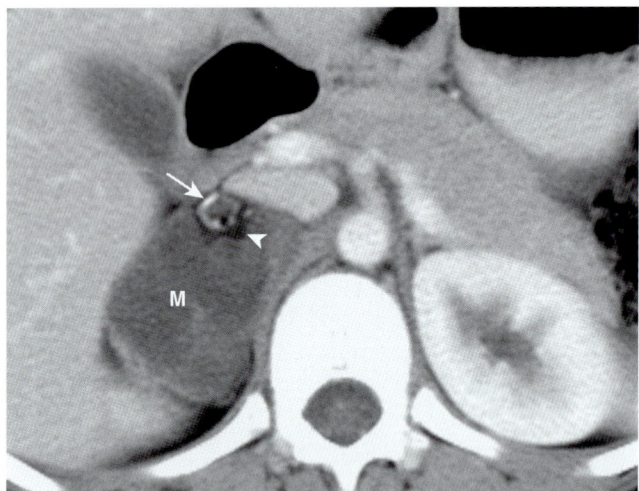

Figure 123-14 Retroperitoneal teratoma in an 11-year-old girl. A contrast-enhanced axial computed tomography image shows a well-defined right suprarenal mass (*M*), with mainly fluid attenuation and some soft tissue septa. Calcification (*arrow*) and fatty attenuation (*arrowhead*) are seen anteriorly within the mass.

Treatment Complete resection of the primary tumor is essential for survival.[10] Chemotherapy has had a major effect on improved outcome. Adenomas clearly have a good prognosis if they are removed completely, but clinical follow-up and imaging follow-up are essential because the histologic differences between adenoma and carcinoma are not clear in all cases.

Other Retroperitoneal Conditions

Overview Apart from pathology arising from the urinary tract and adrenal and sympathetic chains, other less common retroperitoneal conditions include lymphadenopathy (mainly lymphoma or metastatic lymphadenopathy), vascular malformations, hemangiomas, neurogenic tumors (schwannoma, neurofibroma, malignant peripheral nerve sheath tumor), adipocytic tumors, germ-cell tumors (Fig. 123-14), rhabdomyosarcoma, fibromatosis, idiopathic fibrosis, hematomas, and abscesses.

Key Points

Neuroblastoma is the most common extracranial solid neoplasm in children and accounts for almost 10% of all childhood neoplasms.

Metastatic disease in neuroblastoma is present in up to 70% of patients at presentation.

A characteristic imaging feature of neuroblastoma is the displacement of adjacent organs and the displacement or encasement of adjacent major vessels.

Ganglioneuroma cannot be differentiated from neuroblastoma on the basis of imaging appearances alone.

Li-Fraumeni and Beckwith-Wiedemann syndromes are strongly associated with adrenocortical neoplasms.

Suggested Readings

Balassy C, Navarro OM, Daneman A. Adrenal masses in children. *Radiol Clin North Am.* 2011;49:49(4):711-727.

Hiorns MP, Owens CM. Radiology of neuroblastoma in children. *Eur Radiol.* 2001;11:2071-2081.

Lonergan GJ, Schwab CM, Suarez ES, et al. Neuroblastoma, ganglioneuroblastoma and ganglioneuroma: radiologic-pathologic correlation. *RadioGraphics.* 2002;22:911-934.

Paterson A. Adrenal pathology in childhood spectrum of disease. *Eur Radiol.* 2002;12:2491-2508.

Rescorla FJ. Malignant adrenal tumors. *Semin Pediatr Surg.* 2006;15:48-56.

References

Full references for this chapter can be found on www.expertconsult.com.

Chapter 124

Genitourinary Trauma

GEORGE A. TAYLOR

Renal Injury

Overview The kidney is the third most frequently injured abdominal viscus in children and accounts for 1.3% to 15% of injuries in children who suffer blunt abdominal trauma. Children are more susceptible to renal injury during blunt trauma compared with adults because of the relatively increased mobility of the pediatric kidney, less perinephric fat, and reduced protection by a more compliant chest wall. Preexisting renal abnormalities such as a horseshoe kidney (Fig. 124-1) or pelvic kidney, hydronephrosis, cystic renal disease, and tumors may increase the size or alter the location of the kidney leading to an increased susceptibility to injury.[1]

Most children with clinically significant renal injury present with hematuria; the risk of underlying renal injury is markedly higher in patients with gross hematuria (22%) compared with those with lesser amounts of urinary blood (8%). However, the presence of asymptomatic microscopic hematuria is a low-yield sign for the presence of underlying renal injury.[2]

Isolated renal injury in children is relatively uncommon, with associated injuries typically present in the lungs (45%), spleen (33%), and liver (29%).

Imaging Computed tomography (CT) is the preferred modality for initial assessment of hemodynamically stable children with suspected renal injury because of its wide availability, rapid image acquisition, and accuracy. The use of intravenous contrast material is essential for the evaluation of the kidney, and scanning during the mixed venous phase of opacification is recommended. A delayed scan may be helpful for the detection of urinary extravasation. Noncontrast scans are not generally helpful, and they unnecessarily increase radiation dose to the patient. Unstable patients who require immediate evaluation may be examined with ultrasonography at the bedside prior to complete resuscitation or surgery. Routine follow-up imaging can be performed with grey-scale and color Doppler ultrasonography in most patients, and CT can be reserved for selected patients with other associated injury or ambiguous findings on serial ultrasonography.[3]

The most common type of renal injury is parenchymal contusion, which manifests on CT as a focal or diffuse region of absent or delayed contrast enhancement (Fig. 124-2). The contusion is characterized by microscopic areas of hemorrhage and surrounding edema. The involved kidney may also appear larger on CT as a result of the associated edema.

Renal injury may be complicated by perirenal hematoma, which may be subcapsular or perinephric. These two types of hematoma can be differentiated on the basis of CT features. A subcapsular hematoma is limited in its extension by the renal capsule and therefore exerts greater mass effect on the renal parenchyma, whereas a perinephric hematoma is distributed throughout the perirenal space and typically exhibits less mass effect on the renal parenchyma.

Renal collecting system injury results in urinary extravasation of intravenous contrast medium (Fig. 124-3). Urine leakage that remains encapsulated in the perirenal space is termed a *urinoma*. Occasionally, hemorrhage or urinary extravasation may extend into the pelvis owing to direct communication between the perirenal space in the abdomen and the prevesical extraperitoneal space in the pelvis.[1]

The American Association for the Surgery of Trauma has developed an injury scale to categorize the increasing severity of renal injury (Table 124-1). Grade I to grade III injuries are considered low grade, and account for between 69% to 99% of all renal injuries.

Treatment The great majority of renal injuries (69%–99%) are treated nonsurgically with great success. Even in high-grade injuries, no surgical intervention is necessary in 60% to 70%. Early ureteral stent placement may be considered in patients with high-grade injuries who do not demonstrate contrast material in the ipsilateral ureter.[4]

Bladder Injury

Overview Blunt injuries to the bladder typically result from a blow to the lower abdomen when the bladder is distended or when the pelvis is fractured. Fortunately, the incidence of lower urinary tract injury in children is quite low, estimated at 0.2% of pediatric trauma admissions. Although approximately 50% of children with bladder tears have a pelvic fracture, only 0.5% to 3.7% of children with pelvic fractures have associated bladder injuries.[5] High-yield indications for CT cystography include gross hematuria, pelvic fracture, and high-risk mechanisms of injury such as motor vehicle crashes

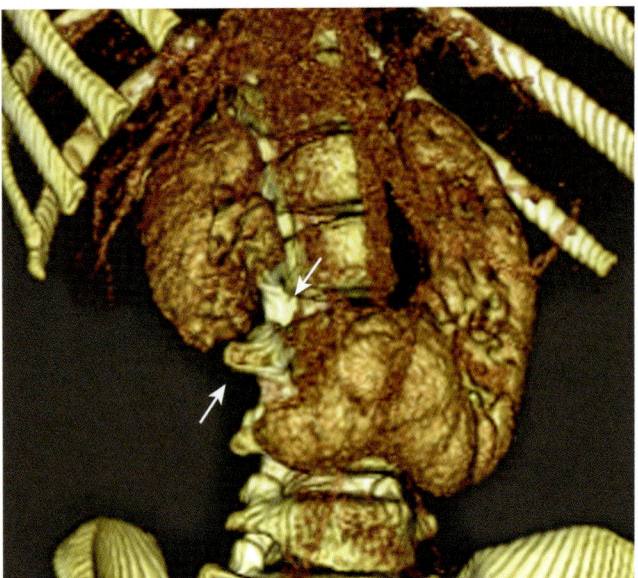

Figure 124-1 Laceration in horseshoe kidney. Oblique three-dimensional volume reconstruction of contrast-enhanced computed tomography shows complete transection (*arrows*) of a horseshoe kidney.

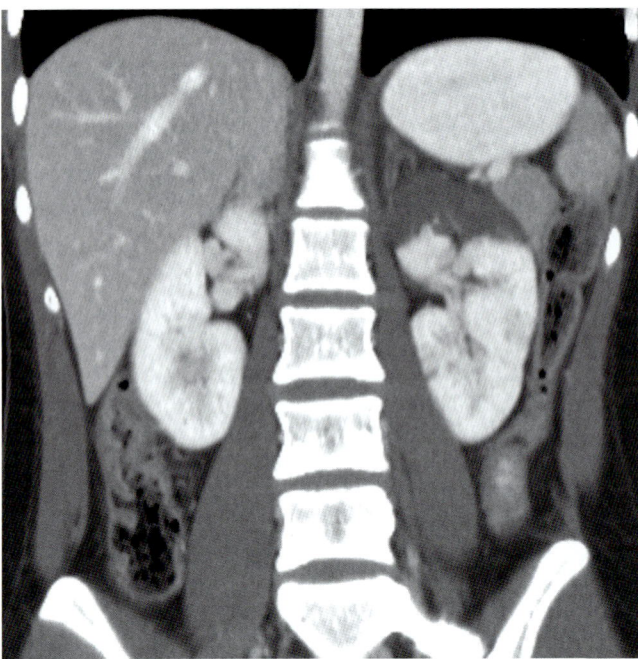

Figure 124-2 Renal contusion. A contrast-enhanced coronal computed tomography image shows markedly diminished enhancement of the upper pole of the left kidney with preservation of renal contour.

and the presence of a seatbelt ecchymosis. Bladder injuries may be classified as intraperitoneal rupture, extraperitoneal rupture, and combined lesions.

Imaging Standard abdominal trauma CT scanning protocols may miss important bladder injuries because of incomplete bladder distention. CT cystography is the preferred technique for the detection of bladder tears with a reported sensitivity and specificity of 95% and 100% respectively.[6] The bladder is filled by low-gravity drip infusion of dilute water-soluble contrast material (125 milliliters [mL] of 60% water-soluble contrast agent in 375 mL of saline) using an age-based estimate of bladder capacity (4.5 × age (0.40) = capacity in ounces).[7]

Intraperitoneal rupture occurs when the bladder is acutely compressed resulting in a sudden increase in pressure and a tear of the dome of the bladder. This results in extravasation of contrast-containing urine into the peritoneum where it fills the cul-de-sac, surrounds the bowel, often extending into the paracolic gutters and subhepatic space (Fig. 124-4 and e-Fig 124-5). In children, intraperitoneal rupture accounts for up to 60% of all bladder tears.

Extraperitoneal rupture is less common in children than in adults, accounting for approximately 40% of all bladder perforations. They are often associated with pelvic fractures that distort and shear the bladder at its attachments near the

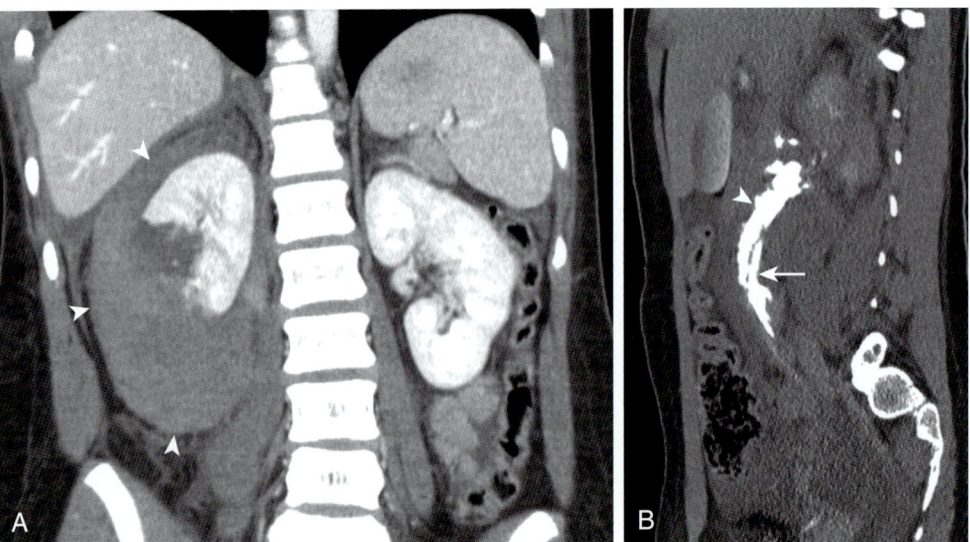

Figure 124-3 Grade IV renal laceration. **A,** Coronal contrast-enhanced computed tomography shows complete transection of right kidney and large perinephric hematoma (*arrowheads*). **B,** A delayed sagittal-reformatted computed tomography scan shows extravasation of contrast-containing urine (*arrowhead*) along the right ureter (*arrow*).

Table 124-1

Renal Injury Scale	
Injury Grade	**Renal Injury**
I	Renal contusion, small, nonexpanding subcapsular hematoma
II	Superficial renal laceration not involving collecting system or deep medulla, nonexpanding perinephric hematoma
III	Deep renal laceration without involvement of renal collecting system, nonexpanding perinephric hematoma
IV	Laceration of renal collecting system, involvement of vascular pedicle
V	Shattered kidney, multiple lacerations, renal fragmentation

trigone, below the peritoneal reflection. On CT cystography, extravasation is usually confined to the perivesical soft tissues (Fig. 124-6 and e-Fig. 124-7), but may extend into the scrotum, superiorly along the anterior abdominal wall or up through retroperitoneal spaces to the level of the kidney.[1,8]

Treatment Intraperitoneal ruptures require immediate surgical repair, whereas extraperitoneal ruptures are usually treated by catheter drainage alone. Combined intraperitoneal and extraperitoneal injuries are uncommon in children and usually identified during surgical exploration. Bladder tears generally have a highly favorable outcome, unless the injury extends longitudinally through the bladder base into the proximal urethra. These injuries frequently lead to incontinence and the need for multiple additional surgeries (Fig. 124-8 and e-Fig 124-9).[9]

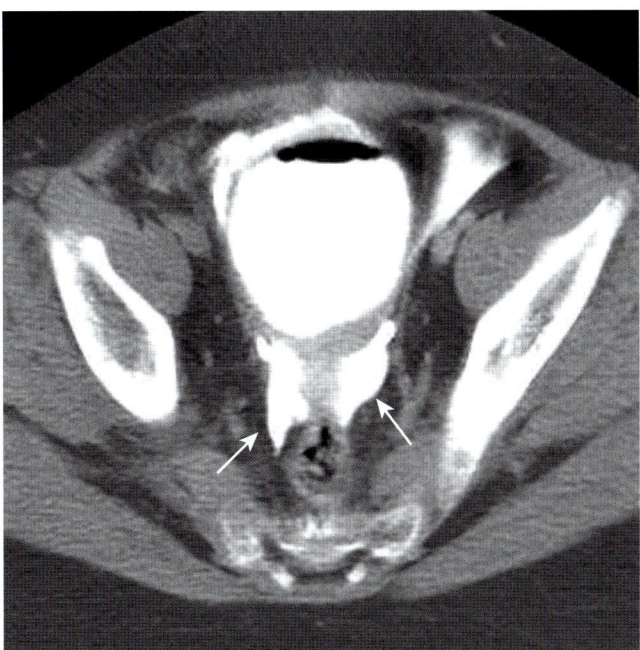

Figure 124-4 **Intraperitoneal bladder rupture.** An axial computed tomography cystogram image through the pelvis shows extravasation of contrast-containing urine into the cul de sac (arrows). See e-Figure 124-5.

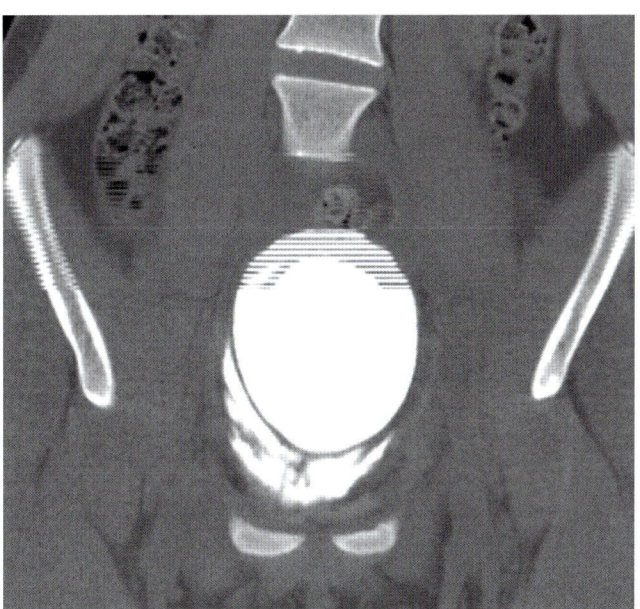

Figure 124-6 **Extraperitoneal bladder rupture.** A coronal computed tomography cystogram image shows contained extravasation of contrast-containing urine into the perivesical spaces. See e-Figure 124-7 for the sagittal view.

Urethral Injury

Overview Urethral injuries can be divided into posterior and anterior urethral injuries. Most posterior urethral injuries are caused by direct blows to the perineum, falls, or motor vehicle accidents, and occur frequently in the setting of pelvic fractures. These injuries usually involve the membranous urethra and are caused by shearing and rupture of the puboprostatic ligaments. Anterior urethral injuries are usually straddle-type injuries that are rarely associated with pelvic fractures (see Fig. 124-8 and e-Fig. 124-9). Although any grade of hematuria may be associated with urethral injury, the strongest clinical sign is the presence of blood at the meatus. No urethral instrumentations should be performed in patients with suspected urethral injury until a retrograde urethrogram is performed to evaluate the integrity of the entire urethra. Attempts to catheterize the bladder may convert a partial urethral tear into a complete transection.[10]

Imaging Retrograde urethrography is performed by inserting the tip of a Foley catheter into the distal urethra. The balloon is slowly inflated in the fossa navicularis, and water-soluble contrast material is injected via a syringe, with the patient positioned in the steep oblique or lateral position. Urethral injuries are manifested by irregular narrowing of the affected urethra and extravasation of contrast into the surrounding tissues (Fig. 124-10).

Although retrograde urethrography is the preferred method of evaluating the urethra, placement of a urinary catheter is common in patients with multiple trauma, and retrograde urethrography may be initially considered only after a CT scan has already been performed. Therefore, familiarity with CT findings associated with urethral injuries is important. These include obliteration of the fat plane around the urogenital diaphragm, obscured contours of the prostate,

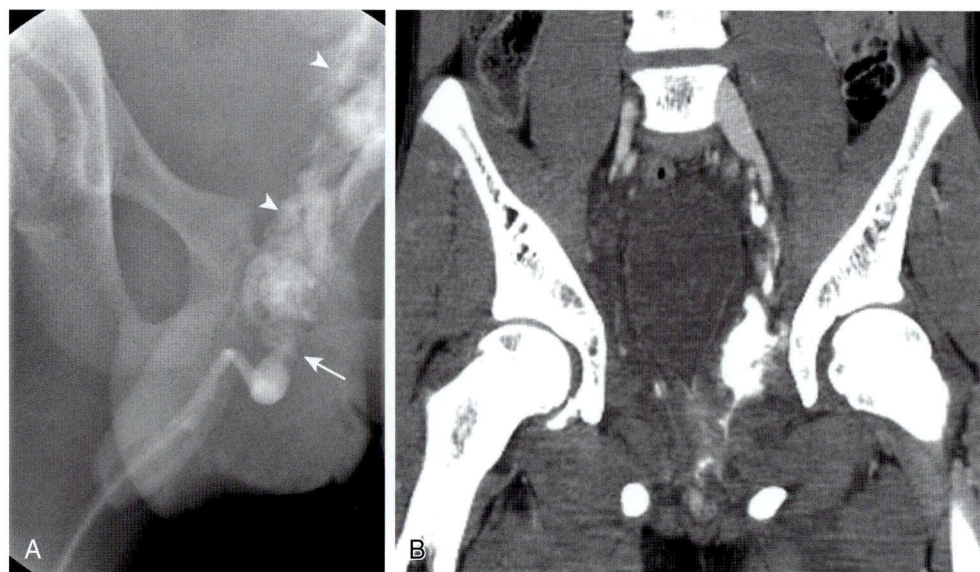

Figure 124-8 Bladder neck and urethral tear. **A,** An oblique retrograde urethrogram shows complete transection (*arrow*) of posterior urethra and bladder neck with extraperitoneal extravasation of contrast (*arrowheads*). **B,** A coronal contrast-enhanced computed tomography image of the pelvis shows elevated bladder base, perivesical "sentinel" hematoma, and extravasated contrast. See e-Figure 124-9 for the sagittal view.

and obturator internus muscle (see Fig. 124-8 and e-Fig. 124-9).[11]

Scrotal Injury

Overview The majority of blunt injuries to the scrotum occur in older boys and are the result of a direct blow to the groin during sport activities (50%), motor vehicle crashes (9%–17%), falls, or straddle injuries. Typical indications for imaging include an acute, painful, or ecchymotic scrotum, and a nonpalpable testis. Although common, scrotal injuries rarely need surgical intervention. Fortunately, over 80% of ruptured testes can be successfully salvaged if surgical repair is performed within 72 hours of injury.[10]

Imaging Ultrasonography is the most effective method of assessing the injured scrotum. High-frequency (7–14 megahertz) linear array transducers should be used to evaluate both testes with grey-scale and color or power Doppler to determine the location and extent of injury. Ultrasonography plays a key role in the identification of testicular rupture allowing for immediate surgical exploration and repair.

Hematomas and hematoceles are the most common findings after scrotal injury. They may be single or multiple and may have a wide range of echogenicities, depending on the time interval between injury and imaging (Fig. 124-11 and e-Fig. 124-12). With time, the contained hemorrhage

Figure 124-10 Straddle injury, membranous urethra. An oblique retrograde urethrogram shows focal urethral narrowing and intraluminal hematoma (*arrow*).

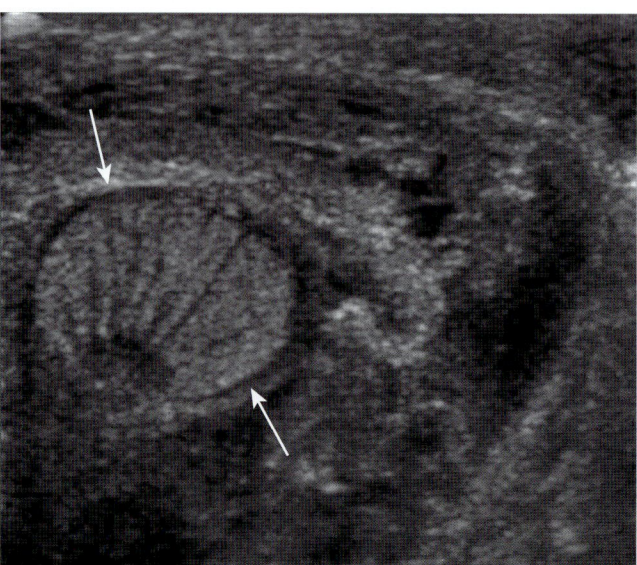

Figure 124-11 Scrotal hematoma. Transverse ultrasonogram of the right scrotum shows an intact testis (*arrows*) surrounded by heterogeneous peritesticular hematoma. See e-Figure 124-12 for the sagittal view.

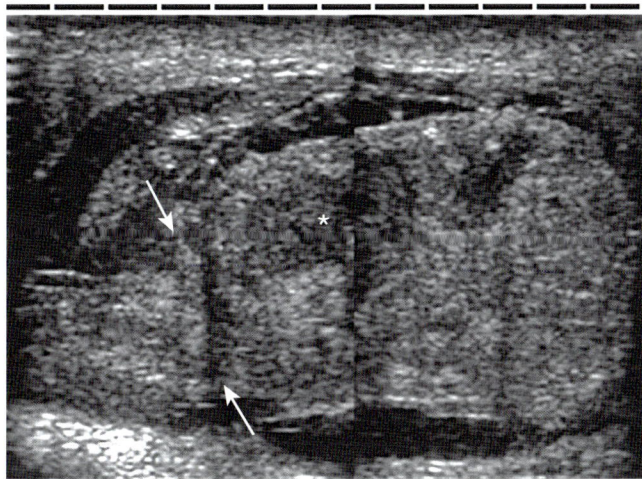

Figure 124-13 Testicular rupture. A sagittal composite scrotal ultrasonogram shows a heterogeneous testis with intratesticular hematoma (*asterisk*) and extrusion of testicular contents through a tear in the tunica albuginea (*arrows*). See e-Figure 124-14.

becomes less echogenic, and the fluid may become more typical of hydrocele.

Testicular fractures may also occur when a break occurs in the testicular parenchyma alone or is associated with a tear in the tunica albuginea (testicular rupture). On ultrasonography, heterogeneous echogenicity to the testicular parenchyma, caused by infarction and hemorrhage is seen. Irregularity of the normally smooth testicular border and, occasionally, nonvisualization of any normal testicular parenchyma are also encountered. Ultrasonographic findings of an abnormal testicular contour and heterogeneous echotexture caused by hemorrhage and extrusion of seminiferous tubules have a high sensitivity and specificity for the diagnosis of testicular rupture (Fig. 124-13 and e-Fig. 124-14).

One must be wary of the possibility that a bizarre heterogeneous echogenicity in a traumatized scrotum may actually be a hematoma that has superiorly displaced a normal testis into the inguinal canal.[10-12] Other extratesticular findings include reactive hydroceles, posttraumatic epididymitis, and testicular torsion.

WHAT THE CLINICIAN NEEDS TO KNOW

- Grade of renal trauma and associated intra-abdominal injuries
- Whether active hemorrhage is present
- Whether bladder rupture is intraperitoneal or extraperitoneal
- Whether urethral injury is present and, if so, whether it is a complete transection
- Whether testicular rupture has occurred

Key Points

Asymptomatic microscopic hematuria is a low-risk indicator of injury.

Delayed scans through an injured kidney should be considered to identify urinary extravasation.

High-risk indicators of bladder injury include the combination of gross hematuria, pelvic fracture, and high-risk mechanism of injury.

A retrograde urethrogram is essential in boys with suspected urethral injury.

Ultrasonographic findings are both sensitive and specific for testicular rupture.

Most genitourinary injuries can be treated nonsurgically. Exceptions include intraperitoneal bladder rupture, urethral transection, and testicular rupture.

50% of children with bladder injury have a fracture of the bony pelvis.

Suggested Readings

Adu-Frimpong J. Genitourinary trauma in boys. *Clin Ped Emerg Med.* 2009;10:45.

Bixby SD, Callahan MJ, Taylor GA. Imaging in pediatric blunt abdominal trauma. *Semin Roentgenol.* 2008;43:72.

Gomez RG, Ceballos L, Coburn M, et al. Consensus statement on bladder injuries. *Br J Urol Int.* 2004;94:27.

Harris AC, Zwirewich CV, Torreggiani WC, et al. CT findings in blunt renal trauma. *Radiographics.* 2001;21:S201-S214.

Ramchandani P, Buckler PM. Imaging of genitourinary trauma. *AJR Am J Roentgenol.* 2009;192:1514.

References

Full references for this chapter can be found on www.expertconsult.com.

Chapter 125

Disorders of Sex Differentiation

HARRIS L. COHEN and VIRENDERSINGH K. SHEORAIN

Embryology, Sex Differentiation, and Gonad Differentiation

Overview The three important precursor components needed for genital system development are the genital ridge and the two sets of internal sex ducts, the müllerian-paramesonephric and the wolffian-mesonephric. Around 7 weeks' gestation, the embryologic genital ridge becomes either an ovary or a testis. The development of the male genital system is an "active" process requiring testes and müllerian inhibiting substance (MIS). The sex-determining region (*SRY* gene) on the Y chromosome's short arm encodes a testis-determining factor. Under this factor's influence (and in the presence of H-Y antigens found in the cell membranes of normal XY males) there is normal testis development with germ cells in the genital ridge differentiating into Sertoli cells and Leydig cells. Sertoli cells secrete MIS, which causes complete müllerian duct system involution. Leydig cells produce testosterone. The enzyme 5a-reductase converts testosterone intracellularly within the target tissues into the powerful androgen dihydrotestosterone (DHT). DHT allows the wolffian duct system to develop into the epididymis, vas deferens, ejaculatory duct, and seminal vesicles. If no Y chromosome exists or if abnormal encoding of testes determining factor is present, the gonad will passively differentiate into an ovary between 11 weeks to 17 weeks' gestation in the presence of two X chromosomes. Absence of two X chromosomes may lead to abnormal or streak ovaries. The ovaries and their hormones, however, are thought to have no apparent role in sex differentiation of the female genital tract. The absence of MIS leads to persistence of müllerian structures, which develop into the fallopian tubes, uterus, cervix, and upper vagina. The wolffian ducts involute in the absence of testosterone. The undifferentiated external genitalia include the urogenital tubercle, urogenital swelling, and urogenital folds. DHT stimulation in males causes these structures to develop into the glans penis, scrotum, and penile shaft, respectively. In females, they develop into the clitoris, labia majora, and labia minora, respectively. The prostate gland develops from the urogenital sinus.[1-6]

Disorders of Sex Differentiation Without Ambiguity of External Genitalia (Box 125-1)

PHENOTYPIC FEMALE

Turner Syndrome (XO Gonadal Dysgenesis)

Overview Classic Turner syndrome (isochromatous 45,XO karyotype pattern) is the most common gonadal dysgenesis associated with an abnormal karyotype in girls and is nonfamilial. A single X chromosome is the probable cause for the presence of streak ovaries (streaks or ridges of connective tissue in the mesosalpinges parallel to the fallopian tubes), rather than normal ovaries. Some functional ovarian elements are present in a few cases. Fallopian tubes, a uterus, and a vagina are present, and no wolffian duct derivatives are found.[1,5,6]

Patients with classic Turner syndrome have several somatic findings. Affected patients are short in stature, with a distinctive facies that includes low-set ears, a low hairline, and a high, arched palate. They have a short, broad, and webbed neck, widely spaced nipples, and a shield chest. Skeletal abnormalities are common—classically short fourth metacarpal, fifth metacarpal, or both. Cystic hygromas of the neck area are noted in fetal life; and the webbed neck is thought to be a residuum. Other variably seen findings include large aortic roots, coarctation of the aorta, renal anomalies (horseshoe kidneys), duplication anomalies, ureteropelvic junction obstruction, and Hashimoto thyroiditis. Patients with Turner syndrome have a history of delayed onset of puberty, no breast development or vaginal mucosal estrogenization (but presence of pubic and axillary hair), infantile internal and external genitalia, and primary amenorrhea.[1,7,8]

Imaging The prepubertal uterus (Fig. 125-1) and vagina are normally formed and will respond to exogenous hormone stimulation. The dysgenetic or streak gonads are difficult to image. When the adnexa are measurable, they are typically less than 1 cm^3 in volume.

Mosaic Turner Syndrome

One fourth of patients with 45,XO Turner syndrome have a so-called chromatin-positive pattern. Their karyotype is a mosaic consisting most often of a mixture of 45,XO and 46,XX chromosomes. Less often, other mosaic patterns (e.g., XO/XXX or XO/XX/XXX) or 46,XX and an abnormal X chromosome are present. In such cases, the gonads may consist of a streak ovary on one side and a hypoplastic or normal ovary on the other side, bilateral hypoplastic ovaries, or essentially normal ovaries. External and internal genitalia are entirely female, without wolffian duct remnants. These patients usually do not have the somatic abnormalities typically attributed to classic Turner syndrome, but many are short.[1] Patients with mosaic Turner syndrome may develop secondary sex characteristics at puberty (found to occur in about 50%), and some may menstruate regularly.[1,9]

Amenorrhea Caused by Hypergonadotropic Hypogonadism

Primary amenorrhea (defined as a lack of menses by age 16 years), with high levels of circulating follicle-stimulating hormone and luteinizing hormone by serum assays, occurs because of ovarian failure; gonadal tissues fail to respond to endogenous gonadotropins. Patients included in this category have classic Turner syndrome, gonadal dysgenesis (including 46,XY and familial 46,XX), and secondary ovarian failure as a result of radiation or chemotherapy or on an autoimmune basis (autoimmune oophoritis).[1,5,6,8]

46,XY Gonadal Dysgenesis

Patients with 46,XY gonadal (X-linked recessive or sex-limited autosomal dominant) dysgenesis are phenotypically female, with streak gonads and infantile internal and external female genitalia. Patients are usually first diagnosed as having an abnormality in adolescence. As with other forms of gonadal dysgenesis, in such patients, the sex chromosome may not be absent but is abnormal. A deletion of the small arm of the Y chromosome (testis-determining factor or MIS) may be present. Mosaicism may lead to the development of ovaries. If a Y chromosome is a component of the karyotype of a patient with gonadal dysgenesis and ovaries, the patient has an increased risk of developing a gonadoblastoma within a dysgenetic ovary. Seminomas also occur in these patients.[1,2]

Familial 46,XX Gonadal Dysgenesis

Patients with familial 46,XX gonadal (sporadic or autosomal recessive) dysgenesis have gonads that consist of bilateral streaks in some cases, whereas in others hypoplastic ovaries or a hypoplastic ovary may be present on one side and a streak gonad on the other. The internal and external genitalia are entirely female, without wolffian duct derivatives. Incomplete puberty may be observed in patients with residual ovarian tissue. Sexual infantilism and primary amenorrhea are typical findings in those patients with bilateral streak gonads.[1,2]

PHENOTYPIC MALES

Klinefelter Syndrome (47,XXY Seminiferous Tubular Dysgenesis)

Seminiferous tubular dysgenesis (Klinefelter syndrome) is the most common aberration of the human sex chromosome. The typical 47,XXY karyotype is found in phenotypic males with primary hypogonadism. It is nonfamilial, occurring in 1 in every 750 to 1000 males. Variants have been described with less common chromosomal abnormalities, including XX/XXY or XY/XXY mosaicism, as well as XXXY, XXXXY, XXYY, or XXXYY sex chromosomal karyotypes. The external genitalia, especially the testes, are small. The testes are usually less than 3 cm in length and are firm. Cryptorchidism and hypospadias are common, with future development of azoospermia and sterility in most patients. The diagnosis is usually not made until after puberty. Gynecomastia develops in almost half of the older patients, and affected patients (particularly those with the classic 47,XXY karyotype) are at an increased risk for breast cancer. Rare cases of testicular and extragonadal germ cell neoplasms have been reported.[1,5,6]

Persistent Müllerian Duct Syndrome

Persistent müllerian duct syndrome is a rare type of sexual differentiation abnormality in males caused by a deficiency of

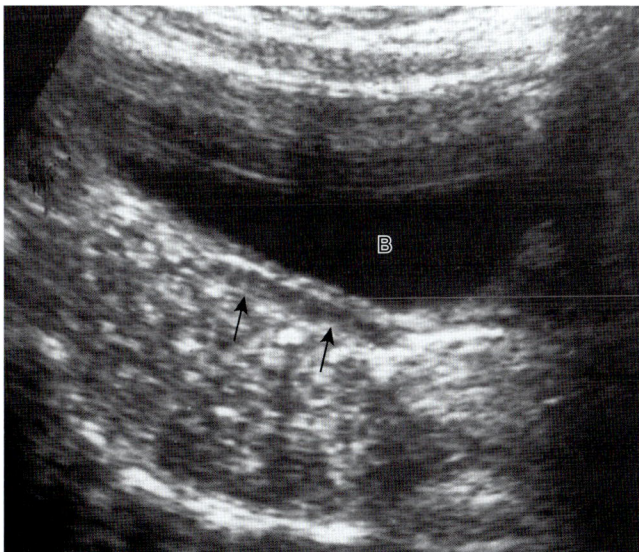

Figure 125-1 Turner syndrome. A longitudinal sonogram of the pelvis shows a small tubular uterus (*arrows*) in this 16-year-old with primary amenorrhea. She was a patient with 45,XO Turner syndrome. Her ovaries could not be definitively identified. *B*, Bladder.

müllerian inhibiting factor (MIF). These patients usually have a normal 46,XY karyotype and are phenotypically male, but they have a small uterus and fallopian tubes and a small vagina connected to the posterior urethra at the level of the verumontanum. Unilateral or bilateral cryptorchidism is common, as are unilateral or bilateral inguinal hernias. A uterus (uteri hernia syndrome), fallopian tubes, or sometimes a testis may be found in the hernia. The disorder, typically sporadic, has been reported in siblings.[1,2,10,11]

Disorders of Sex Differentiation with Ambiguous External Genitalia (Box 125-2)

PSEUDOHERMAPHRODITISM (INTERSEX)

Pseudohermaphroditism or intersex problems are abnormalities in which nonaccord of chromosomal, gonadal, and genital sex is present. Unlike true hermaphroditism, in which two types of gonadal tissue are present, pseudohermaphroditism has nonaccord, but only one gender's gonads are present. By definition, male intersex patients have testes and female intersex patients have ovaries or ovarian tissue.[1]

FEMALE INTERSEX

Overview Female intersex is usually diagnosed in neonatal life in chromosomally normal females (46,XX) with masculinized external genitalia. The cause is usually increased fetal adrenal androgen production, most commonly from congenital adrenal hyperplasia or adrenogenital syndrome. Congenital adrenal hyperplasia (Fig. 125-2) is, by far, the most common cause of abnormal sex differentiation in females, occurring in 1 in 15,000 live births worldwide. It is caused by an inherited deficiency of enzymes involved in adrenocortical hormone biosynthesis. Affected patients have normal ovaries, a uterus, and fallopian tubes and no testicular tissue or internal wolffian duct derivatives. In most cases, the external genitalia are ambiguous (Fig. 125-3), with a prominent penis or partially fused labial scrotal folds.

Imaging A variously sized vagina is connected with the posterior urethra, forming a urogenital sinus, which commonly empties at the base of the penis. No gonads can be palpated in the labioscrotal folds or in the inguinal canal of such patients because they are located within the pelvis. Voiding cystourethrography (VCUG) often shows a male-type elongated urethra (Fig. 125-4). These patients are potentially fertile with external genital reconstruction and correct sex assignment.[1,2]

Box 125-2	Disorders of Sex Differentiation with Ambiguous External Genitalia

- Female intersex (pseudohermaphroditism)
- Male intersex (pseudohermaphroditism)
- Gonadal dysgenesis
- True hermaphroditism

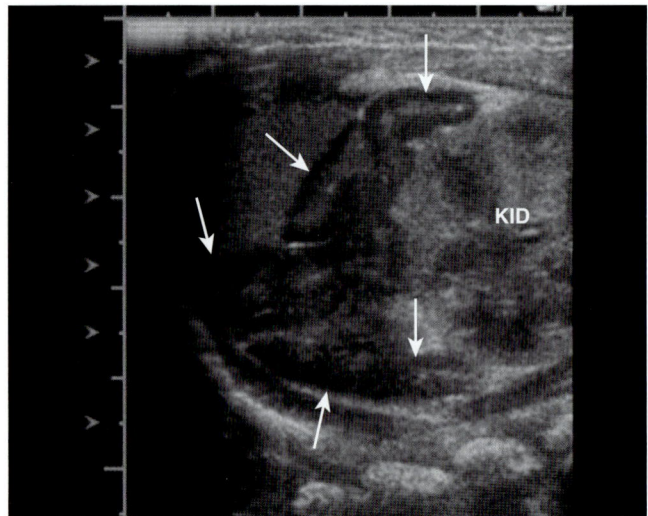

Figure 125-2 Adrenal ultrasound. Sagittal view of adrenal and upper left kidney. A very enlarged adrenal (*arrows*) is seen superior to the upper portion of the kidney. The patient was a newborn with ambiguous genitalia and had three times the normal level of 17 hydroxyprogesterone. Her karyotype proved to be 46,XX. She was diagnosed with salt-wasting 21 hydroxylase deficiency as the cause of her congenital adrenal hyperplasia.

MALE INTERSEX

Male intersex patients are true males with a normal 46,XY male karyotype, present H-Y antigens, normal or mildly defective (and usually undescended) testes, but incomplete masculinization or frank ambiguity of their external genitalia. Decreased testosterone production and a lack of MIF

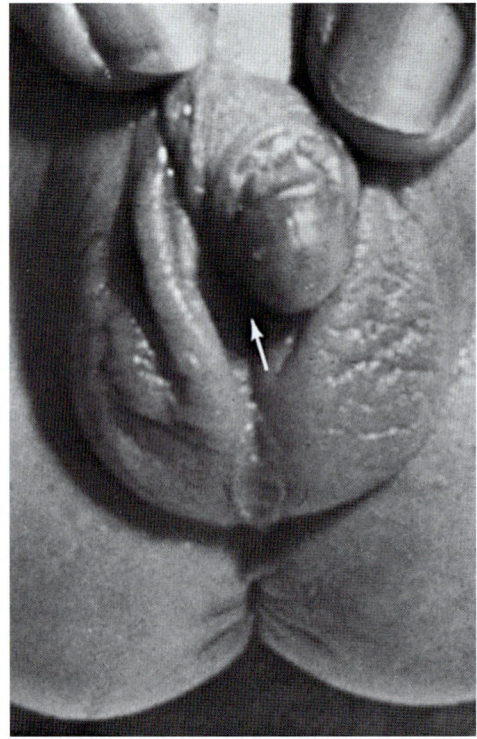

Figure 125-3 Ambiguous external genitalia in a 1-month-old infant. A penis and scrotum are present, but no gonads are palpable. A single perineal opening was found at the base of the penis (*arrow*).

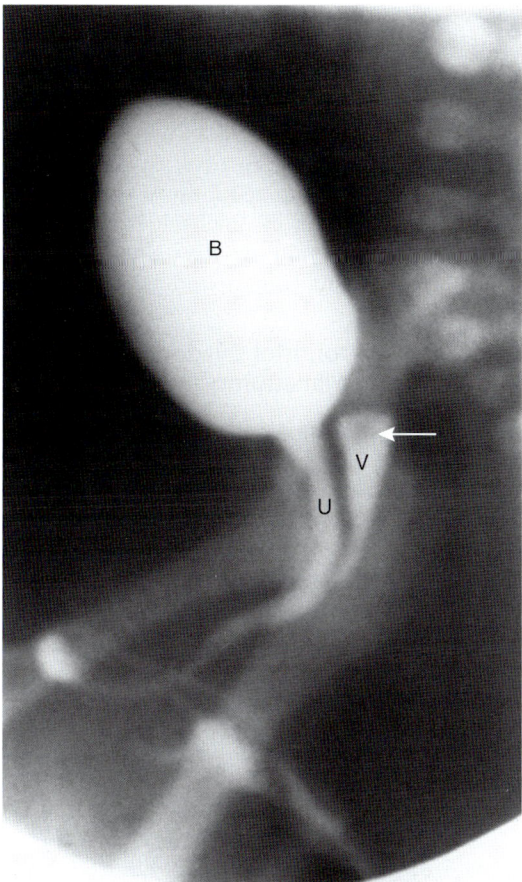

Figure 125-4 Congenital adrenal hyperplasia. Lateral voiding cystoure-thrography image shows a bladder (*B*) with an elongated male-type urethra (*U*). Posterior to it is a vagina (*V*) with a subtle impression (*arrow*) of a cervix superiorly. The patient was a 46,XX neonate from an area in Puerto Rico, where congenital adrenal hyperplasia is common. (From Cohen HL, Haller J. Pediatric and adolescent genital abnormalities. *Clin Diagn Ultrasound.* 1988;24:187-216. With permission. Copyright Elsevier Science USA.)

production results in a karyotypically normal male with a female phenotype (except for partial masculinization of the external genitalia), and incomplete inhibition of the development of müllerian elements such as the uterus, vagina, and fallopian tubes (Fig. 125-5 and e-Fig. 125-6). Such patients usually have no secondary sexual development at puberty and may have an infantile uterus on ultrasonography. If the production of MIF by the testes is not affected, no internal müllerian system structures (uterus and fallopian tubes) will develop. The biochemical defect may be decreased androgen synthesis, decreased DHT production as a result of deficiency of 5a-reductase, or a defect in the androgen receptors. In many cases, the exact etiology remains unknown.[1,2,5,6,12,13]

Testicular Feminization Syndrome (Androgen Receptor Defect)

Testicular feminization syndrome (X-linked recessive) is a form of intersex in which patients with 46,XY karyotype have well-formed testes (usually undescended within the abdomen or inguinal region) that produce androgens and MIF. However, lack of end-organ response to androgens is caused by a defect in a specific cytoplasmic receptor protein

(cytosol receptor) that normally binds DHT to the plasma membrane and transports it to the nuclear chromatin. Müllerian system development is inhibited, and patients do not develop a uterus, fallopian tubes, or the upper two thirds of the vagina. They do develop secondary female sexual characteristics via circulating estrogens (produced from the breakdown of testosterone and adrenal steroids as well as from direct production by the testes). Patients with the complete form of the abnormality appear as phenotypically normal females, although they may have inguinal or labial masses resulting from the undescended testes (Fig. 125-7). They have normal breast development and may or may not have a short, blind-ending vagina behind the urethral opening. They frequently present with amenorrhea and respond to substitutional estrogen therapy. In the incomplete form (10% to 20% of cases) of testicular feminization (incomplete androgen receptor defect), patients present earlier in life compared with those with the complete form and have ambiguous genitalia. Affected patients may have a predominantly female phenotype (incomplete testicular feminization) or a predominantly male phenotype (Reifenstein syndrome).[1,2]

GONADAL DYSGENESIS

Mixed Gonadal Dysgenesis (Dysgenetic Male Pseudohermaphroditism)

Mixed or asymmetric gonadal dysgenesis (also known as XO/XY gonadal dysgenesis) is a relatively common form of abnormal sexual differentiation, usually occurring sporadically. Affected patient karyotypes are most often a mosaic of 45,XO and 46,XX. At times, XO/XYY or other mosaicisms are seen. These patients often have a streak gonad similar to that seen in Turner syndrome on one side and a usually dysgenetic (but occasionally normal) testis on the other. A

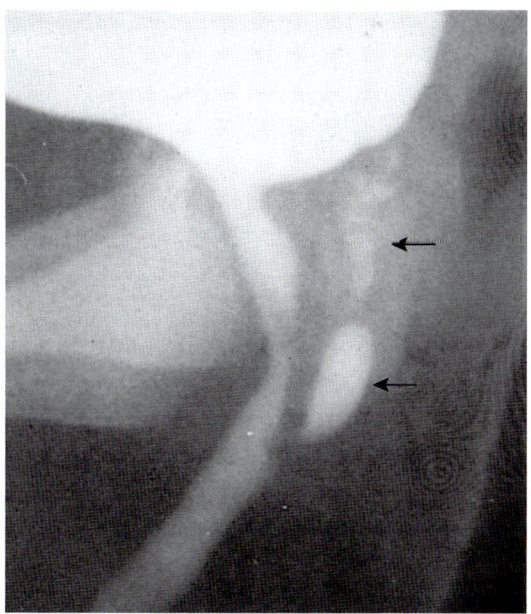

Figure 125-5 A male infant with severe hypospadias (perineal and scrotoperineal), bilateral cryptorchidism, small penis, and unfused scrotal folds. The image shows a utricle or blind vaginal pouch that is very short and extending off the distal aspect of the posterior urethra. Arrows show spermatic ducts emptying into the utricle. The male urethra is somewhat short. See e-Figure 125-6.

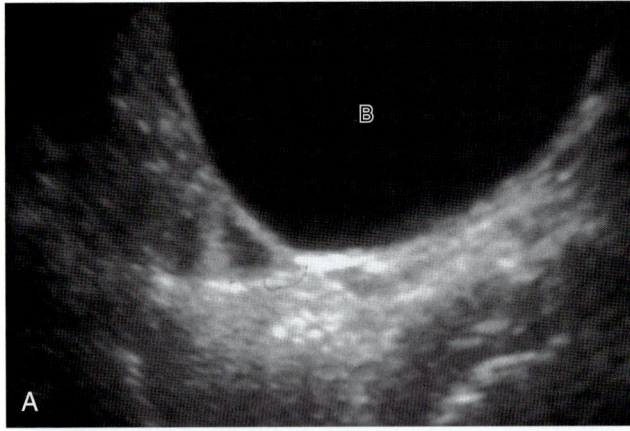

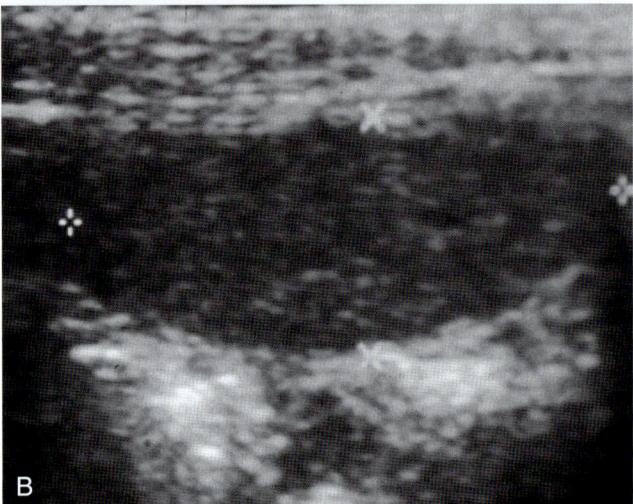

Figure 125-7 Testicular feminization syndrome. **A,** A phenotypically normal 16-year-old girl, who presented with primary amenorrhea. Longitudinal midline sonogram showed no uterus posterior to the bladder (*B*). Ovaries were not seen. Karyotyping showed 46,XY, and the patient was proven to have testicular feminization syndrome. **B,** On examination for primary amenorrhea, this patient was noted to have bilateral inguinal masses. An oval structure (cursors) without contained cysts was found in the patient's left inguinal region on ultrasonography and proved to be an undescended testis. (Courtesy of Joseph Yee, MD.)

fallopian tube is often present on the side of the streak gonad, and a vas deferens may be present on the side of the testis. The testis is usually intraabdominal but can be partially or completely descended. The external genitalia cover a wide spectrum of appearances from that of an almost normal female to that of an essentially normal male with hypospadias. Most patients have ambiguous external genitalia (as seen in other intersex situations), with a penis or clitoris of variable size, unfused labioscrotal folds, and a variously sized vagina connected with the urethra (urogenital sinus) that commonly empties at the base of the penis (Fig. 125-8). A uterus, said to be present in all cases, is usually small or rudimentary. Most patients are raised as females, but at puberty, some virilization may take place (usually without gynecomastia).[1,2]

Familial 46,XY Gonadal Dysgenesis

Familial 46,XY gonadal dysgenesis is an X-linked autosomal dominant trait associated with camptomelic dwarfism. The gonads are variable and may be bilateral streaks, bilateral dysgenetic testes, or a streak on one side and a dysgenetic testis on the other (mixed gonadal dysgenesis). Patients with bilateral streak gonads have a female phenotype with normal fallopian tubes, uterus, and vagina, usually clitoromegaly, and absence of wolffian duct derivatives. Sexual infantilism and amenorrhea are expected at puberty. Patients with bilateral dysgenetic testes or with a mixed form of gonadal dysgenesis typically have ambiguous or incompletely masculinized external genitalia. Müllerian and wolffian duct derivatives are present but may be hypoplastic or rudimentary.[1,5,6]

Drash Syndrome—Gonadal Dysgenesis, Nephropathy, and Wilms Tumor

Drash syndrome is an uncommon form of gonadal dysgenesis and male intersex. Patients most often have a 46,XY karyotype, bilateral gonadal dysgenesis with a variable histologic pattern, ambiguous external genitalia, and intraabdominal testes. They have chronic glomerulonephritis with histologic features similar to those of congenital nephrosis. They develop end-stage renal disease in early life. More than half of these patients develop a Wilms tumor at a young age, with the tumor purportedly occurring only in those patients with a female phenotype. In patients with Drash syndrome, 20% to 30% develop gonadal neoplasia.[14,15]

46,XY Gonadal Agenesis (Vanishing Testes Syndrome)

Patients with this condition are males with a 46,XY karyotype. No gonads are present, and male sex differentiation is absent or incomplete as a result of testicular resorption of

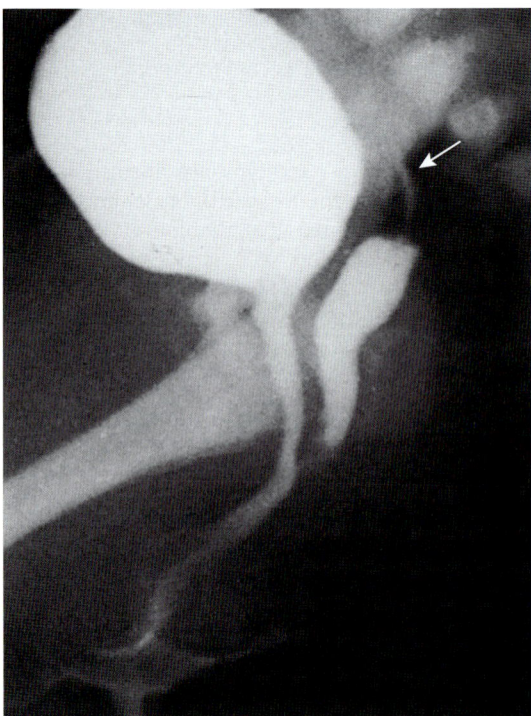

Figure 125-8 Mixed gonadal dysgenesis. A lateral voiding cystourethrography image shows a urogenital sinus with a well-developed vagina in an 11-day-old with ambiguous external genitalia. A cervical imprint is seen, and contrast material opacifies the uterine canal (*arrow*).

unknown cause in early fetal life (13 to 14 weeks' gestation). The external genitalia are ambiguous, and usually, both müllerian and wolffian duct derivatives are completely absent. Vanishing testes syndrome is differentiated from cases of bilateral anorchia (congenital absence of the testes), which are presumably caused by resorption of the testes beyond 13 to 14 weeks' gestational age. Patients with bilateral anorchia have normal male sex development and no residual müllerian structures.[1,16]

XX MALENESS

XX male syndrome (de la Chapelle syndrome) is a very unusual cause of ambiguous genitalia occurring in 4 to 5 cases per 100,000 individuals. Because of errors in meiosis, an unequal interchange of sex chromosomes occurs such that individuals may have one or two X chromosomes containing the male *SRY* gene. Patients are sterile but usually have two small testes, usually descended. Gynecomastia may be present, but more often, the individuals are phenotypically male and have no intraabdominal müllerian tissue despite being genetically female.[1,17]

TRUE HERMAPHRODITISM

True hermaphroditism is a rare condition. It is a sporadic disorder in which the affected patient has both testicular and ovarian tissues in the same or contralateral gonads. More than half such patients have the 46,XX karyotype. Mosaic karyotype patterns with at least one line with a Y chromosome do exist, including XO/XY, XX/XXY, or XX/XY chimerism (30%). Fifteen percent of patients have the 46,XY karyotype. All true hermaphrodites are H-Y antigen positive regardless of karyotype. In patients with the 45,XX karyotype, undetected Y chromosomal material is probably present and transferred to another chromosome. The testes or ovotestes may be intraabdominal, in the inguinal region, in the scrotal area, or in the labia majora. The ovaries of hermaphrodites are almost always intraabdominal. Internal gonadal ducts are usually consistent with the ipsilateral gonad (i.e., a vas on the side of a testis and a fallopian tube on the side of an ovary). In the case of ovotestes, the associated internal gonadal duct is usually a fallopian tube. A uterus is found in almost all cases but is most often hypoplastic and may be bicornuate.[1]

A wide spectrum of external genitalia ranges from normal male to ambiguous to female. Cryptorchidism is common. Inguinal hernia is common as well and, as with normal patients, can contain a gonad with its internal gonadal duct or even a uterus. About 75% of hermaphrodites are brought up as males. At puberty, usually some virilization as well as gynecomastia occurs.[1,2]

Gonadal Neoplasia of Patients with Disorders of Sex Differentiation

The gonads in several intersex disorders (with or without ambiguous genitalia) are at an increased risk for developing neoplasms. Patients with the highest risk of developing gonadal neoplasia are those with XO/XY mixed gonadal dysgenesis and those with 46,XY gonadal dysgenesis. The incidence of a gonadal tumor in both these conditions increases from 3% to 4% by age 10 years to 10% to 20% within the second decade of life and to 70% or more in older patients. Neoplasms are almost always germ cell in type, including seminoma or dysgerminoma and gonadoblastoma. Less commonly, patients may develop a gonadal teratoma, teratocarcinoma, yolk sac tumor, embryonal carcinoma of the adult type, or choriocarcinoma. These neoplasms are rare in patients who do not have a Y chromosome as part of their karyotype. The risk is apparently related to the H-Y antigen.[1,2]

Diagnostic Evaluation of Patients with Ambiguous Genitalia

Overview The discovery of anomalous or ambiguous genitalia in a newborn has been described as an emergency from a social perspective and, hence to many, from a clinical perspective as well. The identification of the uterus, vagina, or urogenital sinus, by using ultrasonography, contrast fistulogram, or vaginogram, is paramount in the decision on how to rear the child. These findings can then be correlated and sexual identification aided by karyotyping, including fluorescent studies for Y chromosomes, specific analysis of the Y chromosome for the testis-determining gene, culture of genital skin fibroblasts for androgen receptor binding, and tests for androgen responsiveness. The appearance of the external genitalia is seldom diagnostic of a specific intersex disorder, but palpable gonads in the inguinal canal, labioscrotal folds, or scrotum can exclude female pseudohermaphroditism in most cases. Sometimes, the definitive anatomic diagnosis is made only at laparoscopy or laparotomy and on the basis of gonadal biopsy. The main role of ultrasonography is identification of the uterus, a relatively easy task in the female newborn.[1,2]

Imaging A detailed radiographic study of the lower genitourinary tract (genitography) is important for diagnosis and as a guide in surgical reconstructive procedures. Patients usually have a urogenital sinus, a common terminal channel for the anterior urethra and posterior vaginal pouch. This sinus usually empties at the base of the penis. VCUG, particularly on lateral view, may outline the entire anatomy needed for evaluation. If the urethral catheter can be advanced only to the vagina, an injection with the catheter in that position may opacify the vagina, the urogenital sinus, and often the proximal urethra. If confusion about the anatomy persists during the VCUG examination, a retrograde injection of contrast material may be attempted through a catheter with the tip placed just inside the "urethral" meatus. At times, a coude catheter (with a curved tip) manipulated under fluoroscopic control into the urethra and bladder or into the vagina may improve contrast study of the area. An effort should be made on the VCUG or vaginogram to determine if a uterine cervix is present. Often, if a uterus (especially if normal) is present, a mass impression of the cervix on the contrast medium–filled vagina (see Fig. 125-4) is evident. A cervical imprint, however, may not be apparent if the vagina is not sufficiently distended or if the uterus is hypoplastic. A uterine cervix is present in all female intersex patients and is a common finding among many patients with mixed gonadal

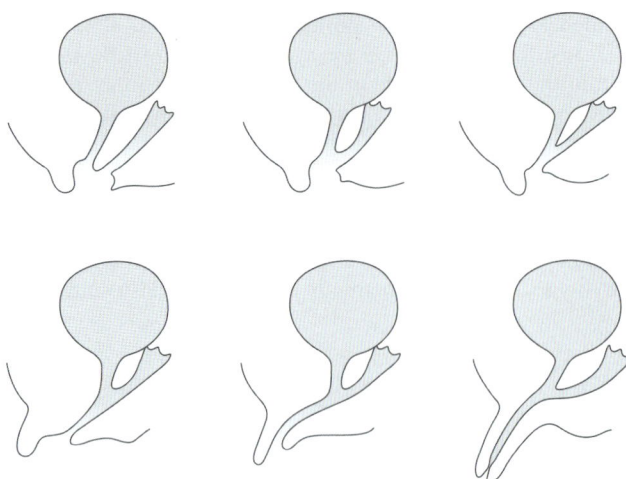

Figure 125-9 Different types of urogenital sinus are arranged in order of increasing masculinization, from an almost normal female pattern to a penile urethra. The urogenital sinus is of variable length, and the vagina may enter the urogenital sinus at various levels.

dysgenesis or true hermaphroditism as well. All members of these groups may have a hypoplastic or rudimentary uterus that may not be noted radiographically. Cervical imprints are not seen in male pseudohermaphroditism or male hypospadias.[1,2]

In some patients evaluated by VCUG or contrast vaginogram, the urogenital sinus is quite short and joined by the vagina very close to the perineal surface (Fig. 125-9). In other patients, it is a much longer channel, joined by the vagina at a much higher level, occasionally near the bladder neck. A very high insertion of the vagina in the urogenital sinus may pose a problem at the time of vaginal reconstruction because of the danger of injuring the external urethral sphincter. In patients evaluated for disorders of sex differentiation or ambiguous genitalia, the vagina may vary in size from a small cavity to an organ of normal size for the patient's age. Occasionally, its distal end is stenosed or is completely obliterated, resulting in hydrocolpos at birth or hematocolpos at puberty (Fig. 125-10).[1]

Pelvic ultrasonography is valuable in evaluating infants with ambiguous genitalia. Ultrasonography is an excellent imaging tool for identification of uterine tissue, although it may be difficult with hypoplastic uteri. The proximal vagina may also be demonstrated, particularly if it contains urine, but the urethra and urogenital sinus cannot be studied by this method. Ultrasonography does not replace genitography, but it is of particular value when genitography is unsuccessful. Ovaries are often seen, but fallopian tubes, unless obstructed, are more difficult to image. Ultrasonography is an excellent tool for the identification of the adrenal gland in the newborn and in the older child. Pelvic magnetic resonance imaging is of great value in evaluating patients with complex anatomy, particularly those with complex müllerian duct system abnormalities, in whom ultrasonography and genitography do not provide sufficient information (Fig. 125-11 and e-Fig. 125-12).[1,18-20]

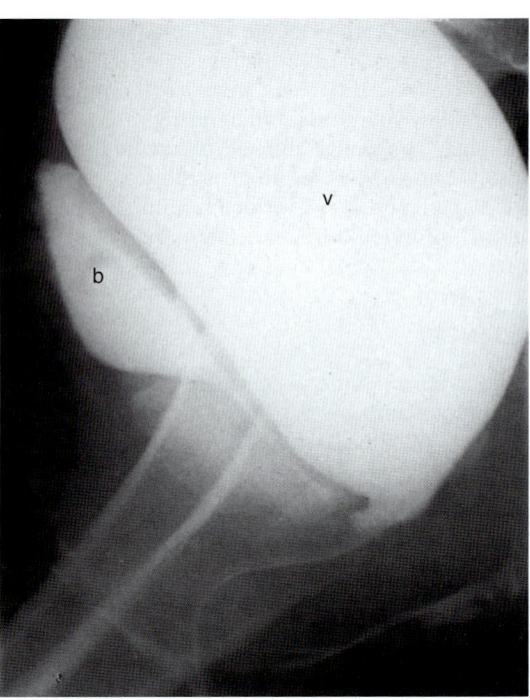

Figure 125-10 Hydrocolpos in adrenogenital syndrome. Lateral view from a retrograde vaginogram of a 14-year-old girl with adrenogenital syndrome, and the urogenital sinus shows a catheter within a large obstructed vagina. She had presented with abdominal pain and a pelvic mass. *v,* vagina; *b,* bladder.

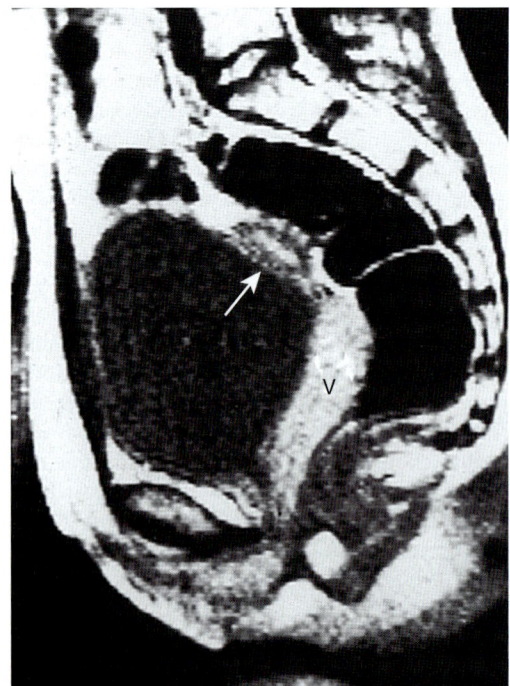

Figure 125-11 Anatomic evaluation of a 13-year-old with known adrenogenital syndrome being evaluated before surgical vaginoplasty. Sagittal T1-weighted magnetic resonance image shows the vagina (*V*) throughout its course posterior to the bladder and anterior to rectum. Uterine tissue (*arrow*) is seen anterosuperior to it.

WHAT THE CLINICIAN NEEDS TO KNOW

- Presence or absence of vagina, uterus, and ovaries on pelvic ultrasonography
- Prepubertal or postpubertal appearance of uterus
- Testicular tissue present or absent
- Presence and classification of urogenital sinus on VCUG
- Cervical impression present at superior margin of vagina on VCUG
- Presence of gonadal mass

Key Points

Abnormal sexual differentiation may be caused by abnormalities of hormone production, end-organ response, chromosomes, or gonads.

The development of a male genital system occurs as an "active" process requiring the presence of testes and their production of MIS.

Turner syndrome is the most common gonadal dysgenesis associated with an abnormal karyotype in girls.

Primary amenorrhea is defined as a lack of menses by age 16 years. Many of the causes may also be linked to causes of delayed sexual development.

Pseudohermaphroditism or intersex problems are abnormalities that have nonaccord of chromosomal, gonadal, and genital sex and the presence of only one type of gonad. Male intersex patients have testes, and female intersex patients have ovarian tissue.

True hermaphroditism is a rare condition. It is a sporadic disorder in which the affected patient has both testicular and ovarian tissues in the same or contralateral gonads.

Patients with several of the intersex disorders are at an increased risk for developing gonadal germ cell neoplasms.

The length of the urogenital sinus and the level of insertion of the vagina are indicators of the degree of virilization but are nonspecific regarding the type of underlying disorder. For this purpose, the presence or absence of a cervical imprint on the vaginogram is more important. A uterine cervix is present in all female intersex patients.

Suggested Readings

Ahmed SF, Rodie M. Investigation and initial management of ambiguous genitalia. *Best Pract Res Clin Endocrinol Metab.* 2010;24(2):197-218.

Barthold JS. Disorders of sex differentiation: a pediatric urologist's perspective of new terminology and recommendations. *J Urol.* 2011;185(2): 393-400.

Chavhan GB, Parra DA, Oudjhane K, et al. Imaging of ambiguous genitalia: classification and diagnostic approach. *Radiographics.* 2008; 28(7):1891-1904.

Choi HK, Cho KS, Lee HW, et al. MR imaging of intersexuality. *Radiographics.* 1998;18(1):83-96.

Cohen-Kettenis PT. Psychosocial and psychosexual aspects of disorders of sex development. *Best Pract Res Clin Endocrinol Metab.* 2010; 24(2):325-334.

Gillam LH, Hewitt JK, Warne GL. Ethical principles for the management of infants with disorders of sex development. *Horm Res Paediatr.* 2010;74(6):412-418.

Lambert SM, Vilain EJ, Kolon TF. A practical approach to ambiguous genitalia in the newborn period. *Urol Clin North Am.* 2010;37(2):195-205.

Vidal I, Gorduza DB, Haraux E, et al. Surgical options in disorders of sex development (DSD) with ambiguous genitalia. *Best Pract Res Clin Endocrinol Metab.* 2010;24(2):311-324.

References

Full references for this chapter can be found on www.expertconsult.com.

Chapter 126

Abnormalities of the Male Genital Tract

HARRIS L. COHEN and VIRENDERSINGH K. SHEORAIN

Overview

Ultrasound, including Doppler imaging in all its forms, is the main diagnostic imaging tool for evaluating the scrotum. Computed tomography (CT) is used predominantly to evaluate metastatic spread of testicular or other intrascrotal tumors. Magnetic resonance imaging (MRI) has been used in the search for undescended testes that remain in an intraabdominal position. MRI, like CT, can be used to analyze metastatic spread of testicular tumor. Its uses in intraabdominal, intrapelvic, and intrascrotal imaging are evolving.[1]

ULTRASOUND TECHNIQUE

Scrotal ultrasound is performed with use of a high-frequency transducer. The superficial position of testes in the normally thin-walled scrotum allows excellent imaging with a transducer of 7.5 MHz or higher. Longitudinal, transverse, and coronal views are taken of each hemiscrotum. Transverse views, with the addition of a convex array transducer (e-Fig. 126-1), allow the best side-by-side comparison of both testes and their adnexa, especially when checking for differences in size, echogenicity, and vascularity (e-Fig. 126-2).[1-6]

NORMAL FINDINGS

The testes should be ovoid, nearly symmetric in size (Box 126-1), and homogeneously echogenic. A highly echogenic linear focus (seen posteriorly and superiorly) represents the mediastinum testis (Fig. 126-3), which is the inward extension of the tightly adherent covering of the testis, the tunica albuginea. Fibrous septa extending from the mediastinum testes divide the testes into more than 250 lobules. The spermatic cord, draining veins, lymphatics, nerves, vas deferens, and a single testicular artery run within the mediastinum testis.[6-9]

The head of the epididymis (e-Fig. 126-4) sits atop the superior pole of each testis. The head is continuous with the epididymal body and tail, which travel inferiorly along the posterolateral margin of the testis. The echogenicity of the epididymis is normally homogeneous. It may be of equal or of slightly greater or lesser echogenicity than that of the testes.[6-9]

The scrotal wall should be between 3 and 6 mm thick. Beneath the scrotal wall are the two layers of the tunica vaginalis (Fig. 126-5), the outer (parietal) and the inner (visceral) layers, which are the residua of the processus vaginalis (i.e., peritoneum that descended with the testis from the abdomen). The visceral layer covers the testis on its anterior border and is attached to the tunica albuginea. Between the tunica's two layers is a potential space that normally may contain as much as 1 to 2 mL of fluid. It is here that the fluid of a hydrocele may accumulate.[6-9]

Three small, persistent, vestigial remnants of the mesonephric and müllerian duct systems occasionally may be seen, usually only when a normal testis is surrounded by hydrocele fluid. These remnants are the appendix testis (e-Fig. 126-6) (a remnant of the müllerian duct), which is attached to the upper pole of the testis (and the most common one to potentially undergo torsion); the appendix epididymis (a remnant of the mesonephron), which is attached to the head of the epididymis; and the vas aberrans (a remnant of the mesonephron), which is attached to the epididymis at the junction of its body and tail.[6-9]

Cryptorchidism

Overview By 32 weeks' gestational age, the testes have descended into the scrotum via the inguinal canal in 93% of all male fetuses. By 6 weeks of age, only 4% of term infants have a nonpalpable testis. Of these infants, 20% have true cryptorchidism (undescended testes). Cryptorchidism is more common on the right (70%) and is bilateral in 10% to 33% of cases. Beyond the age of 1 year, the prevalence of true cryptorchidism is approximately 1%. The etiology of cryptorchidism is not clear; it may be hormonal or mechanical (e.g., lack of proper fixation of the testis or an abnormal gubernaculum), or a combination of the two.[1]

Imaging Ultrasound is the initial procedure for localization of a testis that is not palpable within the scrotum (e-Fig. 126-7). The undescended testes may be smaller and hypoplastic, although usually it is of equal echogenicity compared with the normal testis. MRI with fat-suppression techniques generally is more effective than CT for intraabdominal testes. Normal testes have a homogeneous high signal on T2-weighted images.[1,6,10]

Treatment Surgical treatment for undescended testes is orchiopexy. It is performed, especially in cases of intraabdominal testes, because of the increased risk for the development of testicular neoplasia (a 10 to 40 times greater risk, with a

Box 126-1 Normal Scrotal Volume

Newborn: 1.0 cm length

0-1 year: 2 cm³

1-12 years: 2-5 cm³

13-15 years: 5-10 cm³

15-18 years: 15-25 cm³

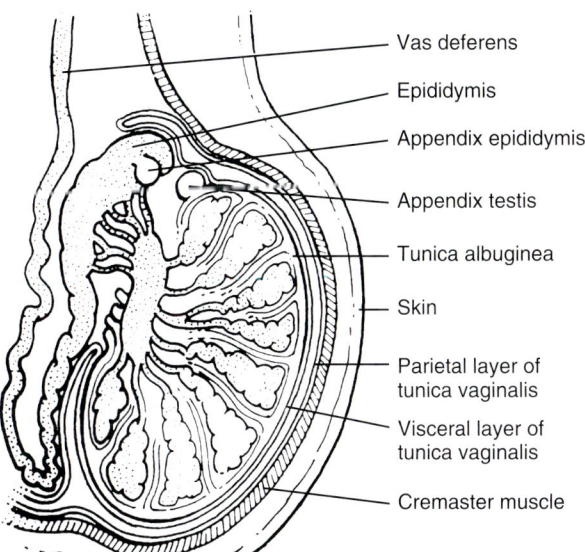

Figure 126-5 A schematic drawing of the scrotum and its contents as seen in the longitudinal plane through a single testis. Note the tunica albuginea surrounding the lobules of the testes. The tunica albuginea, in turn, is surrounded by the visceral layer of the tunica vaginalis and the more superficial parietal layer of the tunica vaginalis. (From Cohen HL, Sivit C, eds. *Fetal and pediatric ultrasound: a casebook approach.* New York: McGraw-Hill; 2001. Reproduced with permission of McGraw-Hill Companies.)

seminoma being the most common neoplasm).[11] Spontaneous descent during the first year of life may occur from an endogenous surge of luteinizing hormone, and thus surgical correction typically is delayed until 18 to 24 months.[1,6,12] After orchiopexy, 53% of the testes are reported to be abnormal by either position, volume, structure, or perfusion.[1,13-16]

Hydrocele

Overview A hydrocele, which is the most common scrotal mass in a child (Fig. 126-8), results from fluid accumulated within the layers of the tunica vaginalis. Several types of hydroceles are identified (Fig. 126-9). The processus vaginalis is closed in 50% to 75% of persons by the time they are born and in most of the remainder of children by the end of the first year of life. Residual fluid from testicular descent is responsible for the noncommunicating hydroceles reported in at least 15% of male fetuses beyond 28 weeks of life. If the processus fails to close, a communicating hydrocele can develop.

In a hydrocele of the cord (a funicular hydrocele), the processus vaginalis is obliterated in its proximal and distal end and the hydrocele is contained in the patent space between these two points. In an inguinoscrotal hydrocele, the processus vaginalis is obliterated only at the internal inguinal ring and the hydrocele extends cephalad from the scrotum into the inguinal canal. In an abdominoscrotal hydrocele (e-Fig. 126-10), closure of the funicular process at the internal

inguinal ring also occurs and forms a dumbbell–shaped cystic mass that protrudes into the extraperitoneal space above the inguinal area.[1,17]

In most cases, the etiology of a hydrocele found in the child or adolescent is idiopathic. Acquired hydroceles occur after scrotal trauma or as a complication of epididymitis-orchitis, testicular torsion, or intrascrotal neoplasm (reactive hydrocele). Increasing size of a hydrocele without an intrascrotal cause suggests a patent processus vaginalis and an associated inguinal hernia.[1]

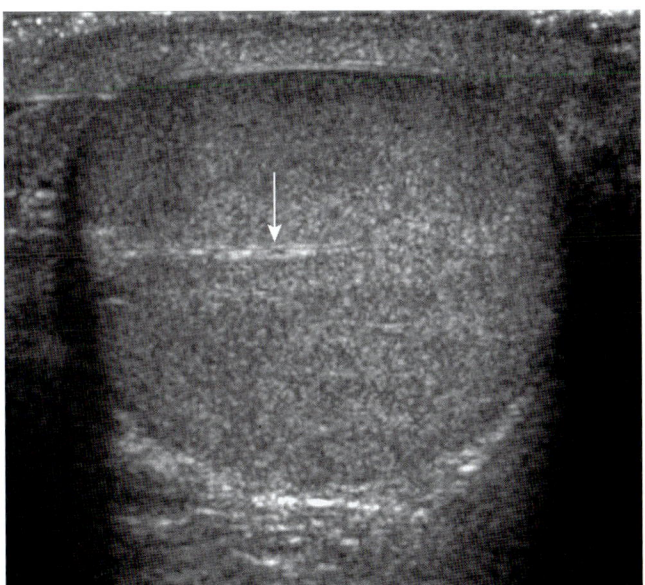

Figure 126-3 Mediastinum testis. A transverse sonogram shows a linear echogenicity (*arrow*) within a normal testis that is the mediastinum testis.

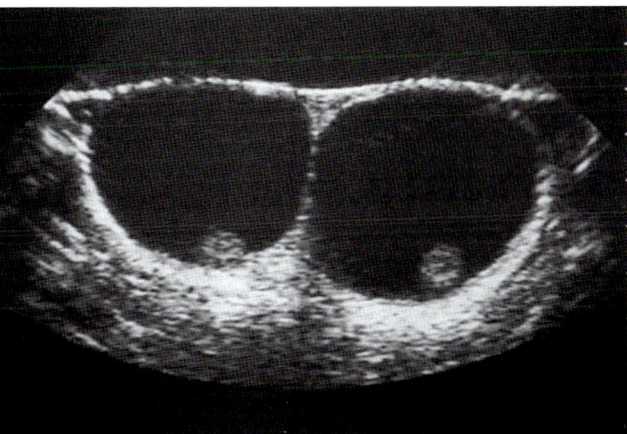

Figure 126-8 Hydroceles. On transverse plane ultrasound, two normal testes are seen as small echogenic structures within a very enlarged scrotum of a young child with large hydroceles. Typically, high-frequency transducers (e.g., 7.5 MHz and greater) are used for improved near-field resolution of superficial structures such as the testes. In cases such as this one with large hydroceles, a lower-frequency transducer may be needed to better penetrate the greater distance between the anterior and posterior scrotal walls to image the testes.

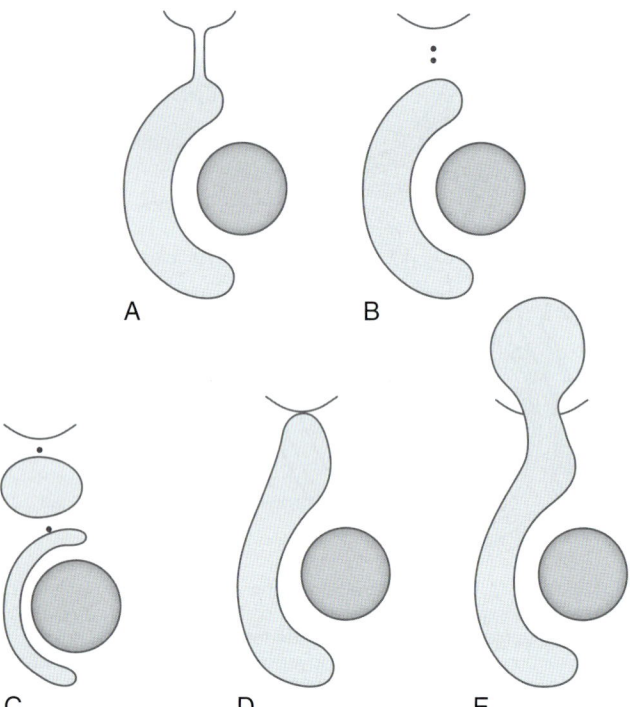

Figure 126-9 Hydrocele types. **A,** Congenital or intermittent hydrocele. **B,** Scrotal hydrocele. **C,** Hydrocele of the cord. **D,** Inguinoscrotal hydrocele. **E,** Abdominoscrotal hydrocele.

Imaging Scrotal ultrasound shows the cystic nature of the hydrocele as it appears to surround the normal homogeneously echogenic testes. Septations and debris may be present, particularly if the hydrocele is infected (i.e., a pyocele) or hemorrhagic (i.e., a hematocele) (e-Fig. 126-11). Echogenic debris (e.g., cholesterol crystals) often is seen in the fluid of chronic hydroceles (Fig. 126-12), along with occasional calcifications.[1]

Treatment After the age of 2 years, a hydrocele is unlikely to resolve, and surgery is required. A high ligation of the patent processus vaginalis should be performed, and the distal fluid collection should be emptied.[18,19]

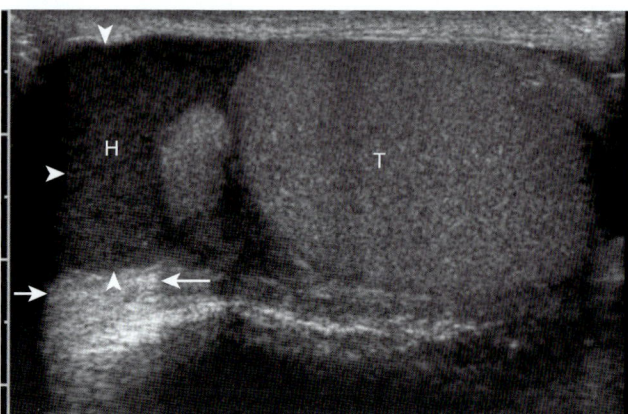

Figure 126-12 Chronic hydrocele (*arrowheads*). Ultrasound in the longitudinal plane. Echogenic debris-filled fluid is seen in a chronic hydrocele (*H*) in the scrotum of a teenager. Excellent through transmission of sound (*arrows*) helps indicate that the echogenic material is complicated fluid rather than solid material. *T,* testicle.

Testicular Torsion

Overview Torsion may occur at any age but is seen most often in adolescent boys between 11 and 18 years of age, perhaps because of the increase in testicular growth and weight during this time. The normal testis is strongly attached to the epididymis, which in turn is applied to the posterior scrotal wall. If these attachments fail to develop properly (the "clapper-in-a-bell" phenomenon), the testis, suspended within the tunica vaginalis, may rotate and the spermatic cord undergoes torsion. A person with acute torsion experiences sudden acute scrotal pain, accompanied by nausea and vomiting. An important finding on physical examination is a change in testicular axis from the normal vertical positioning of the testis in the scrotum to a more horizontal positioning. Within hours of torsion, a reddened scrotum develops, with or without enlargement.[1]

Imaging Ultrasonography is the only diagnostic tool necessary to make the diagnosis of torsion and suggest surgical exploration. The testis is normal-sized to enlarged, with normal to decreased echogenicity (Fig. 126-13). Enlargement and hypoechogenicity are thought to be due to venous congestion. The echogenicity pattern is usually homogeneous. Epididymal enlargement may be an early finding in some cases of torsion. At least 10% of cases of torsion have associated reactive hydroceles. Ultrasound performed more than 48 hours after symptomatology (e-Fig. 126-14) may show a heterogeneous or hyperechoic testis from hemorrhage or hemorrhagic necrosis.[1]

State-of-the-art color or power Doppler imaging methods have made ultrasound the gold standard for the imaging and preoperative diagnosis of testicular torsion. Venous flow is lost before arterial flow ceases. Color flow comparison to the contralateral testis is helpful and necessary, particularly when torsion is incomplete, in which case the diagnosis may be suggested not by absence of arterial flow but by blood flow asymmetry. The spermatic cord always should be seen, and

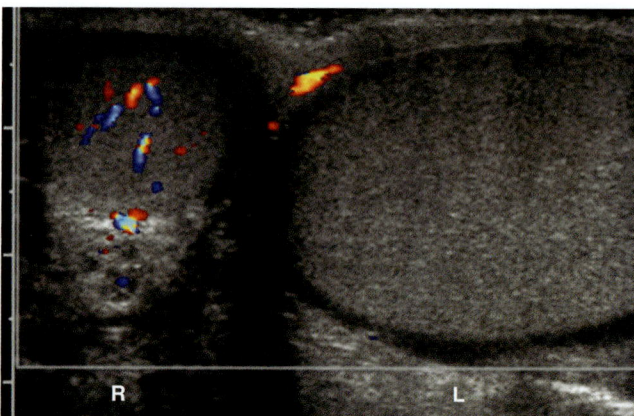

Figure 126-13 Testicular torsion and axis change. A color Doppler ultrasound in the transverse plane shows color flow in the right testicle. The right testicle is oval to circular, because it has been evaluated in the transverse plane. The left testicle is elongated as if it is in longitudinal plane. This axis change is the ultrasound equivalent of the worrisome clinical finding suggestive of torsion when accompanied by a history of sudden pain. Lack of Color Doppler flow in the left testicle confirms a left testicular torsion.

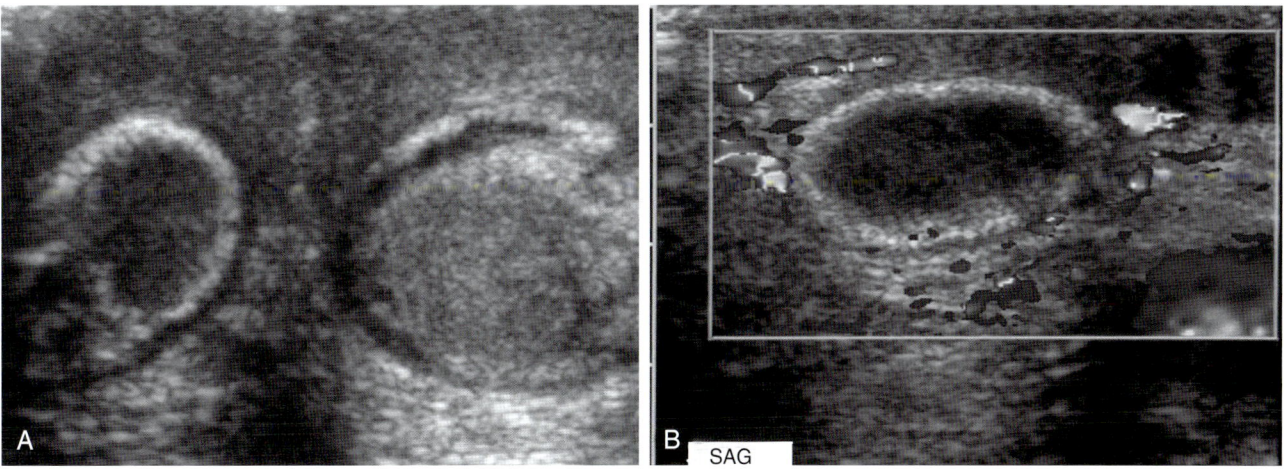

Figure 126-15 Bilateral antenatal testicular torsion. **A,** A transverse sonogram shows two testes with torsion of different ages in a newborn with scrotal swelling. The testes are seen deep to a more superficial thickened scrotal wall. The right testis is hypoechoic with a somewhat hyperechoic periphery, suggesting an old torsion. The grayer left testis does not appear particularly abnormal on this image, although its periphery is more echogenic than the remainder of its parenchyma. Color Doppler imaging showed no flow in either testis. Upon surgery, both testes proved to have undergone torsion. The torsion of the left testis probably occurred later in fetal life. Tiny hydroceles are present bilaterally. Because the scrotum of this newborn was small, it could be seen completely by the high-frequency (14-MHz) linear array probe despite its small footpad. **B,** A longitudinal sonogram of the torsed right testis. No color flow is seen within the hypoechoic parenchyma or the surrounding hyperechoic periphery of this neonate's testis, which underwent torsion during fetal life.

it should be straight. When torsion is present, a spiral twist or Whirlpool sign is seen. Flow may be normal or increased in a torsed testis that spontaneously detorses.[20-23]

Treatment Torsion must be corrected for testicular viability. Surgery within 24 hours leads to 60% to 70% testicular salvage, but after 24 hours salvage is only 20%. Because abnormal testicular fixation is considered a bilateral phenomenon, preventive orchiopexy often is performed on the contralateral nontwisted testis.[16]

TESTICULAR TORSION IN THE FETUS AND NEWBORN

Overview Testicular torsion that occurs in the newborn period usually presents as a painless, firm scrotal mass often associated with bluish-red scrotal discoloration. The affected testis is generally nonviable. If the torsion occurred in intrauterine life, one is imaging the neonatal equivalent of delayed torsion.[1]

Imaging Antenatal torsion may be diagnosed on fetal ultrasound examination. Antenatal torsion must be considered if the fetal testis or testes are heterogeneous in echogenicity or of asymmetric size (Fig. 126-15). Diagnosis in the newborn is made by similar imaging findings.[24-27]

TORSION OF TESTICULAR AND EPIDIDYMAL APPENDAGES

Overview Testicular and epididymal appendage torsion occurs most typically in the 6- to 12-year-old age group. Patients present with localized pain, a pea-sized mass in the area of the upper pole of the testis, and at times, a pinpoint discoloration (the "blue dot" sign) seen through the overlying scrotal skin. The clinical picture may be indistinguishable from that of testicular torsion, albeit in a somewhat younger age group.

Imaging Ultrasound demonstrates an enlarged torsed appendage as a small circular mass (Fig. 126-16) of variable echogenicity near the testis or epididymis of the affected side. Reactive epididymal swelling and hyperemia often is present. Usually the testicular echogenicity and vascular flow are normal.[24,28]

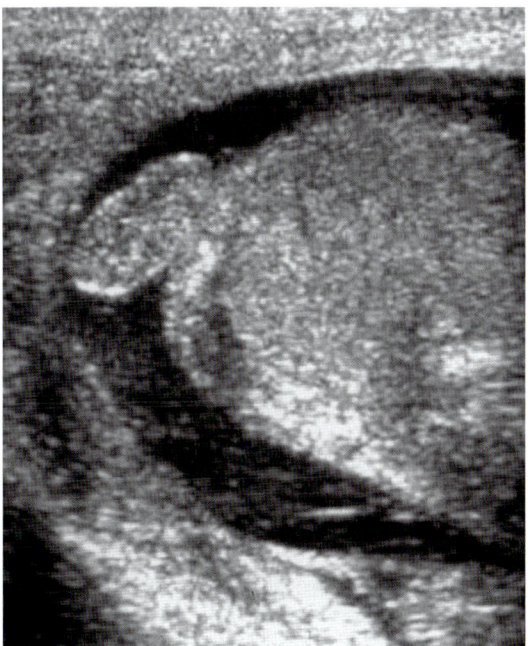

Figure 126-16 A torsed appendix testis. A longitudinal sonogram of the superior portion of the scrotum shows a prominent oval structure superior to the testis of a child who presented with sudden testicular pain. The oval structure is of equal echogenicity to the testis and is an enlarged torsed testicular appendage. Color flow of the testis was normal, proving that no testicular torsion was present. Some debris is present in a small surrounding hydrocele.

Treatment   Twisted appendages generally are a self-limited disorder and respond best to nonsteroidal antiinflammatory medications and comfort measures such as limited activity and a warm compress. As the appendage infarcts and necroses, the pain resolves. Surgical intervention is indicated when the symptoms are prolonged and spontaneous resolution does not occur.[29]

Epididymitis

Overview   Epididymitis is the most common cause of an acute painful scrotum in the postpubescent male. The cause is usually bacterial, although in pediatric and some adolescent patients, epididymitis may be viral (e.g., as a result of mumps). Patients with epididymitis often are febrile, and at least half report dysuria. Pyuria is common, and nausea, vomiting, and leukocytosis may be present. An enlarged epididymis may be palpated, and scrotal edema and tenderness often are present.[1]

The infection usually reaches the epididymis through the spermatic ducts. Causative factors include urinary tract infections, urethral instrumentation and indwelling catheters, distal urethral obstruction, and reflux of urine from the urethra into the seminal ducts as a result of a congenitally patulous orifice, an ectopic ureter draining into the vas deferens, and an ectopic vas draining into the bladder or ureter.

Complications of epididymitis include direct spread of the infection to the testis (i.e., epididymo-orchitis), which can be seen in as many as 20% of cases. Although it is an uncommon complication, an abscess may develop within the scrotum or testes and require drainage. In unusual cases, acute epididymitis may impede testicular blood flow, resulting in focal or diffuse infarction of the testis or epididymis even in the absence of torsion.[1]

Imaging   Ultrasound shows enlargement of the epididymis (e-Fig. 126-17) and commonly a reactive hydrocele or pyocele. Overlying scrotal wall thickening may be present. The echogenicity of the enlarged epididymis may be normal, slightly decreased, or slightly increased. The affected area of epididymis, although enlarged, usually maintains its normal shape. The diagnosis is supported by color Doppler imaging showing increased flow (Fig. 126-18). With epididymo-orchitis, a hypoechoic area of involvement is seen within the testis directly adjacent to the area of involved epididymis (e-Fig. 126-19). Color Doppler imaging usually shows increased flow to the involved portion of adjacent testis and the epididymis. In the prepubescent male, when epididymitis is the result of a congenital anomaly, a voiding cystourethrogram may be performed to detect abnormalities such as reflux of contrast agent into a vas deferens.[30-32]

Treatment   Urine cultures should be obtained for all pediatric patients with epididymitis. Antibiotic therapy is reserved for young infants and those with pyuria and positive cultures.[33]

Henoch-Schönlein Purpura

Overview and Imaging   Henoch-Schönlein purpura is a generalized vasculitis of unknown cause characterized clinically by a purpuric rash, abdominal pain, joint manifestations, and

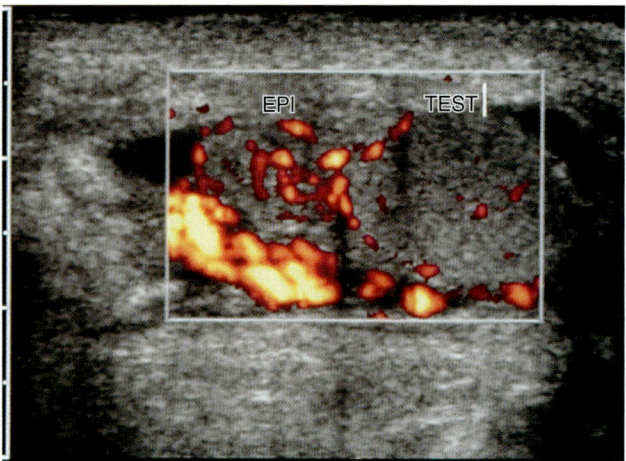

Figure 126-18   A longitudinal color Doppler sonogram shows that flow to the prominent right epididymis (*EPI*) of this 10-year-old child is greater than that to the testis (*TEST*).

often hematuria. Involvement of the epididymis and testis may result in scrotal swelling and tenderness. Most often, however, the scrotum alone is involved by severe purpura and swelling. Imaging may be indicated to exclude testicular torsion. Imaging normal testes with normal flow despite marked edema of the scrotal wall helps suggest the diagnosis and can prevent the need to explore the scrotum surgically.[1,34,35]

Testicular and Paratesticular Neoplasms

PRIMARY TESTICULAR NEOPLASMS

Overview   Testicular neoplasms are uncommon in infants and children, representing only 1% to 1.5% of all childhood malignancies; when they are present, they tend to occur in very young children, with a peak incidence at 2 years of age and with 60% of the cases occurring in children younger than 2 years. Such tumors usually present as a painless, nontender, and firm scrotal mass often of weeks' to months' duration. Scrotal pain and tenderness may occur if associated torsion of the testis occurs. Testicular tumors occasionally are bilateral.[1] Primary testicular tumors are classified according to their tissue of origin (Box 126-2).

Imaging   The predominant imaging tool used to search for and evaluate tumors of the scrotum and its contents is ultrasound. Most testicular neoplasms tend to be hypoechoic

---

Box 126-2   Classification of Primary Neoplasms

Germ cell tumors (yolk sac carcinoma, teratoma, teratocarcinoma, choriocarcinoma, seminoma) occurring as pure histologic patterns or in various combinations (mixed germ cell tumors)

Gonadal stromal tumors (Sertoli–granulosa cell, Leydig cell, or granulosa cell tumors)

Germ cell plus stromal cell tumors (gonadoblastoma)

Tumors of supporting tissues (fibroma, leiomyoma, hemangioma)

(e-Fig. 126-20). Contained anechoic areas within tumors represent either cystic components or more often are evidence of focal necrosis as the tumor outstrips its blood supply. Acute hemorrhage appears echogenic, and echogenic foci with posterior shadowing may be seen with intratumoral calcifications. Reactive hydroceles are associated in at least 15% to 20% of cases. Color Doppler and power Doppler ultrasound demonstrate increased vascularity in the majority of malignant tumors and may help define the mass itself. Abdominal ultrasound, CT, or MRI often is performed for detection of pelvic or retroperitoneal lymph node enlargement and in the search for solid organ metastases. Chest radiographs and CT are used to search for pulmonary metastases.[1,6]

Germ Cell Tumors

Overview and Imaging Most childhood testicular tumors (65% to 75%) are germ cell in origin. Yolk sac tumor is by far the most common malignant germ cell tumor (80% to 90%) in children. Three fourths of yolk sac tumors are diagnosed by 24 months of age. Hemorrhage, particularly after clot dissolution, frequently causes echo-free areas within this typically hypoechoic, somewhat well-circumscribed mass. An elevated serum alpha-fetoprotein level is a tumor marker in approximately 90% of affected patients.[1,6]

Testicular teratomas represent 10% to 15% of childhood germ cell tumors, with 65% of cases diagnosed before 2 years of age. They are composed of elements derived from all three germ cell layers and may contain cartilage, bone, and epidermal elements such as keratin, fibrous tissue, smooth muscle, and fat. Teratomas appear on ultrasound as complex masses with cystic and solid components (Fig. 126-21). Bony and dental elements are echogenic with posterior shadowing on ultrasound, whereas the adipose component appears echogenic but without shadowing. Prepubertal teratomas are said to almost always follow a benign course even if they contain islands of malignant germ cells (15%). Postpubertal teratomas, in contrast, are potentially malignant because of their propensity to develop components of other germ cell tumors, resulting in teratocarcinomas. The serum human chorionic gonadotropin level in these cases usually is elevated.[1,6,36]

Gonadal Stromal Tumors

Overview and Imaging Non–germ cell testicular tumor types represent only 25% to 30% of pediatric testicular tumors. Leydig cell tumors and Sertoli–granulosa cell tumors are very uncommon but represent the most common gonadal stromal tumors of childhood. They almost always are benign adenomas. Almost half (45%) of Leydig cell tumors are diagnosed between the ages of 2 and 9 years, with a peak incidence at 4 years of age. Leydig cell tumors typically are painless but may be associated with premature virilization (Fig. 126-22) if androgen is produced or with gynecomastia if estrogen is produced. Sertoli cell tumors represent 20% of the non–germ cell tumors. Half are diagnosed in the first year of life. Gynecomastia may be caused by estrogen production. Tumors containing a mixture of non–germ cell histologic patterns may occur.[1,6,37,38]

Epidermoid Cyst

Overview and Imaging The epidermoid cyst, also known as a keratocyst, is a benign tumor of germ cell origin representing less than 1% of all testis tumors (Fig. 126-23). It consists of a simple squamous cell–lined echopenic area located within the testicular parenchyma, usually just below the tunica albuginea. The wall is made up of fibrous tissue, and its lumen contains cheesy keratinized material or amorphous debris. Patients usually present with a painless 0.5- to 4-cm nodule that often is picked up incidentally on a routine physical examination. Four basic ultrasound appearances are seen, including a halo with central increased echogenicity, a sharply defined mass with peripheral calcification, and a solid mass with an echogenic rim. The classic appearance is an onion-ring pattern with alternating hyperechoic and hypoechoic rings that typically is avascular.[1,6,39-41]

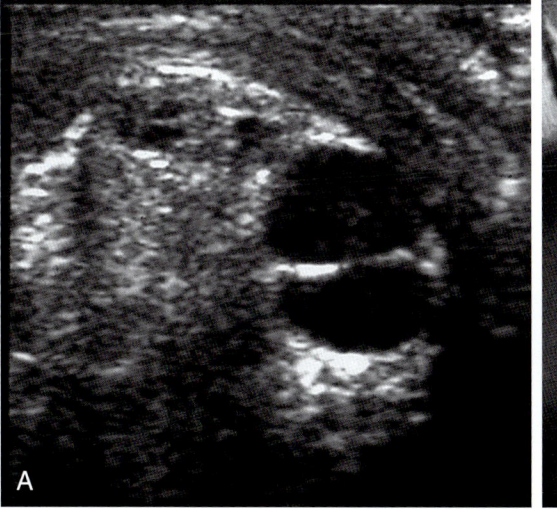 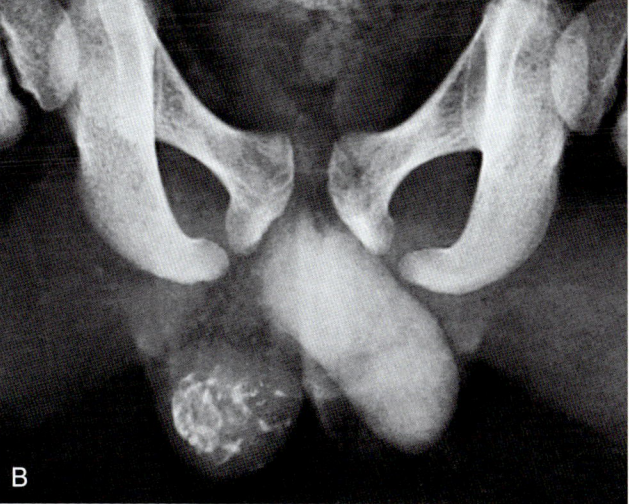

Figure 126-21 A testicular teratoma. **A,** A transverse sonogram of the right testicle shows a complex testicular mass with debris-filled cystic foci and surrounding hyperechogenicity. **B,** A coned radiograph of the lower pelvis identifies a calcified right testicular lesion. (Courtesy Dr. Leslie E. Grissom.)

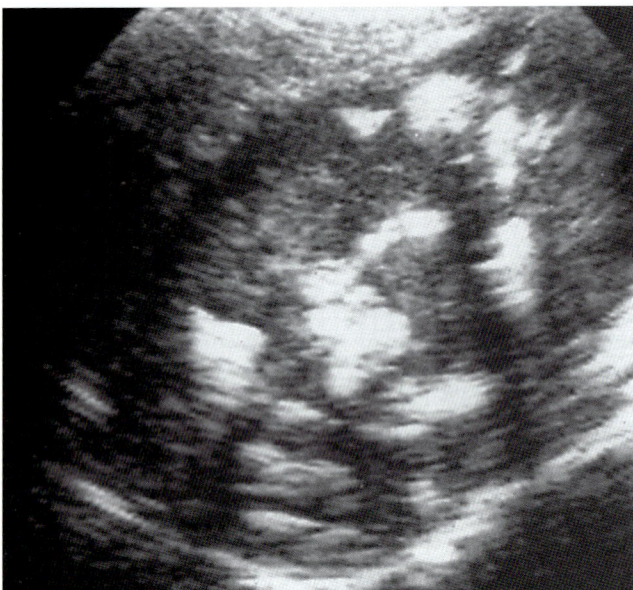

Figure 126-22   A Leydig cell tumor. A longitudinal sonogram in a patient with precocious puberty (i.e., early virilization) shows multiple calcifications (bright echogenicities) scattered in the testicular parenchyma. Shadowing is present beyond one or two of the calcifications. (Courtesy Dr. Kenneth Glassberg.)

SECONDARY TESTICULAR NEOPLASMS

Overview and Imaging   Testicular metastases are rare in children, representing far less than 1% of testicular tumors. Leukemia and lymphoma are the most common causes. Enlarged testes caused by leukemic or lymphomatous infiltration are uncommon but may be the primary manifestation of these diseases or the first sign of relapse after bone marrow remission. The lesions often are bilateral. At least 8% of patients with acute lymphocytic leukemia have testicular involvement at some point during the course of their disease. These enlarged testes have focal (Fig. 126-24) or diffuse areas of decreased echogenicity. Areas of hemorrhage appear echogenic, and lymphatic obstruction may lead to a hydrocele. Color Doppler imaging often shows significant increases in flow, often in an asymmetric pattern related to the position of the infiltrating masses within the testis.[1]

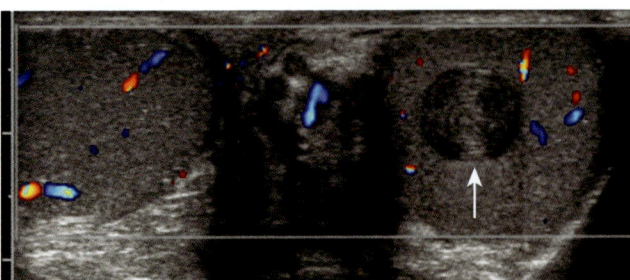

Figure 126-23   A testicular epidermoid. A color Doppler ultrasound in the transverse plane shows that this teenager has a normal right testicle. The left testicle contains a mass (*arrow*) with onion skin layering. This image is typical for a testicular epidermoid. No color flow was seen within the mass, underlining the fact that these masses typically are avascular.

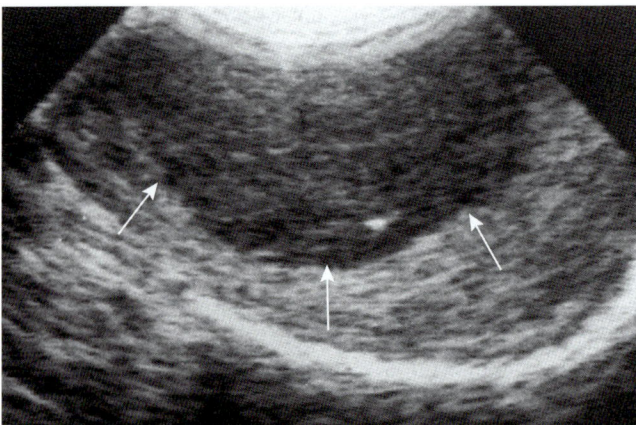

Figure 126-24   A patient with leukemia. A longitudinal sonogram of an enlarged right testis of a teenager with leukemia who was thought to be in remission shows a hypoechoic mass (*arrows*). The echopenic area proved to be due to leukemic involvement of the testis. (From Cohen HL, Sivit C, eds. *Fetal and pediatric ultrasound: a casebook approach.* New York: McGraw-Hill; 2001. Reproduced with permission of McGraw-Hill Companies.)

Adrenal Rests

Overview and Imaging   Adrenal rests are simulators of intratesticular tumors. At times, aberrant cells from the adrenal cortex may travel with gonadal tissue and be incorporated into the testis during fetal life. With high levels of adrenocorticotropic hormone and associated cortical cell stimulation (as in persons with congenital adrenal hyperplasia and Cushing syndrome), these rests may enlarge (Fig. 126-25). Patients present with a testicular mass or enlargement. On ultrasound, several hypoechogenic or hyperechogenic masses generally are seen, usually in both testes. A typical color Doppler ultrasound pattern has been described in which multiple peripheral vessels radiate in a spokelike fashion from the centers of individual rests.[1,41,42]

Testicular Microlithiasis

Overview and Imaging   Testicular microlithiasis is characterized by calcifications within the lumina of seminiferous tubules. It is denoted on ultrasound by individual, tiny (2 to 3 mm), hyperechoic foci without shadowing (Fig. 126-26)

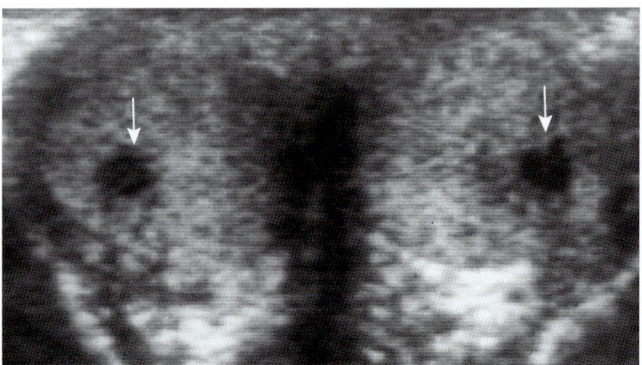

Figure 126-25   Adrenal rests. A transverse sonogram shows single echopenic masses (*arrows*) in both the right and left testes in a boy with congenital adrenal hyperplasia. (Courtesy Dr. Carlos Sivit, Cleveland, OH.)

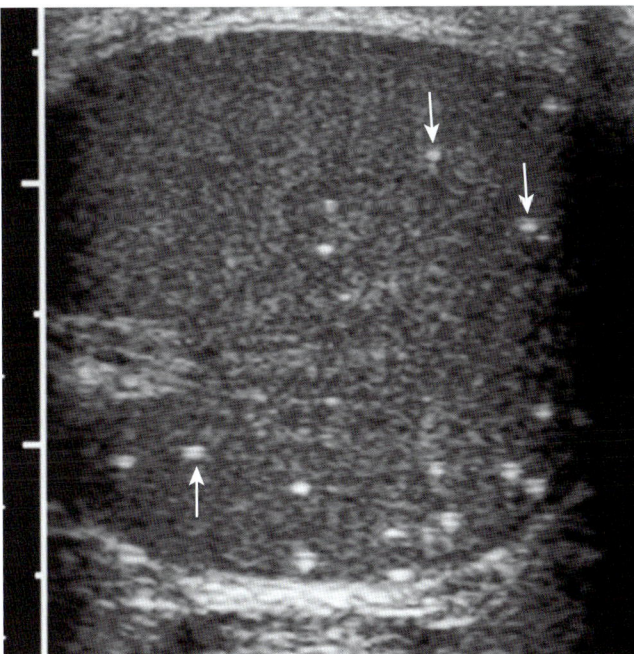

Figure 126-26 Testicular microlithiasis. An ultrasound image in the transverse plane shows several small, nonshadowing, hyperechoic foci (*arrows*) in this right testicle of an older teenager. This incidental finding of testicular microlithiasis was noted in both testes.

within the testicular parenchyma. Some clinicians reserve the diagnosis for cases in which more than five microliths are noted on a single ultrasound image (classic testicular microlithiasis). Testicular microlithiasis is reported in 2.4% of asymptomatic 0- to 19-year-old boys and also has been associated with cryptorchidism, infertility, male intersex, Klinefelter syndrome, and pulmonary alveolar microlithiasis. It usually is an incidental finding; however, there is a debated association between the presence of testicular microlithiasis and the presence or development of testicular neoplasm (reportedly 13 to 21.6 times greater risk), particularly germ cell neoplasia. Because of the association of microlithiasis and tumors, patients with testicular microlithiasis alone are followed up closely both clinically and by ultrasound (with follow-up by 6 months to 1 year) for possible tumor development.[1,43-48]

Intrascrotal Extratesticular Masses

PARATESTICULAR RHABDOMYOSARCOMA

Overview and Imaging Rhabdomyosarcoma is the most common malignant paratesticular mass in children, representing 10% of all intrascrotal tumors of childhood. It originates from the supporting stroma of the spermatic cord, testicular appendages, and paratesticular tunics and often is located superior to the testis. Two incidence peaks are seen for intrascrotal rhabdomyosarcoma, one at 2 to 4 years of age and the other between 15 and 17 years. Rhabdomyosarcomas present as a painless mass, grow rapidly, and frequently are large at presentation. They spread early to regional and retroperitoneal lymph nodes. Venous invasion and distant metastases, especially to the lungs, are not uncommon. On

Box 126-3 Grading of Varicoceles

Grade I (65%): Small varicoceles, appearing as only mild thickening of the spermatic cord

Grade II (24%): Moderate in size and consisting of a mass of veins up to 2 mm in diameter

Grade III (10%): Varicocele made up of individual veins greater than 2 mm in diameter

ultrasound examination, the mass is predominantly echogenic with focal anechoic areas caused by necrosis. As with all extratesticular masses, if the testes are invaded, differentiating the lesion from a mass of testicular origin may be difficult.[1]

VARICOCELES

Overview A common mass found within the scrotum of teenagers is a varicocele, which is composed of dilated veins of the pampiniform plexus. Varicoceles are graded according to their size (Box 126-3). When they are unilateral, 99% of varicoceles are left sided, where the spermatic vein enters the renal vein at a right angle. This anatomic situation is linked to a far greater incidence of venous incompetence compared with the right side, where the right spermatic vein enters the inferior vena cava directly at an oblique angle. The occurrence of bilateral varicoceles is common. However, finding a solitary right-sided varicocele is extremely uncommon, and the examiner must rule out an intraabdominal neoplasm or another mass as a cause.[1,6]

Imaging On ultrasound examination, varicoceles are tortuous, tubular, echo-free structures that typically are situated superior, lateral, and/or posterior to the testis (Fig. 126-27). The diagnosis is confirmed by having the patient perform a Valsalva maneuver, supine or standing, and noting on color Doppler imaging that the tubular vessels, which may not show flow before the maneuver, will fill with color (e-Fig. 126-28).

Treatment Surgical or interventional varicocele ligation is recommended in cases in which ipsilateral testicular volume loss of 2 mL or greater occurs. Histologic analysis of such testes has shown various degrees of tubal hypoplasia, decreased spermatogenesis, focal fibrosis, or arrest of germ cell maturation.[1,6,49-54]

WHAT THE CLINICIAN NEEDS TO KNOW

- Testicular size, symmetry, echogenicity, and lie within the scrotal sac
- The classification of hydroceles
- Nonpalpable testis on physical examination identifiable within the inguinal canal on ultrasound
- Testicular torsion versus a twisted appendage in patients with acute scrotal pain and swelling
- A testicular mass present in patients with painless testicular swelling
- Testicular versus paratesticular masses

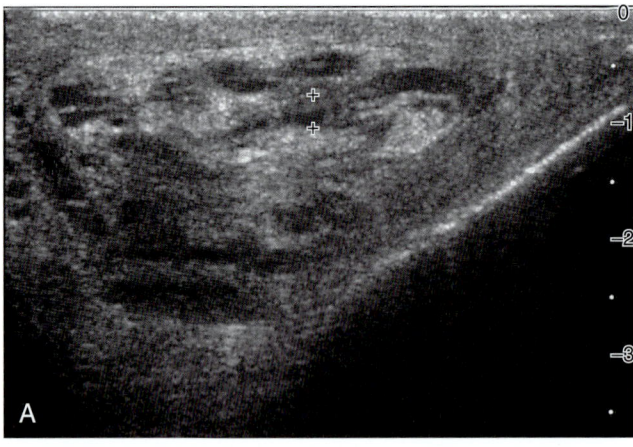
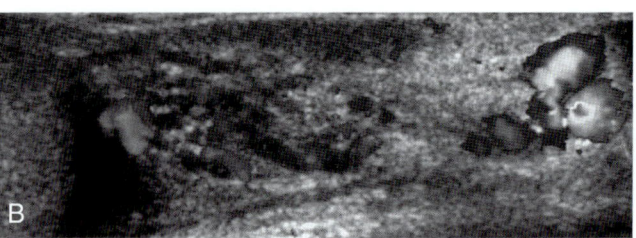

Figure 126-27 A varicocele. **A,** A transverse sonogram shows tubular echoless structures lateral to a teenager's left testis. One (*cursors*) is noted to be 2.7 mm wide. **B,** A color Doppler image during straining by the patient. Color fills several of the tubular structures. A venous spectral pattern was obtained, which proved that they were varicoceles. The normal testis is seen to the reader's left.

Key Points

An undescended abdominal testis has a 10 to 40 times greater risk for a future malignancy.

A hydrocele is the most common scrotal mass in a child.

Testicular (and epididymal) appendages most typically torse in the 6- to 12-year-old age group.

Epididymitis is the most common cause of an acute painful scrotum in the postpubescent male.

Testicular torsion diagnosed in the newborn period usually presents as a painless, firm scrotal mass often associated with bluish red discoloration of the scrotum.

Viable torsed testes undergo orchiopexy; nonviable testes are removed. Preventive orchiopexy is performed on the contralateral normal testis.

Yolk sac tumor is the most common germ cell tumor in children.

Rhabdomyosarcoma is the most common malignant paratesticular mass in children.

Unilateral right-sided varicoceles raise concern for an intraabdominal mass.

Suggested Readings

Ahmed HU, Arya M, Muneer A, et al. Testicular and paratesticular tumours in the prepubertal population. *Lancet Oncol.* 2010;11(5):476-483.

Akbar SA, Sayyed TA, Jafri SZ, et al. Multimodality imaging of paratesticular neoplasms and their rare mimics. *Radiographics.* 2003;23(6):1461-1476.

Coley BD. Sonography of pediatric scrotal swelling. *Semin Ultrasound CT MR.* 2007;28(4):297-306.

Hörmann M, Balassy C, Philipp MO, et al. Imaging of the scrotum in children. *Eur Radiol.* 2004;14(6):974-983.

Karmazyn B, Steinberg R, Livne P, et al. Duplex sonographic findings in children with torsion of the testicular appendages: overlap with epididymitis and epididymoorchitis. *J Pediatr Surg.* 2006;41(3):500-504.

Marulaiah M, Gilhotra A, Moore L, et al. Testicular and paratesticular pathology in children: a 12-year histopathological review. *World J Surg.* 2010;34(5):969-974.

Munden MM, Trautwein LM. Scrotal pathology in pediatrics with sonographic imaging. *Curr Probl Diagn Radiol.* 2000;29(6):185-205.

References

Full references for this chapter can be found on www.expertconsult.com.

Chapter 127

Abnormalities of the Female Genital Tract

HARRIS L. COHEN and ANAND DORAI RAJU

Imaging Techniques

Ultrasound is the key technique used in the analysis of the pediatric gynecologic tract, its diseases, and the simulators of those diseases. Ultrasound provides quick analysis of the uterus, ovaries, and cul-de-sac. Computed tomography (CT) and magnetic resonance imaging (MRI) provide a more global view of the pelvis and abdomen than does ultrasound, and they are preferred for the analysis of tumor extent and metastases. The drawbacks of radiation exposure for CT, less control of the patient's environment for CT and MRI, and sedation needs for MRI are of particular relevance in pediatric patients.[1-3]

Ovarian and Uterine Development

THE NORMAL OVARY

Overview and Imaging The two ovaries are ovoid structures generally located posterior or lateral to the uterus within the mesovarium of the broad ligament. Ovaries may be located anywhere along their embryologic course from the inferior border of the kidney to the broad ligament. Ovaries may be involved in indirect inguinal hernias, 15% of which occur in females. Herniated ovaries can extend as low as the labia (e-Fig. 127-1), the female equivalent of the scrotum.[1-5]

Adnexal volume is determined by ultrasound using the formula for a modified prolate ellipse: $(0.523) \times L \times W \times D$. Length (L) and depth (D) usually are measured on a longitudinal (parasagittal) image, and width (W) is measured on a transverse view (Fig. 127-2). In the first 3 months of life, when gonadotropin levels are highest in children, ovarian volumes average 1.06 cm^3 but have a range of normal as high as 3.6 cm^3. The high end of the range of normal is 2.7 cm^3 for 4- to 12-month-olds and 1.7 cm^3 for 13- to 24-month-olds. The mean ovarian volume reported for children older than 2 years who have not undergone puberty is 1 cm^3. For menstruating females, the mean ovarian volume typically is 6 to 9.8 cm^3.[1,6-10]

Ultrasound routinely identifies follicles or cysts in most children of all ages. Cysts were noted in 80% of the imaged ovaries of a group of healthy children who were newborn to 2 years old, 72% of a 2- to 6-year-old group, and 68% of a 7- to 10-year-old group (Fig. 127-3). Macrocysts occasionally are seen in all age groups. The ovary is not a quiescent organ in childhood but rather is a dynamic organ undergoing constant internal change.[1,11]

THE NORMAL UTERUS

Overview and Imaging The uterus of the newborn has a mean length of 3.5 cm, which decreases to 2.6 to 3 cm by the fourth month of life as gonadotropin levels decrease. On ultrasound examination of a newborn's uterus, it is not uncommon to find either a hypoechoic halo around an echogenic endometrial cavity stripe or endometrial cavity fluid.[1,3,12] The typical newborn's uterus is shaped like a spade, with the anteroposterior diameter of the cervix as much as twice that of its fundus (Fig. 127-4). The newborn's cervix is also longer than the fundus. After the first year of life, the typical uterus is tube shaped and remains that way for several years (e-Fig. 127-5).[1,3,13]

Uterine length increases gradually between 3 and 8 years of age. The mean perimenarchal measurement is 4.3 cm. After puberty, the typical pear-shaped (Fig. 127-6) uterus measures 5 to 8 cm in length. It is said to descend deeper in the pelvis and no longer maintains the typical neutral position of premenarchal life but instead may be anteverted or retroverted.[1,14]

Nonneoplastic Disorders of the Female Pelvis

MÜLLERIAN DUCT ANOMALIES

Overview The müllerian duct system (MDS) develops into the fallopian tubes, uterus, and upper two thirds of the vagina, and the wolffian system degenerates. External genital development proceeds along female lines except in the presence of androgens. By 11 weeks, a Y-shaped uterovaginal primordium has developed into the two fallopian tubes and, with fusion of a large portion of the MDS of both sides, a single uterus and upper two thirds of the vagina. Nonfusion or variably incomplete fusion of the MDS can lead to a wide spectrum of anomalies (Fig. 127-7). The association of uterine and renal abnormalities is quite common, and when a gynecologic anomaly is present, one should evaluate for renal anomalies or agenesis (e-Fig. 127-8) and vice versa.[1,15]

TRANSVERSE VAGINAL SEPTUM AND IMPERFORATE HYMEN

Overview In a person with a transverse vaginal septum, the vagina is obliterated by fibrous connective tissue with vascular and muscular elements lined by squamous epithelium. The

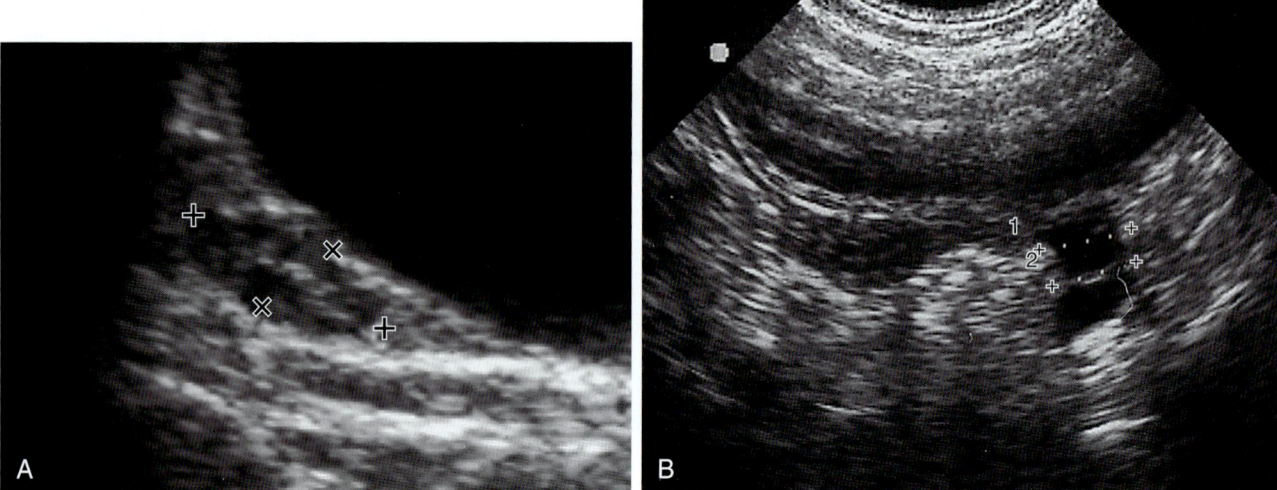

Figure 127-2   A, A normal prepubertal ovary. A longitudinal sonogram shows a normal left ovary (*cursors*). A few echoless follicles are seen within the ovary. **B,** A transverse sonogram in a prepubertal 6-year-old shows two cysts (*cursors*) in an ovary lateral to the uterus. Bladder fluid is filled in by near-field artifact.

area of obliteration may be a thin membrane, but more commonly it involves a segment of the vagina (segmental vaginal atresia). The imperforate hymen is a thin membrane, which forms at the junction of the caudal end of the MDS and the cranial end of the urogenital sinus. Both a transverse vaginal septum and imperforate hymen may present with an obstructed uterus and vagina.[1,12,16-19]

A distended vagina (colpos) or uterus (metros) is filled with secretions (muco), fluid (hydro), or blood (hemato). For example, hematometrocolpos is defined as hemorrhagic material filling a distended vagina and uterus. It is suggested on physical examination by either seeing an interlabial mass or palpating a pelvic mass. Clinical presentation in the teenage years includes amenorrhea (despite normal development of secondary sex characteristics) and cyclic crampy abdominal pains, or a pelvic mass resulting from accumulation of menstrual blood in the proximal vagina (and uterus and tubes).

Complete or partial obstructions may occur in association with various MDS anomalies.[1,15,20-22]

Imaging Ultrasound images are similar in appearance whether seen in a neonate or a menarchal teenager. The distended vagina appears as a tubular mass that usually is midline, often with contained echogenicities either from accumulated cervical mucus secretions or hemorrhage from sloughing of a hormonally stimulated endometrial lining. The uterus can be identified separately from the vagina by the thick muscular uterine wall, whereas the vaginal wall is thin

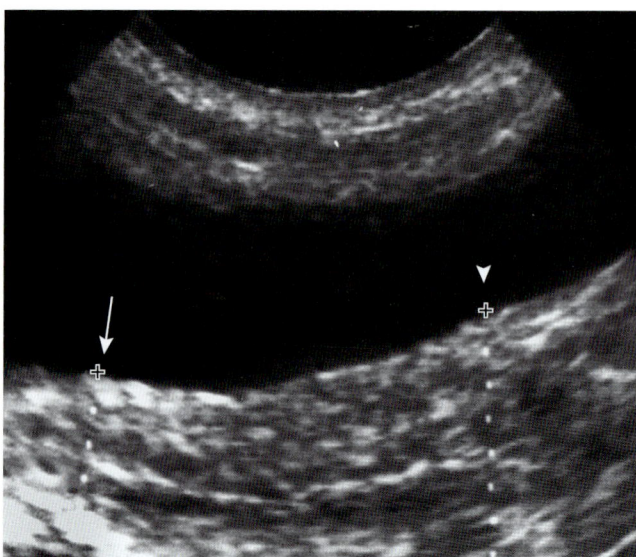

Figure 127-4   A normal neonatal uterus. A longitudinal sonogram shows a spade-shaped uterus posterior to the bladder. Cursors (*arrow*) show a relatively narrow uterine fundus compared with the far wider cervical region (*arrowhead*) of the newborn's uterus. Note the central echogenic line, which is the endometrial cavity. (From Cohen HL. The female pelvis. In: Siebert J, ed. *Syllabus: current concepts: a categorical course in pediatric radiology.* Chicago: RSNA Publications; 1994.)

Figure 127-3   A normal infant ovary. A transverse sonogram shows cursors marking the width of an ovary (*2*) and a contained follicle (*1*), which is common in infants such as this 2-month-old. The left adnexum (*arrow*) also can be seen with contained follicles.

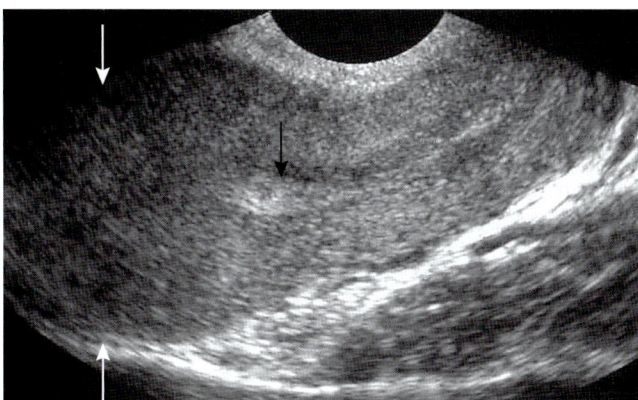

Figure 127-6 A normal postmenarchal uterus. On this transvaginal sagittal sonogram of a sexually active teenager, white arrows mark off the widest part of the uterus, the fundus. The cervix, to the right, is far less wide. A black arrow points to the patient's normal endometrial cavity echogenicity.

(Fig. 127-9). Pelvic MRI in the sagittal or coronal plane can show the dilated vagina as well (Fig. 127-10).[1,15,16,23,24]

Treatment The vaginal obstruction in patients with congenital hydrocolpos is corrected in the newborn period. In patients presenting with hematometrocolpos at puberty, the obstruction should be corrected as promptly as possible to avoid endometriosis as a result of distal obstruction and repeated reverse spillage of menstrual blood into the peritoneal cavity through the fallopian tubes. Hysterectomy is indicated in patients with vaginal agenesis with a rudimentary uterus and a functional endometrium and in patients with cervical atresia occurring as an isolated lesion or in

association with vaginal agenesis (Mayer-Rokitansky-Küster-Hauser syndrome).[1,3,22-25]

INTERLABIAL MASSES IN YOUNG GIRLS

Overview and Imaging The differential diagnosis of interlabial masses is usually made on visual inspection based on the location and external appearance of the mass. Masses associated with the urethral orifice include prolapse of an ectopic ureterocele—identified as a small, reddened, doughnutlike mass with its central opening being the urethral meatus itself—and cystic dilatation of an obstructed paraurethral (Skene) gland, presenting as a mass located on either side of a displaced urethral meatus. Masses associated with the vaginal introitus include prolapse of a vaginal cyst; a remnant of the wolffian or müllerian duct systems or epithelial inclusions originating from elements of the urogenital sinus; an imperforate hymen (e-Fig. 127-11); cystic dilatation of an obstructed Bartholin gland; and prolapse of a sarcoma botryoides or rhabdomyosarcoma of the vagina.[1,3,7]

A cystogram or vaginogram, as well as ultrasound of the bladder and upper genitourinary tract, may be necessary to further define the lesion. CT or MRI may help if continued anatomic questions remain. At times, only surgery is conclusive.[1,7,22]

PELVIC INFLAMMATORY DISEASE

Overview Pelvic inflammatory disease (PID) is the most serious complication of sexually transmitted diseases. PID includes a spectrum of abnormality that ranges from isolated endometritis to extension of infection into the tubes (salpingitis) and ovaries (oophoritis), potentially resulting in a

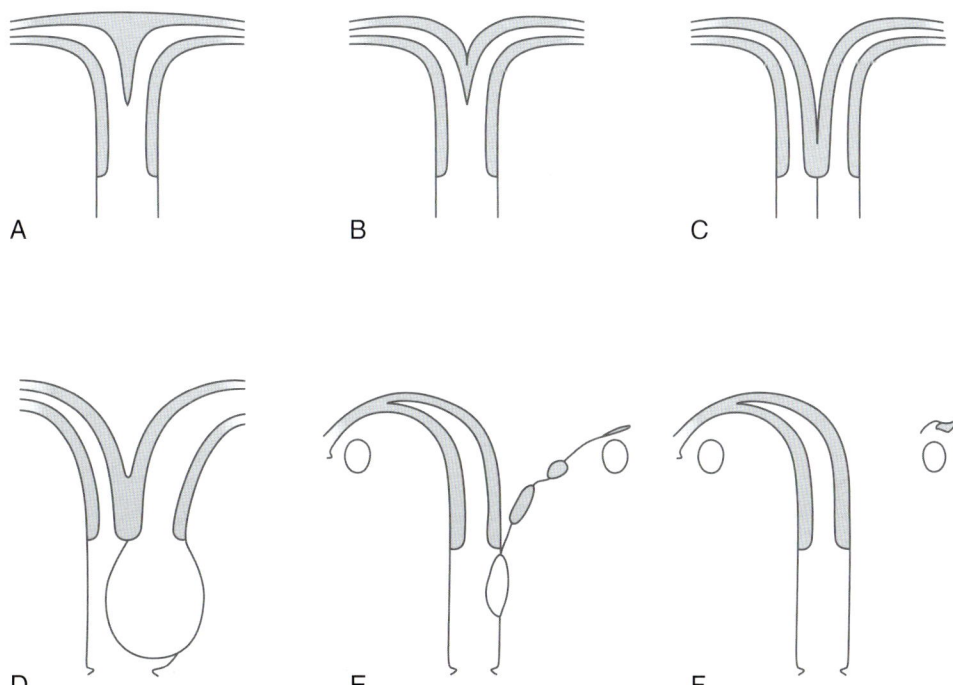

Figure 127-7 Fusion defects of the müllerian ducts (septate vagina with normal uterus not included). **A,** Uterus subseptus (uterus septus if the septum extends to the cervix). **B,** Uterus bicornis unicollis. **C,** Uterus duplex bicornis bicollis and uterus didelphys with a septate vagina. **D,** Uterus didelphys with congenital occlusion of one hemivagina. **E** and **F,** A rudimentary hemiuterus and unicornuate uterus.

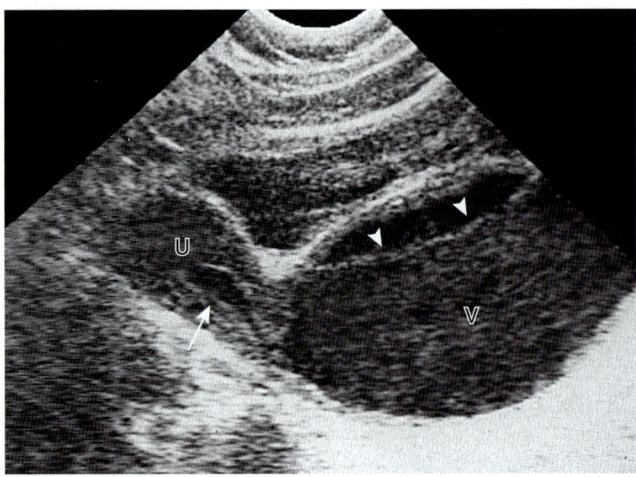

Figure 127-9 Hematometrocolpos. A longitudinal sonogram in this patient with pelvic pain and amenorrhea shows a dilated vagina (*V*). It contains debris with a fluid-debris level (*arrowheads*) anteriorly. The uterus (*U*) has a smaller amount of contained fluid (*arrow*). The uterus can be distinguished from the vagina by its thick muscular wall. The cause in this patient was an imperforate hymen. (From Cohen H, Haller J. Pediatric and adolescent genital abnormalities. *Clin Diagn Ultrasound.* 1988;24:187-216.)

tuboovarian abscess (TOA), and even extension into the peritoneum as disseminated peritonitis. *Neisseria gonorrhoeae* and *Chlamydia trachomatis* are the most common etiologic agents.[1,26,27]

Clinical presentation includes lower abdominal/pelvic pain, purulent vaginal discharge, fever, leukocytosis, and an elevated erythrocyte sedimentation rate. Adnexal tenderness, generally bilateral, and cervical motion tenderness are hallmarks for the clinical diagnosis on bimanual examination.[1,26,27]

Imaging and Treatment Early in the course of PID or salpingitis, no abnormal ultrasound findings may be present, and the diagnosis will be based solely on clinical and laboratory evaluation. A helpful ultrasound finding in cases of salpingo-oophoritis is prominent ovaries that may be adherent to the uterus (e-Fig. 127-12). More advanced cases of acute or, more often, chronic PID may demonstrate evidence of hydrosalpinx, pyosalpinx, or TOA. The affected tubal walls may be thickened with intraluminal linear echoes. The echogenicity of the fluid within the fallopian tube is not a reliable indicator of the presence or absence of infection (Fig. 127-13). TOA appears on ultrasound as partial or complete replacement of the normal ovarian tissue by a heterogeneous mass or an echopenic region with contained debris (Fig. 127-14). The contents (debris filled) of the echopenic areas of a TOA often can be better seen by transvaginal ultrasound examination. TOA usually is treated aggressively with intravenous antibiotic regimens and, if necessary, percutaneous drainage or surgery.[1,27,28]

OVARIAN TORSION

Overview Ovarian torsion is caused by partial or complete rotation of the ovary on its pedicle, compromising first lymphatic, then venous, and finally arterial flow, and leading to hemorrhagic infarction. Torsion of the ovary is most often seen in peripubertal or older girls. Ovarian torsion occurs either in anatomically normal ovaries or in ovaries with an associated ovarian or paraovarian mass or neoplasm.[1,29,30]

Classic ovarian torsion pain is sudden and acute. Associated complaints of nausea, vomiting, or constipation may occur and mislead the clinician. Fever is rare. Leukocytosis with a left shift may be present. At least half of patients with ovarian torsion claim prior bouts of such pain, suggesting previous torsion and detorsion.[1,29,30]

Imaging Ovaries involved in torsion have a variable appearance related to the degree of internal hemorrhage, stromal edema, and infarction that has occurred by the time they are imaged. The ovaries may appear cystic, cystic with septations, cystic with a debris layer, complex with mixed solid and cystic components, or solid. One relatively specific ultrasound image is a unilaterally enlarged solid ovary with multiple peripheral (cortical zone) follicles (Fig. 127-15).[1,31]

An acute ovary that has sustained torsion is larger than a normal ovary. Reported volumes range from only 3.2 to 24 times normal, to ovarian volumes of 150 cm³ or greater in postmenarchal patients. Comparison with the volume and morphology of the contralateral ovary may help make the diagnosis under the appropriate clinical circumstances.[1,30,31]

Color Doppler imaging in the analysis of cases of ovarian torsion is confusing with regard to its reliability. Well-documented cases exist of surgically proven ovaries that had undergone torsion for which color Doppler imaging showed peripheral and even central arterial flow. Other investigators have reported that an assurance of viability can only be made by imaging central venous flow in an ovary that has undergone torsion. An 87% diagnostic accuracy for determining viability is reported by verifying blood flow changes at the twisted vascular pedicle itself. Patients with no blood flow at the twisted pedicle had necrotic ovaries.[1,32-34]

Treatment It is hoped that detorsion and, if necessary, removal of a mass causing torsion will save the gonad and preserve its function. The time from clinical complaint to diagnosis and therapy plays a large role in preserving ovarian function. Doppler imaging may have a role in assessing the recovery of an ovary that has undergone torsion in follow-up studies after surgical treatment.[1,35,36]

OVARIAN MASSES

Ovarian Cysts

Overview and Imaging Nonneoplastic cysts of follicular origin (i.e., functional ovarian cysts) are the most common cause of ovarian enlargement. Beyond puberty, the adolescent ovary is similar to that of the adult, developing several follicles early in the menstrual cycle until a dominant follicle develops and ruptures at midcycle, while the others atrophy and resorb. Occasionally one or more of these follicles fails to resorb and instead enlarges as a functional cyst or as a retention cyst. These cysts can reach a large size but usually are no larger than 3 cm. The classic cyst on ultrasound examination is echoless with a sharp back wall and excellent through-transmission. Most functional ovarian cysts are treated conservatively and resolve spontaneously. A 6-week follow-up evaluation allows analysis of the possible ovarian cyst in the other half of a different menstrual cycle, thus documenting resolution or diminution and thereby helping

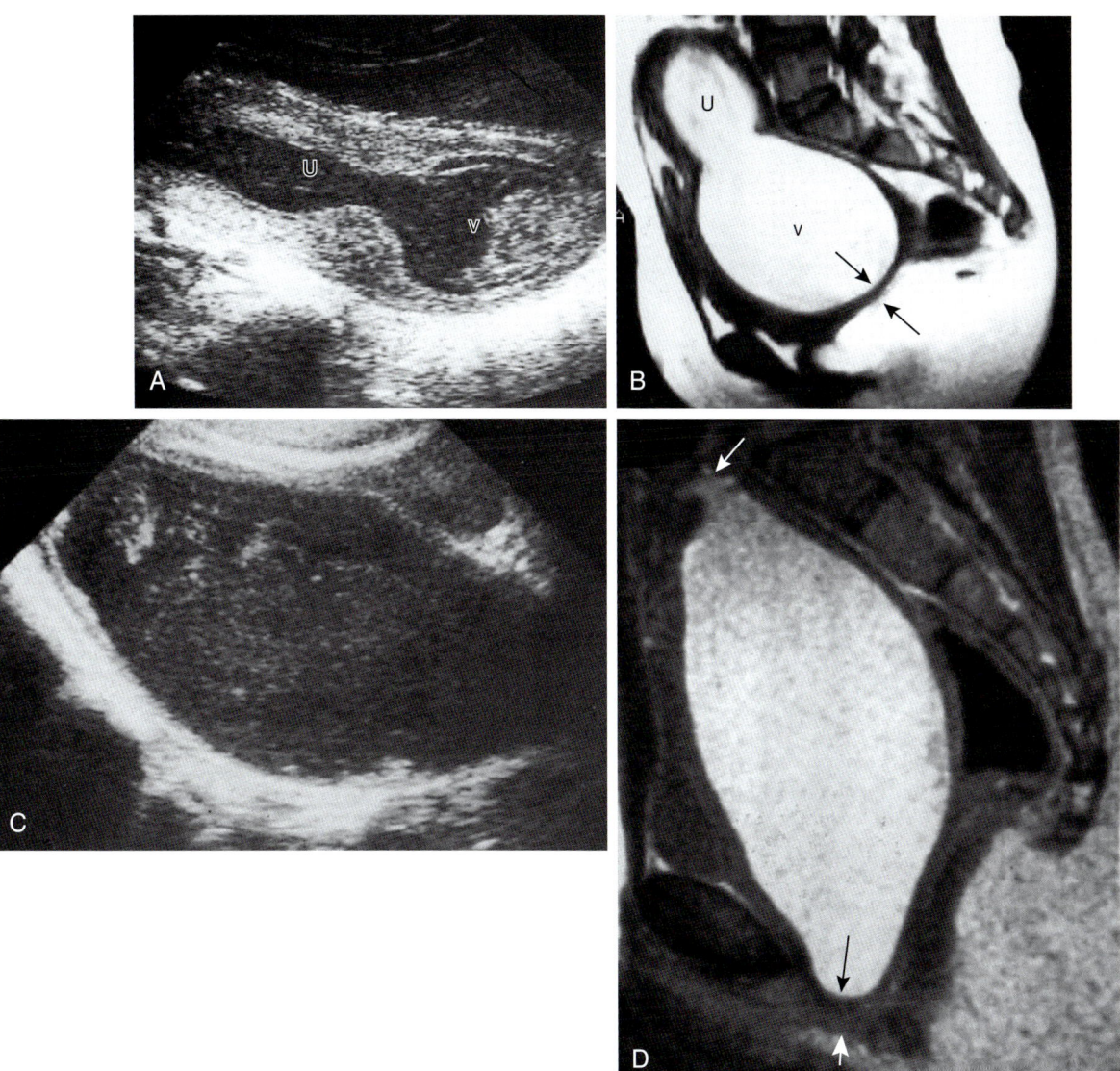

Figure 127-10 Hematometrocolpos from an imperforate hymen. **A,** A longitudinal sonogram shows a large midline cystic structure consistent with a distended vagina (v) and uterus (U). The lower part of the vagina contains echogenic material. The patient is a 13-year-old girl who was evaluated because of crampy abdominal pain and a pelvic mass. The external genitalia appeared normal on inspection. **B,** A midline sagittal T2-weighted magnetic resonance image (MRI) obtained for presurgical planning shows an enlarged vagina (v) and uterus (U) filled with material consistent with old blood. The obstruction is in the distal vagina and measures 0.5 cm in thickness (arrows). At surgery, this was either a very low vaginal septum or a very thick imperforate hymen. **C** and **D**, Hematocolpos from vaginal atresia in a 12-year-old girl who underwent examination because of crampy abdominal pain and a pelvic mass. **C,** A longitudinal sonogram shows a large midline cystic structure containing debris consistent with hematocolpos. **D,** A midsagittal T2-weighted MRI shows a markedly distended vagina filled with material consistent with old blood. The uterus (top arrow) is not enlarged. The occlusion is in the distal segment of the vagina and measures more than 0.5 cm in thickness (bottom arrows). At surgery, the obstruction was found to be a thick vaginal septum or a short zone of vaginal atresia.

to prove that it is a physiologic cyst and helping to disprove the far less likely diagnosis of a cystic neoplasm.[1,37-40]

Hemorrhagic Ovarian Cysts

Overview Functional cysts may develop internal hemorrhage, which occurs when theca interna vessels rupture into the cyst cavity. Such hemorrhagic ovarian cysts can arise from ovarian follicles at any stage in their maturation, even as they involute. The typical clinical presentation of a hemorrhagic ovarian cyst is either sudden, severe, transient lower abdominal pain of 1 to 3 hours' duration or lower abdominal pain

and a palpable mass. The pain is thought to result from sudden distention of the ovarian cyst by the hemorrhage.[1,41]

Imaging Most hemorrhagic ovarian cysts are heterogeneous in echogenicity. They may be hypoechoic or hyperechoic areas separated by thin or thick linear echoes of various orientations (Fig. 127-16), echoless with a contained focal echogenicity of variable size clot, contain fluid-debris levels, or appear as a solid mass when clot fills the hemorrhagic ovarian cyst. A changing ultrasound appearance over time can help confirm the diagnosis as fibrin deposition from acute hemorrhaging dissolves and the clot lyses.[1,38,41]

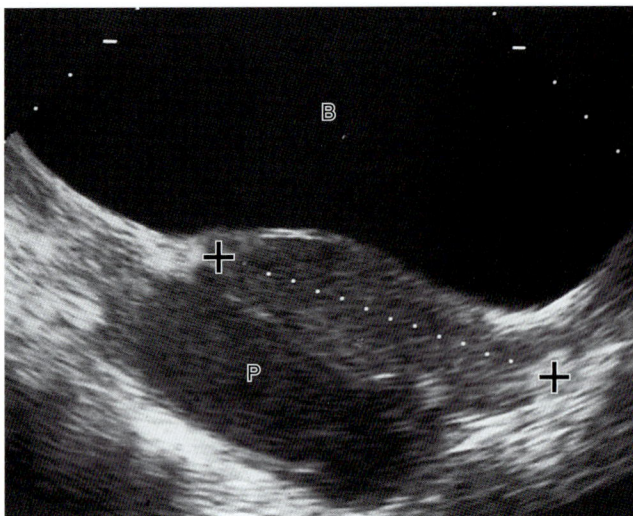

Figure 127-13 Pyosalpinx. A midline longitudinal sonogram shows a fluid-filled tubular structure (*P*), allowing good through-transmission of sound, located posterior to the uterus (*cursors*). It contains debris and was determined to be a pyosalpinx. *B*, Bladder.

POLYCYSTIC OVARY SYNDROME

Overview Polycystic ovary syndrome (PCOS; also known as Stein-Leventhal syndrome) is a hyperandrogenic state with resultant peripheral conversion of larger than normal amounts of estrogen. The chronic hyperestrogenic, hyperandrogenic stimulation leads to chronic anovulation and is responsible for the classic bilaterally enlarged ovaries, which may be asymmetric but usually contain multiple small follicles/cysts. PCOS is the most common pathologic cause of amenorrhea, usually secondary, in adolescents and young adults. Patients often, but far from always, experience the classic triad of obesity (31%), hirsutism (62%), and menstrual abnormalities (80%), including amenorrhea, irregular menses, and prolonged uterine bleeding. Laboratory diagnosis is made by

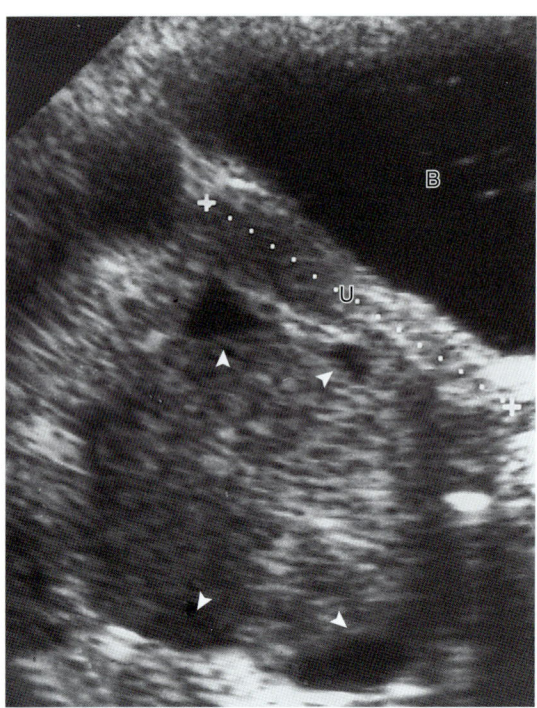

Figure 127-15 Ovarian torsion. A longitudinal sonogram shows a tubular uterus (*U; cursors*) that is posterior to the bladder (*B*) and anterior to a large solid mass with a few peripheral cysts (*arrowheads*). This image is a relatively classic image of early torsion. Infarction or acute hemorrhage would make the internal contents of the ovary that is undergoing torsion more heterogeneous. (From Cohen HL, Safriel YI. Ovarian torsion. In: Cohen HL, Sivit C, eds. *Fetal and pediatric ultrasound: A casebook approach.* New York: McGraw-Hill; 2001:516.)

noting increased luteinizing hormone:follicle-stimulating hormone ratios and elevated androstenedione levels.[1,42]

Imaging A helpful indicator of PCOS is increased ovarian echogenicity, which is thought to be due to ovarian stromal

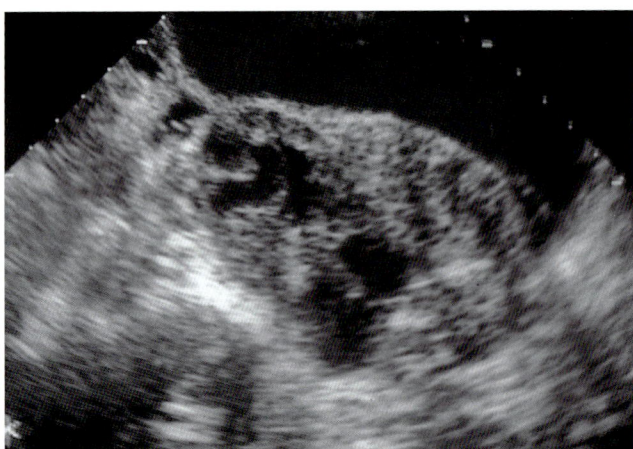

Figure 127-14 A tuboovarian abscess in a teenager with a history of pelvic inflammatory disease. An oblique transverse sonogram of the right adnexa shows a large, heterogeneous, oval structure with contained echoless circular and tubular structures that were not typical of normal follicles or cysts on transverse or longitudinal images. At times a dilated fallopian tube arising from a tuboovarian abscess accounts for part of the contained cystic structure. This scenario is most likely when the structure appears tubular in at least one of the imaged planes.

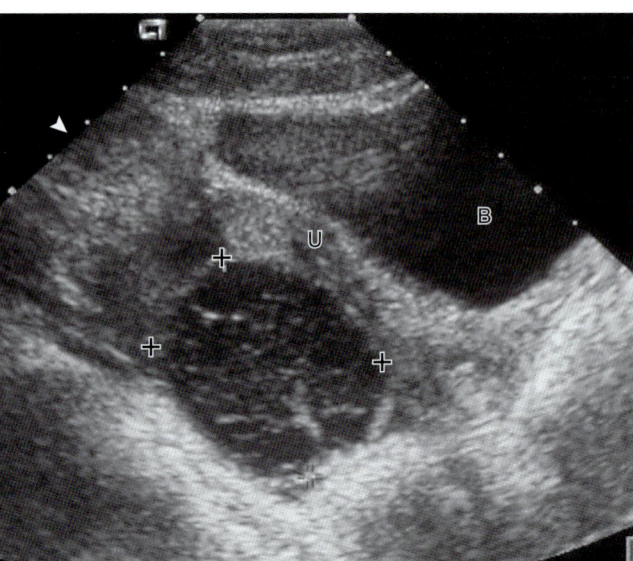

Figure 127-16 A hemorrhagic ovarian cyst. A longitudinal sonogram shows an echopenic mass (*cursors*) containing criss-crossing linear echogenicities in the adnexal area of a 12-year-old with acute abdominal pain. A tuboovarian abscess and endometrioma may look similar but present with different clinical scenarios. *B*, Bladder; *U*, uterus.

hypertrophy, which is considered to be evidence of hyper-androgenism. Persons with PCOS have high numbers of subcapsular follicles in their ovaries (Fig. 127-17). Typically, at least five cysts of 5 to 8 mm in diameter are noted on transabdominal ultrasound evaluation of each ovary. Follicles of classic cases should not be larger than 10 mm in diameter. Larger follicles or the presence of a single large (dominant) cyst makes the diagnosis of PCOS unlikely. Ovarian volumes may or may not be greater than the mean for their control group.[1,43-46]

Neoplasms of the Gynecologic Tract

VAGINA AND UTERUS

Overview and Imaging   Embryonal rhabdomyosarcoma is the most common genital neoplasm in children of both sexes. It generally is seen before the age of 3 years but rarely at birth.

It is rare in older patients. Urogenital sinus remnants are thought to be the origin of some rhabdomyosarcomas, usually originating from the anterior vagina near the cervix. Occasionally they may arise from the cervix. The mass may protrude from the vaginal introitus, often with a polypoid or cluster-of-grapes appearance (botryoid variant). These rhabdomyosarcomas are aggressive tumors that spread rapidly by direct invasion of the vaginal wall and pelvic structures. The tumor may extend to the uterus, bladder, ureters, or rectum. Metastases to regional lymph nodes, the lungs, and other organs may occur. Local recurrence is common.[1,47-49]

Endodermal sinus tumor of the vagina, also known as yolk sac carcinoma or adenocarcinoma of the infant vagina, usually is seen in infants between 8 and 15 months and rarely after the second year. It often originates in the posterior wall of the vagina (e-Fig. 127-18) and may have a polypoid appearance very similar to that of sarcoma botryoides. The tumor spreads to pelvic soft tissues, paraaortic nodes, liver, and lungs.[1,47,49]

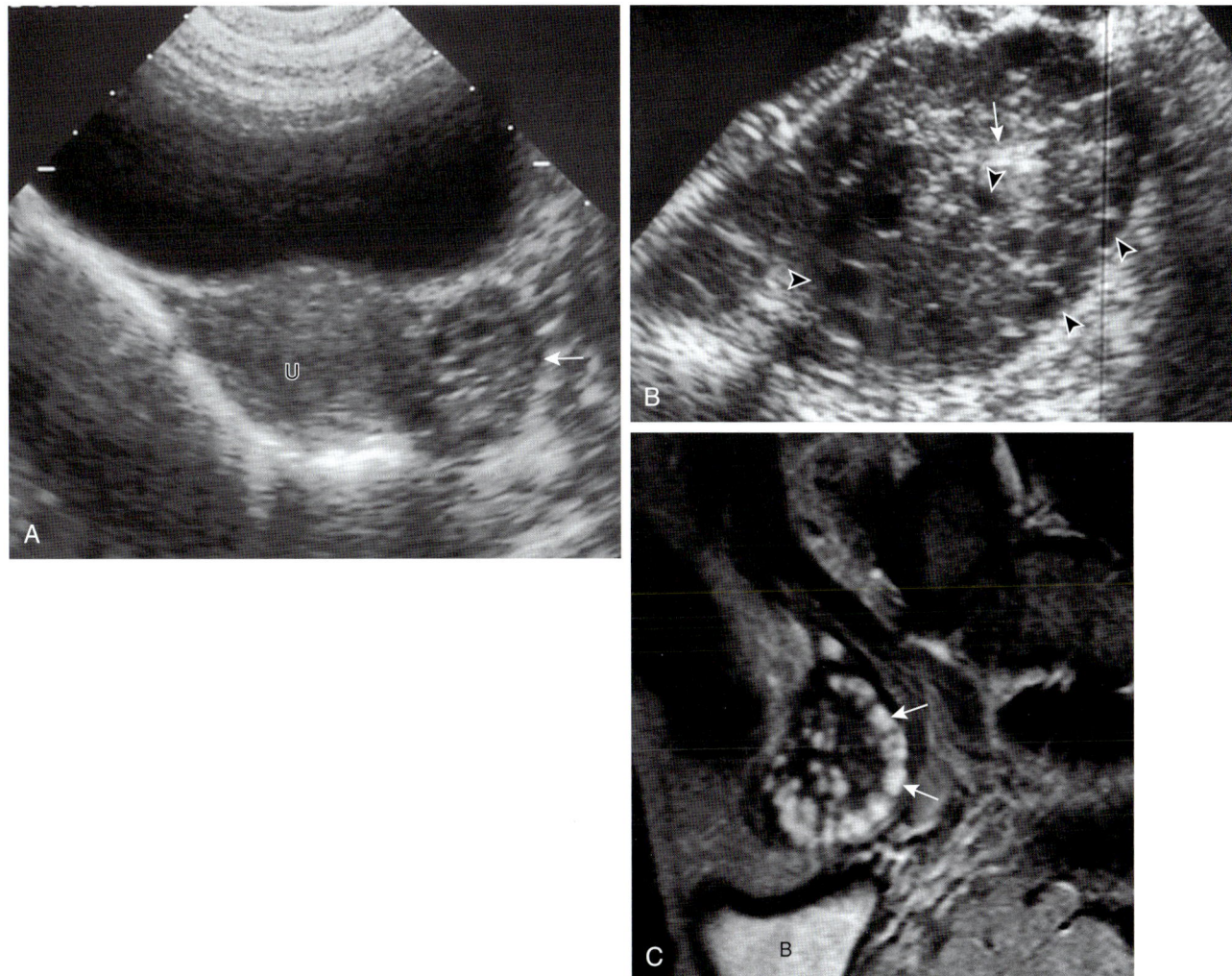

Figure 127-17   Polycystic ovarian disease. **A,** A transverse sonogram shows an enlarged left ovary (*arrow*) containing multiple small follicles is seen adjacent to the uterus (*U*). A similar right ovary was seen in another plane. The echogenicity of the ovarian stroma is increased. **B,** A transvaginal sagittal sonogram shows many small follicles (*arrowheads*) seen within the ovary of a teen with polycystic ovary syndrome. Some bright echogenicity (*arrow*), which is not seen in normal ovaries, is noted in the superior third of this imaged ovary. **C,** A sagittal T2-weighted magnetic resonance image shows multiple cortical cysts, particularly at the periphery of the right ovary of a teenager proved to have polycystic ovary syndrome. The ovary is superior to the bladder (*B*), and its follicles/cysts (*arrows*) have similar high signal intensity. (**A** and **B** from Cohen HL, Ruggiero-Delliturri M. Polycystic ovary syndrome. In: Cohen HL, Sivit C, eds. *Fetal and pediatric ultrasound: A casebook approach.* New York: McGraw-Hill; 2001:496. **C** courtesy Mark Flyer, MD.)

Clear cell (or mesonephric) adenocarcinoma usually originates from the vagina and uncommonly from the cervix. It usually is seen after menarche. In the past few decades, about two thirds of patients with this tumor had a history of maternal exposure to diethylstilbestrol or related substances during the first 3 months of pregnancy. These tumors can become quite large, filling the entire vagina by the time of diagnosis. Tumor spread is via the lymphatics and to pelvic nodes. Local recurrence is common. Pulmonary metastases can occur.[1,47,49]

OVARY

Overview Ovarian neoplasms commonly are divided into groups based on the apparent origin of their cellular components: germ cell tumors, sex cord/stromal tumors, and surface epithelial tumors. Sixty percent of all pediatric ovarian neoplasms are of germ cell origin. Of the germ cell tumors, 70% are teratomas, 25% are dysgerminomas, and 5% are endodermal sinus or yolk sac tumors. Only one fifth of pediatric ovarian tumors are epithelial cell in origin, including cystadenoma (80%) and cystadenocarcinoma (10%). The final 10% of pediatric ovarian tumors are sex cord tumors or tumors of stromal/mesenchymal origin. Fifteen percent of those are arrhenoblastomas and 75% are granulosa/theca cell tumors.[1,47,48]

Overall, one third of ovarian neoplasms are malignant. This percentage decreases with increasing age. Half of hormonally active tumors are malignant. Of the malignant lesions, 85% are germ cell tumors (dysgerminomas, immature teratomas, endodermal sinus tumors, embryonal cell carcinomas, and choriocarcinomas); 10% are stromal (Sertoli–Leydig cell, granulosa/theca cell, and undifferentiated neoplasms); and 5% are epithelial cell tumors (serous and mucinous adenocarcinomas). Malignant neoplasms tend to break through the ovary's capsule and invade adjacent organs. Metastases are most often to the peritoneum, opposite ovary, pelvic and retroperitoneal lymph nodes, omentum, liver, and abdominal organs (e-Fig. 127-19). Involvement of peritoneal and pleural linings may lead to ascites or pleural effusions (Box 127-1).[1,47,50]

Ovarian Teratomas

Overview Mature ovarian teratomas (or dermoid cysts) are the most common ovarian neoplasm in pediatric patients and usually are found in adolescents. The tumors may vary in size from those contained solely within the ovary itself to those that extend 5 to 10 cm beyond the ovary. Almost all dermoids and teratomas are benign, with malignancy found in 2% to 10% of cases or less. Teratomas usually are discovered by chance during pelvic ultrasound examinations performed on adolescents for other reasons; one fourth are bilateral. Occasionally they may be diagnosed by the incidental discovery of calcifications (particularly teeth or bone) in the adnexal area on plain radiograph examination (e-Fig. 127-20).[1,50,51]

Imaging Two thirds of teratomas are sonographically complex cysts with anechoic, hypoechoic, and echogenic components. One third of cases are claimed to be either

---

Box 127-1 Staging for Ovarian Neoplasms
Stage I: Tumor limited to the ovaries
Stage IA: Tumor limited to one ovary, no malignant ascites
Stage IB: Tumor limited to both ovaries, no malignant ascites
Stage IC: Stage IA or IB with malignant ascites
Stage II: Tumor involves one or both ovaries with pelvic extension
Stage IIA: Extension or implants on the uterus or fallopian tubes, no malignant ascites
Stage IIB: Extension to other pelvic tissues, no malignant ascites
Stage IIC: Stage IIA or IIB with malignant ascites
Stage III: Tumor involves one or both ovaries with peritoneal implants outside the pelvis or retroperitoneal lymph node metastasis
Stage IIIA: Microscopic peritoneal metastasis beyond the pelvis
Stage IIIB: Macroscopic peritoneal metastasis beyond the pelvis 2 cm or less
Stage IIIC: Peritoneal metastasis beyond the pelvis more than 2 cm or regional lymph node metastasis
Stage IV: Distant metastasis including liver parenchyma
Based on the American Joint Committee on Cancer and the International Federation of Gynecology and Obstetrics staging of carcinoma of the ovary.

Modified from Emans S, Laufer M, Goldstein D, eds. *Pediatric and adolescent gynecology.* 5th ed. Philadelphia: Lippincott Williams & Wilkins; 2005.

---

purely echoless (perhaps because the solid component is at the mass's periphery and not imaged) or purely echogenic. The classic ultrasound appearance shows a prominent cystic component and at least one contained mural nodule (a dermoid plug or Rokitansky projection) (Fig. 127-21) that often is echogenic, with posterior shadowing as a result of contained fat, hair, sebum, or calcium (e.g., tooth or bone). The shadowing may obscure deeper portions of the mass, a phenomenon called the "tip of the iceberg" sign. The anechoic component of teratomas is made up of serous fluid or sebum, which is in a fluid state when at body temperature. Fat–fluid levels and hair–fluid levels may be seen as part of the cystic component. Similar findings are seen on CT (Fig. 127-22) or MRI. CT may show calcifications that are not seen by other methods. MRI is particularly valuable in demonstrating the fatty components of the mass. Signal characteristics on MRI reflect the composition of a teratoma. Calcium, bone, and hair have low signal intensity on both T1- and T2-weighted images. Fat has a high signal on T1-weighted studies. Fluid has a high signal on T2-weighted studies. Immature, partially differentiated malignant teratomas are uncommon and generally are solid and almost universally unilateral.[1,48,50-53]

Ovarian Dysgerminoma

Overview and Imaging Dysgerminoma is the second most common ovarian neoplasm in children and adolescents after mature teratoma. It is the most common malignant ovarian tumor of pediatric life but is considered a low-grade malignancy. It is said to be the histologic counterpart to the testicular seminoma of boys. Imaging or inspection shows it to

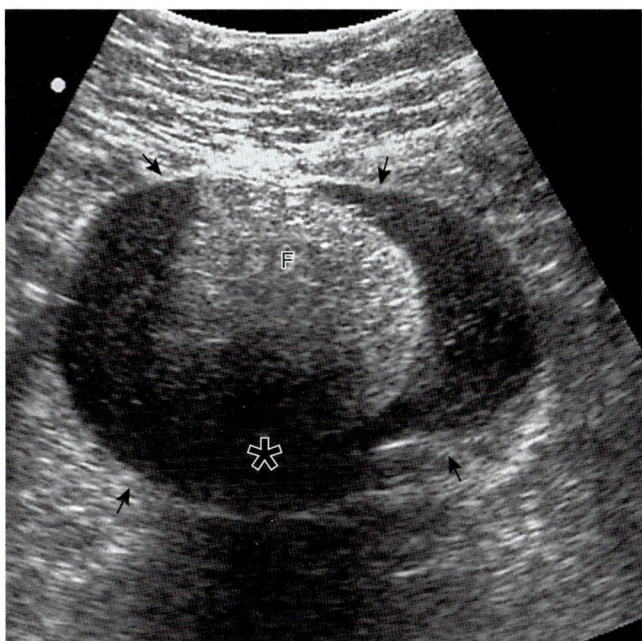

Figure 127-21 An ovarian teratoma. A transverse sonogram shows a large left adnexal mass (*arrows*) with a highly echogenic component (*F*). Shadowing that is present (*asterisk*) distal to the central portion represents a dermoid plug. The echogenicity is predominantly due to fat. Some calcification, which is not evident in this plane, was responsible for the shadowing. The periphery of the mass is fluid with contained debris. (From Ruggierro M, Awobuluyi M, Cohen H, et al. Imaging the pediatric pelvis: role of ultrasound. *Radiologist.* 1997;4:155-170.)

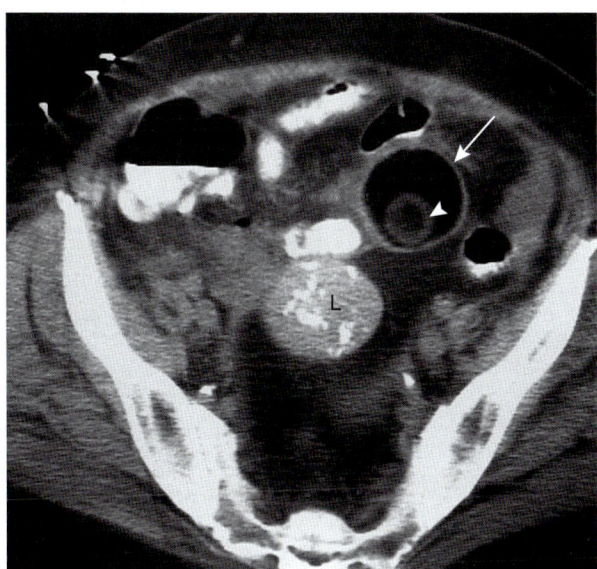

Figure 127-22 Ovarian teratoma. A contrast-enhanced computed tomography (CT) image shows a circular low Hounsfield unit mass (*arrow*) in the anterior left pelvis. The CT technique used makes its predominant component appear to be of the same low density as the air seen within nearby bowel or the fat seen in the posterior pelvis anterior to the sacrum. Its actual Hounsfield measurements were consistent with fat. It contains a mural nodule (*arrowhead*) that has no contained calcification. Incidentally noted is a midpelvic mass (*L*) with calcifications, which was a leiomyoma. (From Cohen HL, Safriel YI. Benign cystic teratomas of the ovaries. In: Cohen HL, Sivit C, eds. *Fetal and pediatric ultrasound: a casebook approach.* New York: McGraw-Hill; 2001:516.)

be solid, smooth, and well encapsulated. These tumors often are large when first diagnosed. One fifth of cases have bilateral involvement. Dysgerminomas may arise in dysgenetic gonads, but this presentation is much less common than with gonadoblastomas. Pure dysgerminomas are nonfunctioning tumors, but function may be observed in germinomas that contain islands of other germ cell tumors. These tumors can spread locally and to retroperitoneal nodes. They are very radiosensitive, and prognosis with treatment is generally good, with an overall survival of more than 90%.[1,50,51]

Endodermal Sinus Tumor

Overview and Imaging An endodermal sinus tumor (e.g., yolk sac tumor, yolk sac carcinoma, or Teilum tumor) is an uncommon malignant neoplasm that can occur at any age. It often is bulky at the time of diagnosis (Fig. 127-23) and is predominantly solid on ultrasound but may contain cystic spaces. In most cases, serum alpha-fetoprotein levels are increased. Some endodermal sinus tumors secrete human chorionic gonadotropin, causing incomplete precocious puberty by stimulating estrogen production by the ovary. This phenomenon can cause menstrual irregularities in post-pubertal girls. The tumor is very radiosensitive. Although the incidence of recurrence is high, the survival rate is high among treated patients.[1,54]

CYSTADENOMAS AND CYSTADENOCARCINOMAS

Overview and Imaging Surface epithelial tumors in children are similar to those in adults and consist predominantly of cystadenomas and cystadenocarcinomas. Cystadenomas are very uncommon before puberty and usually are unilateral. They vary in size from 3 to 30 cm. Of the two types of cystadenomas, serous cystadenomas contain clear watery fluid and the less common mucinous cystadenomas contain mucin,

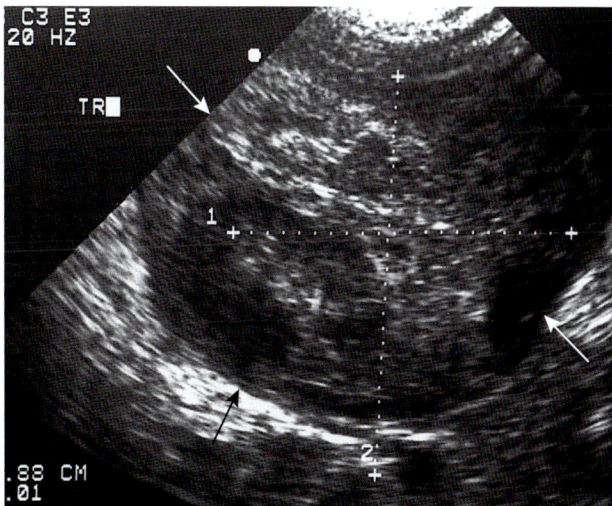

Figure 127-23 An endodermal sinus tumor. A transverse sonogram shows a large solid mass (*arrows*) extending beyond the measurement cursors in this 13-year-old who presented with a distended abdomen. Computed tomography showed significant metastatic disease.

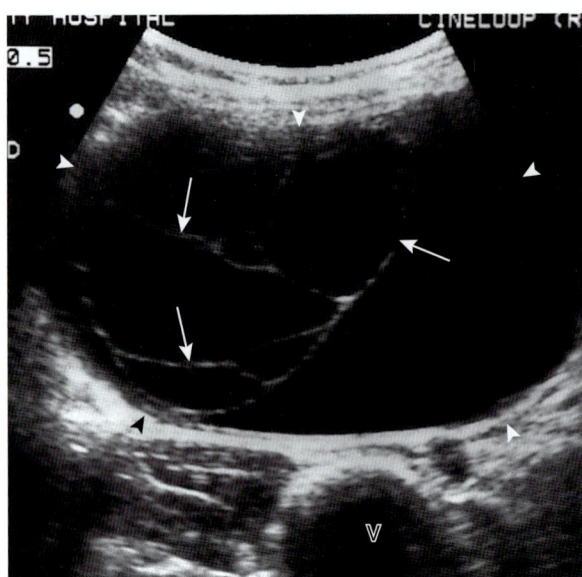

Figure 127-24 An ovarian cystadenoma. A transverse sonogram in a teenager shows a large cystic mass (*arrowheads*) with several intersecting septations (*arrows*). This proved to be an ovarian cystadenoma, which is far more commonly seen in adults than in children. *V,* Vertebral body. (From Ruggierro M, Awobuluyi M, Cohen H, et al. Imaging the pediatric pelvis: role of ultrasound. *Radiologist.* 1997;4:155-170.)

a jellylike material. Most of these tumors are multiseptated cystic masses (Fig. 127-24) when imaged by ultrasound. Cystadenomas are benign neoplasms, but a serous papillary form is reported to be prone to rupture, with spillage of tumor material into the peritoneal cavity, causing a serous papillomatosis. Cystadenocarcinomas are much less common than their benign counterparts. They may appear similar to cystadenomas, but the presence of irregular margins, thick septations, and papillary projections suggests malignancy. Ascites, omental or peritoneal implants, lymphadenopathy, and hepatic metastases indicate malignant spread.[1,47,50]

Granulosa/Theca Cell Tumors

Overview and Imaging Granulosa/theca cell tumors generally are large at the time of diagnosis. They are predominantly solid, but mixed solid and cystic patterns or a predominantly cystic type also are seen. Three fourths of juvenile granulosa cell tumors produce estrogen, which causes isosexual precocious puberty. Nonfunctioning granulosa cell tumors may be discovered incidentally as a mass on physical examination or ultrasound. The vast majority of nonfunctioning granulosa cell tumors are benign, with recurrences and metastases a rarity.[1,47,50]

Arrhenoblastomas

Arrhenoblastomas (Leydig cell tumors) usually are large and unilateral. They may be solid or cystic. They usually are well differentiated and benign, but a poorly differentiated form also occurs. Most arrhenoblastomas produce androgenic substances, causing virilization in prepubertal girls and signs of virilization, hirsutism, and oligomenorrhea or amenorrhea after puberty.[1,55]

Key Points

Ultrasound is the key technique used in the analysis of the pediatric gynecologic tract.

Follicles/cysts exist in the ovaries of most children.

A changing ultrasound appearance over time can help confirm the diagnosis of a hemorrhagic ovarian cyst.

The predominant pelvic mass found in neonates and infants is a distended vagina or uterus filled with secretions, fluid, or blood.

History, clinical findings, and laboratory findings may be necessary to differentiate among TOA, hemorrhagic cyst, and endometrioma, which may look alike on ultrasound.

Ovaries in persons with PCOS show increased ovarian echogenicity and typically at least five cysts of 5 to 8 mm on transabdominal ultrasound.

An acute ovary in torsion is much larger than a normal ovary.

Mature ovarian teratomas and dermoid cysts are the most common pediatric ovarian neoplasm.

Embryonal rhabdomyosarcoma is the most common genital neoplasm in children of both sexes.

One third of all ovarian neoplasms are malignant. As many as half of hormonally active tumors are malignant.

Suggested Readings

Capito C, Echaieb A, Lortat-Jacob S, et al. Pitfalls in the diagnosis and management of obstructive uterovaginal duplication: a series of 32 cases. *Pediatrics.* 2008;122(4):e891-e897.

Chiou SY, Lev-Toaff AS, Masuda E, et al. Adnexal torsion: new clinical and imaging observations by sonography, computed tomography, and magnetic resonance imaging. *J Ultrasound Med.* 2007;26(10):1289-1301.

de Vries L, Phillip M. Role of pelvic ultrasound in girls with precocious puberty. *Horm Res Paediatr.* 2011;75(2):148-152.

Garel L, Dubois J, Grignon A, et al. US of the pediatric female pelvis: a clinical perspective. *Radiographics.* 2001;21(6):1393-1407.

Lang IM, Babyn P, Oliver GD. MR imaging of paediatric uterovaginal anomalies. *Pediatr Radiol.* 1999;29(3):163-170.

Ratani RS, Cohen HL, Fiore E. Pediatric gynecologic ultrasound. *Ultrasound Q.* 2004;20(3):127-139.

Schultz KA, Ness KK, Nagarajan R, et al. Adnexal masses in infancy and childhood. *Clin Obstet Gynecol.* 2006;49(3):464-479.

Schultz KA, Sencer SF, Messinger Y, et al. Pediatric ovarian tumors: a review of 67 cases. *Pediatr Blood Cancer.* 2005;44(2):167-173.

Servaes S, Victoria T, Lovrenski J, et al. Contemporary pediatric gynecologic imaging. *Semin Ultrasound CT MR.* 2010;31(2):116-140.

Shah RU, Lawrence C, Fickenscher KA, et al. Imaging of pediatric pelvic neoplasms. *Radiol Clin North Am.* 2011;49(4):729-748, vi.

Stranzinger E, Strouse PJ. Ultrasound of the pediatric female pelvis. *Semin Ultrasound CT MR.* 2008;29(2):98-113.

Ziereisen F, Guissard G, Damry N, et al. Sonographic imaging of the paediatric female pelvis. *Eur Radiol.* 2005;15(7):1296-1309.

References

Full references for this chapter can be found on www.expertconsult.com.

Chapter 128

Amenorrhea and Abnormalities of Puberty

HARRIS L. COHEN and ANAND DORAI RAJU

Indications for evaluation of the adolescent pelvis usually are reports of abdominal pain, pelvic pain, or a mass. Many of the differential diagnoses for these complaints have been reviewed in Chapter 127. Other clinical symptoms resulting in imaging evaluation in female patients relate to abnormalities of development of secondary sexual characteristics of puberty. These changes may be seen earlier than normal (i.e., precocious puberty), may be delayed (i.e., delayed puberty), or may fail to develop (e.g., hypogonadism and sexual infantilism) in adolescents. The other key reason for adolescent gynecologic evaluation is amenorrhea (lack of menses), whether primary or secondary. Conditions causing pubertal delay also may cause primary or secondary amenorrhea.[1,2]

Puberty

Puberty among girls is the stage of development in between childhood and adulthood when activation of the hypothalamic-pituitary-ovarian-uterine axis produces maturation of the gonads, resulting in an increased production of sex hormones, development of secondary sex characteristics, a growth spurt, and development of reproductive capability. The earliest signs of puberty among girls are breast development (usually occurring between ages 8 and 13 years) and pubic hair growth (at age 8 to 14 years). These signs are followed by a growth spurt (at age 9.5 to 14.5 years), axillary hair development, and menarche (at age 10 to 16 years). Puberty is usually completed within about 4 years.[1,3,4]

Puberty among boys begins between 9 and 14 years of age and is completed in 3.5 to 4 years. It begins with testicular enlargement (usually occurring between age 9 and 13.5 years), followed by the appearance of pubic hair (at age 10 to 15 years), enlargement of the penis (at age 11 to 12.5 years), and development of axillary and facial hair, as well as a growth spurt (at age 10.5 to 16 years).[1,3]

PHYSIOLOGIC CHANGES AT PUBERTY AND THE NORMAL OVULATORY MENSTRUAL CYCLE

Ordinarily, until the age of at least 8 years, an unknown "central restraining mechanism" prevents the pulsatile release of gonadotropin-releasing hormone (GnRH) from the arcuate nucleus of the hypothalamus. Pulsatile release of GnRH appears necessary for ovulation and development of the corpus luteum. In early puberty the pulsatile GnRH release is maximal only at night, but with time the typical adult pattern of continuous pulsatile GnRH secretion develops.[1,4,5]

With the earliest activation of GnRH, most girls undergo ovarian folliculogenesis without ovulation. Unopposed estrogen production leads to progressive uterine growth and endometrial proliferation. Breast budding, physiologic leukorrhea, and accelerated linear growth occur. As the hypothalamic-pituitary-ovarian-uterine axis matures over approximately a 2-year span, cycles with subnormal progesterone production and shortened intermenstrual intervals are replaced by normal corpus luteum function and fertile cycles.[1,4,5]

The typical ovulatory cycle has a 24- to 35-day intermenstrual interval and usually a premenstrual molimina. Longer intervals often are associated with anovulation. Improved nutrition and living conditions are thought to be responsible for the gradual decrease in mean menarchal age during the past century. In North America, the mean menarchal age currently is 12.4 years with a range of 9 to 17 years. Menarche usually occurs 2 to 5 years after breast bud development.[1,5]

PREMATURE THELARCHE AND ADRENARCHE

Overview and Clinical Presentation Premature thelarche and adrenarche are relatively common, self-limited variants of normal pubertal development in girls. Premature thelarche refers to premature breast development without other signs of precocious sexual maturation in girls younger than 8 years of age. It usually is seen between 1 and 4 years of age. A third of the cases resolve spontaneously. Premature adrenarche refers to the appearance of pubic and axillary hair without other signs of precocious sexual maturity. In both premature thelarche and premature adrenarche, bone age and patient height are normal to only slightly increased. The cause of premature thelarche or adrenarche is not certain. The levels of circulating sex hormones usually are normal. Increased end-organ sensitivity to normal levels of estrogen or androgen has been suggested as a possible cause.[1,6,7]

In boys, premature appearance of pubic and axillary hair without other signs or only minor signs of precocious puberty is a relatively common variant of normal development that may be due to an increase in circulating androgens from premature maturation of the adrenal glands of unknown cause. No penile enlargement is present, presumably because the levels of circulating androgens are not sufficiently elevated. The bone age and growth rate are slightly increased. The remainder of pubertal development occurs at a normal age.[1,7]

Precocious Puberty

Precocious puberty refers to the appearance of secondary sex characteristics before 8 years of age in girls and before 9 years of age in boys. Precocious puberty is divided into two main types: (1) complete, central, gonadotropin-dependent, or true precocious puberty and (2) incomplete, peripheral, gonadotropin-independent, pseudoprecocious puberty, or precocious pseudopuberty. Whereas the complete form is characteristically isosexual, with development of secondary sex characteristics that are appropriate for the patient's gender, the incomplete form may be either isosexual or heterosexual. Incomplete heterosexual precocious puberty is manifested by signs of virilization in girls and by gynecomastia or other signs of feminization in boys.[1,6,7]

COMPLETE OR CENTRAL ISOSEXUAL PRECOCIOUS PUBERTY

Overview and Pathophysiology Complete or central isosexual precocious puberty results from premature activation of the hypothalamic-pituitary-gonadal complex with increased production of gonadotropic and sex hormones and an early onset of ovulation or spermatogenesis. Complete precocious puberty may be idiopathic or secondary to organic central nervous system (CNS) lesions.[1,8,9]

Etiology and Imaging The cause of precocious puberty in girls is idiopathic in at least 80% of cases. About 20% of affected girls have a hypothalamic or pituitary lesion. Fewer than 10% of cases of true precocious puberty in boys have an idiopathic cause. A familial tendency to idiopathic early pubertal development is observed in some cases (i.e., constitutional or genetic precocious puberty).[1,8,9]

Possible causes of precocious puberty in either sex include intracranial tumors or cysts, hydrocephalus, sequelae of intracranial inflammatory processes or trauma, and other intracranial lesions that may activate the hypothalamus by pressure or invasion. Of the CNS neoplasms that may cause true precocious puberty, hamartoma of the tuber cinereum (Fig. 128-1) is the most common. This usually small CNS tumor is more common in boys than in girls, is generally benign, and is nonprogressive. The hypothalamic hamartoma secretes GnRH, and the resultant symptoms usually cannot be corrected surgically. The onset of puberty in patients with this lesion is usually at a younger age (2 years) than in patients with idiopathic precocious puberty. Other CNS neoplasms that may cause true precocious puberty in either sex usually are located in or near the hypothalamus and include hypothalamic or optic gliomas, astrocytoma, ependymoma, dysgerminoma, and prolactinoma. Suprasellar dysgerminoma (ectopic pinealoma) in boys also may cause incomplete precocious puberty through tumor secretion of human chorionic gonadotropin (hCG).[1,9,10]

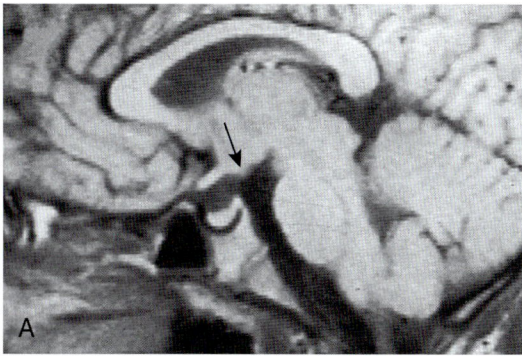
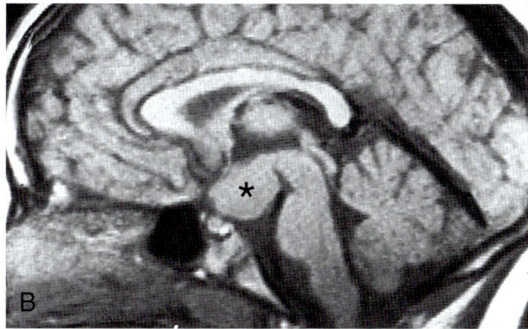

Figure 128-1 Precocious puberty caused by hamartoma of the tuber cinereum. **A** and **B,** On midline sagittal T1-weighted magnetic resonance images of the brain, an arrow points to a small hamartoma in the brain of an 8-year-old and an asterisk indicates an unusually large hamartoma in a 7-year-old, both of whom had a long-standing history of precocious puberty.

True precocious puberty may be observed in some children with long-standing untreated hypothyroidism. The increased production of gonadotropic hormones and prolactin seen in these patients may be due to a hormonal overlap in the pituitary response to thyroid deficiency. Affected patients show little, if any, development of secondary sexual characteristics, especially pubic hair. All of these changes regress with treatment of the hypothyroidism.[1,7]

INCOMPLETE (PSEUDOSEXUAL) PRECOCIOUS PUBERTY IN GIRLS

Overview Pseudosexual (or incomplete) precocious puberty in girls usually presents before 5 years of age. Excess circulating estrogens or related substances develop independent of stimulus by the hypothalamus and pituitary gland. These estrogens usually are produced by the ovaries or adrenal glands or may be from an exogenous source, such as food, parenteral or oral medications, or other substances.[1,6,11]

Etiology and Imaging Gonadotropin levels are low, and the gonads remain immature. The most common ovarian source is an autonomous estrogen-secreting follicular (granulosa-thecal) cyst (Fig. 128-2). Other causes are estrogen-producing ovarian neoplasms, particularly granulosa cell (or granulosa-theca cell) tumors (Fig. 128-3) and rare estrogen-secreting adrenal neoplasms (adenomas or carcinomas).[1,6,11]

McCune-Albright syndrome consists of polyostotic fibrous dysplasia, cutaneous café au lait spots, and precocious puberty. The syndrome is found predominantly in females. Autonomously functioning ovarian cysts are seen in some cases. In

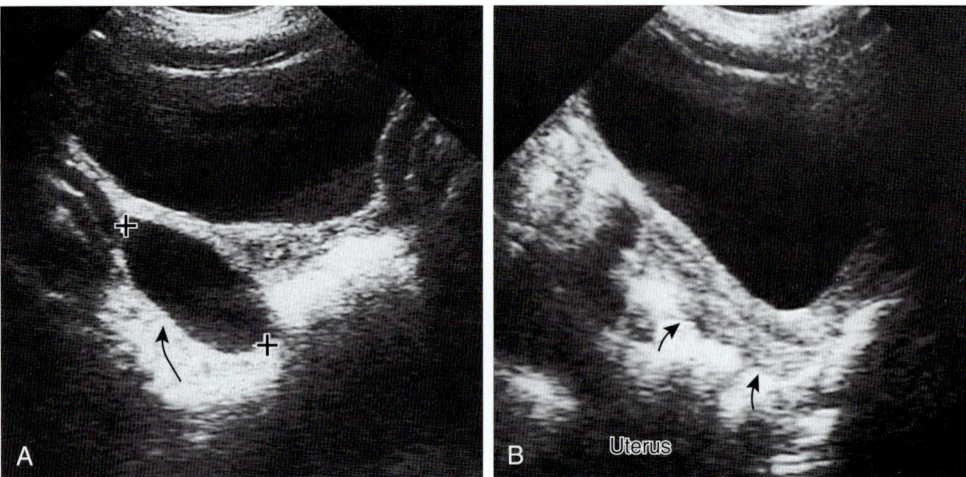

Figure 128-2 Precocious puberty due to an autonomous estrogen-secreting ovarian cyst. **A,** A parasagittal sonogram of the right adnexa (*arrow*) of a 3-year-old with precocious puberty shows a large cyst (*cursors*). This cyst was proved to autonomously secrete estrogen. The left adnexa was normal. **B,** A midline longitudinal sonogram shows that the child's uterus (*arrows*) is longer than normal for her age. It is not the tubular shape typical of childhood but appears almost pear shaped, with an echogenic central endometrial cavity indicating estrogenization.

others, no anatomic cause is noted. McCune-Albright syndrome occasionally presents as complete or true precocious puberty. It has been suggested that the initially partial or incomplete precocious puberty in these patients becomes complete (gonadotropin dependent) as the result of an early maturation of the hypothalamic-pituitary-gonadal complex, which is caused by a long-standing exposure to estrogen.[1,6]

VIRILIZING DISORDERS (HETEROSEXUAL PRECOCIOUS PUBERTY)

Overview and Clinical Presentation Testosterone is produced in normal females by the adrenal gland (25%), by the ovary (25%), and by peripheral conversion of D4-androstenedione

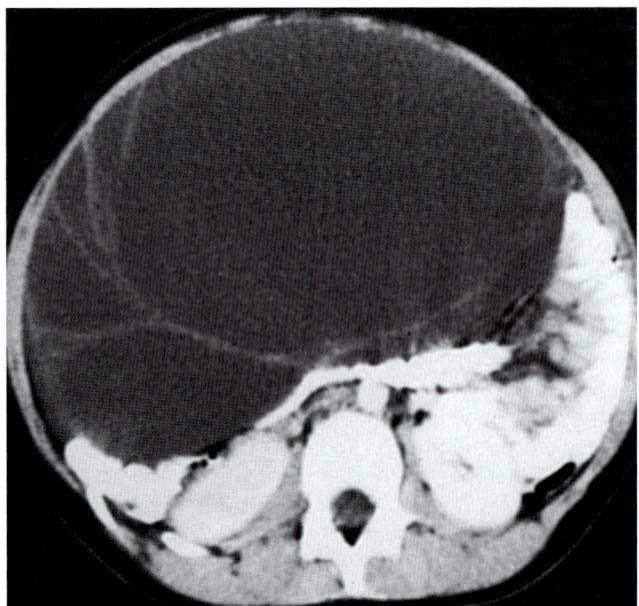

Figure 128-3 Precocious puberty caused by a granulosa cell tumor. Contrast-enhanced computed tomography shows a large, cystic, septated mass occupying most of the abdomen in a 10-year-old girl. The mass proved to be an estrogen-producing juvenile granulosa cell tumor.

(50%), with only 1% typically free and biologically active. A form of pseudosexual precocity may occur in girls when androgen levels are excessive or end organs become excessively sensitive to normal amounts of circulating androgens. Either case may lead to heterosexual pseudoprecocious puberty as the girls undergo virilization and masculine secondary sexual characteristics develop. Clinical findings include increases in body and facial hair (hirsutism), acne, deepening of the voice, clitoromegaly, increased muscle mass, and temporal balding. Menstrual abnormalities are common among affected adolescents.[1,11]

Congenital Adrenal Hyperplasia

Overview and Imaging Congenital adrenal hyperplasia is the most common form of hyperandrogenism. The increased production of androgenic substance is due in most cases to a deficiency of 21-hydroxylase and far less commonly to deficiencies in 11β-hydroxylase, 3β-hydroxysteroid dehydrogenase, or other enzymes involved in cortisol and/or aldosterone synthesis. Imaging of the adrenal gland will show enlargement (Fig. 128-4) that is usually bilateral and diffuse. The normal adrenal shape is maintained.[1,12]

Other Causes of Virilization in Girls

Overview, Etiology, and Pathophysiology Adrenal adenomas or adrenal carcinomas may produce increased levels of androgens and virilization. Signs of Cushing syndrome may be seen as a result of associated tumor secretion of glucocorticoid hormones.[1,12]

Ovarian neoplasms may secrete androgens and cause virilization. These neoplasms include Sertoli-Leydig cell tumors, thecomas (luteoma—a virilizing dysgerminoma that contains theca cells), or gonadoblastomas. Exogenous exposure to androgens or androgen-like substances may cause virilization at all ages. Again, virilization at puberty may develop in some girls with rare anomalies of sex differentiation, such as 46,XY gonadal dysgenesis, even though they are phenotypically normal females at birth.[1,13]

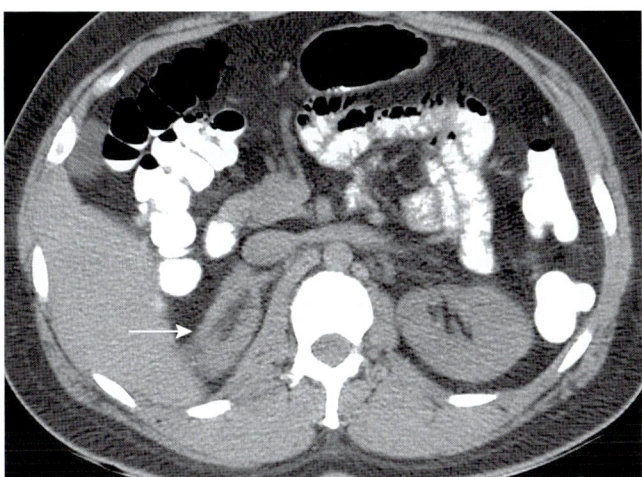

Figure 128-4 Congenital adrenal hyperplasia. A computed tomography scan shows that the right adrenal gland (*arrow*) is thicker than normal in this 24-year-old with simple virilizing congenital adrenal hyperplasia. As is typical with this disorder, the adrenal gland maintains its normal shape.

Idiopathic hirsutism and polycystic ovarian disease also are considered to be among the virilizing disorders of females. Idiopathic hirsutism consists of an increase in body and facial hair (i.e., hirsutism or hypertrichosis) that occurs as the sole or predominant abnormality and is a relatively common problem in otherwise normal pubertal and postpubertal girls. Idiopathic hirsutism may be precipitated by any of the causes of virilization. It may be seen in families or as a result of polycystic ovary syndrome (PCOS) and the increased androgen production by the many small follicular cysts (see Chapter 127). The cause is usually idiopathic and believed to be a result of an altered response of the end organ (hair follicle) to normal levels of circulating androgens.[1,14-16]

INCOMPLETE ISOSEXUAL (PSEUDOPRECOCIOUS) PUBERTY IN BOYS

Overview, Etiology, and Pathophysiology Isosexual pseudoprecocity of sexual development in boys is due to an increase in circulating androgen or androgen-like substances either from production by adrenal glands or testes or from an exogenous source. Congenital adrenal hyperplasia (CAH) is the most common cause for excessive androgen production by the adrenal gland of either sex. Affected males are born with normal external genitalia, but if the CAH is untreated, signs of sexual precocity soon develop. Isosexual pseudoprecocious puberty in males, sometimes associated with signs of glucocorticoid excess, also can occur because of androgen-secreting neoplasms of the adrenal cortex (e.g., adenocarcinoma or benign adenoma). A rare cause of isosexual precocity in boys is an androgen-secreting Leydig cell tumor of the testis (see Chapter 126). Several extrapituitary hCG-secreting tumors also can result in an incomplete form of isosexual precocious puberty by stimulating testosterone production by the Leydig cells of the testis. These tumors include some hepatomas, hepatoblastomas, some teratomas or chorioepitheliomas of the mediastinum and retroperitoneum, and suprasellar germinoma or ectopic pinealoma. A familial form of gonadotropin-independent precocious puberty in boys is caused by premature maturation and sometimes hyperplasia of the Leydig cells of the testis, with production of testosterone. Exposure to exogenous androgens or the administration of hCG for undescended testes may be further causes of incomplete virilization in males.[1,7,12]

ADOLESCENT GYNECOMASTIA AND FEMINIZING DISORDERS IN BOYS

Overview and Etiology Mild breast development may occur transiently in adolescent boys between 13 and 15 years of age. It is usually bilateral, it is idiopathic, and it may be familial. Usually no hormonal abnormality is found. The gynecomastia generally regresses in 2 or 3 years, but in a few cases it may persist into adult life. Pathologic causes of gynecomastia in boys may be exposure to exogenous estrogens, an estrogen-secreting neoplasm of the testis or adrenal cortex, a prolactin-secreting neoplasm of the pituitary gland, Klinefelter syndrome, congenital bilateral anorchia, acquired testicular failure, and other conditions with some biochemical defect in testosterone production or androgen end-organ receptor.[1,17]

CLINICAL AND LABORATORY EVALUATION OF PRECOCIOUS PUBERTY

Overview and Clinical Presentation Physical examination can help determine the correct diagnosis. Physical examination should denote the type and degree of pubertal development as well as the size, shape, and firmness of the testes. In complete precocious puberty, both testes are enlarged; in partial sexual precocity they often are of normal size. Unilateral testicular enlargement suggests a testicular neoplasm. The abdomen should be evaluated for a flank or pelvic mass. The presence of café au lait spots should suggest the diagnosis of fibrous dysplasia or neurofibromatosis. Laboratory studies may include luteinizing hormone, follicle-stimulating hormone, and estradiol levels; gonadotropin response to GnRH; thyroid studies, and a vaginal smear in girls, as well as plasma and urinary testosterone levels.[1,7,18]

IMAGING WORKUP OF PRECOCIOUS PUBERTY

Imaging An anteroposterior film of the left hand, including carpal bones and the distal forearm, is used for bone age determination. Bone age often is advanced in patients with true precocious puberty and in patients with androgenic stimulation. The skeletal length often is increased early in patients with advanced bone age. However, if the precocious puberty is not treated, premature fusion of the epiphyses may develop and result in a decrease in the patient's potential height.[1,7]

Abdominal ultrasound, with emphasis on the adrenals and the ovaries, has become the primary radiologic study in the initial evaluation of patients with precocious puberty. In girls with true precocious puberty, a pelvic ultrasound may show some bilateral enlargement of the ovaries and prominence of the uterus, and in rare cases a large estrogen-secreting ovarian cyst that has resulted in stimulation of the hypothalamic-pituitary complex. Small and multiple ovarian cysts/follicles may be seen in girls with true precocious puberty because of high gonadotropin levels. These cystic ovaries may look and be similar to those seen normally throughout childhood.

Pseudoprecocity caused by the autonomous estrogen secretion of an ovarian cyst or tumor will be denoted by asymmetry of the ovaries of the child, with the autonomous mass being found in the larger ovary (see Fig. 128-2). The finding in prepubertal girls of an increased uterine size and a well-defined central endometrial echo indicates an increase in circulating estrogen from any cause. A skeletal survey is indicated when fibrous dysplasia is suspected.[1,7,19]

Patients with isosexual precocious puberty that is suspected to be of the complete or central type should have magnetic resonance imaging (MRI) of the brain with special attention to the tuber cinereum. Skull radiographs are of limited diagnostic value but may show intracranial calcifications, enlargement of the sella turcica, signs of increased intracranial pressure, or skull changes of fibrous dysplasia.[1,7]

Delayed or Absent Pubertal Development

Puberty is considered to be delayed and should be investigated in girls when secondary sex characteristics fail to appear by 13 years of age, which is considered two standard deviations beyond the norm. Evaluation for pubertal delays in boys is suggested when pubic and axillary hair or other external secondary characteristics, particularly enlargement of the testes and penis, fail to appear by age 14 years. Delayed puberty or failure of puberty to develop may be idiopathic (constitutional) or due to chronic systemic disorders, disorders of the hypothalamic-pituitary complex causing decreased gonadotropin secretion (i.e., secondary or hypogonadotropic hypogonadism), or primary disorders of the gonads with a secondary elevation of gonadotropic hormone secretion (i.e., primary or hypergonadotropic hypogonadism).[1,20,21]

IDIOPATHIC (CONSTITUTIONAL) PUBERTAL DELAY

Overview and Clinical Presentation   In some otherwise normal children, the onset of puberty is delayed for up to several years. When puberty eventually starts, it usually continues to completely normal secondary sexual development. These occurrences underline the fact that there may be constitutional or genetic causes for delay in the maturation of the hypothalamic-pituitary complex. Often, such children may experience a delay in bone age and height development. The ability to differentiate between constitutional pubertal delays in otherwise normal children and true disorders of the hypothalamic-pituitary axis may not be simple.[1,21]

DELAYED PUBERTY IN CHRONIC SYSTEMIC DISORDERS

Overview and Etiology   Delayed puberty may occur on a physiologic basis in patients with chronic diseases. Patients with other long-term debilitating processes, as well as anorexia nervosa, may have delays in pubertal development. Such delays also may be noted in children or adolescents who undergo prolonged and vigorous physical exertion, such as long-distance running or ballet. Puberty may develop or proceed normally in some of these patients after improvement or removal of the precipitating cause. However, any halt in the pubertal development of a patient is a cause for concern and an immediate endocrinologic workup.[1,22,23]

Hypogonadism Caused By Hypothalamic-Pituitary Disorders (Hypogonadotropic Hypogonadism)

Overview and Clinical Presentation   Several disorders of the hypothalamic-pituitary complex result in decreased gonadotropin production and, secondarily, a decrease in gonadal sex steroids. Impaired or absent gonadal function causes an absence of pubertal development. In girls, the uterus remains infantile, menses does not occur, and breast budding and other secondary sexual characteristics do not develop. In boys, the penis and scrotum are infantile and the testes remain immature and smaller than expected for age. Pubic and axillary hair is scanty or absent, the voice remains high pitched, and increased fat deposition often occurs, particularly at the hips, pelvis, abdomen, and breast. Delayed closure of the epiphyses with elongation of the limbs is observed unless an associated growth hormone deficiency is present.[1,21,22]

Etiology and Pathophysiology   Causative abnormalities include intracranial tumors such as craniopharyngioma, hypothalamic and optic gliomas, dysgerminoma, and other tumors of the pituitary gland and hypothalamus or adjacent areas. Other manifestations of pituitary insufficiency, such as diabetes insipidus and short stature, may be present. Primary or secondary hypogonadotropic hypogonadism also may be seen in patients with Langerhans cell histiocytosis and in patients with certain congenital midline defects of the face, the base of the skull, and the CNS (e.g., septo-optic dysplasia or holoprosencephaly), which may be associated with developmental anomalies of the hypothalamus and pituitary gland, resulting in hypogonadism.[1,21]

Functional causes of hypogonadism include idiopathic hypopituitarism, characterized by short stature resulting from growth hormone deficiency, and sometimes other findings associated with deficiencies of other pituitary hormones. Cases of isolated gonadotropic deficiency, sporadic or familial, may occur in association with anosmia or hyposmia and other abnormalities that characterize Kallmann syndrome. Isolated luteinizing hormone deficiency in males, which sometimes is familial, results in failure of pubertal development; it usually is associated with gynecomastia but with the preservation of spermatogenesis (i.e., fertile eunuch syndrome). Hypogonadism, which probably also is related to abnormalities of hypothalamic function, can be observed in Prader-Willi and Laurence-Moon-Biedl syndromes.[1,21]

Hypogonadism Caused By Gonadal Lesions (Hypergonadotropic Hypogonadism)

Overview, Etiology, and Pathophysiology   Certain congenital or acquired lesions of the gonads may result in hypogonadism and failure of pubertal development. Gonadal sex steroids are decreased, and as a result an increased secretion of gonadotropins by the pituitary occurs. Just as in hypogonadotropic hypogonadism, pubertal development is absent in girls or boys. The key gonadal lesions in girls include Turner syndrome, XX gonadal dysgenesis, XY gonadal dysgenesis, and a gonadal dysgenesis with galactosemia and immune oophoritis (often associated with Hashimoto thyroiditis, hypoparathyroidism, adrenal insufficiency, pernicious anemia, chronic active hepatitis, and candidiasis). Hypergonadotropic hypogonadism also can occur among patients with normal karyotypes who experience secondary ovarian failure either by infarction, as with cases of bilateral ovarian torsion, surgical removal of both ovaries, radiation therapy to the pelvis (usually of 800 cGy or greater), chemotherapy, or autoimmune oophoritis.[1,21,24]

Gonadal lesions in boys leading to hypogonadism include congenital bilateral anorchia with otherwise normal external genitalia, which is caused by resorption of the testes after the thirteenth week of gestation (vanishing testes and functional prepubertal castrate syndromes) and acquired testicular atrophy resulting from bilateral testicular torsion, surgical injury during bilateral orchiopexy, radiation, or other causes. Absence of puberty also is observed in some genetic males born with an entirely female phenotype, including those with XY gonadal dysgenesis, and some forms of male pseudohermaphroditism with impaired biosynthesis of active sex steroids as a result of an inherited enzymatic deficiency.[1,25,26]

DIAGNOSTIC AND HISTORICAL CONSIDERATIONS

Overview, Clinical Presentation, and Imaging Important information may be obtained from the patient's family history, medical history, associated medical disorders, and physical examination. At the physical examination, special emphasis should be placed on pubertal staging (Tanner classification), assessment of general growth and maturation, detection of signs and symptoms of CNS disease, and systemic diseases or syndromes. Visual fields testing, gynecologic evaluation, and chromosomal analysis should be carried out if indicated. The hormonal studies include measurements of serum testosterone, estradiol, and gonadotropins; gonadotropic response to GnRH stimulation; and testosterone response to hCG stimulation. Measurements of circulating prolactin and growth hormone, as well as thyroid function tests, may be undertaken. Radiologic procedures include bone age determination, brain MRI, pelvic ultrasound to evaluate the size of the ovaries and uterus, and other studies as indicated.[1,21]

ANALYSIS OF PATIENTS WITH AMENORRHEA

Overview and Etiology Causes of pubertal delay in girls may be similar to causes of primary or secondary amenorrhea. Primary amenorrhea is defined as a lack of menses by age 16 years. Secondary amenorrhea is defined as a cessation of menses at any point in time after menarche and before menopause.[1,27,28]

Primary amenorrhea has many causes and involves several organ systems (Box 128-1). It may be seen in adolescents with normal pubertal development, as well as those with delayed sexual development, delayed menarche with some pubertal development, and delayed menarche plus virilization. Many of its causes have already been reviewed, including hypogonadotropic hypogonadism, hypergonadotropic hypogonadism, pseudohermaphroditism, female adolescents with virilization, PCOS, genital obstruction (e.g., hematometra/hematometrocolpos), and uterine aplasia or hypoplasia. Secondary amenorrhea often is due physiologically to pregnancy and pathologically to PCOS.[1,27,28]

Box 128-1 Etiology of Primary Amenorrhea

Hypothalamus
- Systemic illness
- Chronic disease
- Familial
- Stress
- Competitive athletics
- Eating disorders
- Obesity
- Tumor, irradiation
- Drugs

Pituitary
- Idiopathic hypopituitarism
- Tumor
- Hemochromatosis
- Infarction
- Irradiation, surgery

Thyroid Gland
- Hypothyroidism
- Hyperthyroidism

Adrenal Glands
- Congenital adrenocortical hyperplasia
- Cushing disease
- Addison disease
- Tumor

Ovaries
- Gonadal dysgenesis
- Ovarian failure
- Polycystic ovary syndrome
- Ovarian tumor, Bilateral oophorectomy

Cervix: Agenesis

Vagina
- Agenesis
- Transverse septum

Hymen: Imperforate

Modified from Emans SJ. Amenorrhea in the adolescent. In: Emans S, Goldstein D, eds. *Pediatric and adolescent gynecology.* 5th ed. Philadelphia: Lippincott Williams and Wilkins; 2005.

WHAT THE CLINICIAN NEEDS TO KNOW

- Bone age delayed, normal, or advanced
- Skeletal changes of polyostotic fibrous dysplasia (McCune-Albright syndrome)
- Presence of an intracranial lesion or congenital malformation on MRI/computed tomography that may activate the hypothalamus by pressure or invasion in the setting of central isosexual precocious puberty or result in decreased gonadotropin production in hypogonadotropic hypogonadism
- Presence of an ovarian lesion (cyst or neoplasm) on ultrasound in young girls with pseudosexual precocious puberty
- Presence of a testicular mass on ultrasound in pseudoprecocious puberty in boys
- Presence of enlarged adrenal glands (CAH) or adrenal mass in heterosexual precocious puberty

Key Points

Unopposed estrogen production leads to progressive uterine growth and endometrial proliferation. Axillary and pubic hair development are the result of ovarian and adrenal gland androgen production.

Precocious puberty refers to the appearance of external signs of adolescence before 8 years of age in girls and before 9 years of age in boys.

The cause of precocious puberty is idiopathic in at least 80% of girls but in less than 10% of boys.

Hypothalamic hamartoma is the most common CNS neoplasm to cause true precocious puberty.

Pseudosexual precocious puberty in girls usually presents before 5 years of age. Excess circulating estrogens or related substances develop independent of central stimulation. The most common source is an autonomous estrogen-secreting ovarian follicular cyst.

Congenital adrenal hyperplasia is the most common form of hyperandrogenism; in most cases it is due to 21-hydroxylase deficiency.

Puberty is considered to be delayed when secondary sex characteristics fail to appear by 13 years of age in girls and 14 years of age in boys.

Delayed puberty may occur on a physiologic basis in patients with chronic or debilitating disease, extreme or prolonged exercise, and anorexia nervosa.

Primary or secondary hypogonadotropic hypogonadism may be seen in patients with histiocytosis, congenital midline CNS defects, CNS neoplasms, and primary gonadotropin deficiencies.

Primary amenorrhea is defined as a lack of menses by age 16 years. Secondary amenorrhea is defined as a cessation of menses at any time after menarche and before menopause.

Suggested Readings

Argyropoulos M, Kiortsis D. MRI of the hypothalamic-pituitary axis in children. *Pediatr Radiol.* 2005;35:1045.

Cohen HL, Bober S, Bow S. Imaging the pediatric pelvis: the normal and abnormal genital system and simulators of its diseases. *Urol Radiol.* 1992;14:273.

Garel L, Dubois J, Grignon A, et al. US of the pediatric female pelvis: a clinical perspective. *Radiographics.* 2001;21(6):1393-1407.

Stranzinger E, Strouse PJ. Ultrasound of the pediatric female pelvis. *Semin Ultrasound CT MR.* 2008;29(2):98-113.

Warren MP, Goodman LR. Exercise-induced endocrine pathologies. *J Endocrinol Invest.* 2003;26(9):873-878.

References

Full references for this chapter can be found on www.expertconsult.com.

SECTION 8

Musculoskeletal System

Chapter 129

Embryology, Anatomy, and Normal Findings

J. HERMAN KAN and PETER J. STROUSE

Embryology

Both striated muscle and bone are derived from the mesodermal germ layer. The limb buds form at the end of the fourth week of fetal life. Near the end of the second month of fetal life, the embryonal cartilaginous skeleton is already subdivided into its principal segments, which are the forerunners of bones of the limbs. Primary ossification centers are formed by deposition of calcium in the cartilaginous matrix after hypertrophy and vacuolization of local cartilage cells.[1] In tubular bones, this process occurs at approximately the midpoint of the shaft and is followed by central resorption, which gives rise to the primary marrow cavity. Calcified disks proximal and distal to the primary cavity become preparatory zones of calcification after the development of the advancing, proliferating shaft during growth. Cartilage proximal and distal to the zones of calcification becomes the epiphyses. A layer of cells within the epiphyses near the shaft produces new cells that are interposed between the resting cartilage of the epiphysis and the older cells and calcified cartilage adjacent to the shaft. The matrix around the old cells calcifies and is invaded by capillaries and bone cells from the marrow. Bone is formed on the calcified cartilage, and new bone and cartilage undergo remodeling by osteoclasts and osteoblasts, so that the length of the bone is increased (Fig. 129-1). The girth of the bone and the thickness of the cortex are increased by subperiosteal accretion caused by activity of the subperiosteal osteoblasts. Peripheral resorption of bone at the advancing ends of the shaft maintains the gentle flaring that characterizes normal tubular bone and is the mechanism responsible for what is termed "modeling." Disproportionate osteoclastic activity within the shaft of the bone reams out a marrow cavity. Continued, balanced activity of all these processes permits a small tubular bone to become a large tubular bone while functional shape and relations with adjacent structures are maintained.

Secondary ossification centers appear in the cartilaginous epiphyses and apophyses and enlarge by similar but much slower processes than those that enlarge the shaft. Irregularities in density and discontinuities in the structure of secondary ossification centers are frequent during normal mineralization and simulate the features of disease. The known ages at first appearance and upon fusion of these ossification centers can serve as indicators of physical maturation (Figs. 129-2 and 129-3; Table 129-1).

The epiphyses are terminal remnants of the original cartilaginous models of bone. Longitudinal growth takes place at the junction of the physis and the metaphysis by proliferation of cartilage cells in the physis, calcification of the surrounding matrix, and transformation to bone through the activity of metaphyseal vessels and accompanying osteoblasts and osteoclasts. Ossification centers develop within the epiphyses; growth ceases when these secondary centers fuse, through the physis, with the metaphysis. Apophyses are outgrowths of a bone that develop where muscle tendons originate or insert. Similar to the epiphyses, the apophyses develop ossification centers that eventually fuse with the main body of the underlying bone. Apophyses are different from epiphyses in that they do not contribute to longitudinal growth. Apophyseal and epiphyseal ossification and growth occur related to matrix deposition by the spherical growth plate, which has physiology similar to the physis. When epiphyseal ossification is complete, the spherical growth plate and epiphyseal cartilage are no longer appreciable, and only articular cartilage overlies the epiphyseal bone. This process occurs simultaneously with closure of the physis at skeletal maturity.

Physiology

The bones provide rigid support for the body and sites of insertion for muscles, to which the bones respond as levers. The bones are active physiologically in infants and children, changing size and shape with growth and hormone activity (related to levels of vitamin D, parathyroid hormone, calcitonin, or serum calcium and phosphate levels) and in response to mechanical stresses.[2]

During growth, in addition to its constant increase in length and breadth, the shaft is continuously molded or reshaped to its final form. The mechanism responsible for these changes in shape has been called "modeling" or "tubulation." One of the most conspicuous features of modeling is progressive concentric contraction of the shaft behind the

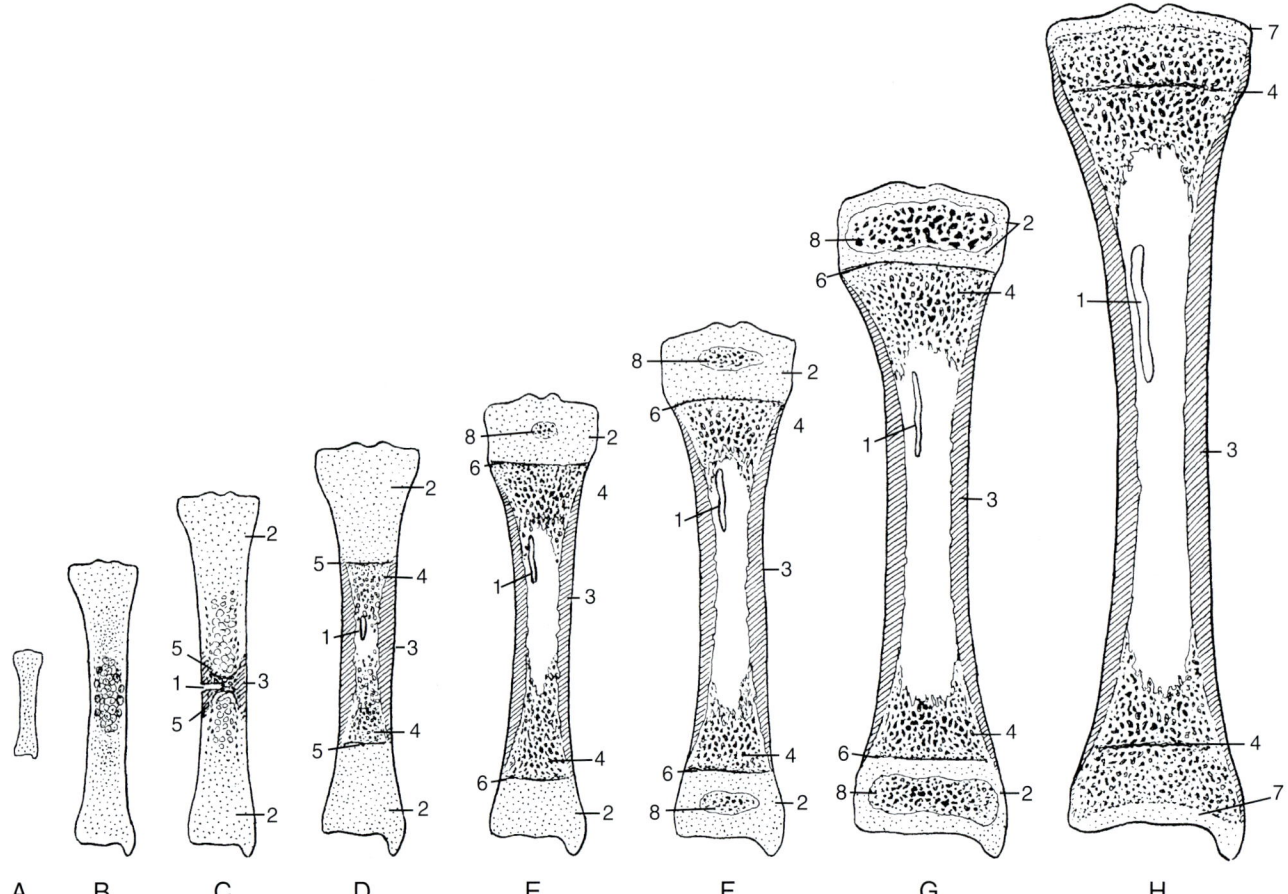

Figure 129-1 Schema of progressive stages in the growth and maturation of the tibia. **A,** The mass of embryonal cartilage that is the anlage of the tibia. **B,** Initial enlargement and multiplication of the central cartilage cells and an increase in cartilaginous matrix—the chondrification center that is the forerunner of the primary ossification center. **C,** The early primary ossification center shows the formation of a central belt of subperiosteal bone (early cortex) and penetration of the cartilaginous matrix by the periosteal elements; the channel of this penetration persists as the nutrient canal. **D,** Extension of ossification toward both ends of the shaft, with central resorption forming the medullary cavity. **E,** The tibia at birth, with a secondary ossification center in the proximal epiphyseal cartilage. **F,** At approximately the fourth postnatal month, ossification centers are seen in both of the epiphyseal cartilages. **G,** The juvenile tibia shows the growth of all components and enlargement of the epiphyseal secondary ossification centers. **H,** The adult tibia, with complete fusion of the shaft and both epiphyses. The narrow plates of articular cartilage that cap each end of the bone persist throughout life. 1, nutrient canal; 2, epiphyseal cartilage; 3, corticalis; 4, spongiosa; 5 and 6, provisional zones of calcification or epiphyseal plates; 7, articular cartilages; 8, secondary epiphyseal ossification centers. (Modified from an original drawing by W. M. Rogers, MD.)

Table 129-1

Epiphyseal Ossification in the Fetus and Neonate: Fifth and Ninety-Fifth Percentiles		
Ossification Center	**Fifth Percentile**	**Ninety-Fifth Percentile**
Humeral head	37th week	16 postnatal weeks
Distal femur	31st week	39th week (female) 40th week (male)
Proximal tibia	34th week	2 postnatal weeks (female) 5 postnatal weeks (male)
Calcaneus	22nd week	25th week
Talus	25th week	31st week
Cuboid	37th week	8 postnatal weeks (female) 16 postnatal weeks (male)

Data from Kuhns LR, Finnstrom O. New standards of ossification of the newborn. *Radiology.* 1976;119:655-660.

wider, advancing terminal segment (Fig. 129-4); this process results in flared ends of bones.

Significant disturbances in configuration of the shafts occur in many of the chronic diseases that affect the growing skeleton. With overtubulation, a diaphysis is abnormally narrow in caliber with accentuation of metaphyseal flaring. This phenomenon usually is seen in children with cerebral palsy or other neuromuscular diseases in which normal muscular stresses are not present. With undertubulation, the diaphysis is abnormally broad in caliber with loss of the normal metaphyseal flaring. Causes may include Gaucher disease, Pyle dysplasia, and osteochondromatosis.

Acute changes related to systemic disease are most commonly seen at the juxtaphyseal metaphysis, which is the most metabolically active component of the growing bone unit, and the location of primary bone deposition (e.g., metaphyseal fraying seen in persons with rickets or juxtaphyseal sclerosis with intervening areas of bony rarefaction in persons with leukemia).

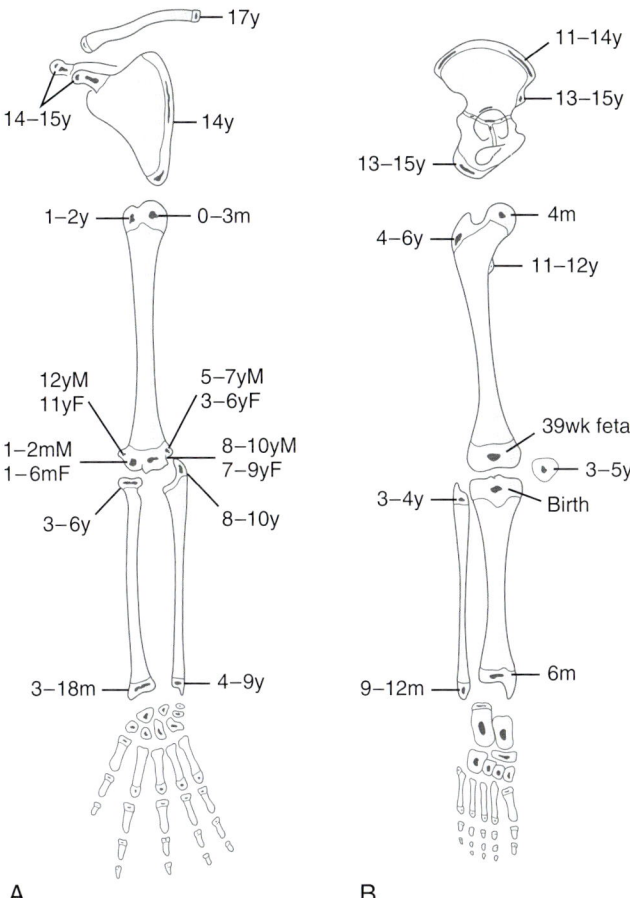

Figure 129-2 Ages of onset of secondary (epiphyseal and apophyseal) ossification of the major bones of the upper (**A**) and lower (**B**) extremity. *F,* Female; *M,* male; *m,* month; *wk,* week; *y,* year. (Reproduced from Ogden JA. *Skeletal injury in the child.* 3rd ed. New York: Springer; 2000.)

Anatomy

Three types of bones are found in the limbs: (1) long and short tubular bones, (2) round bones in the wrists and ankles, and (3) sesamoids, which are small bones in the tendons and articular capsules. Functionally, a growing tubular bone is made up of the following segments: diaphysis, metaphysis, physis, and epiphysis (Fig. 129-5). "Long bones" have epiphyses at both ends. Short tubular bones ("short bones") have epiphyses at one end—generally, where the greater joint motion of the individual bone occurs. In the hands and feet, secondary ossification centers appear in the bases of the phalanges and in the distal ends of the second through fifth metacarpals and metatarsals. Epiphyses for the first metacarpal and first metatarsal are found in the proximal ends of the bones. The location of the secondary centers appears to be related to the sites of maximal joint motion of individual bones. Apparent epiphyseal ossification centers observed at the ends of short bones, where their occurrence is not expected, are termed "pseudoepiphyses."

Normal Findings

DETERMINING SKELETAL AGE

The gestational age of a newborn can be estimated radiographically through several methods. The proximal humeral ossification center appears shortly after birth, with a 95% confidence interval between 37 weeks' gestation and 16 weeks' postnatal life.[3] Because ossification before 37 weeks is unusual, the presence of the proximal humeral ossification center is an indication that a newborn is at term or near term. Teeth appear at a characteristic time; the first deciduous molars form at 33 weeks, and the second deciduous molars form at 36 weeks. The range of values is great for the radiographic appearance of various appendicular bone epiphyseal ossification centers, even in premature infants (see Table 129-1).

Evaluation of bone age is used to estimate biologic maturation relative to chronologic age. Differences in familial, racial, and socioeconomic factors limit the applicability of the standards of Greulich and Pyle (which were developed in the 1940s) to today's children.[4] It is well accepted that maturation

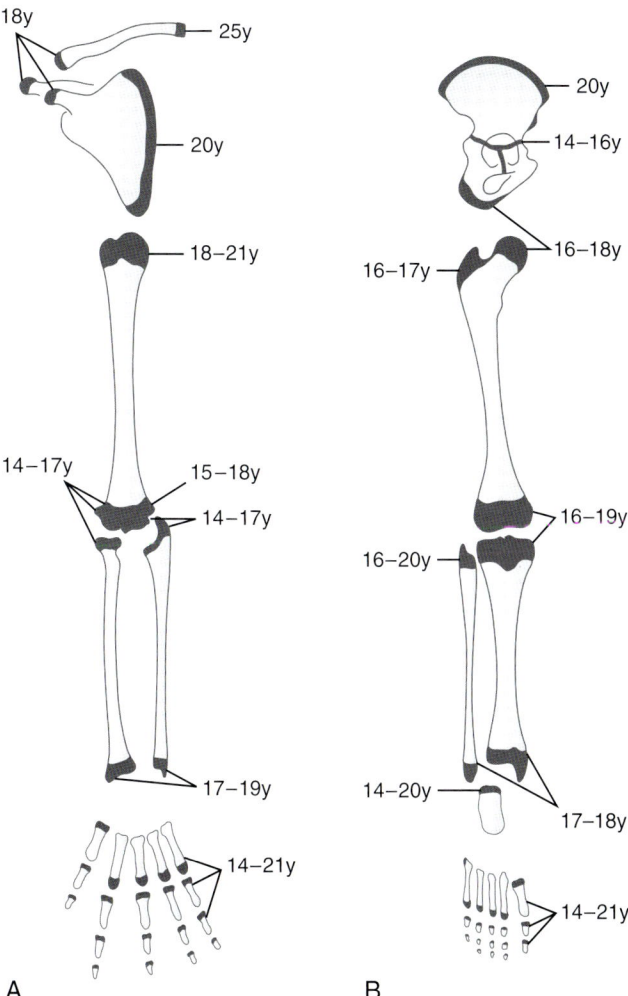

Figure 129-3 Ages of physeal closure of the major bones of the upper (**A**) and lower (**B**) extremities. *y,* Year. (Reproduced from Ogden JA. *Skeletal injury in the child.* 3rd ed. New York: Springer; 2000.)

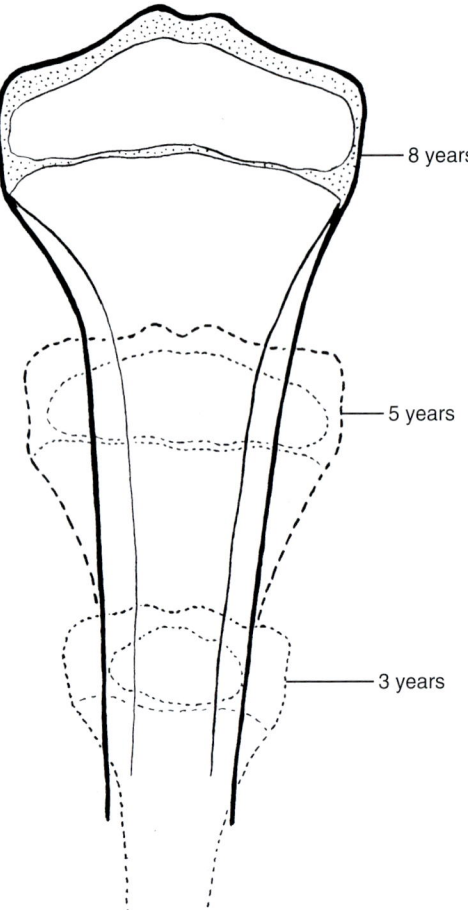

Figure 129-4 Growth and configuration of the tibia with advancing age. The progressive concentric constriction of the shaft away from the wider epiphyseal plate is shown schematically on superimposed tracings of radiographs.

varies between races. For instance, African American children mature faster than do white children.[5] The hand, with its numerous secondary centers in phalanges and metacarpals, and to a lesser degree the wrist, are used as an index of total skeletal maturation. Standard deviations, which are based on chronologic age, are somewhat broad. A bone age within the 5% to 95% confidence interval (or ±2 standard deviations) is considered normal.

In children younger than 2 years, use of the standards of Greulich and Pyle is limited because relatively little change is noted in the ossification centers of the hand and wrist during this period. More rapid changes may be observed in the knee or foot, however. Radiographs of the left knee or left foot—anteroposterior and lateral—therefore are obtained in children younger than 2 years of age and are compared with published standards (for the knee, standards of Pyle and Hoerr [1969][6]; for the foot and ankle, standards of Hoerr, Pyle, and Francis [1962][7]).

The Risser classification can be used to assess skeletal maturation through evaluation of the appearance and state of fusion of the iliac crest.[8] Ossification of the iliac crest begins laterally and proceeds medially: stage 0—no ossification; stage I—up to 25% ossified; stage II—25% to 50% ossified; stage III—50% to 75% ossified; stage IV—75% to 100% ossified; and stage V—fully ossified and fused (e-Fig. 129-6).

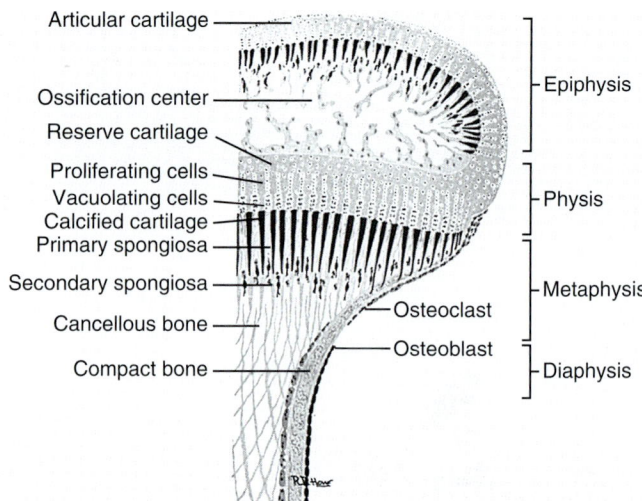

Figure 129-5 Functional components of the growing end of a tubular bone and their anatomic substrate.

Assessment of skeletal age by radiography is useful in many clinical scenarios. Boxes 129-1 and 129-2 list causes of advanced and delayed skeletal maturation, respectively. Menarche typically occurs after fusion of the physes of the distal phalanges. Bone age can be used with long bone measurements to predict adult height. Assessment of bone age is valuable in the planning of orthopedic treatments, including epiphysiodesis, leg-lengthening procedures, and scoliosis management.

ANATOMIC VARIANTS

Experience and knowledge often are the best resources for successfully identifying normal variants. Compendiums of normal variants (e.g., *An Atlas of Normal Roentgen Variants That May Simulate Disease* by Keats and Anderson[9] and *Borderlands of Normal and Early Pathological Findings in Skeletal Radiography* by Freyschmidt et al.[10]) are invaluable resources.

Box 129-1 Advanced Skeletal Maturation

- Acrodysostosis
- Adrenogenital syndrome (adrenocortical tumor or hyperplasia)
- Cerebral gigantism
- Gonadal tumors (androgen or estrogen secreting)
- Growth hormone excess (gigantism)
- Hyperthyroidism (maternal or acquired)
- Hypothalamic tumors
- Idiopathic familial advanced bone age
- Idiopathic isosexual precocious puberty
- Lipodystrophy
- Liver tumors (choriocarcinoma, hepatoma)
- McCune-Albright syndrome (polyostotic fibrous dysplasia)
- Medication with sex hormones
- Pinealoma
- Premature adrenarche
- Premature thelarche
- Pseudohypoparathyroidism
- Various syndromes

Box 129-2 Delayed Skeletal Maturation

- Addison disease
- Chromosomal disorders (e.g., trisomy 21 and trisomy 18)
- Chronic illness
- Chronic renal disease
- Chronic severe anemia (e.g., sickle cell anemia and thalassemia)
- Congenital heart disease (especially cyanotic)
- Congenital malformation syndromes
- Constitutional delay
- Cushing syndrome
- Growth hormone deficiency
- Hypogonadism (e.g., Turner syndrome)
- Hypothyroidism
- Idiopathic causes
- Inflammatory bowel disease
- Intrauterine growth retardation
- Juvenile diabetes mellitus
- Malabsorption syndromes (e.g., celiac disease)
- Malnutrition
- Neurologic disorders
- Panhypopituitarism
- Rickets
- Skeletal dysplasias (most)
- Steroid therapy

Many epiphyseal and apophyseal ossification centers are irregular and fragmented in their early development (Fig. 129-7). When evaluating the significance of irregular ossification in a single area, it is important to remember that normal irregularities of ossification usually are symmetric and accompanied by similar changes in other areas of the skeleton. Normal epiphyseal and apophyseal fragmentary ossification tends to have a smooth, round, and sclerotic appearance. Sometimes epiphyseal fragmentary ossification centers may have a jigsaw configuration. Normal epiphyseal fragmentary ossification should be differentiated from acute fractures that tend to have a linear contour with nonsclerotic margins with accompanying soft tissue swelling and joint effusions.

Physiologic osteosclerosis of the newborn is a common finding. The long tubular bones of fetuses, premature infants, and term newborn infants often appear sclerotic compared with the bones of older children because of proportionately thicker cortical bone and more abundant spongiosa during fetal and neonatal life (e-Fig. 129-8). The sclerotic features disappear gradually during the first weeks of life and resolve by 2 to 3 months of age.

Physiologic periosteal reaction in the newborn also is a common finding that is seen in infants from 1 to 4 months of age and in both premature and term infants. Physiologic periosteal new bone is diaphyseal, smooth, regular, and 2 mm or less in thickness (Fig. 129-9).[11] Physiologic periosteal new bone is most common in the tibia, femur, and humeral diaphysis and occasionally is seen in the radius and ulna. In most infants, physiologic periosteal new bone is symmetric; however, it may be asymmetric in one third to half of patients. Traumatic periosteal new bone tends to be asymmetric, metaphyseal, thicker, and irregular compared with physiologic periosteal new bone.

A variety of normal variants in the metaphyses of infants may simulate injury. It is important to distinguish these findings from the classic metaphyseal lesions of child abuse (see Chapter 145). The most common variant is the subperiosteal bone collar of the juxtaphyseal metaphysis, which has a normal step-off that may mimic a metaphyseal lesion of child abuse (Fig. 129-10).[12]

Gas (nitrogen) commonly is seen in a joint as a result of traction used to position a young child for radiographs. The presence of a vacuum joint on radiography strongly militates against the presence of an effusion.

The following selected, important variants should not be confused with pathology.

Hands and Feet

Ivory Epiphyses

Sclerotic epiphyseal ossification centers of the phalanges are called "ivory epiphyses" (e-Fig. 129-11).[13] They occur in approximately 1 in every 300 patients. Ivory epiphyses usually are found in the distal phalanges and in the middle phalanx of the fifth digit. Maturation may be retarded. Ivory epiphyses also may occur in association with cone-shaped epiphyses in dysplastic syndromes. Ivory epiphyses are more frequently found in the toes compared with the fingers.

Cone-Shaped Epiphyses

Cone-shaped epiphyses of the phalanges (e-Fig. 129-12) occur singly or in combination and most commonly affect the terminal phalanges. When they occur in isolation, they may be related to trauma with resultant central physeal growth disturbance. When they are multiple, they may be seen in association with dysplastic syndromes and metabolic bone disease. Cone-shaped epiphyses are found more frequently in the toes than in the fingers (Fig. 129-13).

Fifth Metatarsal Apophysis

During puberty, a longitudinally oriented, scalelike secondary ossification center appears within the proximal apophyseal cartilage of the fifth metatarsal (Fig. 129-14). Irregular ossification of the apophysis is common. The normal apophyseal ossification center may appear widely spaced from the underlying fifth metatarsal, simulating fracture.[14] The fifth metatarsal apophysis also may be bifid (e-Fig. 129-15). This presentation should be differentiated from a fifth metatarsal avulsion fracture related to the peroneus brevis insertion, which has a horizontal orientation (e-Fig. 129-16) (see also Chapter 143).

Pseudoepiphyses

Pseudoepiphyseal ossification centers may appear in the proximal cartilaginous portion of the growing second through fifth metacarpals and metatarsals and in the distal cartilage of the first metacarpals and metatarsals (Fig. 129-17 and e-Fig. 129-18).[15] They are formed from a thin rod of osteogenic tissue that invades the proximal cartilage from the shaft. The end of the rod enlarges to form a mushroom-shaped mass of bone that appears radiographically as the "pseudoepiphysis." The site of fusion of the pseudoepiphysis with the shaft often

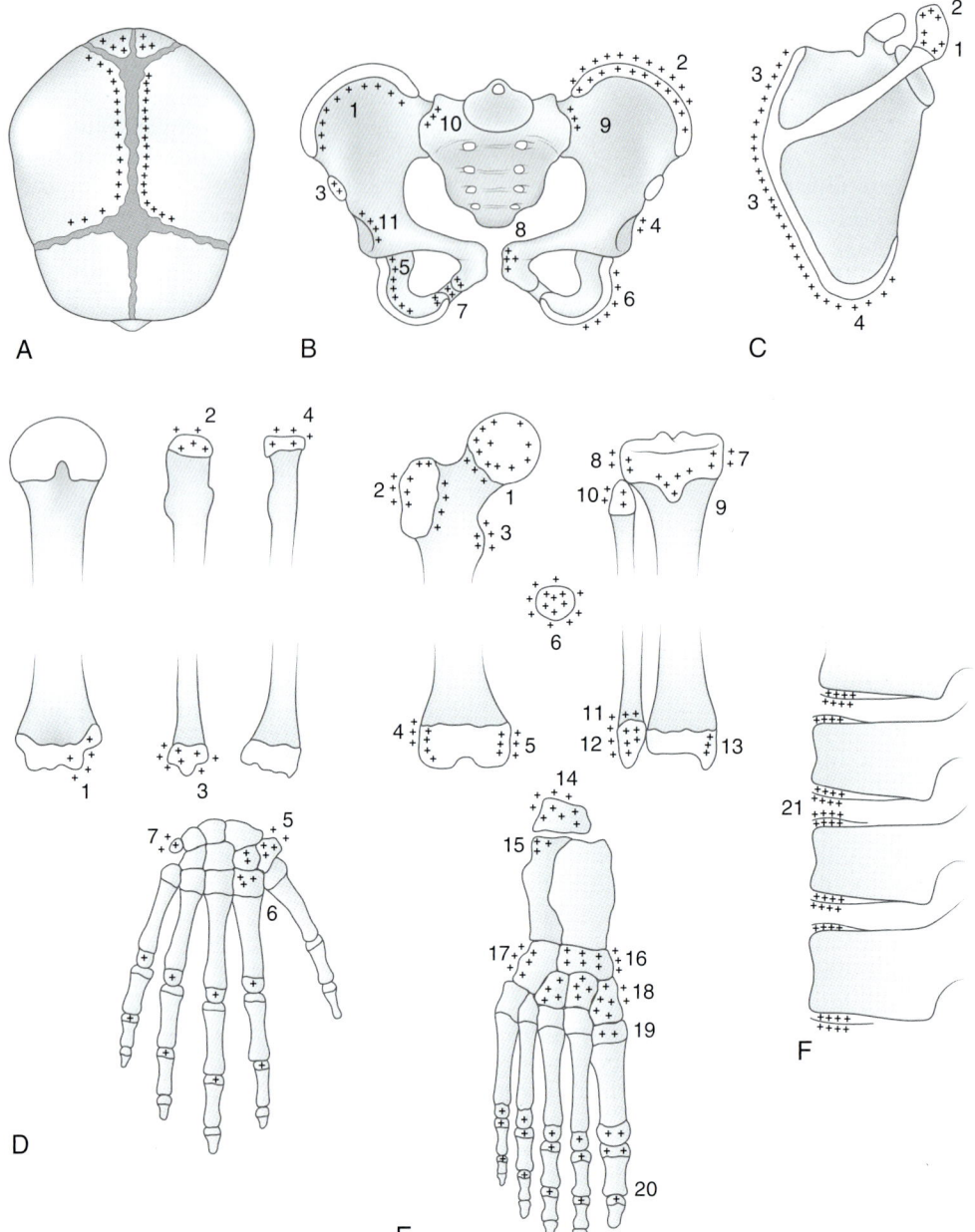

Figure 129-7   Common sites of normally irregular mineralization in the growing skeleton are marked by crosses. **A,** The cranium. During the first weeks of life and continuing for several months, edges of the bones at the great sutures are commonly irregular, and in many infants deep fissures extend from the sutures into the bodies of the bones. Irregularities also are common on the edges of the temporal suture (not shown). **B,** The pelvis: 1, crest of ilium; 2, secondary center in crest of ilium; 3, secondary center of anterior superior spine; 4, os acetabuli marginalis; 5, body of ischium; 6, secondary center of ischium; 7, ischium and pubis at the ischiopubic synchondrosis; 8, body of pubis; 9, ilium at sacroiliac joint; 10, sacrum at sacroiliac joint; 11, iliac edge and roof of the acetabular cavity. **C,** The scapula: 1 and 2, secondary centers of acromion process; 3, secondary center of vertebral edge; 4, secondary center of inferior angle. **D,** The upper limb: 1, secondary center of trochlea, always irregular; 2 and 3, proximal and distal epiphyseal centers of ulna; 4, proximal epiphyseal center of radius; 5, greater and lesser multangulars; 6, inconstant center of second metacarpal (pseudoepiphysis); 7, pisiform. **E,** The lower limb; 1, proximal metaphysis of femur; 2 and 3, secondary center and edges of shaft at greater and lesser trochanters, respectively; 4 and 5, lateral and medial edges, respectively, of distal epiphyseal center of femur; 6, patella; 7 and 8, medial and lateral edges, respectively, of proximal epiphyseal center of tibia; 9, secondary center in anterior tibial process; 10, proximal epiphyseal center of fibula; 11 and 12, distal metaphysis and distal epiphyseal center of fibula, respectively; 13, internal malleolus of distal epiphyseal center of tibia; 14, apophysis of calcaneus; 15, primary center of calcaneus; 16, navicular; 17, cuboid; 18, cuneiform; 19, proximal epiphyseal center of first metatarsal; 20, epiphyseal centers of phalanges. **F,** The spine; 21, marginal centers (end plate apophyses).

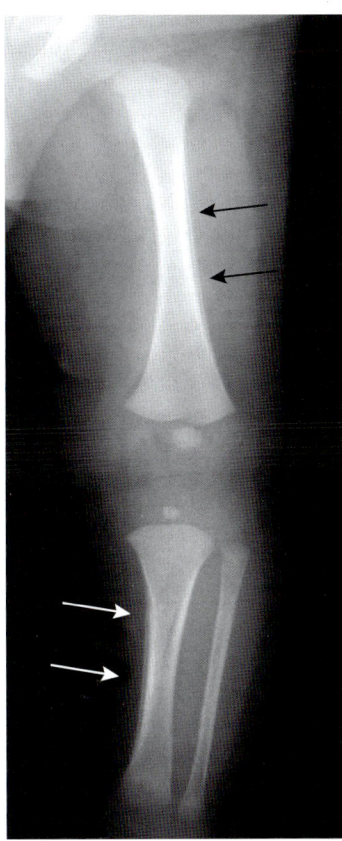

Figure 129-9 Physiologic periosteal new bone on the lateral aspect of the femoral diaphysis and medial aspect of the tibial diaphysis (*arrows*) in a 9-week-old boy.

is indicated by a notch. Pseudoepiphyses are well formed by 4 to 5 years of age and fuse with the underlying shaft at the time of skeletal maturation. Pseudoepiphyses are frequent in children with hypothyroidism and cleidocranial dysplasia.

Sesamoid Bones

Sesamoid bones are present in the foot and hand. Sesamoids of the great toe reside within the medial and lateral slips of the hallux brevis tendon overlying the head of the first metatarsal. The medial great toe sesamoid is bipartite in 4% to 33% of patients (e-Fig. 129-19). Sesamoids of the feet may develop a stress reaction or a complete fracture and may be difficult to distinguish from a bipartite sesamoid on radiographs; magnetic resonance imaging (MRI) may be useful in distinguishing a normal bipartite sesamoid and underlying stress injury. For the first metatarsal phalangeal, stress injury tends to affect the medial sesamoid more frequently than the lateral sesamoid.[16] In addition to the sesamoids, numerous other supernumerary ossicles of the foot and ankle exist (Fig. 129-20).

Irregular Carpal Ossification

Irregular mineralization often occurs in the developing carpal bones (e-Fig. 129-21). The pisiform is the bone most frequently affected (e-Fig. 129-22). In addition, carpal bones sometimes may have wavy cortical contours, which should not be confused with erosions.

Os Styloideum (Carpal Boss)

The os styloideum is a bony protrusion at the dorsum of the wrist between the trapezoid, capitate, and second and third metacarpals.[17] It may be isolated and mobile or fused to an

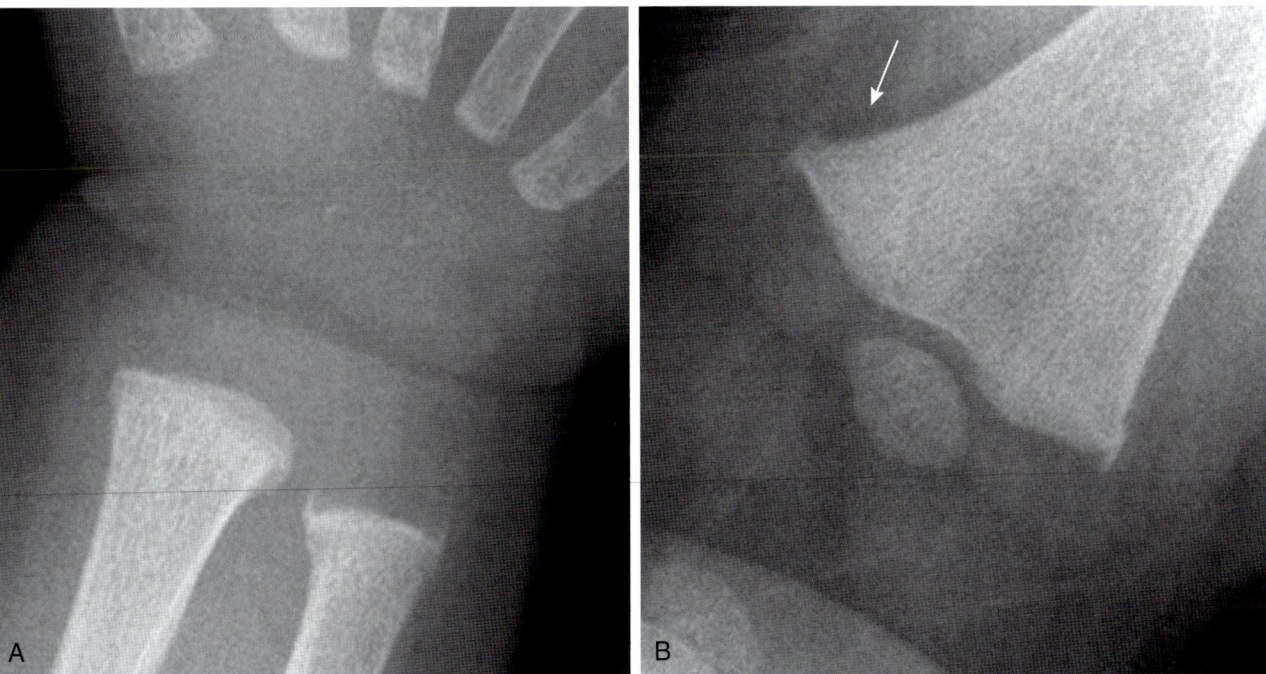

Figure 129-10 Small spurs on the distal ulnar (**A**) and distal femoral (**B**) metaphyses in a 5-month-old girl due to extension of the subperiosteal bone collar beyond the metaphysis. A normal "step-off" also is noted on the distal femur (*arrow*).

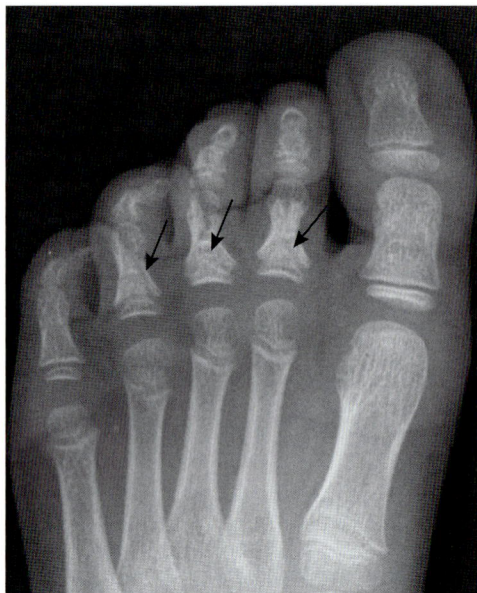

Figure 129-13 Symmetric conical or bell-shaped epiphyseal ossification centers (*arrows*) in the proximal phalanges of the second, third, and fourth toes of an asymptomatic 5-year-old girl. The contiguous distal end of each shaft is recessed to receive its elongated ossification center. The epiphyseal ossification centers in the proximal phalanges of the first and fifth toes are the normal, flat, shallow, transverse disks usually present in all of the phalanges.

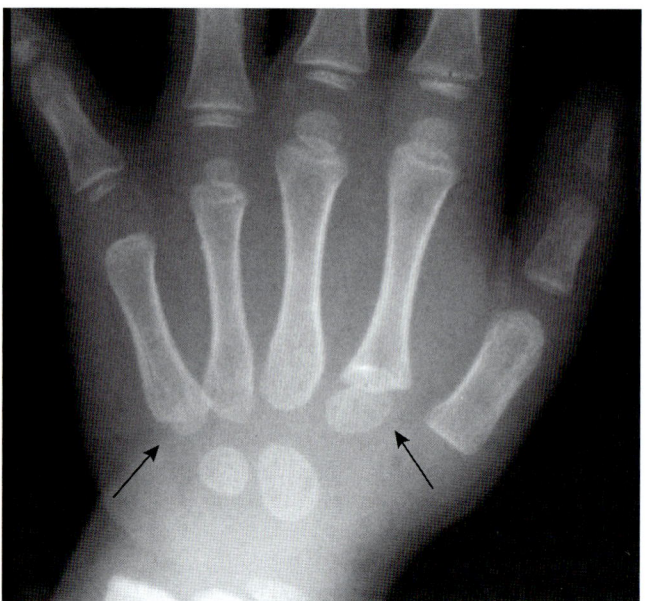

Figure 129-17 Pseudoepiphyses (*arrows*) in the proximal second and fifth metacarpals of a 3-year-old boy.

adjacent bone. The os styloideum is present in 1% to 3% of patients and presents as a palpable mass (Fig. 129-23). The differential diagnosis for a dorsal palpable abnormality along the wrist is an os styloideum versus a dorsal carpal ganglion cyst.

Radial and Ulnar Styloid Processes

Separate ossification centers may appear in the regions of the ulnar (e-Fig. 129-24) and radial (Fig. 129-25) styloid processes before uniting with the main ossification center.

Bifid Epiphyses

Accessory ossification centers may occur in the epiphyses of phalanges and metatarsal bones. Bifid epiphysis is most common in the great toes, where examination before fusion of the centers is complete may simulate fracture (e-Fig. 129-26). The affected epiphysis is relatively sclerotic.[18]

Absent Epiphyses

The phalanges, especially the middle group, frequently lack epiphyseal centers in healthy children; this absence may be associated with symphalangism at the affected joints. Forty percent of the population has a biphalangeal (e-Fig. 129-27) fifth toe[19] that may predispose to hammer or claw toe deformities.

Bifid Calcaneus

The ossification center for the calcaneus is present at birth. Occasionally the body of the calcaneus may ossify from two or more independent centers (Fig. 129-28). This finding is rare as a normal variant. More often it is associated with an underlying disorder such as Down syndrome, mucolipidosis, or Larsen syndrome.

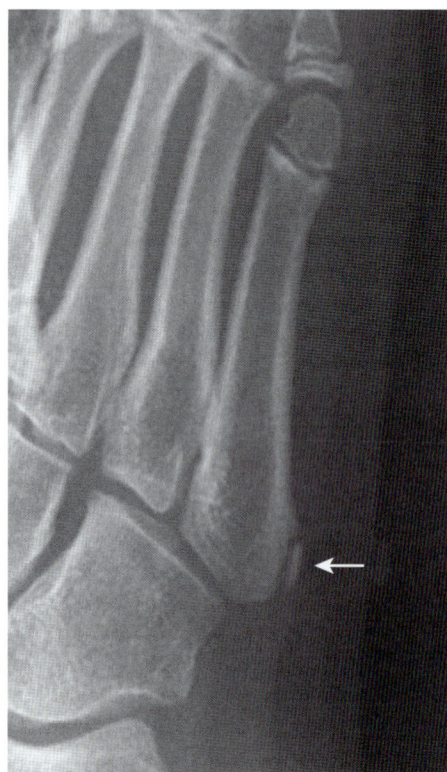

Figure 129-14 Normal apophysis of the fifth metatarsal in a 10-year-old girl (*arrow*). The apophyseal growth plate is longitudinal in orientation, and the apophysis appears "scalelike."

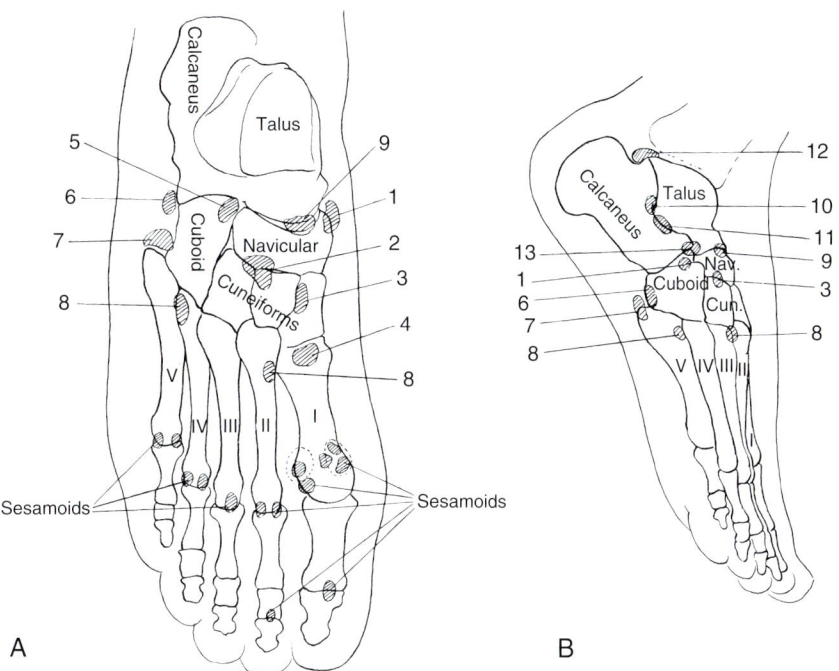

Figure 129-20   Normal supernumerary ossicles of the feet in ventrodorsal (**A**) and lateral (**B**) projections: 1, os tibiale externum; 2, processus uncinatus; 3, os intercuneiforme; 4, pars peronea metatarsalia; 5, os cuboideum secundarium; 6, os peroneum; 7, os vesalianum pedis; 8, os intermetatarseum; 9, accessory navicular; 10, talus accessorius; 11, sustentaculum tali; 12, os trigonum tarsi; 13, calcaneus secundarius.

Calcaneal Apophysis

The calcaneal apophysis appears about the middle of the first decade. It often is fragmented and/or sclerotic well into the second decade until fusion with the body of the calcaneus is complete (e-Fig. 129-29). Calcaneal apophysitis (Sever disease) is a poorly understood cause of heel pain in children, and this diagnosis should not be made on the basis of

radiographs alone.[20] MRI findings of apophyseal edema may suggest the diagnosis; however, Sever disease remains a clinical diagnosis.

Calcaneus Secondarius

The calcaneus secondarius (e-Fig. 129-30) may simulate an anterior process calcaneal fracture. The ossicle is located in

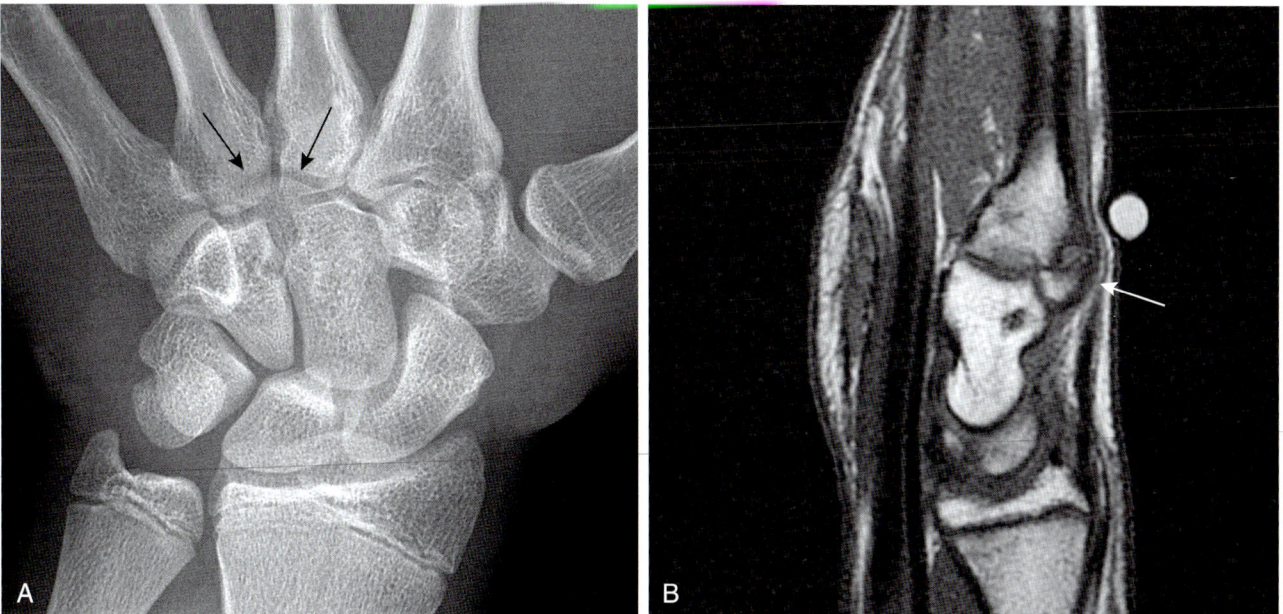

Figure 129-23   Os styloideum (carpal boss) in a 14-year-old boy. **A,** An anteroposterior radiograph; the accessory bone is barely visible (*arrows*). **B,** A sagittal T1-weighted magnetic resonance image shows the accessory ossicle (*arrow*) at the dorsum of the carpometacarpal joint. Note that the ossicle causes a bump on the dorsum of the wrist.

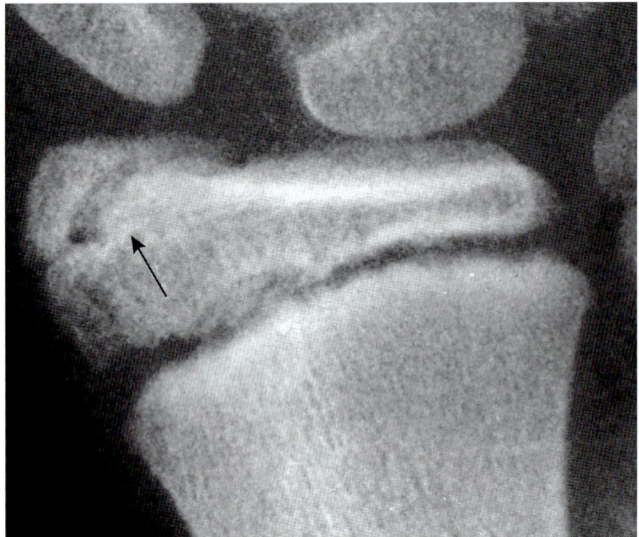

Figure 129-25   A large accessory ossification center (*arrow*) in the styloid process of the radial epiphyseal ossification center of a healthy 13-year-old boy simulates a fracture fragment.

between the anteromedial calcaneus, cuboid, talar head, and navicular. It is rare and of no clinical significance other than possibly being mistaken for a fracture.

Calcaneal Pseudocyst

A pseudocystic triangular area of radiolucency is present in the anterior half of the calcaneal body. At this location, a deficiency of spongy bone is normal. The pseudocyst is of no clinical significance in itself; however, it must be differentiated from true bone cysts or intraosseous lipomas that can develop at this site but tend to have a more round shape. MRI or computed tomography (CT) is helpful for differentiating these lesions when radiographic features are equivocal.

Os Trigonum

An os trigonum is located at the posterior margin of the talus in approximately 15% of persons[21] and may superficially mimic a fracture (Fig. 129-31). Repetitive forced plantar flexion may cause a syndrome of posterior ankle impingement or "os trigonum syndrome." This syndrome occurs most commonly in ballet dancers, soccer players, and

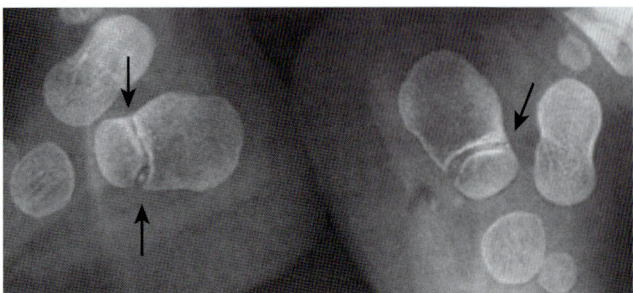

Figure 129-28   Double ossification centers (*arrows*) in the body of the calcaneus on each side of a 20-month-old infant. The infant was normal; films were obtained because of an injury to the left ankle a few hours earlier.

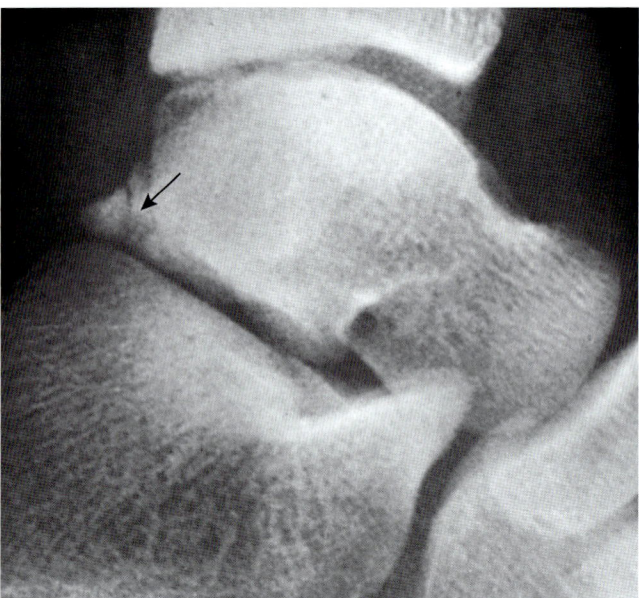

Figure 129-31   A normal apophyseal ossification center (*arrow*) in the dorsal process of the talus in a healthy 11-year-old boy. The radiolucent strip between the body of the talus and the ossification center is a normal synchondrosis, not a fracture line. When the synchondrosis persists after the normal age for its fusion with the body of the talus, the persistent ossification center is called the os trigonum.

basketball players and may cause tendinopathy of the flexor hallucis longus.

Os Supratalare

The os supratalare on the crest of the head of the talus may simulate injury or be simulated by injury (e-Fig. 129-32).

Os Supranaviculare

The center for the navicular bone frequently is irregular up to about 5 years of age and occasionally later (Fig. 129-33). The os supranaviculare (e-Fig. 129-34) is an accessory ossicle that can be confused with an accessory ossification center before the latter fuses with the parent bone; both must be differentiated from fracture.

Accessory Navicular

The accessory navicular is the best known and one of the most important variants in the foot. The accessory navicular is located along the medial aspect of the navicular where the tibialis posterior inserts. Accessory navicular bones are seen in approximately 21% of patients, and 50% to 90% are bilateral.[22] When patients have symptoms related to their accessory navicular, it usually is related to painful flat foot in part as a result of tibialis posterior dysfunction.

The type I variant ("os tibiale externum" or "navicular secundarium") is a true rounded sesamoid bone measuring 2 to 6 mm that lies within the tendon of the posterior tibialis muscle and is approximately 3 mm separate from the navicular bone (e-Fig. 129-35). Type I variants are asymptomatic and do not fuse with the navicular. Type I variants account for 10% to 15% of cases in children.

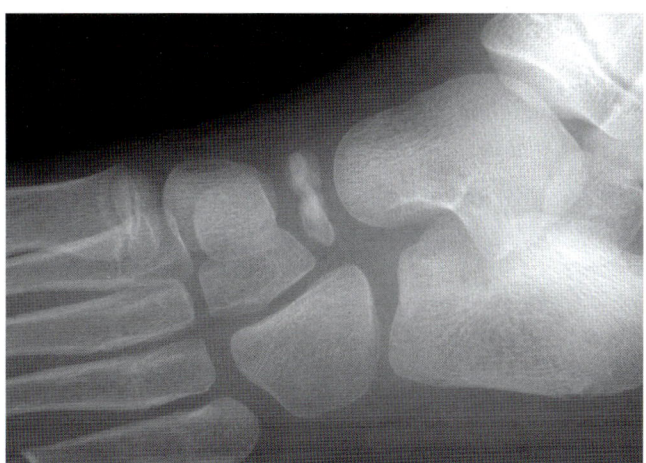

Figure 129-33 Irregular ossification of the navicular in a 2-year-old boy.

Type II variants ("prehallux" or "bifurcated hallux") are united to the navicular by a cartilaginous or fibrocartilaginous bridge and represent an accessory ossification center for the tubercle of the navicular (Fig. 129-36). The ossicle is larger (9 to 12 mm), triangular or heart shaped, and congruent with and closely apposed to the adjacent navicular. It is connected to the navicular by a synchondrosis. Symptoms generally develop in the second decade. Fusion with the navicular bone occurs in most of these cases.

The type III variant is the cornuate navicular. The cornuate navicular represents medial and plantar elongation of the navicular bone without a separate ossicle, which sometimes may result from type II fusion with the navicular bone.

Cuneiforms

The three cuneiforms may ossify irregularly in children who are healthy and have no clinical evidence of local disease in the feet. A bipartite medial cuneiform has a coronal cleft separating it into proximal and distal portions. A duplicate cuneiform may be longitudinal in form (e-Fig. 129-37).

Elbow

The six major ossification centers at the elbow ossify in an expected sequence—capitellum, radial head, internal (medial) epicondyle, trochlea, olecranon, and external (lateral) epicondyle. The sequence of ossification can be remembered with the acronym CRITOE (CRMTOL). If a bony density is seen in one area when an earlier-appearing center is lacking, a traumatic fragment is very likely the cause. This consideration is most important along the medial compartment, and correctly identifying the medial epicondyle and trochlea also is important (Fig. 129-38). The medial epicondyle appears earlier than the trochlea as a rule. Therefore if the medial epicondyle is absent but a trochlear ossification is present, a displaced medial epicondylar fracture should be suspected (e-Fig. 129-39). Rarely, variations in the order of ossification occur. The most common variation is the medial epicondyle appearing before the radial head. The ossification centers of the elbow can appear quite irregular during initial formation, particularly the trochlea (e-Fig. 129-40). The olecranon ossification center (Fig. 129-41) varies considerably in size and should be differentiated from an acute olecranon fracture (e-Fig. 129-42) by the shape of the individual ossifications and the nature of the margins (sclerotic or nonsclerotic).

The lateral epicondyle does not fuse directly with the humeral shaft as the medial epicondyle does but fuses first with the adjacent capitellum; their fused mass then joins with the end of the humeral shaft (Fig. 129-43). With early ossification, the lateral epicondylar ossification center appears as an irregular flake of bone, which is easily mistaken for an avulsion fragment (e-Fig. 129-44). The medial epicondyle occasionally has an irregular, fragmentary appearance (Fig. 129-45). This finding must be differentiated from an avulsion with widening or irregularity, or both, of the medial epicondylar physis (e-Fig. 129-46).

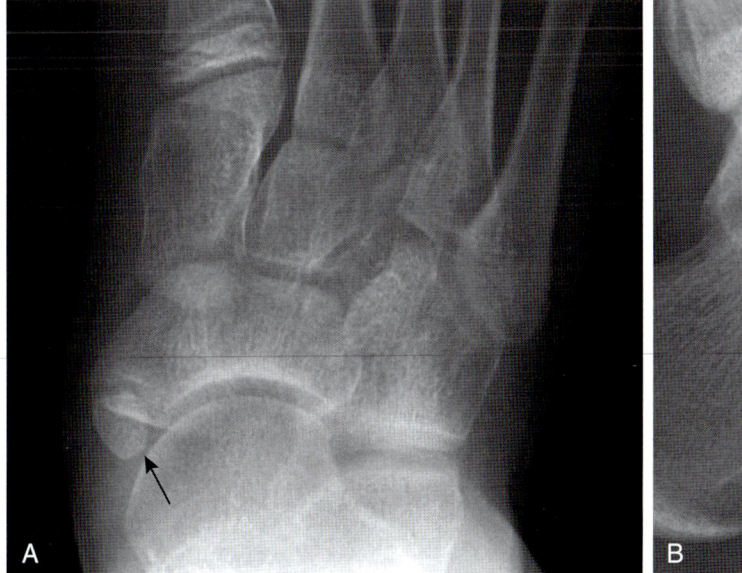
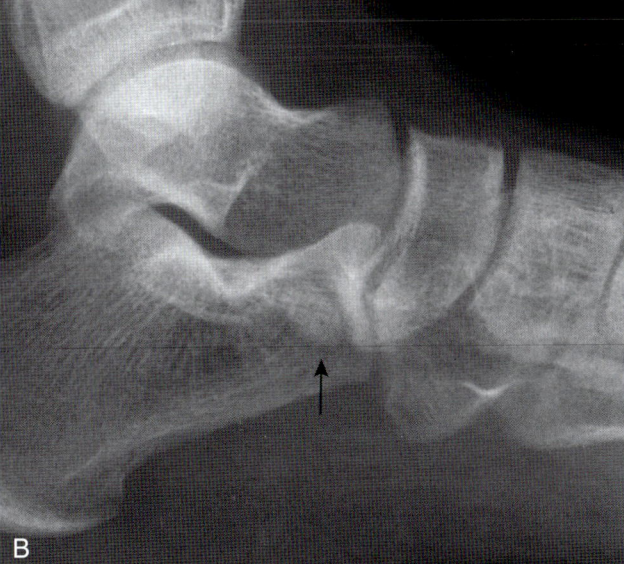

Figure 129-36 Type II accessory naviculars (*arrows*). **A,** An 11-year-old girl. **B,** A 13-year-old girl.

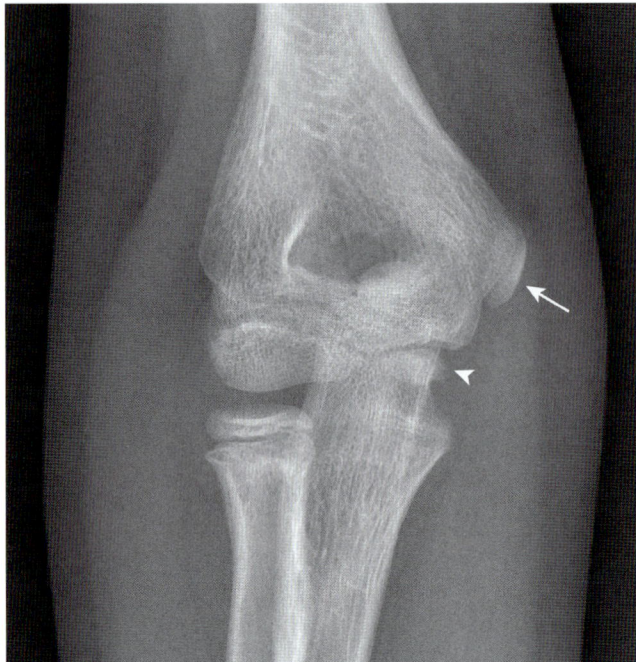

Figure 129-38 An 11-year-old boy with a normal elbow. As a rule, the medial epicondylar ossification center (*arrow*) should appear before the trochlear ossification center (*arrowhead*). If only the trochlear ossification center is present, a medial epicondylar avulsion fracture should be suspected.

Supracondylar Process

The supracondylar process of the humerus is a vestigial structure that projects from the medial aspect of the anterior surface of the humeral shaft 5 to 7 cm proximal to the medial epicondyle (Figs. 129-47 and 129-48).[23] It occurs in 1% of individuals. The supracondylar process may be connected by the ligament of Struthers to the medial epicondyle. Portions of pronator teres and brachioradialis muscles may attach to the process, to the ligament of Struthers, or to both. Occasionally, median nerve neuralgia occurs as a result of

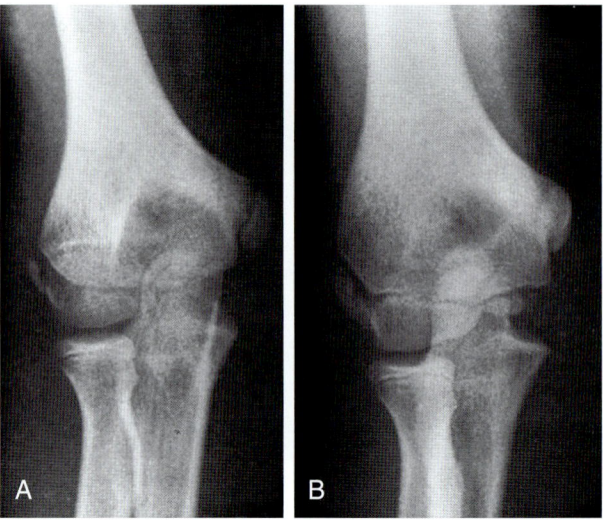

Figure 129-43. The lateral epicondyle center is independent of both the capitulum and the shaft at 11 years (**A**); it already has fused with the capitulum at 12½ years (**B**), and these combined ossification centers will later fuse with the shaft. The medial epicondyle center is fusing directly with the shaft in **A** and **B**. In **B**, the trochlea is normally irregular.

entrapment or compression of the median nerve as it passes through the tunnel created by the supracondylar process, the ligament of Struthers, and associated structures.

Shoulder

Proximal Humeral Epiphyseal Ossification

At the upper end of the humerus, two and occasionally three secondary ossification centers can be observed. The first center (humeral head proper) to appear develops in the

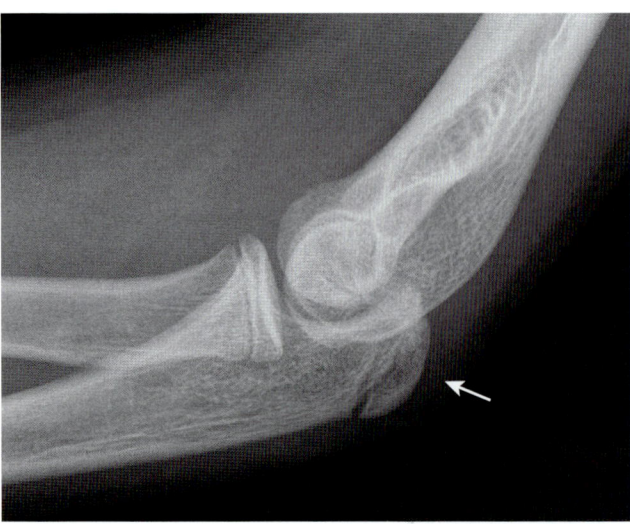

Figure 129-41 A normal smooth, corticated olecranon ossification center (*arrow*) in a 12-year-old boy.

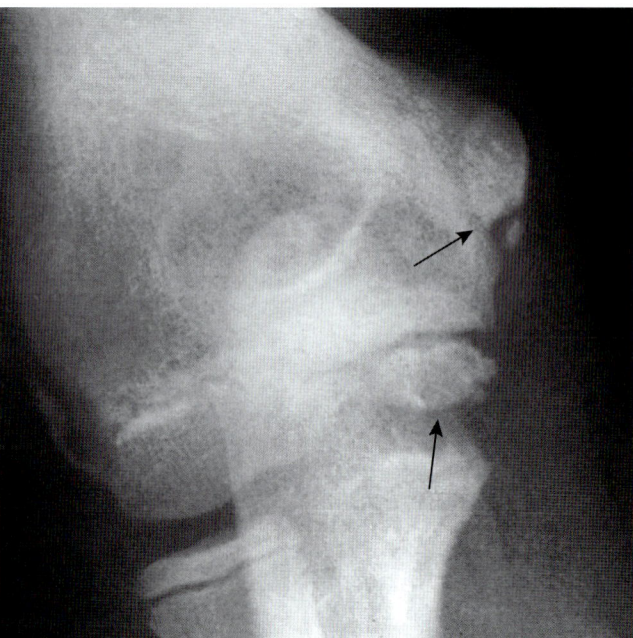

Figure 129-45 An accessory ossification center (*proximal arrow*) at the lower pole of the medial epicondyle of a healthy 12-year-old boy that simulates a fracture fragment. The distal arrow points to the normal irregular edges of the trochlear center of the humerus.

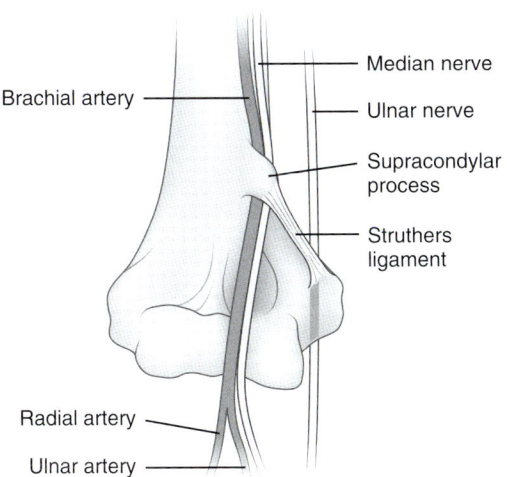

Figure 129-47 A drawing of the supracondylar process on the anterior surface of the humerus that shows the relationship of the process to the brachial artery and its branches and to the median nerve. (From Spinner RJ, Lins RE, Jacobson SR, et al. Fractures of the supracondylar process of the humerus. *J Hand Surg (Am)*. 1994;19:1038-1041.)

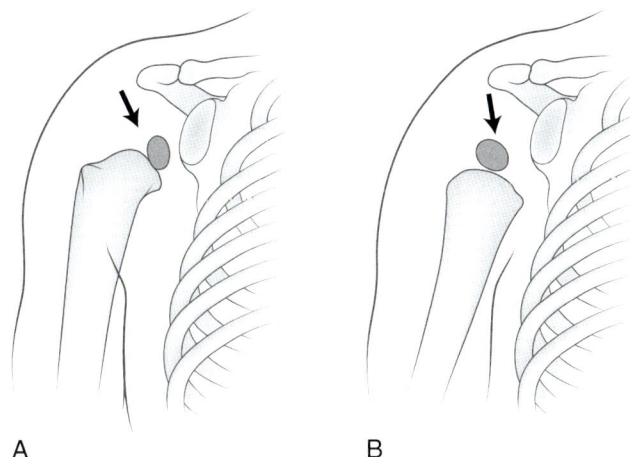

A   B

Figure 129-49 A factitious shift in position (*arrows*) of the normally eccentric proximal ossification center of the humerus caused by rotation of the bone. **A,** The anatomic position of the humerus with the ossification center in the medial segment of the epiphysis. **B,** With the humerus in internal rotation, the ossification center appears to be displaced laterad.

medial half of the epiphysis at about 2 weeks of age; because of its eccentric location, it shifts to a factitious lateral position when the arm is internally rotated (Fig. 129-49). The second center appears laterally in the greater tuberosity during the second half of the first year. A rare third center occurs in the lesser tuberosity during the third year and fuses with the humeral head during the sixth to seventh years. This center may be seen in axillary views of the shoulder and may simulate a fracture fragment.

Proximal Humeral Physis

The proximal humeral physis is tented, with the apex well above the pitched anterior and posterior segments. In rotated positions of the humerus, these segments are projected at different levels and may simulate fracture (e-Fig. 129-50). Offset of the epiphyseal ossification center relative to the lateral metaphyseal margin may simulate a Salter-Harris fracture.

Bicipital Groove

The bicipital groove in the anterior surface of the humerus may simulate local bone destruction or production (e-Fig. 129-51).

Muscular Insertions

Local cortical thickening that resembles a periosteal reaction occurs frequently at sites of insertion of major muscles of the upper arm. This finding is most common at the site of the deltoid insertion at the lateral aspect of the humeral diaphysis (e-Fig. 129-52).

Notched Proximal Metaphysis of the Humerus

The medial cortical wall of the proximal humeral metaphysis may be notched in the absence of disease.[24]

Humeral Head Pseudocyst

When the humeral head is well ossified, the region of the greater tuberosity appears relatively radiolucent and devoid of trabeculation.[25] This appearance may be mistaken for a destructive lesion (e-Fig. 129-53).

Acromion and Coracoid process

The acromion can have a fragmentary appearance during ossification, and superficially it may resemble an acromion

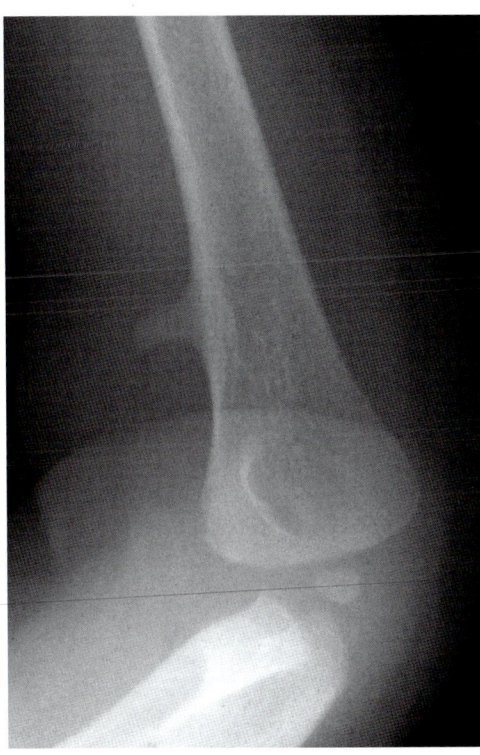

Figure 129-48 The supracondylar process of the distal humerus in a 21-month-old girl.

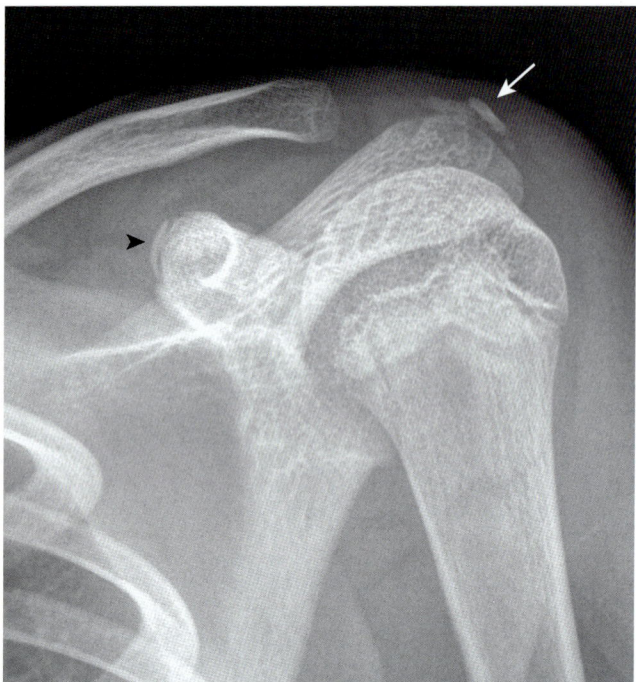

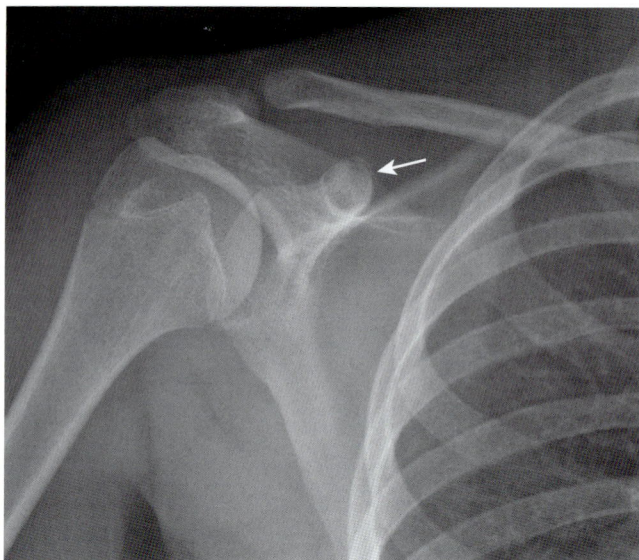

Figure 129-56 In this 15-year-old boy, the normal apophysis of the coracoid process (*arrow*) should not be mistaken for an avulsion injury.

Figure 129-54 Normal acromial fragmentation (*arrow*) and coracoid apophysis (*arrowhead*), which superficially may be mistaken for a fracture in this 12-year-old girl.

fracture (Fig. 129-54). The acromion usually will fuse with the remainder of the scapula by the age of 25 years. When the acromion persists as a separate secondary ossification center beyond 25 years, then it represents an os acromion. Because the acromion in children has a significant cartilaginous component that is radiolucent, the acromioclavicular (AC) joint may appear widened (e-Fig. 129-55). Therefore measurements developed for the AC joint in adult patients as a criterion for determining AC joint injury should not be used in children. The AC joint eventually will narrow as the acromion further ossifies. If AC joint pathology is a concern, comparison with the contralateral asymptomatic side may be helpful.

The coracoid process is the origin of the short head of the biceps tendon and coracobrachialis and is the insertion site of the pectoralis minor muscles. The coracoid process also is the origin and insertion site of various ligaments of the shoulder. The coracoid process apophysis has a complex ossification process with multiple different ossification centers that may develop at various stages and may superficially mimic a fracture (Fig. 129-56). In the beginning of the second decade, a normal lucency is present between the base of the coracoid process and the scapular body that should not be mistaken for a fracture. Later in the teenage years, the tip of the coracoid process may develop a separate ossification center that may superficially resemble an avulsion fracture.

Pelvis

Acetabulum

Irregular ossification of the acetabular roof is a normal phenomenon during growth (e-Fig. 129-57). The regular smooth configuration of the roof develops from a confluence of individual bony foci near the end of the first decade.

Accessory Ossification Centers

Accessory centers of ossification may develop in cartilage in the spine of the ischium and also in the rim of the acetabulum (os acetabuli) just below the anterior inferior iliac spine (Fig. 129-58).[26] An os acetabulae should not be confused with an acetabular rim fracture. These centers usually become visible between the 14th and 18th years, after which they fuse with the main body of the ischium and ilium, respectively. Rarely, an os acetabuli persists as a separate ossicle. The rare os acetabuli centrale is a separate ossification center, or group of centers, that appears during puberty in the central portion of

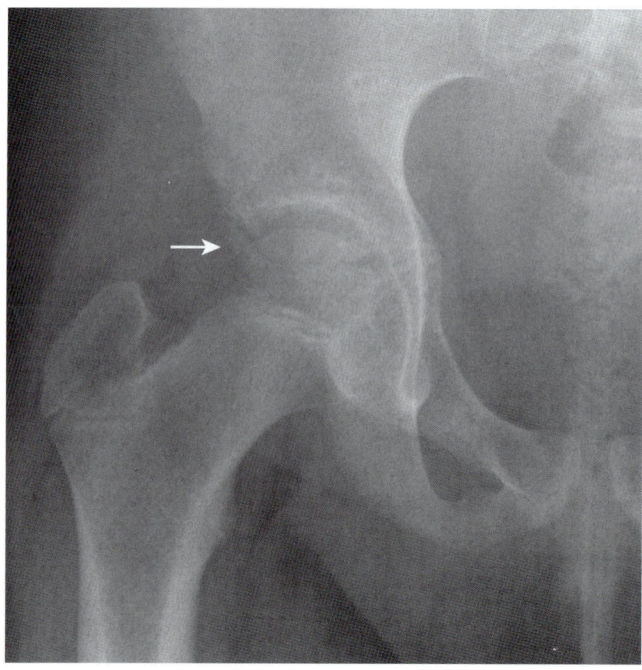

Figure 129-58 Os acetabulae (*arrow*) in a 10-year-old girl.

the triradiate in the wall of the acetabulum.[27] Accessory ossification centers also may form at the pubic symphysis and superior pubic ramus.

Ischiopubic Synchondrosis

Asymmetry of the ischiopubic synchondrosis is a very common normal variant and usually is an incidental finding unrelated to patient symptoms. Ossification of the ischiopubic synchondrosis is extremely variable in both velocity and pattern. The ischiopubic synchondrosis usually is completely fused by the teenage years.

The ischiopubic synchondrosis on the opposite side of the dominant leg usually is more prominent compared with the ischiopubic synchondrosis on the dominant leg.[28] The ischiopubic synchondrosis represents fusion of two metaphyseal equivalent sites: (1) the ischial and (2) pubic component. Therefore it is a potential site for metaphyseal equivalent insults such as osteomyelitis and trauma (Fig. 129-59).

Ischium

Apophyseal irregularities along the posterolateral edge of the ischium also may be observed, usually during preadolescence (e-Fig. 129-60). The apophyseal irregularity of the ischium is the site of origin of the hamstring complex. The two sides may be unequally affected. During growth and before fusion of the body of the ischium, the ischial apophysis is scalelike at the inferior margin of the ischium.

The ischial spine, projecting posteriorly, usually is not visible in frontal radiographs of the pelvis. The lesser sciatic notch lies below it and sometimes appears as an indentation on the lateral margin of the ischium, at the region where the ischial irregularities are most common.

Pubic Rami

Delayed and irregular mineralization of the pubic rami may be present at birth, with subsequent mineralization from several ossification centers.[29] Vertical, radiolucent clefts occasionally noted as incidental findings in pelvis radiographs probably represent bars of nonossified cartilage between expanding ossification centers. The medial edges of the bodies of the pubic bones often are irregularly mineralized during the growth period.

Hip

Asymmetric Appearance of Femoral Head Ossification

A slight disparity in the timing of ossification, the size of the femoral head ossifications centers, or both is normal. In up to 30% of infants 3 to 6 months of age, a disparity of at least 2 mm exists between the two sides.[30]

Irregularity of Femoral Head Ossification

The ossification center for the head of the femur appears at about 4 months of age and enlarges with time. As ossification fills in the hemispheric cartilage of the head, the center may exhibit irregularities of form and density in the absence of disease (e-Fig. 129-61).[31] Ossification may begin with coarse stippling and may progress, as the size increases, to irregularities along the margin. A bifid or split femoral head is a rare variant (Fig. 129-62). A notch (separate from the fovea capitis) at the vertex of the femoral head also may be seen (e-Fig. 129-63). Before the ossification center has rounded out fully, some flattening of the contour may be observed where subsequently the fovea capitis can be recognized. Variations in ossification and contour of the femoral head may mimic avascular necrosis (Perthes disease) or skeletal dysplasia.

Positional Coxa Valga

External rotation of the femur increases the femoral neck-shaft angle and may factitiously suggest coxa valga (e-Fig. 129-64). With true coxa valga (Fig. 129-65), the greater trochanter projects laterally rather than being superimposed on the underlying femur, whereas with external rotation, the greater trochanter is rotated posteriorly and projects over the femur.

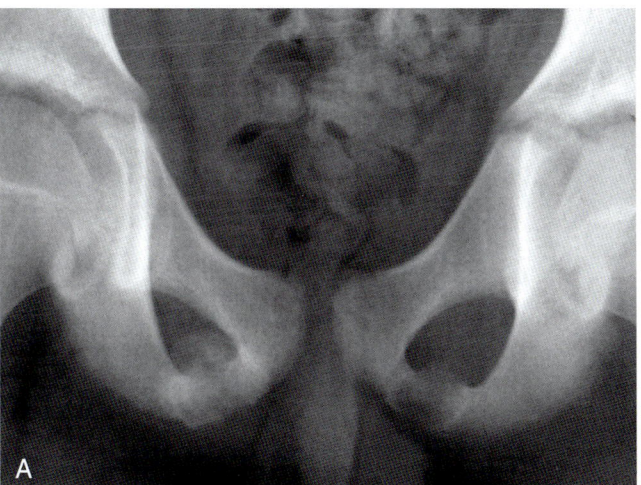
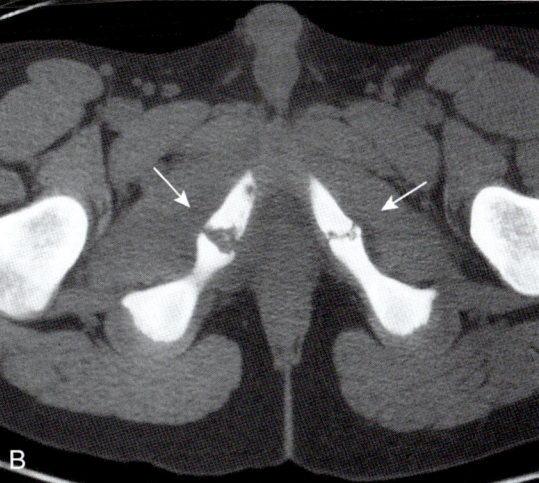

Figure 129-59 **A,** A radiograph showing bilaterally enlarged ischiopubic synchondroses in an 11-year-old male soccer player with right groin pain. The ischiopubic synchondrosis is larger on the symptomatic side. **B,** Irregularity of the ischiopubic synchondroses is seen on computed tomography (*arrows*).

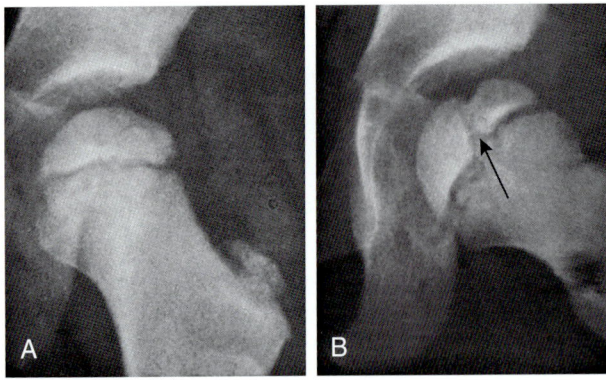

Figure 129-62 Factitious splitting of the femoral head in an asymptomatic 4-year-old girl. **A,** In frontal projection, the femoral head image is normal. **B,** In the lateral, externally rotated position, the femoral head image is divided longitudinally into two unequal segments by a strip of decreased density (*arrow*) that represents the synchondrosis between the two ossification centers that developed one behind the other ventrodorsally.

Trochanters

The centers for the greater and lesser trochanters frequently are irregularly mineralized (e-Fig. 129-66). The physeal equivalent region for the lesser trochanter sometimes appears wide. Avulsions of the lesser trochanter related to the iliopsoas tendon insertion are uncommon, and thus comparison with the opposite, unaffected side may be helpful.

Knee

Cortical Irregularity of the Distal Femoral Metaphysis (Avulsive Cortical Irregularity)

Irregularity of the cortex of the posteromedial distal femoral metaphysis is a common finding that easily can be mistaken for disease (Fig. 129-67 and e-Figs. 129-68 and 129-69).[32] Cystlike cortical defects are common at this location, as are proliferative tuglike lesions, which probably are related to either the adductor muscle insertion or the origin of the medial head of the gastrocnemius muscle. When cystic, these lesions also have been termed "cortical desmoids" and may

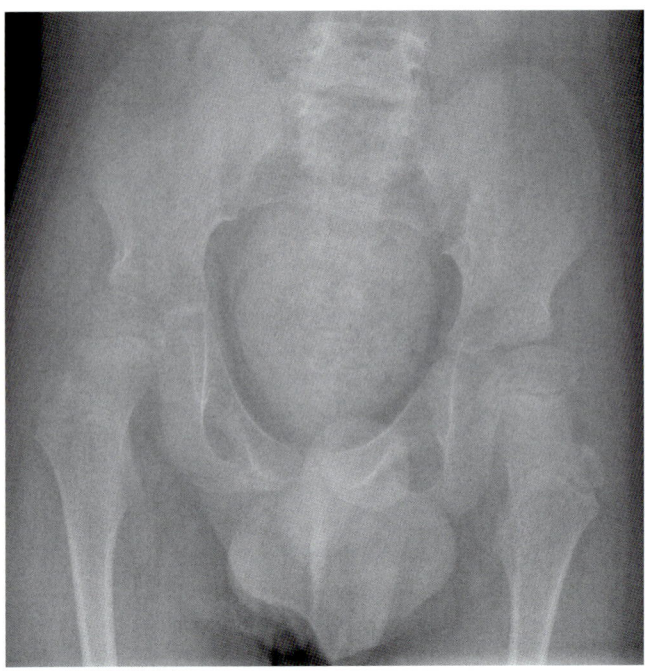

Figure 129-65 An 11-year-old boy with cerebral palsy and coxa valga bilaterally with mild secondary developmental dysplasia of the hip.

be difficult to differentiate from a nonossifying fibroma. Differentiation of these two entities is a nonissue because both are benign and a biopsy is not necessary.

Irregular Ossification of the Distal Femoral Epiphysis

The distal femoral epiphyseal ossification center growth in width occurs rapidly between the second and sixth years. As a result, the lateral and medial margins are commonly irregular and ragged (e-Fig. 129-70). In lateral projection, normal distal femoral ossification centers may have a rough, fringelike margin. Accessory ossification centers may persist at the margins of cartilage-shaft junctions when ossification is almost complete. In older children, marginal mineralization of the

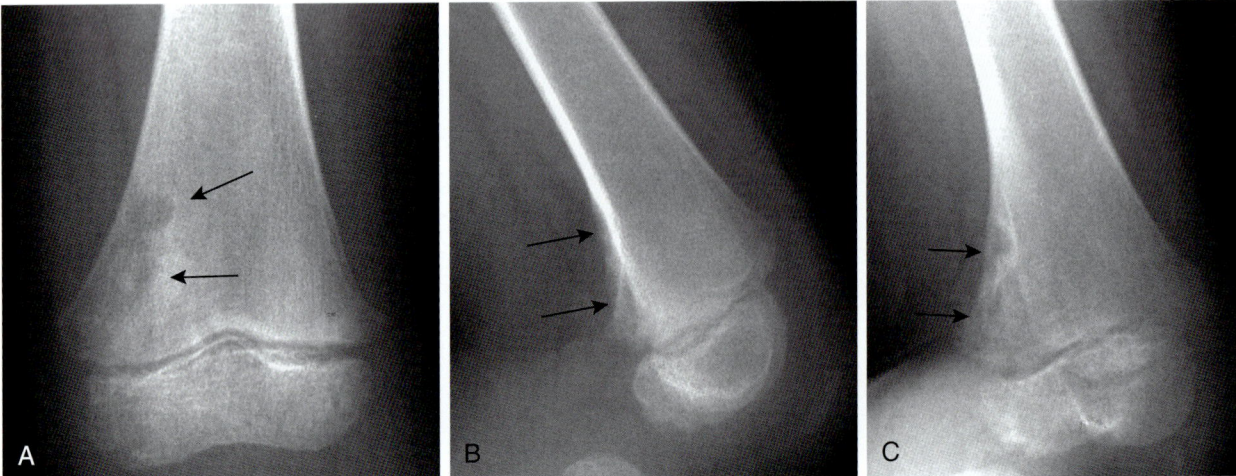

Figure 129-67 Avulsive cortical irregularity (cortical desmoids) of the distal femoral metaphysis in a 4-year-old girl. The defect is posteromedial. **A,** The anteroposterior view shows an ill-defined lucency (*arrows*). **B,** The lateral view shows irregularity (*arrows*) of the posterior margin of the distal femoral metaphysis. **C,** An oblique view shows the cortical lucencies (*arrows*).

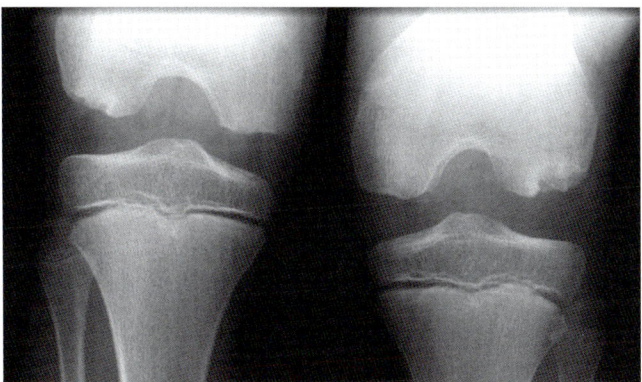

Figure 129-71 Normal developmental irregularity of the posterior aspect of the femoral condyles seen on a notch view in a 10-year-old boy. The defects are most prominent in the lateral condyles.

femoral condyles is characteristically uneven and often is associated with independent ossification centers beyond the edge of the main bony mass.

Subchondral, fragmentary ossification of the femoral condyles may simulate osteochondritis dissecans. Caffey and colleagues found this variant in approximately 30% of healthy children when the knees were examined in tunnel and lateral projections (Fig. 129-71).[33] This defect is much more common on the lateral than on the medial condyle, in contradistinction to osteochondritis dissecans. In addition, these irregularities are seen in children younger than the usual age for this disease.

The posterior margin of the lateral femoral condyle ossification center may be irregular and slightly flattened in appearance. This finding may be evident on radiographs, CT, or MRI. The finding simulates osteochondritis dissecans. Normal developmental irregularity tends to be more posterior and symmetric and occurs in younger children. It is most common at 8 to 10 years of age. The normal variant is differentiated from osteochondritis dissecans on MRI by its position in the inferocentral posterior femoral condyles, an intact overlying cartilage, a large residual cartilage model, accessory ossification centers and spiculation, and absence of adjacent bone marrow edema (e-Fig. 129-72).[34]

Popliteal Groove

The popliteal groove is a normal marginal defect that appears on the posterolateral aspect of the outer condyle in the prepubertal period (e-Fig. 129-73); at times it may be very prominent. This groove carries the tendon of the popliteal muscle and is never visible during infancy or early childhood.

Femoral Condyles

During late childhood, when the intercondylar fossa becomes deeper, lateral projections of the distal femoral epiphysis show the anterior segment to be more radiolucent than the remainder. This phenomenon occurs because the posterior portion of the epiphysis is wider than the anterior, and the x-rays must traverse four layers of cortex (the lateral and medial walls of each of the two condyles) instead of only two layers of cortex anteriorly. The lateral condyle can be differentiated from the medial condyle in lateral projections of the knee because it is relatively flat in comparison with the rounded configuration of the medial condyle.

The Patella and Sesamoid Bones

The patella, lying within the tendon of the quadriceps muscle, is the largest sesamoid bone of the body. The patellar ossification normally develops from several foci. Its edges may be irregular during childhood (e-Fig. 129-74). After fusion of

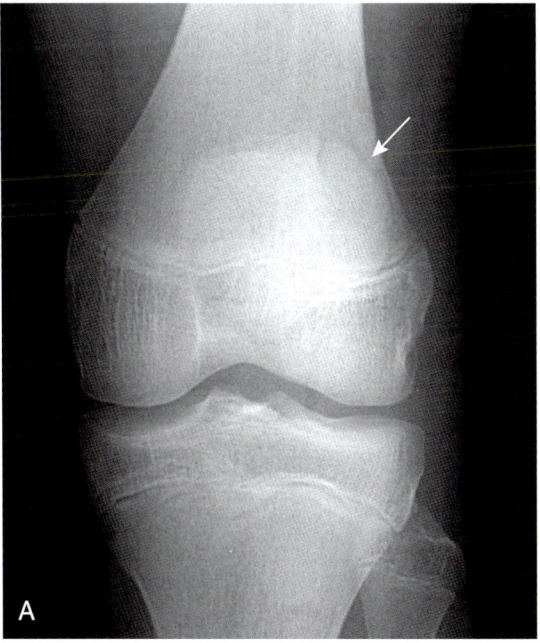
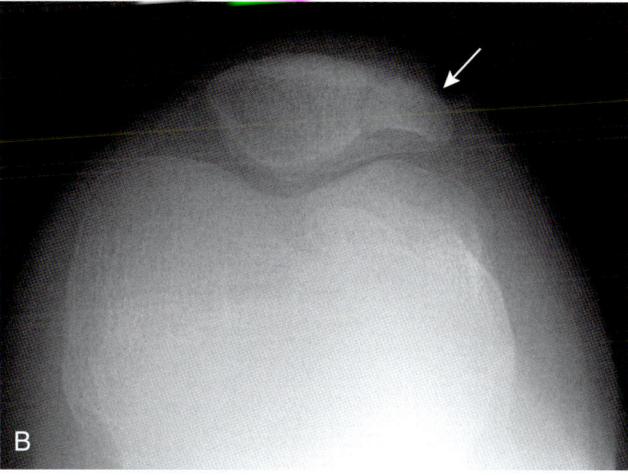

Figure 129-75 Anteroposterior (**A**) and sunrise (**B**) views of a bipartite patella in a 13-year-old boy. The accessory ossification center is superolateral (*arrows*).

the focal centers, another center may develop in the supero-lateral portion of the bone and may persist as a distinct ossicle (Fig. 129-75). This variant, known as bipartite patella, is very common, occurring in 1% to 6% of the population. Ninety percent of persons affected are male, and 40% have bilateral findings. Stress injury or acute fracture may occur at the synchondrosis between the superolateral ossicle and the patellar body, producing symptoms.[35] Bipartite patella may be related to aberrant traction by the vastus lateralis muscle, which inserts into the patella at its upper and outer quadrant. The patella also may be tripartite.

Segmentation of the patella into anterior and posterior components has been described in multiple epiphyseal dysplasia, but it also has been reported without reference to any associated skeletal abnormalities.

Irregular ossification of the lower pole of the patella is a common finding and may be difficult to differentiate from Sinding-Larsen-Johansson syndrome. It may be impossible to distinguish variation in ossification from old traumatic avulsion. Acute patellar sleeve injuries will be symptomatic and will have a linear nonsclerotic fracture fragment and accompanying soft tissue swelling.

Two other sesamoids of the knee occur as normal variants, the fabella and cyamella. The fabella (which is more common) forms in the tendon of the lateral head of the gastrocnemius muscle. The cyamella (which is less common) forms in the tendon of the popliteus muscle. A fabella is best seen on a lateral view (e-Fig. 129-76). The cyamella is found at the edge of the lateral condyle of the femur in the popliteal groove. Fabella syndrome is characterized by intermittent pain at the posterolateral knee accentuated by extension and localized tenderness over the fabella accentuated by compression.[36]

Dorsal Defect of the Patella

Dorsal defects of the patella may be seen along its superolateral aspect and usually are asymptomatic (Fig. 129-77). On

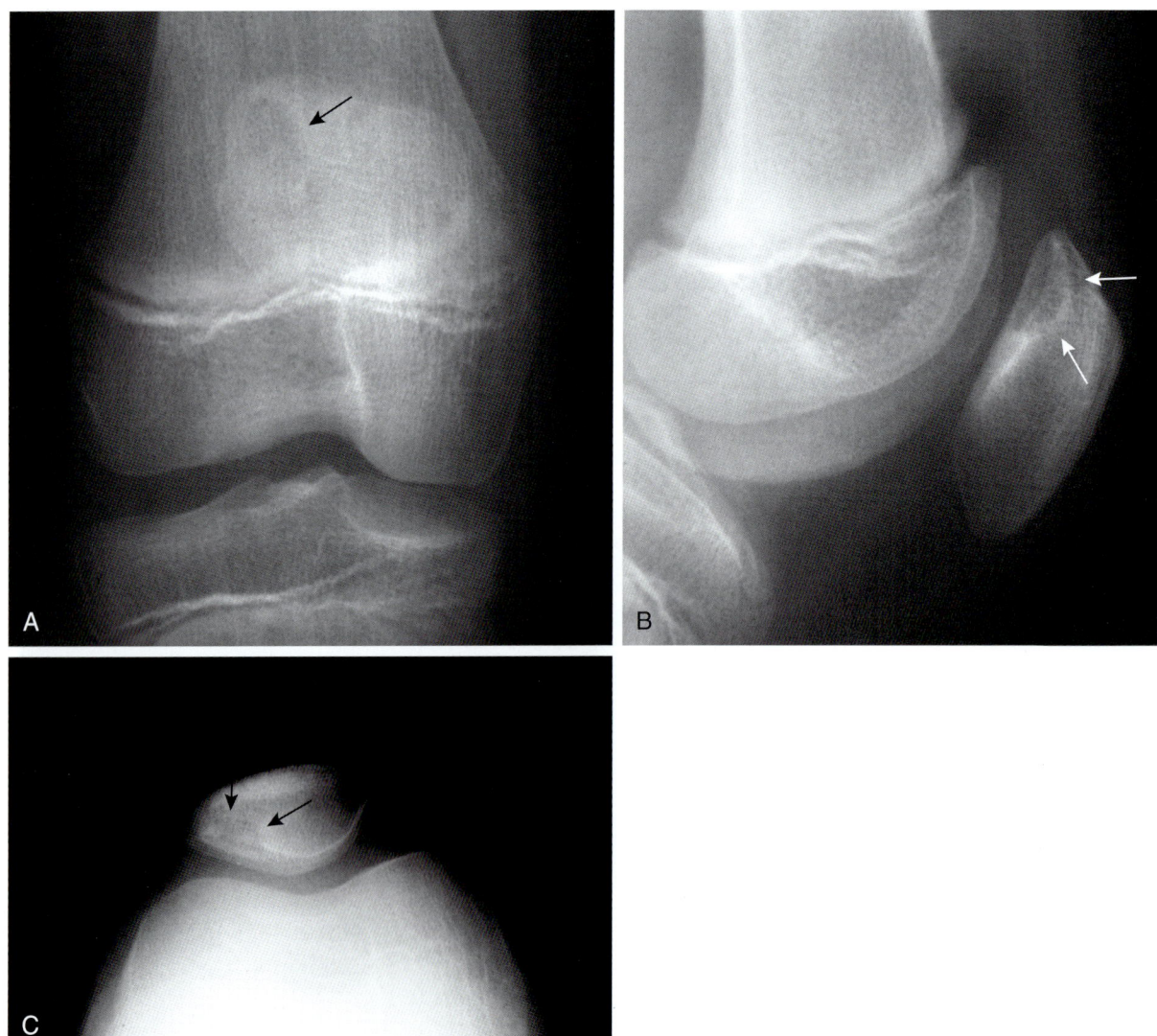

Figure 129-77 A dorsal defect of the patella. Anteroposterior (**A**), lateral (**B**), and sunrise (**C**) views of an 11-year-old girl with a dorsal defect of the patella. The defect is at the posterior aspect of the superolateral portion of the patella (*arrows*).

MRI, overlying cartilage is intact. A dorsal defect of the patella may be seen concomitantly with a bipartite patella.[37] Dorsal patella defects should be differentiated from osteochondritis dissecans of the patella, which usually affects the inferior aspect of the patella bone.

Tibia and Fibula

Tibial Tuberosity

A step-like notched defect appears in the upper anterior border of the tibia in lateral projection before ossification proceeds into the cartilaginous anterior tibial tubercle from the main proximal tibial ossification center. The tubercle also may be ossified from multiple fragmentary accessory centers that, before union, may simulate avulsed fragments of bone. When ossification of the anterior tibial process is nearly complete, the radiolucent cartilage still separating the process from the shaft may appear as a notch or a horizontal strip (e-Fig. 129-78).

A fragmentary appearance of the tibial tuberosity is a normal finding in persons who are skeletally immature. However, when accompanied by focal tenderness on palpation, edema in adjacent Hoffa's fat pad, and pretibial edema, a diagnosis of Osgood–Schlatter disease should be suggested.

Variations in Tibial and Fibular Contour

Irregularity of the interosseous membrane may produce undulations of the lateral tibial or medial fibular cortex that mimic a periosteal reaction, particularly on the oblique lateral view. The proximal fibular metaphysis may have a flanged appearance, possibly as a result of muscular tug.

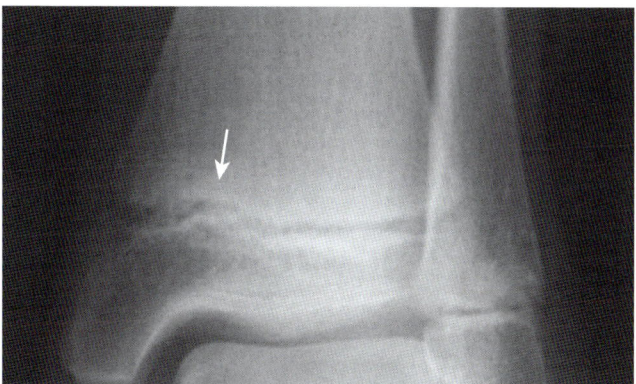

Figure 129-81 Accessory ossification centers (os subfibulare) of the lateral malleolus (*arrow*) in a 14-year-old boy.

Irregular Ossification of the Medial and Lateral Malleoli

The medial and lateral malleolus are initially fully cartilaginous and may superficially mimic soft tissue swelling (Fig. 129-79). Fragmentary ossification of both the medial and lateral malleoli is a normal finding in the skeletally immature and should not be confused with fracture.[38]

Separate accessory ossification centers are common in the cartilage of the medial malleolus (os subtibiale) and less common in the lateral malleolus (os subfibulare) (e-Fig. 129-80 and Fig. 129-81). At each location, the differential diagnosis is an avulsed fragment. Acute avulsed fragments will have an irregular shape and a sharp, noncorticated margin. A common pitfall is to mistake an acute avulsion fracture of the anterior talofibular ligament with an os subfibulare.

Fibular Ossicle

The provisional zone of calcification in the distal fibular metaphysis may be notched upward, and a tiny extra ossicle may develop in the notch. The notching is usually bilateral.

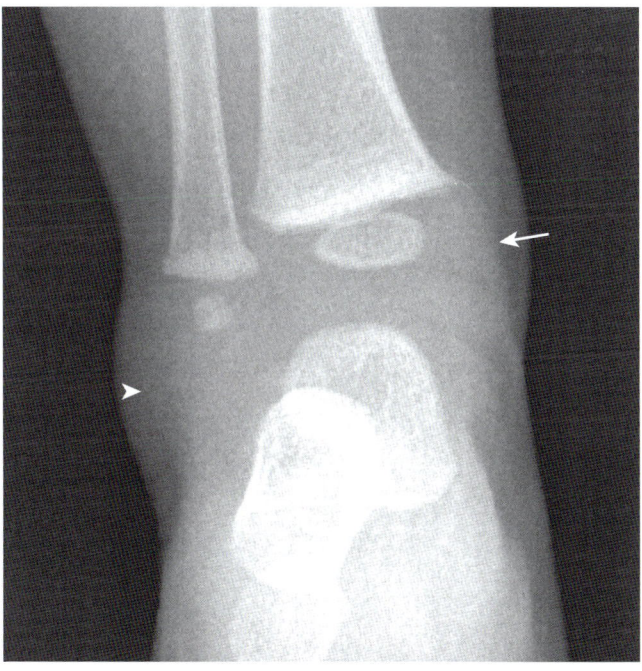

Figure 129-79 Medial (*arrow*) and lateral (*arrowhead*) cartilaginous epiphyses may superficially mimic ankle soft tissue swelling in this 9-month-old girl.

Key Points

The spherical growth plate is responsible for epiphyseal ossification, and its physiology is similar to that of the physis.

The subperiosteal metaphyseal bone collar should not be confused with classic metaphyseal lesions of child abuse.

The ischiopubic synchondrosis can close asymmetrically and superficially mimic a fracture and a tumor. The irregular side is usually contralateral to the dominant foot.

Epiphyseal ossification can be quite fragmentary in the femoral condyles and should not be mistaken for fractures.

The acromion process is mainly cartilaginous, particularly in the first decade, and may cause pseudowidening of the AC joint, superficially mimicking AC joint diastasis. Imaging the unaffected side may be helpful for comparison.

Os acetabulae is a normal ossification center along the acetabular rim and should not be confused with acetabular rim fractures or anterior-inferior iliac spine avulsion fractures related to the rectus femoris origin.

The medial epicondyle of the elbow appears before the trochlear ossification. If only a trochlear ossification is present, a displaced medial epicondylar avulsion fracture should be suspected.

Suggested Readings

Duncan AW. Normal variants—an approach. In: Carty H, Brunelle F, Stringer D, et al, eds. *Imaging children.* 2nd ed. Philadelphia: Elsevier; 2005.

Greulich WW, Pyle SI. *Radiographic atlas of skeletal development of the hand and wrist.* 2nd ed. Stanford, CA: Stanford University Press; 1959.

Hoerr NL, Pyle SI, Francis CC. *Radiographic atlas of skeletal development of the foot and ankle.* Springfield, IL: Charles C Thomas; 1962.

Ogden JA. Diagnostic imaging. In Ogden JA, ed. *Skeletal injury in the child.* 3rd ed. New York: Springer; 2000.

Pyle SI, Hoerr NL. *A radiographic standard of reference for the growing knee.* Springfield, IL: Charles C Thomas; 1969.

References

Full references for this chapter can be found on www.expertconsult.com.

Chapter 130

Imaging Techniques

J. HERMAN KAN and PETER J. STROUSE

Pediatric musculoskeletal radiology is a broad field that requires an understanding of normal growth and developmental variations, fracture patterns unique to the immature skeleton, skeletal dysplasias, and knowledge of unique tumor and tumor-like conditions. Advanced imaging has improved our ability to arrive at a precise diagnosis. However, it also has created the need for additional expertise within the field of pediatric imaging to learn how to properly use these tools to arrive at a diagnosis and provide information beyond that of the humble radiograph. This section will cover the spectrum of pediatric musculoskeletal disorders from a multimodality imaging approach. Key images are provided in the printed version and an expanded, comprehensive image library is provided in the electronic version.

Imaging Technique Overview

RADIOGRAPHY

Radiography remains the initial tool for the evaluation of acute trauma, inflammatory arthritis, infection, suspected primary bone neoplasms, and skeletal dysplasias.

In the setting of acute trauma, nonarticular long bones should be imaged with at least two views (frontal and lateral). Osteoarticular regions should be imaged with three views (frontal, lateral, and oblique). Dedicated imaging of the digits is preferred rather than general imaging of an entire hand or foot when a patient has a single symptomatic digit. The radiograph should be the initial screening tool before computed tomography (CT) or magnetic resonance imaging (MRI) is performed in the setting of acute injuries. For alignment disorders, including scoliosis and foot deformities, weight-bearing views should be obtained routinely. In cases of suspected child abuse, a dedicated skeletal survey should be performed. Bone scintigraphy and MRI are complementary tools in the evaluation of child abuse, but they may miss the classic metaphyseal corner fracture.[1]

In the setting of infection, radiography should be performed before advanced imaging, although a normal radiograph should not preclude referral for MRI for suspected acute osteomyelitis. Radiographs are helpful for initial screening before the use of MRI to ensure that symptoms of suspected infection are not a result of an underlying fracture or primary bone neoplasm.

For primary bone neoplasms, radiographs are key to determining coverage by MRI; they also complement the MRI diagnosis. Radiographs may help with the final diagnosis because the matrix and pattern of bone destruction are better delineated by radiography than by MRI.

ULTRASONOGRAPHY

Musculoskeletal ultrasound has three primary roles: evaluation of dysplasias, of soft tissue masses, and of pyogenic and nonpyogenic arthritis.

Sonographic evaluation of dysplasias includes developmental dysplasia of the hip, glenohumeral dysplasia related to brachial plexopathy, and selected congenital foot deformities. For developmental dysplasia of the hip, the optimal time of imaging is before the capital femoral epiphyseal ossification center appears, which usually is at 4 to 6 months of age and younger. Sonography can image through cartilage but not bone. Sonography can evaluate the relationship of the humeral head with respect to the glenoid in the setting of suspected glenohumeral dysplasia and subsequently can be used to calculate a glenoid version angle. Sonography also is useful for certain congenital foot disorders and can determine the relationship between the nonossified navicular and talus in the setting of congenital vertical talus.

Sonography is useful in determining solid or cystic soft tissue lesions. However, a positive or negative sonographic result does not preclude the need for additional imaging. Sonography may be the end point for imaging when a ganglion cyst is identified, and the tail can be definitively followed to a tendon sheath or joint space. However, sonography is nonspecific when a solid soft tissue mass is seen and should be used with caution in differentiating benign and malignant etiologies.

Identification of the presence or absence of a joint effusion of any region is straightforward with sonography. However, the etiology is predicated on clinical history. It is not possible to differentiate pyogenic, nonpyogenic, and posttraumatic causes based on sonography alone.

COMPUTED TOMOGRAPHY

The three primary roles for musculoskeletal CT include fracture assessment, including orthopedic hardware failure; assessment of alignment disorders, including physeal bar assessment; and evaluation of tumor matrix and tumor recurrence in the setting of an existing neoplasm or a resected neoplasm with hardware in place.

A low kVp technique may be used because of the inherent contrast of bone. However, when orthopedic hardware is present, a high mAs and kVp technique is required to image through the hardware to minimize artifact. Multiplanar and volume-rendered reformats should be performed routinely for all musculoskeletal CT applications.

Fracture assessment by CT should be performed when radiographs do not fully define the fracture. Alternatively, CT should be performed when radiographs are negative and a high clinical concern exists for fracture and relative contraindications exist for MRI. Indications for CT when radiographs already demonstrate a fracture include fully defining the intraarticular component of the fracture, identifying additional fractures, determining exact measurements of fracture diastasis, which is particularly important at the articular surfaces, and identifying intraarticular loose bodies that may not be visible by radiography.

Alignment disorders that can be evaluated by CT include determination of acetabular and femoral version, tibial torsion, glenohumeral dysplasia, and patellofemoral tracking disorders. Patellofemoral tracking disorders usually are dynamic studies in which the knee is placed in varying degrees of flexion to evaluate lateral patellar dislocation. CT leg-length surveys have limited utility because they are performed in the supine position, and thus alignment cannot be assessed.

MAGNETIC RESONANCE IMAGING

The volume and varying applications of musculoskeletal MRI in the pediatric population has grown because of the popularity of youth sports and subsequent injuries. MRI plays a useful role in oncologic, metabolic, and sports medicine imaging. For oncologic imaging, the child should be referred for CT imaging if orthopedic hardware related to tumor resection and graft placement is in place.

Four basic sequence types may be used for musculoskeletal MRI. These types include an anatomy sequence (usually T1, proton density); a fluid-sensitive sequence (proton density with fat saturation, T2 with fat saturation, short tau inversion recovery, and a fluid-weighted gradient echo sequence); a contrast sequence (postgadolinium T1 with or without fat saturation); and a susceptibility sequence (any gradient echo sequence).

The purpose of the anatomy sequence is to evaluate marrow replacement, trabecular anatomy, and ligamentous abnormality. In general, a T1W sequence usually is required to evaluate the marrow in children younger than 10 years. When children are older than 10 years, marrow abnormalities can be evaluated with a fluid-sensitive sequence. However, a T1W sequence still should be included in all oncologic or metabolic imaging, including children who are older than 10 years. Proton density sequences without fat saturation are useful for evaluating trabecular anatomy for fractures and to evaluate ligamentous, labral, and cartilaginous anatomy.

Fluid-sensitive sequences are used to evaluate marrow edema, ligamentous anatomy, and cartilage. Spin echo fluid-sensitive sequences are superior to gradient echo sequences in the evaluation of pediatric cartilage. Spherical growth plate, epiphyseal cartilage, articular cartilage, and physis can be differentiated on a spin echo sequence, whereas all four types of cartilage have the same signal intensity on a gradient echo sequence.

A susceptibility sequence is an optional sequence for most musculoskeletal protocols. Its role is to evaluate for anything that will cause a susceptibility artifact, including loose bodies and blood. When conventional anatomy and fluid-sensitive sequences show no abnormality, the susceptibility sequence adds little additional information.

Postcontrast sequences are useful for determining tumor vascularity, defining granulation tissue versus abscess in the setting of infection, and evaluating the synovium. Normal noninflamed synovium eventually enhances and should not be mistaken for pathology.[2] The relative thickness of the synovium as depicted by contrasted sequences is what is important in the setting of a joint effusion if pyogenic or nonpyogenic inflammatory arthritis is suspected. When initial precontrast images are entirely normal, postcontrast images have limited additional value.

In general, girls who are older than 6 years and boys who are older than 8 years may be able to undergo the magnetic resonance (MR) study without the need for sedation. MR sedation should be handled by a dedicated and qualified team.

NUCLEAR IMAGING

Skeletal scintigraphy has a higher sensitivity relative to skeletal radiography for bone pathology that exhibits osteoblastic activity including fractures, tumors, and infection. The radiopharmaceutical agent that is most commonly used is technetium-99m methylenediphosphonate. Images obtained after injection of this compound reflect a combination of pathophysiologic functions (blood flow and bone turnover) but are nonspecific and do not provide exceptional anatomic detail. Images therefore should be interpreted in the context of the patient's clinical presentation and relevant radiologic findings. The anatomic areas that are most difficult to image and interpret accurately are the growth centers. Before closure of the physes, these rapidly growing areas display especially high uptake that may mask the activity associated with an adjacent pathologic lesion. Single-photon emission CT helps in localization of such lesions because it improves the spatial resolution of activity in contiguous and overlapping structures.

Indications for skeletal scintigraphy are varied and include investigation of bone pain and diagnosis of early and chronic osteomyelitis, osteonecrosis, and occult trauma, including nonaccidental trauma and stress fractures. Improvements in the diagnostic accuracy of CT and MRI have usurped skeletal scintigraphy in many clinical settings; however, bone scanning remains a very useful imaging tool.

Positron emission tomography (PET) imaging with fluorine-18-deoxyglucose (FDG) offers improved spatial resolution and greater sensitivity for detection of aggressive bone neoplasms. FDG-PET is particularly effective in detecting an active tumor. Because of its high sensitivity, increased signal on PET is nonspecific. The fusion of PET with CT or MRI allows for better spatial localization of lesions and improves the characterization of lesions. PET also is an effective method of determining response of malignant bone tumors to therapy.

References

Full references for this chapter can be found on www.expertconsult.com.

Chapter 131

Prenatal Musculoskeletal Imaging

CHRISTOPHER I. CASSADY

Overview

Evaluation of the fetal skeleton is one of the more challenging aspects of prenatal imaging for a variety of reasons. It is such a rapidly changing system in gestation that ossification varies in extent and distribution from week to week; ultrasonography, the primary fetal imaging modality, does not clearly demonstrate the full morphology of a bone because of lack of sound penetration; and many skeletal pathologies that become increasingly obvious with growth are, at best, subtle in the fetus. Still, some techniques are available to overcome some of these barriers, and these include indirect evaluation of bone contour abnormalities and proportions by using ultrasonography or magnetic resonance imaging (MRI). Musculoskeletal abnormalities in the fetus are diagnosable in the following categories:

1. Skeletal dysplasias
2. Limb reductions and amniotic band syndrome
3. Primary anomalies of the spine
4. Neuromuscular disorders, including clubfoot
5. Tumors

Skeletal Dysplasias

Etiology Dysplasias are often the result of genetic mutations that encode for proteins important to development of the growth plate.[1,2] Current clinical application of "skeletal dysplasia testing panels" is, however, very limited. Both the range of included mutations and the sensitivities of their detection are expected to increase with time. In utero testing in sporadic cases remains controversial.[3]

Imaging Over 450 dysplasias have been described in the literature. Only a small percentage is considered diagnosable in utero with imaging, the first investigation for which is ultrasonography.[3,4] Because of the lack of specificity of many of the findings, which have generally to do with abnormal bone shape (formation) or length (growth), efforts at prenatal evaluation have focused on identification of cases in which the neonates are not expected to survive. Identification of these fetuses allows counseling and for the parents and appropriate care planning. To this end, various ultrasonography criteria have been suggested to separate those conditions that are thought to be lethal from those that are not, with very high reliability (Box 131-1).[5-11] Most of these criteria

correlate limb length with survival. Emphasis is also placed on measures predicting lethal pulmonary hypoplasia. For example, the thoracic circumference is measured in the axial plane at the level of the four-chamber view of the heart; a thoracic circumference at or below the lower limit of the 95% confidence interval for gestational age is considered predictive of lethality in the setting of a micromelic bone dysplasia.[12,13] Other findings that may be detected in association with lethality and that increase diagnostic certainty are polyhydramnios and nonimmune hydrops fetalis. It is important to avoid making a diagnosis of lethality in borderline cases and to use the criteria in combination for the most accurate discrimination. The fetus with intrauterine growth retardation should not be assigned a diagnosis of generalized skeletal dysplasia on the basis of proportionate but short bones. Questionable cases in either category deserve follow-up ultrasonography for interval growth.

The three most common lethal dysplasias are (1) thanatophoric dysplasia, (2) achondrogenesis, and (3) osteogenesis imperfecta type II. These three diagnoses together constitute the majority of cases. Therefore, a familiarity with their ultrasonographic features is essential (Box 131-2).[14,15]

Certain skeletal morphologic findings on ultrasonography suggest particular diagnoses in the setting of a suspected dysplasia. Long bone fractures, for example, are indicative of osteogenesis imperfecta or hypophosphatasia, and rib fractures are rarely seen with other diagnoses (Fig. 131-1). Kleeblattschadel, or cloverleaf skull, may be present in several of the acrocephalosyndactyly syndromes (Apert, Carpenter, Crouzon, and Pfeiffer syndromes), campomelic dysplasia, osteocraniostenosis, and thanatophoric dysplasia type II (Fig. 131-2). Hypoplastic scapular bodies are a feature of campomelic dysplasia and Antley-Bixler syndrome.[16] However, many findings such as platyspondyly are not specific and must be considered in relation to other features (short ribs, abnormal mineralization, solid organ malformations) to arrive at a more narrow differential diagnosis (Fig. 131-3).[17] Three-dimensional ultrasonography can be very helpful when an appropriate volume of fluid is present around the fetus to display the morphology of specific segments, including the face, hands, and feet.[18]

Fetal MRI, in general, has not been pursued routinely in the evaluation of fetal dysplasia because of the difficulty in imaging the signal-poor ossified skeleton. However, it may have a role in quantification of fetal lung volumes in cases in which ultrasonography has limitations.[19] In addition, fetal MRI has been used successfully to make the diagnosis of

Box 131-1 Proposed Ultrasonography Criteria for Lethal Dysplasia

- Micromelias >4 standard deviation behind expected lengths
- Femur length >5 mm below 2 standard deviation in second and third trimesters
- Femur length or abdominal circumference <0.16
- Thoracic or abdominal circumference <0.6
- Thoracic circumference < lower limit of the 95% confidence interval for gestational age
- Chest to trunk ratio <0.32

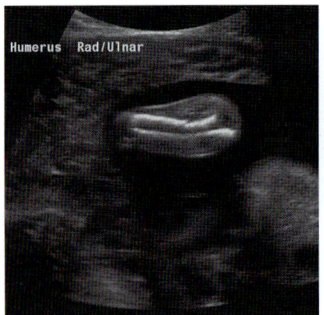 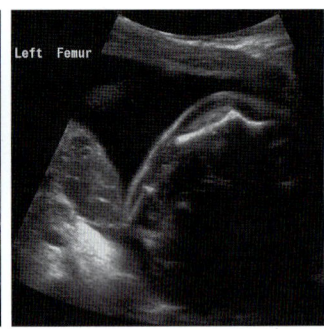

Figure 131-1 Long bone fractures in a fetus with severe micromelia. Diagnosis is osteogenesis imperfecta type II.

dysplasias that primarily involve the epiphyses, taking advantage of the high water content and, therefore, the high T2-weighted signal characteristics of cartilage.[20]

The use of ionizing radiation is avoided during pregnancy unless the need to make a diagnosis is critical to patient care. In such a circumstance, low-dose computed tomography techniques have been used to reconstruct highly detailed three-dimensional models of the fetal skeleton (Fig. 131-4).[21,22] The features described would be compared with an atlas of postmortem radiographs in identified syndromes to aid in diagnosis.[23] This strategy can be offered at radiation doses of 3 to 5 millisievert with superb resolution of individual skeletal components.[22]

Treatment and Follow-up When a lethal skeletal dysplasia is detected by using ultrasonography, the parents and fetal care team can make informed decisions about the continuation of the pregnancy and the circumstances of delivery. An opportunity exists for neonatal hospice care coordination, when appropriate. Even though ultrasonography is reliable at separating lethal dysplasias from nonlethal dysplasias, neonatal

physical examination and radiographs, appropriate genetic testing, and autopsy, if relevant, are crucial in arriving at a specific diagnosis, which, in turn, is necessary for accurate family counseling.

Amniotic Band Syndrome and Limb Reductions

Etiology Limb reductions may be caused by a variety of insults. Some of these are from amputation, such as in the amniotic band sequence spectrum. Although the initiating event in this sequence has not been incontrovertibly established, the most commonly supported theory is that a tear is made in the amnion, exposing the fetus to the more adhesive chorion, with subsequent loss of tissue or the development of a constrictive band.[24] In other cases, primary vascular insults are blamed for segmental limb loss, and teratogens (e.g., thalidomide) are highly associated in some instances.[25,26] Limb reduction abnormalities can be chromosomal, particularly with Trisomy 18.[27] Proximal focal femoral deficiency is a particular form of reduction that affects the femoral head and neck and is associated with fibular aplasia or hypoplasia. It may be unilateral or bilateral (Fig. 131-5).

Box 131-2 Imaging Features of the Most Common Lethal Dysplasias*

Thanatophoric Dysplasia

- "Telephone receiver" shaped femurs
- Depressed nasal bridge, macrocephaly
- Platyspondyly
- Short ribs
- Trident hand
- Clover leaf skull in type II
- Oversulcation of the inferomedial temporal lobes

Achondrogenesis

- Deficient vertebral ossification, ± calvarial
- Short, flared ribs ± fractures
- Hydrops (25% of cases)
- Micrognathia, midface hypoplasia

Osteogenesis Imperfecta Type II

- Multiple long bone fractures
- Hourglass-shaped thorax (from fractures), normal rib lengths (two thirds the way around chest)
- Increased conspicuity of brain anatomy on ultrasound (decreased mineralization)
- Skull deformity with pressure

*All have marked micromelia.

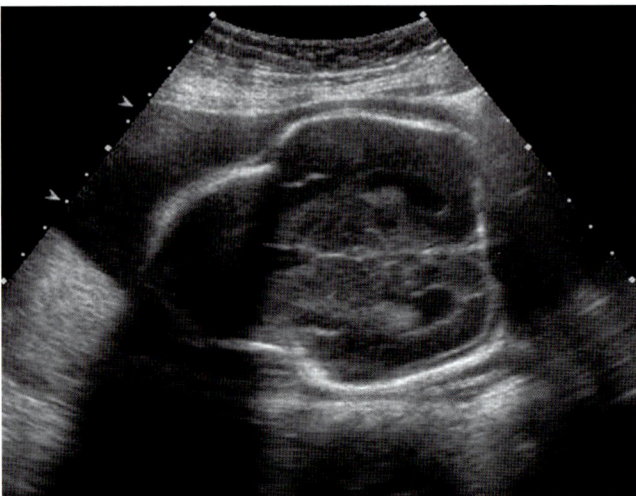

Figure 131-2 Kleeblattschadel, or cloverleaf skull (pancraniosynostosis). In the setting of a lethal bone dysplasia, the differential diagnosis includes thanatophoric dysplasia type II, campomelic dysplasia and osteocraniostenosis.

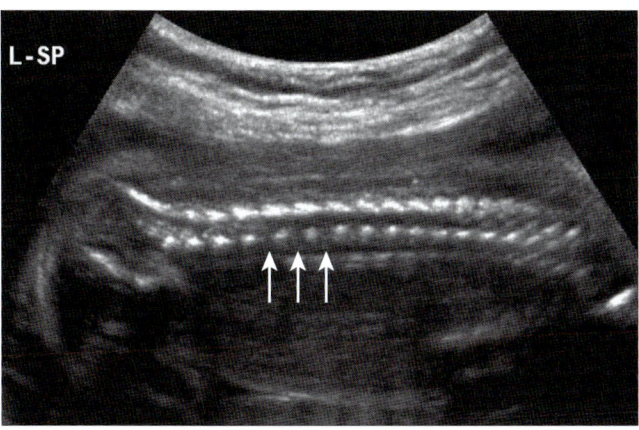

Figure 131-3 Platyspondyly. Disc spaces (*arrows*) are wider than the ossification centers for the vertebral bodies.

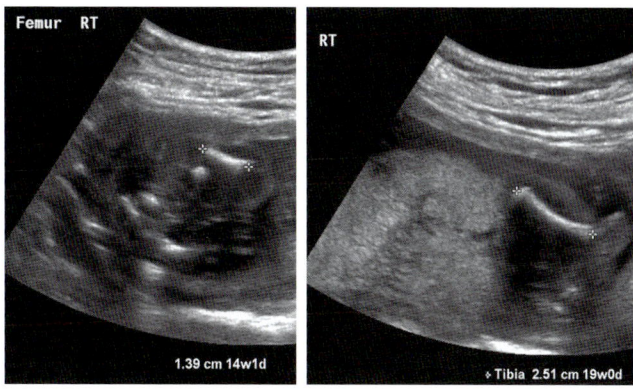

Figure 131-5 Proximal focal femoral deficiency with fibular aplasia. Fetus at 20 weeks gestational age shows a short femur associated with a single long bone in the distal leg.

Imaging Limb reduction anomalies may be subtle in the case of isolated, very distal defects involving fingers or toes. Ultrasonography can characterize the shape of the affected limb well and is diagnostic, and MRI is usually not necessary (Fig. 131-6). Associated findings may include edema of the extremity distal to a constricting band (Fig. 131-7 and Video 131-1). Cine ultrasound sequences can capture the abnormal motion that is a consequence of subluxation or dislocation if the affected segment involves a joint. Random, multiple defects are more likely secondary to amniotic band sequence than are symmetric defects, which tend to be related to chromosomal abnormalities or syndromes (Fig. 131-8).[28] As amniotic bands can cause defects in any body part, a thorough evaluation of the entire fetus and its umbilical cord is indicated. Umbilical cord involvement is often overlooked but has consequences because of the risk of cord occlusion.[29]

Treatment and Follow-up Successful cases of fetoscopic lysis of amniotic bands have been reported when it has been thought that release could improve blood flow to and consequent growth of an affected limb segment.[30] Otherwise, plastic surgery consultation is sought for limb salvage following delivery of the fetus.

Primary Anomalies of the Spine

Etiology Primary anomalies of the spine are some of the more common antenatally detected skeletal abnormalities. These anomalies typically manifest as an unusual curvature, either scoliotic or kyphotic. Care must be taken to ensure that this finding is a fixed abnormality and not positional or the result of a lack of space (e.g., in anhydramnios). Fixed scoliosis is abnormal and may be the result of tethering, as

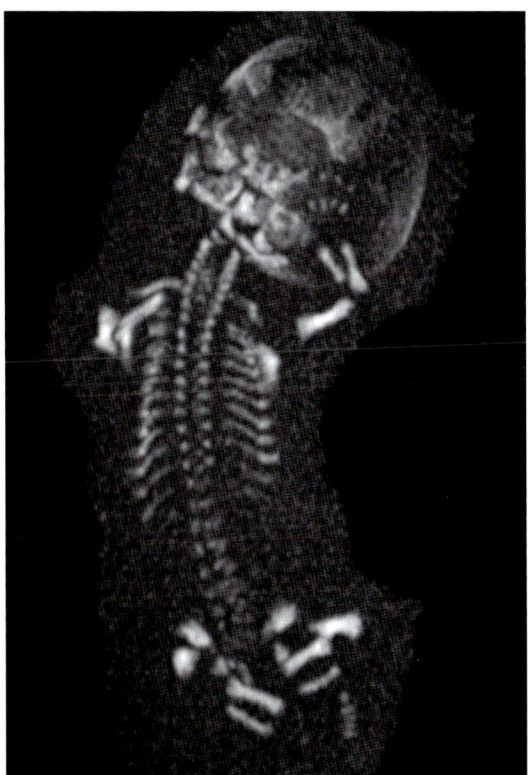

Figure 131-4 Thanatophoric dysplasia type I. Three-dimensional volume set acquisitions allow reconstructed computed tomography projections in any plane. Radiation dose to the 21-week fetus was 3.9 millisievert. Gene testing confirmed an *FGFR* mutation. (Courtesy of Teresa Victoria, MD.)

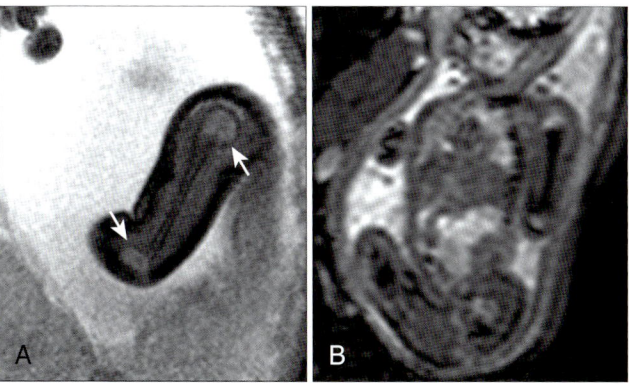

Figure 131-6 **A,** Sagittal steady-state free precession gradient-recalled echo image at 33 weeks' gestation. The higher-signal cartilage (*arrows*) is distinct from the ossified diaphysis in the humerus. **B,** Coronal gradient-recalled echo-planar imaging at 27 weeks. Echo-planar imaging is more reliable for bone morphology than other sequences at younger gestational ages.

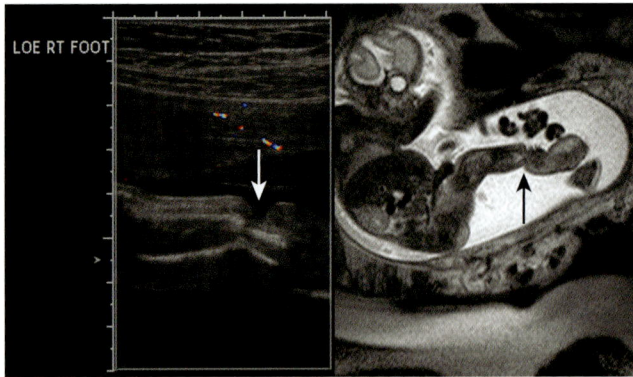

Figure 131-7 *Amniotic band syndrome.* Ultrasound and sagittal T2-weighted single-shot fast spin echo images show focal constriction of both soft tissue and bone (*arrows*) at the distal leg, with edema of the ankle and foot.

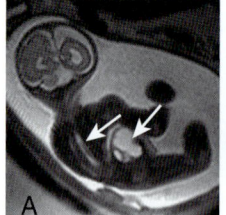 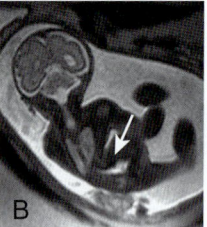 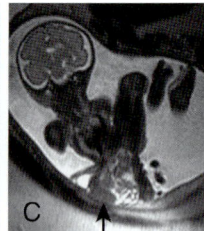

Figure 131-9 *Limb–body wall complex.* Multiple images had shown fixed scoliosis and contortion in a fetus with extrusion of abdominal contents adherent to the amnion (*black arrow*). White arrows indicate the spinal canal in this fetus, who also has a closed neural tube defect.

with limb–body wall complex (Fig. 131-9), a severe and lethal form of amniotic band sequence; rib fusions, as in Jarcho-Levin syndrome (Fig. 131-10); or fetal akinesia or hypokinesia.[31] Often, the finding is subtle and secondary to segmentation anomalies of the spine, such as hemivertebrae or butterfly vertebrae (Fig. 131-11). Complex spinal anomalies can be seen with neural tube defects and with the Currarino triad, which is a heritable complex of anomalous sacrum, presacral mass, and anorectal malformation.[32] Absence of the sacrum, with variable involvement of the more proximal spine, occurs in caudal regression syndrome, which is significantly associated with elevated glucose levels in the fetus of a mother with diabetes.[33]

The most common spinal anomaly in the fetus involves the dysraphism of posterior elements in a neural tube defect. This group of lesions is discussed in detail in Chapter 42.

Imaging A spinal anomaly may be an isolated fetal finding, but it does prompt a careful search for associated syndromic abnormalities, including the various components of the VACTERL complex (*v*ertebral anomaly, *a*norectal atresia, *c*ardiac lesion, *t*racheo*e*sophageal fistula, *r*enal anomaly, *l*imb defect) (Fig. 131-12). The presence of an anal dimple can be confirmed on ultrasonography, where attention is also directed specifically to the size of the stomach and the morphology of the radial ray segments. Devoted echocardiography is recommended in suspicious cases. MRI has been used to examine for a distended esophageal pouch, although this is seen inconsistently. A higher sensitivity may be present for transient esophageal distension using repetitive dynamic steady-state free precession (SSFP) sequences in the sagittal midline.[34] The use of the multiplanar capabilities of MRI may be advantageous in sorting out the components of complex spinal anomalies (Fig. 131-13). T2-weighted sequences, whether single-shot fast spin echo or gradient-echo SSFP, are most useful. Fast T1-weighted gradient sequences may help identify ectopic fat.

Treatment and Follow-up Correlation with imaging and physical examination after delivery is critical to confirm the suspected anomaly and to guide therapy. Because both ultrasonography and MRI have limitations in the evaluation of the spine, prenatal imaging findings may not be straightforward, and it should not be assumed that the most complete diagnosis has been described antenatally.

Neuromuscular Disorders

Etiology Several conditions that cause generalized hypotonia in the fetus and neonate are heritable: the most important,

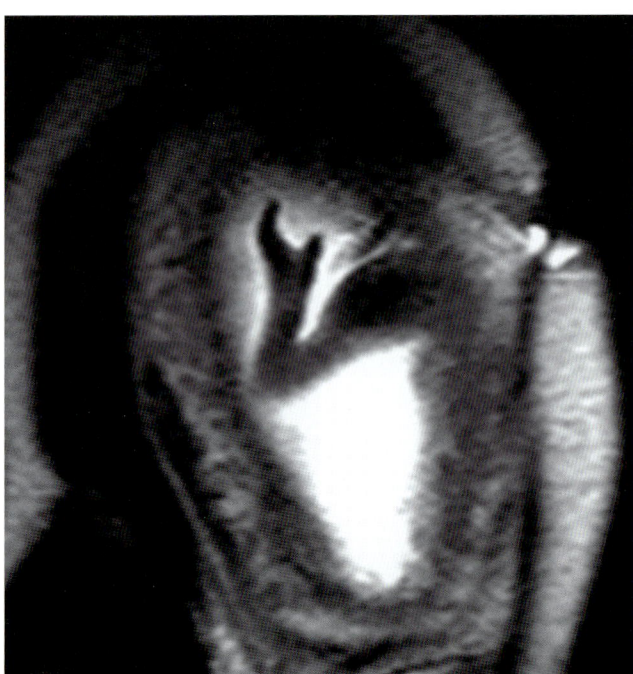

Figure 131-8 *Brachmann-DeLange syndrome.* This 30-week fetus had bilateral ectrodactyly (split hand-foot malformations), with only two digits on each hand.

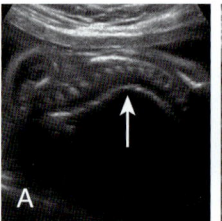 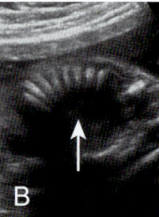 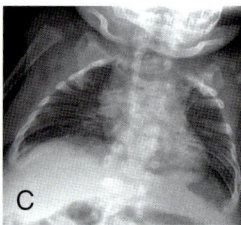

Figure 131-10 **A** and **B,** Fixed scoliosis associated with thoracic restriction, with ribs fanning out from a central fusion. **C,** Typical chest appearance of spondylocostal dysostosis (Jarcho-Levin syndrome).

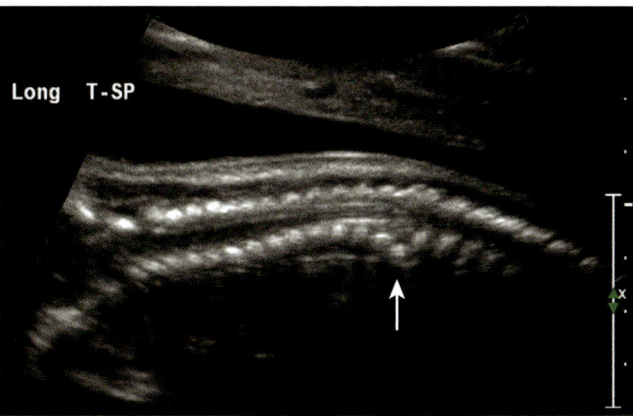

Figure 131-11 Focal interruption in the continuity of vertebral body ossification centers, signifying a segmentation anomaly (hemivertebra, *arrow*).

at least from the point of view of obstetric management, is congenital myotonic dystrophy. This is an autosomal dominant muscular disease, in which expansion of abnormal genomic repeats inserted during cell division will be greater in an affected child than in the carrier parent. Milder cases in adults often go undiagnosed, and a carrier mother may not display obvious manifestations of muscular insufficiency until administered respiratory-depressant anesthetics, to which these patients are exquisitely sensitive. Sudden death from cardiac conduction abnormalities during sedation has also been reported.[35] Therefore, if myotonic dystrophy is suspected as part of the differential diagnosis in a fetus, maternal genetic testing should be performed and a meticulously careful anesthetic strategy planned for the delivery.[36,37]

Most of the time, a specific diagnosis is difficult to establish for a fetus with limited movement, fixed position of the extremities, multiple contractures, or all of these. An unsatisfactory term, *arthrogryposis multiplex congenita*, has been used to describe this combination of findings, but the etiologies are likely to be multiple and various. Muscular, neurologic, and connective tissue disorders may all play roles. Differential considerations include multiple pterygium syndrome, in which skin webs tend to tether the limbs at the joints and restrict fetal movement. The major cause of arthrogryposis is

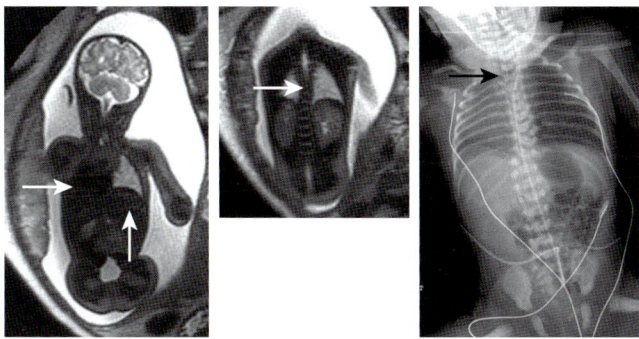

Figure 131-12 VACTERL complex (*vertebral anomaly, anorectal atresia, cardiac lesion, tracheoesophageal fistula, renal anomaly, limb defect*). Coronal T2-weighted single-shot fast spin echo images show a right-sided heart, absence of fluid in the stomach, and thoracic scoliosis from hemivertebrae (*white arrows*), with subsequent neonatal image. Note the Repogle tube in the proximal esophageal pouch (*black arrow*).

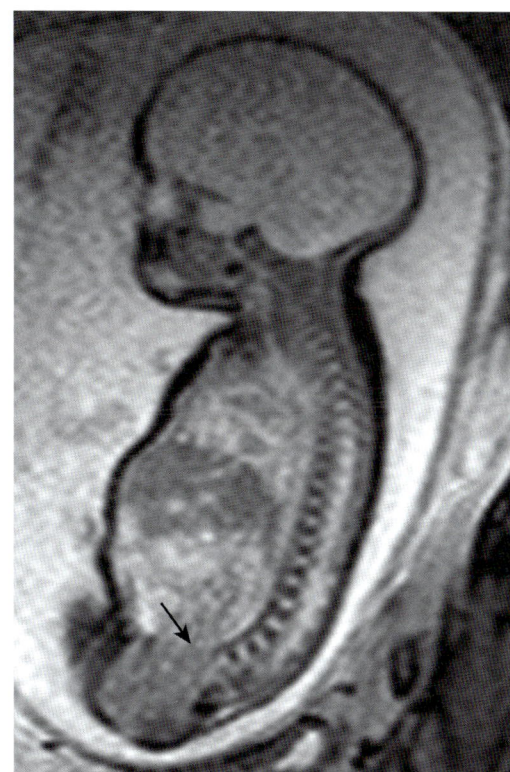

Figure 131-13 **Caudal regression sequence.** Sagittal gradient-recalled echo image at 31 weeks' gestation. The spine terminates abruptly without a sacrum (*arrow*).

fetal akinesia sequence, which has been associated with Pena-Shokeir syndrome (pseudo-trisomy 18), nemaline rod myopathy, and maternal myasthenia gravis.[38-40]

"Clubfoot" is a term that tends to be used generically to describe abnormal foot position relative to the leg; the more accurate term is *talipes*, the most common presentation of which is fixed plantar flexion with internal rotation at the ankle (talipes equinovarus, or clubfoot), though several forms of talipes (combinations of calcaneo- or equino- varus/valgus) are described.[41] If unilateral, it is often an isolated finding with a low likelihood of syndromic association. Bilateral clubfoot, however, is typically secondary to spinal cord abnormalities such as meningomyelocele; anhydramnios or oligohydramnios, as with fetal renal or bladder obstruction; fetal akinesia; or genetic anomalies. Rocker-bottom foot (congenital vertical talus, or rigid flatfoot) is nearly always bilateral and is highly associated with aneuploidy (Trisomies 9, 13, or 18), though most cases are associated with neurologic disorders such as myelomeningocele (Fig. 131-14).[42]

Imaging Most fetuses move during ultrasonography, and assessment of fetal posture and movement is an essential part of determining fetal well-being.[43,44] Those that do not move as expected may be just sleeping and therefore are reimaged after a time interval to avoid further unnecessary evaluation. Movement limitation should be determined as generalized versus focal, and an effort should be made to look for tethering, constricting bands or a neural axis lesion, and muscle bulk should be assessed. Polyhydramnios is likely if the fetus is not swallowing; a lack of breathing will result in a small chest and pulmonary hypoplasia. Fetal MRI may be indicated

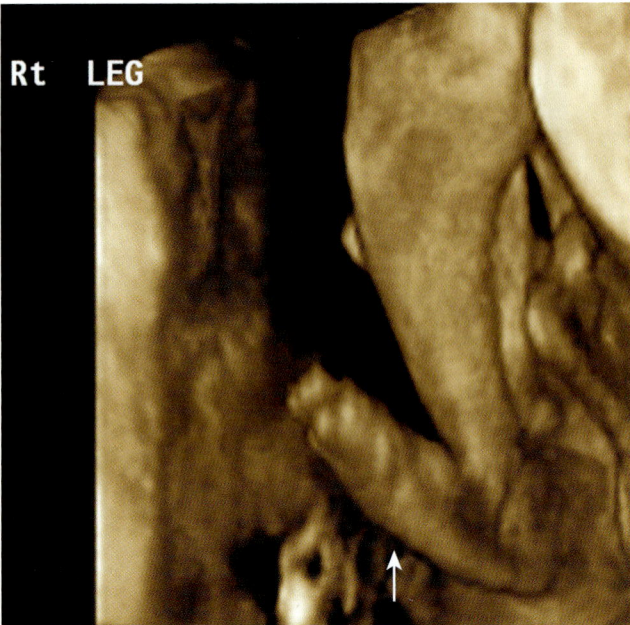

Figure 131-14 Congenital vertical talus (rocker-bottom foot). Three-dimensional ultrasound reconstruction using surface rendering. Note the fixed dorsiflexion of the foot (*arrow*).

to evaluate the neural axis for a cause of generalized hypotonia or contractures and can help measure lung volumes. Alterations on MRI of muscular contour, thickness, and signal have suggested atrophy from neuromuscular disease.[45]

Clubfoot is diagnosed on ultrasonography or MRI when both the foot and leg are imaged in a coronal plane together (Fig. 131-15). Care should be taken to ensure that this is a fixed position over time; spontaneous flexion at the ankle on real-time ultrasonography suggests the finding is positional.

Treatment and Follow-Up Neonatal treatments for hypotonia, arthrogryposis, or both are supportive. No fetal treatments are described, though testing for myotonic dystrophy should be undertaken in appropriate cases to avoid maternal complications. Treatment for clubfoot is generally started in the first days of life, and surgery depends on the success of manipulation and casting.[46]

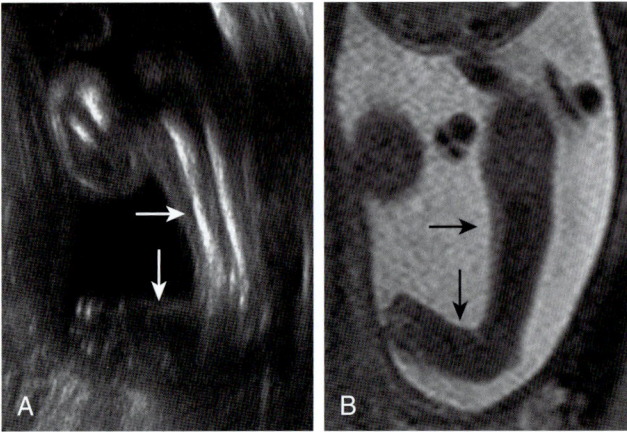

Figure 131-15 Congenital clubfoot. Ultrasonography (**A**) and T2-weighted magnetic resonance imaging (**B**) scans with a view of the foot (*vertical arrows*) in the same coronal plane as the leg (*horizontal arrows*).

Tumors

Etiology Tumors of the fetal musculoskeletal system are extraordinarily rare, except for sacrococcygeal teratoma (SCT). Still, this entity is uncommon, with a reported incidence of only 1 per 40,000.[47] SCT is thought to arise from primitive cells associated with the fetal coccyx, which must be removed in entirety with the tumor at excision to prevent recurrence. The Altman classification of SCT applies to the fetus but may change during gestation (Box 131-3).[48]

Imaging As with teratoma anywhere in the fetal body, tumors are characteristically mixed cystic and solid, with arterial vessels identifiable in the solid components. Ultrasonography is excellent for identifying the abnormal mass at the pelvis and involvement of superficial soft tissue just dorsal to the anus, which is invariably displaced ventrally when an external tumor component is present. Color Doppler interrogation is used to assess the vascularity of the tumor. Because of tumoral vascular shunting, a fetus may develop signs of high cardiac output failure, with the typical findings of hydrops fetalis that occurs if intervention is not undertaken. Close-interval follow-up with serial ultrasonography for the evolution of cardiac dysfunction and hydrops is indicated in a fetus with SCT if intervention is to be considered.[49] Because pelvic bones may interfere with clear visualization of the deep structures on ultrasonography, MRI is advantageous for better defining the extent of a lesion, its relationship to the bladder and rectum, and calculating a tumor–body weight ratio that some institutions use for prognosis (Fig. 131-16).[50] Both single-shot T2- and T1-weighted sequences for meconium–rectal position and hemorrhage may be helpful. Fetal MRI can supplant neonatal MRI in some cases. Although much more rare, neuroblastoma in the low pelvis has been reported to mimic the appearance of SCT.[51]

Rhabdomyoma, rhabdomyosarcoma, fibrosarcoma, or myofibroma (myofibromatosis) are extraordinarily rare in the fetus. These are, when prospectively diagnosed, characteristically solid masses with some internal heterogeneity that grow on serial examination; they are typically found in the fetal neck or pelvis but may be in the extremities, retroperitoneum, or chest wall.[52-58] They may be confused with vascular tumors such as a kaposiform hemangioendothelioma, although the latter are typically more infiltrative. Lymphatic malformation may also be infiltrative and multicompartmental and may have both solid (microcystic) and cystic (macrocystic) components. The differential diagnosis for solid tumors includes teratoma (which is more common, generally has some cysts, and might be distinguished by a fat component) and potentially neuroblastoma. Either of these tumors can contain calcifications.

Box 131-3 Altman Classification of Sacrococcygeal Teratoma

Type 1: Tumor entirely external to the pelvis

Type 2: Tumor larger in volume externally than in the pelvis

Type 3: Tumor larger internally, extends above the true pelvis into the abdomen

Type 4: Tumor without an external component

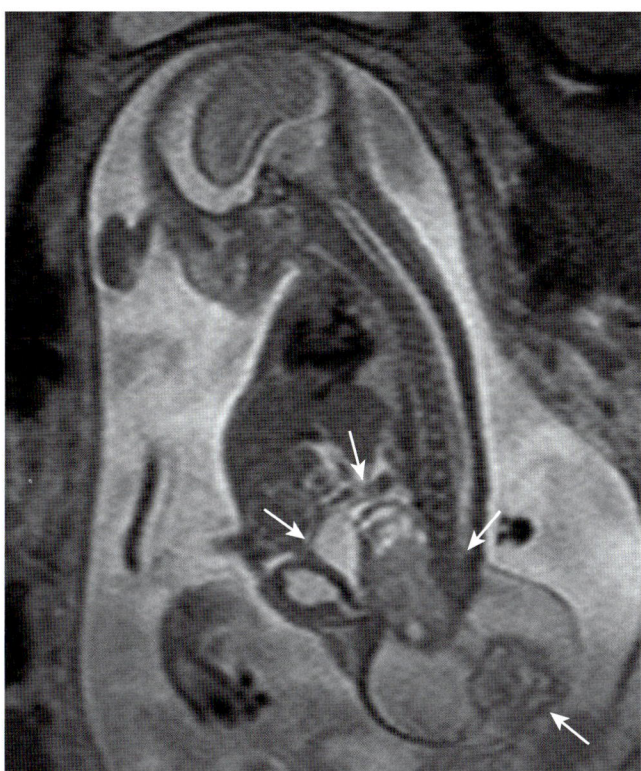

Figure 131-16 Sacrococcygeal teratoma. Mixed cystic-solid mass in the fetal pelvis between the bladder and the spine, extending externally (*arrows*).

Treatment and Follow-up Prior to viability, should a fetus develop cardiac failure and hydrops fetalis, in utero surgical resection of SCT has been offered in some centers as an alternative to inevitable demise. The procedure involves a hysterotomy with partial delivery of the fetus, tumor resection, and return of the fetus to the uterus with myometrial closure. A significant complication is preterm labor, and efforts are therefore being directed toward less invasive surgeries.[59] This is clearly a rare circumstance, but it has been successfully managed. After the age of viability, a fetus in distress could be delivered for further ex utero treatment options.

Treatment for SCT in the neonate is complete surgical excision of the tumor; the risk of malignancy is lowest with fetal or neonatal presentation and therapy.[60] Recurrence rates are negligible as long as the coccyx is also removed with the tumor.[61]

WHAT THE CLINICIAN NEEDS TO KNOW

- If limb lengths are abnormal, degree of suspicion of lethality (small chest)
- Distribution and extent of limb defects
- Presence of fixed scoliosis or abnormal posturing of neck, trunk, or limbs
- An assessment of vascularity to an organ of origin of any mass
- Associated anomalies

Key Points

- Marked thoracic restriction portends lethality in cases of skeletal dysplasia.

- The majority of lethal skeletal dysplasias are one of three diagnoses: thanatophoric dysplasia, achondrogenesis, or osteogenesis imperfecta type II.

- Thorough evaluation of the fetus and its environment, including the umbilical cord, is indicated when a limb defect is detected.

- Fetal posture should be assessed for fixed or abnormal positions.

- Fetal musculoskeletal tumors are rare; SCT is the most common and can cause fetal cardiac high-output failure due to arterial shunting.

Suggested Readings

Avni FE, Massez A, Cassart M. Tumours of the fetal body: a review. *Pediatr Radiol.* 2009;39:1147-1157.

Avni FE, Rypens F, Zappa M, et al. Antenatal diagnosis of short-limb dwarfism: sonographic approach. *Pediatr Radiol.* 1996;26(3):171-178.

Cassart M. Suspected fetal skeletal malformations or bone diseases: how to explore. *Pediatr Radiol.* 2010;40:1046-1051.

Dighe M, Fligner C, Cheng E, et al. Fetal skeletal dysplasia: an approach to diagnosis with illustrative cases. *RadioGraphics.* 2008;28:1061-1077.

Teele R. A guide to the recognition of skeletal disorders in the fetus. *Pediatr Radiol.* 2006;36(6):473-484.

References

Full references for this chapter can be found on www.expertconsult.com.

Chapter 132

Congenital Anomalies of Bone

TAL LAOR and J. HERMAN KAN

Regardless of origin, abnormal limb development tends to fall into patterns that can be recognized clinically and radiographically (Fig. 132-1). Most classification systems of congenital malformations are based on osseous structures, but it is well recognized that anomalous conditions of surrounding soft tissues are certain to be present. Although one deficiency is usually dominant, dysplasia often involves the entire limb.

Congenital deficiencies are more common than acquired amputations in children. Frantz and O'Rahilly developed a system of classification that is still commonly used to evaluate congenital anomalies of the extremities.[1] Each malformation is defined by the part that is deficient. For example, the fibula is deficient in fibular hemimelia. The abnormality is considered terminal if the deformity extends to the distal aspect of the extremity; it is intercalary if the limb distal to the deformity is normal. For example, in fibular hemimelia, if the foot is abnormal, the deficiency is terminal, and if the foot is normal, it is intercalary. Likewise, a defect may be classified as longitudinal (paraxial) or transverse. The malformation is paraxial if only the fibular side is affected. If both the tibia and the fibula are affected, the deformity is considered transverse.

The cause of reduction malformations is known in only a small number of cases. A few abnormalities are heritable, but most are sporadic. Environmental factors are implicated infrequently. Medications such as thalidomide induced malformations that were reduction deformities, ranging from severe amelias to mild muscular hypoplasia.[2] Most malformations were on the radial or tibial side, and the upper limbs were affected more often than were the lower extremities. Infrequently, excess deformities such as polydactyly were observed.

Extremity Deficiencies

PROXIMAL FEMORAL FOCAL DEFICIENCY

Etiology Proximal femoral focal deficiency (PFFD) refers to abnormalities that range from mild shortening and hypoplasia of the femur to severe deficiency of the bone and dysplasia of the acetabulum. The defect is thought to be a result of altered proliferation and maturation of the chondrocytes of the proximal femoral physis in utero, which in turn results in underdevelopment of the ipsilateral acetabulum. A child with PFFD usually presents in infancy with a short extremity and an unstable hip.[3] A well-formed acetabulum implies the presence of a femoral head, which might be cartilaginous and therefore is not apparent radiographically early in life. Most cases are sporadic; however, the combination of bilateral femoral deficiencies and abnormal facies, known as the femoral hypoplasia–unusual facies syndrome, is thought to be an autosomal-dominant disorder.

PFFD should be distinguished from developmental dysplasia of the hip, infantile coxa vara, and congenitally short femur. In the setting of developmental dysplasia of the hip, proximal femoral neck and head hypoplasia may be present. The subtrochanteric region of the femur is normal and distal congenital anomalies are absent, and the deformities at the level of the acetabulum are more severe than the deformities at the level of the femoral head and neck. Persons with infantile coxa vara have a normal subtrochanteric region and distal bones, and the femur is normal length, accounting for bowing. Unlike PFFD, infantile coxa vara is discovered after weight bearing occurs.[4] A congenitally short femur may be unilateral or bilateral and often is associated with reduction defects elsewhere in the same limb. Most cases are sporadic, but several external factors have been implicated in more complex deformities. Known causes include drugs (such as thalidomide), trauma, irradiation, infection, and focal ischemia.[5] Unlike patients with PFFD, patients with a congenitally short femur have a stable hip.

Imaging The most commonly used classification for PFFD was proposed by Aitken (Fig. 132-2).[6] The least severe type is class A, which refers to an adequate or only mildly dysplastic proximal femur and acetabulum. The femoral head is present but is separated from the shortened distal femoral segment. With age, a fibrous connection between the head and the distal femoral segment ossifies—usually, not completely. A subtrochanteric varus deformity invariably is present. Class C deformities have a residual acetabulum present (Fig. 132-3). In the most severe form, class D, most of the femur and the ipsilateral acetabulum are absent.

PFFD is associated with other ipsilateral deformities, including fibular hemimelia (in more than 50% of affected children), shortening of the tibia, equinovalgus deformity of the foot (more often than equinovarus deformity), and deficiency of the lateral rays of the foot. PFFD is bilateral in 15% of affected children.[7]

Sonography can be used to delineate radiographically inapparent structures at an early age. If a cartilaginous femoral

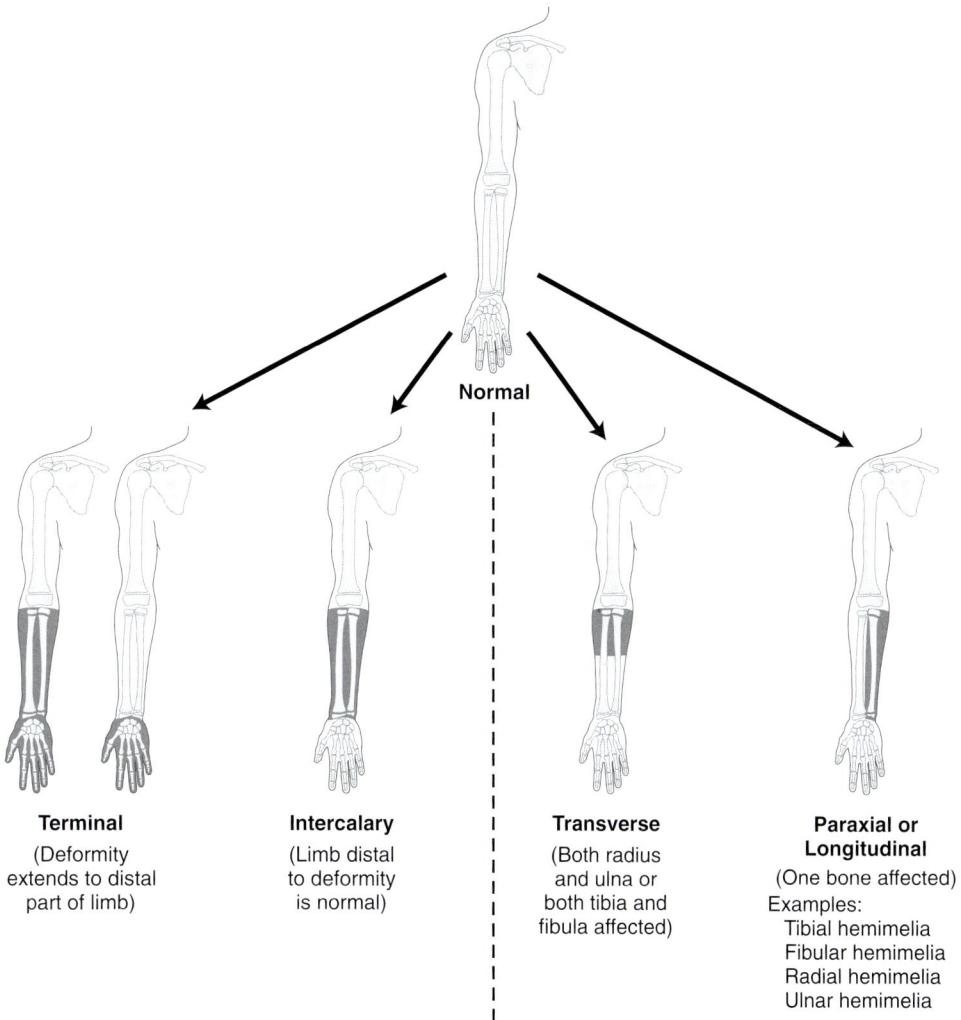

Figure 132-1 Skeletal deformities of the limbs. The shaded, blackened areas indicate deficient parts.

head and its connection to the femoral shaft can be shown, the stability of the hip joint is likely greater than is implied from radiographs. Similar to sonography, magnetic resonance imaging (MRI) is useful for defining the anatomy of the hip joint and associated deformities of the limb,[8] allowing for appropriate early classification of deformity. Although the acetabulum might appear developed, even the least severe forms of PFFD are associated with acetabular deficiency. In contrast to the predominantly anterior deficiency of developmental acetabular dysplasia, the acetabulum in PFFD usually has an insufficient posterior wall. Most of the muscles about

the affected hip are hypoplastic when compared with the contralateral normal side, with the exception of the sartorius muscle, which often is hypertrophied. This situation results in the characteristic flexion deformity of the hip and knee. MRI also defines the anatomy of soft tissues that can guide surgical exposure and preparation of the limb stump for fitting of a prosthesis.

Treatment and Follow-up Therapy for children with PFFD is based on the severity of the deficiency and projection of growth and final limb length discrepancy at maturity.

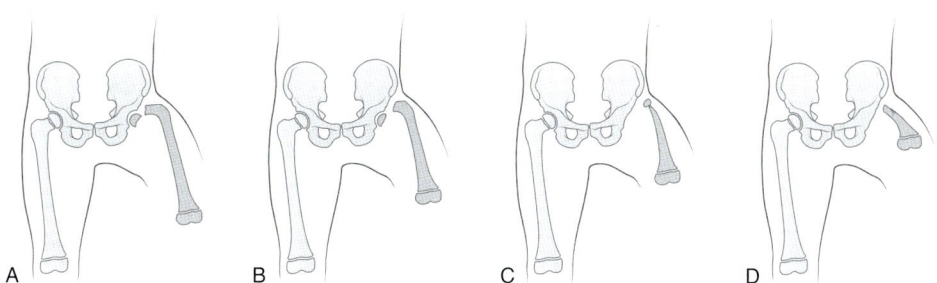

Figure 132-2 Aitken classification of proximal femoral focal deficiency.

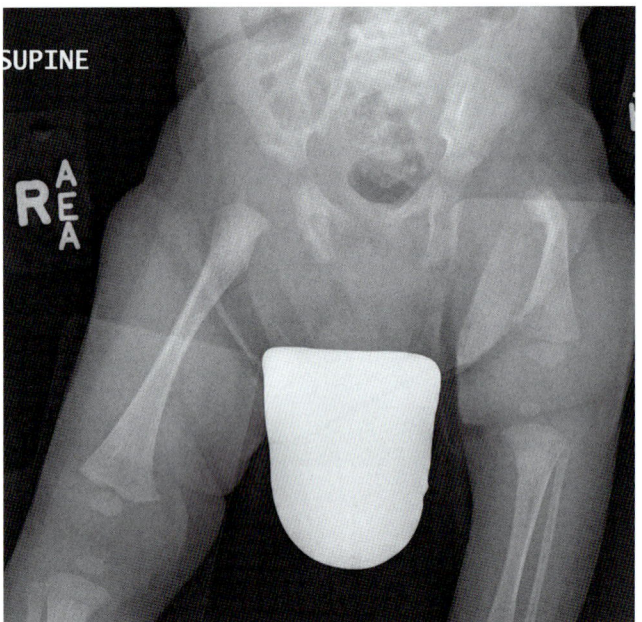

Figure 132-3   Aiken type 3 proximal femoral focal deficiency of the left hip in a 4-week-old boy. The femur is substantially short and the left acetabulum is severely dysplastic. Mild developmental dysplasia of the right acetabulum is present.

Objectives for treatment are to maximize the length of the extremity, to promote stability of the hip, knee, and ankle, and to optimize anatomic alignment. Mild deformities may not require surgery. Stabilization of the upper femoral defect is controversial and usually is indicated if a deformity is progressive. Children with severe deformities benefit from amputation of the foot and fusion of the knee. Rotationplasty of the tibia, in which the foot is rotated 180 degrees (so that the toes face posteriorly and the ankle now serves as a knee joint), allows the ankle and foot to control a distal prosthesis.[9] Intact sensory feedback from the foot provides proprioceptive control of the knee. Thus it is imperative to assess the morphology of the proximal femur and acetabulum, the cartilaginous epiphyses of the knee, and the supporting soft tissue structures. For example, instability of the knee can result from absence of the anterior cruciate ligament. In the rare case of bilateral PFFD, amputation is contraindicated and therapy is based on extension prostheses that enhance the child's height.

FIBULAR HEMIMELIA

Etiology   Fibular hemimelia is the most common hemimelia and the most common congenital anomaly of the fibula. It also is referred to as congenital short tibia with absent fibula syndrome. Unilateral absence is more frequent than bilateral deformity. A band of strong connective tissue may replace all or most of the fibula.[10] Fibular hemimelia is associated with a short, bowed tibia, absence of lateral rays of the foot, tarsal abnormalities (particularly coalitions), and femoral shortening or deficiency in 15% of patients. Caskey and Lester[11] reported a clubfoot deformity in 16% of patients with fibular hemimelia. Other associations include small, subluxed, or dislocated patellae, hypoplastic femoral condyles, and ligamentous deficiencies of the knee.

Imaging   Fibular hemimelia ranges from mild deficiency of the proximal end of the bone to complete absence accompanied by multiple malformations of neighboring structures (Fig. 132-4). MRI can document associated abnormalities, particularly if surgery is contemplated, including associated ligamentous deficiencies of the knee.

Treatment and Follow-up   The talipes equinovalgus deformity of the foot and severe shortening of the limb associated with fibular hemimelia result in poor function of the limb. Children with extensive abnormalities involving the fibula, ipsilateral tibia, femur, and foot benefit the most from early amputation of the foot and often the more proximal structures.[12] If the deformity is less severe, lengthening of the affected side, realignment of the tibiotalar articulation, and epiphysiodesis of the contralateral limb often are undertaken. Attempts at lengthening a severely dysplastic limb often are unsatisfactory.

TIBIAL HEMIMELIA

Etiology   Most cases of tibial hemimelia are sporadic, although reported forms (particularly bilateral deformities) display an autosomal-dominant inheritance pattern. Jones et al.[13] classified the spectrum of tibial dysplasia into four groups. In type I, which is the most severe form, the tibia is not recognized radiographically at birth. Lack of ossification of the distal femoral epiphysis implies that no proximal tibia is present. The least severe form, type IV, includes congenital tibial diastasis. In children with this form, the tibia is short and

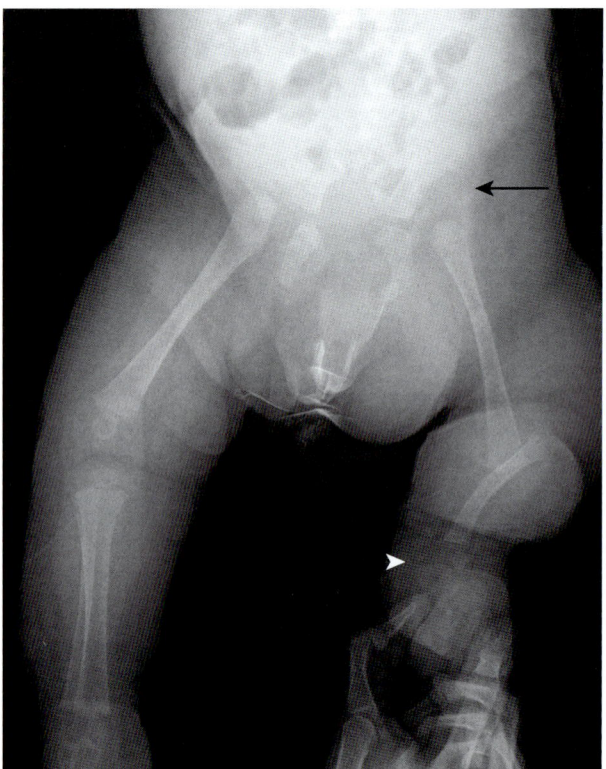

Figure 132-4   Left fibular hemimelia in a 5-month-old girl. The left knee is dislocated and the tibia is short and bowed. The left femur is short, the distal epiphysis is not yet ossified, and the acetabulum is dysplastic (*arrow*). The talus is small (*arrowhead*).

diverges from the fibula at the ankle. The talus is displaced proximally. No normal distal tibial articulation surface is present.

Imaging Radiography of tibial hemimelia (Fig. 132-5) ranges from absence of a portion of the distal tibia to complete absence with multiple malformations of neighboring structures. MRI can document associated abnormalities, including associated muscular and ligamentous deficiencies, which is important if surgery is contemplated. MRI may identify a cartilaginous tibial remnant that may not be identified readily on radiography.

Treatment and Follow-up Treatment of tibial hemimelia varies with the severity of the deformity. A knee disarticulation is recommended for complete tibial absence. Brown pioneered centralization of the fibula with a Syme amputation of the foot in children with complete tibial hemimelia.[14] This approach produces adequate results in the rare cases in which the quadriceps muscles are well developed. When the quadriceps mechanism is abnormal, the patella often is absent. MRI can be used to assess deficiencies preoperatively, allowing the clinician to discern who will function better with primary knee disarticulation (most patients) rather than knee reconstruction.

RADIAL DEFICIENCY (RADIAL DYSPLASIA, RADIAL CLUBHAND)

Etiology Conditions associated with radial deficiency are listed in Box 132-1.[15] Usually the entire limb is involved to

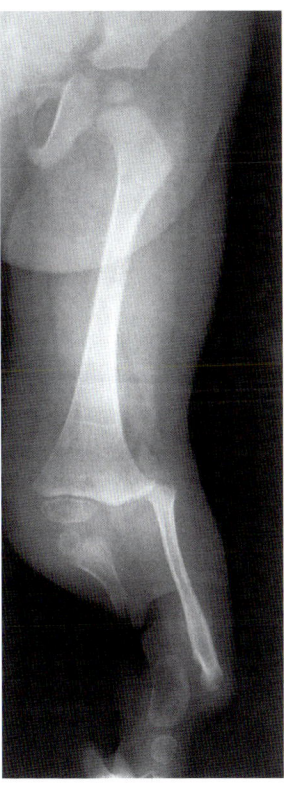

Figure 132-5 **A 2-year-old girl with tibial hemimelia.** A dysplastic proximal tibial remnant is evident. The fibula is short and subluxed laterally, and multiple tarsal bones are absent.

Box 132-1 Conditions Associated with Radial Deficiency (Dysplasia)

Syndromes Associated with Congenital Heart Disease
- Holt-Oram syndrome

Syndromes Associated with Blood Dyscrasias
- Fanconi anemia (pancytopenia–dysmelia syndrome)
- Thrombocytopenia—absent radius syndrome

Syndromes Associated with Intellectual Disability
- Brachmann-de Lange (Cornelia de Lange) syndrome
- Seckel syndrome

Syndromes Associated with Chromosomal Abnormalities
- Trisomy 13
- Trisomy 18

Syndromes Associated with Teratogens
- Thalidomide embryopathy
- Varicella embryopathy

Other
- VACTERL association

VACTERL, Vertebral, anal, cardiac, tracheal, esophageal, renal, limb. Modified from Goldberg MJ, Bartoshevsky LE. Congenital hand anomaly: etiology and associated malformations. *Hand Clin.* 1985;1:405-415.

---

some degree, which often results in joint dysfunction of the shoulder, elbow, wrist, carpus, and small joints of the hand. Associated muscular deficiencies also are proportionate to the degree of skeletal abnormality. Neurovascular abnormalities include an absent radial artery and superficial radial nerve.

Whether radial deficiency is isolated or is associated with a syndrome, the primary malformation is likely the result of a vascular abnormality in the embryo that occurred before differentiation of mesenchyme into muscle and bone.[16] Most cases are sporadic, but some autosomal-dominant and autosomal-recessive inheritance patterns are reported. Other cases are likely the result of various environmental insults from viruses, chemicals, radiation, and drugs during limb bud development.

Imaging Congenital radial deficiency ranges from hypoplasia of the thumb to various degrees of radial hypoplasia. Complete absence is the most common longitudinal deficiency. This deformity usually is accompanied by radial and volar deviation of the hand, which results in part from unopposed pull by the flexor carpi radialis and brachioradialis muscles.

In most cases of radial aplasia, the forearm is bowed to the radial side and the distal ulna is prominent (Fig. 132-6). The forearm is short (usually approximately two thirds the length of the normal contralateral side) and remains proportionately so throughout growth. Often, only the capitate, hamate, and triquetral bones and the metacarpals and phalanges of the four ulnar rays are present and normal. The trapezium, scaphoid, and first ray often are deformed or absent. If a remnant of the radius is present proximally, it usually is fused to the ulna, which is curved, shortened, and thickened. Bilateral deficiency occurs in approximately 50% of affected children.[15] The degree of deformity of the hand is related to the severity of deficiency of the forearm.

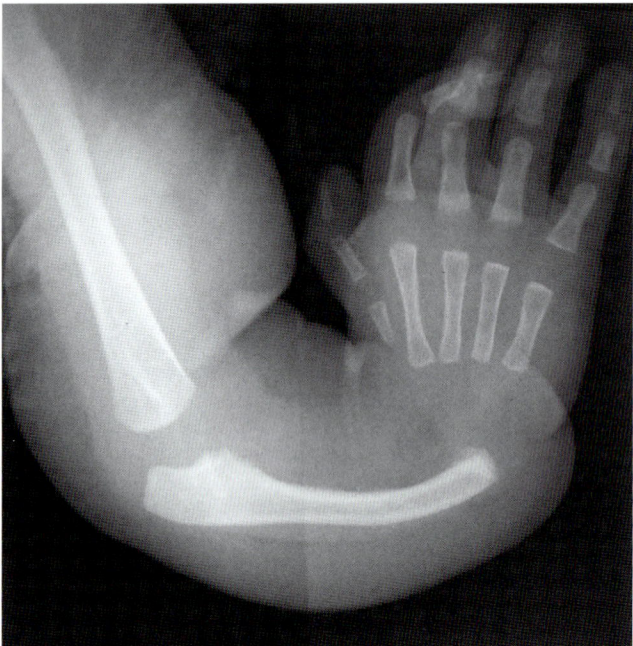

Figure 132-6 Radial deficiency (radial clubhand) in a 10-month-old boy with complete absence of the radius. The ulna is short and bowed, and the thumb is hypoplastic.

Treatment and Follow-up Treatment of a longitudinal radial deficiency begins with serial casting and splinting intended to improve radial deviation by stretching the soft tissues. This treatment often is followed by surgical centralization of the hand over the ulna to improve function and appearance.[17] Thumb reconstruction and pollicization of the index finger often are indicated.

ULNAR DEFICIENCY (ULNAR DYSPLASIA, ULNAR CLUBHAND)

Etiology Deficiency that occurs along the ulnar or postaxial border of the upper extremity is known as ulnar deficiency or ulnar clubhand. It is a relatively uncommon disorder that occurs much less frequently than radial deficiency (radial clubhand). Approximately 48% of cases have anomalies of the contralateral limb.[18] Most cases are sporadic, but associations with many other syndromes have been reported, most commonly Brachmann-de Lange syndrome.

Imaging In persons with ulnar deficiency, coexisting abnormalities almost always are present in the carpal, metacarpal, and phalangeal rays (e-Fig. 132-7). The pisiform is always absent, and the hamate frequently is not detected. Syndactyly, carpal fusion, and radiohumeral fusion are frequent. The forearm is shortened and bowed, with a concavity to the ulnar side. The hand is deviated in an ulnar direction, and elbow abnormalities are common. Hypoplasia of the shoulder girdle and the upper arm can coexist with ulnar deficiencies. Anomalies of the contralateral upper limb and the lower limbs (such as PFFD) have been reported.

Treatment and Follow-up Treatment for ulnar deficiency includes early correction of ulnar deviation of the hand, which is achieved with serial casting. Surgical treatment is reserved for cases with significant limitation of function.[19] Forearm instability and associated hand deformities must be addressed.

Generalized Anomalies

CONGENITAL CONSTRICTION BANDS

Etiology Constriction bands are thought to result from intrauterine rupture of the amnion and subsequent mechanical constriction of fetal limbs.[20] Various body parts become entangled in the amnion as it separates from the chorion. In some instances, adjacent structures are pulled together by the bands and ultimately become fused, producing a soft tissue syndactyly. Bony syndactyly is very rare. The earlier the amnion ruptures, the more severe are the malformations. Limb abnormalities range from slight soft tissue grooves to transverse intrauterine amputations. Acrosyndactyly, craniofacial and visceral anomalies, and fetal death are part of the spectrum of congenital constriction band syndrome. Sporadic congenital constriction band syndrome is estimated to occur at an incidence of 1 : 1200 to 1 : 15,000 births.

An alternative explanation is the intrinsic theory, which suggests that an inherent defect leads to bands during limb embryogenesis.[20]

Imaging Radiography may underestimate the degree of soft tissue compromise, and associated anomalous vascular anatomy may not be recognized. Typical conventional radiographic findings include a tethered appearance of fingers with a characteristic tight distal waist with soft tissue syndactyly (Fig. 132-8). MRI can be used to evaluate the depth of the constriction band, the degree of resultant lymphedema, and the integrity of the involved musculature.

Treatment and Follow-up Surgical treatment usually is cosmetic, although it may be needed to relieve massive edema distal to a constriction band or to improve neurovascular function. Intervention for patients with acrosyndactyly may result in partial correction of the deformity and improved longitudinal growth.

ARTHROGRYPOSIS

Etiology Arthrogryposis is a descriptive term used loosely to refer to conditions that result in congenital contractures involving two or more joints, such as those that limit intrauterine movement.[21] The earlier in gestation that movement is limited and the longer the restriction lasts, the more severe will be the contractures at birth. Normal in utero motion is necessary for normal development of joints.

Arthrogryposis may result from abnormal muscles (such as myopathies), abnormal nerve function or innervation, abnormal connective tissues, or mechanical limitation of movement (such as oligohydramnios or multiple fetuses). Other possible causes include genetic defects, mutagenic agents, mitotic abnormalities, and toxic chemicals or drugs (Box 132-2).

Imaging Contractures that are present at birth often are symmetric and most commonly affect distal parts of limbs. Clubfoot deformities often are present. The lower extremities

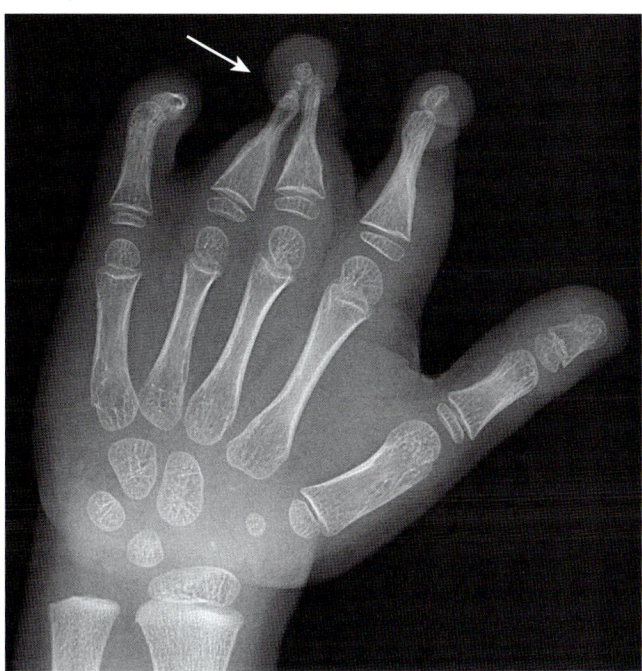

Figure 132-8 Constriction bands in a 3-year-old girl with a "tight waist" appearance (*arrow*) and multiple distal digital amputations.

are usually involved, but more than half of patients have upper limb abnormalities as well. Rigid joints and hypotonia contribute to frequent perinatal fractures. Soft tissue dimples may be seen over the affected joints, and muscle mass is decreased in affected limbs (e-Fig. 132-9). Affected muscles are partially or completely replaced by fatty or fibrous tissue. In many children, a scoliosis eventually develops. MRI can be used to assess joint integrity when surgery to maximize joint function is planned.

Treatment and Follow-up The long-term prognosis for most children with arthrogryposis is good. However, children with associated central nervous system abnormalities usually have a limited life span. A neuromuscular workup is recommended for all children with arthrogryposis. Early therapy, including manipulation to increase range of motion, as well as surgery, is advocated for best results.[22]

Fusion Deformities

TARSAL COALITION

Etiology Tarsal coalition is a congenital failure of segmentation of the primitive mesenchyme that results in the union of two or more tarsal bones. A preadolescent or adolescent child with pain in the midfoot and hindfoot that is associated with lack of motion in the subtalar region should be suspected of having a tarsal coalition. Prevalence in the U.S. population is approximately 1% or less. At least 50% of patients with coalitions have bilateral findings.[23] An autosomal-dominant inheritance pattern with a high level of penetrance is reported, although the coalition need not involve the same joint. Although it typically presents during the second decade of life, tarsal coalition may not manifest until adulthood.

Tarsal coalition is defined on the basis of anatomic location and completeness of ossification. A complete ossific bar forms a synostosis, a cartilaginous bar forms a synchondrosis, and a fibrous union is termed a syndesmosis. The most common fusions are talocalcaneal and calcaneonavicular. The middle facet is the most common location for a talocalcaneal coalition. Talocalcaneal coalitions often may extend posteriorly, with involvement of the junction of the middle and posterior facet. Talonavicular (e-Fig. 132-10) and calcaneocuboid coalitions are much less common. Synostoses can occur between other bones of the foot but frequently are associated with other limb abnormalities, such as fibular hemimelia or short femur, or disorders such as Apert syndrome.

Symptoms from a tarsal coalition present with advancing ossification. Pain with activity usually is the presenting symptom. The child may have a peroneal spastic flatfoot, which involves pain and rigid valgus deformity of the hindfoot and forefoot, along with peroneal muscle spasm. This condition is not a true spasticity but reflects peroneal shortening to adjust for heel valgus and to maintain a less painful position for the subtalar joint.

Imaging A 45-degree lateral oblique radiograph of the foot directly shows a calcaneonavicular coalition. The secondary radiographic features of calcaneonavicular coalitions visible on a lateral radiograph include pes planus, anteater sign (Fig. 132-11), and talar beak sign (e-Fig. 132-12). A reverse

---

Box 132-2 Causes of Arthrogryposis: Causes of Limited Fetal Joint Mobility

Neurologic
- Disorders of cerebrum
- Anterior horn cell deficiency
- Abnormalities of nerve function or structure (central or peripheral)

Muscular
- Abnormal formation or function
- Congenital muscular dystrophy
- Mitochondrial disorders

Connective Tissue or Skeletal
- Primary disorders

Vascular Compromise
- Severe bleeding
- Monozygotic twins
- Amniotic bands

Mechanical Compression
- Fetal crowding from multiple births
- Oligohydramnios
- Uterine fibroids/other tumors
- Amniotic bands
- Trauma

Maternal
- Diabetes mellitus
- Hyperthermia
- Infection
- Drug use and abuse

Modified from Jones K. *Smith's recognizable patterns of human malformation.* 5th ed. Philadelphia: WB Saunders; 1997.

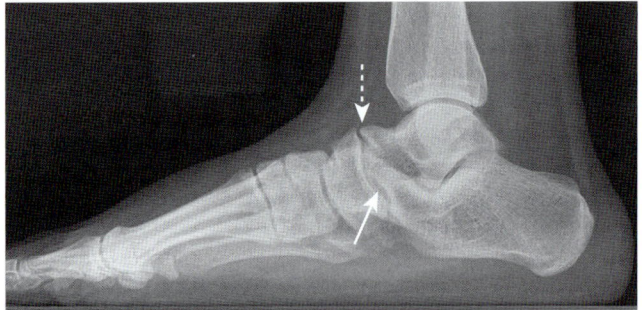

Figure 132-11 The anteater sign in a child with a calcaneonavicular coalition (*arrow*) and talar beak (*dotted arrow*). Elongation of the anterior calcaneus resembling the nose of an anteater is present.

anteater sign is seen on the anteroposterior (AP) view of the foot and is defined as diminished AP height of the lateral portion of the navicular (compared with the medial navicular), with the navicular extending far lateral with respect to the talar head.

Radiographic features of talocalcaneal coalitions include the C sign (Fig. 132-13, *A*), talar beak, an ovoid, enlarged sustentaculum tali (see Fig. 132-13, *A*), and broadened lateral process of the talus.

The talar beak associated with tarsal coalitions is a dorsal extension of the talar head (see e-Fig. 132-12). A talar beak should not be confused with a talar ridge. The talar ridge represents bony proliferation related to the insertion of the anterior tibiotalar capsule and is located along the more proximal dorsal talar neck rather than at the distal talar head.[24]

A ball-and-socket articulation of the distal tibia and talus is an uncommon association with tarsal coalition. However, this configuration at the ankle joint is nonspecific and may be associated with congenital long bone deficiencies, as well as tarsal coalitions.[25]

Computed tomography (CT) and MRI help to define the nature and cross-sectional area of a fusion. CT is more cost-effective if the clinical suspicion for coalition is high (Fig. 132-13, *B*). If other causes of pain and limited hindfoot mobility are considered, then MRI may be indicated. MRI may directly show bony, cartilaginous, and fibrous unions. Bone marrow edema often is noted adjacent to the fused articulation (Fig. 132-14).

Treatment and Follow-up Casting and nonsteroidal antiinflammatory medications often are the initial treatment for symptomatic children. Steroid injections and physical therapy also may be used. If symptoms are not relieved and no degenerative changes have occurred, then surgical resection of the abnormal tarsal bridging often is attempted.[23] Regrowth of a calcaneonavicular coalition can be halted by interposition of the extensor digitorum brevis tendon. Fat frequently is interposed after resection of a subtalar coalition. Subtalar fusion or triple arthrodesis may be indicated in refractory cases.

CARPAL FUSION

Isolated fusion of the carpal bones is a normal variant that is seen in approximately 0.1% of the white population and approximately 1.6% of the African American population (e-Fig. 132-15).[26] Carpal fusion is seen most frequently between the lunate and triquetrum. Fusion between bones of the proximal and distal carpal rows usually is associated with a syndrome. Fusions also may be acquired, as in juvenile idiopathic arthritis or after trauma.

SYNDACTYLY

Fusion between adjacent digits resulting from intrauterine failure to separate is termed *syndactyly* (also referred to as "webbed toes" or "webbed fingers"). These fusions may involve only soft tissue (simple syndactyly), or they also may involve bone (complex syndactyly). If the entire length of the digit is involved, syndactyly is termed complete, and if only a partial length is bridged, it is incomplete. Fusion may be unilateral or bilateral and usually involves the second, third, and fourth digits. Syndactyly may be isolated or may be associated with congenital disorders such as Poland, Apert (Fig. 132-16), and Carpenter syndromes. Poland syndrome includes symbrachydactyly (brachydactyly and syndactyly) and ipsilateral chest wall anomalies, most commonly pectoralis muscle hypoplasia or aplasia. Apert syndrome includes syndactyly, craniosynostosis, and facial bone anomalies. Carpenter syndrome includes polysyndactyly, craniosynostosis, and facial bone anomalies. Syndactyly is thought to have an autosomal-dominant inheritance pattern.[27] Surgery is performed early in life to improve function and appearance

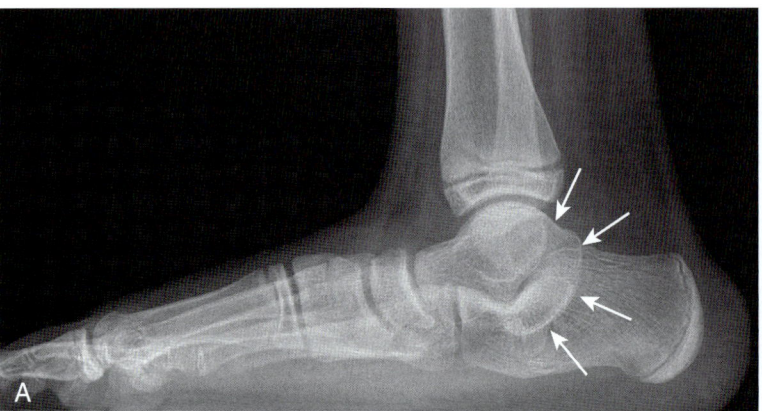
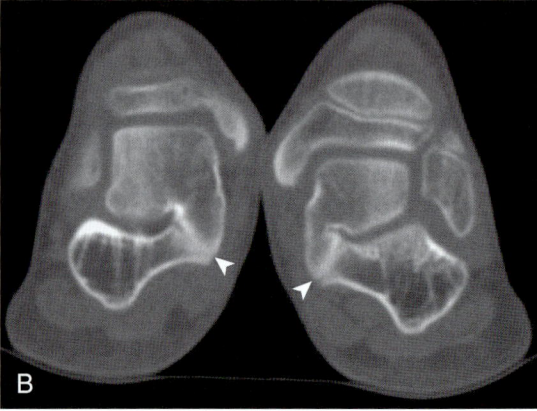

Figure 132-13 Talocalcaneal coalition. **A,** A lateral radiograph demonstrates the C sign (*arrows*), ovoid, elongated sustentaculum tali, and pes planus. **B,** Computed tomography with coronal reformats in a different patient demonstrates bilateral middle facet subtalar coalitions (*arrowheads*).

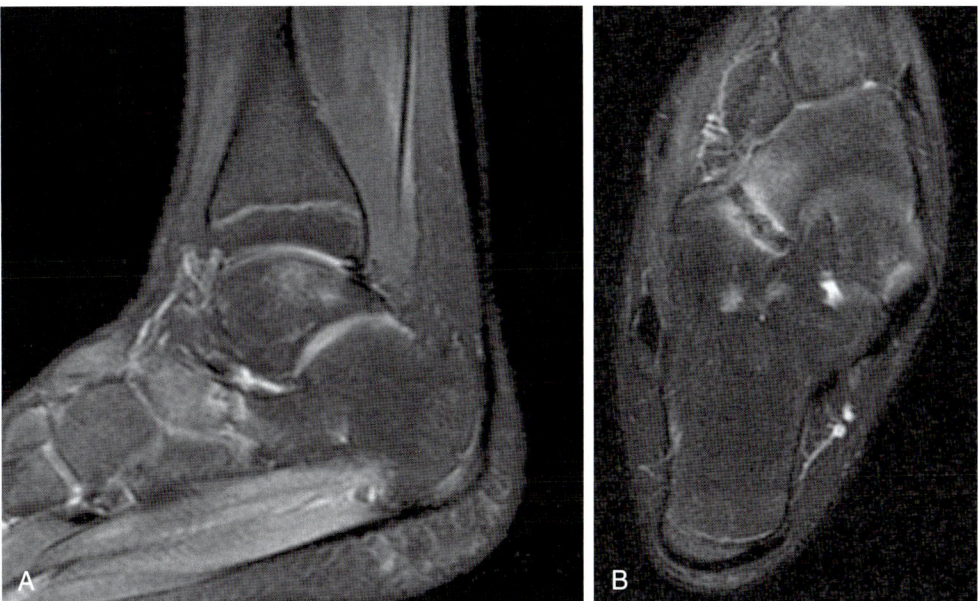

Figure 132-14 Talonavicular coalition in a 12-year-old girl. Short Tau inversion recovery sagittal (**A**) and T2 fat-saturated axial magnetic resonance (**B**) images demonstrate marrow edema on both sides of a fibrous coalition.

when the hand is involved. Surgery is rarely indicated for the foot.

SYMPHALANGISM

Symphalangism is an uncommon autosomal-dominant disorder of fusion of the interphalangeal joints of the hands and feet (Fig. 132-17). Although proximal interphalangeal joint fusion is more common, fusion also can be more distal.[28] The anomaly is usually bilateral, and the little finger and little toe are affected most often. Fusion may not be recognized radiographically until later in childhood. Despite the radiographic appearance of the digits, seldom is disability or loss of function of the hand reported. Symphalangism may be associated with other skeletal abnormalities, various digit deformities (e.g., brachydactyly, clinodactyly, and camptodactyly), radioulnar fusion, hip dislocation, tarsal coalition, and spinal anomalies.

RADIOULNAR SYNOSTOSIS

Etiology   Congenital radioulnar synostosis anomaly is due to failure of longitudinal segmentation between the radius and the ulna.[29] In utero, cartilaginous anlagen of the humerus, radius, and ulna are connected. Normal separation progresses from the distal end of the forearm to the proximal end. An insult to segmentation during early in utero development can lead to bony or fibrous synostosis. Radioulnar synostosis is associated with disorders such as Apert and Carpenter syndromes, as well as with other upper extremity abnormalities such as polydactyly, syndactyly, and carpal coalition.

On clinical examination, the child often may have a fixed degree of pronation and a mild degree of flexion at the elbow. Pain usually occurs during the teen years, when progressive and symptomatic radial head subluxation may be seen.

Imaging   Osseous coalition is best seen on AP radiographs (Fig. 132-18). Radioulnar synostosis may lead to secondary radial head dysplasia (see Fig. 132-18, *B*) because of the lack of articulation between the radial head and capitellum needed for normal development. Posterior dislocation of the radial head also may be seen (e-Fig. 132-19).

Treatment and Follow-up   Surgical treatment usually is reserved for patients with a severe pronation deformity or symptomatic radial head subluxation, particularly when it involves the dominant hand. A both bone extraarticular derotational osteotomy through the forearm to improve supination may be performed.[30] Resection of the proximal synostosis is complex and may not lead to improved forearm and hand function.

Other Congenital Malformations

CLINODACTYLY

Clinodactyly is a curvature of the finger in a radial or ulnar direction (in the mediolateral plane) away from the axis of joint flexion and extension. Although it may involve any digit, clinodactyly most often refers to radial curvature of the distal interphalangeal joint of the fifth digit (Fig. 132-20).[31] Clinodactyly is associated with a short middle phalanx and usually is bilateral. It may be seen in the normal population as a sporadic variant but also can be inherited in an autosomal-dominant pattern. It has been described in numerous syndromes (most commonly Down syndrome), in bone dysplasias, after trauma, and in many miscellaneous conditions. The curvature deformity may occur in the setting of a normal phalanx, as a result of physeal growth disturbance, or related to a longitudinal epiphyseal bracket deformity. Treatment is undertaken for cosmesis or for excessive scissoring of the digits.

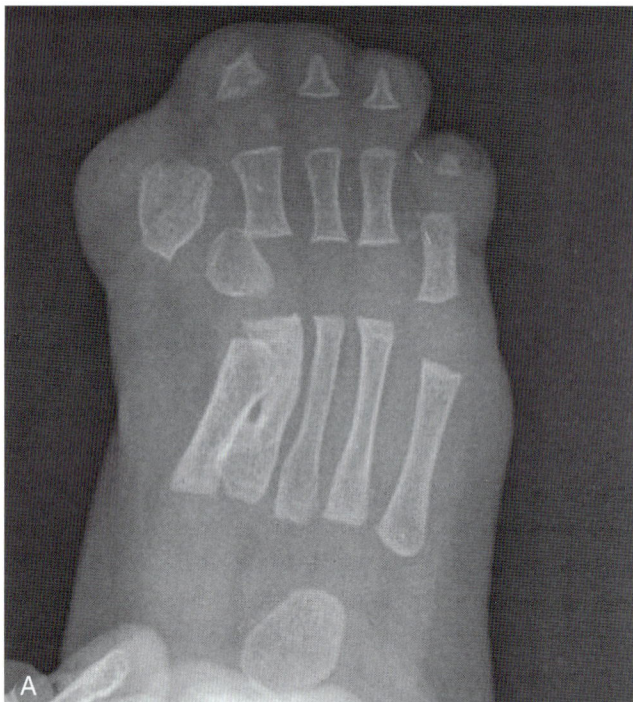

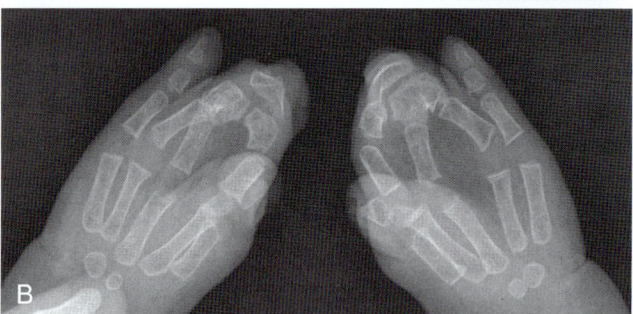

Figure 132-16   A 1-year-old child with Apert syndrome. **A,** A frontal view of the foot shows syndactyly of the digits. Hypoplasia of many bones of the foot is seen with absent middle phalanges. The first and second metatarsals are partially fused. **B,** A frontal radiograph of both hands of the same child shows syndactyly, synostosis, and symphalangism bilaterally.

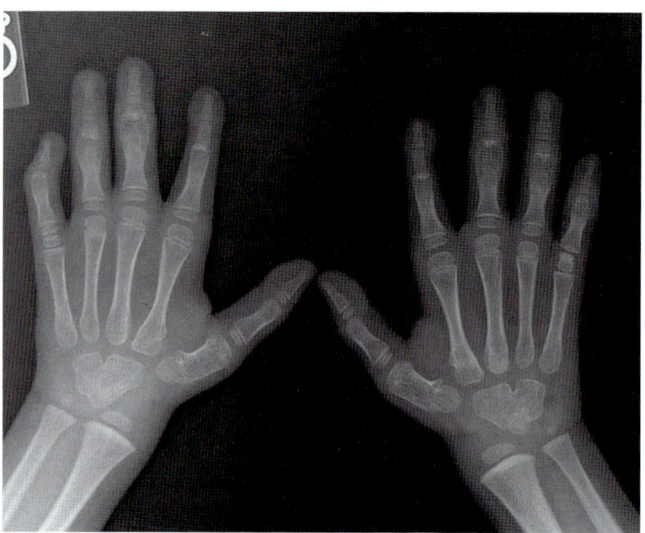

Figure 132-17   Bilateral symphalangism involving multiple rays associated with carpal coalitions in a 3-year-old girl.

CAMPTODACTYLY

Camptodactyly refers to a congenital or acquired flexion contracture of the finger. It usually is located at the proximal interphalangeal joint of the fifth finger but also can involve the second through fourth digits (Fig. 132-21).[31] Occasionally the distal interphalangeal joints may be affected. The cause remains unknown but may relate to abnormal insertion of the lumbrical muscles or the flexor digitorum superficialis tendon. Similar to clinodactyly, camptodactyly may be sporadic or may show an autosomal-dominant inheritance pattern. Occasionally it is associated with a chromosomal abnormality, a bony dysplasia, or another syndrome. Treatment includes bracing or, infrequently, surgical release.

KIRNER DEFORMITY

Palmar bending of the distal phalanx of the fifth digit is termed *Kirner deformity*.[31] It usually is an isolated abnormality that is bilateral and symmetric. The long axis of the distal

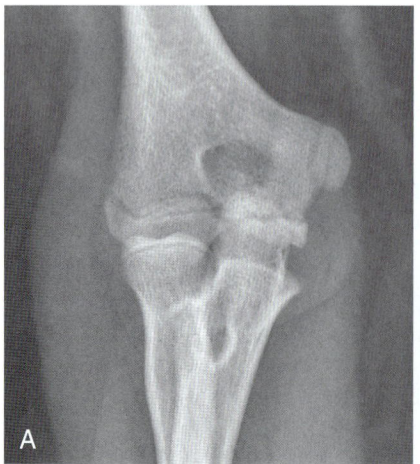

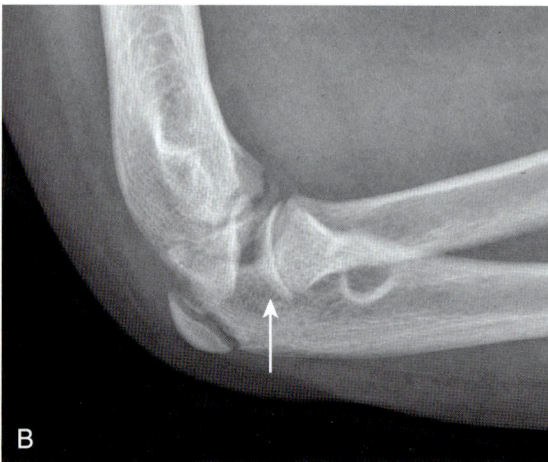

Figure 132-18   Radioulnar synostosis in a 12-year-old boy. **A,** Anteroposterior radiographs demonstrate osseous synostosis. **B,** A lateral radiograph demonstrates a convex-appearing radial head (*arrow*) related to secondary radial head dysplasia.

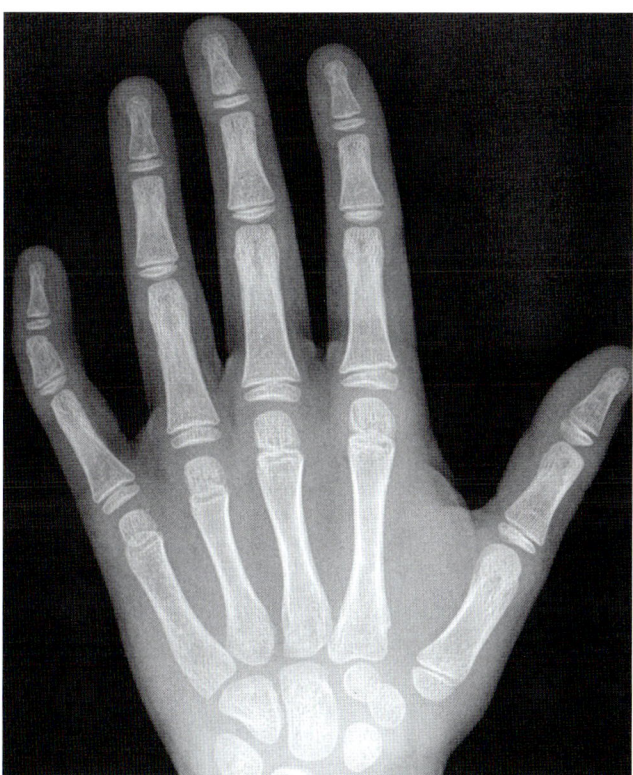

Figure 132-20   A 7-year-old girl with clinodactyly of the fifth digit. Medial bending of the finger and a short middle phalanx are noted.

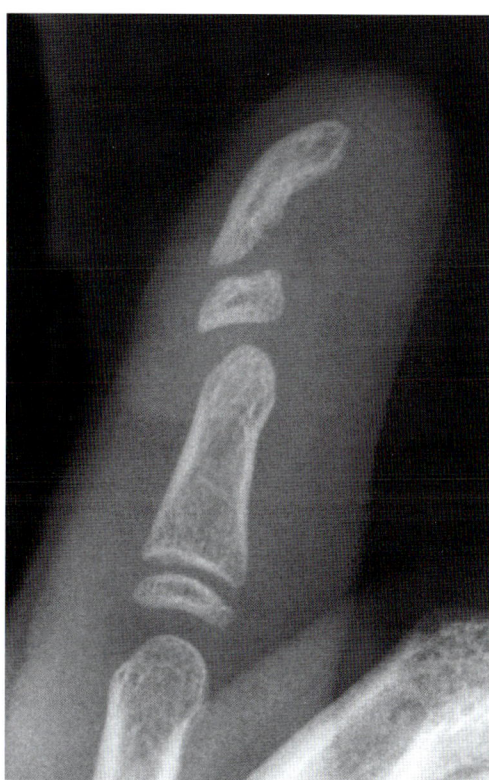

Figure 132-22   A girl with Kirner deformity. Palmar bending of the distal phalanx of the fifth digit is revealed. The epiphysis is in a normal position. (From Oestreich AE, Crawford AH. *Atlas of pediatric orthopedic radiology.* New York: Thieme; 1985:166.)

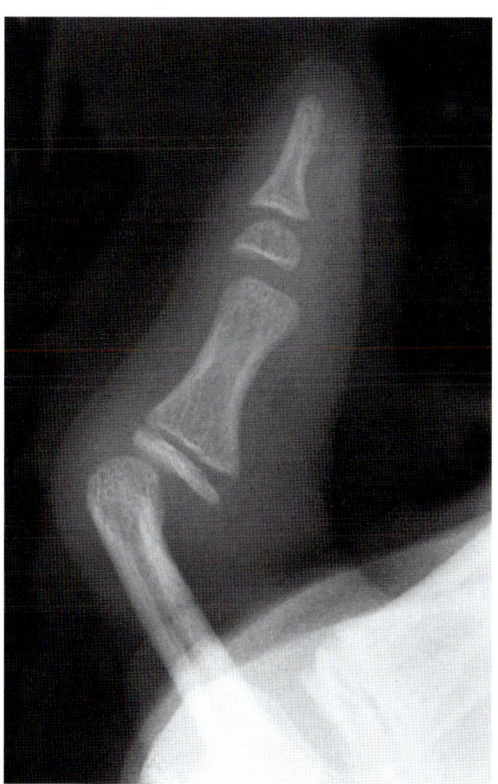

Figure 132-21   Child with camptodactyly. Flexion of the proximal interphalangeal joint is present with palmar subluxation of the middle phalanx of the little digit. The child has no skin crease.

phalanx is bent toward the palm, and the epiphysis is normally oriented (Fig. 132-22). The physis is widened. With skeletal maturation, the physis fuses on an angle. The distal phalanx exhibits a permanent palmar curvature. Similar to the other digit deformities, Kirner deformity can be a sporadic or an autosomal-dominant inherited anomaly.

BRACHYDACTYLY

Brachydactyly is a descriptive term that describes hypoplasia or complete aplasia of phalanges of the hands or feet (e-Fig. 132-23). Morphologically the affected bone may appear normal but just abnormally shortened compared with the other digits. The most commonly affected level is the middle phalanges. Brachydactyly may coexist with other processes such as longitudinal epiphyseal bracket and symphalangism. Brachydactyly may be sporadic or may be inherited in an autosomal-dominant fashion. Brachydactyly also may be seen with syndromes such as Apert and Poland syndromes.

LONGITUDINAL EPIPHYSEAL BRACKET (DELTA PHALANX)

Etiology   Longitudinal epiphyseal bracket is a congenital deformity that affects the short tubular bones that normally develop a proximal epiphyseal ossification center (e.g., phalanges, first metacarpal, and first metatarsal). The deformity may be sporadic or may occur in association with conditions such as Rubinstein-Taybi syndrome and fibrodysplasia ossificans progressiva. The cause is likely incomplete development of the primary ossification center of the bone during early fetal growth. The growth disturbance relates to the longitudinally oriented cartilaginous bracket, which causes growth to follow a "C-shaped" curve.[32]

Imaging   The involved bone is trapezoid or triangular in shape (Fig. 132-24). The diaphyseal–metaphyseal osseous unit is bracketed along the longitudinal side by a physis and an epiphysis. The physis is arclike (see Fig. 132-24, *B*), extending from the medial proximal surface along the longitudinal margin of the bone to the distal medial surface, and is similar in configuration to a bracket. The thumb usually is affected. Other anomalies of the digits frequently are associated with the longitudinal epiphyseal bracket.

Treatment and Follow-up   Corrective splinting in infancy is not effective. Early surgical intervention, often a wedge osteotomy, is recommended to allow for remodeling and to facilitate longitudinal growth of the bone.[33]

SPLIT HAND-FOOT MALFORMATIONS

Etiology   Split hand-foot malformation (SHFM) refers to the congenital splitting of the hands or feet into two halves. SHFM is attributed to hypoplasia or aplasia of the phalanges, metacarpals, or metatarsals of one or more fingers or toes. The deformity also is referred to as ectrodactyly, cleft hand or cleft foot, or lobster or crab claw deformity.

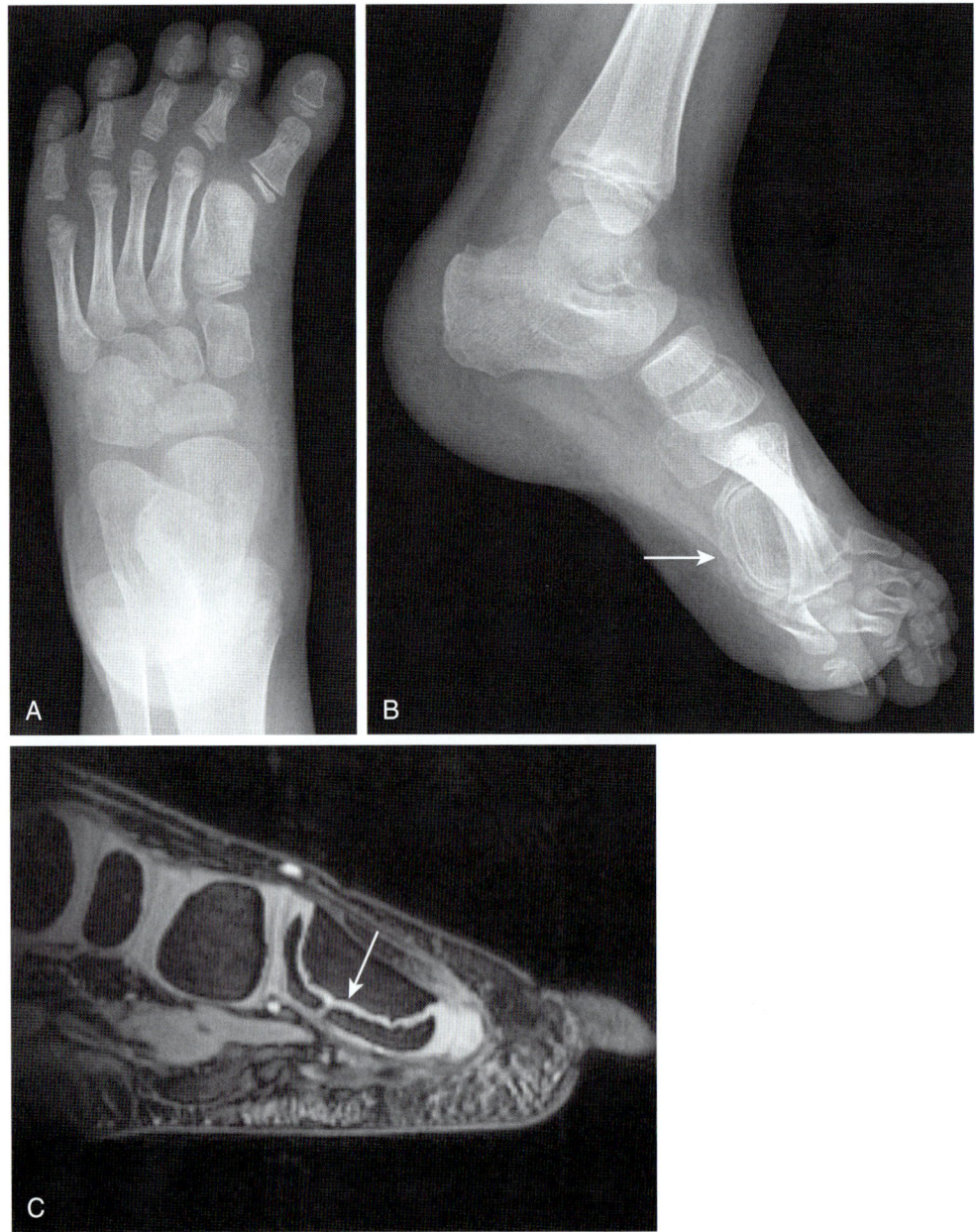

Figure 132-24   A longitudinal epiphyseal bracket. **A,** A frontal radiograph of the foot of a 4-year-old girl. The first metatarsal is short and widened and has a shorter medial than lateral length, forming a trapezoidal shape. **B,** A lateral radiograph of the same child shows the C-shaped epiphysis and physis of the first metatarsal (*arrow*). **C,** A sagittal gradient echo image shows a high-signal intensity C-shaped physis (*arrow*) and adjacent epiphysis.

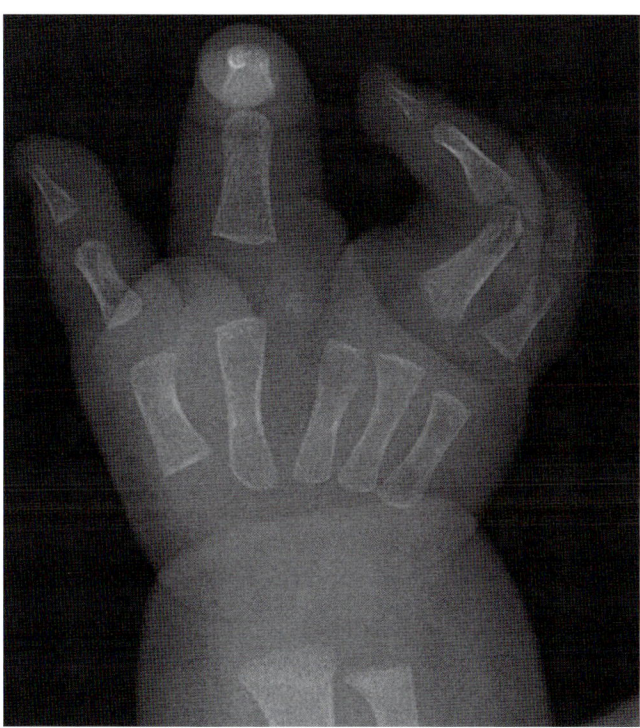

Figure 132-25 Split hand-foot malformation in a 6-month-old boy. The child has near complete absence of the long digit.

SHFM may be isolated or associated with congenital constriction band syndrome, or, most commonly, it may occur as a component of the ectrodactyly–ectodermal dysplasia–cleft lip/palate syndrome.[34] More than 75 syndromes have been associated with SHFM. Ectrodactyly–ectodermal dysplasia–cleft lip/palate syndrome usually has an autosomal-dominant inheritance pattern with incomplete penetrance and variable expression, although autosomal-recessive forms have been described. SHFM has been detected on prenatal ultrasonography, which can guide counseling and reconstructive efforts.

Imaging SHFM is highly variable in presentation. It can range from mild digital changes to the most severe monodactyly with only the fifth digit remaining. Two distinctive clinical forms have been described—typical and atypical forms. The typical form has an autosomal-dominant inheritance pattern and involves the lack of phalanges and metacarpals, resulting in a deep V-shaped cleft with the two halves resembling a lobster claw (Fig. 132-25). The much less frequent atypical form is sporadic and results in a much wider cleft, which forms a U-shaped central defect. The atypical form rarely involves the feet. Vascular disruption has been implicated as the cause. In most forms the digits frequently curve in toward the cleft, and a reduction in the number of digits may occur. Syndactyly or synostosis often is present.

Treatment and Follow-up Patients affected by SHFM usually have good functional use of their extremities and therefore surgical intervention usually is not indicated.

CONGENITAL RADIAL HEAD DISLOCATION

Etiology Congenital radial head dislocation is the most commonly identified congenital abnormality of the elbow. More than half of cases are associated with other conditions, such as anomalies of the lower extremities, scoliosis, and various syndromes (e.g., Klippel-Feil).[35] Whether it is an isolated abnormality or is associated with other conditions, congenital radial head dislocation is believed to have an autosomal-dominant inheritance pattern. The deformity can be unilateral or bilateral.

Imaging Congenital radial head dislocation is associated with a small, underdeveloped forearm, a flattened and hypoplastic capitellum, and a short ulna. The proximal ulnar diaphysis often may have a posterior apex bowing (Fig. 132-26, *B*). The radial head is dysplastic with an elongated, thinned, and convex articular surface instead of the normal

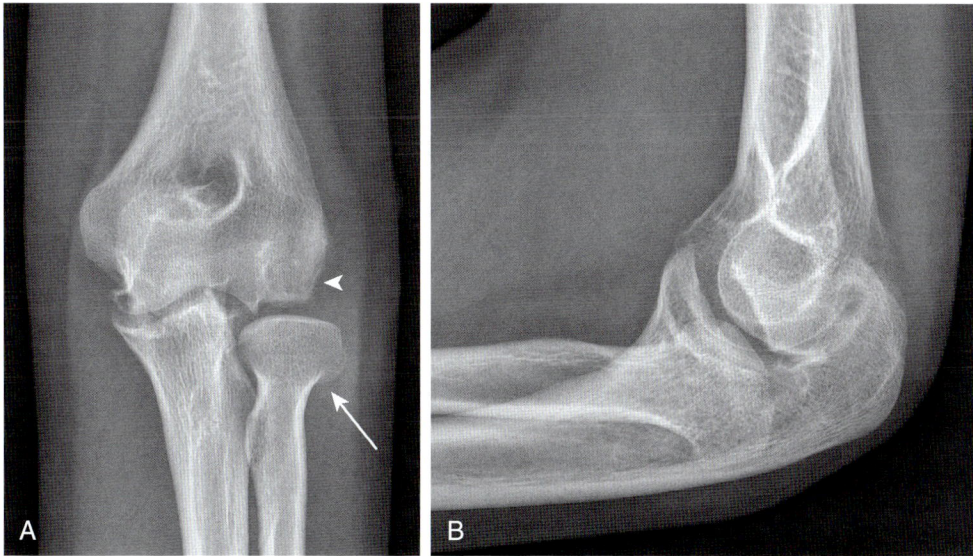

Figure 132-26 Congenital radial head dislocation in a 12-year-old girl. Anteroposterior (**A**) and lateral (**B**) radiographs show a dysplastic convex-shaped radial head (*arrow*) with posterior dislocation as well as posterior bowing of the proximal ulnar diaphysis. Note the presence of a capitellar osteochondral lesion (*arrowhead*) and medial compartmental osteoarthritis, which likely is related to abnormal elbow biomechanics.

concave shape. The radial head is most commonly dislocated posteriorly (see Fig. 132-26). The degree of radial head dysplasia is correlated with the severity of dislocation. Radiographs should be carefully evaluated for concomitant radioulnar synostosis.

Treatment and Follow-up Asymptomatic dislocations are not treated. If the child has pain, the radial head can be excised. However, excision of the radial head frequently is accompanied by pain from abnormal mechanics at the wrist. Recent work suggests that open reduction of the proximal radius at an early age may be beneficial.

TIBIAL BOWING DEFORMITIES

Etiology Posteromedial congenital bowing affects the tibia, fibula, and soft tissues of the lower extremity. The origin and pathogenesis remain uncertain and may be related to abnormal early embryologic development rather than to abnormal fetal positioning or intrauterine fracture. Fetal vascular insufficiency also may play a role. After examination of a fetus with congenital bowing, De Maio and associates suggested that compressive events associated with amnion rupture may be responsible.[36] As the child grows, tibial bowing and shortening often partially resolve.

Posteromedial congenital bowing should be differentiated from congenital tibial dysplasia (CTD). Other terms for CTD include anterolateral tibia bowing or congenital pseudoarthrosis of the tibia. It is a rare anomaly but does occur in a small number of patients with neurofibromatosis type 1 (NF1). Approximately 20% to 50% of patients with CTD do not have NF1.[37]

CTD presents as anterolateral bowing or fracture of the tibia, often before other manifestations of NF1 present. Lack of involvement of the fibula suggests that the bowing will resolve spontaneously. Pathologic studies show abnormal, highly cellular fibrovascular tissue with variable amounts of fibrocartilage and hyaline cartilage within the tibia. Bone growth and repair are abnormal. The pattern of abnormal fibrous tissue results in the dysplastic or cystic changes characteristic of the disorder.

Imaging With posteromedial congenital bowing, the tibia and the fibula show marked posteromedial bowing at the middle or distal one third of the shaft (Fig. 132-27). Rarely is the bowing lateral. At birth, the foot is held in a calcaneovalgus (dorsiflexed) position.

Radiographic changes seen with CTD are variable and include anterolateral bowing of the tibia, fracture, pseudarthrosis, hourglasslike constriction of the midshaft of the tibia, cystic changes usually at the junction of the upper and middle thirds of the tibia, sclerosis that narrows the medullary canal, and, infrequently, involvement of the fibula alone (Fig. 132-28).

Treatment and Follow-up Treatment for posteromedial congenital bowing of the tibia is conservative; for example, corrective casts or splints may be used to hold the foot and support the leg during growth and remodeling. If a severe persistent deformity continues beyond toddler age, a leg length discrepancy, usually on the order of 3 to 7 cm, may result that requires osteotomies and lengthening procedures.

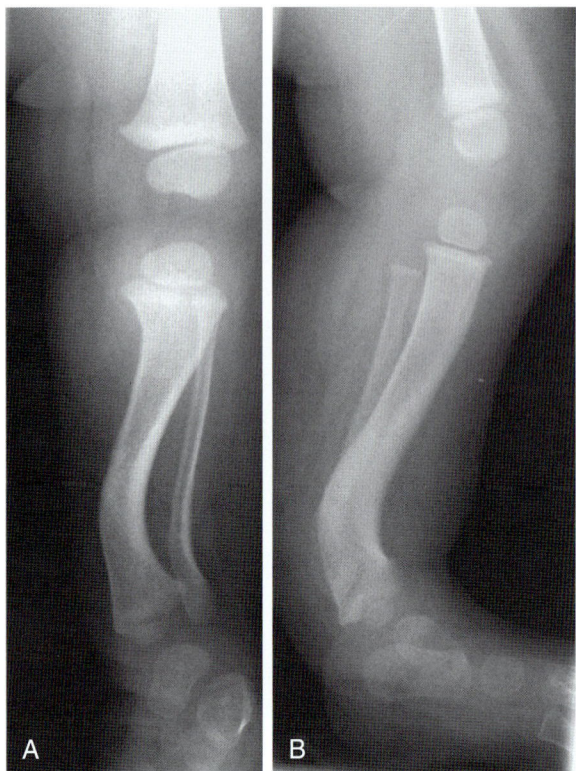

Figure 132-27 A 1-year-old girl with congenital posteromedial bowing. **A,** On the frontal radiograph, medial bowing is seen at the junction of the middle and distal one third of the tibia. The fibula is similarly bowed. **B,** The posterior component of the bowing is seen on the lateral radiograph.

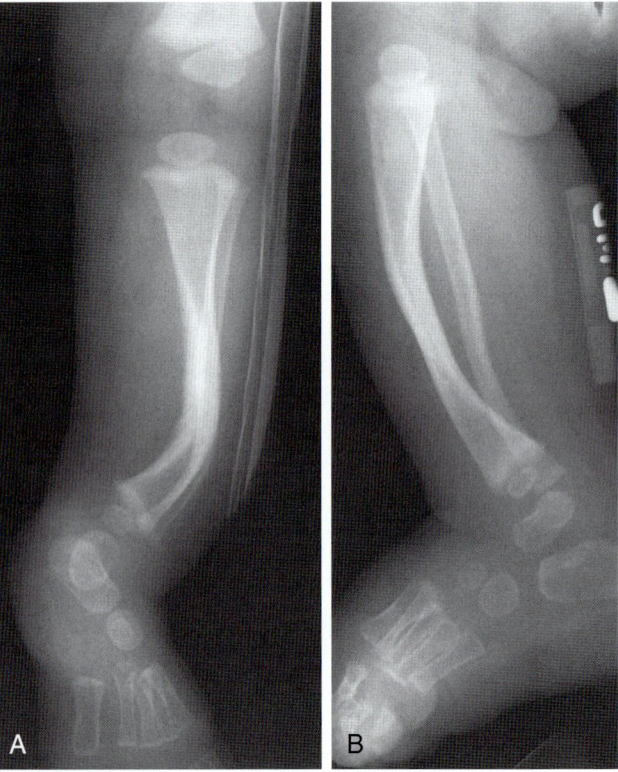

Figure 132-28 A child with congenital tibial dysplasia and neurofibromatosis type 1. Anteroposterior (**A**) and lateral (**B**) radiographs show anterolateral tibial bowing. The medullary canal is nearly obliterated, but no fracture is apparent.

Occasionally, epiphysiodesis of the contralateral side may be needed.

In persons who have anterolateral bowing associated with NF1, fracture and refracture rates are very high. Limb length inequality is frequent and results from disuse atrophy and abnormal growth at the distal tibial physis. Often a valgus deformity is noted at the ankle. Surgical management can be frustrating because nonunion or pseudarthrosis after osteotomy is frequent.

Key Points

For PFFD, the femoral head and acetabular deformities are related; the more dysmorphic the femoral head, the more severe the acetabular deformity.

Fibular hemimelia often has coexisting deformities at the level of the knee and foot.

The most commonly affected facet in subtalar coalitions is the middle facet.

A complete ossific bar forms a synostosis, a cartilaginous bar forms a synchondrosis, and a fibrous union is termed a syndesmosis.

Symphalangism most commonly affects the fifth ray of the hand and foot.

Congenital radial head dislocation is associated with a convex radial head, whereas traumatic radial head dislocation shows the normal radial articular surface convexity.

Suggested Reading

Poznanski A. *The hand in radiologic diagnosis*. 2nd ed. Philadelphia: WB Saunders; 1984.

References

Full references for this chapter can be found on www.expertconsult.com.

Chapter 133

Skeletal Dysplasias and Selected Chromosomal Disorders

JERRY DWEK and RALPH LACHMAN

As opposed to just a decade ago, the study of congenital syndromes is no longer an exercise in the rote memorization of seemingly disconnected syndromes. Instead, the unveiling of the intricacies of the genetic code has made apparent relationships among many inborn syndromes that had been previously unsuspected. What has emerged is that a relatively few genes are the cause of a multitude of syndromes, and by grouping syndromes and dysplasias into families based on the gene at fault, a taxonomy has emerged and has allowed a framework within which we can understand the relationships among a number of dysplasias and syndromes.

The abridged form of the International Skeletal Dysplasia Society skeletal dysplasia classification serves as the organization of this chapter (Box 133-1).[1] The full nosology text can be found at http://isds.ch/uploads/pdf_files/Nosology2010.pdf (accessed August 12, 2012). The major genetic families are presented with a short description of the salient unifying characteristics of the diseases within each group. When known, the gene and protein involved are considered and the impact of the mechanism of action discussed. The major members of each group are then expanded on to provide a clear picture for the reader.

In this chapter, the terms *syndrome* and *dysplasia* are used somewhat loosely. A syndrome is a set of characteristic findings that occur together and suggest a particular diagnosis, although the cause may not be known. A dysplasia is a set of characteristic findings in which the cause and effect are known. The distinction now has lost its value, as the cause of many "syndromes" are now known, and the term *dysplasia* is used to indicate not just purely a grouping of symptoms but the actual disease entity.

Radiologic Assessment

In the history of the delineation of many of the specific skeletal dysplasias, radiologic assessment plays a major role. By using an orderly approach to the radiographic analysis, the general type of the dysplasia may be elucidated. Many of the skeletal dysplasias and syndromes have distinctive radiographic features that will allow an exact diagnosis when even one of those distinctive features is identified and used as a search criterion in textbooks on skeletal dysplasia. Two such texts are Taybi and Lachman's *Radiology of Syndromes, Metabolic Disorders and Skeletal Dysplasias*, which includes an excellent gamuts section, and *Bone Dysplasias, An Atlas of Genetic Disorders of Skeletal Development* by Spranger and colleagues, in which the images are particularly helpful.[2,3] In the online version of Taybi and Lachman's book, the gamut search may be built iteratively, with the diagnoses becoming more selective as findings are added to the search criteria. Internet searches can also be performed on the Online Mendelian Inheritance in Man database, which is accessed through the U.S. Library of Medicine portal at http://www.ncbi.nlm.nih.gov/pubmed/.

STEP I: ASSESSMENT OF DISPROPORTION

Micromelia is overall shortening of the extremities. *Rhizomelia* is relative shortening of the femurs and humeri. *Mesomelia* is relative shortening of the radii, ulnae, tibiae, and fibulae. *Acromelia* is relative shortening of the bones of hands and feet.

Classification of the shortened appendicular segment is helpful for diagnosis. Rhizomelia may be very helpful to confirm the specific diagnosis of the rhizomelic form of chondrodysplasia punctata. Very significant mesomelia suggests a group of specific disorders loosely classified as the mesomelic dysplasias. Acromelia is found in many disorders; when it occurs by itself, several specific dysplasias are suggested, including acrodysostosis, acromicric dysplasia, or pseudohypoparathyroidism.

The pattern of brachydactyly may facilitate diagnosis. For instance, brachydactyly type E manifests with variable shortening of the metacarpals and distal phalanges, and brachydactyly type A4 manifests with shortening restricted to the second and fifth middle phalanges. Even the absence of acromelia may be helpful. The lack of significant hand and foot shortening is a significant feature of spondyloepiphyseal dysplasia congenita (SEDC), a type 2 collagenopathy.

STEP II: ASSESSMENT OF EPIPHYSEAL OSSIFICATION

If epiphyseal ossification is delayed or if the ossified epiphyses are very small, irregular for age, or both, then an epiphyseal dysplasia of some sort is present. Carpal and tarsal bones are often affected. In diseases that can be considered pure

Box 133-1 Nosology and Classification of Genetic Skeletal Disorders

FGFR3 Group
- Thanatophoric dysplasia type 1 and 2
- Homozygous achondroplasia
- Achondroplasia
- Hypochondroplasia

Type 2 Collagen Group
- Achondrogenesis type 2
- Spondyloepiphyseal dysplasia congenital
- Kniest dysplasia

Type 11 Collagen Group
- Stickler syndrome type 2
- Marshall syndrome
- Oto-spondylo-mega-epiphyseal dysplasia

Abnormal Sulfation Group
- Achondrogenesis type 1b
- Diastrophic dysplasia
- Multiple epiphyseal dysplasia: Multilayered patellae/brachydactyly/clubfeet

Filamen Group
- Oto-palato-digital syndrome type 1 and 2
- Larsen syndrome

TRPV4 Group
- Metatropic dysplasia
- Spondylometaphyseal dysplasia Koslowski type

Short Rib Dysplasias
- Short rib-polydactyly
- Asphyxiating thoracic dysplasia
- Chrondroectodermal dysplasia

Multiple Epiphyseal Dysplasia and Pseudoachondroplasia Group
- Multiple epiphyseal dysplasia
- Pseudoachondroplasia

Metaphyseal Dysplasia Group
- Jansen-type metaphyseal chondrodysplasia
- Schmid-type metaphyseal chondrodysplasia
- McKusick-type metaphyseal chondrodysplasia
- Shwachman-Diamond dysplasia

Spondylometaphyseal Dysplasia Group
- Spondyloenchondromatosis

Acromelic/Acromesomelic Dysplasia Group
- Trichorhinophalangeal syndrome types I and II
- Acromesomelic dysplasia of Maroteaux

Mesomelic Dysplasia Group
- Dyschondrosteosis

Bent Bone Dysplasia Group
- Campomelic dysplasia

Chondrodysplasia Punctata Group
- Rhizomelic type

Increased Bone Density Group (Without Modification of Bone Shape)
- Osteopetrosis
- Pyknodysostosis
- Osteopoikilosis
- Osteopathia striata
- Melorheostosis

Increased Bone Density Group with Metaphyseal and/or Diaphyseal Involvement
- Craniometaphyseal dysplasia
- Craniodiaphyseal dysplasia
- Pyle disease

Osteogenesis Imperfecta and Decreased Bone Density Group
- Osteogenesis imperfecta

Abnormal Mineralization Group
- Hypophosphatasia

Lysosomal Storage Diseases
- Hunter syndrome or Hurler syndrome
- Morquio syndrome
- Mucolipidosis type II (I-cell disease)

Osteolysis Group
- Hajdu-Cheney dysplasia

Overgrowth Syndromes with Skeletal Involvement
- Marfan syndrome
- Congenital contractural arachnodactyly
- Proteus syndrome

Cleidocranial Dysplasia and Isolated Cranial Ossification Defects Group
- Cleidocranial dysplasia

Dysostoses with Predominant Vertebral Involvement
- Currarino triad

Brachydactylies
- Rubinstein-Taybi syndrome
- Poland anomaly

Limb Hypoplasia Reduction Defects Group
- Brachydactyly A-E
- Brachmann-De Lange syndrome
- Holt-Oram syndrome

Miscellaneous Syndromes and Chromosomal Disorders
- Fetal alcohol spectrum disorder
- Noonan syndrome

VATER/VACTERL
- Klinefelter syndrome
- Trisomy 13
- Trisomy 18
- Trisomy 21
- Chromosome X monosomy

VACTERL, vertebral, anorectal, cardiac, tracheoesophageal, renal, limb.

epiphyseal dysplasias such as multiple epiphyseal dysplasia and pseudoachondroplasia, carpal and the tarsal bones are markedly crenellated and small (Fig. 133-1). Another excellent location for epiphyseal analysis is the ring apophyses of the vertebral bodies, which exhibit delayed and irregular epiphyseal ossification in epiphyseal dysplasia. Central anterior vertebral body protrusions (central tongues or beaking) noted in Morquio syndrome and pseudoachondroplasia are also disorders related to abnormalities of the ring apophyses.

STEP III: ASSESSMENT OF METAPHYSES AND PHYSES

Fraying and irregularity of the physes and abnormal flaring of the metaphyses indicate disturbed endochondral ossification. Marked irregularity of the physes is characteristic of the pure metaphyseal dysplasias such as metaphyseal dysplasia, Jansen or Schmid type. When the metaphyses are merely flared and the physes are fairly normal, endochondral ossification may be slowed but the actual process of endochondral ossification progresses normally. This occurs in achondroplasia. The metaphyses are flared, whereas the physis and the zone of provisional calcification (ZPC) are sharply defined (Fig. 133-2).

It must be kept in mind that rickets also disturbs the physis. In rickets, the physis is frayed and cupped. Except in healing rickets, the ZPC is inapparent. In metaphyseal chondrodysplasias, the ZPC is present, although it is markedly irregular (Fig. 133-3). Analysis of the sclerotic line of the ZPC is frequently an excellent differentiating feature. Other factors include prominent osteopenia in rickets with blurring of the trabeculae; clinical data are also very helpful.

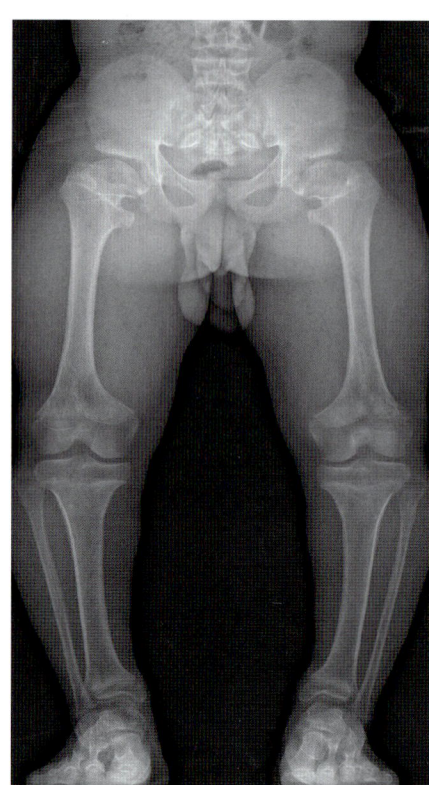

Figure 133-2 A 14-year-old boy with achondroplasia. The long bones are short and thick. Note the normal, sharp-appearing physes.

STEP IV: ASSESSMENT OF THE DIAPHYSES

Diaphyseal abnormalities primarily include bent bones and thickened sclerotic bones. The classic bent bone dysplasia is campomelic dysplasia. Others include hypophosphatasia and kyphomelic dysplasia. Thickened and sclerotic diaphyseal cortices may indicate one of the craniotubular dysplasias.

STEP V: ANALYSIS OF THE VERTEBRAL BODIES

Decreased height of the vertebral bodies is termed *platyspondyly*. The lumbar vertebral bodies are the best level to analyze compared with the cervical level, especially in infancy. The cervical vertebral bodies tend to appear relatively hypoplastic compared with other levels in the normal infant. This is because ossification occurs later in cervical vertebral bodies compared with vertebral bodies elsewhere. In addition to platyspondyly, other vertebral body changes are important. In the lumbar spine in normal children, the interpediculate distance usually widens on a frontal film moving inferiorly. Narrowing of the interpediculate distance is a feature of fibroblast growth factor receptor 3 (FGFR3) abnormalities such achondroplasia and thanatophoria.

Anisospondyly is when the vertebral body shape varies wildly (e-Fig. 133-4). Multiple ossification centers may also be present. Although rare, this is a specific finding in dyssegmental dysplasia.

STEP VI: ASSESSMENT OF BONE MINERALIZATION

Bone mineral density should be assessed by not only examining the actual "whiteness" of bones but also by determining

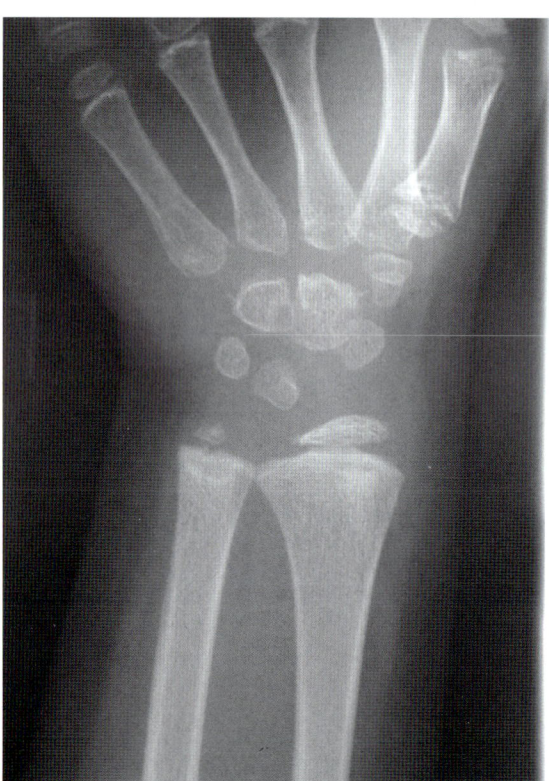

Figure 133-1 An 8-year-old boy with multiple epiphyseal dysplasia. Note the small and crenellated carpal bones.

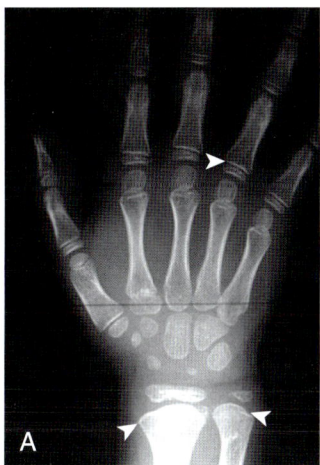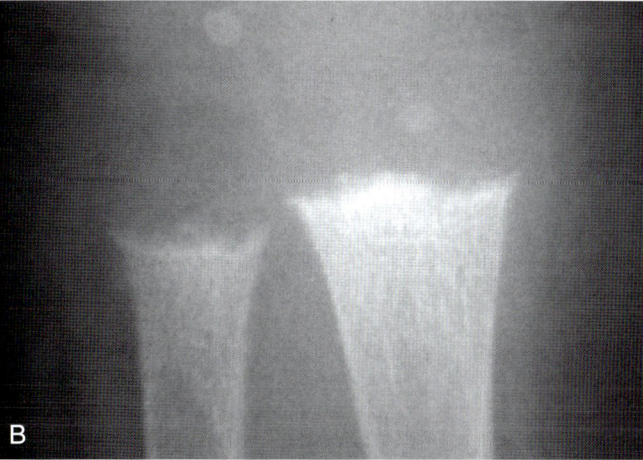

Figure 133-3 An 8-old boy with Schmid metaphyseal chondrodysplasia. **A,** Note the presence of zone of provisional calcification (*arrowheads*). Normal laboratory values help confirm the diagnosis. **B,** A 15-month-old girl with rickets. The physes are frayed with mild metaphyseal cupping. The bright white line of the zone of provisional calcification is not evident.

the relative thickness of the cortices relative to the medullary cavity and the coarseness of the trabecula. Osteopenia, especially when severe, indicates defective bone mineralization, as seen in rickets, hypophosphatasia, and osteogenesis imperfecta. Abnormally dense bones may indicate one of the craniotubular disorders such as pyknodysostosis and osteopetrosis. In the neonate, bones are normally sclerotic and the medullary cavity narrowed. Distinguishing abnormally dense bones from normal neonatal sclerosis can be difficult.

STEP VII: ASSESSMENT OF JOINTS

Multiple joint dislocations are a salient and persistent feature of some dysplasias. A standard skeletal survey frequently includes only frontal views of the skeleton, which may make it difficult to identify joint dislocations, especially in the infant. The elbow is frequently involved in the setting of dislocations secondary to a dysplasia. Dedicated lateral views are recommended when dislocation is clinically suspected.

STEP VIII: SUMMATION

After all radiologic findings have been established, a gamut search of some or all of these abnormalities, in conjunction with the clinical findings, may lead to the specific diagnosis. If the "group" of dysplasias has been established, then the specific diagnosis can often be made by referring to a differential diagnosis table such as that developed by Taybi and Lachman.[2]

Selected Skeletal Dysplasias and Syndromes

FIBROBLAST GROWTH FACTOR RECEPTOR TYPE 3 GROUP

Overview   This group includes thanatophoric dwarfism and achondroplasia. The former is probably the most common lethal skeletal dysplasia and the latter the most common

skeletal dysplasia. The group includes the milder variant called hypochondroplasia, and homozygous achondroplasia, which is similar to thanatophoria.[4]

A common genetic locus (*4p16.3*) is involved. Differing allelic mutations are the cause of the variable severity of expression. The protein encoded is FGFR3, which governs the velocity of endochondral growth. Although long believed that achondroplasia and thanatophoria were caused by loss of function mutations, the mutation in this group actually results in an upmodulation of FGFR3 activity, which is inversely related to the velocity of endochondral growth. FGFR3 mutations have been linked to advanced paternal age, with mutations theoretically accumulating during spermatogenesis.[5]

Several common radiologic threads run through this group. FGFR3 slows endochondral bone growth, so long bones are short. However, it does not affect overall bone thickness because of membranous ossification. Therefore, long bones are relatively thick. The fibula is usually longer than the tibia. Femoral necks are short and broadened and have a peculiar scooped-out appearance. It is seen as an ovoid lucency of femoral necks, as if an ice cream scoop was radiographed en face. The finding can be seen in all forms of thanatophoria. It is well seen in achondroplasia but not in most forms of hypochondroplasia.

In the normal individual, on a frontal radiograph, the horizontal distance between the pedicles of the vertebral bodies should widen moving inferiorly. FGFR3 group abnormalities exhibit narrowing in the interpediculate distance in the lumber spine. The decrease in the velocity of endochondral ossification also causes platyspondyly. Brachydactyly of all the bones of the hand is present. Since soft tissues are relatively unaffected, fingers are splayed into the "trident configuration."

COMMON FEATURES IN FGFR3 GROUP

- Platyspondyly
- Narrow sacrosciatic notch
- Interpediculate narrowing
- Short thick long bones

- Ovoid lucency at femoral necks (scooped out appearance)
- Frontal bossing
- Trident hands
- Fibula longer than tibia

THANATOPHORIC DWARFISM

Given the lethality of this dysplasia, it is aptly named after Thanatos, the Greek god of death (*Thantophoria*, meaning "death loving"). Although it is nearly uniformly fatal, rare cases of survivors have been reported.

Type 1 includes "cloverleaf skull," caused by in utero craniosynostosis, and curved long bones. The femurs have a "French telephone receiver" appearance. The type 2 variant has straight long bones and no craniosynostosis.

Platyspondyly is severe. They are described as U-shaped or H-shaped on an anteroposterior projection.

Radiographic Findings (Fig. 133-5)

1. *Skull:* proportionately large skull in relation to the body, narrow skull base, cloverleaf skull (type 1 only)
2. *Thorax:* long, narrow trunk; very short ribs; handlebar clavicles
3. *Spine:* severely flattened, small vertebral bodies with round anterior ends
4. *Pelvis:* small, flared iliac bones; very narrow sacrosciatic notches; flat, dysplastic acetabula
5. *Extremities:* generalized micromelia; ovoid lucency of femoral necks, round proximal femoral metaphyses with medial spike, curved long bones (type 1 only)

ACHONDROPLASIA

Patients with achondroplasia have normal mentation and a normal or near normal lifespan. As in other members of the FGFR3 family, long bones are short and thick. Interpediculate narrowing is present. In infancy, femoral necks have a scooped out appearance. Since the sacrosciatic notches are narrowed, the pelvic inlet has an appearance of a wide-mouthed champagne glass.

Except for the portions of the occipital bone that form the margin of the foramen magnum, all the bones of the skull are formed by membranous ossification.[6] This results in an enlarged forehead and is termed *frontal bossing*. In contrast, the foramen magnum is narrowed and can cause cervicomedullary compression. Symptoms may include occipitocervical pain, ataxia, incontinence, apnea, paralysis, and respiratory arrest.[7]

Radiologic Findings (Fig. 133-6 and e-Fig. 133-7)

1. *Skull:* enlarged, with significant midface hypoplasia; hydrocephalus rarely present; small skull base with tight foramen magnum
2. *Thorax:* small; shortened and anteriorly splayed ribs
3. *Spine:* short pedicles with decreased interpediculate distance most marked in the lumbar spine moving downward; posterior vertebral body scalloping, gibbus deformity.
4. *Pelvis:* round iliac wings with lack of flaring (elephant ear–shaped), flattened acetabular roofs, narrow sacrosciatic notches with champagne glass shaped pelvic inlet

5. *Extremities:* rhizomelic micromelia
6. *Hands:* brachydactyly with trident hands
7. *Knees:* Central deep notch in growth plates (Chevron deformity)
8. *Hips:* proximal femoral ovoid lucency (infancy); hemispheric capital femoral epiphyses, short femoral necks
9. *Legs:* prominent tibial tubercle apophyseal region, fibula overgrowth
10. *Arms:* Cortical hyperostosis at deltoid insertion on anterolateral humerus

HYPOCHONDROPLASIA

In hypochondroplasia radiographic and clinical findings are less severe compared with achondroplasia, and the diagnosis can be challenging. Stature is slightly shortened but is highly variable and may be normal given the range of normal stature in society. Radiographically, aside from shortening of the long bones, interpediculate narrowing is a very sensitive finding (Fig. 133-8).[8]

TYPE 2 COLLAGEN GROUP

Overview Defects in chromosome 12q13.1-13.3 result in abnormalities of type 2 collagen. Type 2 collagen is present in cartilaginous epiphyses and in the *vitreous humor*. Therefore, abnormalities of collagen 2 manifest with platyspondyly due to lack of normal growth at the ring epiphysis, a general delay in epiphyseal ossification, and myopia. Cleft palate completes the phenotypic picture.

The more common members of the group include, in order of severity, achondrogenesis type 2, hypochondrogenesis, spondyloepiphyseal dysplasia, Kniest dysplasia, spondyloepimetaphyseal dysplasia, Strudwick type, Stickler syndrome type 1, and spondyloperipheral dysplasia.

COMMON FEATURES IN TYPE 2 COLLAGENOPATHY GROUP

- Platyspondyly
- Delay in epiphyseal ossification most apparent in femoral heads
- Cleft palate
- Myopia
- Short stature
- Occipitoatlantal or atlantodental instability

ACHONDROGENESIS TYPE 2

The most severely affected member of the group, achondrogenesis type 2 is invariably lethal. Patients with less severe hypochondrogenesis die in the first few months of life.

Radiologic Findings (Fig. 133-9)

1. *Skull:* proportionately large
2. *Thorax:* very small and short ribs
3. *Spine:* almost complete lack of mineralization; cervical and sacral posterior elements also often unossified
4. *Pelvis:* small iliac wings with concave inferior and medial margins; absence of ischia, pubic bones, and sacral elements

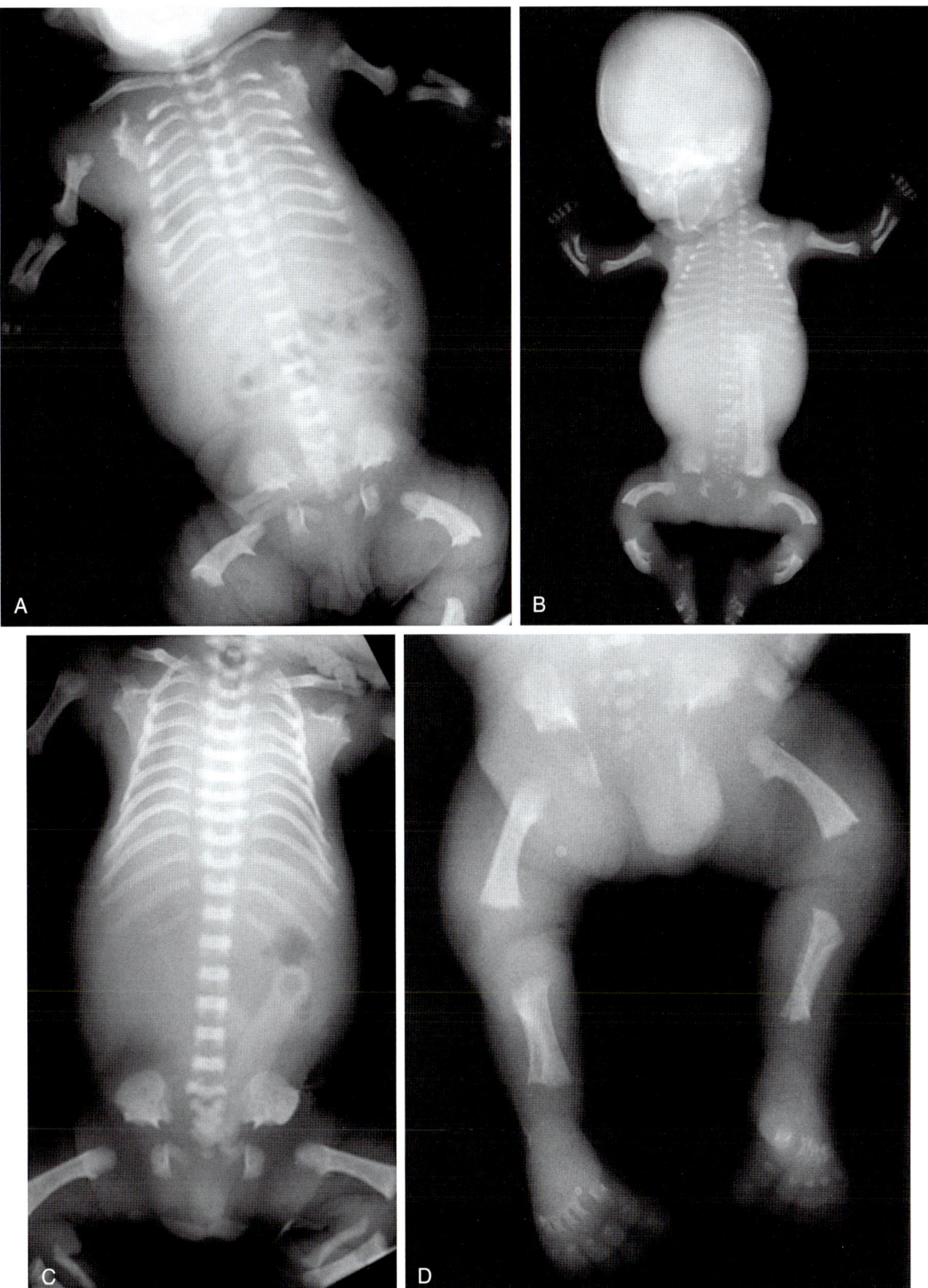

Figure 133-5 Thanatophoric dysplasia. **A** and **B,** Radiographic findings in thanatophoric dysplasia type I. In an affected fetus of 30 weeks' gestation (**A**), a long, narrow trunk; very short ribs; severe platyspondyly are seen. Note the H and U shapes of bodies are caused by angle of incidence of the x-ray beam; small, flared iliac wings; narrowed sacrosciatic notches; dysplastic (trident) acetabular roofs; and French telephone receiver–shaped femurs. At 22 weeks' gestation in another affected fetus (**B**), a proportionally large skull, micromelia, and other findings similar to those in **A** are seen. **C** and **D,** Radiologic findings in thanatophoric dysplasia type II. An affected preterm fetus (**C**) exhibits findings similar to those in type I except for taller vertebral bodies and straighter femurs. Another affected fetus (**D**) also shows the same findings as in type I but with straighter femurs.

Continued

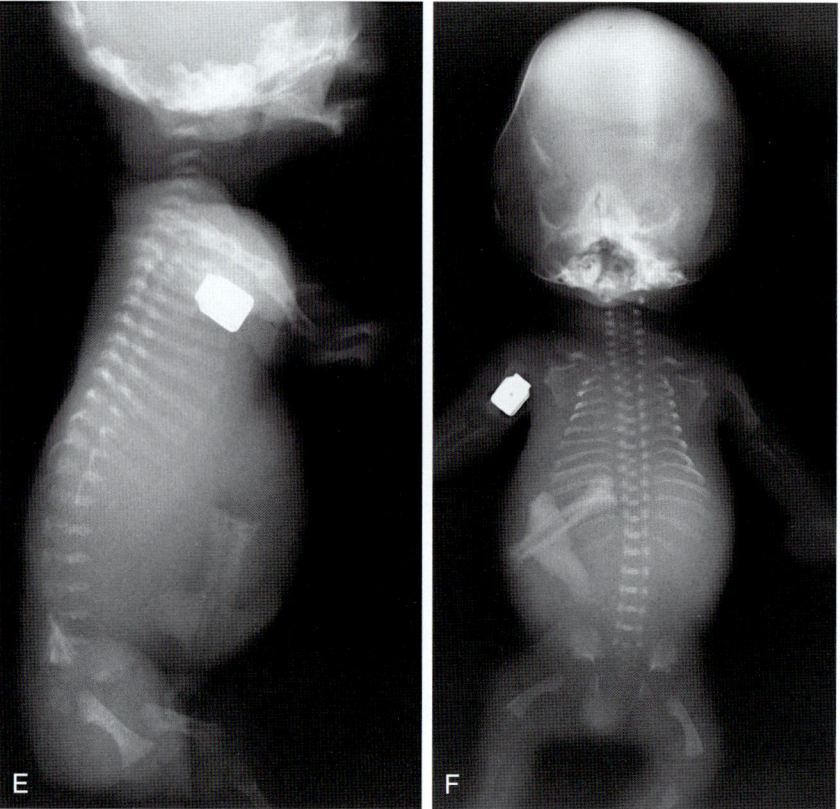

Figure 133-5, cont'd. **E,** Radiograph of affected infant with severe platyspondyly, anteriorly rounded vertebrae, straight femurs, and severely constricted skull base. **F,** Cloverleaf skull and almost straight femurs; otherwise, radiographic findings are similar to those in **C.** Note the ovoid lucency at the femoral necks in all cases.

5. *Extremities:* micromelia, mostly rhizomelia and mesomelia, with relative sparing of hands and feet; metaphyseal flaring; absence of talus and calcaneal ossification (epiphyseal equivalents)

HYPOCHONDROGENESIS

Radiologic Findings

1. *Thorax:* larger, with longer ribs
2. *Spine:* more vertebral body ossification (hypoplasia and platyspondyly)

Note: Hypochondrogenesis is otherwise similar but milder form of achondrogenesis type 2.

SPONDYLOEPIPHYSEAL DYSPLASIA CONGENITA

The combination of platyspondyly and short long bones make spondyloepiphyseal dysplasia congenita (SEDC) a good example of short-limbed, short-trunk dwarfism. It is also a good model for an epiphyseal dysplasia. Ossification in the vertebral bodies begins in the fetus at the lower thoracic spine and progresses superiorly and inferiorly. The cervical spine ossifies last. The normal cervical spine vertebrae at birth are slightly dorsally wedged and are small. In infants with SEDC, the cervical vertebral bodies show little or no ossification. Thoracic and lumbar bodies are, however, small, dorsally wedged, and anteriorly rounded (pear or oval shaped), similar in appearance to the cervical spine in the normal infant. In childhood, characteristic central beaks, typical of epiphyseal

delay, may be seen. In the adult, vertebral bodies are flattened with irregular end plates.

At birth, no ossification of the talus, calcaneus, or the epiphyses at the knee is present. Normally, the talus and the calcaneus ossify at 20 to 24 weeks' gestation and the epiphyses at about 36 weeks' gestation.

One salient feature is that the hands and feet in patients with SEDC are normal, apart from carpal, midfoot, and hindfoot ossification delay.

Radiologic Findings (Fig. 133-10)

1. *Thorax:* small; short ribs
2. *Spine:* dorsally wedged or oval vertebral bodies (at birth); anteriorly rounded platyspondyly (later)
3. *Pelvis:* absent pubic ossification (at birth and during infancy), vertical ischia with short ilia
4. *Extremities:* normal tubulization with mild micromelia, significant generalized ossification delay (early) and hypoplastic-appearing or dysplastic epiphyses (later), unossified talus or calcaneus in the newborn, normal hands and feet with ossification delay (epiphyses or carpal, tarsal)

KNIEST DYSPLASIA

The same delay in epiphyseal ossification is seen along with platyspondyly. Cloudlike dystrophic calcification is present in abnormally enlarged epiphyses as the child gets older. On magnetic resonance imaging (MRI), the areas of calcification

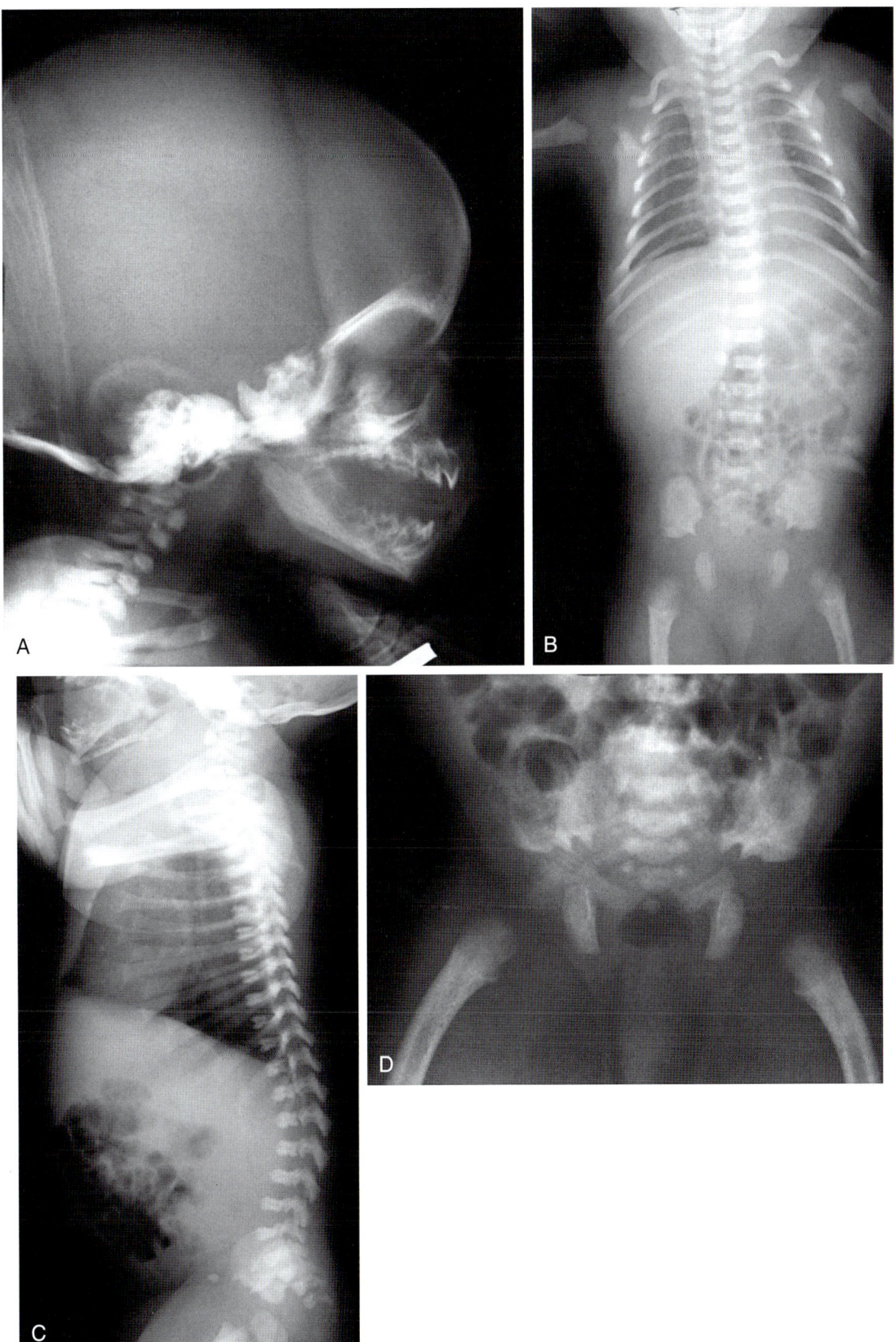

Figure 133-6 Achondroplasia. **A** to **D,** Radiographs of an affected newborn. **A,** Severe midface hypoplasia. **B,** Thorax: small thorax and short ribs. **C,** Thorax: short ribs with anterior scalloping and bullet-shaped vertebrae. **D,** Pelvis: rounded ilia (elephant ear–shaped) iliac bones, narrow sacrosciatic notches, flat acetabular roof, and proximal femoral ovoid lucency. Achondroplasia.

Continued

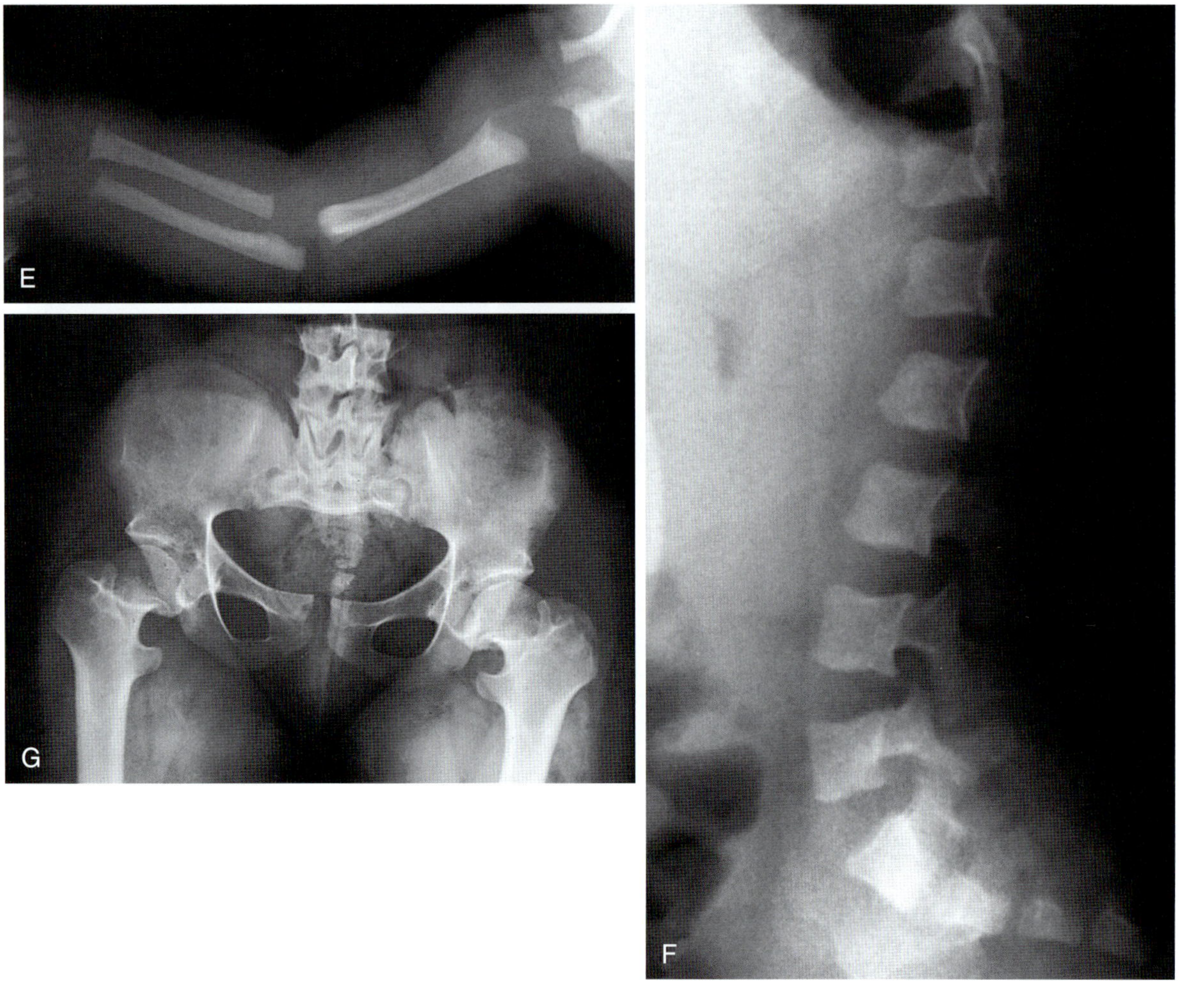

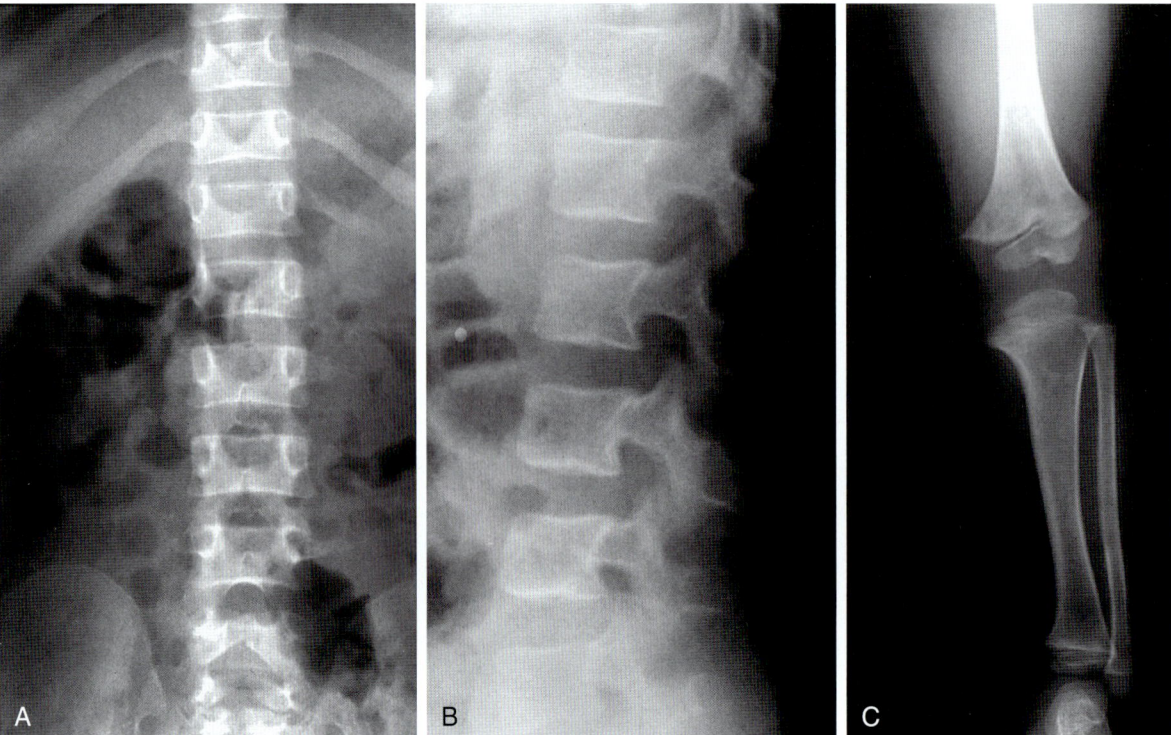

Figure 133-6, cont'd. E, Extremities: rhizomelia and mesomelia. **F,** Radiograph in an affected 1½-year-old with classic vertebrae with short pedicles, posterior scalloping, and somewhat short vertebral bodies. **G,** Radiograph in an affected woman with flat acetabular roofs, elephant ear–shaped iliac wings, and short femoral necks (compare with **D**). (**G,** From Silverman FN: Achondroplasia. *Prog Pediatr Radiol.* 1973;4:94-124.)

Figure 133-8 Radiographs in a 3-year-old with hypochondroplasia. **A,** Lumbosacral interpediculate narrowing. **B,** Posterior vertebral body scalloping with normal pedicles. **C,** Proximal and distal fibular overgrowth. Mild chevron deformities in the distal femur are seen.

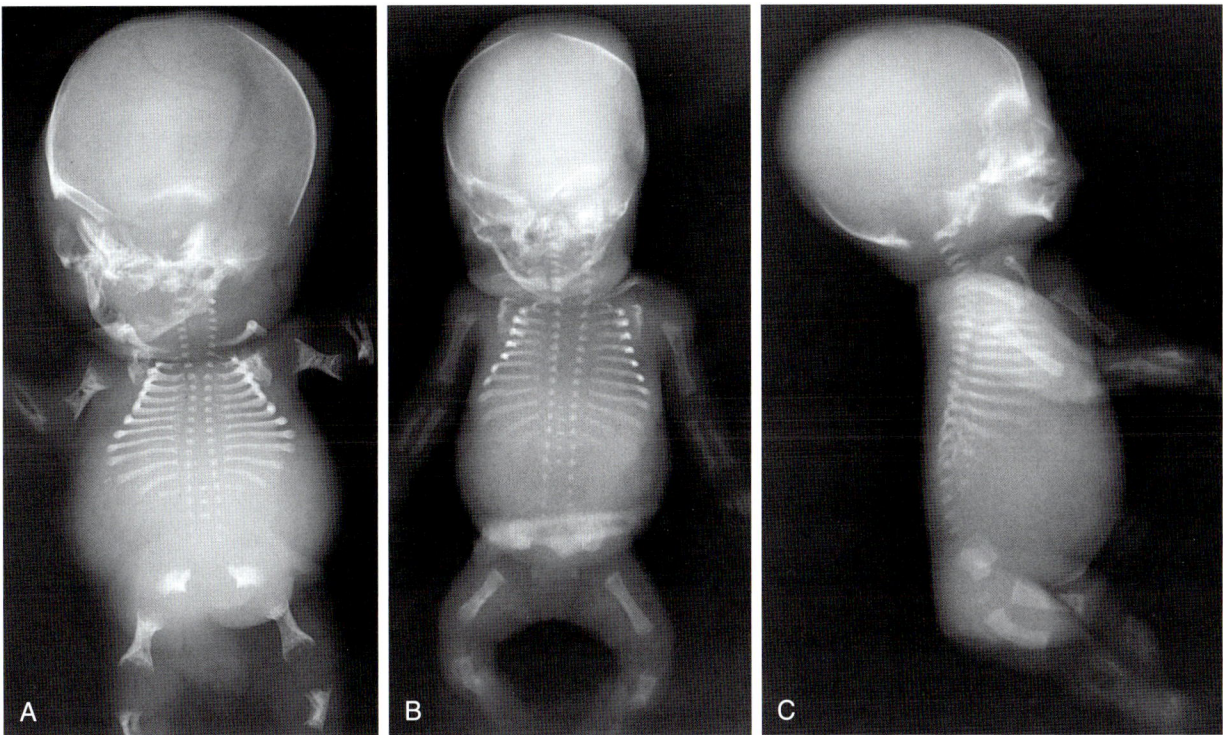

Figure 133-9 A, Radiograph from a stillborn infant with achondrogenesis type II. Findings include an enlarged skull; a tiny thorax with short ribs; almost no vertebral body ossification with lower pedicle ossification deficiency; small wide ilia, notched acetabular roofs, and absence of ischial and pubic ossification; micromelia; and normally modeled femurs with metaphyseal flaring and cupping. **B** and **C,** Radiographs from a fetus of 21 weeks' gestation with hypochondrogenesis, revealing better vertebral ossification, with better defined bone modeling.

have prolonged T2 values that are likely related to the degeneration of abnormal collagen matrix.[9]

Radiologic Findings (e-Fig. 133-11)
1. *Thorax:* small to normal
2. *Spine:* coronal clefts (at birth and during infancy), platyspondyly with endplate irregularity (later)
3. *Extremities:* dumbbell femurs; generalized ossification delay, epiphyses becoming hypoplastic or dysplastic and then later even mega-epiphyses, cloudlike irregular calcification in physeal plate regions (in late childhood and early adulthood); hands with bulbous joints (metaphyseal flaring or epiphyseal fragmentation) mimicking rheumatoid arthritis

Note: In the newborn, Kniest syndrome is radiographically identical to SEDC except for coronal clefts and dumbbell femurs.

TYPE 11 COLLAGENOPATHY GROUP

Overview Members of this group include Stickler syndrome type 2, Marshall syndrome, oto-spondylo-mega-epiphyseal dysplasia (OSMED) autosomal-dominant type (Weisenbach-Zweymuller phenotype, and Stickler type 3).

The multiple synonyms and names applied to the different members of the group cause some confusion. Stickler syndrome type 2 is a type 11 collagenopathy and has a similar appearance to Stickler syndrome type 1 (see type 2 collagenopathy above) with milder ocular changes and more severe auditory changes. It is autosomal recessive. Marshall syndrome is very similar to Stickler syndrome type 2 and may be considered, for all practical purposes, the same entity.

OSMED autosomal-dominant type is a type 11 collagenopathy as well. It is also called *nonocular Stickler syndrome* or *Stickler syndrome type 3*. Osseous changes in OSMED are usually worse with greater shortening of the long bones and platyspondyly. OSMED may be also called *Weisenbach-Zweymuller syndrome.*

Adding to the confusion is a very similar form of Stickler syndrome, which is a type 9 collagenopathy. The similarity is not coincidental. Type 11 and type 2 collagens along with type 9 collagen form collagen fibrils so that the phenotypic expression of a type 2, type 11, or type 9 collagenopathy may be similar. This is an important point in the phenotypic expression of genetic abnormalities. Since the tissues of the body are constructed of multiple elements, differing genetic and biochemical abnormalities may have similar outcomes when considering the end results of the tissues produced.

In practice, when faced with a case with a resemblance to a mild or intermediate severity type 2 or type 11 collagenopathy, both paths should be investigated.

Common Features in Type 11 Collagenopathy Group

- Similar to type 2 collagenopathy
- Cleft palate
- Sensorineural hearing loss

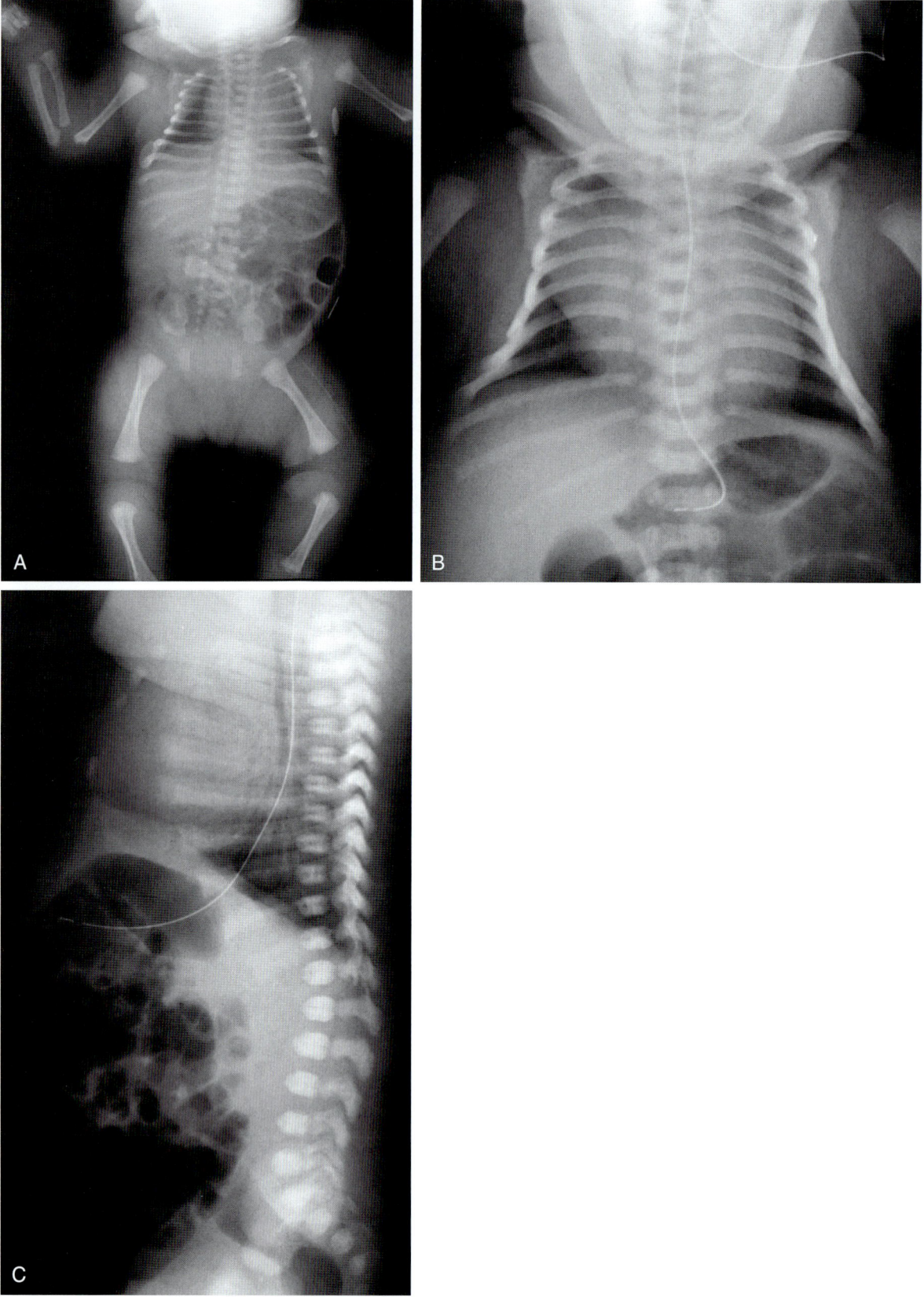

Figure 133-10 Spondyloepiphyseal dysplasia congenita. **A,** Radiograph in an affected newborn with a small thorax, rounded iliac wings, vertical ischia, absence of pubic ossification, short femurs, and metaphyseal rounding of long bones. **B,** Radiograph in an affected newborn with bell-shaped chest, short ribs, and elongated clavicles. **C,** Radiograph in an affected newborn with moderately short ribs with mild anterior splaying and anteriorly rounded vertebral bodies with minimal flattening and no coronal clefts.

- Myopia (except for Stickler type 3)
- Epiphyseal dysplasia (may be large or mildly flattened)
- Early arthritis
- platyspondyly

ABNORMAL SULFATION GROUP

The abnormal sulfation group is a molecularly defined group of disorders with a defect in the sulfate transporter gene on chromosome 5 coding for the diastrophic dysplasia sulfate transporter (DTDST) protein. This group comprises not only diastrophic dysplasia but also multiple epiphyseal dysplasia MED–multilayered patellae/brachydactyly/clubfeet, as well as achondrogenesis type IB and atelosteogenesis type II.[10] These conditions are all autosomal recessive, and the severity of the phenotype is inversely related to the level of sulfation.[11,12]

Common Features in Abnormal Sulfation Group

- Platyspondyly
- Scoliosis
- Proximally placed and short first metacarpal ("hitchhiker thumb")
- Clubfoot
- Short thick long bones

ACHONDROGENESIS TYPE I

Achondrogenesis type I is actually two separate disorders that appear almost identical radiographically. Achondrogenesis type IB belongs to this diastrophic dysplasia (molecular) group.[11] In achondrogenesis type IA, a molecular or gene abnormality has not yet been identified. Clinically, the two types appear identical: proportionately large skull; micromelic, hydropic, pear-shaped trunk; polyhydramnios; and lethality.

Radiologic Findings (Fig. 133-12)

1. *Skull:* decreased ossification
2. *Thorax:* tiny; very short ribs with anterior splaying
3. *Spine:* absent or minimal vertebral body ossification
4. *Pelvis:* short iliac bones with concave acetabular roofs, absent pubic (ischial) ossification
5. *Extremities:* severe micromelia with broadened ends of limbs, trapezoidal or wedge-shaped femurs

Note: Radiographic findings in achondrogenesis type IA include multiple fractured, beaded ribs, and wedged femurs. Achondrogenesis type IB shows no rib fractures or beading and has trapezoidal femurs.

DIASTROPHIC DYSPLASIA

Diastrophic dysplasia is, like all the other disorders of this group, is an autosomal-recessive condition. It is commonly identifiable at birth and usually nonlethal.

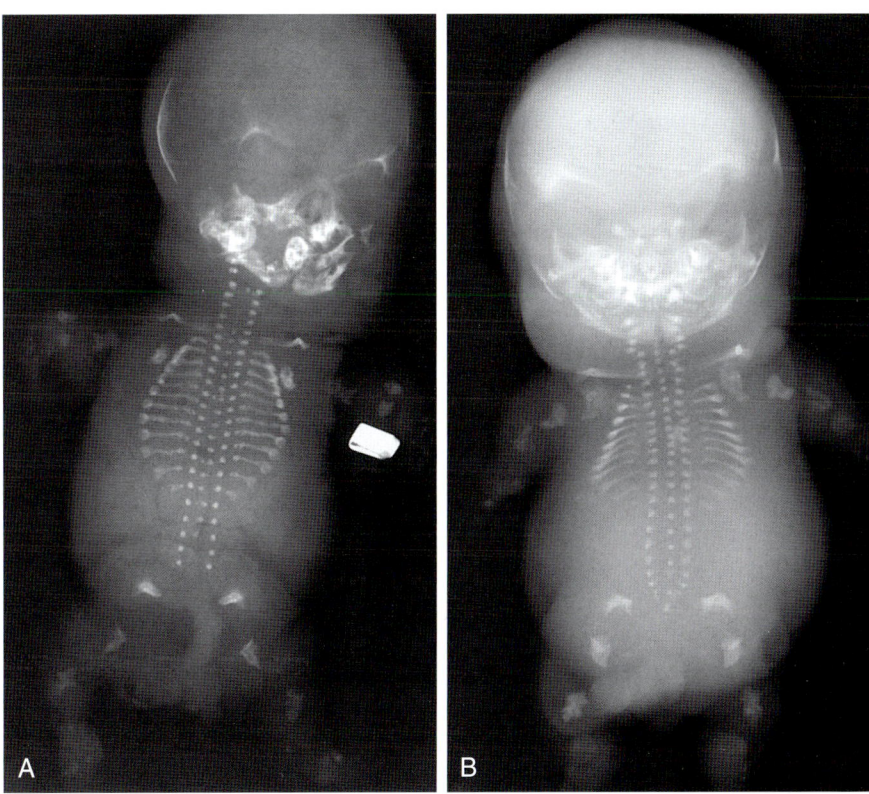

Figure 133-12 **Achondrogenesis. A,** Radiograph from a stillborn infant with type IA achondrogenesis demonstrates a tiny thorax; short, anteriorly cupped ribs with beading; micromelia; wedged femurs; and poor to absent vertebral body ossification. **B,** Radiograph from a stillborn infant with type IB achondrogenesis. Findings are similar to those in type IA but with arched iliac wings, no rib beading, and trapezoidal femurs

Radiologic Findings (Fig. 133-13)

1. *Head:* ear pinna calcification, cleft or high arched palate
2. *Thorax:* moderately small
3. *Spine:* progressive scoliosis, kyphosis, upper cervical subluxation (odontoid hypoplasia), cervical kyphosis, posterior process clefting (cervical and sacral)
4. *Extremities:* often micromelia; short, thick tubular bones; generalized brachydactyly; short ovoid first metacarpal delta phalanx causing proximal placement of thumb (hitchhiker thumb), twisted metatarsals, accessory and irregular carpal bones; epiphyseal dysplasia with multiple joint contractures

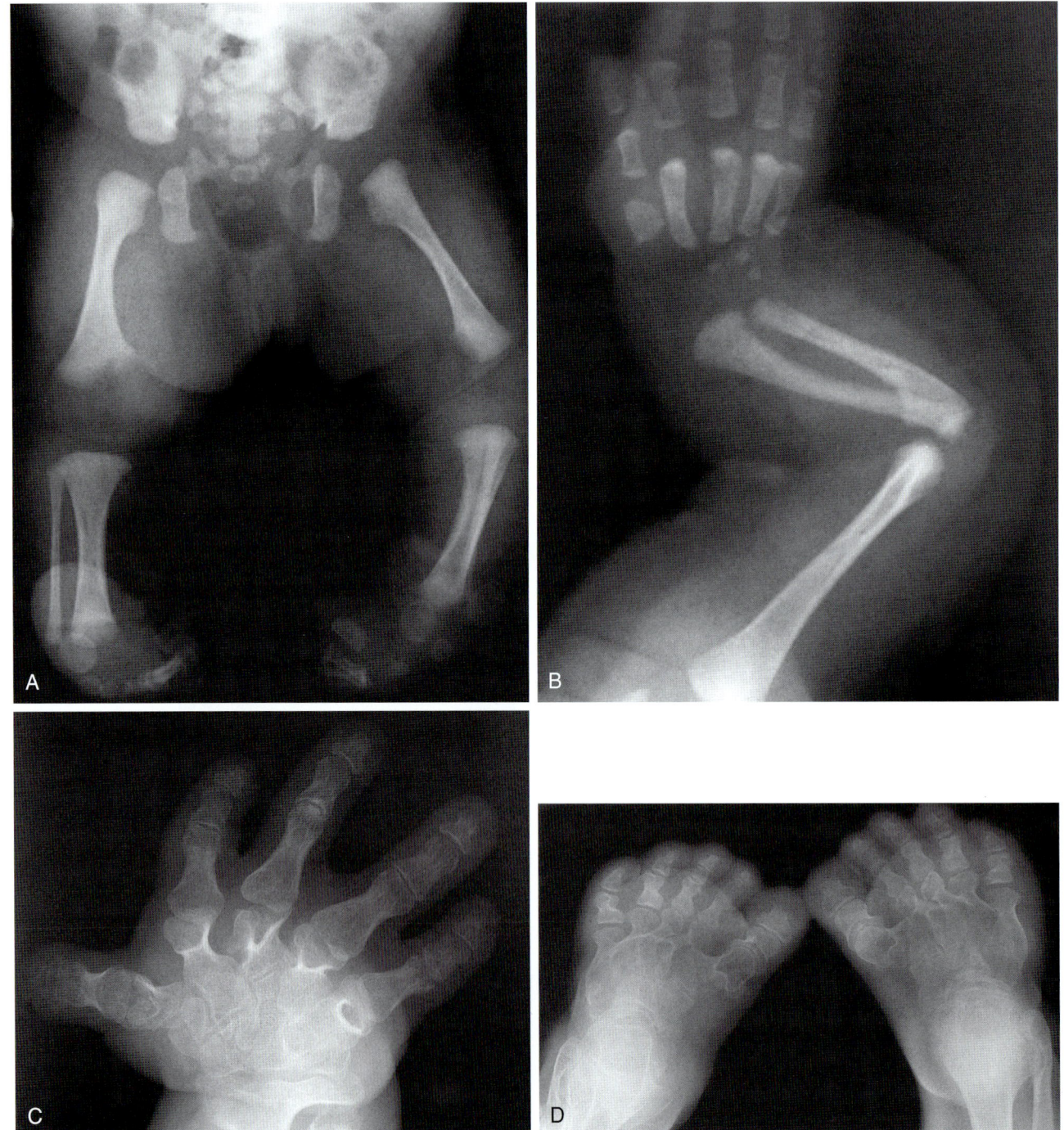

Figure 133-13 Diastrophic dysplasia. **A** and **B,** Radiographs from an affected newborn. **A,** Lower extremities: rhizomelia and mesomelia and severe clubfeet deformities. **B,** Upper extremity: elbow dislocation and short, ovoid first metacarpal. **C** and **D,** Radiographs from an affected 21-year-old. **C,** Upper extremity: hitchhiker thumb, ovoid first metacarpal, brachydactyly, and irregular and extra carpal bones. **D,** Lower extremities: unusual clubfoot and twisted metatarsals

5. *Other sites:* precocious costochondral and laryngeal area cartilage calcification; multiple sternal and patella centers

MULTIPLE EPIPHYSEAL DYSPLASIA: MULTILAYERED PATELLAE/BRACHYDACTYLY/CLUBFEET

In some cases of MED, *DTDST* gene abnormalities exist. Radiographs reveal MED changes, but patients also exhibit mildly short or normal stature, clubfeet, and additional deformities due to the *DTDST* gene abnormality.

Radiologic Findings Extremities show the following: epiphyseal dysplasia, especially at hips (half- or quarter-moon–shaped); double-layered or multilayered patella (visible on lateral knee radiograph); mild brachydactyly; clubfeet or twisted metatarsals; mildly shortened long bones, some with mild undertubulation.

Filamin Group

The filamin group combines a wide group of dysplasias that have in common an abnormality in the number and configuration of carpal, tarsal, and vertebral bones with joint dislocations. The identification of the group is another triumph in the study of molecular genetics, as it reclassifies correctly a group of disorders described as "syndromes" within a common framework of genetically determined diseases no different from other skeletal dysplasias.[13,14] The group includes oto-palato-digital (OPD) syndrome types 1 and 2, Larsen syndrome, frontometaphyseal dysplasia, Melnick-Needles osteodysplasty, and spondylo-carpal-tarsal synostosis.

COMMON FEATURES IN THE FILAMIN GROUP

- Sensorineural hearing loss
- Carpal and digital anomalies
- Joint dislocation
- Skull thickening

OPD SYNDROME

OPD syndrome causes hearing loss, cleft palate, and deformity of the digits, especially the first digit. Hearing loss is caused by malformation of the auditory ossicles. Multiple carpal bone abnormalities, including accessory carpal bones and fusion of carpal bones, are present. The capitate may be malformed, with its long axis in the transverse plane. The trapezoid is commonly fused to the base of the second metacarpal, although the finding may not manifest until skeletal ossification nears maturity in late adolescence. The distal phalanx of the thumb is short and wide. The same deformity is present in the foot, where the hallux is short. Prominence of the frontal and occipital bones is present, with a prominent supraorbital ridge. In the more severe type 2 variety, rib shortening is marked. The radial head is usually dislocated.

Radiographic Findings in OPD (e-Fig. 133-14)
1. *Head:* prominent supraorbital ridge
2. *Spine:* small pedicles with wide interpediculate distance

3. *Extremities:* accessory carpal bones, double ossification center of lunate, fusion of carpal bones especially trapezoid and scaphoid, fusion of the second metacarpal to trapezoid in adolescence, similar findings in feet; short first metatarsal and phalanges of great toe, and short and wide distal phalanx of thumb; radial head dislocation

LARSEN SYNDROME

In Larsen syndrome, multiple joint dislocations are present. In keeping with the common theme of filamin abnormalities, supernumerary carpal bones are common along with other digital changes. A doubled calcaneal ossification center is a helpful clue to accurate diagnosis. Scoliosis is common. This is a filamin type B abnormality. A similar filamin type B abnormality causes spondylo-carpal-tarsal synostosis syndrome, whose name describes the pattern of skeletal involvement.[15]

Radiographic Features (Fig. 133-15 and e-Fig. 133-16)
1. *Spine:* cervical spine kyphosis
2. *Extremities:* multiple joint dislocations, double or triple calcaneal ossification center, accessory carpal bones, broad irregular metacarpals

TRPV4 Group

TRPV4 (transient receptor potential cation channel, subfamily 5, member 4) is a calcium permeable nonselective cation channel that appears to play an important role in chondrogenesis. This channelopathy is also the cause of several other nonskeletal syndromes such as Charcot Marie-Tooth disease, scapula-peroneal spinal muscular atrophy, and congenital distal spinal muscular atrophy.[16,17]

The key to this group is the appearance of the vertebral bodies on a frontal view. Because of a relatively wide but flat vertebral body, the pedicles appear "overfaced." This means that the pedicle outline projects completely within the contour of the vertebral body instead of at the margin of the body overlying the superior end plate. The appearance has been also described as an" open staircase." Additionally, the major members of the group—metatropic dysplasia, brachyolmia (autosomal-dominant type), and spondylometaphyseal dysplasia (SMD) Koslowski type—also manifest delay in carpal bone ossification. Although brachyolmia primarily affects the vertebral bodies, subtle metaphyseal changes are seen as they are in metatropic dysplasia and SMD Koslowski type. It may be very difficult to differentiate between metatropic dysplasia and SMD Koslowski type.

COMMON FEATURES IN THE TRPV4 GROUP

- Platyspondyly with overfaced pedicles
- Carpal ossification delay
- Metaphyseal or physeal irregularity

METATROPIC DYSPLASIA

Metatropic dysplasia, or metatropic dwarfism, is evident in the newborn with a relatively long trunk and markedly

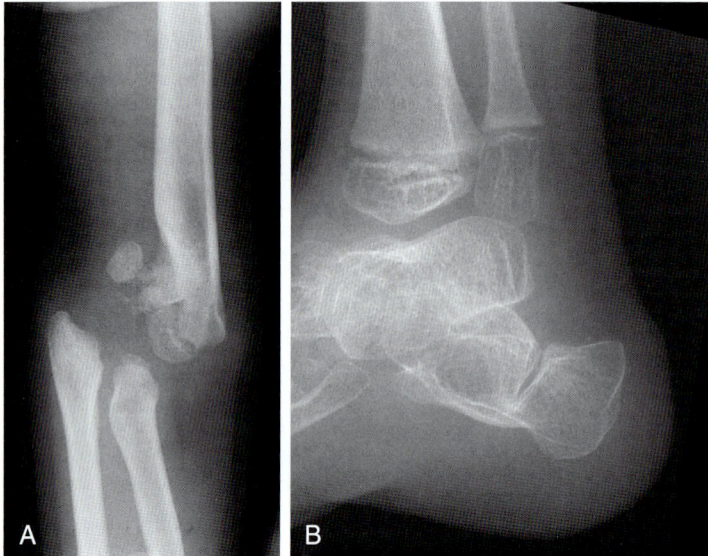

Figure 133-15 A 5-year-old girl with Larsen syndrome. **A,** Anteroposterior elbow radiograph shows chronic dislocation with epiphyseal deformities. **B,** Lateral radiograph of an ankle in a 5-year-old boy shows a bifid calcaneus and deformity of the talus and distal tibial epiphysis.

shortened limbs. This "changing" dysplasia over time produces a short-trunk or short-limb form of dwarfism with a "tail." Although heterogeneous, most cases are nonlethal and are autosomal dominant.

Radiologic Findings (Fig. 133-17)

1. *Thorax:* small; short ribs
2. *Spine:* dense wafer vertebral bodies (newborns), reconstituted platyspondyly (children and adults), scoliosis (adults)
3. *Pelvis and hips:* short, squared iliac wings; flat, irregular acetabular roof; narrow sacrosciatic notches; widening of proximal femoral metaphyses with a pronounced medial aspect about lesser trochanter (halberd (hunting ax)–shaped proximal femurs)
4. *Extremities:* flared metaphyses (trumpet shaped), with epiphyseal dysplasia and shortening (dumbbell shape).

SPONDYLOMETAPHYSEAL DYSPLASIA KOSLOWSKI TYPE

Characteristic radiographic findings (e-Fig. 133-18) include severe platyspondyly with overfaced pedicles. The extremities show sclerosis, flaring, and irregularity at the metaphyses. Carpal bone ossification is delayed and may not be apparent until age 5 to 6 years.

Short Rib–Polydactyly Group

The short rib dysplasias with or without polydactyly (short rib–polydactyly [SRP]) group of disorders is a diverse group, linked only radiologically by extreme rib shortening.

The group consists of all the SRP disorders (types I through IV), asphyxiating thoracic dysplasia (ATD, various types), and chondroectodermal dysplasia. All are autosomal recessive.

Some members of this group are now known to be ciliopathies.[18] Several types of SRP and types of ATD are

caused by mutations in genes encoding for normal dynein heavy chains or other aspects of the ciliogenesis.[19,20] It is interesting to note that situs abnormalities are a feature of these dysplasias attesting to the important role cilial transport plays in body situs. In patients with primary cilial dyskinesia (immotile cilia syndrome), approximately 50% have situs inversus (Kartagener syndrome).

SHORT RIB–POLYDACTYLY DYSPLASIA

SRP dysplasia is a subgroup of disorders that are typed largely on radiographic grounds. Types I and III are quite similar, as are types II and IV. The role of the pediatric radiologist is to make the diagnosis of this subgroup as separate from ATD and chondroectodermal dysplasia. To that end, it is important to note the SRP dysplasias have the shortest ribs of any of the skeletal dysplasias.

Radiologic Findings (Fig. 133-19)

1. *Thorax:* small; very short horizontal ribs
2. *Spine:* relatively normally shaped
3. *Pelvis:* small, dysplastic ilia
4. *Extremities:* micromelia; medial and lateral spurs at metaphyses; ovoid or tiny, normal-shaped tibias; severe brachydactyly with hypoplastic middle and distal phalanges; polydactyly commonly present

ASPHYXIATING THORACIC DYSPLASIA (JEUNE SYNDROME)

ATD is a genetically heterogeneous disorder with a mixed prognosis. Many affected patients die in the perinatal period from respiratory complications related to a small chest. Survivors may die from renal complications (progressive nephropathy) later in life. Other internal organs may also be involved. Sometimes, postaxial polydactyly is present. Definite radiographic (but not clinical) similarities to chondroectodermal dysplasia are evident. An allelic relationship has been considered but remains unproven.[21] Some cases are so alike

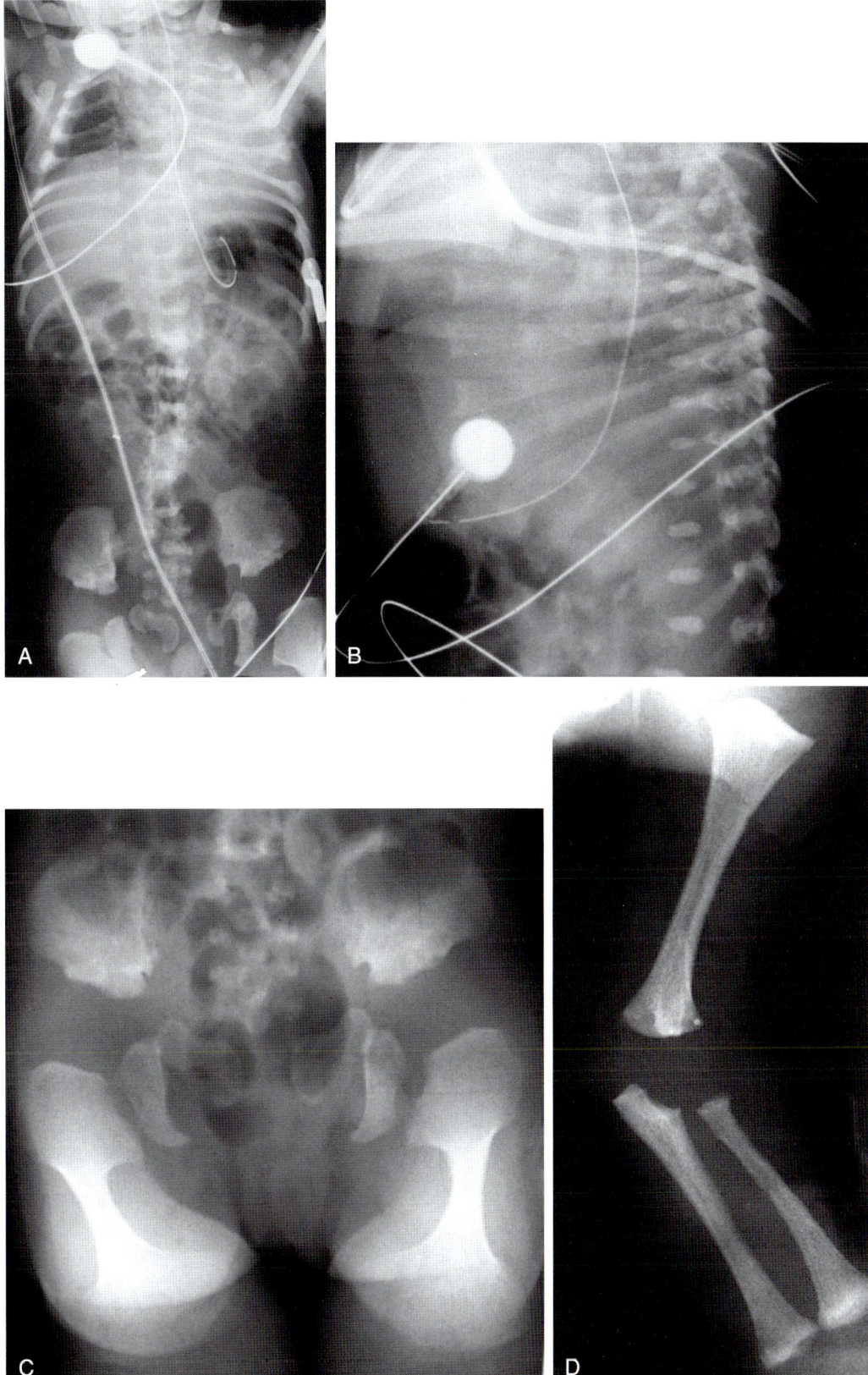

Figure 133-17 A newborn with metatropic dysplasia. **A,** Thorax: long trunk and small chest. **B,** Spine: dense wafer vertebral bodies and short ribs with anterior splaying. **C,** Pelvis: short iliac wings, narrow sciatic notches, irregular acetabular roofs, and rounded, enlarged proximal femoral metaphyses (halberd shaped) with markedly flared distal metaphyses (trumpet-shaped) **D,** Upper extremities: flared proximal humeral and distal radial and ulnar metaphyses; shortened long bones.

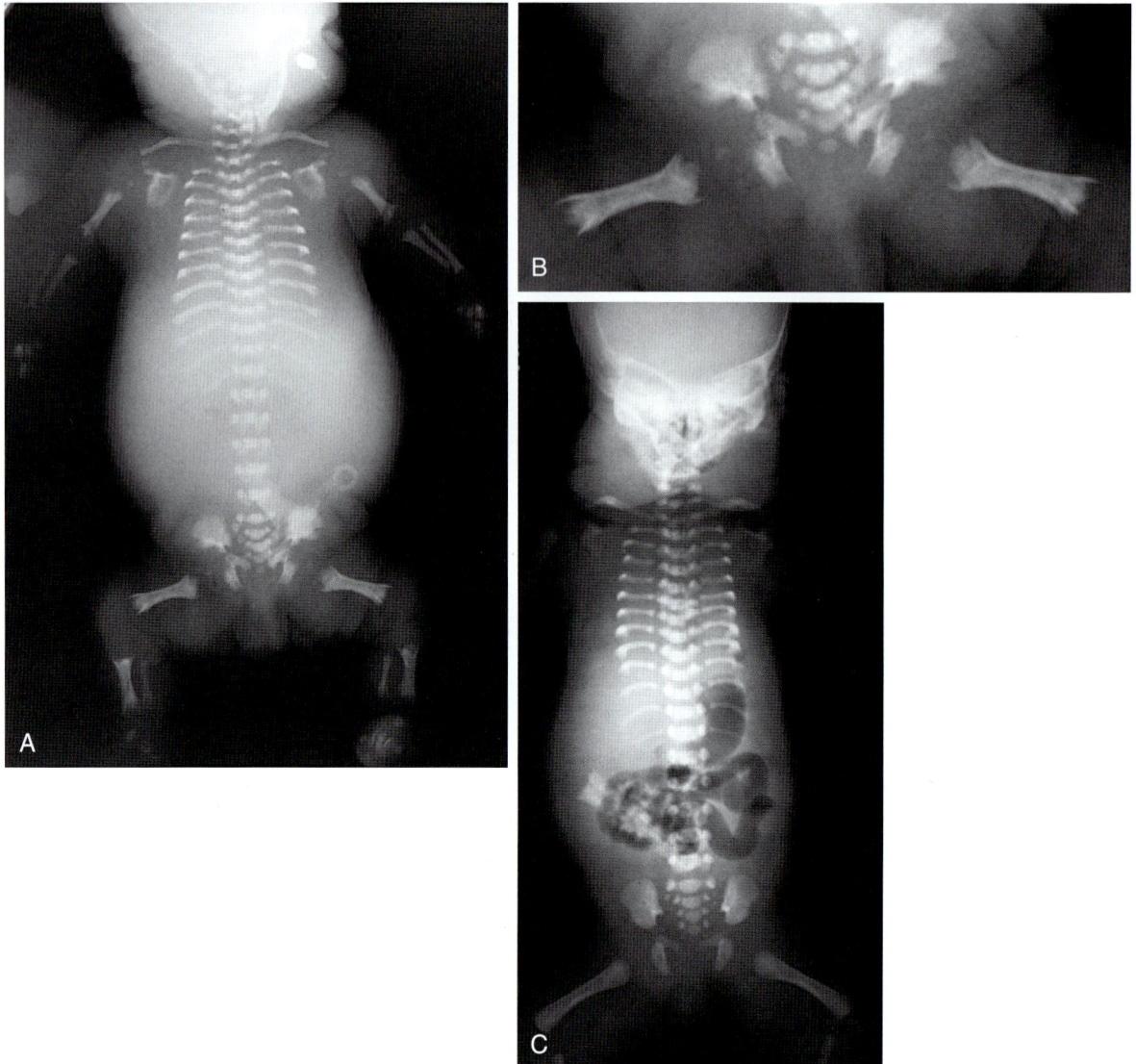

Figure 133-19 Short rib–polydactyly dysplasia. **A,** Radiograph from a stillborn infant with type I/III form, demonstrating very short ribs and, handlebar clavicles. **B,** Magnified, coned view of pelvis shows hypoplastic pelvis with notched acetabula, and metaphyseal-spiked femurs. **C,** Radiograph from a stillborn infant with short rib–polydactyly dysplasia type II. Findings are similar to those in type I/III but with round-ended femurs and hypoplastic acetabula.

radiologically that they are best termed *ATD/Ellis–van Creveld syndrome complex.*

Radiologic Findings (Fig. 133-20)
1. *Thorax:* long and barrel-shaped, handlebar clavicles, short horizontal ribs with bulbous anterior ends
2. *Spine:* normal
3. *Pelvis:* small; short, flared iliac wings; trident acetabular roof; narrowed sacrosciatic notches
4. *Extremities:* generalized shortening, precocious proximal femoral epiphyseal ossification, cone-shaped epiphyses in hands, metaphyseal flaring with irregularity(more pronounced in child)

CHONDROECTODERMAL DYSPLASIA (ELLIS–VAN CREVELD SYNDROME)

Chondroectodermal dysplasia is a nonlethal skeletal dysplasia. The nonskeletal involvement in this disorder is extremely important in defining this condition and distinguishing this lesion from ATD. Signs include hair, nail, and teeth abnormalities, as well as congenital heart disease. Polydactyly is almost invariably present. The radiologic findings are very similar to those of ATD. The genes involved in this autosomal recessive condition have been identified (*EvC* genes 1, 2), located at chromosome 4p16.

Radiologic Findings (e-Fig. 133-21)
1. *Thorax:* small; moderately short ribs
2. *Pelvis:* small; short, flared iliac wings; trident acetabula; narrowed sacrosciatic notches
3. *Spine:* almost normal
4. *Extremities:* generalized shortening with more mesomelia and acromelia; premature ossification of capital femoral epiphyses; delayed ossification of proximal tibial epiphyses; humeral and femoral bowing; exostosis of proximal/medial portion of tibia

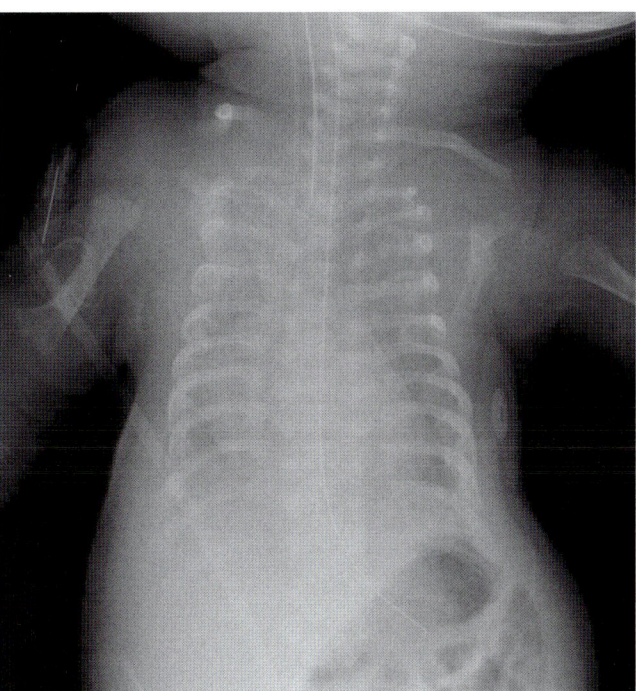

Figure 133-20 Newborn with asphyxiating thoracic dysplasia. Note the short ribs (although not as short as ribs in short rib–polydactyly (see Fig. 133-19) and metaphyseal flaring and irregularity in proximal humeri.

5. *Hands:* characteristic postaxial polydactyly, capitate/hamate (and other carpal) fusions, extra carpal bone, cone-shaped epiphyses
6. *Feet:* polydactyly

Multiple Epiphyseal Dysplasia and Pseudoachondroplasia Group

Pseudoachondroplasia and some cases of typical multiple epiphyseal dysplasia (MED) are cartilage oligomeric protein (COMP) gene defects on chromosome 19 (70%) and share some commonality of radiographic findings. However, many other cases of MED (with the same apparent radiologic abnormalities) represent type IX collagen defects on chromosome 1, or matrilin 3 defects. It appears that all the described entities within this group are autosomal-dominant disorders, except for MED-multilayered patellae/brachydactyly/clubfeet, which is autosomal recessive.

MULTIPLE EPIPHYSEAL DYSPLASIA

Historically MED was divided into the milder Ribbing form and the more severe Fairbanks form. Although the classification does not agree with molecular genetics data, the distinction is helpful from a clinical point of view. Ribbing MED may entail only hip involvement and can be confused with bilateral Legg-Calvé-Perthes disease and Meyer dysplasia. Differentiation from these entities is possible because almost all patients with MED have clinically significant short stature. Many patients with MED later go through an asymptomatic phase of avascular necrosis of the capital femoral epiphyses. This makes differentiation of MED from Legg-Calvé-Perthes

disease very difficult if old radiographs are not available. The Fairbanks form has involvement of all the long bone epiphyses to some degree. MED manifests after about 2 years of age but is most commonly diagnosed in an adolescent or young adult. Involvement is always bilateral and symmetric. The shortening is quite mild.

It is possible to suggest the molecular defect from the radiologic changes. The COMP group has a greater resemblance to pseudoachondroplasia. Those affected by the COMP gene locus have tiny capital femoral epiphyses, irregular and poorly formed acetabula, mushroomlike flaring at the knees, brachydactyly with proximally rounded metacarpals and central protrusions in the vertebral bodies caused by delayed ossification of the ring apophyses. As noted elsewhere in this chapter, the presence of central vertebral body protrusions is a good radiologic marker for epiphyseal dysplasia.

The MED multilayered patella form includes a multilayered ossific center of the patella, clubfoot and brachydactyly.

Radiologic Findings (Fig. 133-22 and e-Fig. 133-23)
1. *Spine:* in young adults, disk herniations into vertebral end plates (Schmorl nodes)
2. *Extremities:* small, irregular, flattened ossification centers (epiphyses); small, irregular carpal (and tarsal) centers

PSEUDOACHONDROPLASIA

This short-limb, short-trunk form of skeletal dysplasia was referred to at first as "achondroplasia with a normal face." In actuality, the affected individual usually has the most beautiful or the most handsome face in the family.

Radiologic Findings (Fig. 133-24)
1. *Skull:* normal
2. *Thorax:* mild anterior rib widening
3. *Spine:* superiorly and inferiorly rounded vertebral bodies, anterior central tongue (unossified ring epiphyses), normalization of vertebrae (later)
4. *Pelvis:* rounded iliac wings; hypoplastic, poorly formed acetabular roofs
5. *Extremities:* mini-epiphyses in the hips, moderate to severe generalized epiphyseal "dysplasia" (small, irregular, poorly ossified), mushroomlike metaphyseal widening and irregularity in the knees, proximally rounded metacarpals with mini-epiphyses in hands, irregular carpal and tarsal bones

Metaphyseal Chondrodysplasia Group

Metaphyseal chondrodysplasias (MCDs) are also a heterogeneous group of disorders that have common radiologic features. Members of this group include Jansen-type MCD, Schmid-type MCD, McKusick-type MCD, and Shwachman-Diamond dysplasia. Spines are usually normal except in Schmid-type MCD, in which mild platyspondyly may be seen. Immune deficiencies are notable in Shwachman syndrome and Mckusick-type MCD (Cartilage-Hair hypoplasia).

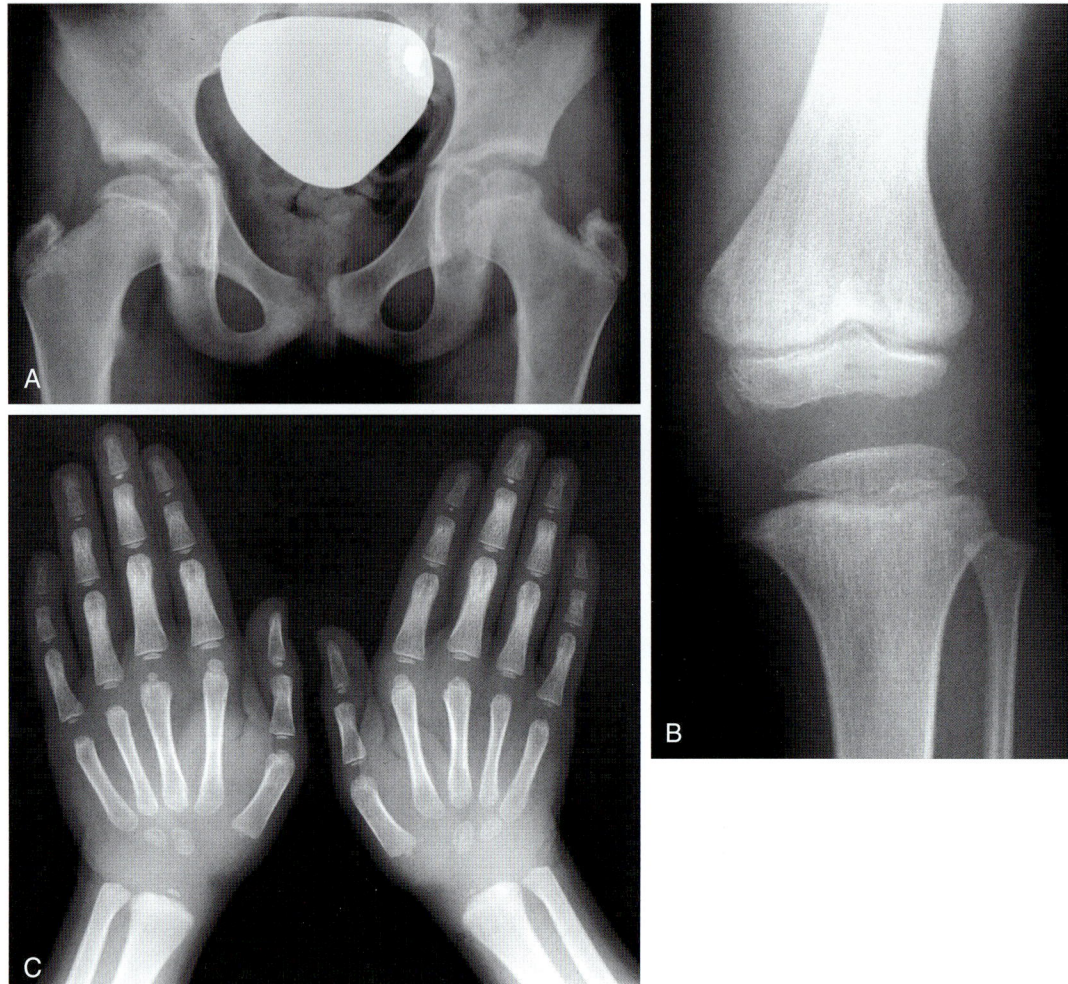

Figure 133-22 Fairbanks-type multiple epiphyseal dysplasia. **A,** Radiograph from an affected 10-year-old with small ossified proximal femoral epiphyses (ossification defect). **B** and **C,** Radiographs from an affected 6-year-old. **B,** Similar epiphyseal ossification defects in the knee. **C,** Small epiphyses of the short tubular bones of the hands and carpal ossification delay (epiphyseal equivalents), but no brachydactyly.

JANSEN-TYPE METAPHYSEAL CHONDRODYSPLASIA

This is the severest form of MCD. The presentation is in the neonatal period or during late infancy, with marked short stature and a waddling gait. This is a distinct autosomal-dominant disorder with an abnormality in a parathyroid receptor gene (*PTHR*), leading to hypercalcemia and its complications.[22] However, the radiographic findings in the skeleton are not those of typical hyperparathyroidism or hypoparathyroidism.[23]

Radiologic Findings (Fig. 133-25)
1. *Skull:* brachycephaly, platybasia, underdeveloped mandible
2. *Thorax:* normal size; expanded irregular anterior rib ends
3. *Extremities:* extensive irregularity of markedly expanded metaphyses involving all metaphyseal regions; hands exhibit wide separation of epiphyses from metaphyses

Note: As in other parathyroid abnormalities, pathologic fractures (in 45% of affected patients) and subperiosteal bone resorption (in 50%) are common.

SCHMID-TYPE METAPHYSEAL CHONDRODYSPLASIA

This form of MCD is an autosomal-dominant condition caused by a specific defect in collagen type X, the gene for which is located on chromosome 6. This disorder is the mildest of the MCDs. Presentation is usually at about 2 years of age or later with a waddling gait or bowed legs, or both. Mild short stature is present.

Radiologic Findings (Fig. 133-26)
1. *Thorax:* widened anterior rib ends
2. *Spine:* mild platyspondyly
3. *Extremities:* metaphyseal flaring, cupping and fraying, especially at the knees; rounded capital femoral mega-epiphysis with widened growth plate; usually no hand involvement

MCKUSICK-TYPE METAPHYSEAL CHONDRODYSPLASIA

Cartilage-hair hypoplasia, as this entity is also known, is an autosomal recessive disorder. The genetic defect is at the 9p

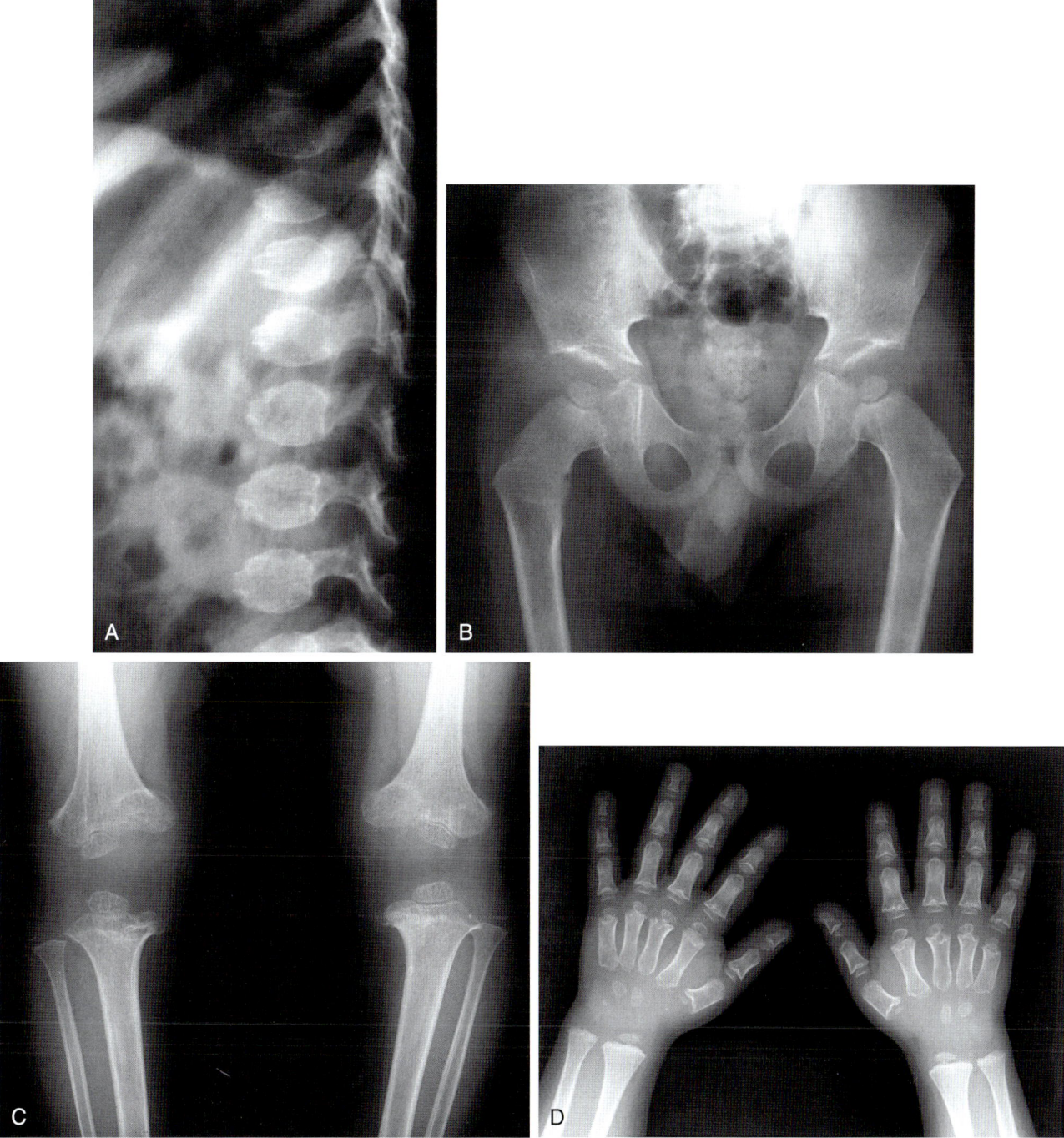

Figure 133-24 Pseudoachondroplasia. Radiologic findings at ages 3 years (**A** and **C**) and 4 years (**B** and **D**). **A,** Central anterior tonguing and superior and inferior rounding of vertebral bodies. **B,** Acetabular roof hypoplasia and mini-epiphyses. **C,** Small knee epiphyses and metaphyseal widening with ossification defects. **D,** Proximal metacarpal rounding, small epiphyseal centers, metaphyseal widening and irregularity, and carpal ossification delay.

region (*RMRP* gene), with a high frequency among the Amish and Finnish populations.[24-26] The presentation is of variable short-limbed dwarfism in early childhood. Significant clinical features indicate the diagnosis and are important for medical management: sparse, thin, light-colored hair; Hirschsprung disease; immunological problems; and increased incidence of malignancy.

Radiologic Findings (e-Fig. 133-27)

1. *Thorax:* anterior rib widening/flaring
2. *Spine:* slightly small square vertebral bodies

3. *Extremities:* flaring, cupping, and fragmentation of metaphyses (especially knees), hips usually spared; brachydactyly with cone shaped epiphysis

SHWACHMAN-DIAMOND DYSPLASIA

This rare autosomal-recessive disorder is also known as MCD. Major clinical findings include pancreatic insufficiency and cyclic neutropenia. It manifests in infancy with recurrent infections and failure to thrive. The skeletal radiographic features are quite mild. The defect, involving the

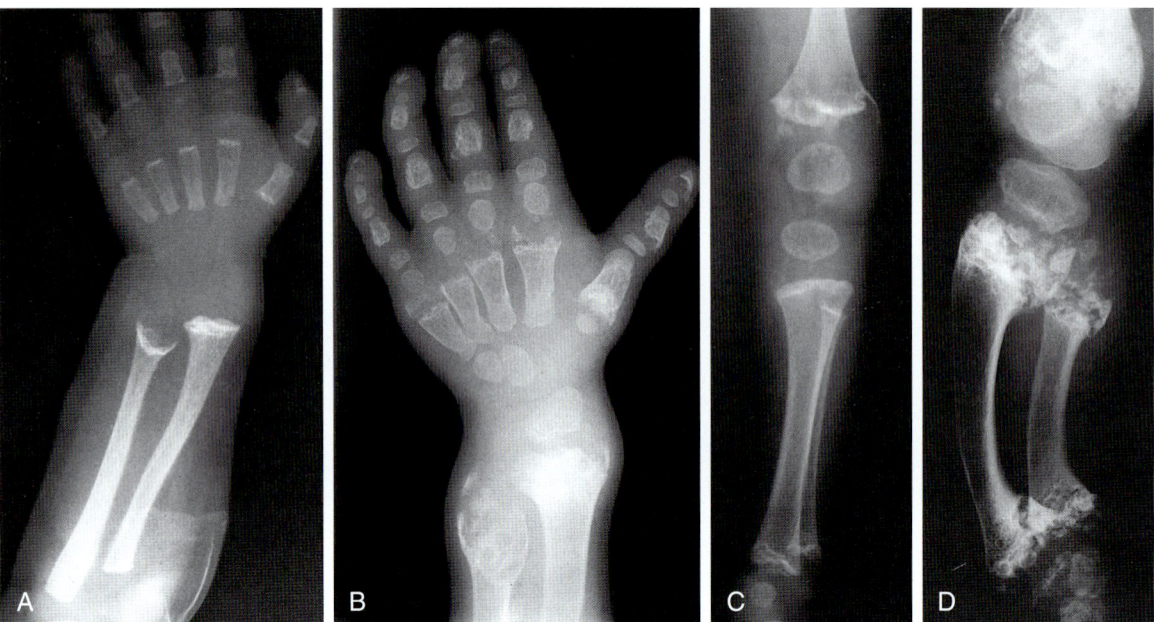

Figure 133-25 Radiographic findings in Jansen-type metaphyseal chondrodysplasia. **A,** At 1 year, severe metaphyseal cupping and splaying are present at the wrists and also in the hand bones. **B,** At 7 years, increasing metaphyseal change is seen at the wrists with enlarged epiphysis; enlarged epiphyses with wide epiphyseal plates are also present in the hands. **C,** At 1 year, severe metaphyseal irregularities at the knees and ankles (femur, tibia, and fibula) and enlarged, rounded epiphyses are present. **D,** At 7 years, severely fragmented, sclerotic metaphyses, wide epiphyseal plates, and enlarged epiphyses are present.

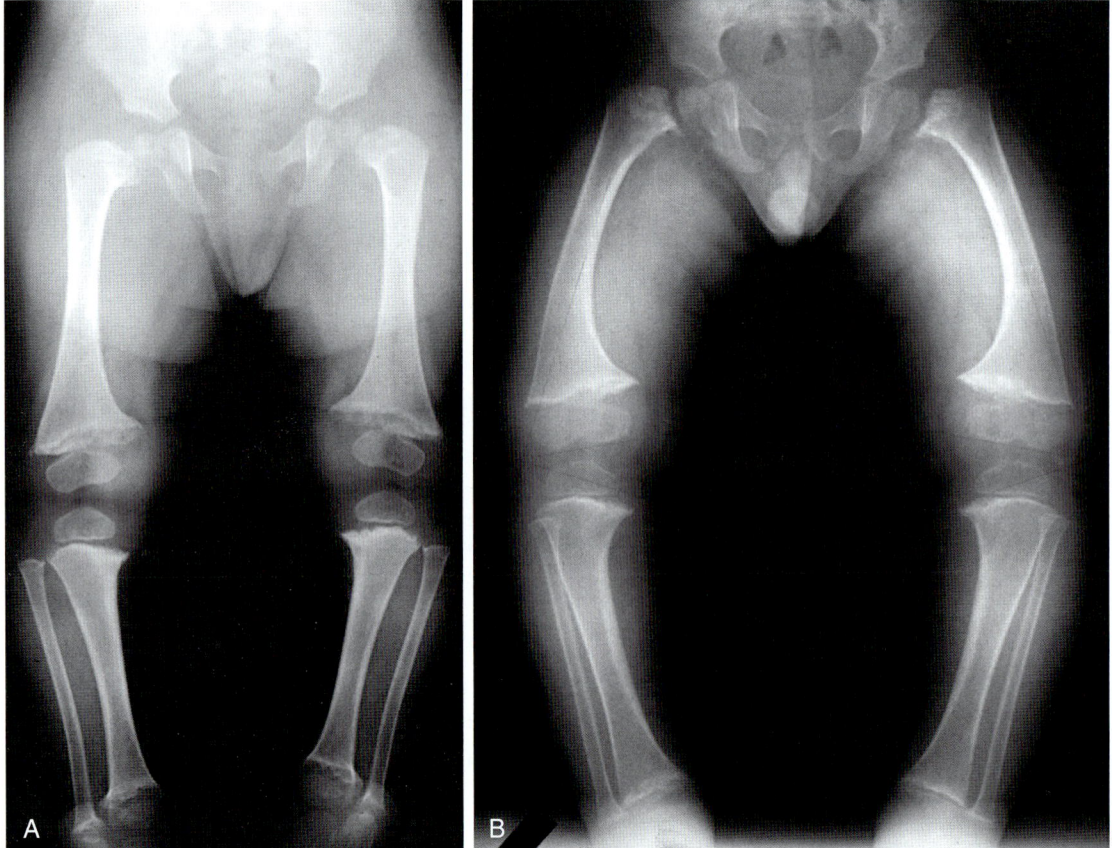

Figure 133-26 Schmid-type metaphyseal chondrodysplasia. **A,** Radiograph from an affected 19-month-old with severe coxa vara and moderate metaphyseal changes (cupping irregularity, widening) at the knees (and, not pictured here, ankles). **B,** Radiograph from an affected 3-year-old with coxa vara, genu varum, and moderate metaphyseal changes at hips and knees (widening, irregularity).

Shwachman–Bodian–Diamond syndrome (*SBDS*) gene, is located on chromosome 7q11.

Radiologic Findings (e-Fig. 133-28)

1. *Thorax:* anterior rib irregularity or splaying
2. *Extremities:* metaphyseal irregularity and sclerosis, especially at knees and hips
3. *Gastrointestinal:* malabsorption pattern on small bowel examination; lipomatosis of pancreas

Spondylometaphyseal Dysplasia Group

SPONDYLOENCHONDROMATOSIS

This autosomal-recessive disorder is also known as *spondylo-enchondrodysplasia*, characterized by low-normal or mild short stature, with kyphosis, lordosis, or both. Prominent joints may be apparent.

Radiologic Findings (e-Fig. 133-29)

1. *Spine:* severe platyspondyly with endplate irregularity
2. *Extremities:* enchondromatosis in long bones, but rarely involving hands and feet

Acromelic/Acromesomelic Dysplasia Group

The acromelic/acromesomelic dysplasia group consists of a large, heterogeneous collection of disorders. For a number of these dysplasias, the molecular defect has been delineated. Only trichorhinophalangeal syndrome (TRPS) types I and II, and acromesomelic dysplasia of Maroteaux (acromesomelic dwarfism) are detailed.

TRICHORHINOPHALANGEAL SYNDROME TYPES I AND II

Both of these disorders have been located on the long arm of chromosome 8. The gene implicated in TRPS type I (also known as *Giedion syndrome*) is *TRPS1*. TRPS type II (also known as *Langer-Giedion syndrome*) is slightly more complicated. TRPS type II is the result of a contiguous gene abnormality resulting from the loss of not only *TRPS1* but also *EXT1*, a major cause of multiple hereditary exostoses located distal to *TRPS1*. TRPS type I is autosomal dominant, whereas most cases of TRPS type II are sporadic. The clinical manifestations of both disorders include mild short stature; sparse, slow-growing hair; pear-shaped nose ("hose nose"); and short, crooked fingers. The contiguous gene abnormality explains the added features in TRPS type II, which include multiple exostoses and mental retardation.[27]

Radiologic Findings (Fig. 133-30)

1. *Extremities:* Perthes-like changes at the hips, brachydactyly with multiple cone-shaped epiphyses in the phalanges of both hands. With TRPS type II, multiple exostoses are also present.

ACROMESOMELIC DYSPLASIA OF MAROTEAUX

This skeletal dysplasia is actually a misnomer in that the changes in this disorder are hardly just acromelic and mesomelic. Significant spinal abnormalities are also present. The disorder is autosomal recessive with a defect in *NPR2*, which maps to chromosome 9p and is involved in regulation of skeletal growth. Abnormalities are discoverable at birth but are quite significant by 1 year of age. Clinical findings include moderate short stature, short forearms, stubby hands and feet, and short lower legs.

Radiologic Findings (e-Fig. 133-31)

1. *Spine:* oval vertebral bodies (early), anterior beaking and posterior wedging (later), gibbus, kyphoscoliosis, or all of these ultimately
2. *Extremities:* shortening of all tubular bones, especially radius or ulna and tibia or fibula; brachydactyly of hands and feet with cone-shaped epiphyses but with relatively large great toes

Mesomelic Dysplasia Group

The mesomelic dysplasia (mesomelic dwarfism) group consists of a large number of disorders involving shortening of the middle segment bones. Milder shortening of other segments may also be noted. The most common entity in this group is dyschondrosteosis.

DYSCHONDROSTEOSIS

This skeletal dysplasia, also known as *Leri-Weill syndrome*, is an autosomal-dominant condition. It consists of a pseudoautosomal homeobox gene (*SHOX* gene) found on the short arm of the X chromosome. Dyschondrosteosis manifests with mild to moderate short stature, usually with both forearm and calf shortening. Madelung deformity is the major marker for this disease. Interestingly, Madelung deformity is also common in Turner syndrome because of the lack of two copies of *SHOX* since only one X chromosome is present (see discussion of Turner syndrome).

MRI is important here from a therapeutic point of view. A thickened ligament has been described by Vickers and Nielsen, which appears to tether the medial radial physis.[28] It can be found on the volar side of the joint and may be an abnormally thickened volar radiolunotriquetral ligament. Operative lysis of this structure if performed early can ameliorate the Madelung-type deformity. Radiographically, the ligament should be suspected when a triangular lucency is seen at the medial aspect of the distal radial metaphysis. On MRI, the ligament is clearly visible as a thick hypointense band of tissue originating at the medial radial physis.[29]

Radiologic Findings (Fig. 133-32)

1. *Extremities:* symmetric bowing and shortening of both radii, shortened ulnas, radiographic Madelung deformity changes, variable tibial and fibular shortening; short stature with abnormal upper to lower segment ratio

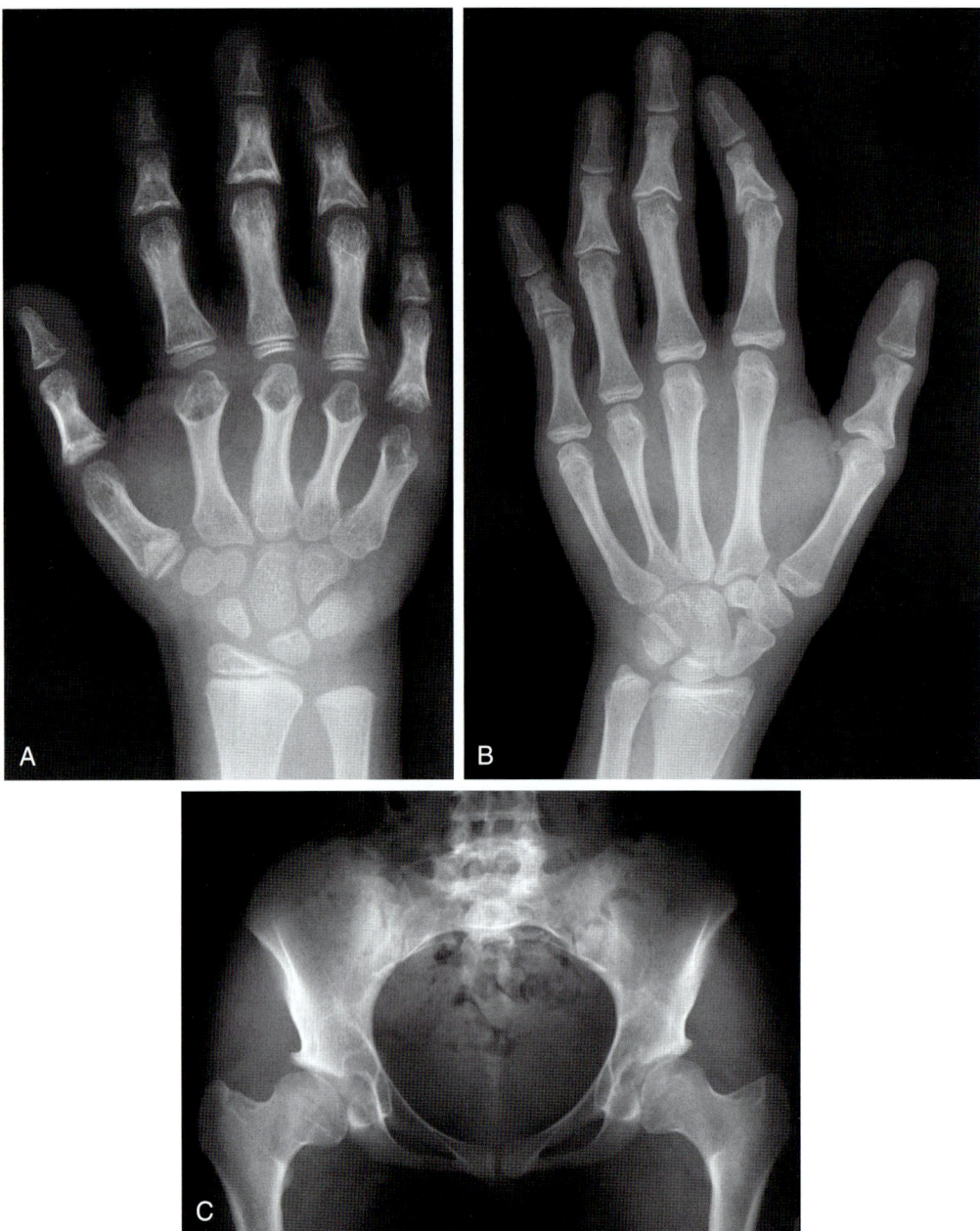

Figure 133-30 Radiographic findings in trichorhinophalangeal syndrome type I. **A,** In an affected 8-year-old, cone-shaped epiphyses involving the first metacarpal, the proximal fifth phalanx, and all middle phalanges and metacarpals in the second through fifth digits (early fusion) are present. **B,** The radiograph from an affected 18-year-old shows similar changes. **C,** In an affected young adult, coxa vara and small capital femoral epiphyses are present.

Chondrodysplasia Punctata Group

The chondrodysplasia punctata (stippled epiphyses) group is very diverse, united by the radiographic commonality of epiphyseal stippling. Several but not all of these entities are related to each other. The rhizomelic form of chondrodysplasia punctata is a peroxisomal enzyme abnormality; the Conradi–Hünermann type is associated with a gene on the long arm of the X chromosome (*EBP* gene defect); and the brachytelephalangic type is on the short arm of the X chromosome (a defect in the *ARSE* gene).

RHIZOMELIC CHONDRODYSPLASIA PUNCTATA

This is a distinct form of chondrodysplasia punctata and has an autosomal-recessive inheritance pattern. It is a symmetric rhizomelic skeletal dysplasia manifesting in the neonatal period. Affected infants usually die in the first year of life. Associated clinical findings include cataracts, skin lesions, alopecia, and joint contractures. Later manifestations are severe psychomotor retardation and spasticity. These infants appear to be in constant pain. Thus far, abnormalities in three genes (*PEX7, DHPAT, AGPS*) have been noted.

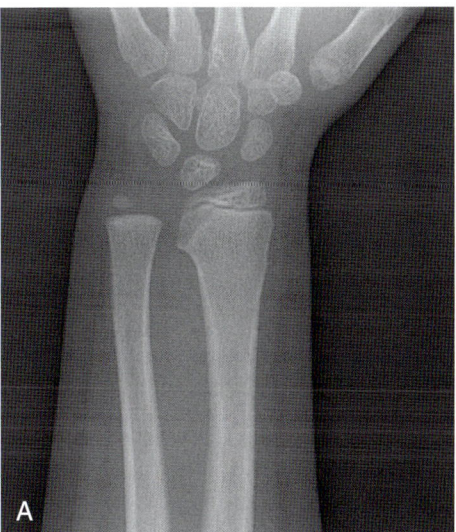
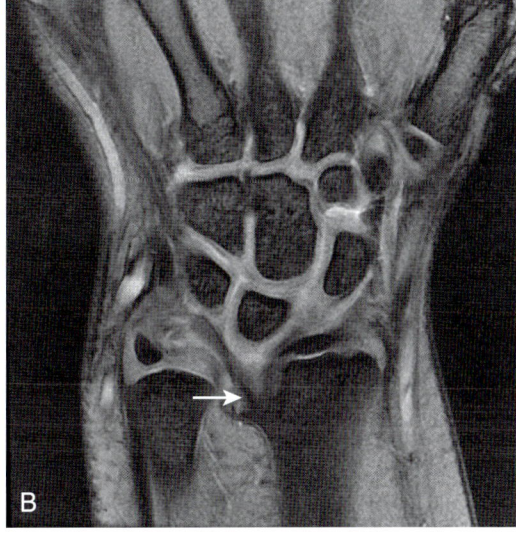

Figure 133-32 A 7-year-old girl with dyschondrosteosis. **A** and **B**, Madelung deformity is present on conventional radiography. Note the triangular lucency in the distal radius. The Vickers ligament (*arrow*) is shown inserting by magnetic resonance imaging onto the triangular lucency tethering physis.

Radiologic Findings (Fig. 133-33)

1. *Spine:* coronal clefting, anteriorly rounded vertebral bodies
2. *Extremities:* stippled epiphyseal ossification, symmetric bilateral shortening of femurs (and humeri) with less severe shortening of all the remaining long bones

Bent-Bone Dysplasia Group

The bent-bone dysplasia group of disorders is a rather small but diverse group, with campomelic dysplasia (campomelic dwarfism) having been well described molecularly. These dysplasias have been grouped together because of their radiographic expression.

CAMPOMELIC DYSPLASIA

This unusual entity is an autosomal-dominant disorder diagnosable at birth, manifesting as bent thighs, clubfeet, respiratory distress, and unusual small facies. Sex reversal is often present. All the extremities are moderately short. Neonatal or perinatal death occurs in most cases. The molecular defect is a homeobox gene abnormality called *SOX9*, found on chromosome 17. Radiographically the combination of kinked femora with severe hypoplasia of the blade of the scapula makes for an easy diagnosis.

Radiologic Findings (Fig. 133-34)

1. *Skull:* enlarged, narrow with a small face
2. *Thorax:* mildly short ribs, numbering 11; severe hypoplasia of the bodies of the scapulae
3. *Spine:* nonossification of thoracic pedicles, cervical kyphosis, hypoplasia of cervical vertebral bodies
4. *Pelvis:* narrow, tall iliac wings
5. *Extremities:* proportionately long, bowed femurs with shortened bowed tibias; shortened upper extremity long bones

Disorders of Increased Bone Density Without Modification of Bone Shape

The disorders of increased bone density without modification of bone shape include several entities of interest. These disorders are grouped by their radiographic expression but have in common either diffuse or focal areas of bone sclerosis.

OSTEOPETROSIS

Our understanding of osteopetrosis has evolved considerably and no less than 13 general mutation loci have been described. For clinical purposes, the disease can be distinguished by age at onset. The types with onset in infancy are the most severe.

The very severe precocious or malignant type is autosomal recessive. Patients with this type present in infancy with hepatosplenomegaly, pancytopenia, multiple infections (osteomyelitis), and leukemia. Early death is common. The delayed type (late-onset form) is autosomal dominant. Lifespan is normal, and the condition is frequently diagnosed when a radiograph is obtained after minor trauma causes a fracture. Individuals with this type sustain multiple fractures and are at increased risk of osteomyelitis, particularly in the mandible.

The condition known as *osteopetrosis with renal tubular acidosis (carbonic anhydrase II deficiency)* is a rare entity localized to chromosomal locus 8q and gene *CA2* (carbonic anhydrase II). Diffuse dense cerebral calcifications suggest the correct diagnosis.

An intermediate form is also recognized with onset within the first decade, and although significant clinical abnormalities, including hematologic disease, are present, findings are milder than in the infantile form.

Although multiple genes are involved, the defect ultimately leads to osteoclast dysfunction because of

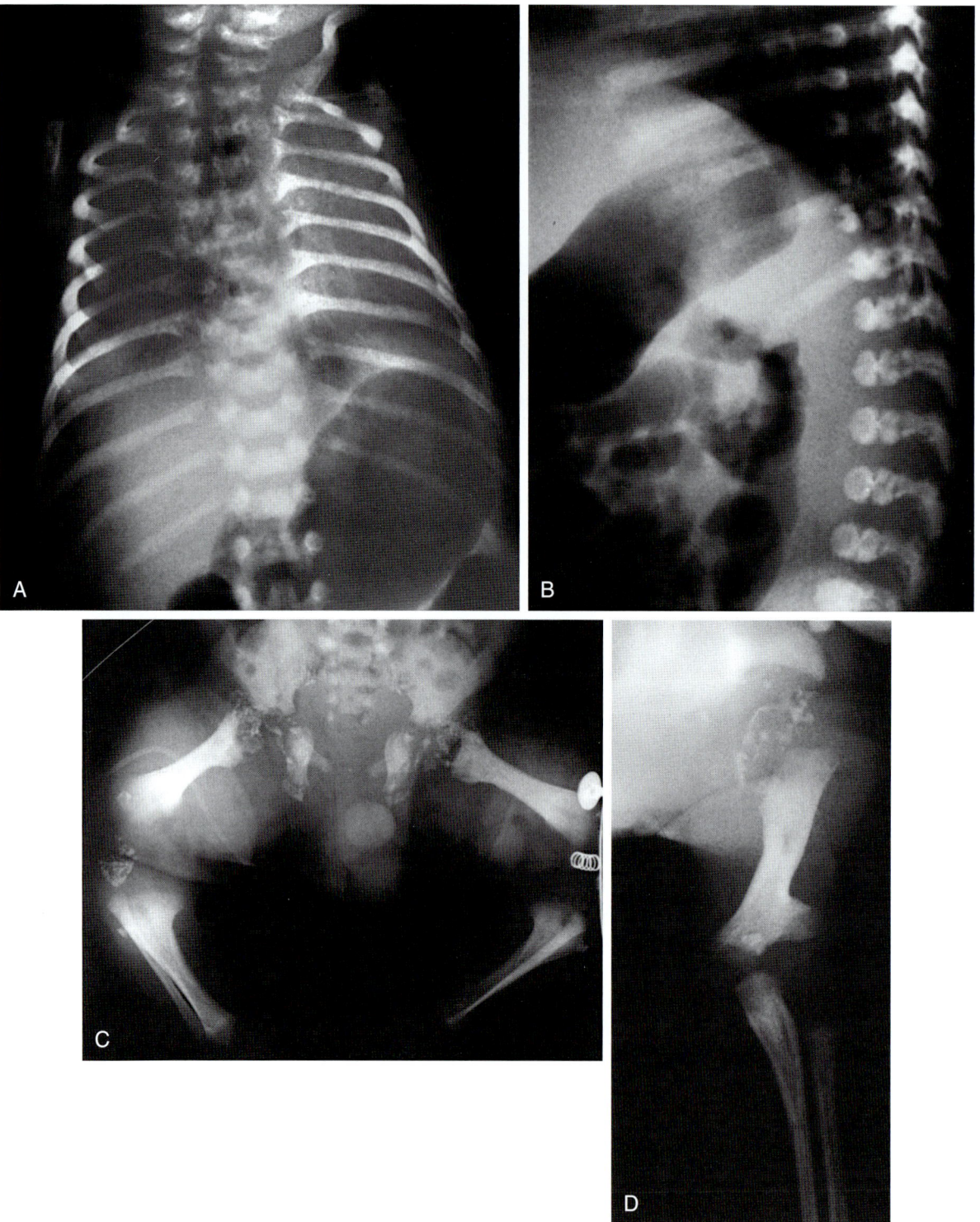

Figure 133-33 A newborn with rhizomelic chondrodysplasia punctata. **A** and **B,** Radiographs reveal a small thorax, punctate vertebral body ossification, and coronal clefting. **C** and **D,** Diffuse stippling in epiphyseal regions and rhizomelia (femurs and humeri).

unresponsiveness to parathyroid hormone. Without the remodeling activity of normal osteoclasts, bone becomes sclerotic and brittle. Long bone fractures are common.

Of importance is the seemingly contradictory presentation of osteopetrosis with rickets. This occurs in the severe malignant form. With this combination, dense osteopetrosis changes are seen in conjunction with rickets physeal changes.

It can be understood when considering that 99% of the calcium store is bound in highly calcified dense bone. Without osteoclast function, that calcium is unavailable for correct physeal growth and mineralization, and a relative calcium deficiency is present.

Bone marrow transplantation is curative as it repopulates the marrow with normally functioning osteoclasts.

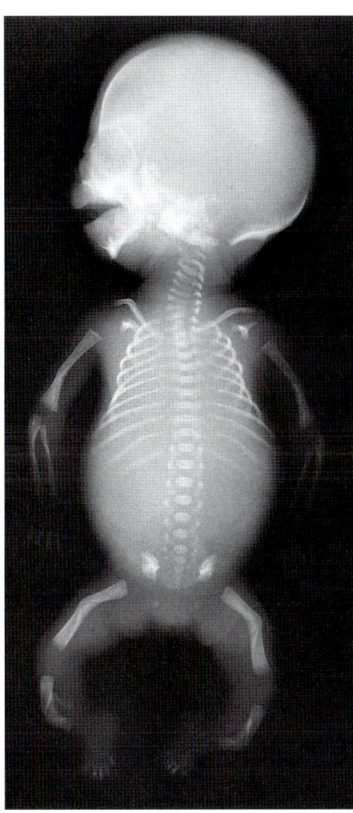

Figure 133-34 A fetus of 21 weeks' gestation with campomelic dysplasia. Radiographic findings include a large skull with a small face; hypoplastic or absent scapular bodies; 11 ribs; poorly ossified thoracic pedicles; tall, narrow iliac wings; and short extremities with proportionately long, bent femurs.

Radiologic Findings (e-Fig. 133-35 and Fig. 133-36)
1. Generalized increased bone density
2. *Skull:* thick and dense, especially at the base
3. *Thorax:* splayed anterior ribs
4. *Spine:* "sandwich" vertebral bodies, "picture frame" vertebral bodies
5. *Extremities:* splayed metaphyses, bone–within–bone configuration, dense metaphyseal bands
6. *Central nervous system:* carbonic anhydrase II deficiency has diffuse dense cerebral calcifications

PYKNODYSOSTOSIS

Pyknodysostosis is an autosomal-recessive disorder that often manifests in infancy. Clinical findings include short-limbed dwarfism, micrognathia, fractures, and short fingertips. The impressionist painter Toulouse-Lautrec likely had this condition.[30]

Radiologic Findings (Fig. 133-37)
1. Generalized osteosclerosis
2. *Skull:* marked delay in closure of fontanels and sutures, wormian bones, obtuse or absent mandibular angle, dense skull
3. *Thorax:* resorbed acromial ends of clavicles
4. *Extremities:* resorbed phalangeal tufts mimicking acro-osteolysis

OSTEOPOIKILOSIS

This is an autosomal-dominant condition caused by mutations in LEMD3.[31] The gene function and its relationship to this disease are not clear. It is often asymptomatic and identified on routine radiographs. These lesions often show increased uptake on bone scans. When skin lesions of dermatofibrosis are also present, the combination is called Buschke-Ollendorff syndrome.

Radiologic Findings (Fig. 133-38)
1. Small foci of bone sclerosis (round, oval, lenticular) located primarily in cancellous bone areas

OSTEOPATHIA STRIATA

This is an asymptomatic sporadic condition, but when associated with cranial sclerosis, it is an X-linked dominant disorder. It is often identified on routine radiographs as a "normal variant." It can be seen, however, as a manifestation of other discrete disorders such as the dysplasia of spondylar changes, nasal anomaly, and striated metaphyses (SPONASTRIME).

Radiologic Findings (Fig. 133-39)
1. Vertical, fine, dense, linear striations
2. Most common at the ends of the long tubular bones, skull and clavicles unaffected
3. No uptake on bone scan

MELORHEOSTOSIS

This is often sporadic but can be seen as an autosomal dominant entity in families with an *LEMD3* gene mutation, similar to osteopoikilosis. Patients can experience bone pain and joint stiffening, as well as limb asymmetry.

Radiologic Findings (Fig. 133-40)
1. Monostotic or polyostotic usually affecting the same extremity
2. Linear dense cortical hyperostosis following the long axis of bones that resembles melting or dripping candle wax
3. Can cross joint space
4. Increased uptake on bone scan

Increased Bone Density Group with Metaphyseal and Diaphyseal Involvement

This group includes the craniotubular dysplasias. The hallmark is sclerosis of the long bones with either a diaphyseal or a metaphyseal focus and abnormal calvarial thickening and sclerosis. Craniodiaphyseal dysplasia, craniometaphyseal dysplasia, and Pyle dysplasia are described here.

CRANIODIAPHYSEAL DYSPLASIA

This rare autosomal-recessive condition manifests in early infancy with progressive facial and calvarial thickening.

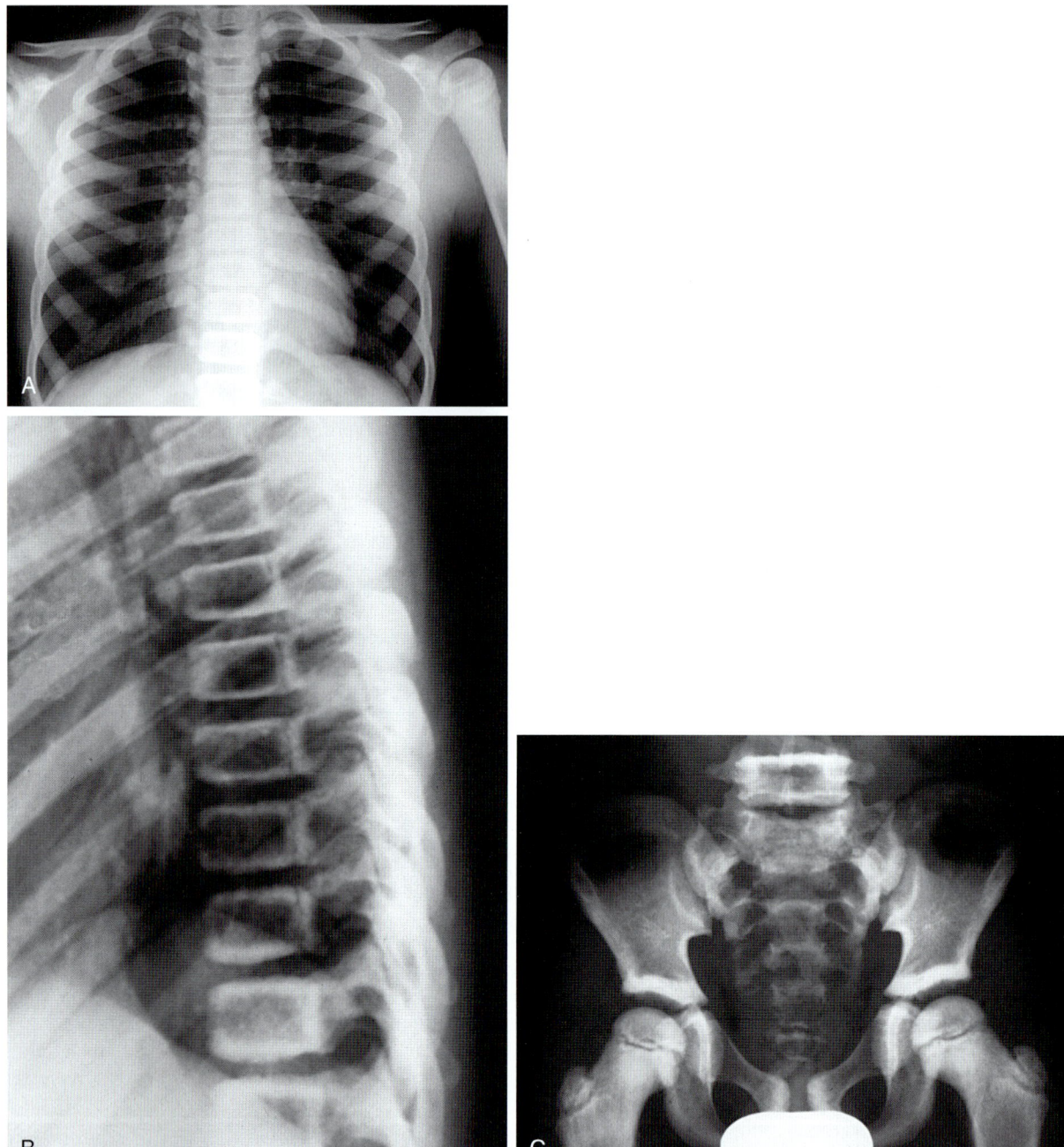

Figure 133-36 An 8-year-old with delayed-type osteopetrosis (autosomal dominant). **A,** Radiographs reveal dense thoracic bones without medullary encroachment of left humerus. **B,** "Sandwich," almost "picture frame" vertebral bodies (dense outer borders). **C,** Increased bone density outlining ileum, including supraacetabular regions, and pubic symphysis region, as well as dense proximal femoral epiphyses and femoral necks with sparing of lower medullary space.

Sudden death, as the result of cranial foraminal narrowing, is frequent.

Radiologic Findings (Fig. 133-41)
1. *Skull:* marked thickening and sclerosis of calvaria and facial bones, obliteration of foramina and sinuses
2. *Thorax:* diffusely widened, sclerotic ribs and clavicles
3. *Extremities:* straightened, undermodeled long bone with diaphyseal widening with metaphyseal sparing; "flame" sclerosis (cortical thickening) of the short-tubular bones (hands)

CRANIOMETAPHYSEAL DYSPLASIA

Two forms of this disease are described on two different gene loci. Both are similar but the autosomal-recessive form is more severe and manifests as cranial and facial thickening, often with nasal obstruction. Improvement may occur with

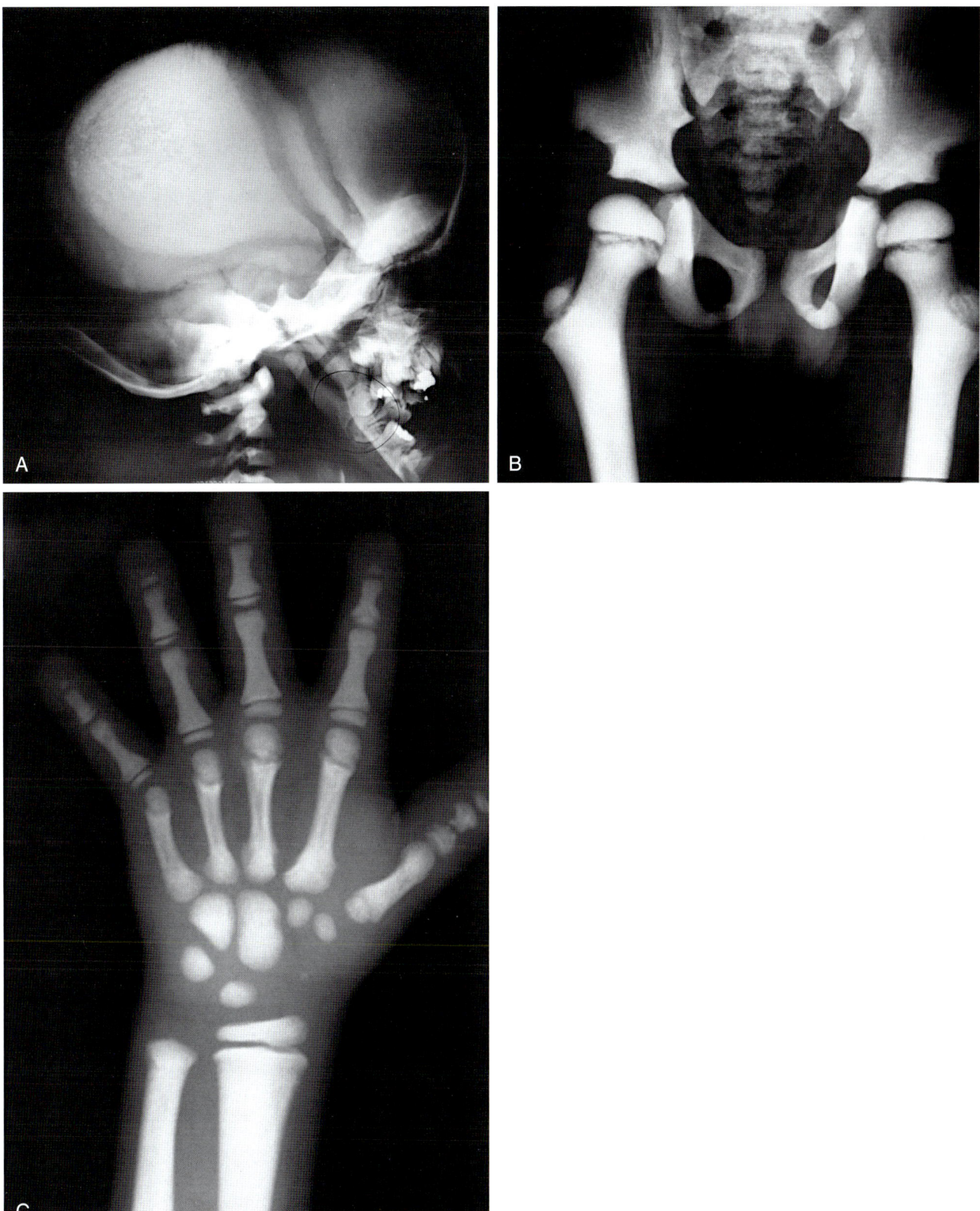

Figure 133-37 An 8-year-old with pyknodysostosis. **A,** Radiographis reveal dense skull convexity and base, widely separated sutures with open fontanel, and absence of mandibular angle. **B,** Hip and pelvis: generalized increased bone density with long, overmodeled (resorbed) femoral necks. **C,** Hands: dense bones, overmodeled metacarpals and phalanges, phalangeal tuft resorption.

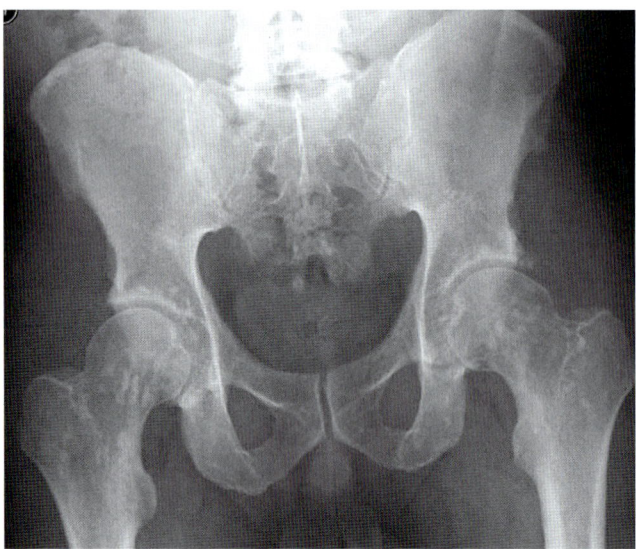

Figure 133-38   Radiographic findings in osteopoikilosis. The anteroposterior view of the pelvis and hips reveals scattered small sclerotic lesions involving the proximal femurs, ilia, and ischia in an affected man.

age. Cranial encroachment–induced neurologic abnormalities may develop.

Radiologic Findings (Fig. 133-42)

1. *Skull:* diffuse hyperostosis of cranial vault base and facial bones, obliterated paranasal sinuses
2. *Extremities:* sclerosis of diaphyses with normal metaphyseal modeling (early), undermodeled flared metaphyses of long bones with normal diaphyses (later)

PYLE DYSPLASIA

This autosomal-recessive entity, also known as *familial metaphyseal dysplasia*, is somewhat similar to craniometaphyseal dysplasia but differs in its minimal craniofacial involvement. Patients are often asymptomatic or develop genu valgum (knock knee).

Radiologic Findings (Fig. 133-43)

1. *Skull:* mild skull and facial involvement, minimal base-of-skull sclerosis, prominent supraorbital ridging
2. *Thorax:* mildly thickened clavicles and ribs, mild platyspondyly
3. *Pelvis:* thickened ischium and pubis
4. *Extremities:* marked undertubulation of long bones, especially distal femurs (Erlenmeyer flask deformity);

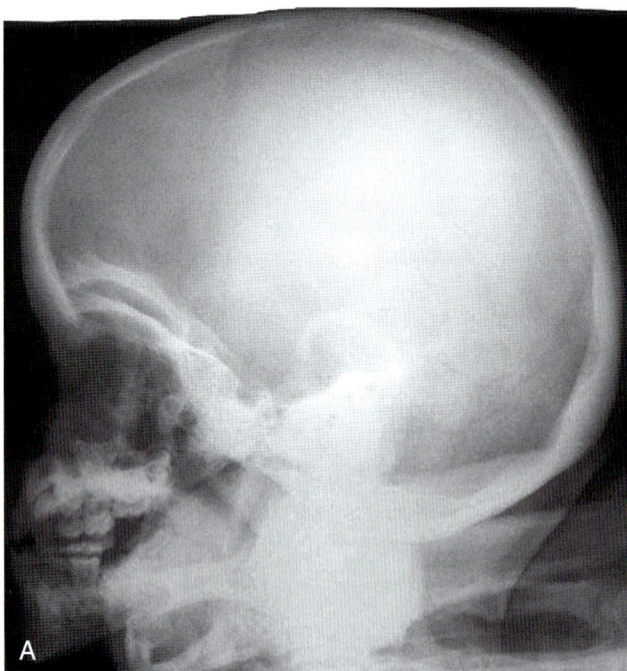

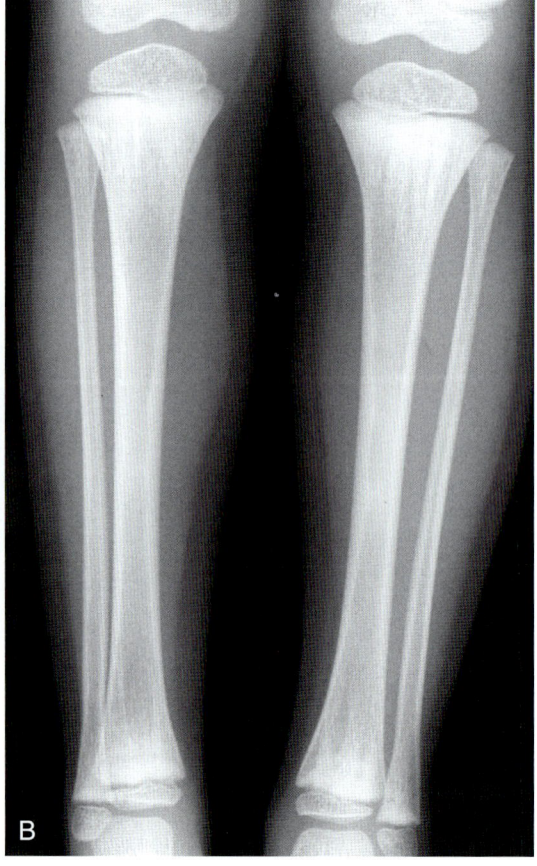

Figure 133-39   Radiographic findings in osteopathia striata with cranial sclerosis. **A,** Lateral skull film revealing dense thickening of the calvaria with increased basilar and orbital sclerosis. **B,** An anteroposterior radiograph of the lower extremity reveals linear striations of the metadiaphyseal regions of both ends of the tibias and fibulas.

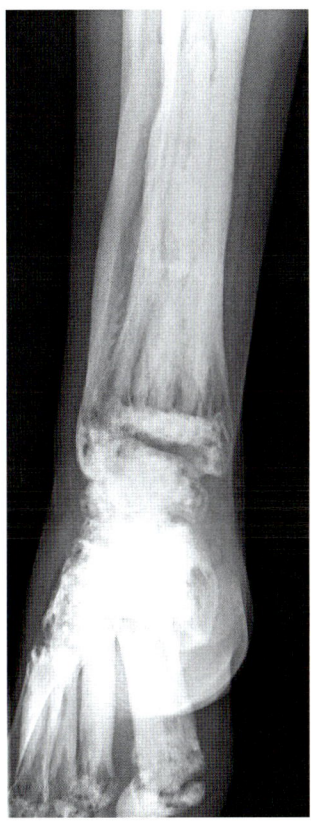

Figure 133-40 Radiographic findings in a 14-year-old boy with melorheostosis. The image of the tibia and fibula and the ankle shows dense "candle-wax dripping" changes involving both tibia and fibula, extending into the epiphyses and across the joint into the tarsal-metatarsal bones.

distal flaring of metacarpals and proximal flaring of phalanges

Osteogenesis Imperfecta and Decreased Bone Density

The cardinal feature of osteogenesis imperfecta (OI) is increased bone fragility. Clinically, a bluish hue to the sclerae may be seen.

The initial classification of OI was divided into the congenita and tarda forms. With the recognition that all forms are genetically determined, the congenita/tarda system was discontinued. Since 1979, OI is classified according to the Sillence classification. Originally including only four types, this system has now grown to eight types (Table 133-1). The Sillence classification describes a spectrum of disease rather than a strict system based on objective scientific identities such as molecular genetics. In fact, we know now that multiple allelic mutations affect collagen I and cause OI, although other OI types are unrelated to collagen I abnormalities.

Radiologic Findings, Severe Type (Fig. 133-44)
1. *Skull:* very poor to no ossification
2. *Thorax:* small, narrow chest; beaded ribs from healing fractures
3. *Spine:* severe deossification, collapsed vertebral bodies
4. *Extremities:* generalized osteoporosis with or without fractures; shortened, widened long bones with thin cortices; accordion–shaped femurs

Radiologic Findings, Mild Types (e-Fig. 133-45)
1. *Skull:* abnormal number of wormian bones (>8 to 10), variable decrease in ossification

Table 133-1

Osteogenesis Imperfecta Classification System				
Type 1	Mild	Mild bone fragility	Autosomal dominant	Abnormal type I collagen
Type 2	Severe, lethal	Minimal cranial ossification Short accordion femurs with multiple fractures in long bones, beaded ribs	Autosomal dominant	Abnormal type I collagen
Type 3	Severe	Multiple fractures even at birth Short stature deformed long bones Scoliosis	Autosomal dominant	Abnormal type I collagen
Type 4	Moderate, variable severity	Multiple fractures with deformity Not as severe as type 3	Autosomal dominant	Abnormal type I collagen
Type 5	Moderate severity	Calcification of interosseous membrane of forearm Hypertrophic callus at fracture sites Metaphyseal dense bands	Autosomal dominant	Unknown
Type 6	Moderate severity, very rare	Multiple long bone and vertebral fractures	Autosomal recessive	Mineralization defect of osteoid on bone biopsy Error in pigment epithelium derived factor
Type 7	Severe	Multiple long bone and vertebral fractures	Autosomal recessive	Error in cartilage associated protein (*CRTAP*) gene
Type 8	Severe	Multiple long bone and vertebral fractures	Autosomal recessive	Severe deficiency of prolyl 3-hydroxylase activity due to mutations in the *LEPRE1* gene

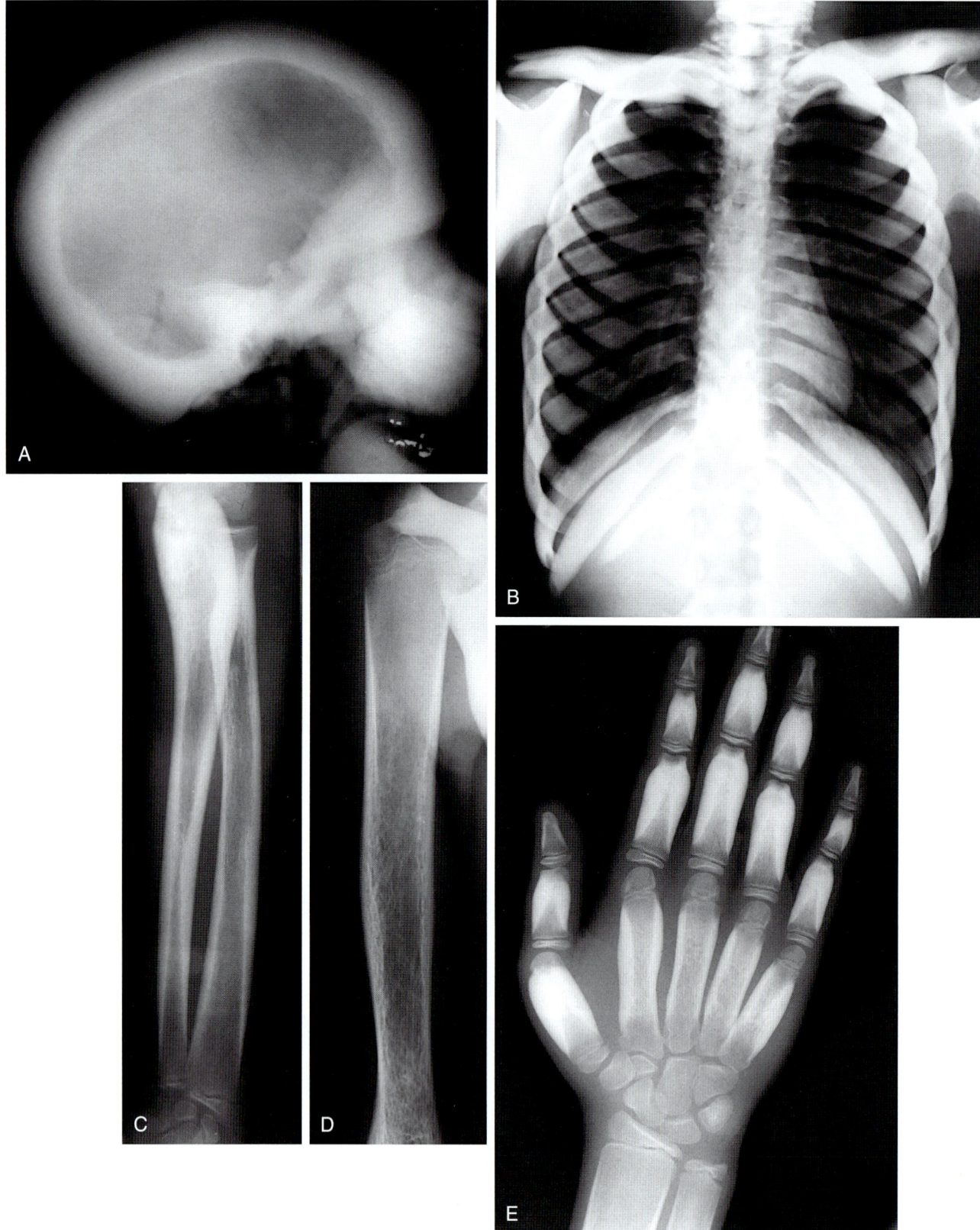

Figure 133-41   Radiographic findings in a 13-year-old with craniodiaphyseal dysplasia. **A,** Extremely dense bone filling in the facial region and thickening the diploic space. **B,** Diffusely dense, thickened ribs and clavicles. **C** and **D,** Diffuse cortical long bone diaphyseal thickening and diaphyseal undermodeling. **E,** "Flame" sclerosis (cortical thickening) of the tubular bones of the hand.

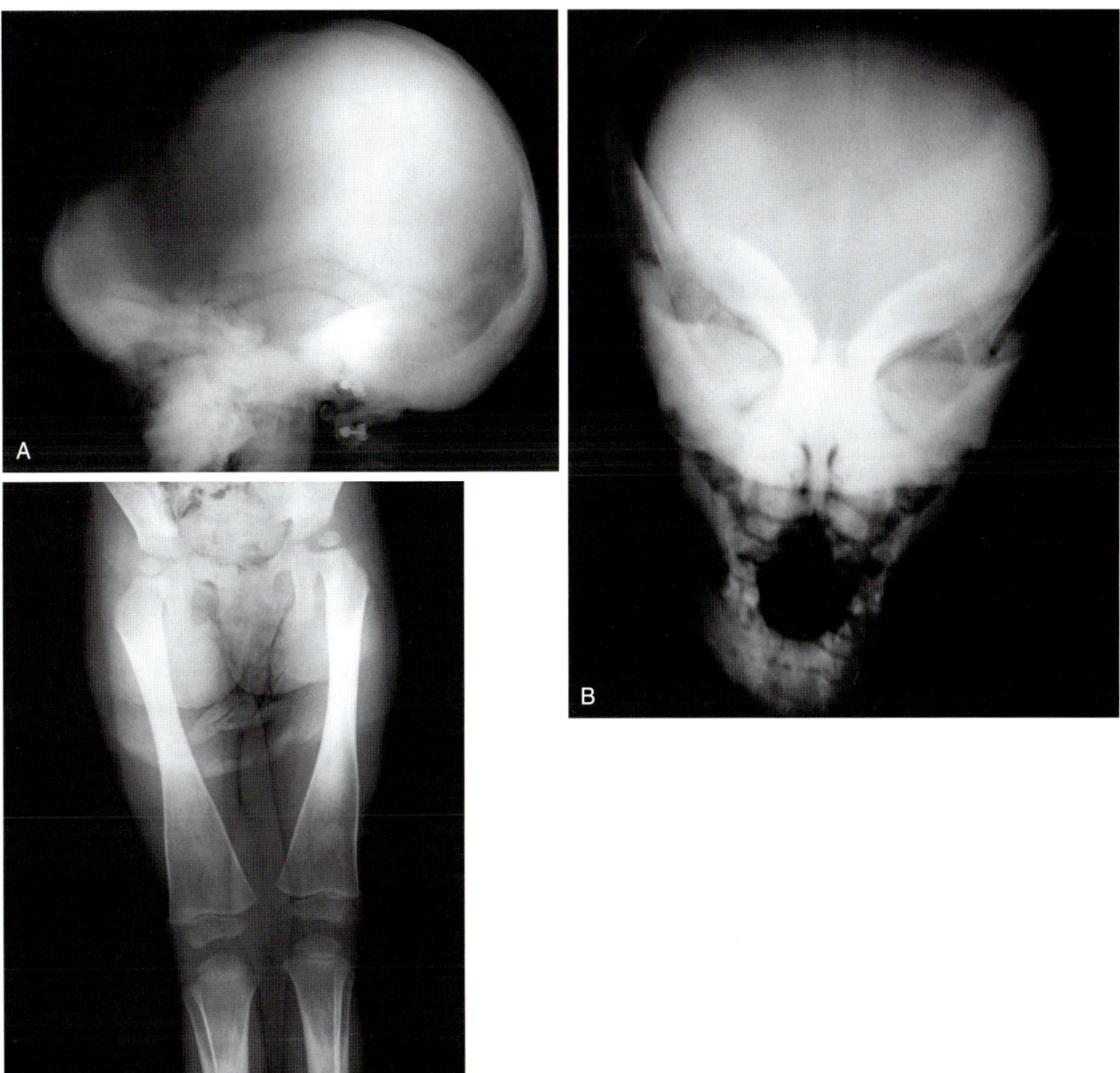

Figure 133-42   Radiographic findings in a 2-year-old with craniometaphyseal dysplasia. **A** and **B,** Marked increased bone density of cranial base and vault, and dense facial bones with obliteration of sinuses. **C,** Undermodeled flared metaphyses (Erlenmeyer flask deformity) of distal femurs.

2. *Spine:* wedged or collapsed vertebrae
3. *Extremities:* at least some osteoporosis, variable number of fractures (especially pathologic fractures)

Abnormal Mineralization Group

Among the dysplasias with defective mineralization, one important entity to recognize and discuss is hypophosphatasia.

HYPOPHOSPHATASIA

The two distinct genetic forms of hypophosphatasia are (1) the autosomal-recessive perinatal lethal or infantile type and (2) a later-onset autosomal-dominant adult type. Both result from an abnormality of the enzyme alkaline phosphatase. The chromosome loci for both conditions are 1p36.1–34 and involve *TNSALP*. The perinatal or lethal form appears to represent autosomal-recessive inheritance, whereas the adult form is probably autosomal dominant. As a consequence of

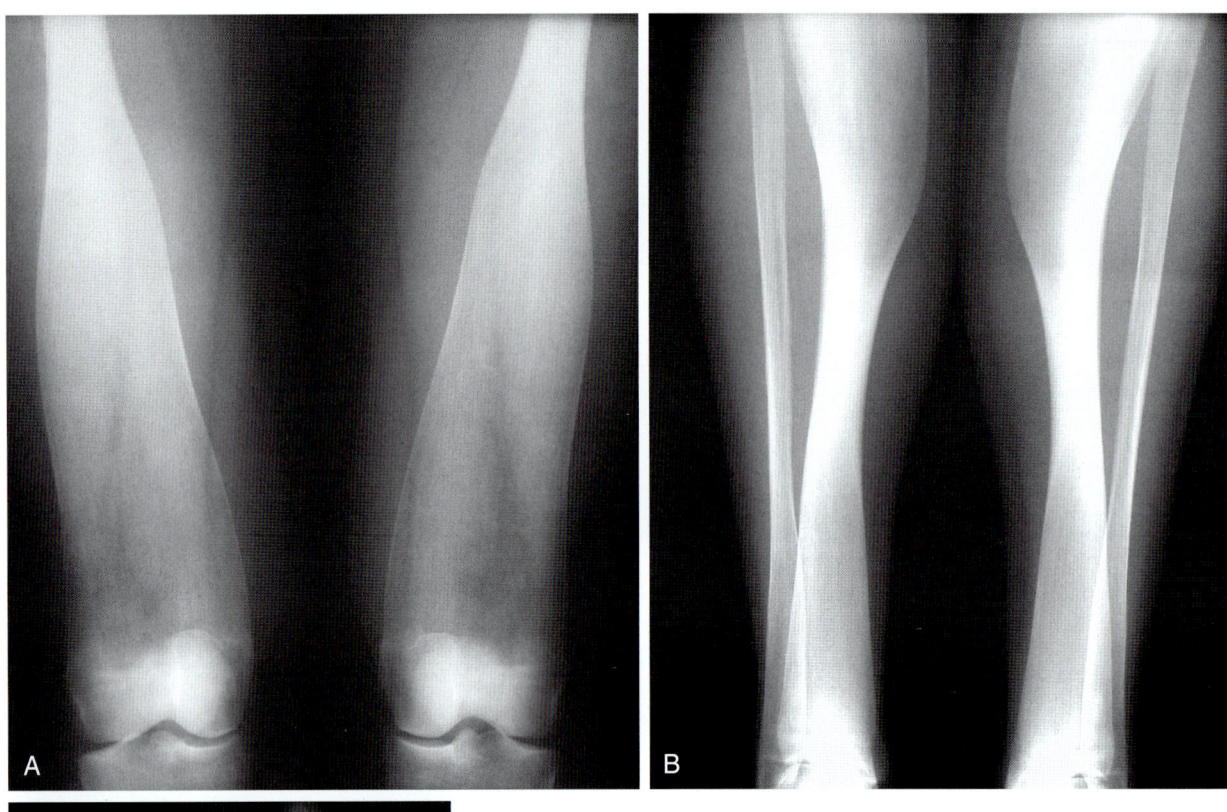

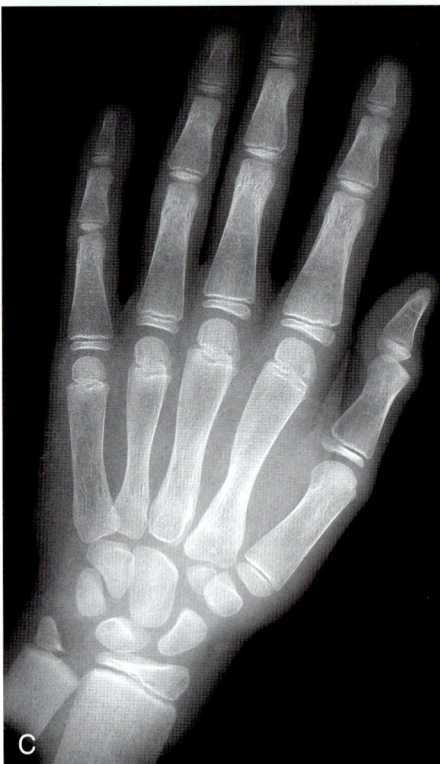

Figure 133-43 Radiographic findings in pyle dysplasia. **A** and **B,** In an affected 17-year-old, markedly broad, undertubulated distal femurs (**A**) and markedly broad, undertubulated proximal and distal tibias with mild medial bowing proximally (**B**). **C,** In a different patient, distal flaring of metacarpals and proximal flaring of phalanges are seen. The distal radial and ulnar metaphyses are broadened.

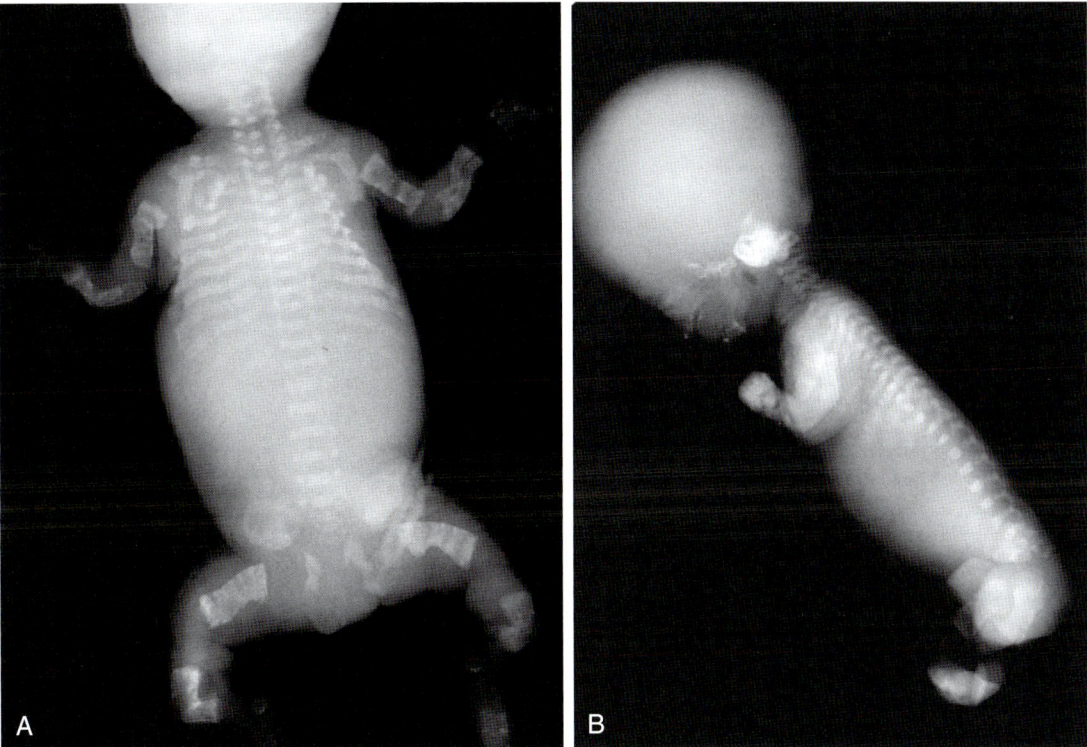

Figure 133-44 Radiographic findings in a stillborn full-term fetus with osteogenesis imperfecta type II. **A** and **B,** Findings include generalized osteoporosis, absence of skull ossification, beaded ribs, and crumpled long bones.

defective alkaline phosphatase, bone formation is impaired because of local increase in phosphate, impaired hydroxyapatite formation, and hypercalcemia with resultant Rickets-like changes.

Radiologic Findings (e-Fig. 133-46)
Perinatal lethal/infantile form:
1. *Skull:* decreased ossification with single island-like centers for frontal occipital and parietal bones
2. *Thorax:* poorly ossified ribs; thin, wavy, fractured ribs; clavicles not affected
3. *Spine:* sporadic unossified vertebral bodies, dense and osteopenic vertebrae, sporadic platyspondyly, butterfly-shaped vertebral bodies, sporadic missing pedicles
4. *Extremities:* generalized decreased ossification, chromosome-shaped femurs, metaphyseal cupping and irregularity, central lucent defect, "campomelic femurs," sporadic "missing" short tubular bones of hands and feet

Adult form:
1. Generalized osteopenia
2. *Extremities:* metaphyseal widening (rickets-like changes), punched-out metaphyseal lesions, pathologic fractures
3. Heterotopic calcifications

Lysosomal Storage Diseases

The dysostosis multiplex group contains all the mucopolysaccharidoses (MPSs), mucolipidoses, and multiple other storage diseases that produce a skeletal dysplasia. The abnormalities in this entire group consist of well-described enzymatic defects that can be diagnosed by appropriate urine, blood, or fibroblast culture analyses. These diseases act similarly on the skeleton to produce a abnormalities of varying severity, termed dysostosis multiplex. The real role of the radiologist is to suggest the likelihood of one of these disorders; the geneticist biochemically determines which exact dysplasia it is. Hurler or Hunter syndrome (MPS types IH and II) may be used as stereotypical examples of this group. Morquio syndrome (MPS types IVA and IVB) can often be differentiated from other MPS entities radiographically, as it has very prominent epiphyseal changes. In Hurler or Hunter syndrome, inferior beaking of the vertebral bodies with kyphosis is centered on the thoracolumbar junctions. This is known as *gibbus type abnormality* and is related to hypotonia in affected patients. This is a secondary effect from chronic pressure and stress on the vertebral bodies at the thoracolumbar junction and causes delay in ossification of the inferior portion of the T12 and L1 disk spaces. In Morquio syndrome, the central tongue or beaked appearance is caused by the primary dysplasia from a delay in epiphyseal ossification and causes a delay in ossification at the lower and upper end plates.

HURLER OR HURLER SYNDROME (MUCOPOLYSACCHARIDOSIS TYPE IH & II)

The enzyme abnormality is alpha-L-l-iduronidase, located on chromosome 4p. As with all the other members of this group, the inheritance pattern is recessive. Most of the MPS entities manifest clinically in late infancy or early childhood.

Radiologic Findings (Dysostosis Multiplex) (Fig. 133-47)

1. *Skull:* enlarged neurocranium, abnormal J-shaped sella
2. *Thorax:* short, thick clavicles; paddle (oar)–shaped ribs; hypoplastic glenoid
3. *Spine:* gibbus, superior notched (inferior beaked) thoracolumbar vertebral bodies, upper cervical subluxation
4. *Pelvis:* flared, small iliac wings with inferior tapering; steep acetabular roofs
5. *Extremities:* diaphyseal widening of long bones; hands characteristically exhibit brachydactyly, proximal metacarpal "pointing," diaphyseal widening of metacarpals and proximal or middle phalanges, small irregular carpal bones

MORQUIO SYNDROME (MUCOPOLYSACCHARIDOSIS TYPES IVA AND IVB)

The enzyme abnormality is in galactose-6-sulfatase, resulting in the accumulation of excess MPS material in multiple organ systems, including the skeletal system. MPS IVB patients usually have more mild radiographic and clinical findings compared with MPS IVA.

Radiologic Findings (Differentiating Features from Other Mucopolysaccharidoses) (Fig. 133-48)

1. *Skull:* no J-shaped sella
2. *Thorax:* widened, not oar shaped, ribs

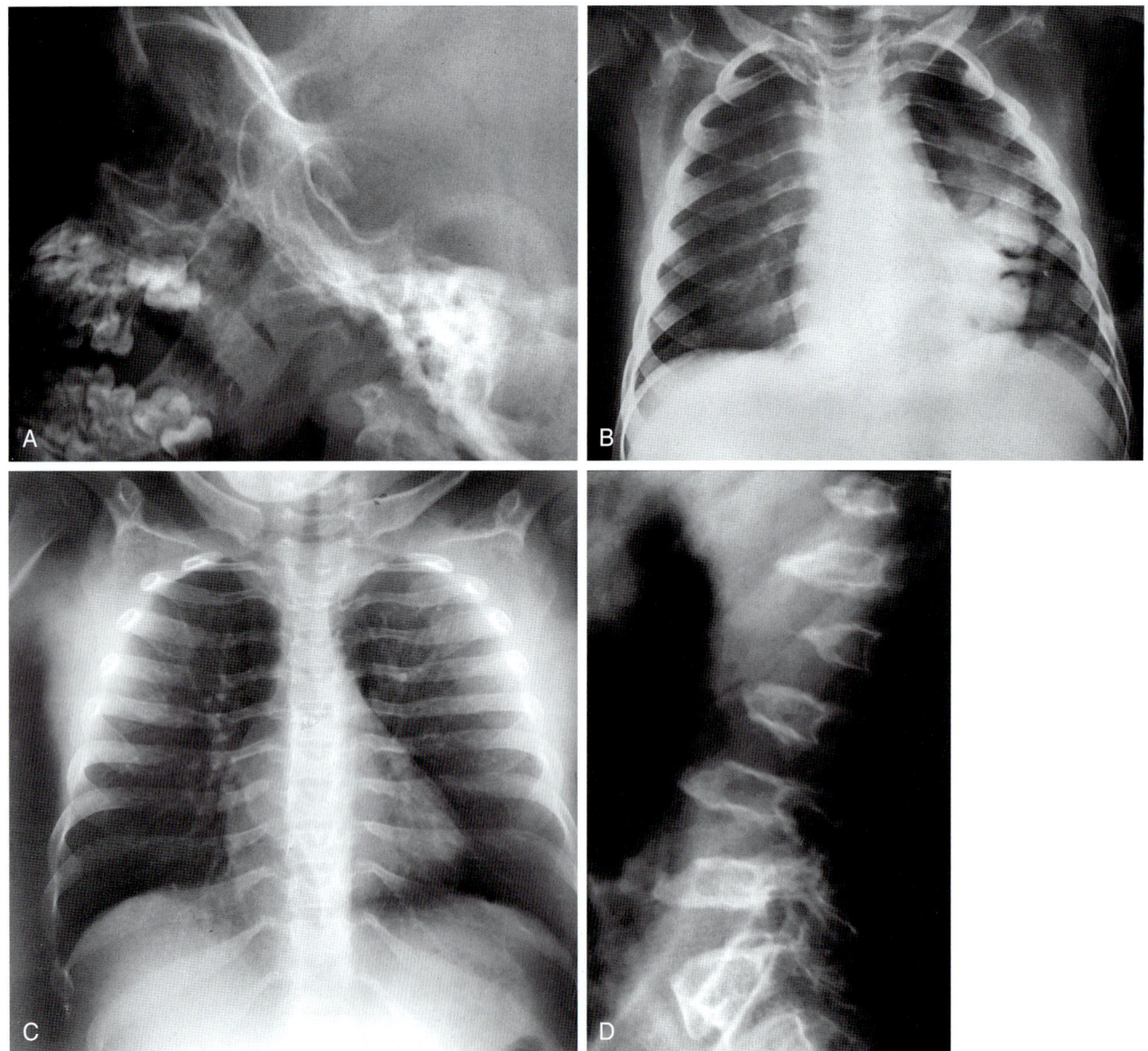

Figure 133-47 Hurler syndrome (mucopolysaccharidosis type IH). **A,** Skull of an affected 3-year-old with abnormal, excavated J-shaped sella turcica. **B** and **C,** Thoraces of an affected 3-year-old (**B**) and an affected 8-year-old (**C**) with thick clavicles and paddle-shaped ribs (thin posteriorly and thick anteriorly). **D,** Spine of an affected 8-year-old with superiorly notched (inferiorly beaked) vertebral bodies. Radiographic findings in Hurler syndrome (mucopolysaccharidosis type IH).

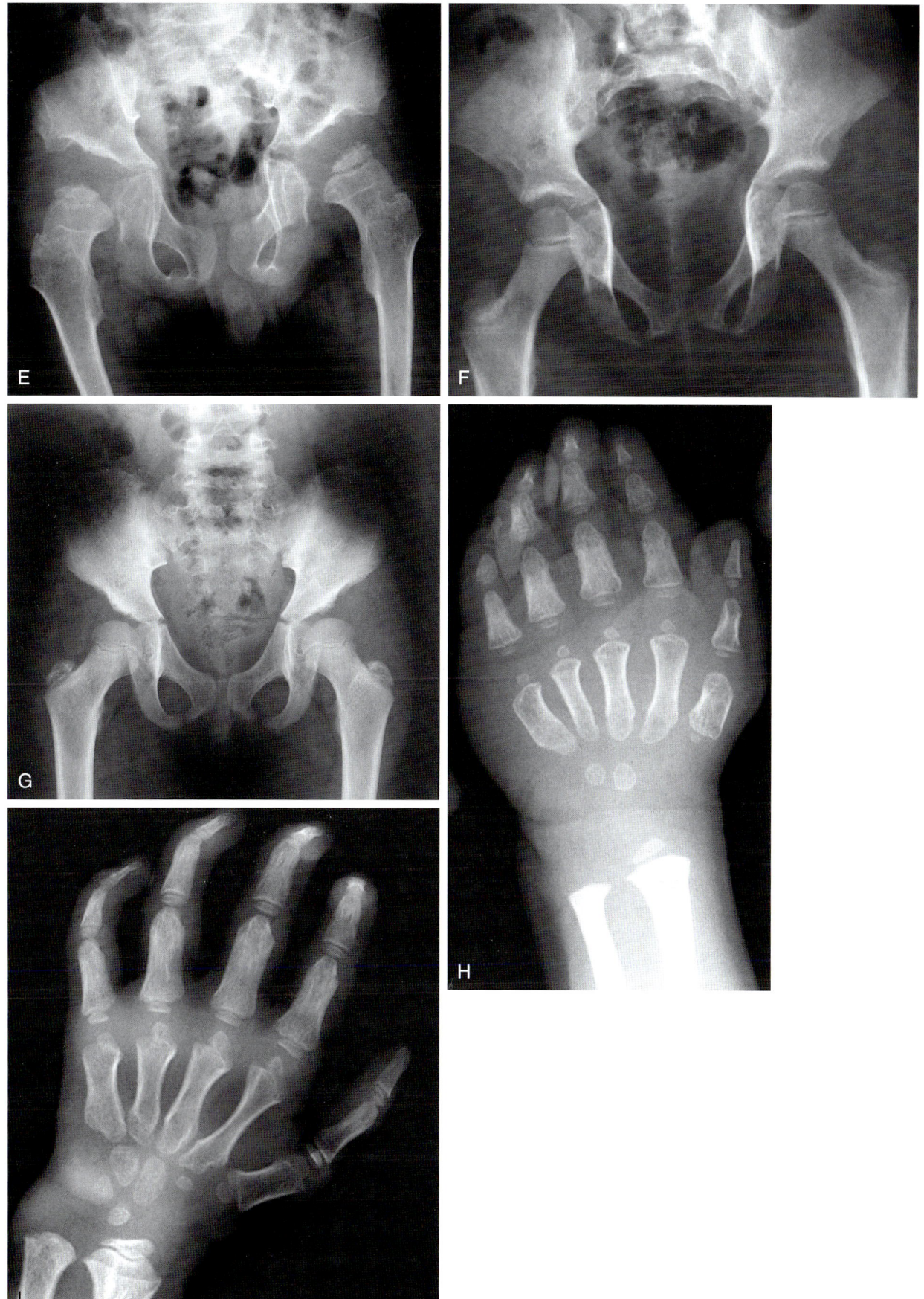

Figure 133-47, cont'd.   **E** to **G,** Pelvis of an affected 8-year-old (**E**), another affected 8-year-old (**F**), and an affected 12-year-old (**G**) with small iliac wings with inferior tapering, and a slanted, irregular acetabular roof (**E** and **G**). **H** and **I,** Hands of an affected 6-year-old (**H**) and an affected 10-year-old (**I**) with proximal metacarpal pointing and epiphyseal ossification delay.

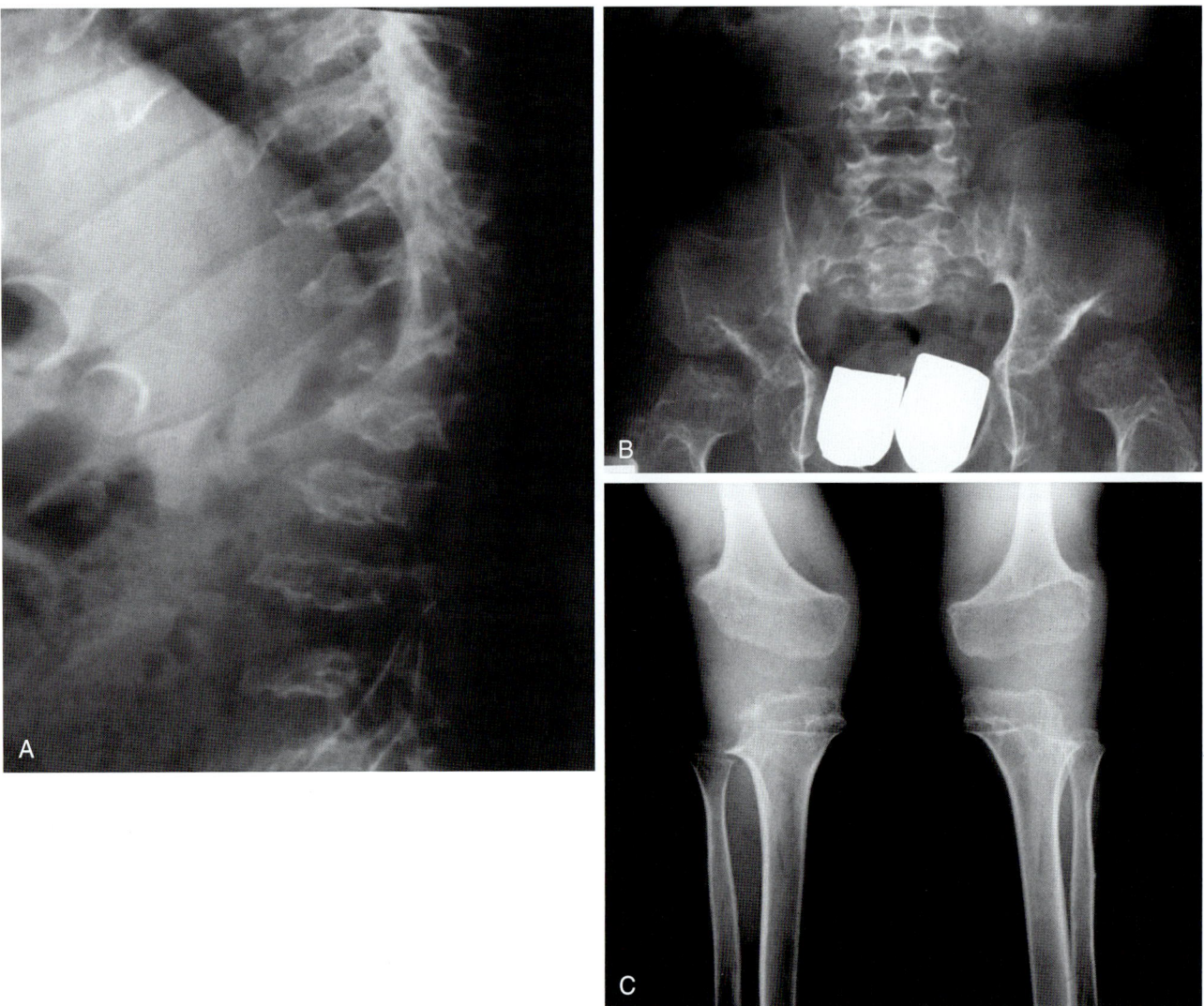

Figure 133-48 Morquio syndrome (mucopolysaccharidosis types IVA and IVB). **A,** Radiograph from an affected 7-year-old with platyspondyly with central beaking (tongue). **B,** Radiograph from an affected 18-year-old with severe capital femoral epiphyseal and acetabular dysplasia but no inferior iliac tapering. **C,** Radiograph from an affected 15-year-old with lateral distal femoral and proximal tibial epiphyseal ossification defects with genu varum.

3. *Spine:* central vertebral beaking or tongue; odontoid hypoplasia and cervical instability
4. *Pelvis:* no tapering of ileum, steep acetabular roofs
5. *Extremities:* proximal metacarpal rounding, genu valgus; epiphyseal dysplasia especially at carpal bones and femoral heads

MUCOLIPIDOSIS TYPE II (I-CELL DISEASE)

Mucolipidosis type II is an enzyme abnormality, of N-acetylglucosamine phosphotransferase, the gene for which is found on chromosome 4q. It clinically and radiographically manifests in the newborn and can be seen prenatally. Most affected patients die in infancy. Certain radiographic features are quite unique.

Radiologic Findings (e-Fig. 133-49)

1. *Extremities:* severe osteopenia with metaphyseal cupping and fraying, poorly defined cortices, "periosteal cloaking" or reaction seen diffusely with areas of cortical bone destruction; diaphyseal expansion
2. *Pelvis:* wide iliac flare with hypoplastic lower iliac segment, steep acetabular roofs
3. *Spine:* biconvex end plates with anterior concavity of the vertebral bodies
4. The changes of dysostosis multiplex occur later

Osteolysis Group

This group includes a range of syndromes all with varying degrees of osteolysis present. The separate syndromes are best classified according to their primary sites of involvement.

1. Multicentric hands and feet
   a. Multicentric carpal or tarsal osteolysis with or without nephropathy
   b. Torg syndrome or Winchester syndrome or nodulosis with arthropathy syndrome

2. Acro-osteolysis
   a. Hajdu-Cheney syndrome (HCS)
   b. Mandubuloacral syndrome
3. Diaphyseal and metaphyseal
   a. Familial expansile osteolysis

Hadju-Cheney Syndrome

Distinctive transverse (bandlike) acro-osteolysis is present; skull features, including persistence of the skull sutures, a J-shaped sella, and wormian bones, characterize HCS. More important, however, is the progressive osteoporosis that occurs and can lead to vertebral body fractures. Many patients with confirmed HCS have an elongated and gracile twisting fibula and polycystic kidneys. Serpentine fibula polycystic kidney syndrome had been considered a separate genetic syndrome, but recently, the same genetic defect in the NOTCH2 signaling pathway has been found to cause both syndromes, unifying the picture.[32]

NOTCH2 is interesting for its effects on the skeleton and tumorogenesis. The defect in HCS causes an upmodulation in NOTCH signaling, which inhibits endochondral growth and osteoblastic differentiation resulting in osteopenia[33]. Errors in the NOTCH signaling pathway have been associated with T-cell leukemia and lymphoma (NOTCH1).[34] Dysregulated NOTCH signaling is known to occur in multiple myeloma. Recently, enhanced NOTCH2 signaling has been associated with osteosarcoma and is associated with greater tumor invasiveness.[35]

Radiologic Findings (Fig. 133-50)
1. *Skull:* wormian bones; cranial sutures remain open through adult life, hypoplastic sinuses, edentulous mandible
2. *Extremities:* bandlike acro-osteolysis; progressive osteopenia

Overgrowth Syndromes with Skeletal Involvement

Important members of this group include Marfan syndrome, congenital contractural arachnodactyly (CCA), and Proteus syndrome.

MARFAN SYNDROME AND CONGENITAL CONTRACTURAL ARACHNODACTYLY

These two congenital syndromes are caused by errors in fibrilin. Fibrilin is a glycoprotein that functions as a structural scaffold for elastic microfibrils. It can be found in abundance in the connective tissues of the walls of large vessels, lungs, bones, and eyes. The marfanoid body habitus is a constant feature along with long spidery fingers (hence the term *arachnodactyly*) and tall stature. The loss of normal fibrilin may allow liberation of transforming growth factor-β from the connective tissues, thereby allowing greater expressivity as tall stature.[36,37]

Dislocation of the lens of the eye occurs since fibrilin is found in the supportive connective tissues of the lens. The

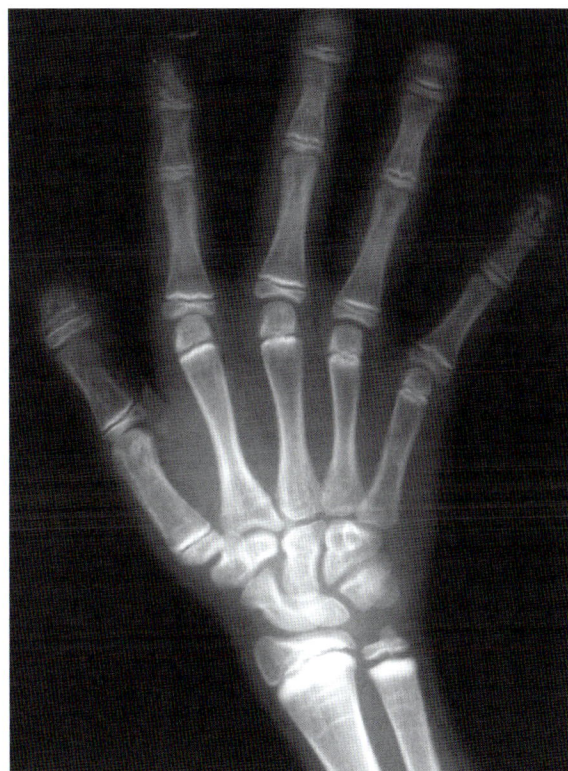

Figure 133-50 Hajdu-Cheney syndrome in a 14-year-old boy. The anteroposterior view of the hand shows transverse acro-osteolysis of the distal phalanges. Note the dense sclerosis at metaphyses—the patient takes bisphosphonates to enhance bone mineral density.

lack of normal fibrilin damages the elastic walls of the large vessels. Aortic root dilatation and rupture are the leading cause of death.

Marfan syndrome is a fibrilin 1 abnormality, whereas CCA is a fibrilin 2 abnormality. The two are phenotypically similar, each manifesting the typical marfanoid body habitus. However, patients with CCA also have joint contractures at the proximal interphalangeal joints, elbows, and knees. Although joint contractures can occur in Marfan syndrome, it is not a hallmark.

Radiographic Features (e-Fig. 133-51)
1. *Skull:* dolicocephaly, arched palate
2. *Thorax:* scoliosis, pectus deformities, dural ectasia
3. *Pelvis:* acetabular protrusion deformity
4. *Extremities:* dolichostenomelia (long thin limbs or bones), arachnodactyly, joint hyperextensibility, osteopenia
5. *Other:* aortic root dilatation, spontaneous pneumothorax

PROTEUS SYNDROME

Proteus syndrome is named for the Greek god Proteus, who was able to change his shape at will. Proteus syndrome is a congenital hamartomatous disorder, which may be autosomal dominant. Affected patients have overgrowth of the hands and feet, limb asymmetry, gross cranial hyperostosis, and facial asymmetry leading to a frequently grotesque appearance. Patients with Proteus syndrome may also have mixed vascular malformations. Some have suggested that Joseph Merrick, also known as "the elephant man," may have had Proteus syndrome rather than neurofibromatosis as was originally thought.

The radiographic findings of Proteus syndrome reflect what is seen clinically, namely, overgrowth of limbs and digits from both bone and soft tissues. Several types of tumors are associated with Proteus syndrome, including lipomas that tend to grow aggressively, ovarian cystadenoma, monomorphic parotid adenoma, testicular tumors, and central nervous system tumors (especially meningiomas).

Radiologic Findings (e-Fig. 133-52)
1. *Skull:* macrocrania with cortical hyperostosis, dolichocephaly, and facial asymmetry
2. *Thorax:* scoliosis, kyphosis, large and asymmetric vertebral bodies
3. *Extremities:* asymmetric bone and soft tissue overgrowth
4. *Other:* mixed vascular malformations, hydrocephalus, emphysematous lung disease (12%)

Other Disorders

CLEIDOCRANIAL DYSPLASIA

In this autosomal-dominant disorder, the chromosome locus is at 6p21 coding for a gene called *CBFA1* (core binding factor a1), also known as *RUNX2*. This dysplasia is quite common, with marked clinical variability and is often diagnosable at birth. The clinical findings include enlarged skull with large, late-closing fontanels; dental abnormalities; drooping, hypermobile shoulders; mild short stature; and a narrow chest.

Radiologic Findings (Fig. 133-53)
1. *Skull:* large, brachycephalic; wormian bones; wide sutures; persistently open anterior fontanel
2. *Thorax:* absence or hypoplasia of clavicles, mildly shortened ribs with downward slope, 11 ribs
3. *Spine:* significant posterior wedging of thoracic vertebrae
4. *Pelvis:* high narrow iliac wings, absence or hypoplasia of pubic bones
5. *Extremities:* numerous pseudoepiphyses of metacarpals and tapered distal phalanges in the hands

CURRARINO TRIAD

Currarino triad (hereditary sacral agenesis syndrome) consists of imperforate or stenotic anus, osseous sacral defect, and a presacral mass.[38] The presacral mass may be a teratoma (two thirds of cases), a lipoma, a dermoid cyst, an enteric cyst, or an anterior meningocele. The first sacral segment is not affected. The remainder of the sacrum is deformed into a sickle shape because of partial agenesis. Life-threatening meningitis and sepsis may occur, particularly with presacral anterior meningoceles. Moreover, approximately 50% of presacral tumors communicate with the spinal canal in Currarino triad, making surgical repair difficult without neurologic complications. The syndrome is another homeobox type mutation, this one at 7q36 affecting the *HLXB9* homeobox gene.

Radiologic Findings (e-Fig. 133-54)
1. Congenital anal stenosis or low imperforate anus
2. Sickle or scimitar hemisacrum
3. Presacral mass (teratoma, lipoma, dermoid cyst, enteric cyst, or anterior meningocele)[39]

BRACHYDACTYLY GROUP

Rubinstein-Taybi Syndrome

Rubinstein-Taybi syndrome is characterized by short stature, distinctive facial features, mental retardation, and broad, short thumbs and great toes. It is caused by sporadic mutations, the majority affecting the CREB-binding protein, which plays an important role in embryonic development. In slightly more than half of the patients, a cytogenetic abnormality can be identified. Radiographically, a delta-phalanx (longitudinal epiphyseal bracket) is seen at the first proximal phalanx (Fig. 133-55). The first distal phalanx is short and broad. At times, it may have a central lucency indicating an attempt at duplication. Other findings include congenital heart defects, agenesis of the corpus callosum, and vertebral and sternal anomalies. Patients have an increased risk of tumors, mainly meningioma, leukemia, and lymphoma.

Poland Syndrome

Poland syndrome includes a spectrum of abnormalities that includes absence or hypoplasia of the pectoralis major muscle and variable deformities of the ipsilateral upper extremity. In the mildest form, absence or hypoplasia of the pectoralis major muscle is seen. In the most severe presentations in the chest, absence of some ribs, scoliosis, absence of the latissimus dorsi, and mammary hypoplasia are seen. The entire hemithoracic cavity may be shortened with a low-riding clavicular head and high-riding insertion of the rectus abdominus. In the hands, ipsilateral shortening of fingers 2 to 4, with cutaneous syndactyly, is seen.

The cause is thought to be an interruption of the embryonic vascular supply during the sixth week of gestation, at a time when the chest wall musculature and hand are differentiating Generally, the sternal head of the pectoralis major muscle is affected, as the clavicular head is known to form first and is, therefore, usually present.

Radiologic Findings (Fig. 133-56)
1. Hyperlucent hemithorax and absent axillary fold related to absence of the pectoralis major muscle
2. Syndactyly and polydactyly of ipsilateral upper extremity
3. Brachymesophalangy (brachydactyly of the middle phalanges)

LIMB HYPOPLASIA—REDUCTION DEFECTS GROUP

Brachydactyly A-E

The brachydactyly classification system most commonly used was described by Bell in 1951 and refined by Temtamy and McKusick in 1978.[40-42] Since these descriptions, the genetic loci associated with many of the types of isolated brachydactyly have been elucidated. Some of the patterns of shortening of the bones of the hand will be easily recognized by the practicing radiologist. Brachdactyly type A3 in which the fifth

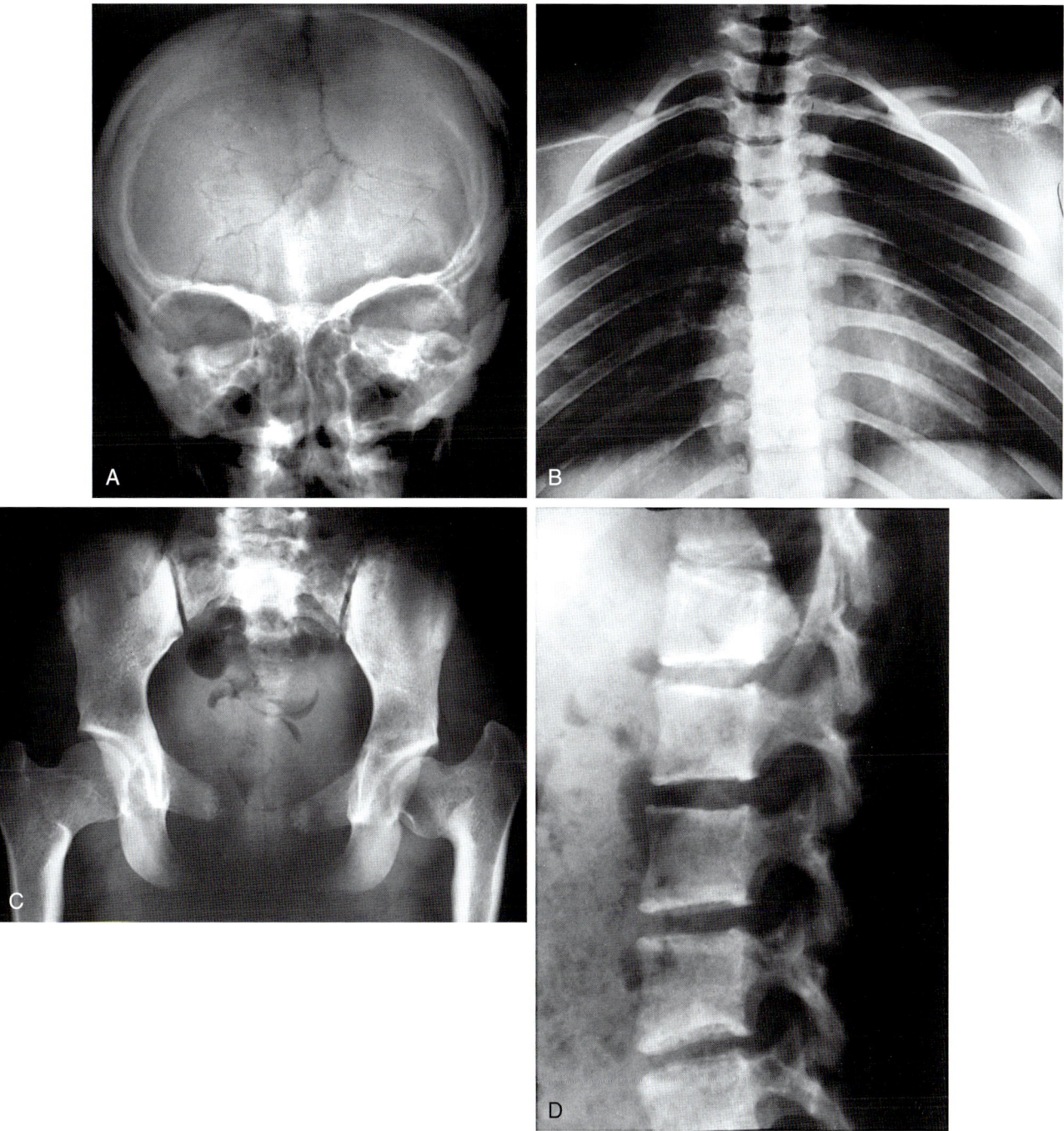

Figure 133-53 A 15-year-old with cleidocranial dysplasia. **A,** Skull: large open anterior fontanel and multiple wormian bones. **B,** Thorax: asymmetric hypoplastic or absent clavicles and downward-sloping ribs. **C,** Pelvis: tall, narrow ilia and hypoplastic pubic bones. **D,** Spine: posteriorly wedged but otherwise normal vertebral bodies.

middle phalanx is short is especially common. This can be differentiated from (1) Kirner deformity, with radial bowing of the distal phalanx, and (2) camptodactyly, with a flexion contracture of the interphalangeal joints.

Brachydactylies are usually isolated genetic abnormalities, but some may have associated syndromes or metabolic conditions. Variable shortening of the metacarpals is classified as brachydactyly type E which most commonly affects the fourth and fifth rays. A short fourth metacarpal is also a well-known feature of many syndromes, including Turner syndrome and pseudohypoparathyroidism or pseudopseudohypoparathroidism (PHP/PPHP). Many patients with brachydactyly type E are short and, as such, may be indistinguishable from those with PHP/PPHP.

Brachmann-De Lange (Cornelia De Lange) Syndrome

Brachmann-De Lange syndrome is characterized by multiple congenital anomalies, including microcephaly, limb anomalies, digital anomalies, marked mental retardation and a distinctive facial appearance.

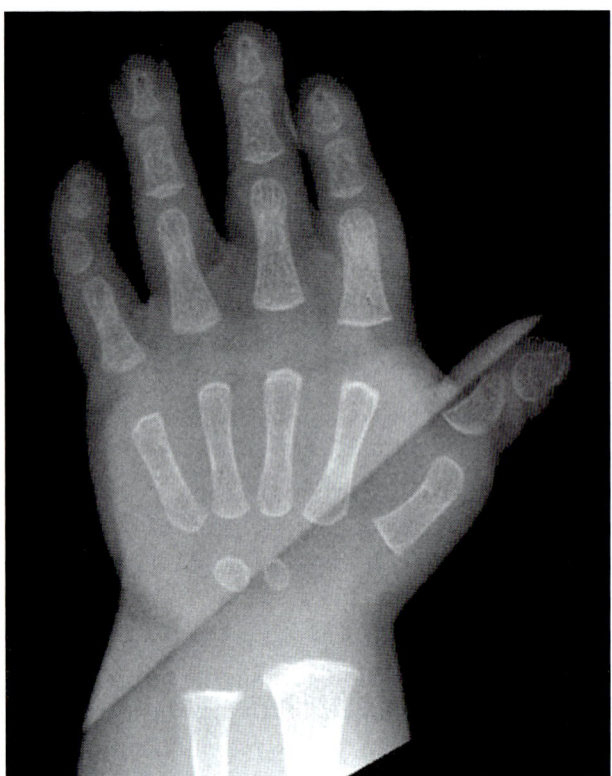

Figure 133-55 Rubinstein-Taybi syndrome in an 8-month-old boy. The anteroposterior view of the hand exhibits the classic delta phalanx at the first proximal phalanx.

The head is small with a single confluent eyebrow. The nose is upturned, and the upper lip is downturned, giving the philtrum a flat and elongated appearance that echoes fetal alcohol spectrum disorder. Congenital heart defects, urinary anomalies, and congenital diaphragmatic hernias have been reported.

Limb anomalies include micromelia, phocomelia, and hemimelia. Whereas the radius may be absent in many other syndromes, in this case, it is the ulna that is deficient. The radial head may be dislocated. Digital findings include syndactyly, oligodactyly, small digits, and proximally placed thumbs. Skeletal maturation is retarded. The chest is small and the ribs are slender and have an undulating appearance.

Radiologic Findings (Fig. 133-57)

1. *Skull:* microcephaly
2. *Thorax:* slender small ribs
3. *Extremities:* Limb anomalies including phocomelia, radial head dislocation, absent ulna, syndactyly with proximally places thumbs

Holt-Oram Syndrome

Holt-Oram syndrome, also called *heart–hand syndrome*, is caused by a completely penetrant mutation involving *TBX5* at 12q2. *TBX5* encodes a protein that plays a role in heart development and limb identity and patterning. It is part of the T-box gene family, which encodes transcription factors important in body development.

The disease is familial in 60% to 70% of cases; new mutations account for the remainder. Limb anomalies range from phocomelia with absent or hypoplastic humerus (10% of patients in some series) to triphalangeal thumbs. The most common limb anomalies are radial ray anomalies. These include absence of hypoplasia of the radius, bipartite or hypoplastic scaphoids of abnormalities of the thumb. Since radial ray abnormalities commonly involve the most distal part of the radial ray, the syndrome is well marked for the common occurrence of the triphalangeal thumb. The triphalangeal thumb is an interesting anomaly. In the normal first metacarpal, the epiphysis is proximal in contrast to the metacarpals 2 to 5, in which a distal epiphysis is seen. In the phalanges, however, the epiphyses are always proximal. In the most common form of triphalangeal thumb, in which the so-called "five-fingered hand" is seen, the thumb recapitulates fingers 2 to 5 with a distal metacarpal epiphysis and three phalanges each with basilar epiphyses. In this form, the thumb is frequently not opposable and articulates in the same plane as fingers 2 to 5.

The most common heart defects are septal defects, both atrial (58%) and ventricular (28%). *TBX5* appears to play a significant role specifically in the septation of the heart into four chambers. In addition, it plays a role in determining electrical conductive pathways between the chambers, giving rise to occasional conduction defects (18%).

Miscellaneous and Chromosomal Disorders

FETAL ALCOHOL SPECTRUM DISORDER

Fetal alcohol spectrum disorder (FASD) combines characteristic facies with predominantly neurologic abnormalities. The distinctive facies include thin palpebral fissures, a smooth philtrum, midface hypoplasia, and a thin upper lip. Neurologic abnormalities include microcephaly, agenesis of the corpus callosum, cerebellar hypoplasia, and migrational anomalies. Even in the face of no observable structural changes in the brain, intelligence may be drastically reduced. FASD is thought to be the leading known cause of intellectual disability in the developed world. Interestingly, the level of severity of the syndrome is directly related to the degree of exposure and the more characteristically abnormal the facies, the more brain damage is suspected; that is, the face predicts the brain.

A wide range of anomalies may be present. Skeletal changes include vertebral body segmentation and fusion anomalies, radiolunar synostosis, tibial exostoses, and hand anomalies, including ectrodactyly, brachydactly, and carpal fusions. Cardiac defects include septal defects, tetralogy of Fallot, and aortic arch interruption.

Urogenital anomalies associated with FASD include horseshoe kidneys, ureteral duplications, and renal aplasia. Gastrointestinal tract abnormalities include esophageal atresia with tracheoesophageal fistula, anal and small bowel atresias, and diaphragmatic hernia. Hepatobiliary abnormalities include hepatic dysfunction, biliary atresia, and hepatic fibrosis.

NOONAN SYNDROME

Noonan syndrome is a relatively common autosomal-dominant disorder caused by mutations in any one of these

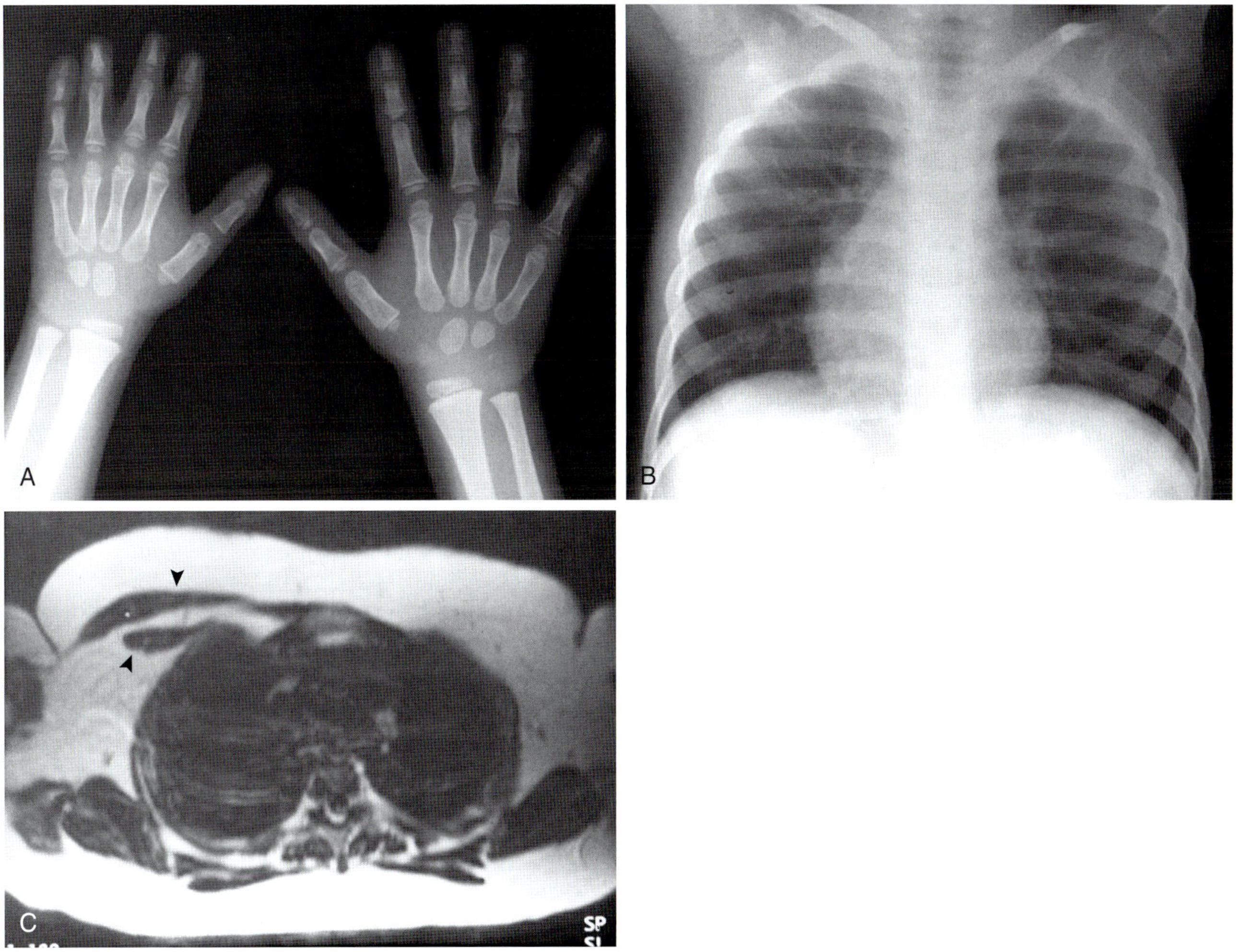

Figure 133-56 Poland syndrome. **A,** A hand radiograph shows generalized hypoplasia of the right hand, with soft tissue syndactyly affecting the second through fourth digits. **B,** The anteroposterior chest radiograph on a different patient shows relative lucency of the left hemithorax with loss of the pectoral shadow. **C,** An axial T1-weighted magnetic resonance imaging scan shows absence of the left anterior chest wall musculature (*arrowheads* indicate normal musculature on the right).

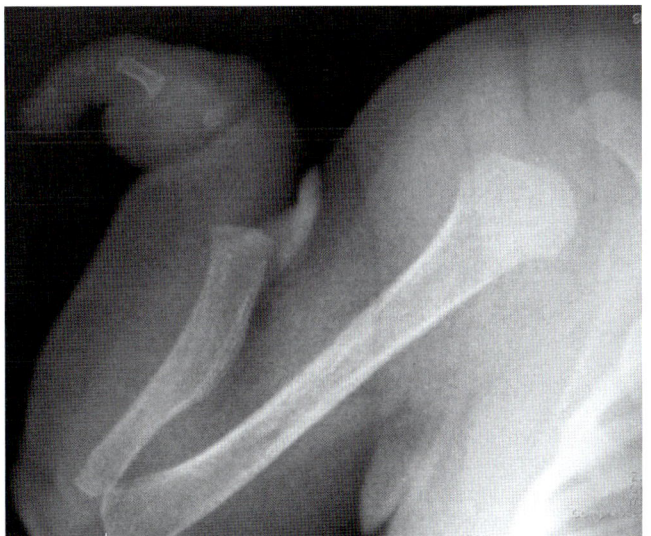

Figure 133-57 Brachmann-de Lange (Cornelia de Lange) syndrome. The radiograph of the right upper extremity shows absent ulna, shortened radius, and a single digit, the thumb.

four genes: *KRAS, PTPN11, RAF1,* and *SOS1.* About half of the patients have affected *PTPN11.* Those with *KRAS* mutations are more severely affected. Noonan syndrome used to be thought of as a "male Turner syndrome," and although the two syndromes are genetically distinct, the paradigm has validity as a memory tool.

Short stature, abnormal facies, and distinctive congenital heart defects are seen, typically pulmonic stenosis and hypertrophic cardiomyopathy. In about 20% of patients lymphatic abnormalities are present and echo Turner syndrome. These include lymphangiectasia and lymphedema. Bleeding diathesis occur in about 50% of patients.

VACTERL ASSOCIATION

VATER association, now expanded to VACTERL association, refers to a specific combination of anomalies in multiple organ systems which is believed to represent a developmental defect arising during the fifth week of gestation. The acronym indicates the following:

V: vertebral (fusion and segmentation anomalies)

A: anorectal (imperforate anus)

C: cardiac (septal defects, tetralogy of Fallot, transposition of the great vessels)

T: tracheoesophageal (esophageal atresia)

R: renal (agenesis, hypoplasia, horseshoe kidney)

L: limb (especially radial ray anomalies)

VACTERL is referred to as an association rather than a syndrome, indicating that the cause is uncertain. The various organ defects occur together and are associated. They are probably caused by a problem in blastogenesis around the fifth week of gestation. It is not associated with facial dysmorphism, learning disability, growth failure, or abnormal head size or shape. If any of these features is present, a genetic condition associated either with esophageal atresia such as Feingold syndrome or CHARGE association or with imperforate anus such as Townes-Brocks syndrome needs to be excluded.

In those patients with imperforate anus, sacral anomalies, and posterior spinal fusion defects, including tethered cord and lipomyelomeningocele, are common.

Hydrocephalus associated with the VACTERL association is known to have a high rate of recurrence in subsequent pregnancies. This is referred to as VACTERL-H association, with hydrocephalus added to the acronym. VACTERL-H is frequently an X-linked disorder, particularly when aqueductal stenosis is present and the prognosis is poor. (Fig. 133-58)

KLINEFELTER SYNDROME

The addition of one or more X chromosomes in the male results in Klinefelter syndrome. Affected patients have greater expression of female characteristics, including gynecomastia, a feminine body fat distribution, small testes, and elevated

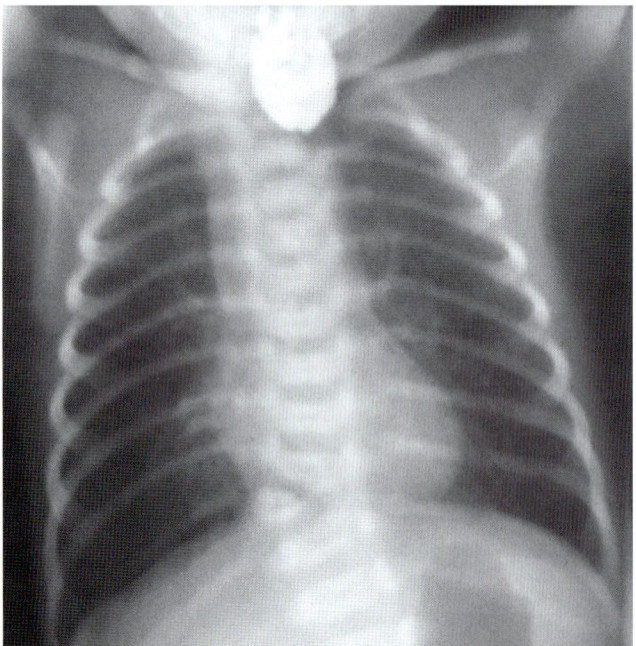

Figure 133-58 VACTERL association (vertebral, anorectal, cardiac, tracheoesophageal, renal, limb). The chest radiograph of a newborn with tracheoesophageal fistula and esophageal atresia. Contrast medium is in the proximal esophageal pouch. Air in the stomach indicates the presence of a distal tracheoesophageal fistula. A hemivertebra is noted. The patient also had a pelvic kidney.

levels of follicle-stimulating hormone. An increased incidence of male breast cancer, mediastinal germ cell tumor, leukemia, non-Hodgkin lymphoma, and lung cancer is seen, but the risk of prostate cancer is decreased.

Osseous changes are inconstant and include kyphoscoliosis, radioulnar synostosis, and a short fourth metacarpal. Skeletal findings are more apparent when more than two X chromosomes are present.

Other organ systems also may be affected. The risk of lupus, diabetes mellitus, mitral valve prolapse, bronchiectasis and emphysema, and situs inversus is increased.

TRISOMY 13 (PATAU SYNDROME)

Trisomy 13 occurs as a pure trisomy as well as a mosaic syndrome. Survival beyond the age of 10 years is rare and most die in infancy. Severe intracranial abnormalities, including holoprosencephaly, Dandy-Walker malformation spectrum, agenesis of the corpus callosum, and anencephaly, are often present. Congenital heart disease with various renal anomalies are often present. Additional components of the syndrome include congenital vertical talus (rocker-bottom foot), digital anomalies, micropthalmia, micrognathia, and cleft palate.

TRISOMY 18 (EDWARDS SYNDROME)

Abnormalities in trisomy 18 include severe central nervous system changes such as holoprosencephaly and nonspecific migrational disorders, congenital heart disease, clubfeet or rocker-bottom feet, and digital anomalies. The hands are clenched in utero, and at birth, the first finger is adducted, and the second finger overlaps the third. Multiple other organ systems, including genitourinary, gastrointestinal, and biliary systems, are also affected. Life expectancy is short. Very few cases survive childhood. Mosaics may be less affected.

TRISOMY 21 (DOWN SYNDROME)

Trisomy 21 is the most common chromosomal syndrome. A host of anomalies involving virtually all organ systems are well described. The most common cause of trisomy 21 is a nondisjunction event during gametogenesis, usually in the mother. At times, a trisomy 21 mosaic situation can occur when the nondisjunction event occurs in an embryo during early cell division. Rarely, trisomy 21 can occur as a result of an unbalanced translocation in one parent when the long arm of chromosome 21 attaches to the long arm of chromosome 14.

Both occipitoatlantal and atlantoaxial instability is found in Down syndrome. Anteroposterior occipitoatlantal instability is defined as more than 2 mm of motion on extension of the occipitoatlantal joints. If present, a neck MRI is recommended to evaluate for signal changes in the cord. An atlantoaxial distance of 4.5 mm or less is considered normal. With a distance from 4.5 to 10 mm and a normal neurologic exam, avoidance of high-risk sports (diving, football) is recommended. If more than 4.5 mm and with a neurological deficit, activities are restricted and MRI recommended to evaluate for cord changes.[43] However, the poor reproducibility of findings and both intraobserver and interobserver variability may make it difficult to base surgical and clinical treatment protocols for upper cervical spine instability on measurements alone.

The brains of trisomy 21 patients have smaller than normal volumes, but no other consistent changes occur. The level of intellectual performance of affected individuals varies, but many are able to function normally in society with some assistance.

Clinical and Imaging Findings

- *Skull:* brachycephaly
- *Spine:* occipitoatlantal and atlantoaxial instability
- *Thorax:* hypersegmented manubrium, 11 rib pairs, small bell shaped chest with short ribs
- *Pelvis:* flared iliac wings, flat acetabular roofs
- *Gastrointestinal tract:* duodenal atresia, Hirschsprung disease, malrotation, tracheoesophageal fistula, imperforate anus
- *Cardiac:* endocardial cushion defect most common but other types also occur
- *Other:* increased risk for leukemia (acute lymphoblastic leukemia)

TURNER SYNDROME

Turner syndrome is most commonly caused by a 45,XO chromosomal pattern. In 15% of cases, one full X chromosome is present as well as an X isochromosome that contains only the long arms of chromosome X. Although originally it was thought that in the normal 46,XX female, complete inactivation of the second X chromosome occurs, some genes on the short arm of the inactivated X chromosome remain activated and are necessary for proper development, which explains why a patient with an X isochromosome and the classic XO are phenotypically similar.[44] The locus involved on the short arm of the X chromosome is in the pseudoautosomal region at Xp22 at a gene termed the *short stature homeobox gene* (*SHOX*). *SHOX* was originally determined to be associated with some patients with idiopathic short stature syndrome who have a significantly short stature (>2 SDS), a persistently low growth rate for age and no identifiable cause of a specific metabolic growth retarding condition. Subsequently, *SHOX* has been found to be active in Turner syndrome.[45] Later, homozygous loss was found to be the cause of Langer mesomelic dysplasia and heterozygous loss the cause of dyschondrosteosis (Leri–Weill syndrome).[46,47] In each of these last three conditions, the common thread of short stature, a short fourth metacarpal, and a varying degree of Madelung deformity is present.

Turner syndrome, or monosomy X, was initially described as a triad of infertility, webbing of the neck, and cubitus valgus deformity of the elbow. Since that time, a multitude of associated radiographic findings have been described involving most organ systems:

1. *Skull:* brachycephaly
2. *Spine:* platyspondyly
3. *Thorax:* pectus carinatum, thin lateral clavicles
4. *Pelvis:* sacral hypoplasia

5. *Extremities:* elbow valgus, overtubulation of long bones, flattening of the medial femoral condyle and patellar dislocation, proximal tibial exostosis, phalangeal abnormalities

Hand radiographs demonstrate typical changes with osteopenia, shortening of the fourth and fifth metacarpals, delayed maturation, phalangeal predominance, a V-shaped deformity of the distal radiocarpal joint (Madelung deformity), and drumstick-shaped distal phalanges.

The classic cardiovascular finding is postductal coarctation of the aorta, but septal defects, aortic coarctation and dissection, and mitral valve prolapse are also common. Renal anomalies include rotational anomalies, bifid renal pelvis, horseshoe kidney (common), and multicystic dysplastic kidney. Autoimmune conditions, including hypothyroidism, diabetes, and juvenile rheumatoid arthritis, have been associated with Turner syndrome. Genital abnormalities, best evaluated with pelvic ultrasound or MRI, include ovarian and uterine absence or hypoplasia. Vascular abnormalities also include intestinal telangiectasia, lymphedema, and an increased incidence of vascular tumors (hemangioma, lymphangioma).

Key Points

An ordered segmental approach to the radiographs of a patient with skeletal dysplasia is the key to proper diagnosis.

Abnormalities should be generally classified as to the area of abnormality. Are the epiphyses or metaphyses involved? Is there vertebral body involvement? Are the findings rhizomelic, mesomelic, or acromelic?

Following a general classification, a search should be made for any more peculiar or specific changes.

After appropriate analysis, consultation with any of the excellent referral texts included in this chapter will be very helpful.

Suggested Readings

Alman BA. Skeletal dysplasias and the growth plate. *Clin Genet.* 2008;73(1):24-30.

Ikegawa S. Genetic analysis of skeletal dysplasia: recent advances and perspectives in the post-genome-sequence era. *J Hum Genet.* 2006;51(7):581-586.

McAlister WH, Herman TE. Osteochondrodysplasias, dysostoses, chromosomal aberrations, mucopolysaccharidoses, and mucolipidoses. In: Resnick D, ed. *Bone and joint disorders.* 4th ed. Philadelphia, PA: Elsevier; 2002.

Superti-Furga A, Bonafe L, Rimoin DL. Molecular-pathogenetic classification of genetic disorders of the skeleton. *Am J Med Genet.* 2001;106(4):282-293.

Rimoin DL, Cohn D, Krakow D, et al. The skeletal dysplasias: clinical-molecular correlations. *Ann N Y Acad Sci.* 2007;1117:302-309.

References

Full references for this chapter can be found on www.expertconsult.com.

Chapter 134

Alignment Disorders

PETER J. STROUSE

Overview

Malalignment of bony components of the extremities may be congenital or acquired. A defect that results in malalignment may be primary to bone or secondary to soft tissue or neuromuscular disorders. Malalignment is often seen with congenital deformities characterized by embryologic failure of development, discussed in Chapter 128. One of the most common alignment disorders is developmental dysplasia of the hip, discussed in Chapter 133.

Upper Extremities

ERB PALSY

Etiologies, Pathophysiology, and Clinical Presentation Erb palsy is caused by birth trauma to the C5 and C6 nerve roots. It is associated with prolonged, difficult delivery (dystocia) and with larger infants. Infants present soon after birth with decreased motion of the involved extremity. Children with a persistent defect will hold their arms in internal rotation with pronation of the forearm and flexion of the wrist. The brachial plexus injury is the primary insult leading to secondary glenohumeral dysplasia.

Imaging At birth, radiographs serve to exclude fractures of the clavicle and humerus. Ultrasonography and magnetic resonance imaging (MRI) have been used to directly evaluate the brachial plexus;[1,2] however, the primary goal of advanced imaging is to evaluate orthopedic anatomy to determine function and orthopedic treatment since primary repair of the brachial plexus injury is difficult.

Progressive deformity with secondary glenohumeral dysplasia manifests as a small, flattened humeral head, which may sublux, usually in the posterior direction relative to a small, shallow, abnormally retroverted glenoid (Fig. 134-1).[3] In normal shoulders, the glenoid is mildly retroverted by approximately 5 degrees posteriorly relative to a line perpendicular to the axis of the scapular body.[4] With Erb palsy, glenoid retroversion averages 25 degrees. The scapula is hypoplastic and elevated; the acromion is tapered and inferiorly directed, as is the coracoid; the clavicle is shortened. Many of these findings are seen on radiography; however, computed tomography (CT) or MRI can be used to quantify

the degree of glenoid retroversion, deformity of the glenoid and humeral head, glenoid–humeral head congruence, and relative muscle volume and quality of the affected shoulder.[5-9] The glenoid normally has a concave shape. With glenohumeral dysplasia, the glenoid becomes progressively flat, convex, or biconvex with a pseudoarticulation with the humeral head. MRI is preferred in young children (<5 years old) (e-Fig. 134-2) and CT in older children. To determine glenoid version, the articular cartilage should be used when MRI is performed; the glenoid cortical bone should be used when CT is performed. In infants, ultrasonography may be used to assess instability of the glenohumeral joint.[10-12]

Treatment Microsurgery techniques may be attempted to address the underlying traumatic neural injury.[13] Controversy exists as to their role and proper timing. The main focus of treatment is on the reconstructive surgical techniques of the shoulder, elbow and forearm, and hand and wrist, aimed at preserving joint integrity and maximizing function.[13,14] Therefore, imaging optimization should be tailored for orthopedic anatomy rather than the brachial plexus.

MADELUNG DEFORMITY

Etiologies, Pathophysiology, and Clinical Presentation In Madelung deformity, the radius is short and its distal articular surface tilted toward to ulna.[15] In most cases, the cause of Madelung deformity is unknown. Madelung deformity occurs more often in girls.[16] Patients may have pain; however, treatment is more often sought because of deformity or limited range of motion. With an underlying syndrome, the deformity is more likely to be bilateral. Madelung deformity is occasionally seen with Turner syndrome and is a characteristic in dyschondrosteosis (Léri-Weill syndrome) (Fig. 134-3).[15] Among these cases, 10% to 15% are familial. A Madelung-like deformity may also be seen in patients with hereditary osteochondromatosis or enchondromatosis, also suggesting a defect in normal distal radial maturation. Madelung deformity may occur as a complication of infection or trauma that results in medial and volar radial physeal growth disturbance.[17]

Imaging The distal articular surface of the radius is tilted in an ulnar and volar direction.[18,19] The radius is short and bowed dorsally and laterally ("bayonet deformity").

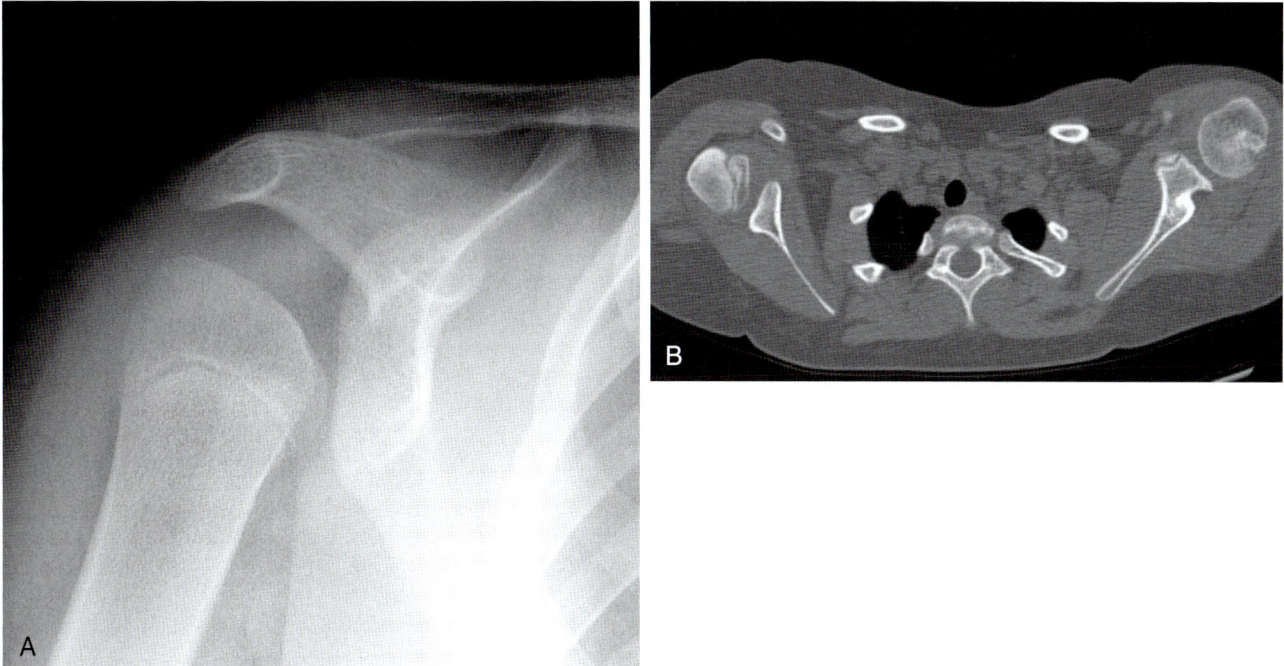

Figure 134-1 Erb palsy in a 9-year-old girl. **A,** On radiography, the humeral head appears small and abnormally contoured, the glenoid margins are indistinct, and the acromion is curved. **B,** Axial computed tomography shows the right glenoid to be small and retroverted. The right humeral head is small and squared in contour but appears normally located relative to the glenoid. Note the asymmetric muscle volume of the right shoulder girdle compared with the left shoulder girdle.

Secondary distortion of the carpus is observed with an abnormally narrow carpal angle and proximal lunate migration.[18,19] The distal ulna is subluxed. The distal radial growth plate may prematurely fuse along its ulnar aspect. CT or MRI may be used to assess the extent of distal radial physeal fusion.[20]

Treatment Treatment is aimed at relieving pain caused by ulnocarpal impingement and improving wrist mobility.[17]

Ulnar shortening and radial wedge osteotomies are common techniques.[17]

ULNAR VARIANCE

Etiologies, Pathophysiology, and Clinical Presentation Trauma, infection, inflammatory disease (juvenile idiopathic arthritis) or other causes of premature fusion may lead to shortening

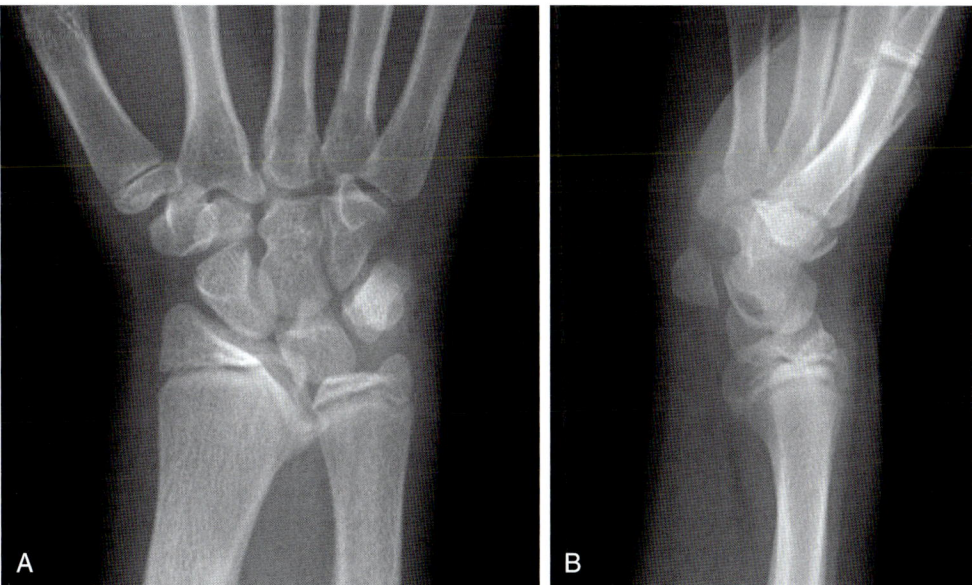

Figure 134-3 Madelung deformity in a 10-year-old girl who presented with right wrist pain. **A,** Posteroanterior radiograph shows medial tilt of the distal radial articular surface and physis with thinning of the medial aspect of the distal radial epiphysis. **B,** Lateral radiograph shows anterior tilt of the distal radial articular surface with mild anterior displacement of the carpus.

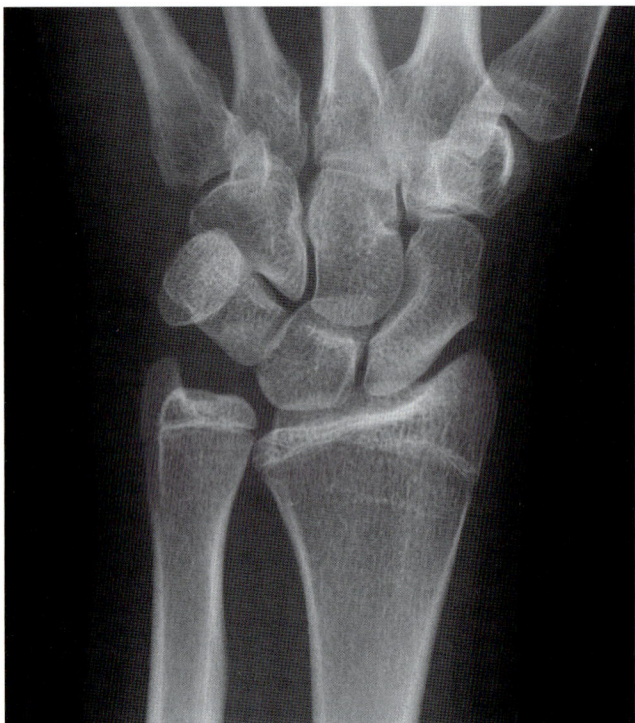

Figure 134-4 Positive ulnar variance in a 14-year-old girl with a history of prior osteomyelitis of the ulna. Presumably, resultant overgrowth of the ulna occurred. The patient required ulnar shortening because of clinical evidence of ulnar impaction syndrome.

of the ulna relative to the radius (negative ulnar variance) or shortening of the radius relative to the ulna (positive ulnar variance) (Fig. 134-4).[21] Most cases are idiopathic. Processes associated with hyperemia, for example, fracture healing, infection and vascular lesions, may lead to over growth of one of the bones.

Imaging At skeletal maturity, the distal radial and ulnar articular surfaces are nearly at the same level, and the radial styloid projects 9 to 12 mm distal to the ulnar articular surface.[21,22] With negative ulnar variance, the ulna ends more proximally, and with positive ulnar variance, the ulna ends more distally (e-Fig. 134-5).[21,23] Ulnar variance may be exaggerated with forearm pronation and decreased with forearm supination.

Treatment Osteotomy with ulnar or radial shortening may be indicated to reduce symptoms and avoid sequelae. Negative ulnar variance is associated with the development of avascular necrosis of the lunate (Kienböck disease).[24] Positive ulnar variance is associated with ulnolunate impaction syndrome (Fig. 134-6) and triangular fibrocartilage complex degeneration.

Lower Extremities

HIP/FEMUR

Coxa Vara

Etiologies, Pathophysiology, and Clinical Presentation The normal neck-shaft angle of the proximal femur is

approximately 150 degrees at birth and decreases to 120 to 130 degrees in adulthood.[25] External or internal rotation of the hip or femoral anteversion may affect measurement.[26]

Functional coxa vara occurs with disorders that result in femoral neck shortening, as in trauma, infection, or epiphyseal osteonecrosis.[27] True coxa vara occurs as a congenital anomaly that is caused by bone softening (e.g., rickets, osteogenesis imperfecta, fibrous dysplasia) or to abnormal growth (e.g., spondyloepiphyseal dysplasia congenita, spondyloepimetaphyseal dysplasia, cleidocranial dysplasia).[28,29] Children with developmental coxa vara present with a limp (unilateral deformity) or a waddling gate (bilateral deformities). Coxa vara may occur as the result of abnormal growth at the proximal femoral physis that results in abnormal angulation of the physis. Congenital coxa vara occurs with a congenital short femur (i.e., proximal focal femoral deficiency) and does not spontaneously resolve.[28] With infantile or developmental coxa vara, the hip is normal at birth, and deformity is noted when the child begins to walk.[28,30] Infantile coxa vara may be self-limited. Acquired coxa vara is caused by another process such as trauma.[28]

Imaging In coxa vara, the femoral neck-shaft angle is decreased from normal. A measurement below 110 degrees is considered coxa vara.[31] Fragmentation and sclerosis may be seen at the medial margin of the proximal femoral metaphysis (Fig. 134-7).[30] The Hilgenreiner epiphyseal angle is the angle between the Hilgenreiner line and a line drawn through the physis (e-Fig. 134-8).[28,31] If it is less than 45 degrees, progression is unlikely. If over 60 degrees, progression is likely. If 45 to 60 degrees, prognosis is less predictable.

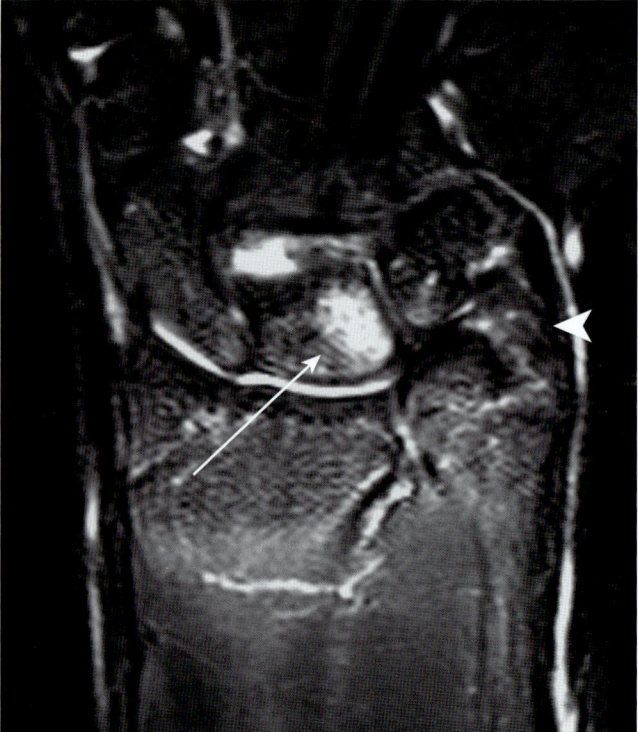

Figure 134-6 A 14-year-old boy with ulnolunate impaction syndrome. Inversion recovery coronal sequence demonstrates elongated ulna (*arrowhead*) with lunate edema (*arrow*) caused by ulnolunate impaction syndrome.

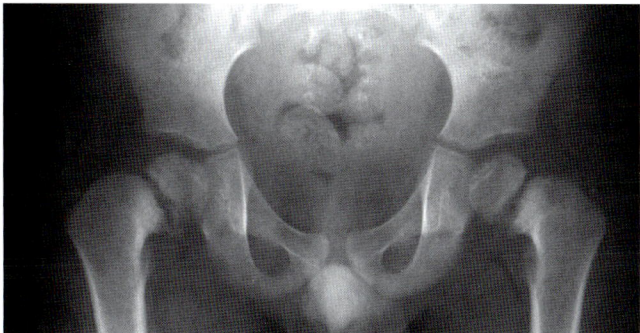

Figure 134-7 Bilateral congenital coxa vara in a 4-year-old boy. Proximal femoral growth plates are tilted, medial side down. Slight fragmentation is noted at the medial aspect of each proximal femoral physis.

Treatment Surgical management may be warranted for progressive disease, especially if asymmetric or associated with pain, leg length discrepancy, or both.[28] Valgus osteotomy is performed, and physeal fixation or tendon transfers may also be performed to deter progression and improve mechanical function.

Coxa Valga

Etiologies, Pathophysiology, and Clinical Presentation With coxa valga, the neck-shaft angle of the proximal femur is increased.[32] Coxa valga is most often seen in patients who are nonambulatory and nonerect, such as those with cerebral palsy and other neuromuscular disorders (Fig. 134-9).[26,33]

Imaging The femoral neck-shaft angle is measured on radiographs. External rotation may mimic coxa valga and can be differentiated through the positioning of the greater trochanter.[26] With external rotation, the greater trochanter projects through the femur, whereas with true coxa valga, it is located laterally. Increased femoral anteversion may cause the femoral neck-shaft angle to be overestimated.[32] Acetabular dysplasia and femoral subluxation are frequently concomitant findings.[32]

Treatment Varus osteotomy and iliac osteotomy are often performed together in patients with cerebral palsy to better direct the femoral head into the acetabulum.

Femoral Anteversion

Etiologies, Pathophysiology, and Clinical Presentation Increased femoral anteversion may hinder proper localization of the femoral head relative to the acetabulum. Increased femoral anteversion is seen in hip deformity caused by developmental dysplasia of the hip, Legg-Calvé-Perthes disease, and cerebral palsy.[32] With increased anteversion, in-toeing of feet is noted.

Femoral version is the angulation of the femoral neck in the transverse plane measured relative to the femoral condyles distally (Fig. 134-10). If the femoral neck is anteriorly angulated with respect to the femoral condyles, the femur is anteverted. If the femoral neck is posterior with respect to the femoral condyles, the femur is retroverted. Normal femoral anteversion is 35 to 50 degrees at birth, decreasing steadily to 10 to 15 degrees in adulthood (Fig. 134-11).[27]

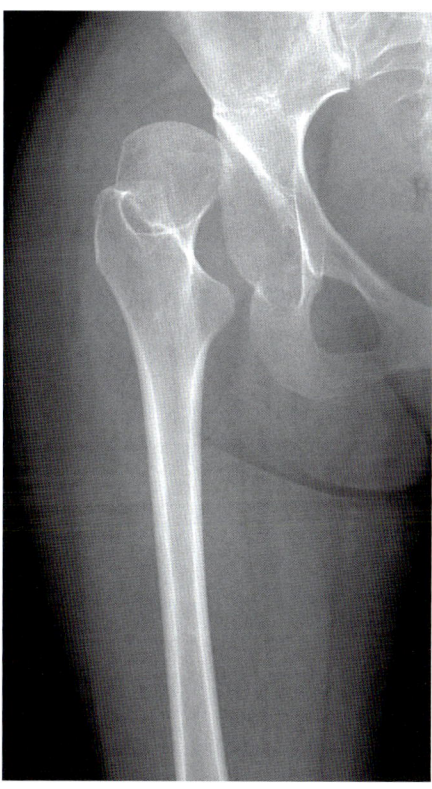

Figure 134-9 A 15-year-old girl with cerebral palsy. The acetabulum is markedly dysplastic. The femoral head is subluxed. Coxa valga is noted, and the lesser trochanter is disproportionately larger compared with the femoral head.

Imaging On CT, femoral anteversion is the angle between the axis of the femoral neck and the transcondylar axis at the distal femur (Fig. 134-12).[34-36] Limited low-dose axial images are usually performed; however, axial oblique or three-dimensional images may improve measurement.[37,38]

Treatment Most children with increased femoral anteversion are managed conservatively. Surgical indications for treatment include symptomatic in-toeing secondary to excessive femoral anteversion. Femoral rotational osteotomy may be performed to optimize femoral version.

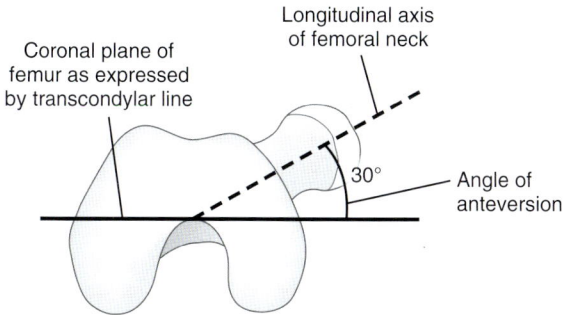

Figure 134-10 Schematic diagram of the right femur as viewed from below. The femoral neck is angulated anterior (anteversion) relative to the transcondylar axis of the distal femur. (Modified from Greenspan A. *Orthopedic imaging: a practical approach.* 4th ed. Philadelphia, PA: Lippincott Williams & Wilkins; 2004.)

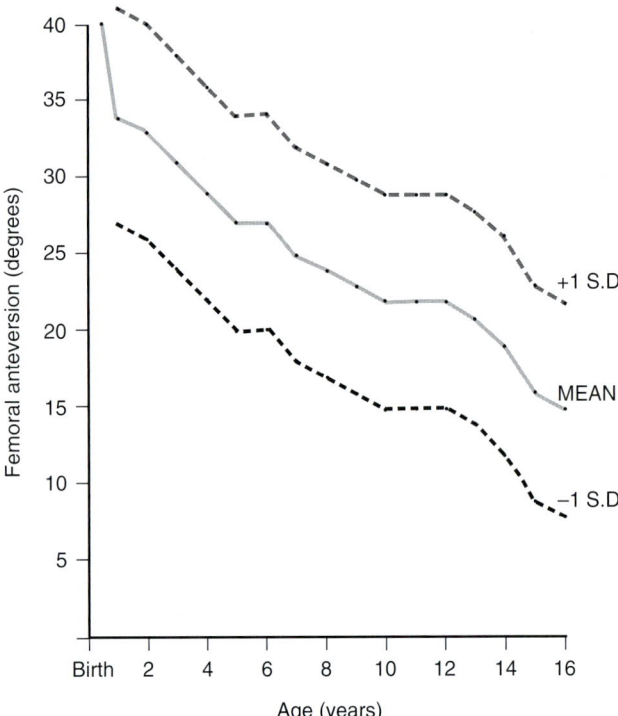

Figure 134-11 Normal femoral anteversion. The mean value is an average of those reported by Shands and Steele (1958), Crane (1959), and Fabry and associates (1973). Standard deviations are only an approximation and are based on the range of those determined by Fabry and associates. *(From Ozonoff MB: Pediatric orthopedic radiology. 2nd ed. Philadelphia: WB Saunders; 1992.)*

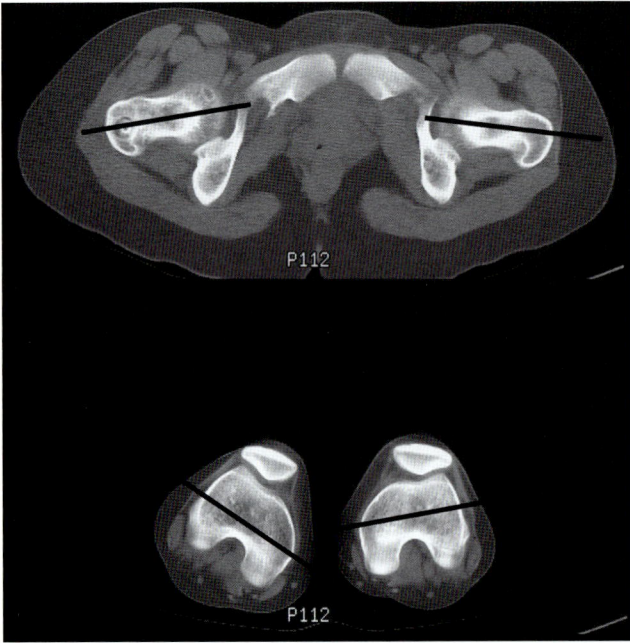

Figure 134-12 Computed tomography method for assessing femoral anteversion in a 17-year-old girl with a history of right femoral fracture. Lines denote the axes of the femoral necks and the transcondylar axes of the distal femora. An angle of 49 degrees of anteversion was measured on the right and an angle of 14 degrees was measured on the left.

LEG

Tibial Torsion

Etiologies, Pathophysiology, and Clinical Presentation Tibial torsion is the degree of rotation of the distal end of the tibia relative to the upper end of the tibia. Newborns have internal tibial torsion relative to older children and adults. Lack of normal progression results in in-toeing. Internal tibial torsion is the most common cause of in-toeing in the preschool age group.

Imaging Assessment of tibial torsion is often performed with assessment of femoral version. Limited axial low-dose CT images are obtained through the proximal and distal tibias.[41] Tibial torsion is best measured as the angle between the posterior epiphyseal cortical margin of the tibia proximally and a bimalleolar line distally. Normal values are 5 degrees of external rotation in a newborn, which progresses to 15 to 20 degrees of external rotation in an adult.[40,42]

Treatment Surgery is rarely needed as more than 95% of cases resolve spontaneously, usually by 8 years of age. Tibial rotational osteomy may be performed to optimize tibial alignment.

Bowleg (Genu Varum)

Etiologies, Pathophysiology, and Clinical Presentation Bowleg deformity manifests as separation of the knees, with the legs in anatomic position. Pathologic causes include rickets, osteogenesis imperfecta, neurofibromatosis, skeletal dysplasias (i.e., campomelic dysplasia, achondroplasia), focal fibrocartilaginous dysplasia, congenital bowing, Blount disease, and, occasionally, growth plate trauma.[43-46] Recently, greater prevalence of bowleg and tibia vara has been noted in some adolescent athletes, most notably soccer players.[47-49] Repetitive stress on the proximal tibial physis may play a role in this.[48] Most lateral bowing in otherwise normal infants and children younger than 2 years of age is normal and developmental ("physiologic") and resolves without treatment.[44,50-52] Similar to Blount disease, exaggerated physiologic bowing is seen in early walkers, African Americans, and heavier children.[44]

Imaging Ozonoff described the following findings as characteristic of physiologic lower extremity bowing: (1) The tibia is abducted relative to the femur, and both bones are intrinsically bowed laterally; relative tibial torsion produces external rotation of the upper tibia relative to the distal tibia; (2) margins of the distal femoral and proximal tibial metaphyses are mildly accentuated with small beaks; (3) medial cortices of the tibia and femur are thickened; (4) distal femoral and proximal tibial epiphyses are not well ossified medially and are wedge shaped; (5) the distal tibial growth plate may be tilted lateral.[53]

Radiographically, the femur and the tibia are also mildly bowed anteriorly, with beaking occurring posteriorly (Fig. 134-13). Physiologic bowing is usually more marked in the tibias. Occasionally, lateral bowing may almost exclusively be seen in the distal femur (e-Fig. 134-14). The varus deformity is common in normal infants and converts to valgus between 18 and 36 months of age. Degree of valgus reduces spontaneously by 6 to 7 years of age to a mild degree that remains

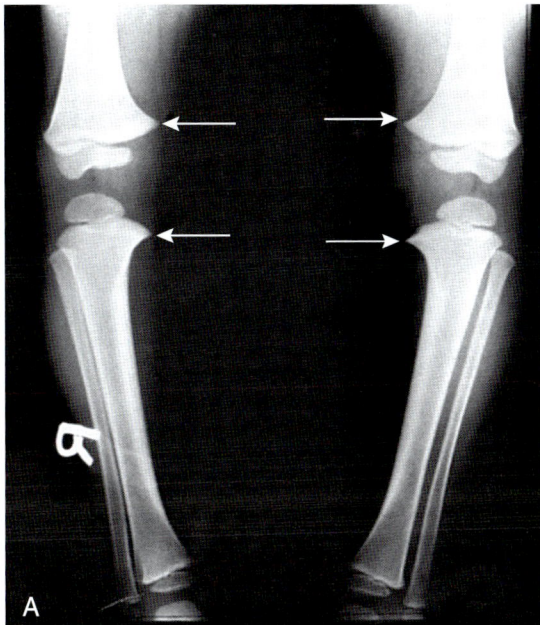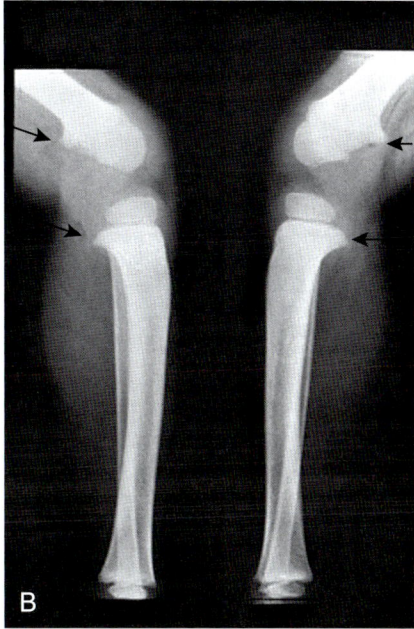

Figure 134-13 Bilateral idiopathic bowed legs in a 22-month-old boy. **A,** Frontal projection. *Arrows* point to the medial beaking of the femoral and tibial metaphyses at the knees. The increased stress of weightbearing has thickened the medial and dorsal cortical walls of the tibias inward. The medial femoral epiphyseal ossification centers are too small, which are under greater stress of weightbearing when the legs are bowed. **B,** Lateral projection. Arrows point to dorsal beaking of the femoral and tibial metaphyses. After correction of bowed legs, these "stress" phenomena disappear after several months.

throughout life. Approximate normal angles are 17 degrees varus in a newborn, 9 degrees varus at 1 year, 2 degrees valgus at 2 years, 11 degrees valgus at 3 years, and 5 to 6 degrees valgus at 13 years (e-Fig. 134-15).[52,54,55]

Radiographs should be taken with the patient bearing weight as soon as he or she is able to stand (Fig. 134-16). The radiographs may suggest an underlying disorder such as rickets or a dysplasia.

Treatment   Persistent varus with delayed conversion to valgus may indicate a higher likelihood of Blount disease (tibia vara). In the second year, it may be difficult to distinguish normal physiologic bowing from Blount disease.[56] Exaggerated varus during the second year is likely developmental or physiologic and does not require treatment.[50,51,54] Any varus at the knee after 2 years of age should raise concern. Such patients must be monitored to exclude progression to Blount disease.[55,57] Realignment surgery is rarely needed in isolated bowleg without underlying dysplasia, metabolic bone disease, or Blount disease.

Blount Disease (Tibia Vara)

Etiologies, Pathophysiology, and Clinical Presentation   Blount disease (tibia vara; osteochondrosis deformans tibiae) is a progressive deformity affecting the proximal tibia (Fig. 134-17).[58-60] It is theorized that stress on the posteromedial proximal tibial physis causes growth suppression.

The infantile form of Blount disease, which develops in children between 1 and 3 years of age, must be differentiated from developmental bowing.[61] Infantile Blount disease may represent normal developmental bowing that fails to correct and progresses. The diagnosis is made when progressive clinical bowing is seen in the presence of characteristic

radiographic changes in the proximal tibia.[61] The disease is typically bilateral (60% to 80%) but often asymmetric and occasionally unilateral (Fig. 134-18). A family history is often reported. The disorder is more common in early walkers, African Americans, and obese children.[44,60,62]

Adolescent or late-onset tibia vara is a separate entity from the infantile form. It occurs in children 8 to 14 years of age; obese African American males of normal height are at particular risk (Fig. 134-19).[43] Adolescent tibia vara is commonly unilateral but may be bilateral. Adolescent Blount disease is slowly progressive and probably results from the repetitive trauma of weight bearing on the medial physis of the proximal tibia.[43] Patients often present with knee pain.

Imaging   The characteristic radiographic feature of infantile Blount disease is deformity of the medial metaphysis of the proximal tibia (Fig. 134-20).[44] Irregularity with a more vertically oriented growth plate creates a beaked appearance. The severity of radiographic changes has been described by the six-stage Langenskiöld classification (e-Fig. 134-21).[63] Higher stage denotes greater abnormality; bone bridging between the diaphysis and the metaphysis is seen with stage IV and higher. The medial portion of the epiphyseal ossification center is often smaller than the lateral portion. The tibia may subluxate laterally.

The metaphyseal–diaphyseal angle is measured by drawing a single line through the widest portion of the proximal tibial metaphysis (between the medial and lateral beaks) and another line perpendicular to the long axis of the tibia.[51] With physiologic bowing, this angle measures approximately 5 degrees, whereas with Blount disease, average angle measurement is 16 degrees (e-Fig. 134-22). A metaphyseal–diaphyseal angle greater than 11 degrees suggests Blount disease.[44-51] However, several studies have questioned the

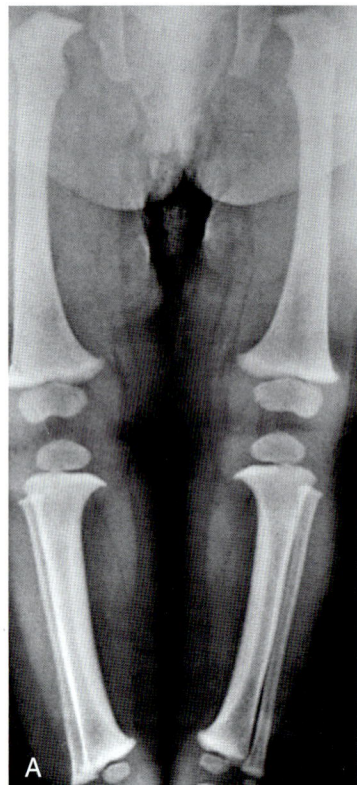
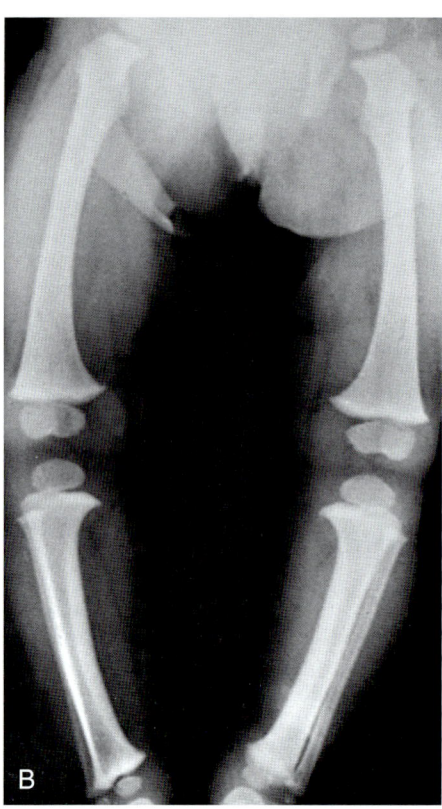

Figure 134-16 Bowed legs of a 12-month-old girl who started to walk at 8 months. **A,** In recumbent position, the tibias and femora are bowed, but the legs are not bowed because the knees and ankles are in apposition. **B,** In erect position, during weightbearing and with ankles in apposition, the legs are bowed, with a gap of 12 cm at the knees. The real clinical deformity of bowed legs is shown most accurately when the patient is erect and is bearing weight.

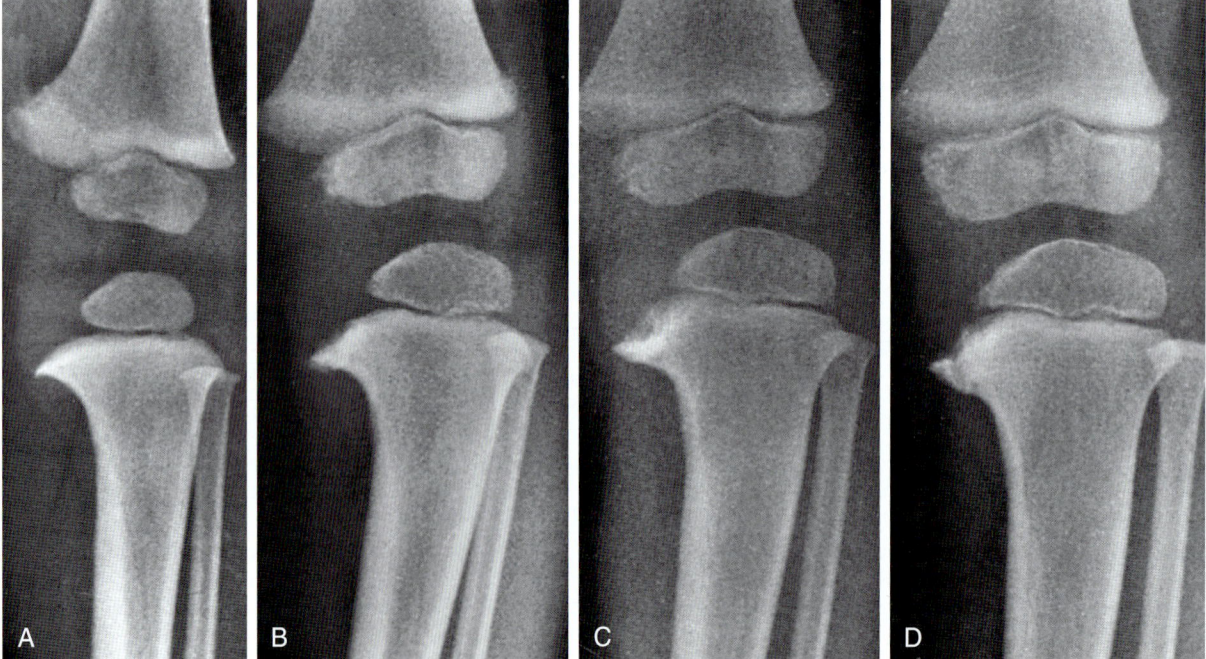

Figure 134-17 Progressive changes in Blount tibia vara. **A,** At 17 months, the medial segment of the tibial metaphysis is widened and sharpened into a short beak or spur that is bent slightly caudad. **B,** At 26 months, the spur is longer, sharper, and more bent; a radiolucent strip on its upper edge represents noncalcified cartilage. **C,** At 32 months, the amount of cartilage is increased and the spur thickened. **D,** At 38 months, the beak of the spur is displaced caudad, possibly owing to trauma; the medial edge of the ossification center is flattened, and the femur has shifted mediad in relation to the tibia.

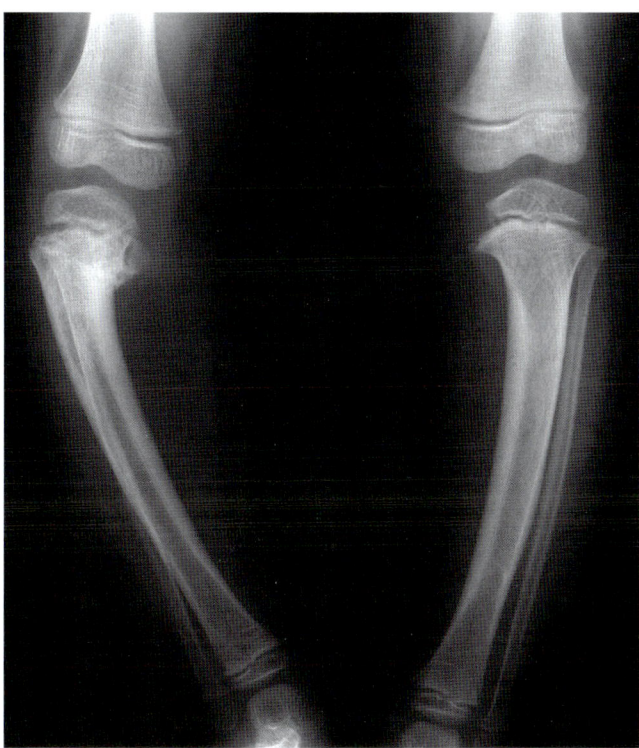

Figure 134-18 Bilateral Blount disease in a 3-year-old girl. Abnormality is greater on the right, where more sclerosis and irregularity of the proximal tibial metaphysis are evident.

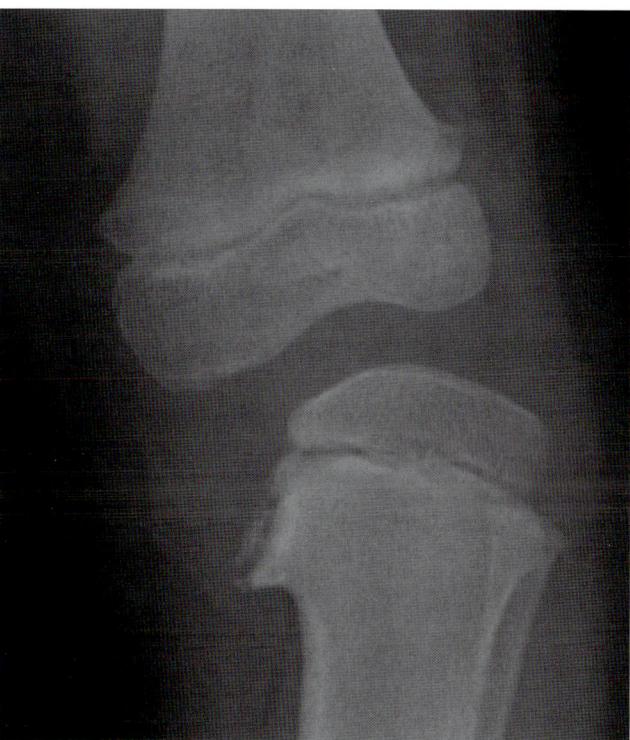

Figure 134-20 Infantile Blount disease in a 4-year-old girl. Unlike adolescent Blount disease, sharp metaphyseal angulation, beaking, and markedly diminished and near-absent medial epiphyseal ossification of the proximal tibia are seen.

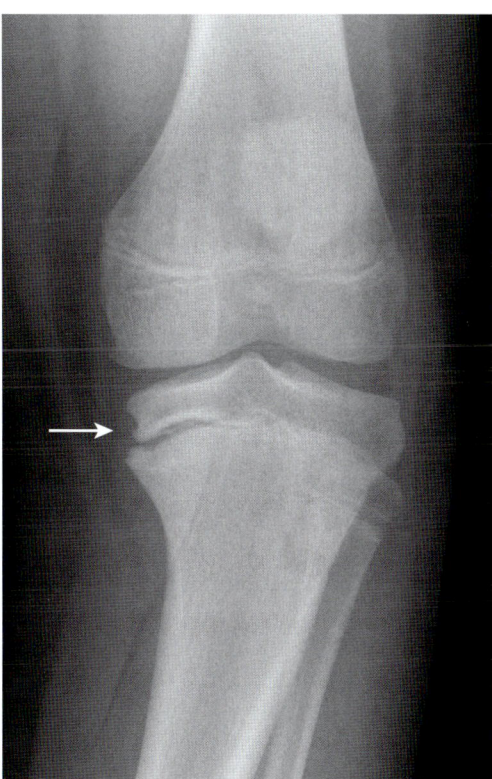

Figure 134-19 Adolescent Blount disease in a 13-year-old boy. Note the medial tibial physeal widening, metaphyseal fraying, and diminished medial epiphyseal height (*arrow*).

validity of the metaphyseal–diaphyseal angle, and measurement may be affected by tibial rotation.

Changes related to infantile Blount disease should be distinguished from those of adolescent Blount disease (see Figure 134-19). The metaphyseal angular deformities, diminished medial epiphyseal height, and degree of tibia vara are less severe with adolescent Blount disease.

CT or MRI can assess the degree of proximal tibial growth plate fusion and epiphyseal cartilage abnormalities (e-Fig. 134-23).[64,65] Cartilage-sensitive MRI sequences display the cartilage model of the proximal tibial epiphysis.[65]

Treatment Although spontaneous resolution of infantile Blount disease is reported in some instances, treatment with bracing is begun usually between ages 18 and 24 months and is continued during waking hours for an average of 2 years. If conservative management fails, the patient may undergo a realignment osteotomy, which is most effective when performed before 5 years of age. For adolescent Blount disease, a lateral tibial epiphyseodesis may be performed if sufficient growth still remains. If the proximal tibia physis are near fused, a proximal tibial valgus osteotomy to produce normal alignment may be performed.[60]

Knock-Knee (Genu Valgum)

Etiologies, Pathophysiology, and Clinical Presentation Genu valgum is a normal developmental phase that lasts from 2 to 12 years of age and is most apparent at 3 to 4 years of age in normal children.[52,54,55,66] Persistent knock-knee can be related to pathologic causes such as trauma, skeletal dysplasia, obesity, metabolic disease, or laxity of muscles and ligaments.

Imaging In knock-knee, the legs deviate laterally when in anatomic position. Wide separation is noted at the ankles (Fig. 134-24). Radiographs may show evidence of an underlying disorder or complicating process.

Treatment Treatment is conservative, particularly for children with physiologic knock-knee. Bracing is occasionally employed. Rarely, surgical osteotomies are performed for realignment.

Leg Length Discrepancy

Overview A leg length discrepancy of less than 1 cm is considered within normal limits; however, in most normal individuals, the legs are within 1 mm of each other in length. The presence of a leg length discrepancy may reflect overgrowth of the long limb or decreased size or growth of the short limb. Leg length discrepancy is often of clinical significance because of associated alteration of gait and resultant pelvic tilt. With significant pelvic tilt, secondary compensatory scoliosis may develop.

Etiologies, Pathophysiology, and Clinical Presentation The differential diagnoses for overgrowth and undergrowth is lengthy. Overgrowth is associated with a number of syndromes and vascular abnormalities. Mild overgrowth may

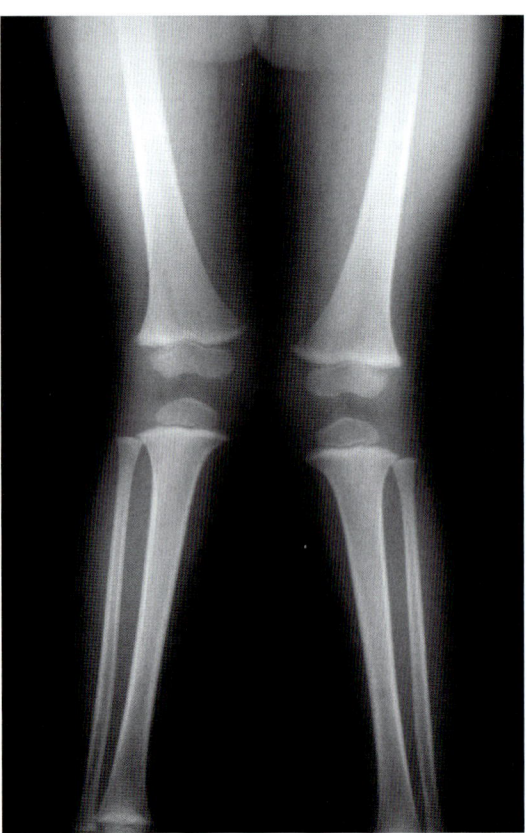

Figure 134-24 **Physiologic knock-knee in a 3-year-old girl.** In follow-up, the child's legs were seen to have straightened normally, without treatment.

occur as the result of fracture healing. In many cases, the cause is unknown. Undergrowth may be caused by hypoplasia or aplasia of a segment of the limb. Acquired shortening most often occurs as a consequence of premature growth plate fusion due to trauma, infection, or vascular insufficiency.

Imaging Radiographic techniques seek to determine bone lengths in a manner that minimizes magnification and other technical factors. Orthoroentgenography ("scanogram") uses three separate exposures collimated to the hip, knee, and ankle with a radiopaque ruler.[67] CT digital scout images may be used to measure bone length.[68,69] It is preferable to quantify length and alignment abnormalities with standing radiographs.

In addition to determining quantitative length and discrepancies in length of the lower extremities, leg-length studies should also be evaluated and comments should be made with regard to the alignment of the hips, knees, and ankles. Any underlying cause of the leg length discrepancy such as physeal growth disturbance or abnormal nonosteoarticular bowing deformities should also be discussed.

Treatment Mild leg length discrepancy does not warrant treatment. The type of treatment varies with age, amount of projected growth remaining, site of abnormality, and degree of leg length discrepancy. Treatment may be aimed at halting growth on the longer side (i.e., epiphyseodesis) or lengthening the shorter side (i.e., lengthening osteotomy procedure).[70] With a lengthening osteotomy procedure, bone on either side of a diaphyseal corticotomy is distracted slowly utilizing an external frame. New bone forms within the gap to add length.

FEET

Overview Alignment disorders of the feet may be idiopathic or caused by an underlying disorder. The standard method of radiologic evaluation of the foot involves weight bearing or simulated weight bearing anteroposterior (dorsoventral) and lateral views. Diagnosing alignment abnormalities of the feet should be approached with caution when nonweightbearing radiographs are obtained.

The talus is more proximal and is considered fixed at the ankle because it has no musculotendinous attachments of its own. The calcaneus is linked to the midfoot and forefoot and moves as a unit with these structures relative to the talus. In a normal foot, on the anteroposterior view, the axis of the talus extends through the base of the first metatarsal (Fig. 134-25). With hindfoot varus, the more distal calcaneus is angulated inward, and the axis of the talus passes lateral to the base of the first metatarsal. With hindfoot valgus, the more distal calcaneus is angulated outward, and the axis of the talus passes medial to the base of the first metatarsal.[81] The normal lateral talocalcaneal angle is approximately 45 degrees, decreasing to 30 degrees in older children and adults.[71-73] With hindfoot varus, the lateral talocalcaneal angle is decreased, whereas with hindfoot valgus, the angle is increased.

Normal elevation of the middle metatarsals relative to the fifth metatarsal reflects the transverse arch of the foot. The anterior calcaneus is slightly inclined upward. Accentuation

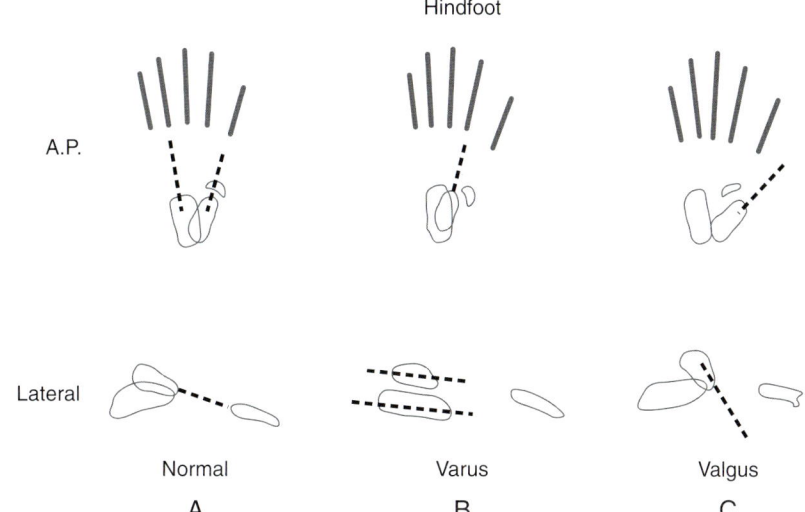

Hindfoot

A.P.

Lateral

| Normal | Varus | Valgus |
| A | B | C |

Figure 134-25 Hindfoot and forefoot relationships in the anteroposterior and lateral projections. **A,** Normal hindfoot. The talar axial line intersects or points slightly medial to the first metatarsal base. The navicular is situated directly opposite the head of the talus. The calcaneus points toward the fourth metatarsal base, forming a definable angle with the talus. On the lateral projection, the anterior portion of the talus is slightly plantarflexed, and the calcaneus is slightly dorsiflexed. The talar axial line points down the shaft of the first metatarsal. **B,** Hindfoot varus. The talocalcaneal angle is decreased, with these two bones more parallel to each other and actually superimposed. The navicular is medially displaced, and the axial talar line points lateral to the first metatarsal base. On lateral projection, the calcaneus and the talus are more horizontal and parallel to each other. **C,** Hindfoot valgus. The talocalcaneal angle is increased, with the navicular and other midfoot bones displaced lateral to the talus. The talar axial line passes medial to the first metatarsal base. On lateral projection, the talus is more vertical than normal. (From Ozonoff MB. *Pediatric orthopedic radiology.* 2nd ed. Philadelphia: WB Saunders; 1992.)

of this upward inclination is called "calcaneus" position of the hindfoot. Equinus is downward inclination of the distal calcaneus. Normal calcaneal tilt and normal slight downward tilt of the distal metatarsals create slight longitudinal concavity in the osseous contour of the bottom of the foot.

Clubfoot

Etiologies, Pathophysiology, and Clinical Presentation Talipes ("talus" = ankle; "pes" = foot) equinovarus, or clubfoot, is a common congenital anomaly that is clinically obvious at birth. The principal components of clubfoot deformity include plantar flexion of the ankle (equinus), inversion of

the heel (varus), and adduction of the forefoot (varus) (Fig. 134-26). Abnormal intrauterine pressures contribute to the development of clubfoot.[74] Genetics also appear to play a role.[74]

Imaging Radiographs are obtained with true or simulated weight bearing, as this is the position of best correction.[74] An anteroposterior radiograph shows superimposition and parallelism of the talus on the calcaneus with the talar axis directed lateral to the first metatarsal (hindfoot varus). Parallelism of the talus and calcaneus is also seen on a lateral view. The lateral view shows plantar flexion of the calcaneus (equinus) and a step-ladder arrangement of the metatarsals, with the

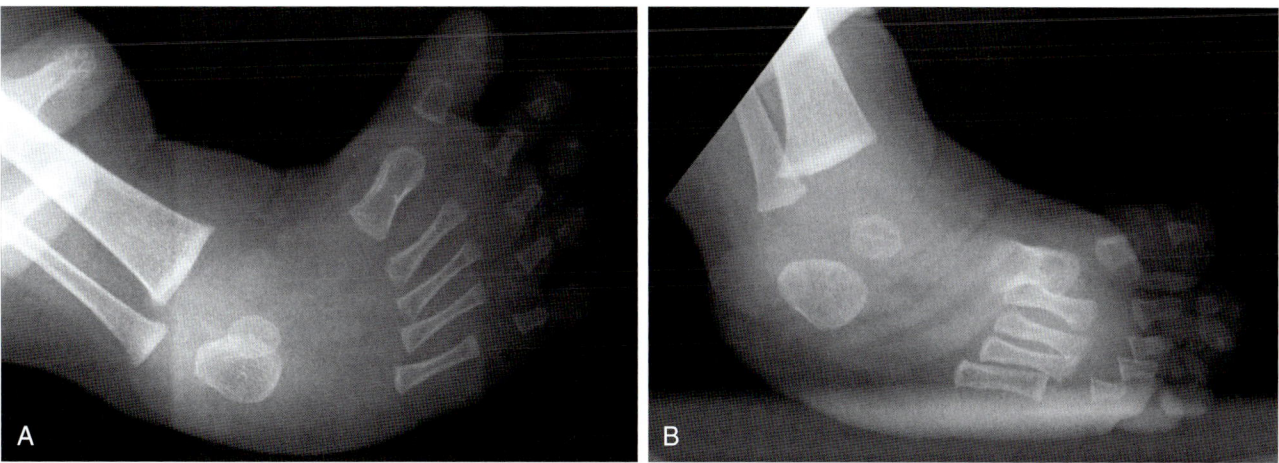

Figure 134-26 Radiographs of congenital clubfoot obtained with simulated weightbearing. **A,** Note the inversion and forefoot adduction in the anteroposterior view. **B,** Inversion on the lateral view shows "laddering" of the metatarsals. Equinus of the hindfoot and parallelism of the talus and calcaneus are evident.

first metatarsal highest and the fifth metatarsal at the weight-bearing surface of the foot. Ultrasonography has been used in select centers to assess the flexibility of clubfoot and to guide therapeutic decision making (e-Fig. 134-27).[75-78]

Treatment Approaches to treatment include serial casting for supple clubfoot deformity, and casting followed by surgical correction for rigid clubfoot deformity.[74,79,80] Anatomic deformities persist after treatment of clubfoot and should be recognized as children grow. Many treated clubfeet have small, squared tali with flattened heads, decreased talocalcaneal angles, subtalar joint changes, and medial displacement of the navicular. Valgus deformity may result from overcorrection.

Congenital Vertical Talus

Etiologies, Pathophysiology, and Clinical Presentation Congenital vertical talus (congenital rigid flatfoot) may be an isolated condition or may be seen in association with various syndromes (e.g., trisomies) or other systemic abnormalities (i.e., central nervous system defects, arthrogryposis, and neurofibromatosis).[81,82]

Imaging The talus is almost completely vertical in this condition (parallel with the longitudinal axis of the tibia), and the calcaneus is fixed in plantar flexion (equinus) (Fig. 134-28). In the anteroposterior projection, the talar axis is medial to the base of the first metatarsal (valgus). The navicular dislocates dorsally, and clinically, a pronated rocker-bottom foot is present. After the navicular ossifies, its abnormal position helps to distinguish congenital vertical talus from severe planovalgus or flatfoot deformity. Prior to ossification,

the position of the navicular can be determined by ultrasonography.[83]

Treatment Congenital vertical talus is initially managed with conservative measures, followed by surgical correction for recalcitrant cases.[82]

Rocker-Bottom Foot

Etiologies, Pathophysiology, and Clinical Presentation Rocker-bottom foot is seen with congenital vertical talus and severe cerebral palsy with hindfoot valgus, and it occurs as a complication of incorrectly treated clubfoot with persistent equinus.

Imaging In rocker-bottom foot, the calcaneus is in equinus position and the metatarsals are dorsiflexed, producing a convex surface on the bottom of the foot.

Metatarsus Varus (Adductus)

Etiologies, Pathophysiology, and Clinical Presentation Metatarsus adductus is a cause of in-toeing that is usually seen in children younger than 5 years of age. Forefoot adduction differs from clubfoot in that midfoot and hindfoot relationships are normally maintained. The affected foot has a C-shaped contour on examination. Forefoot adduction simulating metatarsus adductus may occur as a result of excessive internal tibial torsion or increased femoral neck anteversion.

Imaging The metatarsals are adducted and hindfoot alignment is normal.

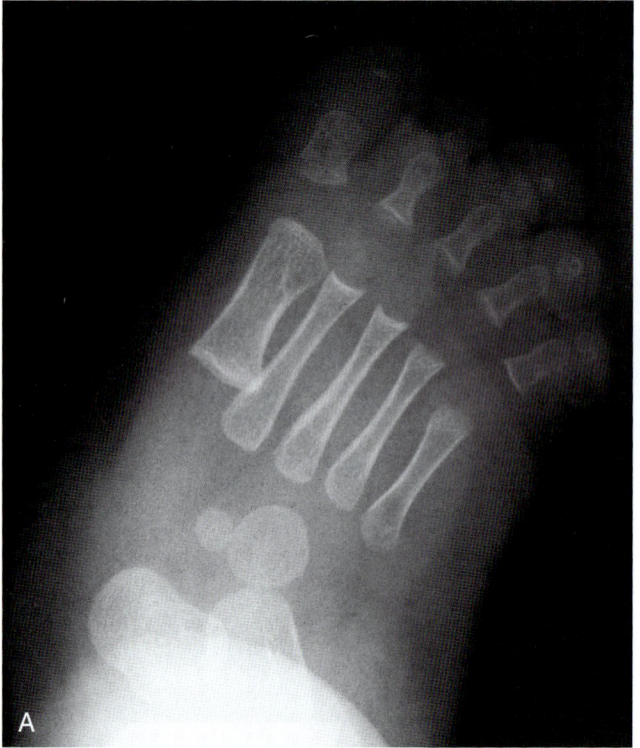

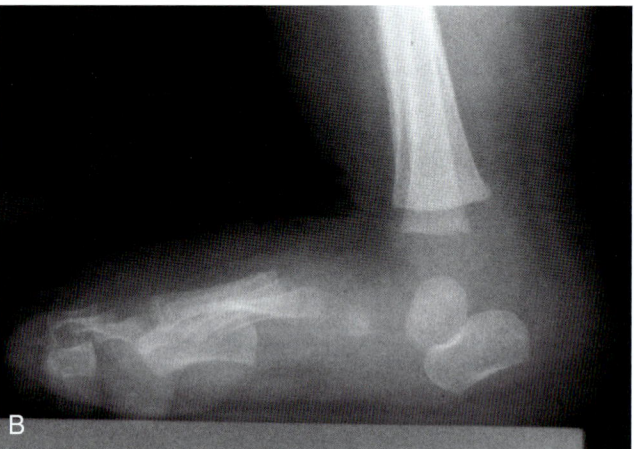

Figure 134-28 Congenital vertical talus in 7-month-old boy. **A,** In the anteroposterior view, the axis of the talus projects well medial to the base of the first metatarsal, consistent with hindfoot valgus. **B,** In the lateral view, the talus is nearly vertical in orientation, and the calcaneus is plantarflexed.

Treatment Metatarsus adductus commonly resolves with normal maturation and no treatment.[84]

Skewfoot

Etiologies, Pathophysiology, and Clinical Presentation Skewfoot (Z-foot; serpentine metatarsus adductus) is considered a severe form of metatarsus adductus. It is not a congenital deformity but develops in the young child idiopathically or may result from the treatment of other congenital foot deformities such as treated clubfoot or vertical talus. Skewfoot occurs in children with cerebral palsy and with some dysplasias and in otherwise normal children as well.[85]

Imaging In skewfoot, the forefoot is adducted, the midfoot is abducted, and the hindfoot is in valgus, resulting in a "Z"-like distortion of the bones of the foot (Fig. 134-29).[85]

Treatment Conservative management suffices in most idiopathic cases, with resolution of the abnormality. A variety of surgical techniques have been applied to reduce deformity in children with fixed or progressive deformity.[84,85]

Flatfoot (Pes Planus)

Etiologies, Pathophysiology, and Clinical Presentation Flatfoot (pes planus) is a descriptive term. The differential diagnosis of pes planus includes flexible planovalgus foot, peroneal spastic (rigid) flatfoot related to tarsal coalition, congenital vertical talus (congenital rigid flatfoot), and congenital

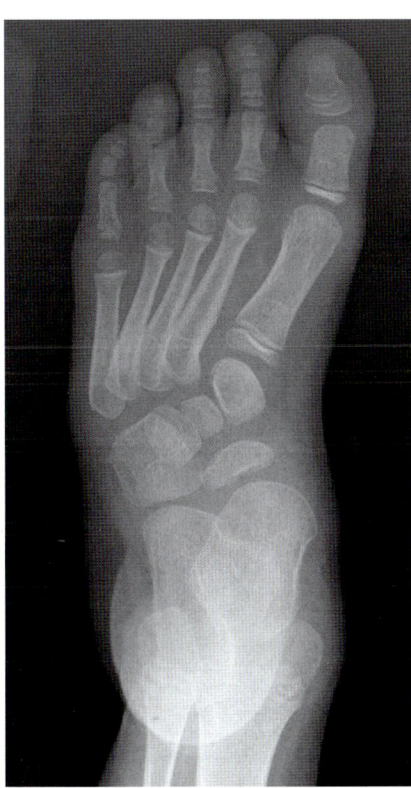

Figure 134-29 Skewfoot in a 6-year-old girl. The forefoot is adducted, midfoot is abducted, and the hindfoot is in valgus, resulting in a Z-shaped appearance of the feet.

calcaneovalgus (congenital flexible flatfoot).[81,86-88] Tarsal coalition is discussed in Chapter 128.

The common flatfoot is a painless, flexible planovalgus foot.[91] Variable degrees of hindfoot valgus, plantar arch flattening, and forefoot pronation occur. Pathology is thought to involve excess ligamentous laxity, which allows the calcaneus to shift into a valgus position under the talus. Abduction and eversion result from loss of calcaneal support. Patients may develop peroneal muscle spasm and pain caused by irritation.

Imaging With flexible planovalgus foot, the anteroposterior projection shows hindfoot valgus with an increased talocalcaneal angle and the midtalar line passing medial to the first metatarsal. On the lateral projection, hindfoot valgus causes the talus to be more vertical than normal. The navicular subluxes dorsally and laterally with respect to the talar head. The calcaneus and metatarsals are horizontal longitudinally, and loss of the plantar arch is noted.[81] Similar deformity may occur in some children with cerebral palsy (e-Fig. 134-30). With a rigid or painful flatfoot (peroneal spastic flatfoot), CT may be performed to detect an underlying subtalar coalition.

Treatment Therapy for pes planus depends on the etiology and type of deformity.[86] Flexible planovalgus deformity is managed conservatively.[88] Rigid (spastic) flat foot with tarsal coalition requires surgery.[87]

Calcaneovalgus

Etiologies, Pathophysiology, and Clinical Presentation Calcaneovalgus feet are reflective of intrauterine positioning. A total of 30% to 50% of newborns have mild calcaneovalgus deformity.[91] In severe congenital calcaneovalgus, the foot is dorsiflexed with respect to the talus. The defect is flexible and correctable.

Imaging Radiographs show the hindfoot in severe valgus position with a plantar flexed talus. The navicular is not dislocated. The defect is flexible and correctable.

Treatment Calcanovalgus foot is treated conservatively with physical therapy.

Cavus Foot

Etiologies, Pathophysiology, and Clinical Presentation An idiopathic congenital form of cavus foot exists, but more commonly, the finding is related to neuromuscular abnormalities, including peroneal muscular atrophy (Charcot-Marie-Tooth disease), Friedreich ataxia, myelomeningocele, poliomyelitis, and other paralytic conditions.[89,90] A cavus foot may also result from treated clubfoot deformity.

Imaging In pes cavus, the longitudinal plantar arch is increased. The anterior calcaneus is abnormally dorsiflexed and the metatarsals are plantarflexed (Fig. 134-31).

Treatment Treatment may involve conservative measures and surgery (soft tissue and plantar fascia release, osteotomy, tendon transfers).[89]

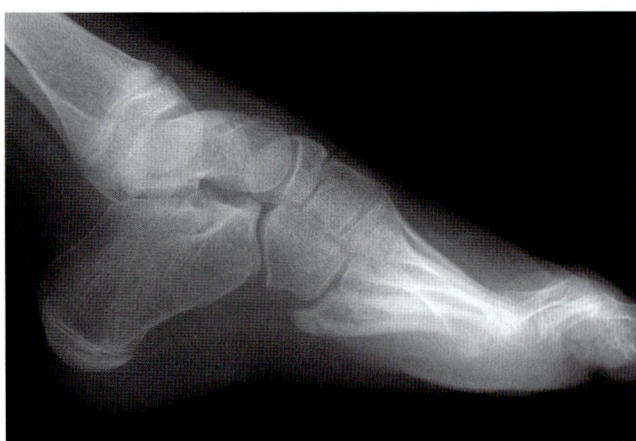

Figure 134-31 Marked pes cavus in an 11-year-old girl with Charcot-Marie-Tooth peroneal muscular atrophy. The talocalcaneal angle is increased, and the longitudinal arch is elevated. The metatarsophalangeal joints are extended, and the interphalangeal joints are flexed (hammertoe deformity).

Hallux Valgus

Etiologies, Pathophysiology, and Clinical Presentation Hallux valgus deformity begins to develop and may occasionally present in childhood.[91] Hallux valgus affects females ten times as frequently as males. Patients present with pain and deformity which may interfere with proper shoe fitting.

Imaging The upper normal limit of medial angulation of the proximal phalanx of the great toe to the first metatarsal is 14 to 16 degrees. Higher angles are considered hallux valgus (e-Fig. 134-32). With increasing angulation, the medial margin of the first metatarsal head may become more uncovered and protuberant.

Treatment First metatarsal osteotomy may be performed to correct alignment.[91]

Generalized Disorders

CEREBRAL PALSY

Overview Children with cerebral palsy are afflicted with multiple orthopedic disorders requiring radiographic investigation and surveillance.[102,103] Variable manifestations of cerebral palsy are caused by variation in severity and location of the original insult.[102] In most cases, cerebral palsy is the consequence of fetal or perinatal insult to the brain, usually hypoxic–ischemic or hemorrhagic in nature. Cerebral palsy also occurs as the result of injury to the brain matter that occurs during early childhood.

Etiologies, Pathophysiology, and Clinical Presentation The orthopedic disorders of cerebral palsy are caused by imbalanced muscular forces. Although cerebral palsy is a static encephalopathy, the resultant musculoskeletal disease may be progressive, even after skeletal maturity.

Imaging About 25% of cerebral palsy patients have scoliosis.[32,104] Scoliosis is more prevalent and severe with greater neurologic deficit. Scoliosis occurs as the result of imbalanced forces on the two sides of the spinal column. As opposed to the S-shaped curves of idiopathic scoliosis, curves in cerebral palsy often have a long C-shaped contour, and the curves may progress after skeletal maturation.[32,94] Associated findings may include accentuated thoracic kyphosis or lumbar lordosis, spondylolysis or spondylolisthesis, and pelvic obliquity. Nonambulatory patients also show caninization of the vertebral bodies (narrow anteroposterior diameter) caused by lack of weightbearing forces during development.

Upper extremity defects include radial head dislocation (Fig. 134-33) and contractures at the elbow, wrist, and fingers.[95,96] Kienböck disease and negative ulnar variance are of increased incidence in cerebral palsy, but a link between the two findings has not been shown in these patients.[97] Accelerated degenerative changes in the elbow and wrist are common in older patients with cerebral palsy.[95]

Abnormalities at the hip include coxa valga caused by lack of weightbearing, increased femoral anteversion, prominence of the lesser trochanter caused by external rotation forces by the iliopsoas tendon, femoral head subluxation or dislocation, acetabular hypoplasia and dysplasia, and flattening of the femoral head (see Fig. 134-9).[32,98] Posterior and superior acetabular deficiency is seen. Patients may experience pain with progressive hip subluxation, which progresses to dislocation. The "windswept" pelvis is seen when one hip has an adductor contracture and the other hip has an abductor contracture, reflecting the asymmetric neuromuscular defects often seen in nonambulatory patients with severe spasticity. Older patients with cerebral palsy show evidence of superimposed degenerative disease at the hips.

At the knee, flexion contractures may be present. The patella is often high (patella alta) and elongated.[32,99] Tug lesions are common at the lower pole of the patella, producing a fragmented appearance.[32,100] The tibial tuberosity may appear elevated and irregular. Genu recurvatum may be seen with rectus femoris contracture. Valgus is seen at the ankle, and equinus and hindfoot valgus are common in the foot (see e-Fig. 134-30).[32,101] Osteopenia predisposes patients with cerebral palsy to fracture.[102]

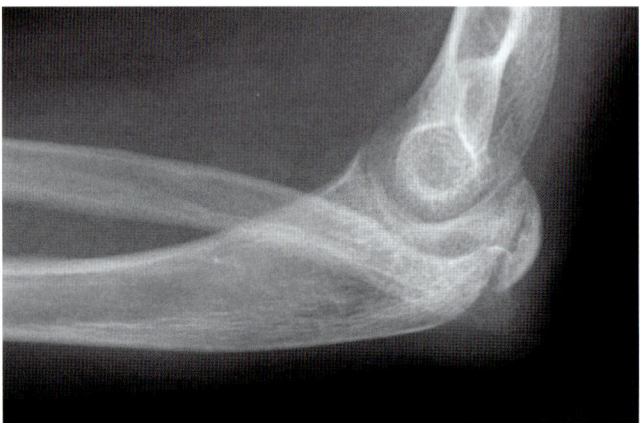

Figure 134-33 Chronic radial head dislocation in a 14-year-old boy with cerebral palsy. The radial head is displaced posteriorly and has a rounded contour. The radius is bowed anteriorly. Similar findings were present on the opposite side.

Treatment Treatment of orthopedic conditions in cerebral palsy is aimed at maximizing function and limiting the progression of deformity.

MYELOMENINGOCELE

Overview Children with myelomeningocele and related spinal disorders may be afflicted with multiple orthopedic disorders of the spine and lower extremity requiring radiographic investigation and surveillance.[103,104] Variable manifestations of myelomeningocele relate to the level of the defect. Children with other spinal pathologies, including those suffering injury to the spinal cord at a young age, may develop orthopedic disorders similar to those with myelomeningocele.

Etiologies, Pathophysiology, and Clinical Presentation Orthopedic disorders in myelomeningocele patients are caused by lack of normal muscle development and function. This leads to scoliosis and joint malalignments.

Imaging Scoliosis in patients with myelomeningocele may be congenital or developmental and progressive.[104] In 20% of patients with myelomeningocele, congenital scoliosis is often caused by vertebral segmentation errors. Congenital kyphosis is most common at L1-L2. Kyphosis may also be acquired.[104] Lumbar lordosis is commonly accentuated.

One third to one half of patients with myelomeningocele have hip dysplasia. The hips are occasionally dislocated at birth; however, more often, dysplasia develops over time as the result of paralysis of the hip extensors and abductors with unopposed hip flexors and adductors (e-Fig. 134-34).[104] Coxa valga and increased femoral anteversion are common.[104] Excessive external tibial torsion with out-toeing or internal tibial torsion with in-toeing may be seen. In all, 80% to 95% of patients have foot deformities. Equinovarus (clubfoot), congenital vertical talus, and other foot deformities may also be seen in these patients.[104]

Infants with myelomeningocele have an increased incidence of fracture of a lower extremity during birth.[105] A higher incidence of fracture is seen with contractures and higher levels of spinal defect. Patients with myelomeningocele may develop neuropathic injuries as the result of osteoporosis and lack of sensation.[104,106,107] Fractures are most commonly metaphyseal or diaphyseal, but they may occur through a physis. Periosteal new bone and callous may be exuberant because of delayed diagnosis without immobilization and abundant subperiosteal hemorrhage.[104,106] Such injuries may be mistaken for tumor or infection.

Treatment Treatment of orthopedic conditions in patients with myelomeningocele is aimed at maximizing function and limiting the progression of deformity.

✓ **WHAT THE CLINICIAN NEEDS TO KNOW**

- Whether the alignment disorder is caused by an underlying bone disorder or dysplasia, affecting treatment
- Accurate measurements of bone length, angulation, and displacement
- Degree of physeal fusion within the involved bones
- Progression of abnormality from the previous examination
- Complications of treatment

Key Points

Radiography plays a key role in the diagnosis and surveillance of disorders of alignment. Proper positioning of the patient facilitates evaluation.

Radiography may show findings of an underlying disorder or complications of treatment, either of which might be clinically unsuspected.

Bowleg and knock-knee may be physiologic, depending on the age of the patient and the degree of abnormality.

Radiographic assessment of the foot requires a clear understanding of normal anatomic relationships.

Orthopedic disorders are common in cerebral palsy. Deformity may continue to progress after skeletal maturity because of imbalanced muscular forces.

Suggested Readings

Driscoll SW, Skinner J. Musculoskeletal complications of neuromuscular disease in children. *Phys Med Rehabil Clin North Am.* 2008;19:163-194.

Kling TF. Angular deformities of the lower limbs in children. *Orthop Clin North Am.* 1987;18:513-527.

Morrell DS, Pearson JM, Sauser DD. Progressive bone and joint abnormalities of the spine and lower extremities in cerebral palsy. *Radiographics.* 2002;22:257-268.

Ozonoff MB. *Pediatric orthopedic radiology.* 2nd ed. Philadelphia: WB Saunders; 1992.

Oestreich AE. *How to measure angles from foot radiographs: a primer.* 1st ed. New York: Springer-Verlag; 1990.

References

Full references for this chapter can be found on www.expertconsult.com.

Chapter 135

Scoliosis

SUMIT PRUTHI

The term *scoliosis* is defined as a structural lateral curvature of the spine in a coronal plane greater than 10 degrees, as measured by the Cobb method on a standing radiograph.[1] Curves less than 10 degrees are termed *spinal asymmetry*. The lateral curvature is often accompanied by abnormalities in the axial and the sagittal planes rendering it a three-dimensional abnormality, an important concept that influences assessment and management. Scoliosis is classified into various categories, according to etiology, curve location, age at onset, and curve type. The Scoliosis Research Society has classified scoliosis into the following broad subcategories:[2]

1. Idiopathic (infantile, juvenile, and adolescent)
2. Congenital (osteogenic and neuropathic)
3. Neuromuscular (neuropathic and myopathic)
4. Developmental syndromes (dysplasias and dysostosis)
5. Tumor associated (vertebral and intraspinal)

Biomechanics and Pathogenesis

Scoliosis is a three-dimensional deformity involving the coronal, sagittal, and axial planes. The initiation and progression of the scoliotic curve is commonly thought to result from the effect of Hueter-Volkmann law, which states that epiphyseal growth (ring apophysis of the vertebral body) in the skeletally immature is inhibited when a compressive force acts on it and stimulated when a distraction force is applied.[1,3] An initial abnormality in the axial plane leads to more compressive forces on the ventral aspect of vertebral body or disc and less on the posterior aspect. This discrepant growth of the anterior part versus the posterior part of the spine is accentuated over time, particularly during rapid skeletal growth, leading to eventual differential growth of the left and right sides of the spine, with suppression of growth on the concave side and excessive growth on the convex side eventually leading to scoliosis.[3] This asymmetric growth not only forms the genesis of the curve but may also have significant surgical implications, as the pedicles on the concave side become asymmetrically smaller, posing a surgical challenge in pedicle screw for spinal fixation.[4]

Terminology

An understanding of the nomenclature and methods of measurement used to describe scoliosis on radiographs is essential for radiologists (Fig. 135-1). Identification of the curve apex or the apical vertebra, significant vertebrae, and central sacral vertebral line (CSVL) is not only crucial for denoting the curve type, assessing curve stability, and selecting the surgical approach and instrumentation system but also for determining the optimal level for fusion.[5,6]

- *CSVL:* CSVL is a vertical line that is drawn perpendicular to an imaginary tangential line drawn across the top of the iliac crests bisecting the sacrum. This is used to identify the stable vertebrae, evaluate coronal balance, and determine the curve type, independent of the curve classification system applied.[5-7]
- *Apex: Apex* is defined as the vertebra or the disc that is farthest from the CSVL and the most rotated and horizontal vertebra.
- *End vertebrae:* The vertebrae with the maximum tilt or angulation toward the apex or concavity of the curve. They usually demarcate the proximal and distal vertebral bodies of the curve and are used to measure the Cobb angle.
- *Stable vertebra:* The vertebral body at the distal and proximal aspect of the curve that is bisected or nearly bisected by the CSVL.
- *Neutral vertebrae:* These represent the most nonrotated vertebrae and may be at the same level as end vertebrae or proximal or distally within the curve.
- *Plumb line:* This represents the vertical line drawn downward on standing radiographs from the center of the C7 vertebral body to assess coronal and sagittal balance. Measuring the distance between the CSVL and the plumb line assesses coronal balance. Sagittal balance is evaluated by measuring the distance between the posterosuperior aspect of the S1 vertebral body and the plumb line. An abnormal coronal and sagittal balance is defined if the distance is greater than 2 cm. A plumb line located to the right of the CSVL reflects positive coronal balance and a line located to the left of the CSVL reflects negative coronal balance. Similarly, a plumb line that is anterior to the posterosuperior aspect of the S1 body is considered positive sagittal balance, whereas a plumb line that is posterior to the posterosuperior aspect of the S1 body is considered negative sagittal balance.[5-8]
- *Sagittal balance:* The primary sagittal curves, which are present since birth, include the thoracic and sacral kyphoses. The secondary curves, which are acquired to

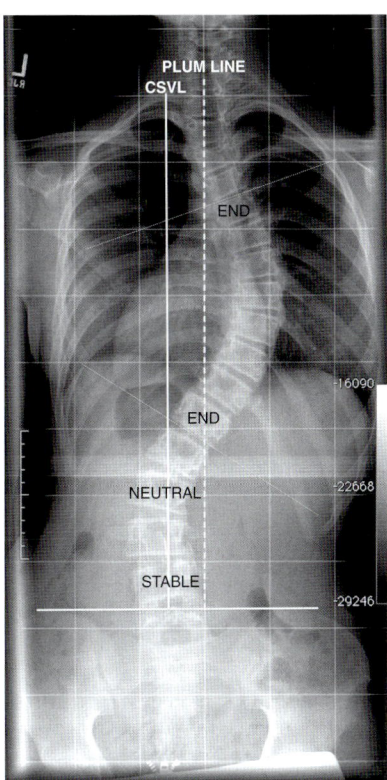

Figure 135-1 **Nomenclature.** Standing posteroanterior radiograph from a patient with scoliosis: central sacral vertebral line (CSVL) (*solid line*) is a line that is perpendicular to a tangent across the iliac crest, bisecting the sacrum. The stable vertebra is the vertebra that is bisected or nearly bisected by the CSVL. The end vertebrae are the vertebra that are most tilted along the curve. Tangents (*thin dotted-dash line*) are drawn along the superior end plate of superior end vertebra and inferior end plate of inferior end vertebra to calculate the Cobb angle. A neutral vertebra is one that is not rotated. The plumb line is a line that is drawn from the center of the C7 vertebral body and is parallel to the edge of the image. If the distance between the CSVL and the plumb line is 2 cm or greater, it indicates coronal imbalance.

assume bipedal stance, include the cervical and lumbar lordoses. This normal mature pattern of sagittal alignment is established by age 6 years.[9,10] Thoracic kyphosis ranges between 10 and 50 degrees and is measured from T5 to T12 with apex usually at T6-T8. Lumbar lordosis ranges from 35 to 80 degrees when measured from L1 to L5, with apex between L3 and L4.[1,11,12] In scoliosis, the thoracic kyphosis is mainly influenced by the spinal deformity, whereas lumbar lordosis is mainly influenced by pelvic configuration.[13] Most thoracic idiopathic scoliosis is associated with a decrease in normal thoracic kyphosis. A true kyphotic component may indicate a congenital or neuromuscular origin; however, some idiopathic cases may have a true kyphotic component.[1,6,13] Positive sagittal balance is more significantly associated with pain and disability than curve magnitude, curve location, or coronal imbalance.[13,14]

- *Curve location:* This is defined on the basis of the location of the apical vertebra and is classified as *cervical* (apex between C2 and C6), *cervicothoracic* (C7–T1), *thoracic* (T2–T11), *thoracolumbar* (T12–L1), *lumbar* (L2–L4), or *lumbosacral* (L5 and below).[1,6,13]
- *Curve types:* The curve is classified broadly as *primary* (major) or *secondary* (minor) *curves*, or *structural* or

nonstructural curves. Primary curves are the first to appear and are the largest abnormal curves. Secondary curves usually develop later to stabilize the position of the head and pelvis.[6,13-15] A structural curve is a curve that is not correctable on side-bending views or on traction and is accompanied by vertebral rotational abnormalities. A nonstructural curve usually corrects on bending views and may be secondary curves or functional curves (curves related to posture, secondary to leg length discrepancy, muscle spasm, etc.).[13] Curves that are 25 degrees or greater on the standing anteroposterior radiograph and do not decrease to less than 25 degrees on the side-bending radiographs should be considered structural.[16] A curve less than 25 degrees on the standing anteroposterior radiograph may be deemed structural if the regional sagittal profile reveals a kyphosis +20 degrees or greater.[16] If a curve is considered structural, it should be included in the fusion surgery.

- *Classification of curves:* Various different classification systems exist describing the curve types preoperatively. The importance of classification systems is that they help guide the surgical approach and help compare the efficacy of different treatment methods.[6,13] The Lenke classification system is the most recent and widely used classification system, replacing the established King-Moe classification system. The Lenke system is considered more comprehensive, complete, and reliable and takes into account the three-dimensional nature of scoliosis as opposed to the two-dimensional approach of the King-Moe classification.[6,13,16,17] The Lenke system divides curves on the basis of location and type, differentiates structural from nonstructural curves, includes lumbar and sagittal modifiers, and proposes that only major curves and minor structural curves should be included in spinal arthrodesis.[16,17] For unknown reasons, the typical curve in adolescent idiopathic scoliosis is usually a thoracic curve with right-sided convexity.

Idiopathic Scoliosis

Idiopathic scoliosis constitutes 80% of the patients with spinal deformity and is a diagnosis of exclusion.[1] A judicious use of various imaging is a necessary prerequisite to exclude other underlying causes of scoliosis before labeling any case as idiopathic.

Etiologies, Pathophysiology, and Clinical Presentation The reported prevalence of idiopathic scoliosis in children and adolescents ranges from 0.5 to 3 per 100.[1,18,19] In the mild curves (<20 degrees), the female-to-male ratio is 1:1, but, when greater and progressive curves are evaluated (>30 degrees), females predominate with a 5:1 to 7:1 ratio. Only 0.2% of children have severe curves (>30 degrees).[1,19,20]

Idiopathic scoliosis is further divided into the following types based on age at diagnosis: *infantile* (0-3 years); *juvenile* (4-10 years); *adolescent* (11-17 years); and *adult* (≥18 years). Age at onset has prognostic significance both in terms of underlying neuraxis abnormality as a cause of scoliosis and the natural history of the curve. Whether juvenile scoliosis is truly a separate entity, is debatable because of the high prevalence of associated abnormalities in preadolescent scoliosis by magnetic resonance imaging (MRI).[2] Moreover, the demarcation is further obscured by the possibility of early existence of the established adolescent curve. Hence the terms *early onset* and *late onset* are increasingly being used to classify scoliosis after the age of 5 years.[2,21] The rationale behind this distinction is the increased risk of cardiopulmonary compromise in children before age 5 years with larger curves.[2,22]

Imaging The role of imaging in scoliosis is early detection and characterization of the type of curve and its severity, assessment of disease progression, definition of the need and timing of the surgery, monitoring of changes related to treatment, and identification of those cases in which an underlying structural anomaly is present.[23] The extent and type of imaging is also governed by the category of scoliosis. Cross-sectional imaging is extensively used in congenital scoliosis to identify and characterize structural anomalies, whereas radiography is principally utilized in idiopathic scoliosis to monitor curve progression.[2]

Screening Upright, standing, posteroanterior radiograph of the entire spine is the standard initial screening examination, once the deformity is suspected clinically. The radiograph should include the cervicothoracic junction, enough of the pelvis to show the iliac crest in full extent, and the triradiate cartilage to enable assessment of skeletal maturity. Although standing radiography is preferred, sitting or supine radiography may be the only alternative in young patients, patients with congenital scoliosis, or patients with severe neuromuscular disorders. The rationale behind standing radiography is that treatment methods are based on standing views and the magnitude of the curve is greatest in the standing position. This is an important consideration in congenital and infantile scoliosis when young patients with scoliosis start to ambulate. It is easy to mistake change in curvature as curve progression if the upright radiograph is compared with a prior supine radiograph.[1] The patient should stand with the feet placed shoulder width apart, looking straight ahead with the elbows bent and knuckles in the supraclavicular fossa bilaterally, allowing visualization of the upper thoracic region on the lateral radiographs.[24] A lateral radiograph is not required at the time of screening but should be obtained in patients with documented scoliosis to assess sagittal balance. Radiographic techniques should minimize radiation exposure, especially to sensitive organs (e.g., breast, thyroid, and lens of eyes). A posteroanterior technique involves less radiation to the breast compared with an anteroposterior technique. The image may have a grid that helps identify deviations of the spine from the plumb line. When surgical treatment is considered, side-bending radiographs are acquired to differentiate between structural and nonstructural minor curves to help guide the optimal level of fusion. Various techniques used to obtain side-bending radiographs include supine bending, standing bending, and bending over a bolster.

Curve Magnitude: The Cobb angle is the accepted standard for assessing the magnitude of the scoliotic curve. It is defined as the angle formed by the intersection of two lines, one parallel to the end plate of the superior end vertebra and the other parallel to the end plate of the inferior end vertebra. Alternatively, pedicles may be used to calculate the Cobb

angle when the end plates are poorly defined because of radiographic technique or obscured because of the severity of the curve. Although the Cobb angle provides limited assessment of the deformity and does not take rotation into account, it is still the foundation for diagnosis, follow-up, and treatment.[1] The angle may be plotted manually or digitally with equal reliability.[25] It is important to note that multiple factors, including patient positioning, radiographic techniques, known diurnal variation of 5 degrees, and interobserver and intraobserver variability, may affect the reproducibility of the angle.[26-30] A progressive curve is usually defined by a Cobb angle increase of 5 degrees or more between consecutive radiographic examinations.[1,2,6] The Cobb angle may decrease because of prone positioning and anesthesia during surgery, which sometimes leads to a postoperative rebound effect, with loss of correction when the patient returns to the standing position.[6,13] Despite multiple caveats, measurements of the Cobb angle are usually considered reproducible, particularly when measuring end plates, patient positioning and techniques are kept constant.

Assessing Curve Progression: Prognosis and management in scoliosis is highly specific to the case and the surgeon but is usually governed by three important factors: (1) etiology, (2) magnitude and the type of the curve at presentation, and (3) speed of curve progression. The risk of progression is directly related to the spinal growth remaining, the severity of the curve at presentation, and the gender of the patient.[1,10,19,31,32] Various clinical tools to assess residual growth potential include chronologic age, menarche in girls, serial height measurements, and Tanner staging.[10,19,33-37] In general, the onset of the adolescent growth spurt occurs at 13 years in boys and 11 years in girls, with menarche indicating the declining phase of the growing peak and a low risk of progression for idiopathic curves under 30 degrees.[1,10,33,35] Various radiographic parameters may indicate remaining potential growth. Development of the iliac bone apophysis, quantified by Risser, has become a universally accepted sign (Fig. 135-2). Despite the wide use of the Risser grade as a measure of maturity, the appearance of the iliac apophysis generally occurs after the most important period of rapid growth.[1,33,34] Given the inaccuracies related to the Risser grade, other radiographic parameters are used to assess bone maturation. Bone age may be assessed from a hand and wrist radiograph; however, use of bone age becomes less accurate in the juvenile age group secondary to the larger standard deviation and suffers from interobserver variability.[1,38] Assessment of pelvic triradiate cartilage is considered more accurate than the Risser grade. The triradiate cartilage closes around age 11 years in girls at the time of peak growth velocity.[1,23] The physis of the olecranon of the elbow closes at age 13 years, shortly before menarche and may also be used to assess remaining skeletal growth.[23] Unfortunately, many of the above-mentioned markers of maturity are quite variable and may be difficult to put in proper context without an accurate record of prior growth performance. Sometime, more than one imaging parameter is taken into consideration for accurately assessing skeletal maturation.

With regard to *curve patterns*, curves with an apex above T-12 are more likely to progress compared with isolated lumbar curves.[1] With regard to *curve magnitude*, Risser stage 0 or 1 patients with an initial curve of 5 to 19 degrees progressed in 22% of cases, compared with curve progression in

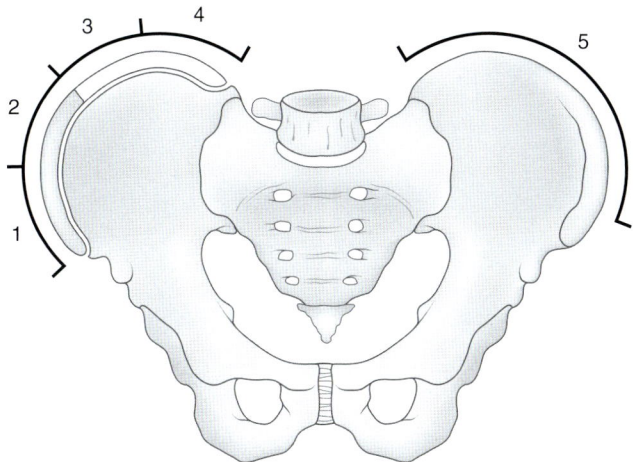

Figure 135-2 Risser grade. The Risser grade proceeds from grade 0 (no ossification) to grade 4 (all four quadrants show ossification of the iliac apophysis). When the ossified apophysis fuses completely to the ilium (Risser grade 5), the patient is skeletally mature. (From Herring JA, ed. Scoliosis. In: Herring JA, ed. *Tachdjian's pediatric orthopedics. vol 1.* 3rd ed. Philadelphia: WB Saunders; 2002:213-321.)

68% of cases with initial curve magnitude of 20 to 29 degrees.[32] The rate of curve progression increased to 90% when the initial curve was 30 to 59 degrees.[1]

Most idiopathic scoliosis cases do not require imaging beyond radiography. Evidence does not support the usefulness of MRI in an otherwise normal adolescent with scoliosis.[1,6] The use of MRI in idiopathic scoliosis is restricted to unusual curve patterns, alarming clinical manifestations, or both.[1,6] The prevalence of central nervous system abnormalities in patients with presumed adolescent idiopathic scoliosis is very low, ranging from 2% to 4%.[39,40] Hence, the use of MRI for presurgical screening of neural axis abnormality in patients who have presumed idiopathic scoliosis with a typical curve pattern but no pain or a neurologic deficit is still controversial with no clear consensus.[1,2,6,41]

Indications for using MRI in scoliosis include infantile group; juvenile group; left thoracic curve; abnormal neurologic examination, including abnormal sensory evoked potentials; painful scoliosis; hyperkyphotic sagittal alignment; and rapidly progressing curves.[1,2,6,39,40,42]

Treatment and Follow-up Treatment in idiopathic scoliosis varies on a case-by-case basis and is highly surgeon specific. The majority of patients with idiopathic scoliosis present with curves less than 20 degrees, with very minimal risk of progression even without treatment. These patients usually are monitored with clinical and radiographic follow-up only.[1,6]

Bracing: Bracing (e-Fig. 135-3) is generally indicated when a scoliotic curve progresses from 25 to 30 degrees with a documented annual curve progression of at least 5 degrees, with the upper limit of curve magnitude being 45 degrees.[1,43] Bracing modifies spinal growth by applying an external force and is usually effective in patients with substantial spinal growth remaining (Risser 2 to 3 or less).[1,2,6] The use of bracing may be altered on the basis of the clinical circumstance, with early bracing being used by surgeons when a strong positive family history for progressive scoliosis is present. Bracing may be useful for limiting curve progression but usually does not stop or improve the curve.

Risser Casting: In some cases, a Risser cast or molded cast is applied as an alternative to bracing to provide more corrective force than can be applied by bracing alone (e-Fig. 135-4). The primary indication for Risser casting is in patients who have progressive scoliosis and are too small for rigid instrumentation prior to fusion or in those who have severe deformities and are too young to undergo fusion. The idea behind casting is to avoid repeated surgery as much as possible that may follow application of a growing rod instrumentation system.[1] Similar to bracing, Risser casting only *limits* curve progression but does not stop or reduce the curve.

Surgery: The primary goal of surgical treatment is stabilization of curve progression, the secondary goals being improvement in the spinal alignment and balance of the body.[1,6] The indications for surgical correction are multifaceted and include the degree of curve magnitude, risk for progression, skeletal maturity, and curve pattern. Moreover, the cosmetic perception of the deformity by the patient or the patient's family may also greatly influence the decision for surgery.[1]

Thoracic curves of the Cobb angle greater than 40 to 50 degrees in skeletally immature patients are usually surgically corrected; in skeletally mature patients, surgical correction is reserved for curves of 50 degrees or more.[1] However, a wide range of Cobb angles may act as a threshold for surgery secondary to the reasons mentioned above. The surgical treatment includes corrective instrumentation plus anterior or posterior fusion of the spine, with the aim of correcting both the coronal and sagittal deformities, which include decreased thoracic kyphosis and lumbar lordosis in most cases. The surgical goal is to achieve a stable bony fusion mass to maintain the correction over time, with the hardware serving as internal struts while fusion proceeds (Fig. 135-5). Earlier hardware for spinal fusion included Harrington rods, which corrected coronal plane imbalance at the expense of decreased thoracic kyphosis and flattening of the lumbar spine. As most idiopathic scoliosis patients have a hypokyphotic component, placement of Harrington rods led to a flat back deformity.[1] Because of these reasons, Harrington rods are no longer used and have been replaced by multiple hooks and rod systems addressing the coronal imbalance while maintaining the sagittal balance.[1,44] Instrumentation without fusion (as with growing rods) is sometime used as a temporary method in young children with rapidly progressing curves. The vertical expandable prosthetic titanium rib (VEPTR) is one such method, which is more commonly used in the treatment of infantile and juvenile types of idiopathic scoliosis.

The length of fusion varies according to the curve type and the associated lumbar modifiers.[17] In broad perspective, to improve surgical outcomes, the segment to be fused should be as short as possible but long enough to minimize residual disease. Usually, the stable vertebra, that is, the point where the CSVL bisects the spine, broadly defines the lower limit of fusion.[13] Efforts are made to avoid nonstructural curves and to spare as many mobile segments of the lower lumbar spine.[6]

Follow-up Imaging No standard guidelines are available to monitor patients with idiopathic scoliosis. It is generally recommended that patients with idiopathic scoliosis be monitored every 4 to 12 months, depending on age and growth rate. Those in the rapid phases of growth are seen at more

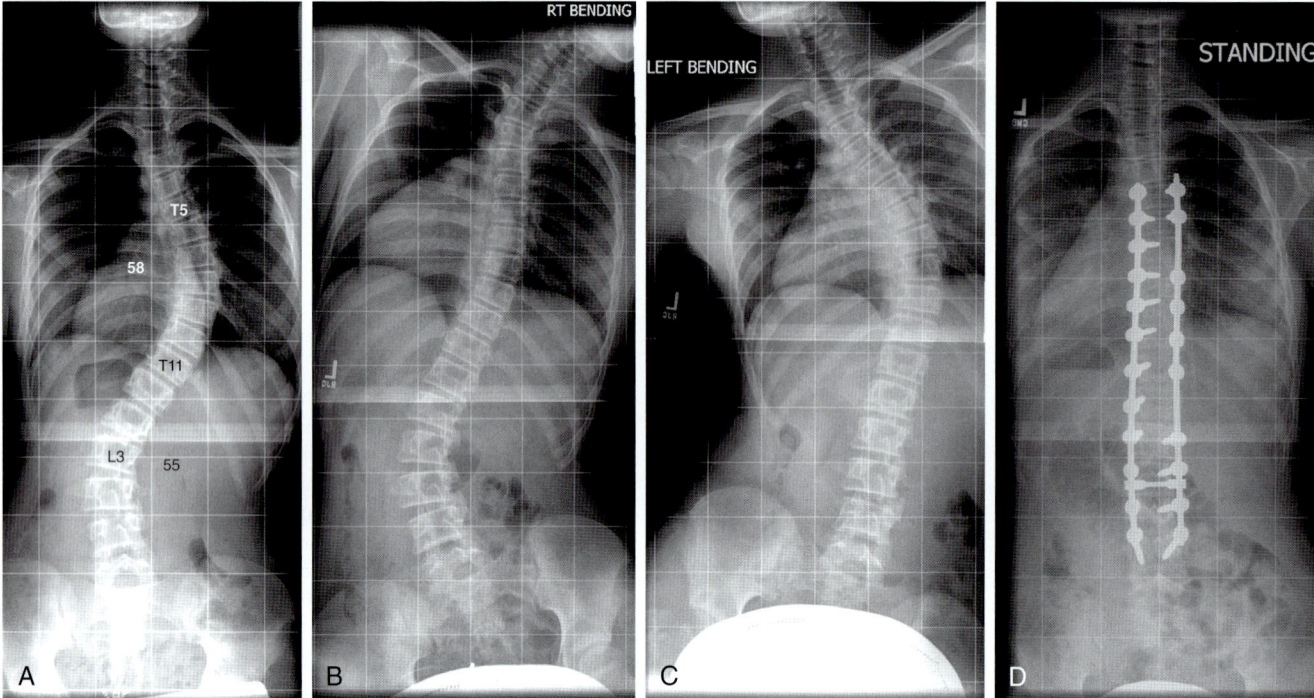

Figure 135-5 Idiopathic scoliosis. A posteroanterior radiograph (**A**) shows a right main thoracic curve with the largest Cobb angle of 58 degrees with its apex at the level of the T8-T9 disk and its end vertebrae at T5 and T11. Rightward-bending anteroposterior (AP) radiograph (**B**) shows some improvement of the main thoracic curve; however, the Cobb angle remains more than 25 degrees, a finding consistent with structural curve based on the Lenke classification. Leftward-bending AP radiograph (**C**) shows that the Cobb angles of the proximal thoracic and lumbar curves do not exceed 25 degrees, indicating nonstructural curves. A postoperative radiograph (**D**) shows posterior spinal fusion extending from T5 through L3 level.

frequent intervals (every 4 to 6 months).[1,6] After the cessation of spinal growth, only curves with Cobb angles greater than 30 degrees should be monitored for progression. Follow-up imaging usually is performed every 5 years, although the follow-up interval depends on the patient's symptoms and the severity of the curvature.[1]

Follow-up usually involves not only monitoring curve progression but also the efficacy of nonsurgical treatment such as bracing. Effective bracing should achieve about 30% correction of the Cobb angle.[45] Subsequent to fixation, patients are usually followed up until the fusion has matured to ensure that the fixation is secure, to exclude the development of pseudoarthrosis, and to exclude recurrence of the deformity.[45]

Congenital Scoliosis

Congenital scoliosis results from disordered embryologic or intrauterine spine development, presumably during somitogenesis between weeks 5 and 8 of gestation.[46] Vertebral malformations are often associated with coexistent nonspinal, musculoskeletal malformations. Multiple recognized syndromes are associated with congenital scoliosis. The two most common known coexisting conditions are VACTERL (*v*ertebral anomaly, *a*norectal atresia, *c*ardiac lesion, *t*racheo*e*sophageal fistula, *r*enal anomaly, *l*imb defect) association and Klippel-Feil syndrome.[46] Scoliosis as a spectrum of skeletal dysplasia is considered separate from congenital scoliosis. Anomalies in skeletal dysplasia result from failure of normal bone growth and development and are not caused by

early failures of vertebral segmentation or formation as in congenital scoliosis. Although labeled as congenital, it is important to note that the clinical deformity may not be apparent at birth and usually develops with spinal growth presenting later in childhood.[46,47]

Etiologies, Pathophysiology, and Clinical Presentation Congenital scoliosis is caused by failures of vertebral segmentation, formation, or a combination of the two. Classifications by Winter et al. and McMaster (Fig. 135-6) are helpful in describing anomalies and predicting which will be progressive.[47-50] If the failure of formation or of segmentation occurs on the right or left side of the vertebral body, scoliosis results. If the segmentation anomaly occurs along the anterior or posterior vertebral body, then congenital kyphosis or lordosis results, respectively.[46] Most cases are combinations of both coronal and sagittal plane deformities, emphasizing the three-dimensional nature of the deformity.

The most common underlying spinal abnormality is a hemivertebra, seen in about 40% of cases, usually resulting from unilateral complete failure of formation and by the absence of a contralateral-paired pedicle.[46,51] Hemivertebrae may be further classified as fully segmented, semisegmented, or nonsegmented on the basis of the relationship to the cranial and caudal vertebrae. Wedged vertebrae result from a unilateral partial failure of formation with presence of two pedicles. "Butterfly vertebrae" are presumed to originate from failure of anterior midline fusion between somite pairs. Complete anterior and posterior failure of segmentation creates a block vertebra, whereas unilateral anterior and posterior failure of segmentation causes a unilateral bar.[46]

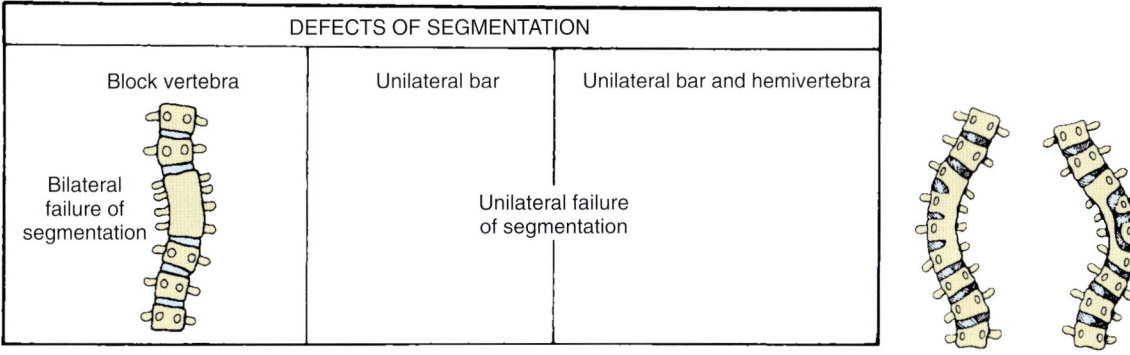

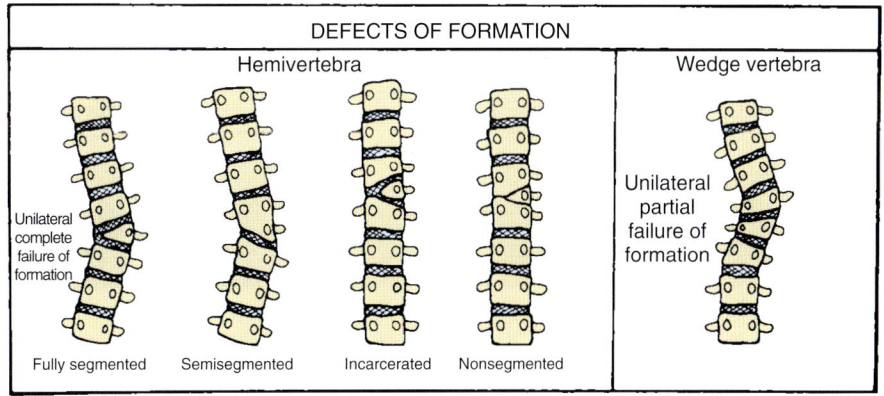

Figure 135-6 Forms of congenital scoliosis. Various types of congenital scoliosis based on defects of segmentation versus defects of formation. (From McMaster MJ. Congenital scoliosis. In: Weinstein SL, ed. *The pediatric spine*. Philadelphia: Lippincott Williams & Wilkins; 2001:161-177.)

Natural history and the risk of progression in congenital scoliosis are related to multiple elements: (1) type of anomaly, (2) site, (3) age at presentation, (4) single versus multiple curves, and (5) associated nonspinal abnormalities.[52] Curve progression has been strongly related to the type of vertebral abnormality (Table 135-1), with unilateral unsegmented bars with contralateral hemivertebrae having the poorest prognosis, a less severe progression with hemivertebrae, and the least severe progression with block and wedge vertebrae (Fig. 135-7).

Imaging Fetal imaging modes, including ultrasonography and MRI, allow early and more comprehensive detection of fetal spinal anomalies, but the significance of earlier detection and prognosis is still being debated.[46] The postnatal diagnosis of congenital scoliosis is usually made with the use of radiography. Findings suggestive of congenital scoliosis include absence of spinous processes, rib fusions, joined pedicles, or absent or narrowed disc spaces.[46] In the majority of cases, identification of the type of anomaly is possible with radiography. Absolute Cobb angle magnitude is of much less

Table 135-1

Median Yearly Rate of Deterioration (in Degrees) without Treatment, for Type of Single Congenital Scoliosis in Each Region of the Spine						
			Hemivertebra		Unilateral Unsegmented Bar	Unilateral Unsegmented Bar and Contralateral Hemivertebrae
Site of Curvature	Block Vertebra	Wedge Vertebra	Single	Double		
Upper thoracic	<1-1†	*-2†	1-2‡	2-2.5§	2-4§	5-6§
Lower thoracic	<1-1†	2-2	2-2.5‡	2-3§	5-6.5§	5-8§
Thoracolumbar	<1-1†	1.5-2†	2-3.5‡	5-*§	6-9§	7-14§
Lumbar	<1-*†	<1-*†	<101‡	*	>5-*§	*
Lumbosacral	*	*	<1-1.5§	*	*	*

*, Too few or no curves; †, no treatment required; ‡, may require spinal surgery; §, requires spinal fusion. Ranges represent the degree of deterioration before and after 10 years of age.
Modified from McMaster MJ, Ohtsuka K. The natural history of congenital scoliosis: A study of 251 patients. *J Bone Joint Surg Am*. 1982;66:588-601. McMaster MJ. Congenital scoliosis caused by a unilateral failure of vertebrae segmentation with contralateral hemivertebrae. *Spine*. 1998;23:998-1005. and McMaster MJ. Congenital scoliosis. In: Weinstein SL, ed. *The pediatric spine*. Philadelphia, PA: Lippincott Williams & Wilkins; 2001:161-177.

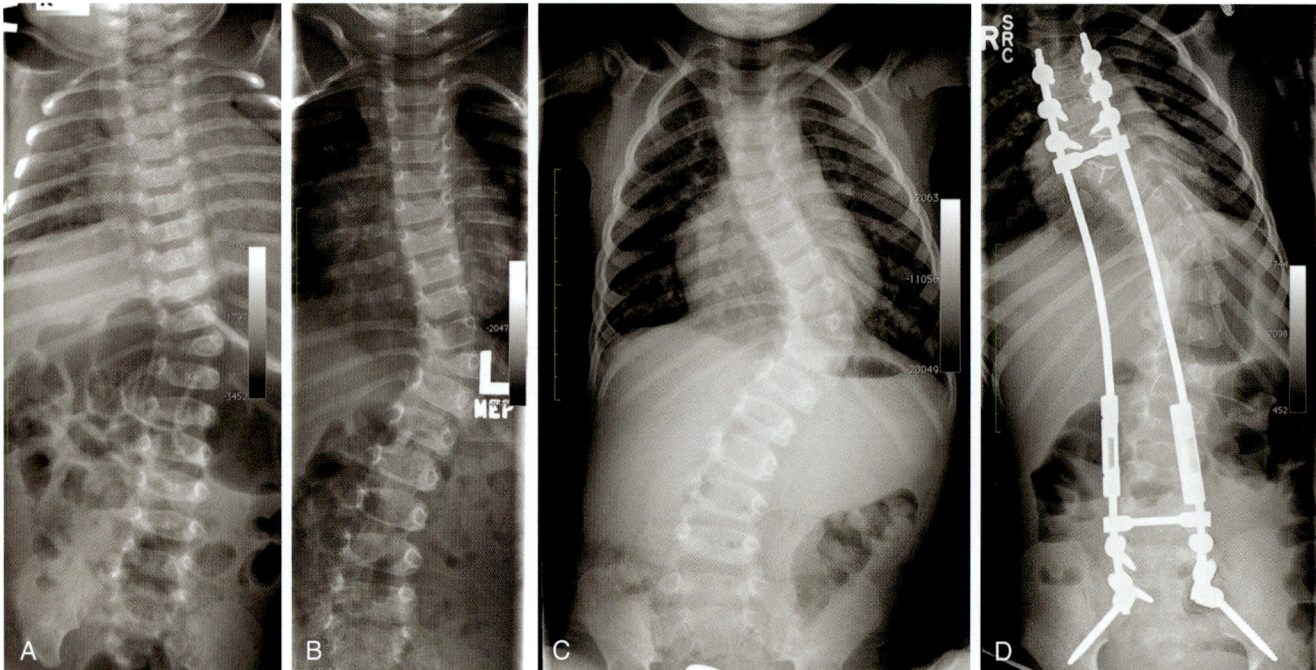

Figure 135-7   *Congenital scoliosis.* Rapid progression of curve in a patient with fully segmented hemivertebra from 32 months (**A**) to 3 years of age (**B**) to 4 years of age (**C**). A postoperative radiograph (**D**) shows placement of expandable posterior spinal fusion hardware, which still allows some continued growth of the abnormal spine with maintaining or controlling the deformity. Curve progression in congenital scoliosis is strongly related to the type of underlying vertebral abnormality, with a poor prognosis associated with unilateral unsegmented bars with contralateral hemivertebrae and fully segmented hemivertebrae, as in this case.

significance than the overall deformity and the change in that deformity over time with growth. Documentation of radiographic change with growth is the mainstay of observation and surgical decision making.[46]

Radiography is very useful if both anterior and posterior structures of anomalous vertebrae correspond to each other. However, it is not uncommon to have differences between the anterior and posterior structures often leading to a complex unclassified pattern of abnormality.[46,51] These characteristics make independent evaluation of the malformation in each vertebra extremely difficult with radiography, which highlights the role of three-dimensional computed tomography (CT) in the evaluation of complex malformations, particularly the posterior elements. Radiography has difficulty in accurately identifying the deformities that will be progressive, which has called for a newer three-dimensional classification of congenital scoliosis.[51] CT is currently restricted as a preoperative evaluation tool. CT may be especially helpful when planning the surgical excision of an anomalous vertebra, as CT may depict unexpected osseous anomalies not clearly depicted on radiography. Preoperative CT angiography may also be useful for determining coexistent vascular anomalies and to assess the relationship of the aorta to the spine.

Imaging in congenital scoliosis not only demands detailed evaluation of the spine but also exclusion of extraspinal anomalies, mainly cardiovascular and genitourinary anomalies.[46] Associated intraspinal or neural axis abnormalities with congenital scoliosis may occur in 20% to 37% of patients, mandating screening (Fig. 135-8).[46,53,54] The most common associated abnormalities include syrinx, Chiari I malformation, cord or spinal canal tumors, diastematomyelia, and low conus medullaris.[46] Spinal ultrasonography may be effective

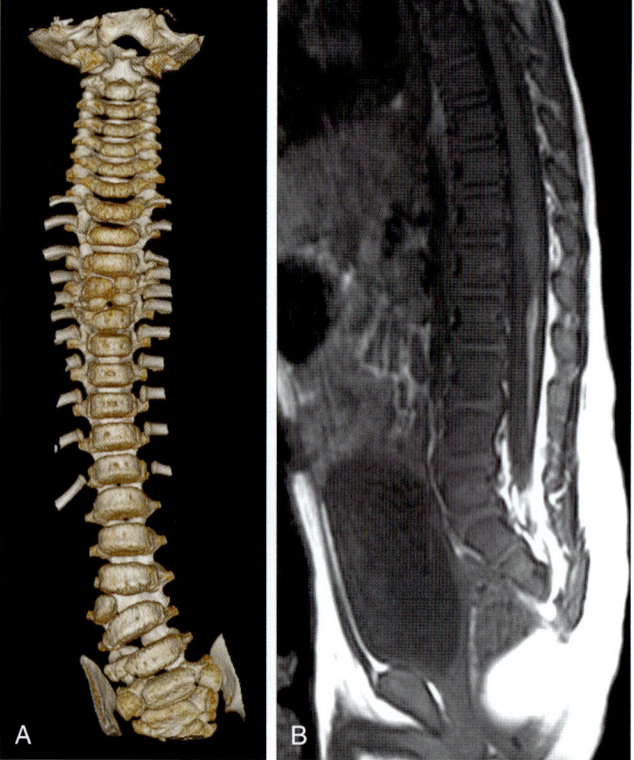

Figure 135-8   *Neural axis abnormality in congenial scoliosis.* A coronal three-dimensional, surface shaded reformatted image of the spine (**A**) clearly demonstrates a lumbar hemivertebra with butterfly vertebrae involving the midthoracic spine. A sagittal T1 magnetic resonance image of the lumbar spine (**B**) in the same patient shows a low-lying cord with an associated filum lipoma. Intraspinal abnormalities in congenital scoliosis are not uncommon, and magnetic resonance imaging of the neural axis is a routine prerequisite before any treatment is contemplated.

for initial screening. The role of MRI as a screening tool in all congenital scoliosis cases is controversial, with some experts believing that MRI should be restricted to presurgical evaluation. If not addressed preoperatively, major associated intraspinal abnormalities, including cord tethering, may lead to progressive deformity and progressive or acute neurologic loss.[46,54]

Treatment Surgery is the mainstay in the treatment of congenital scoliosis, as nonoperative measures provide no definite efficacy; early surgical treatment is preferred to late treatment. If an underlying spinal cord abnormality is found, it should be corrected prior to scoliosis surgery. The various surgical options are complex and beyond the scope of this discussion; however, the traditional approach still includes early fusion to avoid the development of more severe deformities.[46] In some patients, expansion thoracoplasty with the use of the VEPTR device (Fig. 135-9) is used instead of early fusion.[55] This technique is usually utilized in patients with shortened spines, which would necessitate fusion of a long portion of spine at an early age, especially in those with associated chest wall anomalies. The VEPTR technique allows some continued growth of the abnormal spinal elements while still controlling the deformity. A major disadvantage of this treatment is the need for repetitive lengthening procedures, but it may be an appropriate temporary choice in certain children.[46]

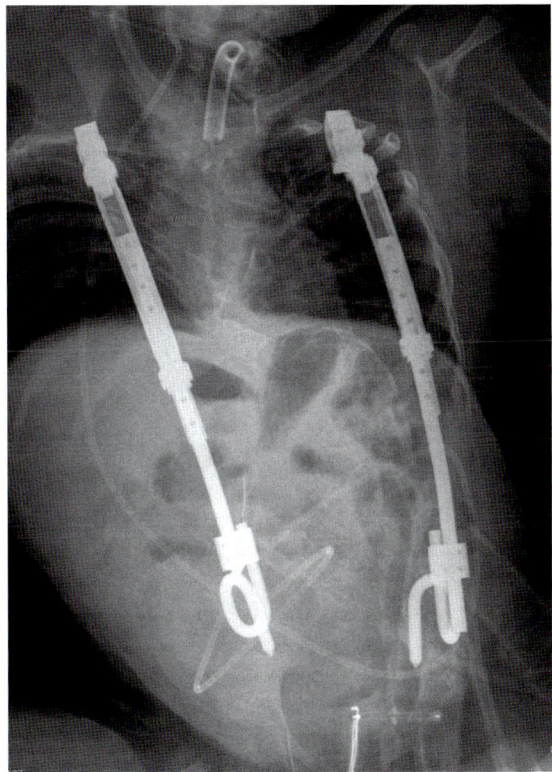

Figure 135-9 A 7-year-old girl with multiple thoracolumbar segmental fusion anomalies presented with severe thoracolumbar scoliosis. A vertical expandable prosthetic titanium rib, extending from the upper ribs and anchored along the iliac crests, was placed.

Neuromuscular Scoliosis

Neuromuscular scoliosis is caused by a defect in the neural pathways through which the central nervous system controls and coordinates muscle activity.

Etiologies, Pathophysiology, and Clinical Presentation The Scoliosis Research Society further classifies neuromuscular scoliosis into neuropathic and myopathic scoliosis.[10] The first group includes include neurologic disorders such as cerebral palsy or spinomuscular dystrophies, and the second group includes muscular disorders such as the muscular dystrophies.

Imaging The characteristic curve pattern in neuromuscular scoliosis is an early onset long C-shaped curve (e-Fig. 135-10) with rapid progression, which continues beyond skeletal maturity. Curve patterns similar to adolescent idiopathic scoliosis may also be seen. Affected children also often present with severe kyphosis or lordosis in the sagittal plane, with multiple additional comorbidities related to their primary disease.[10] Because of non-weight bearing status, the vertebral bodies are often tall and slender. Additional findings include diminished lumbar lordosis with a single, broad-based thoracic kyphosis. In addition, because of the underlying disease entity, these children often have coexisting hip dislocation caused by pelvic muscle imbalance and non–weight bearing status.

Treatment Bracing is usually reserved for nonsevere flexible curves, immature children, and ambulatory patients, and usually does not prevent curve progression.[56] Surgical fusion is the mainstay of the treatment. The objectives of curve correction in neuromuscular scoliosis are to restore seating balance, to facilitate wheelchair use, to control pain, and to support the trunk so as to reinforce respiratory function.[10] Postoperative complications occur more frequently in patients with neuromuscular scoliosis than in those with idiopathic scoliosis, ranging from 44% to 62%, likely related to the presence of multiple comorbidities.[57]

Scoliosis and Radiation

The radiographic examination of children with scoliosis has historically involved a relatively high radiation dose, particularly to the breast, and may increase the risk of subsequent breast cancer.[58] The issues are twofold: (1) Initially, scoliosis radiographs were done in the anteroposterior projection, exposing the adolescent breast to maximum dose; and (2) many patients with scoliosis are adolescent girls with pubertal growth spurt and rapid breast development. Radiography for scoliosis must entail optimization to minimize radiation risk. This includes the use of posteroanterior positioning, high tube voltage, high-speed screen film combinations, contoured filtration, shielding of breasts (if anteroposterior positioning is used, that is, in nonambulatory children who have sitting anteroposterior scoliosis studies), replacement of antiscatter grids with air gap techniques, and appropriate techniques to balance the need for adequate visualization and the use of the lowest possible radiation dosage. The radiation dose may be further reduced by using CT and digital imaging systems.[59,60]

Key Points

Sagittal balance is an important concept in normal spinal stability. All efforts are made to maintain normal thoracic kyphosis and lumbosacral lordosis while treating patients with scoliosis.

Curve measurement is usually performed by using the Cobb method. Wide interobserver and intraobserver variations exist with this technique, but measurements are reproducible if the levels measured and patient positioning are kept constant.

CT imaging is mainly utilized for visualization of complex scoliotic deformities. CT with three-dimensional reconstructions is often utilized in preoperative assessment and planning.

MRI is often utilized in the setting of congenital, infantile, and juvenile idiopathic scoliosis because of higher incidence of associated neural axis abnormality. It is also used in the setting of painful scoliosis or scoliosis associated with specific neurologic or clinical abnormalities.

Surgical treatment is usually resorted to in curves greater than 45 in patients with remaining spinal growth.

Suggested Readings

Cassar-Pullicino VN, Eisenstein SM. Imaging in scoliosis: what, why and how? *Clin Radiol.* 2002;57(7):543-562.

Goethem JV, Campenhout AV, Hauwe LVD, et al. Scoliosis. *Neuroimag Clin North Am.* 2007;17:105-115.

Kim H, Kim HS, Moon ES, et al. Scoliosis imaging: What radiologists should know. *RadioGraphics.* 2010;30:1823-1842.

Lenke LG, Betz RR, Harms J, et al. Adolescent idiopathic scoliosis: a new classification to determine extent of spinal arthrodesis. *J Bone Joint Surg Am.* 2001;83-A(8):1169-1181.

Lenke LG, Edwards II CC, Bridwell KH. The Lenke classification of adolescent idiopathic scoliosis: how it organizes curve patterns as a template to perform selective fusions of the spine. *Spine.* 2003;28(20): S199-S207.

References

Full references for this chapter can be found on www.expertconsult.com.

Chapter 136

Developmental Dysplasia of the Hip

SABAH SERVAES

Developmental dysplasia of the hip (DDH), formerly referred to as *congenital dislocation of the hip*, was first described thousands of years ago. Hippocrates is credited with ascribing intrauterine pressure as a possible etiology for this entity.[1] This chapter covers the etiology, multimodality diagnostic imaging, and its implications in the treatment of DDH.

Etiology DDH is a spectrum that may vary from a normal congruent hip with normal appearing acetabula with ligamentous laxity, to a structurally abnormal hip with joint incongruity related to primary acetabular dysplasia. Usually, DDH is a result of a combination of both structural and ligamentous laxity leading to an abnormal incongruent hip. Ultimately, the precise underlying etiology of DDH is not known. Purported in utero developmental factors and fetal crowding may result in DDH. During week 7 of gestation, hip joint cleavage occurs.[2] The lower extremity rotates medially during week 12 of gestation and hip muscles develop during week 18. However, it has been suggested that only 2% of cases result from intrauterine factors at this early phase of development and that the remaining 98% of cases are caused by changes to a normal hip during the last 4 weeks of pregnancy or in the immediate postnatal period.[2] Postnatal factors are also hypothesized to have a role in DDH, including tight swaddling or the use of cradle boards that force the legs into extension and adduction.

Structural causes leading to DDH are related to a primary acetabular dysplasia with secondary changes that may affect the femoral head leading to joint incongruity. Ligamentous laxity is often related to exposure to maternal hormones, particularly in female infants, leading to capsular, ligamentum teres, and transverse ligament laxity and subsequent hip joint incongruity. Proper development of the acetabulum and femoral head requires close approximation of the articular surfaces. Therefore, with untreated DDH with hip joint incongruity, acetabular dysplasia and secondary femoral head dysplasia may result, and DDH changes may become more severe over time.

Epidemiology Being the first born, breech birth, oligohydramnios, being large for gestational age, skull-molding deformities, female gender, and positive family history have all been associated with DDH. DDH is more common on the left.[2] The theory of many of these factors relating to the cause of DDH reflects constricted in utero space. The uterus of a primiparous woman has less give. The hips are subjected to increased pressure and hyperflexion in breech presentations. With frank breech presentations, the risk is even greater. Decreased amniotic fluid or a large gestation also results in increased constriction. The most common fetal presentation is cephalic, with the fetal spine aligned to the mother's left. This causes the left hip to be wedged against the maternal spine, which limits abduction and leads to a higher incidence of DDH on the left. Females are thought to be more affected because they are more sensitive to the circulating maternal hormone relaxin, resulting in ligamentous laxity.[2]

DDH is associated with myelodysplasia, arthrogryposis, multiple syndromes (such as Mobius and Poland syndromes), and chromosomal abnormalities. DDH is associated with talipes equinovarus or clubfoot, torticollis (fibromatosis colli, with a reported incidence of 5.5%), and congenital knee dislocation.[3,4]

The prevalence of DDH is reported up to 28.5 per 1000, depending on the population studied.[5] Variation in rates may result from expertise of the examiners and inclusion of children with isolated ligamentous laxity. The incidence of DDH increases with family history: 6% chance with an affected sibling, 12% chance with one affected parent, 36% chance with both parents affected.[2] During the first 2 weeks of life, physiologic instability exists, but it dissipates with increasing muscle tone and resolving ligamentous laxity as maternal hormones decrease.

Natural History If undiagnosed or left untreated, DDH may result in permanent acetabular dysplasia in children of walking age, typically having a shallow acetabular roof (sourcil) with anterior undercoverage related to increased acetabular version. Similarly, the femoral head may become secondarily dysplastic and lose its normal sphericity related to eccentric loads because of an incongruent hip, with resultant spherical growth plate disturbance and modeling changes.[6] The femoral head must be seated within the acetabulum for normal development to occur. If the femoral head is dislocated, the transverse acetabular ligament and inferior capsular fibers become interpositioned, inhibiting hip congruity. Pulvinar (fibrofatty tissue) may also interpose between the femoral head and acetabulum, interfering with hip congruity. Hypertrophy of the fibrocartilaginous labrum often compensates for a shallow bony acetabular roof, and this has historically been referred to as a *limbus*.[2] Long-term sequelae include incomplete coverage of the femoral head, excessive femoral anteversion, coxa

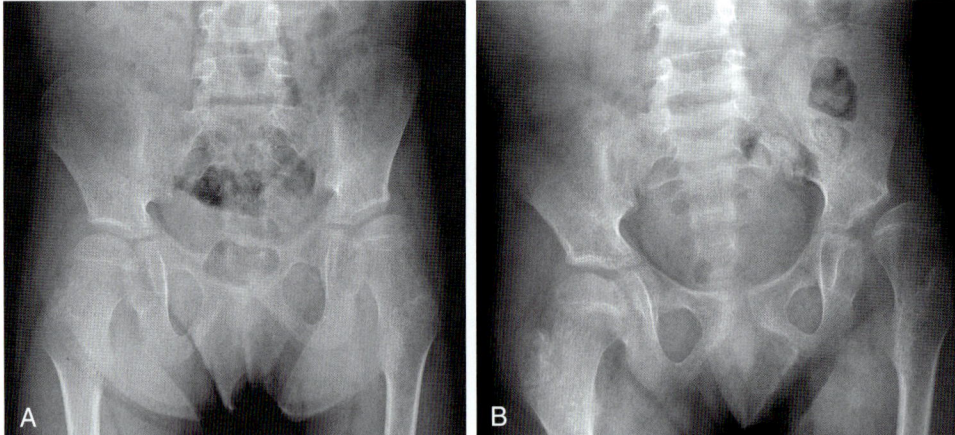

Figure 136-1 Frontal radiographs of the pelvis demonstrating late presentation, and progression of developmental dysplasia of the hip of the left hip. **A,** At presentation, in this 11-year-old boy, the left hip is dysplastic, with an upsloping sourcil and mild undercoverage of the femoral head. The femoral head is already noted to be aspherically shaped. **B,** Three years later, progressive lateral uncovering of the femoral head and progressive secondary dysplastic changes of the femoral head are seen, and the greater trochanter overlies the femoral neck despite proper positioning, indicative of excessive femoral anteversion.

valga, and coxa magna with muscle tightness (with the greatest impact on the adductors)[7] (Fig. 136-1). As a result of these morphologic features, individuals with untreated DDH may develop premature degenerative changes of the hip joint and a permanent limp. Excessive femoral anteversion will lead to in-toeing. Hip degenerative changes are caused by loss of cartilage and labral tears secondary to abnormal eccentric joint contact pressure from chronic incongruent acetabular and femoral head articulation; rupture of the ligamentum teres has also been described.[8] Degenerative changes caused by hip subluxation typically appear before women reach the age of 40 years and before men reach the age of 55 years; however, symptoms may become apparent during adolescence.[2] With completely dislocated hips, many patients may function very well even into late adolescence with a neoacetabulum that forms along the iliac wing.[2]

Physical Examination The physical examination to diagnose DDH consists of maneuvers described by Ortolani, a pediatrician, and by Barlow, an orthopedic surgeon. Ortolani described the hip click in 1937, although hip instability had been reported in 1879 and the clinical test described by Le Damany and Saiget in 1910.[5] Barlow described his technique to demonstrate laxity of the dysplastic hip in 1961.

In the Ortolani maneuver, forward pressure is applied to each femoral head with the infant in the supine position and the hips flexed to abduct the hip and to reduce a subluxated or dislocated femoral head. If subluxation or dislocation exists, an audible "clunk" is heard as the femoral head is reduced into the acetabulum. In the Barlow maneuver, backward pressure is applied to each femoral head with the in the infant supine position and the hips flexed to subluxate the hip.[9-11] Both these maneuvers may fail to diagnose bilateral irreducible hip dislocations.

Asymmetrical thigh skin creases, limited abduction, leg length discrepancies, and isolated hip clicks have also been suggested as signs of DDH. The Galeazzi sign may help diagnose DDH in older children. Unequal height of the knees in a supine child with flexed hips and knees means a positive result; however, the result is negative if both hips

are abnormal. Older children may have a limp as the only symptom of DDH.

Imaging

Radiography The infant's lower extremities should be positioned in neutral extension with longitudinal symmetry. For symmetric imaging, the central ray should be directed above the pubic symphysis in the midline. In the presence of abnormality such as dislocation of the femoral head, a frog-leg view may be useful to evaluate reduction of the femoral head and may provide an opportunity for a second look at acetabular morphology. Positioning the thigh in abduction and internal rotation with a 45-degree angle (the von Rosen view) provides similar information as a frog-leg lateral view.[12]

Several lines may be drawn to assist in the assessment of hips, but attention should be made to the overall configuration rather than to the measured angles, which could have varying rates of interobserver and intraobservor variability. The Hilgenreiner line passes horizontally through the superior aspect of the triradiate cartilages. The Perkin line is the vertical line extending from the lateral margin of the acetabulum. The expected location of the femoral head is in the medial, inferior quadrant of the intersection of the Hilgenreiner and Perkin lines (Fig. 136-2, *A*). The Shenton line curves along the lesser trochanter, femoral neck, and inferior margin of the pubis or obturator foramen and should be smooth (Fig. 136-2, *B*)

The acetabular index is the angle between the acetabulum (from the superolateral margin of the acetabulum and the superolateral margin of the triradiate cartilage) and the Hilgenreiner line. The acetabular index changes with age: 28 degrees in newborns, 23.5 degrees at age 6 months, 22 degrees at age 1 year, and 20 degrees at age 2 years. The maximal normal measurement for the acetabular index is 30 degrees up to age 4 months and 25 degrees up to age 2 years. The orientation of the pelvis on the radiograph impacts this measurement.[13,14]

Hips should be in slight flexion during radiographic evaluation. Concavity of the acetabulum, which occurs as a result of pressure from the femoral head, should be noted.

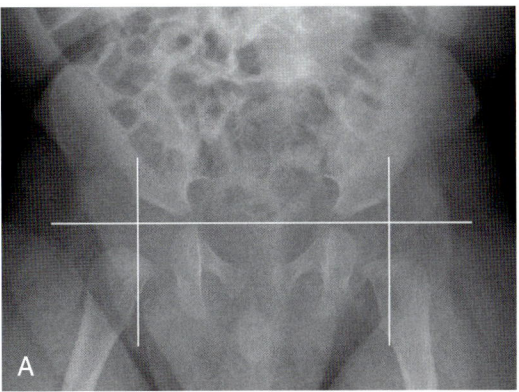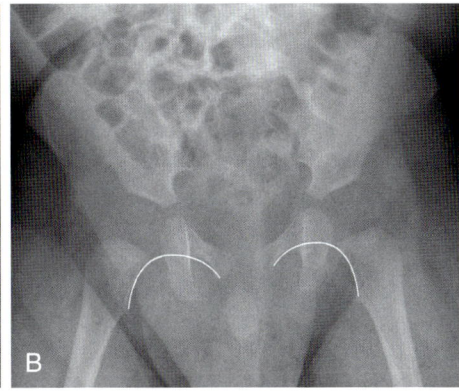

Figure 136-2   **A,** Frontal radiograph of the pelvis with the horizontal Hilgenreiner and vertical Perkin lines. The expected location of the femoral head is in the medial, inferior quadrant of the intersection of the Hilgenreiner and Perkin lines. **B,** The Shenton lines are drawn on this same pelvic radiograph. Disruption of this line will occur if the hip is dysplastic with either a subluxation or a dislocation.

Typically, sclerosis develops in this region of pressure forming the sourcil, which is most prominent in the middle third of the acetabulum. The sourcil should normally have a rounded or arched configuration.

In the preschool children and older children, the center edge angle may be calculated, and this measures the relative acetabular coverage of the femoral head. To determine the center edge angle, one line is drawn between the center of both femoral heads. Next, a vertical line is drawn 90 degrees at the center of the femoral head, and this serves as one reference line. Next, a line from the femoral head is drawn to the lateral acetabulum, and this serves as the second reference line. Now the center edge angle can be determined. This measurement is used in children over age 5 years. DDH should be suspected when the center edge angle is less than 19 degrees in children aged 6 to 13 years and less than 25 degrees in those over age 13 years.[13,15]

Radiographs are utilized to screen for DDH after age 4 to 6 months, when ultrasonography becomes more challenging and less reliable because of ossification of the femoral heads. Radiographic findings of DDH include an upward slanting sourcil, small capital femoral epiphysis, and superolateral subluxation of the femoral head (Figs. 136-3 and 136-4). Anteroposterior views are sufficient for screening. When abnormal, a frog-leg lateral view or a von Rosen view may be obtained to assess whether the femoral head reduces with hip abduction. When chronic, untreated DDH exists, the ipsilateral capital femoral epiphysis may become disproportionately smaller (Fig. 136-5). Without concentric apposition of two bones of a joint, as may occur with untreated DDH, epiphyseal ossification will be delayed.

Ultrasonography   An orthopedic surgeon, Graf, described the use of ultrasonography in the assessment of the anatomy of the infant hip in 1980.[16] Four years later, a group of radiologists including Harcke, described the dynamic technique to assessing infant hips.[17] Ultrasonography has the advantages of absence of ionizing radiation, widespread availability, and the feasibility of a dynamic examination.

The examination is typically performed with a linear array transducer using the highest frequency that provides adequate

Figure 136-3   An anteroposterior radiograph in an 8-month-old girl demonstrates bilateral developmental dysplasia of the hip, with the left hip worse than the right hip. Note the upward slanting sourcil bilaterally. The right femoral head is concentrically located within its dysplastic acetabula. The left femoral head is superolaterally dislocated.

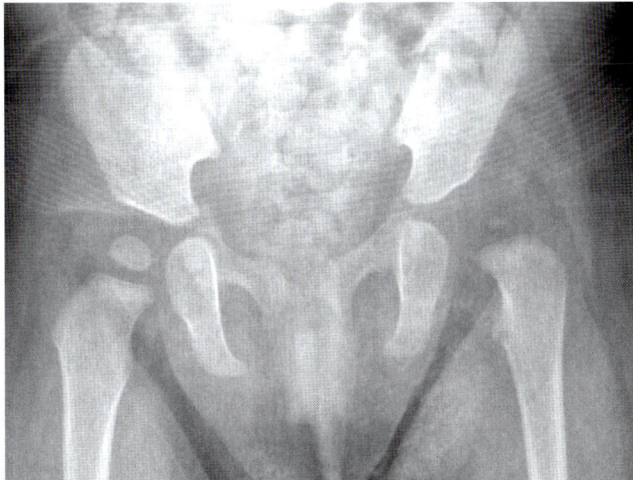

Figure 136-4   An anteroposterior radiograph in a 1-year-old girl demonstrates left-sided developmental dysplasia of the hip, with upward slanting sourcil, a superolaterally subluxed femoral head, and delayed ossification of the left capital femoral epiphysis.

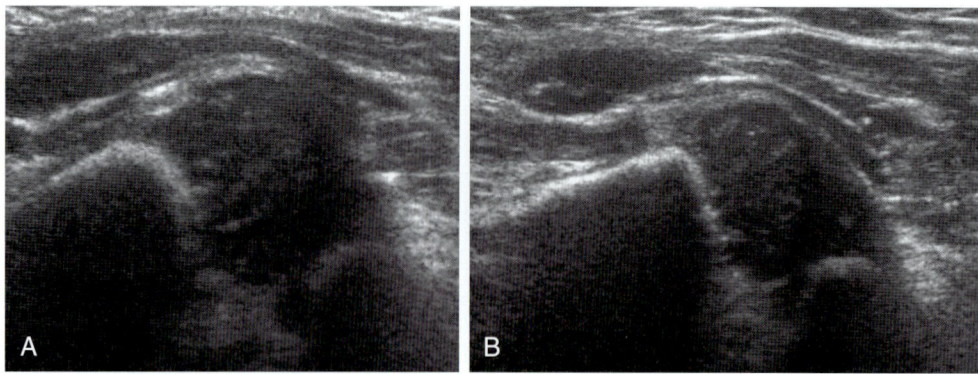

Figure 136-5   An ultrasonographic scan of subluxable hip. **A,** In the transverse plane with adduction, the hip is in neutral and is concentrically located. **B,** With stress maneuvers, the hip posterolaterally subluxes.

penetration (often 12 megahertz [MHz]). The transducer is placed over the lateral aspect of the hip in either the coronal plane, with the hip in neutral or flexed positions, or in the transverse or axial plane, with the hip in adduction or abduction (e-Fig. 136-6). The infant should be placed in the lateral decubitus or supine position. In the coronal plane, the ilium should appear as a horizontal line, the midportion of the acetabulum visualized to its maximal depth, and the middle of the fibrocartilaginous labrum seen. Without technical accuracy, a normal hip may appear abnormal; the converse is not true. The femoral head should be in close apposition with the acetabulum with at least 50% of the femoral head covered by the acetabulum. Subluxation is present if the femoral head is less than 50% covered but in contact with the acetabulum. In the absence of contact between the femoral head and acetabulum, the hip is dislocated. The hip may reduce with changes in position, typically in abduction and flexion.

The alpha-angle, which is the slope of the posterior and superior acetabulum relative to the iliac line on the coronal view, should be greater than or equal to 60 degrees (Fig. 136-7). Until age 3 months, 50 to 60 degrees may be physiologic. The majority of these hips develop normally without treatment, but maturation should be confirmed with a follow-up study. The beta-angle, which is the slope of the anterior cartilaginous roof relative to the iliac line on the coronal view, should be less than 55 degrees; the beta-angle is not as significant as the alpha-angle in diagnosis or treatment.

In addition to the abnormally lateral and superior positioning of the femoral head and the abnormal angle of the acetabulum seen with DDH, the labrum may become thick and echogenic. The acetabular rim in normal hips has a sharply defined corner at the intersection of the anterior iliac line and sourcil (see Fig. 136-7). With progressive acetabular dysplasia, this corner becomes rounded and dysplastic (Fig. 136-8, *A*). The deformed labrum and pulvinar may be interposed between the acetabulum and femoral head (see Fig. 136-8, *A*).

The femoral head ossification centers become apparent with the use of ultrasonography prior to detection with radiography. Unless a delay occurs in the formation of the ossification of the femoral heads, ultrasonography of the hips to evaluate DDH is not practical beyond age 1 year and not often used beyond ages 6 to 8 months.

Dynamic examination includes the use of stress maneuvers, which correspond to the physical tests of Ortolani and Barlow. Normally, the femoral head is well seated within the acetabulum at rest and while stress maneuvers are applied. If laxity exists or if the hip is dislocatable, the femoral head moves posterolaterally when stress is applied. The transverse view is excellent for visualization of this movement during the stress maneuver (e-Fig. 136-9). These maneuvers are not performed if the patient is undergoing therapy with a harness.[18]

Because of the physiologic laxity normally present during the first 2 weeks of life, hip ultrasonography is not recommended during this period. Some have recommended waiting until 6 weeks of life for mild clinical findings or history because of the possibility of the likelihood of spontaneous

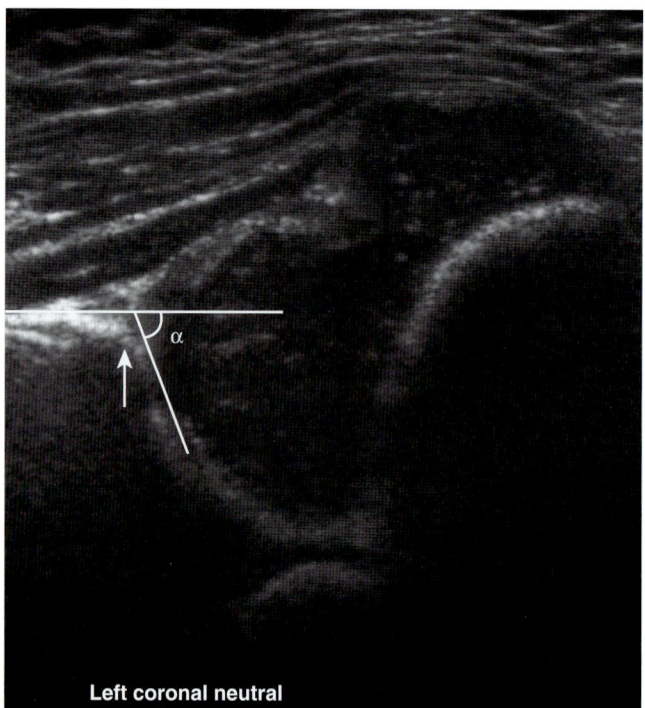

Left coronal neutral

Figure 136-7   Ultrasonographic depiction of a normal hip in the coronal plane with the hip in neutral position and the alpha-angle measured along the iliac bone and the acetabular roof. The alpha-angle is normal, measuring 64 degrees in this example. The acetabular roof is mature, with a sharply angulated acetabular margin (*arrow*).

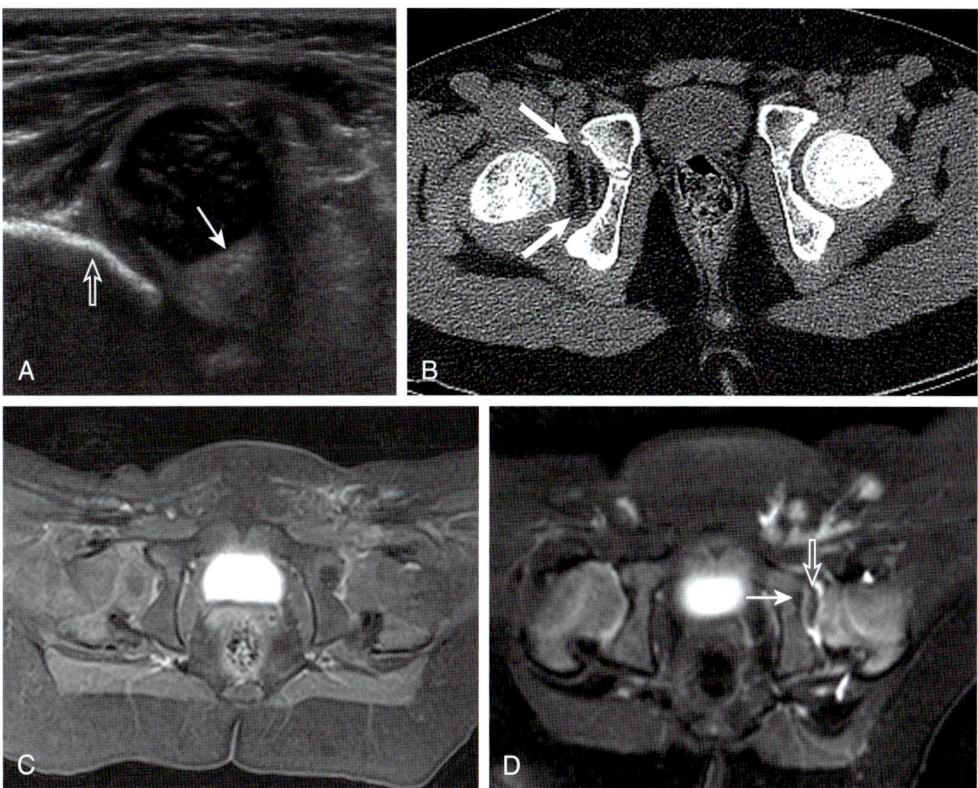

Figure 136-8 Obstacles to hip reduction. **A,** A coronal ultrasonographic image of a dysplastic hip with echogenic pulvinar (*solid arrow*). Note the dysplastic shallow acetabula with blunted obtuse margin (*open arrow*). **B,** Low-dose axial computed tomography demonstrating fatty pulvinar (*arrows*) within the right hip joint. **C,** An axial T1-weighted 3T magnetic resonance image demonstrates pulvinar, thickened posterior labrum and ligamentum teres within the dysplastic left hip, which was successfully reduced. Symmetric enhancement is seen in this postcontrast image. **D,** An axial magnetic resonance image with pulvinar between the femoral head and acetabulum (*arrow*) and thickened ligamentum teres (*open arrow*).

resolution. If clear dislocation is apparent on physical examination, ultrasonographic examination is not necessary. Ultrasonography is necessary if the findings of the examination are questionable, if risk factors are identified with a negative examination result, and for treatment follow-up evaluation.

Screening Some advocate for screening of all newborns for DDH and some for screening only those with risk factors or a positive or equivocal clinical examination. Many studies have been published describing the merits of each approach.[19-34] General screening may help prevent delayed diagnosis and the need for surgical intervention but may also increase costs and lead to unnecessary treatment. The benefits of screening all newborns are not yet clear, and the current practice in the United Sates is to screen with ultrasonography only patients with an abnormal physical examination result or those who have positive risk factors for DDH.[34-36]

Computed Tomography Primarily used for patients who have undergone treatment or will undergo open surgical repair with orthopedic hardware for DDH, rather than as a means of obtaining a diagnosis, computed tomography (CT) provides excellent spatial resolution for determining femoral and acetabular version.[37] CT may be performed immediately following surgical reduction of DDH and is ideally performed using the low-dose technique and a small scan extent (Fig. 136-10). CT screening after surgical reduction is reserved for patients who have undergone a periacetabular osteotomy or

proximal femoral osteotomy or for those who have had orthopedic hardware placed within 2 cm of the hip joint line, thereby precluding the ability to perform magnetic resonance imaging (MRI). Artifacts from metallic hardware are decreased by using higher peak kilovoltage (increasing the penetration of x-rays) and increasing tube current (allowing enough photons to reach the detector); this parameter needs to be manually changed to overcome automatic exposure controls.

Displacement and subluxation should be described in both the coronal and axial planes. Identification of any orthopedic hardware failures such as pin extrusion into the joint line, migrated interposition bone grafts and identification of any intrinsic or extrinsic causes of failed reduction should be made. The gluteus maximus should have a clear fat plane anteriorly between the muscle and a line tangent to the posterior aspect of the ischia on axial imaging; this fat plane will be interrupted, displaced posteriorly, or both, if the hips are not adequately reduced. Reconstructions of CT data may assist in demonstrating anatomic relationships and are often particularly helpful to the surgeon. Coronal reconstructions are excellent in depicting the acetabular roof.[18,37]

As part of surgical planning for older patients (usually in their second decade or older) with DDH, measurement of femoral and acetabular version by CT is obtained after scanning the pelvis and distal femurs. In addition, preoperative CT is also used to provide additional details of bone quality and joint morphology for potential periacetabular

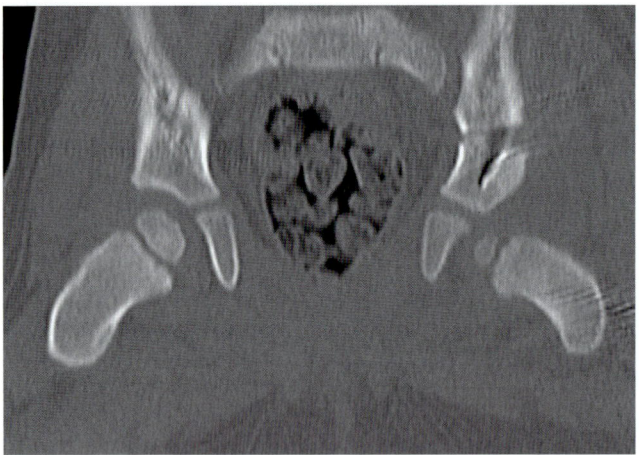

Figure 136-10 A coronal computed tomography image reformatted in a 2-year-old boy following Salter osteotomy for treatment of left-sided developmental dysplasia of the hip. Note that the bilateral femoral heads are concentrically located. The left femoral head is small, an expected finding in the setting of developmental dysplasia of the hip.

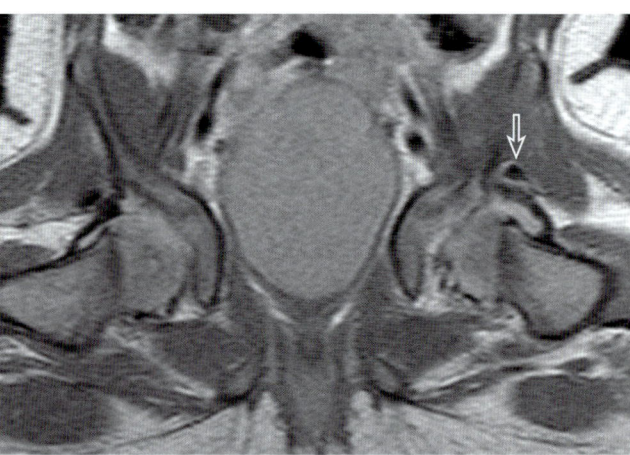

Figure 136-13 Magnetic resonance spica proton density imaging sequence in a 6-month-old girl demonstrates a floating superior labrum after reduction (*arrow*). Note the hyaline cartilage lateral sourcil margin, as the superior labrum has been displaced. Normal right superior labrum for comparison.

osteotomies and femoral osteotomies to help with hip joint containment.

CT should still be the first line of postoperative imaging in children with DDH who have orthopedic hardware placement or have undergone periacetabular osteotomies to determine bone graft quality and position[18,38-40]

Magnetic Resonance Imaging Following reduction and placement of a spica cast, MRI is increasingly being utilized as an evaluation of the anatomy because of lack of ionizing radiation and the ability to perform the study without sedation (Fig. 136-11).[41-46] In addition to providing anatomic

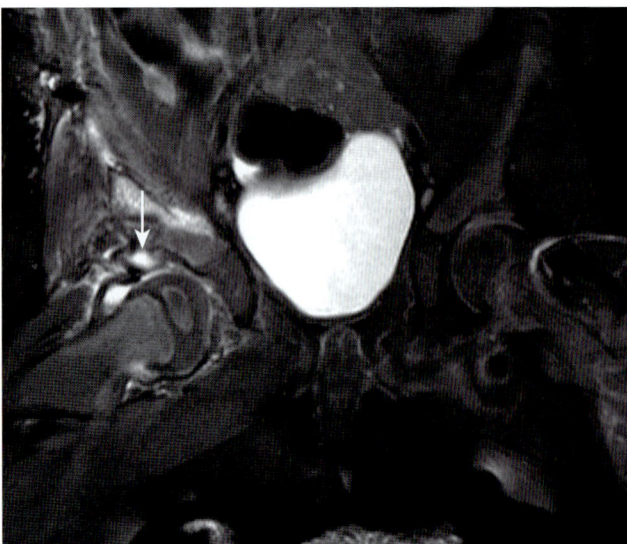

Figure 136-11 A T2-weighted fat-saturated coronal magnetic resonance image of the hips in a patient who underwent acetabuloplasty of the right hip and is in a spica cast. No sedation was used for this study. The femoral head is concentrically located. There is globular increased signal within the superior labrum at the chondro-osseous junction (*arrow*) related to labral injury incurred during reduction.

information regarding the relationship between the femoral head and the acetabulum, obstacles to reduction may be visualized better than with CT (e-Fig. 136-12). Fatty pulvinar, thickened or inverted labrum, transverse acetabular ligaments, and hypertrophied ligamentum teres (see Fig. 136-8) may be present in the hip joint preventing successful reduction. Sometimes, the labrum may be displaced altogether because of trauma from intraoperative femoral head relocation into the acetabular fossa (Fig. 136-13). An abnormal shape of the acetabulum or the capital femoral epiphysis may also be obstacles to reduction. Extrinsic obstacles to reduction include shortened external rotator and adductor muscles, interpositioning of the iliopsoas muscle, and capsular adhesion to the ilium.[47] The most useful sequences include T1-weighted and proton density–weighted sequences in the axial and coronal planes.[48-50]

With the administration of contrast, MRI can detect ischemia within the femoral head and possibly identify patients at risk for epiphyseal osteonecrosis, which is the most common serious complication of hip reduction and may occur to some degree in more than 70% of cases. The risk of epiphyseal osteonecrosis is increased with greater hip abduction, which has led to the concept of the "safe zone," which is the amount of abduction that is large enough to prevent redislocation and small enough to prevent avascular necrosis, usually at 55 degrees maximal hip abduction.[46] Abduction may compromise the blood supply to the femoral head, as the blood supply arises primarily from the deep medial femoral circumflex vessels. This ischemia may be detected by low-signal on postcontrast T1-weighted images (Fig. 136-14). Because of the lack of intraepiphyseal vascular anastomoses, regions of poor enhancement are often well delineated by immediately adjacent well-perfused areas. Performance of this examination immediately after reduction is currently the recommended practice.[45]

Treatment The objective of DDH treatment is concentric reduction of the femoral head into the acetabulum. The method of achieving this outcome depends on the age of the patient as well as the severity of the presentation. Up to age

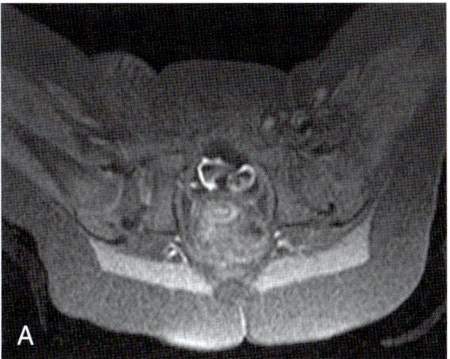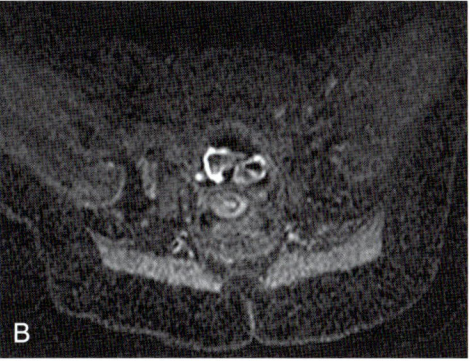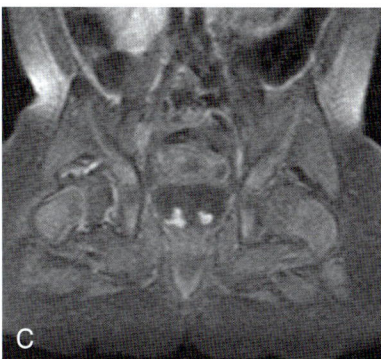

Figure 136-14 Magnetic resonance imaging of the hips obtained in a 1.5 Tesla magnet after placement of a spica cast without sedation. **A,** An axial T1-weighted, fat-suppressed image demonstrates lower signal in the right femoral head. **B,** A subtraction image more clearly demonstrates the asymmetric perfusion of the femoral heads. **C,** A coronal T1-weighted, fat-suppressed image demonstrates decreased perfusion on the right.

6 months, orthoses, often a Pavlik harness, are used to place the hip in flexion and abduction. This treatment aids in developing the acetabulum along the lateral edge. The risk of epiphyseal osteonecrosis increases with greater hip abduction, as discussed above. The harness is often worn for 3 to 6 weeks following successful reduction; both clinical examination and ultrasonography are performed to evaluate the effectiveness of therapy. In the patient in a harness, stress maneuvers are not performed during ultrasonography.

Children over 6 months but less than 2 years of age are often treated with a spica cast following closed or open reduction. Intraoperative arthrography is often performed to assess for structures that my impede reduction and to assess the anatomy (e-Fig. 136-15). A total contrast volume of 3 to 4 milliliters is typically all that is required; too much contrast may give the impression of capsular laxity.[18] Positioning of the femoral heads following placement of the cast may be ascertained with CT or MRI, with MRI having the advantages of no radiation and the possibility of assessing perfusion of the femoral head. Radiography may also detect late features of avascular necrosis. Recurrent dislocation may occur in up to 8% of patients and is more common in those with bilateral or right-sided DDH, decreased abduction in the spica cast, and large pelvic width.[51]

DDH that is diagnosed late or that persists despite treatment may require surgical osteotomy. For patients with persistent subluxation and mild to moderate acetabular dysplasia, an innominate or Salter osteotomy may be indicated. This technique includes a horizontal osteotomy of the ilium superior to the acetabulum to create a wedge, which is filled with bone from the iliac crest (e-Fig. 136-16). Frequently utilized in children with cerebral palsy caused by posterolateral deficiency, the Dega osteotomy is made in the lateral ilium and cannot be distinguished from the Pemberton osteotomy radiographically (e-Fig. 136-17). Patients over 8 years of age may require a Chiari osteotomy, which increases the size of the acetabulum with a supraacetabular osteotomy. For adolescents and adults, the Ganz or periacetabular osteotomy may be necessary to improve anteversion and redirect the acetabulum.

For children older than 2 years, shortening of the femur is often required with derotational osteotomy. Children with cerebral palsy, for example, may have spasticity at the hip, which may result in coxa valga and limit the ability to reduce the femur. Adductor tenotomy may be performed to overcome this obstacle.

WHAT THE CLINICIAN NEEDS TO KNOW

- Identifying and stratifying infants into three categories of patients during screening ultrasonography (infants <6 months) or radiography (for infants >6 months): normal with no need for follow-up, borderline that requires follow-up imaging or orthopedic examination, or abnormal and requires orthopedic referral and treatment
- Identifying postreduction complications including epiphyseal osteonecrosis or identifying inhibitors to successful reduction such as an inverted labrum

Key Points

In the United States, screening for DDH is done on the basis of clinical findings such as asymmetric leg creases and hip clicks and with history such as breech birth.

Ultrasonography provides a dynamic examination to evaluate the location of the femoral head and the shape of the acetabulum, as well as to identify obstacles to reduction

CT is typically used in older patients requiring surgical repair or in infants after spica reduction with orthopedic hardware within 2 cm of the hip joint line.

MRI is used to evaluate the level of success of spica closed reduction and may help to determine if the hip is at risk for epiphyseal osteonecrosis.

Suggested Readings

Dezateux C, Rosendahl K. Developmental dysplasia of the hip. *Lancet.* 2007;369:1541-1552.

Grissom L, Harcke HT, Thacker M. Imaging in the surgical management of developmental dislocation of the hip. *Clin Orthop Relat Res.* 2008;466:791-801.

Karmazyn BK, Gunderman RB, Coley BD, et al. ACR Appropriateness Criteria on developmental dysplasia of the hip—child. *J Am Coll Radiol.* 2009;6:551-557.

Shipman SA, Helfand M, Moyer VA, et al. Screening for developmental dysplasia of the hip: a systematic literature review for the US Preventive Services Task Force. *Pediatrics.* 2006;117:e557-e576.

Tiderius C, Jaramillo D, Connolly S, et al. Post-closed reduction perfusion magnetic resonance imaging as a predictor of avascular necrosis in developmental hip dysplasia: a preliminary report. *J Pediatr Orthop.* 2009;29:14-20.

References

Full references for this chapter can be found on www.expertconsult.com.

Chapter 137

Arthritis and Differential Inflammatory Joint Disorders

ANDREA SCHWARZ DORIA and PAUL BABYN

Rheumatologic conditions in children are myriad in presentation, with overlapping imaging features that may sometimes superficially mimic infection. Rheumatologic conditions in children do not follow the typical course and presentation compared with their counterparts in adults. As a consequence, the International League of Associations for Rheumatology (ILAR) formulated a revised nomenclature to describe the various pediatric rheumatologic conditions (Box 137-1).[1] In this chapter, we discuss imaging of pediatric arthritis from the point of view of noninfectious synovial proliferation using the ILAR classification, including juvenile idiopathic arthritis (JIA) and its differentials: hemophilic arthropathy, lipoma arborescens, synovial chondromatosis, pigmented villonodular synovitis, and reactive synovitis (Box 137-2). Subtypes of JIA, enthesitis-related arthritis and psoriatic arthritis, will be discussed in their own subsections because of their unique presentation and imaging findings.

Juvenile Idiopathic Arthritis

CLINICAL OVERVIEW

JIA, which occurs worldwide, is the most frequent cause of chronic musculoskeletal pain in youths and the most common chronic musculoskeletal disease of childhood.[2-4] It is a nonmigratory, chronic, monoarticular or polyarticular arthropathy of childhood.[2]

The diagnostic criteria for JIA include disease onset before the age of 16 years, the presence of arthritis in one or more joints for at least 6 weeks, onset type defined by type of disease in the first 6 months of diagnosis (Box 137-1), and exclusion of other forms of juvenile arthritis.[1] JIA may be associated with systemic manifestations that include fever, erythematous rashes, nodules, leukocytosis, and, less commonly, iridocyclitis, pleuritis, pericarditis, anemia, fatigue, and growth failure.[5] At the time of presentation, other causes of inflammation should be excluded. JIA differs from the adult type of rheumatoid arthritis because of the age of presentation, its preference for large joints, its tendency to generate joint contractures and muscle wasting, and its association with extraarticular clinical manifestations.[6]

A new internationally accepted classification system was established in 1995[1,7] and revised in 2001[1] (Box 137-1). The previously used terms "juvenile chronic arthritis" and "juvenile rheumatoid arthritis" were incorporated under the term JIA.

The early diagnosis of JIA is essential to interrupt or delay the course of the disease, which results in joint deformity, severe functional impairment, and chronic pain if the disease is not treated at its early stage.

The clinical and laboratory tests that are currently available for assessment of JIA are poor for characterization of early inflammatory, hypoxic, and vascular changes, which are the primary physiologic events involved in the disease.[8] Hence because the clinical and laboratory diagnosis of early joint changes in JIA is suboptimal,[9,10] imaging becomes an ideal noninvasive method for early diagnosis and outcome measure during follow-up of joint changes in persons with this disease.

Box 137-1 Classification of Juvenile Idiopathic Arthritis

Onset <16 years

Duration: 6 weeks

Other unknown conditions are excluded

Subtypes

1. Systemic arthritis
2. Oligoarthritis

Persistent

Extended

3. Polyarthritis (rheumatoid factor negative)
4. Polyarthritis (rheumatoid factor positive)
5. Psoriatic arthritis
6. Enthesitis-related arthritis
7. Other undifferentiated arthritis
   a. Does not meet any criteria for categories 1-6
   b. Meets criteria for more than one of the categories 1-6

From Petty RE, Southwood TR, Manners P, et al. International League of Associations for Rheumatology classification of juvenile idiopathic arthritis: second revision, Edmonton, 2001. *J Rheumatol.* 2004;31: 390-392.

Box 137-2 Differential Diagnosis of Juvenile Idiopathic Arthritis

Noninfectious Disorders

Synovial Disorders

Pauciarticular

Acute
- Early rheumatic disease
- Arthritis associated with chromosomal abnormalities—Down, Turner syndromes
- Seronegative spondyloarthropathy
- Acute transient synovitis

Chronic
- Rheumatic diseases
- Arthritis associated with chromosomal abnormalities—Down, Turner syndromes
- Synovial masses
- Nodular synovitis
  - Pigmented villonodular synovitis
  - Synovial hemangioma (venous malformation)
  - Lipoma arborescens
  - Synovial osteochondromatosis

Other
- Foreign body arthritis
- Hemophilic arthropathy
- Sarcoidosis
- Intra articular osteoid osteoma

Polyarticular

Seronegative spondyloarthropathy
- Connective tissue disorders
  - Systemic lupus erythematosus
  - Sarcoidosis

Inherited disorders

Familial hypertrophic synovitis

Hemophilic arthropathy

Immunodeficiency

Nonsynovial Disorders

Pauciarticular

Acute
- Malignancy
- Leukemia
- Neuroblastoma

Chronic
- Noninflammatory disorders
- Avascular necrosis
- Slipped capital femoral epiphysis and dysplasias

Other
- Juvenile osteoporosis
- Multifocal osteolysis

Polyarticular

Metabolic or inherited disorders

Diabetic arthropathy

Turner syndrome

Lysosomal storage disease

Kniest syndrome

Winchester syndrome

Chondrodysplasias

Frostbite

Goldbloom disease

Infectious Disorders

Pauciarticular

Infectious arthritis

Septic arthritis

Reactive arthritis

Tuberculous arthritis

Postinfectious arthritis

Polyarticular

Infectious arthritis

Lyme disease

Reactive arthritis

EPIDEMIOLOGY

The incidence and prevalence of JIA, respectively, is between 5-18 and 30-150 per 100,000 children younger than 16 years in Europe and North America.[11] Twice as many girls as boys have JIA.[12] Although few data are available on geographic or racial groups of persons with JIA, studies suggest that in the United States, proportionately fewer African American than white children have JIA.[13] The onset of JIA before the age of 6 months is distinctly unusual; nevertheless, the age at onset is often quite young, with the highest frequency occurring between 1 and 3 years.[14]

Radiographic changes are seen most frequently in patients with JIA who have a polyarticular course.[15,16] Large joints are most commonly affected in persons with this disease. The knee is the most frequently affected joint, followed by the ankle. Occasionally, changes may develop in the cervical spine or temporomandibular joint.[17] It has been suggested that patients with JIA who have polyarthritis and wrist disease are at high risk of experiencing radiographic progression.[18]

The wrist is the most vulnerable site for early radiographic changes in patients with JIA.[16,19]

PATHOPHYSIOLOGY

Although the etiology of JIA is unknown, some investigators believe that it is multifactorial given the heterogeneity of presentations and course of the disease.[20] JIA is characterized by an acute synovitis that leads to synovial proliferation and formation of a highly cellular pannus.[21] The pannus erodes the adjacent articular cartilage and subchondral bone, leading to centripetal articular destruction; that is, the articular damage starts at the periphery of the joint and progresses toward its center. Inflammatory changes also can involve tendon sheaths and bursa and can give rise to periostitis. With prolonged inflammation, more extensive joint changes including cartilage destruction, bone erosions, and joint malalignment often are present.

Despite the fact that JIA is usually transient and self-limited, without active synovitis in adulthood, up to 10% of children become severely disabled in adulthood. Despite therapy, 28% to 54% of children have progressive disease and experience cartilage or bone erosions, with a median onset of radiographic findings between 2.2 to 5.4 years after the initial disease presentation.[22] The disease process leads to joint instability, subluxation, and ankylosis.[23,24] Disturbance of joint growth can be consequent to the disease itself and/or to the treatment.[17]

IMAGING

Imaging often plays a key role in establishing the presence, severity, and extent of joint disease, and it can also help monitor for disease complications, exclude other diagnoses, and assess treatment response. Imaging can provide early diagnosis and visualization of inflammatory abnormalities, including synovitis and osteochondral damage.[25-27]

Radiographs are the standard imaging tools for the diagnosis of JIA; however, they have low sensitivity (50%) and moderate specificity (85%) for detection of cartilage destruction.[8]

Both magnetic resonance imaging (MRI) and ultrasound can detect synovial hypertrophy, cartilage erosion and joint effusion in peripheral joints, and clinically meaningful response to treatment in children with JIA. Ultrasound is less sensitive than MRI for assessment of both soft tissue findings (sensitivity, 62%) and superficial cartilage loss (sensitivity, 60%).[8] Overall, MRI is the imaging modality of choice for evaluation of joints in children with JIA. However, ultrasound can be an excellent initial imaging tool for evaluation of young children who otherwise would require sedation for MRI.[8]

Radiography

Conventional radiography is not effective in the evaluation of soft tissue abnormalities, which are precursors of cartilage degeneration in persons with JIA.[26] Moreover, available radiographic scoring systems for assessment of JIA have poor internal consistency and poor criterion and construct validity because they do not take into consideration patients' sex and age.[28] Despite the aforementioned limitations and the strong evidence for low sensitivity (50%) and moderate specificity (85%) in the detection of cartilage destruction,[8,28] in many centers this technique remains the standard practice for imaging evaluation of disease progression in persons with JIA, with an expanding role for ultrasound and MRI.[29]

A variety of radiographic features can be encountered with joint disease. Specific joint findings will depend on the underlying abnormality, the chronicity of the disease, and the response to therapy. A systematic approach to the imaging interpretation of any joint is highly recommended. One popular approach is the "ABCDS" of joint disease, featuring assessment of joint Alignment, Bone density and other bone changes, Cartilage loss, Distribution of joint disease (whether monoarticular, oligoarticular, or polyarticular) and Soft tissue abnormalities (Box 137-3).

The earliest abnormalities include soft tissue swelling, osteopenia, and effusion. Periosteal reaction occasionally may be seen. Typically, the osteopenia is initially periarticular (Fig. 137-1), becoming more diffuse with time. Osteopenia may be subtle and better recognized by comparison with the contralateral extremity (if it is unaffected). With long-standing

---

Box 137-3 Radiographic Features of Juvenile Idiopathic Arthritis

Alignment Examples
- Atlantoaxial subluxation
- Coxa valga or varus
- Finger deformities including boutonniere or swan neck deformity
- Knee valgus
- Hallux valgus

Bone Density
- Juxtaarticular osteoporosis
- Diffuse osteoporosis (late)
- Metaphyseal lucent band (rarely)
- Periosteal reaction adjacent to affected small joints

Cartilage and Joint Spaces
- Erosions (late), may appear corticated
- Cartilage space narrowing (late)
- Ankylosis (especially spine, wrists)

Distribution
Monarticular, oligoarticular, or polyarticular

Growth Abnormalities
- Affected small bones are shorter than normal
- Overgrowth (lengthening) of affected long bones
- Advanced maturation of affected epiphyses
- Large epiphyses
- Micrognathia (may have mandibular notching)
- Protrusio acetabuli
- Small fused cervical vertebrae
- Angular carpal bones
- Square patella
- Intercondylar notch widening (also a feature of hemophilia)

Soft Tissues
- Effusions and joint distension
- Nodules
- Periarticular calcification (probably due to corticosteroid injections)

From Johnson K, Gardner-Medwin J. Childhood arthritis: classification and radiology. *Clin Radiol.* 2002;57:47-58.

---

disease, uniform bone loss may occur with a thin cortex. Uncommonly, a linear subphyseal demineralization can be observed, but this finding is nonspecific and can also be seen in persons with other conditions such as leukemia.[30]

Joint effusions are encountered commonly and can be seen in inflammatory or noninflammatory joint disease. A sign of knee effusions is fullness in the suprapatellar region, which is best seen on the lateral view. In the elbow, knee, and ankle, adjacent fat lines and fat pads are displaced. Periosteal reaction, when present, is commonly seen in the phalanges, metacarpals, and metatarsals but also can occur in the long bones. Joint space narrowing may be caused by cartilage loss (Fig. 137-1). In persons with JIA, the joint space narrowing is usually uniform. In some patients with rheumatoid factor positive polyarthritis or systemic arthritis, early erosive disease can occur (Fig. 137-2).

Bone erosions are typically located at joint margins in the bare areas but also may occur at tendinous insertions. Bone

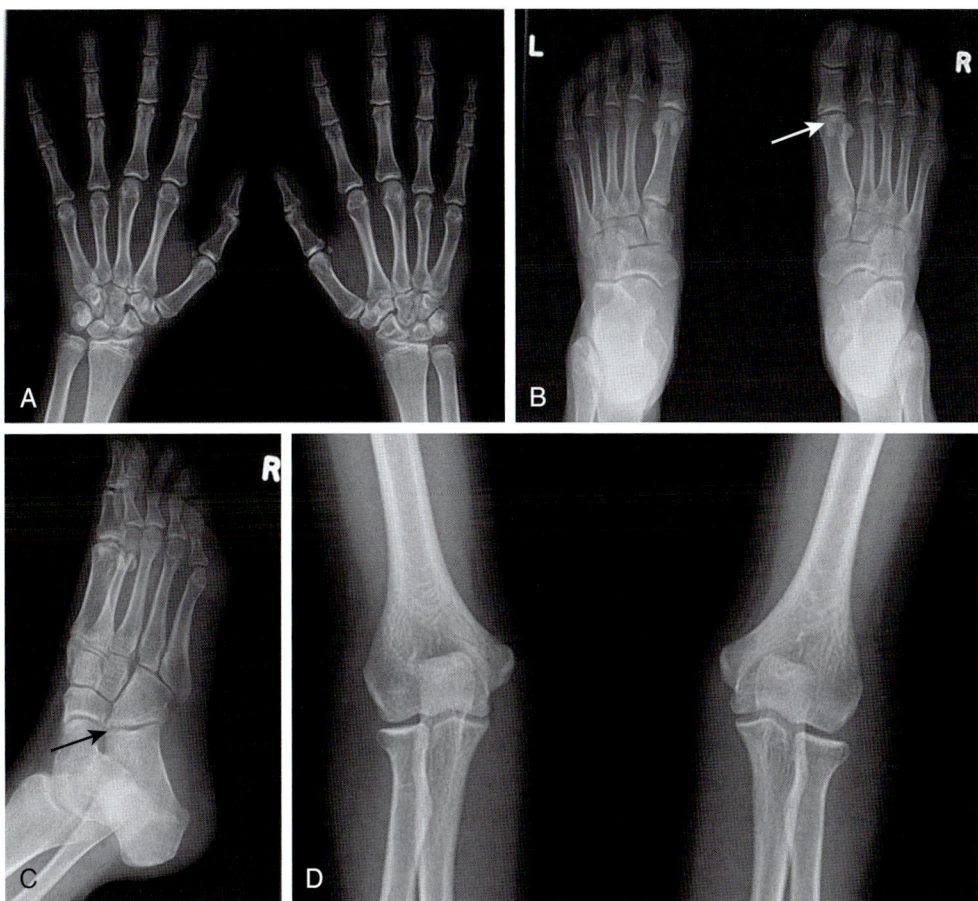

Figure 137-1 A 15-year-old girl with polyarticular juvenile idiopathic arthritis. A frontal radiograph of the hands and wrists (**A**) shows periarticular osteopenia, erosive changes in the scaphoid, capitates, hamate, and triquetrum bilaterally, and joint space narrowing at the radiocarpal and carpal-metacarpal joints of the second and third digits. Radiographs of the feet (**B** and **C**) show flattening and subchondral sclerosis of the metatarsal head of the first right toe, suggesting avascular necrosis (*arrow,* **B**), and a right calcaneocuboid joint space narrowing (*arrow,* **C**) that was believed to be related to underlying inflammatory changes. A frontal radiograph of the elbows (**D**) demonstrates overgrowth of epiphyses (medial humeral epicondyles and radial heads) bilaterally.

erosions also can be seen in persons with septic arthritis or hemophilic arthritis related to the inflammatory reaction caused by intraosseous hemorrhage. Large erosions can be seen in the camptodactyly arthropathy coxa vara pericarditis syndrome[31] (e-Fig. 137-3). Deformity of the fingers, whether with boutonniere (proximal interphalangeal [PIP] flexion with distal interphalangeal [DID] extension) or swan neck (PIP extension with DIP flexion) deformity, can be seen in a variety of disorders, including JIA (Fig. 137-4), camptodactyly arthropathy coxa vara pericarditis syndrome, or systemic lupus erythematosus. Enlarged or irregular epiphyseal ossification centers can be seen in persons with hemophilia, JIA, and tuberculous arthritis. Atlantoaxial subluxation or cervical vertebrae pseudosubluxation and ankylosis (e-Fig. 137-5) may be noted in persons with JIA, the arthropathy of Down syndrome, dysostosis multiplex, and systemic lupus erythematosus.

In contrast to adult patients with inflammatory arthritis, bone erosions are less commonly seen in children because the epiphyseal ossification center is surrounded not only by articular cartilage but also by epiphyseal cartilage and the spherical growth plate. As a result, significant cartilage loss must occur before osseous erosions are visible with radiography. Therefore the role of MRI is relatively more important in children compared with adults to detect erosions in articular or epiphyseal cartilage before actual bony erosions are visible on radiography.

Changes in bone growth and maturation with changes in the normal size of ossification centers and alteration of normal bone modeling can be seen in persons with JIA and in persons with infections and hemophilia. Enlargement of ossification centers and epiphyses (Fig. 137-4), contour irregularity, trabecular changes, and squaring (typically of the patella) can be seen. Tibiotalar slant (ankle valgus) also can be noted in persons with JIA.[32]

Late sequelae of JIA include epiphyseal deformity, abnormal angular carpal bones, widening of the intercondylar notch of knees (Fig. 137-4), and premature fusion of the growth plates. Growth disturbances are more frequent if disease onset is early. Joint space narrowing and osseous erosions are usually late manifestations. At the hip, protrusio acetabuli (Fig. 137-4), premature degenerative changes, coxa magna, and coxa valga can be seen. Joint space loss can progress to ankylosis, particularly in the apophyseal joints of the cervical spine (Fig. 137-5) and wrist. Rarely, ankylosis also can be seen in larger joints, including the hips. Subluxation of the joints, especially at the wrist, may be evident. Growth disturbance of the temporomandibular joint may lead to micrognathia and temporomandibular disk abnormality.[32]

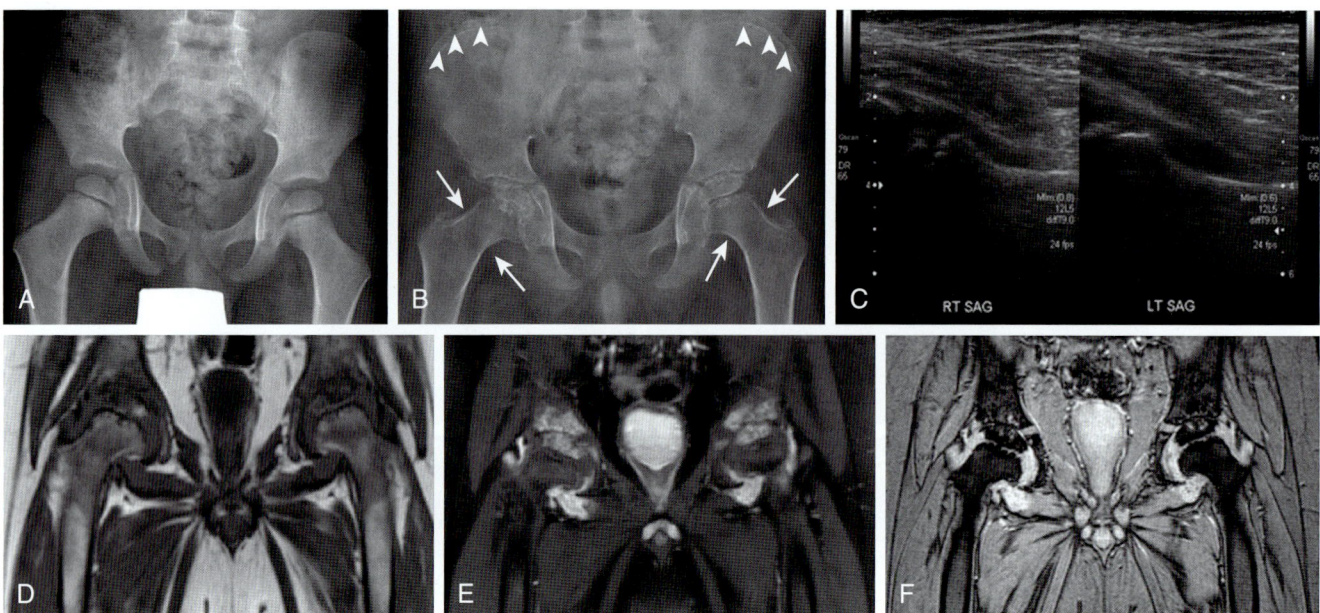

Figure 137-2 A patient with systemic juvenile idiopathic arthritis after having multiple hip infections. At the age of 4 years, only slight irregularity of the contour of the proximal femoral epiphyses is noted on a frontal radiograph (**A**) representing a variation of normal, with preserved joint spaces. At the age of 11 years, extensive erosive changes are seen in the femoral heads and acetabula with further joint space loss at the hips bilaterally, as seen on radiographs (**B**). Interval increased sclerosis is noted along the acetabular roof bilaterally. Nonspecific periosteal reaction is seen along the medial aspect of the femoral necks bilaterally (*arrows*). Sclerotic lines are shown along the iliac wings (*arrowheads*) compatible with previous bisphosphonate therapy. Gray-scale ultrasound images (**C**) obtained at the age of 11 years, 1 month before the corresponding magnetic resonance (MR) imaging scan, demonstrate moderate left hip joint effusion and mild right joint effusion. On an unenhanced multiplanar gradient recalled acquisition MR image (**D**), a contrast-enhanced coronal T1-weighted spectral presaturation inversion recovery MR image (**E**), and a multiplanar gradient recalled acquisition MR image (**F**) at the age of 11 years, markedly thickened, lobulated, heterogeneously enhancing synovium is seen in both hip joints. Enhancing signal abnormality, subchondral cysts, and surface irregularity are seen along the superior compartment of the hip joints. Marked reduction in the hip joint spaces is seen bilaterally, with flattening of femoral heads. The findings are likely to represent severe progression of inflammatory arthritis with diffuse pannus formation. Bilateral secondary avascular necrosis of the femoral heads is noted.

Although radiography should be used initially in evaluation of joints, cross-sectional imaging techniques have provided a significant improvement in anatomic delineation and diagnosis.

Magnetic Resonance Imaging

MRI is an optimal tool for evaluation of both soft tissues and osteochondral abnormalities with superb tissue contrast.[33,34] Contrast-enhanced MRI is extremely sensitive for detecting active disease and for early detection of cartilage loss, bone erosions, and synovial hypertrophy in children and adolescents.[34] MRI can define vascular anatomy, often without the need for intravenous contrast.[35] Higher cost, limited availability, and more frequent need for sedation in younger patients have limited its more widespread use. MRI provides multiplanar evaluation with a combination of available imaging sequences, including T1 and fast spin echo T2-weighted sequences, gradient echo sequences, and postcontrast studies all tailored to the specific clinical problem.[36-38]

Three-dimensional (3D) isovolumetric sequences also can be obtained, making it possible to reformat images in any desired plane. Cartilaginous structures including the growth plate are well visualized with gradient-recalled echo techniques[39] or fat-suppressed fast proton density sequences. Gadolinium-enhanced MRI can help differentiate physeal from unossified epiphyseal cartilage and can visualize normal vessels present within the chondroepiphysis.[40] MRI also is helpful in detecting synovial abnormalities within the joint[41]

and can be used to assess for changes in the synovium with therapy.[42] Additionally, MRI can be used to demonstrate muscle pathology, typically demonstrating nonuniform increased signal intensity on T2-weighted images and normal signal on T1-weighted sequences. These findings are not specific but may help in the selection of a biopsy site.

Without use of contrast material, proliferating synovium on MRI appears as soft tissue thickening with an intermediate T1- and T2-weighted signal (Fig. 137-6). It may have slightly higher signal intensity than adjacent fluid on unenhanced T1-weighted images. Pannus appears as a thickened intermediate to dark signal intensity on T2-weighted images and is best seen when outlined by bright signal joint fluid. Its variable signal intensity reflects the relative amount of fibrous tissue and hemosiderin. Intravenous administration of gadolinium-based contrast agents improves visualization of thickened synovium, especially with use of fat-suppression techniques. Proliferating synovium appears as enhancing linear, villous, or nodular tissue. Images should be obtained immediately after contrast injection because diffusion of contrast material from the synovium into joint fluid occurs over time. Hypervascular inflamed pannus enhances significantly (see Fig. 137-2, *E*), whereas fibrous inactive pannus shows much less enhancement. Subchondral cysts and bone erosions (see Fig. 137-2) appear as low signal areas on T1-weighted sequences,[36] with overlying articular and epiphyseal cartilage loss better delineated on fluid-sensitive sequences. Meniscal hypoplasia can be seen in some cases of JIA (e-Fig. 137-7).[34]

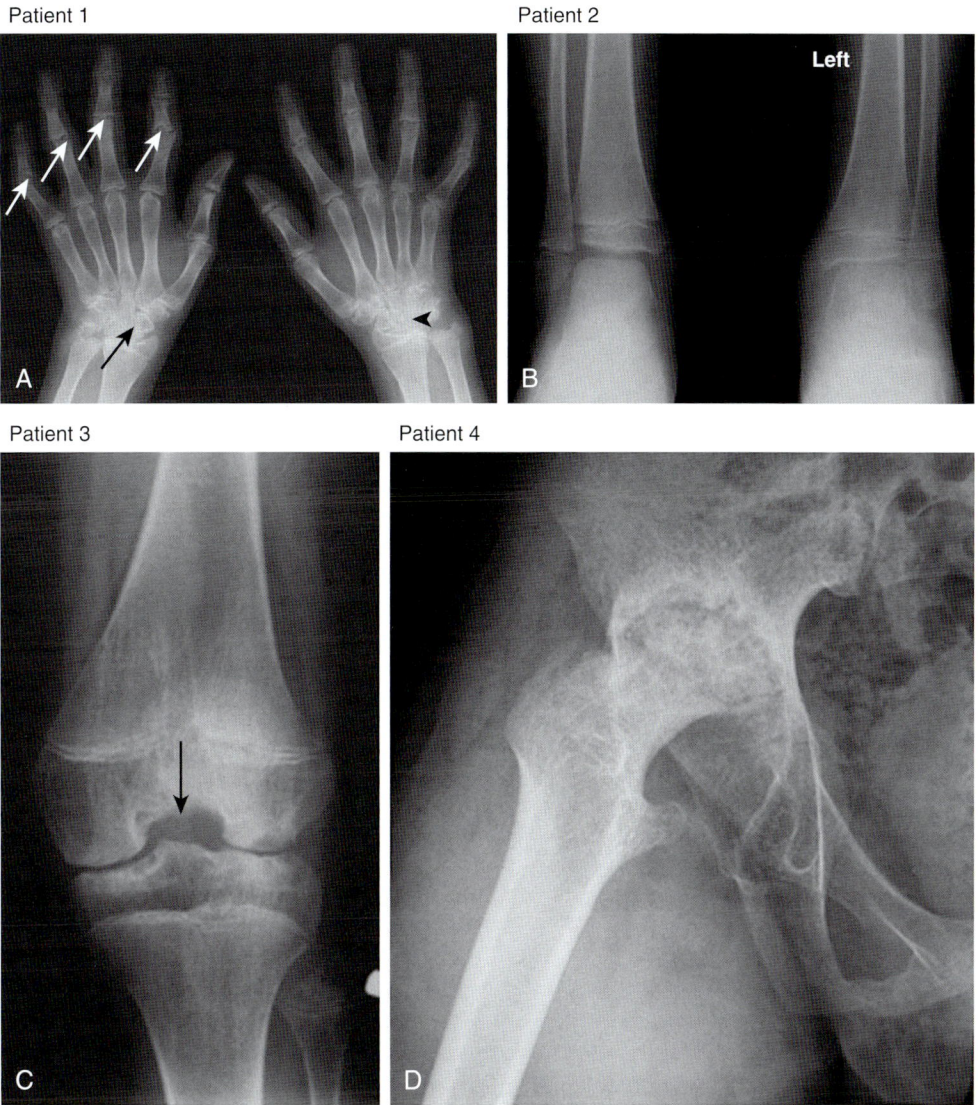

Figure 137-4 Radiographic findings of advanced juvenile idiopathic arthritis in the peripheral skeleton in different patients. **A,** Patient 1: Deformity of the digits as a result of erosive changes is seen at the phalangeal heads and bases (*white arrows*) and metacarpal and carpal bones (*black arrow*), along with joint space narrowing, carpal ankylosis (*arrowhead*), and array subluxation. **B,** Patient 2: A radiograph shows joint space narrowing, advanced maturation, and epiphyseal overgrowth (shown in the distal left tibia and fibula in comparison with normal-appearing right counterparts). **C,** Patient 3: Widening of intercondylar notch of the knee. **D,** Patient 4: Protrusio acetabuli.

Quantitative techniques have been developed for synovial volume.[43,44] MRI is more sensitive than clinical evaluation in detecting some specific joint involvement, including the temporomandibular joint, which often demonstrates inflammatory change in the absence of clinical symptoms.[45]

With prolonged synovial inflammation, well-defined intraarticular nodules termed "rice bodies" (Fig. 137-8) may be present. Rice bodies likely arise from detached fragments of hypertrophied synovial villi. On MRI, rice bodies have dark signal on T2-weighted images because of their fibrous tissue composition and are associated with joint effusion, synovial hypertrophy, and synovial enhancement after gadolinium administration.[46] Bone marrow edema is represented by areas of low T1-weighted and high T2-weighted signal intensity (e-Fig. 137-9) and should be differentiated from normal marrow speckling seen on fluid-sensitive sequences, most frequently in the ankle and foot.

Recently, studies in adults[47-49] have shown an association between presence of subchondral bone marrow edema in persons with inflammatory arthritis and radiographic erosive progression.

Although MRI has being extensively investigated for use in persons with JIA,[8,50] standardized measures for data acquisition and interpretation are not currently available[51]; hence this technique is underutilized both in clinical practice and in research. In addition, the imaging evaluation of growing joints is challenging because thinning of articular cartilage can be either a physiologic or a pathologic process. As a result, early subchondral abnormalities can be masked in joints of young children on MRI because of the greater thickness of epiphyseal cartilage in these joints, which makes evaluation less accurate.[8] Very few MRI scales have been designed to specifically assess morphologic changes with JIA.[52,53]

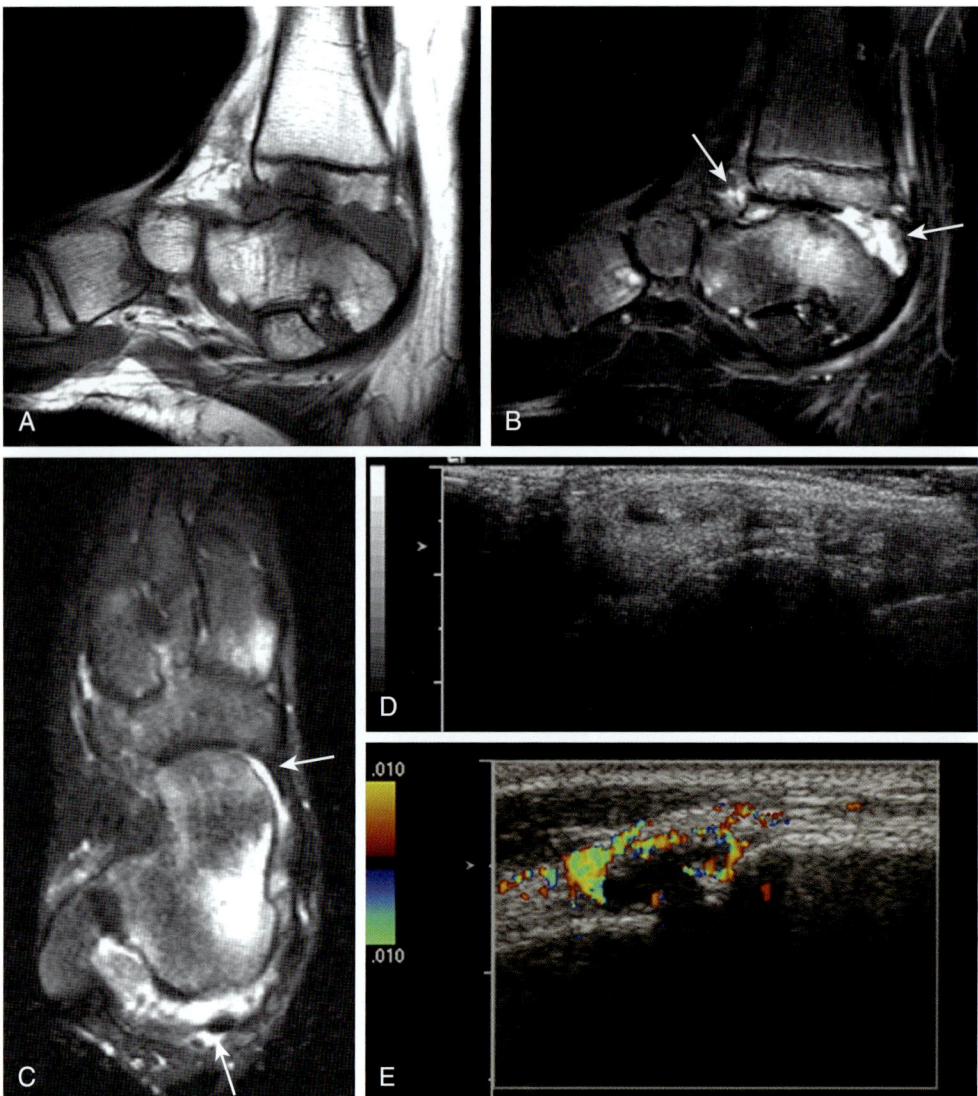

Figure 137-6 A 14-year-old girl with juvenile idiopathic arthritis and symptomatic tenosynovitis. Sagittal T1-weighted (**A**) and fat-saturated T2-weighted (**B**) magnetic resonance (MR) images of the right ankle show synovial overgrowth within the tibiotalar (*arrows*) and intertarsal joints. Extensive erosive changes and bone marrow edema are noted at the tibiotalar joint (**A** and **B**). A small amount of fluid is seen within the synovial sheaths of the tendons of the medial aspect of the right foot, including the tibialis posterior (*long arrow*) and flexor hallucis longus (*short arrow*) on axial T2-weighted MR images, suggesting tenosynovitis (**C**). Longitudinal gray-scale (**D**) and color Doppler (**E**) ultrasound scans demonstrate a small amount of fluid noted within the synovial sheaths of the tendons of the medial aspect of the right foot (**D**) with associated local hyperemia (**E**).

Novel MRI Techniques

A number of novel MRI techniques are under evaluation for improved assessment of synovial, cartilaginous, or osseous abnormalities (Table 137-1). These MRI techniques include diffusion-weighted imaging (DWI) and perfusion imaging, delayed gadolinium-enhanced cartilage imaging, and T2 quantification. DWI evaluates the translational movement (Brownian motion) of water molecules that occurs in all tissues, including synovium and cartilage. Alteration of normal diffusion can occur in diseases including infection, inflammation, and infarction.[54] Diffusion tensor imaging (DTI) is a variant of DWI and has been used to study the structure of ordered biological tissue.[55] DTI-derived metrics correlate with inflammatory cytokines and adhesion molecules and holds potential to delineate synovial inflammation; however, it is not superior to conventional MRI in the detection and assessment of therapeutic response.[56] Despite the contrast-free

characteristics of DWI and the possibility of using 3D steady-state sequences to enable imaging of short-T2 species with high signal-to-noise ratio, the use of DTI to assess cartilage in knee joints is limited because of the short T2 relaxation time of cartilage (30 to 70 msec).[57]

Contrast-enhanced perfusion MRI assesses blood flow using intravenously administered paramagnetic contrast agents and may be helpful in characterizing ischemic or hyperemic areas. Potential uses of this technique include recognition of epiphyseal ischemia and quantification and monitoring of synovial inflammation.[58] The rate of synovial enhancement depends in part on tissue vascularization and capillary permeability, both of which are highly correlated with synovial inflammation.[59,60] Rapid enhancement suggests active synovial inflammation, whereas gradual delayed enhancement suggests subacute/chronic synovial inflammation.

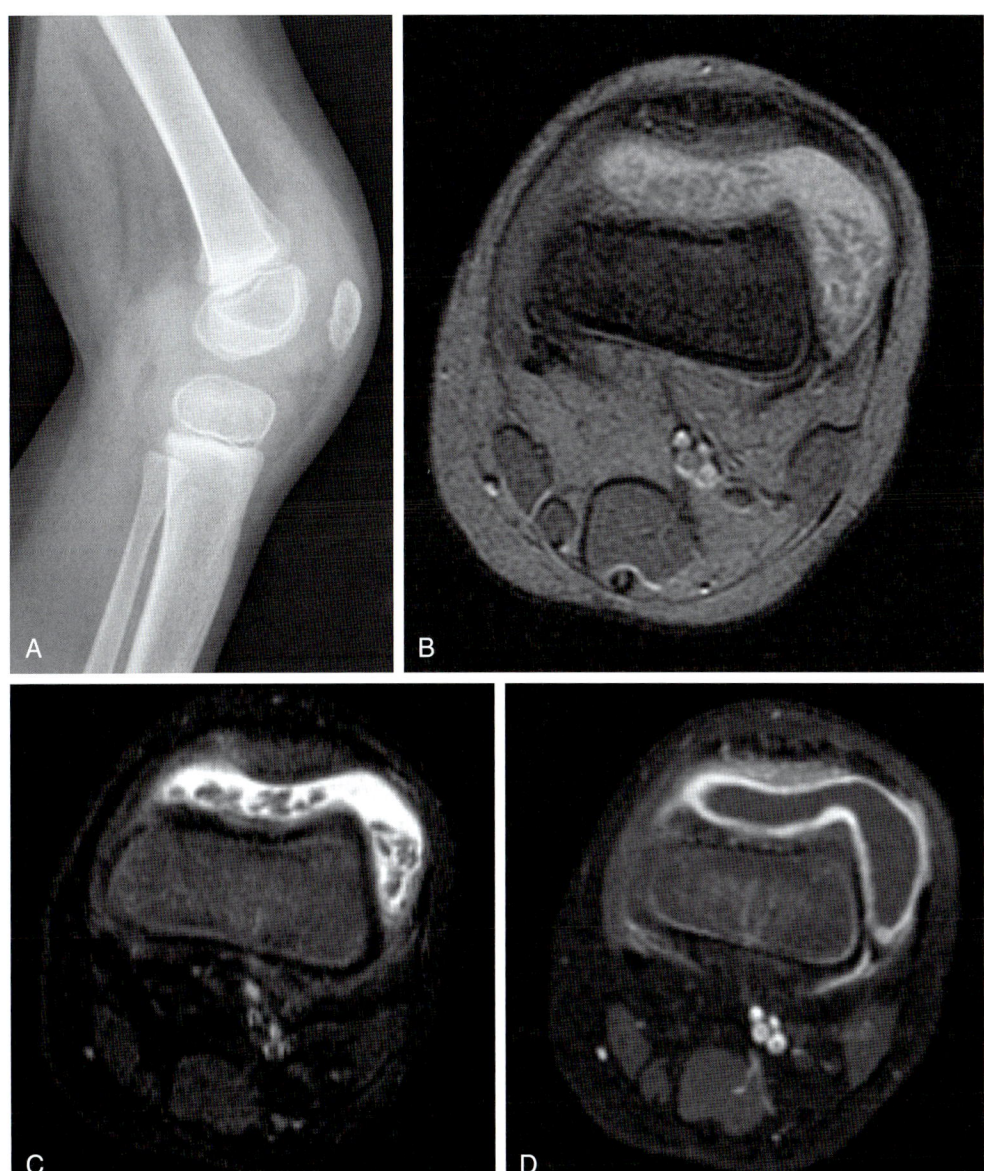

Figure 137-8   Rice bodies. A 3-year-old boy had persistent knee pain 1 month after sustaining a trauma. The lateral radiograph view (**A**) shows moderately large joint effusion distending the suprapatellar bursa. Intraarticular elongated bodies are seen on axial multiplanar gradient-recalled acquisition (**B**) and T2-weighted fat-saturated (**C**) and contrast-enhanced T1-weighted fat-saturated (**D**) magnetic resonance images; these bodies, which extend into the recesses of the joint space and layer in dependent portions, are so-called "rice bodies." Marked synovial enhancement also is noted. These findings suggest an underlying inflammatory arthritic process without associated joint destruction.

Table 137-1

Matching of Magnetic Resonance Imaging Sequences to Tissue of Interest		
Tissue	**Measurement**	**MRI Sequence/Technique**
Synovium	Fluid	T2-weighted fast spin echo MRI
	Rate of transfer of contrast between plasma and extravascular extracellular space	Dynamic contrast-enhanced MRI
	Restricted water motion (inflammation proxy)	Diffusion tensor imaging
Cartilage	Cartilage hydration and collagen orientation	T2-mapping MRI
	Glycosaminoglycan content	Delayed gadolinium-enhanced MRI
	Proteoglycan depletion	23Na MRI
	Proteoglycan content	T1 rho MRI
Bone	Erosions	T1-weighted MRI
	Bone marrow edema	T2-weighted fast spin echo or short tau inversion recovery MRI

Modified from Borrero CG, Mountz JM, Mountz JD. Emerging MRI methods in rheumatoid arthritis. *Nat Rev Rheumatol.* 2011;7:85-95.

The use of pharmacokinetic modeling for quantitative mapping of the perisynovial tissue[61,62] can add information to subjective synovial assessment. In this physiologically based model, signal enhancement time courses are described by a plasma compartment and the extracellular extravascular space. Pharmacokinetic parameters that are representative of tissue signal enhancement have been shown to decrease in children with arthritis under treatment over time and provide specific information on synovial inflammation.[62]

Because cartilage is one of the earliest sites of damage in persons with JIA, it is an important area to be evaluated with MRI. Cartilage has bright signal on both fast spin echo and fat-suppressed proton density sequences; hyaline cartilage has the highest intensity[40] and can be differentiated from epiphyseal and physeal cartilage. Articular cartilage should be assessed for areas of altered signal, thinning, erosions, or deep cartilage loss that may extend to the subchondral bone. The development of a variety of fast imaging methods with increased signal-to-noise ratio provide greater cartilage-synovial fluid contrast and have improved the MRI evaluation of cartilage morphology. Fat-suppressed 3D spoiled gradient-recalled echo imaging provides excellent contrast because cartilage has a bright signal compared with adjacent structures, but it is limited in differentiating epiphyseal, articular, and physeal cartilage. Other valuable sequences in cartilage assessment include driven equilibrium Fourier transform, dual-echo steady-state imaging, Dixon water-fat separation technique, and steady-state free precession.[35]

Delayed gadolinium-enhanced MR cartilage imaging is a sensitive technique for assessing cartilage proteoglycan content using the negative charge of the intravenously administered paramagnetic MR contrast agent.[63] The contrast agent distributes into cartilage inversely to the fixed charge density of negatively charged glycosaminoglycan (GAG). T1 relaxation time in the presence of gadolinium agent is approximately linearly related to GAG content. Delayed gadolinium-enhanced MR cartilage imaging may be used to assess early cartilage injury with depletion of GAG before anatomic changes are visible by conventional cartilage sequences.

Cartilage assessment can also be provided by mapping T2 relaxation time measurements. These measurements may help characterize the structural integrity of the cartilaginous tissue and quantitatively assess the degree of cartilaginous hydration and collagen orientation.[64] Typically an overall decrease in T2 relaxation from the cartilage surface to the deeper layers occurs.[65,66] In persons with JIA, increased cartilage T2 relaxation time is thought to be an early marker of disease progression in JIA, because it can identify microstructural changes before damage becomes visible.[67] In a longitudinal study evaluating patients with JIA from 3-month to 2-year follow-up, the clinical assessments improved, whereas T2 maps showed increased T2 values.[68] This increase likely represents progressive microstructural changes, even though clinical symptoms improved with treatment.

Another alternative MRI method is Na23 MRI,[69,70] which identifies areas of proteoglycan depletion through bonding of the positively charged sodium with negatively charged GAG molecules.[71] The major limitation of this technique is the low overall sodium content in cartilage, which limits the signal-to-noise ratio. MRI protocols using higher strength field MRI scanners (7 tesla) have been devised to try to overcome this technical challenge.[72-74] With the improved signal-to-noise ratio of higher strength field MRI scanners and dedicated transmit-receive radiofrequency coils, signal-to-noise ratio can be increased while specific absorption rate is reduced, which should facilitate imaging of small joints.[75,76]

Ultrasonography

Recent advances in ultrasonography, including better transducers and more pediatric musculoskeletal experience, have stimulated increased use of ultrasound in the assessment of pediatric joint disease. Ultrasound is ideal for assessing the pediatric musculoskeletal system largely because of its ability to visualize intraarticular structures such as cartilage and thickened synovium without the need for radiation. Ultrasound is very sensitive in detecting joint effusion, particularly in the hip (see Fig. 137-2, C) and shoulder, where radiographs are insensitive.[77] Intraarticular masses also may be detected with ultrasound, although their appearance is often nonspecific. Tendons and ligaments also can be assessed with higher frequency transducers.[78] Fluid within the synovial sheath appears as an anechoic halo surrounding the tendon (Fig. 137-10), whereas synovial thickening appears as a hypoechoic thickening around the tendon. Vascular anatomy can be assessed by combining sonography with Doppler. Synovial hyperemia leads to increased Doppler signal.[79] Power Doppler has been shown to detect residual disease activity more sensitively than clinical examination and/or MRI both in active disease and when JIA is in remission[80,81] and could be used to predict short-term relapse in patients with JIA who appear to be in remission clinically.[82]

Sonography can also be used to assess other periarticular soft tissue abnormalities, including popliteal cysts (e-Fig. 137-11) or other soft tissue masses, and to guide aspiration or injection of joints.[83]

Disadvantages of ultrasound include lack of standardization of ultrasound techniques for assessment of growing joints and normative literature data, lack of capability to visualize the central aspect of some joints, and difficulty in assessing some joints, such as the temporomandibular joints (Fig. 137-12).[45,84] Data on the diagnostic accuracy of ultrasound in children with JIA are limited. Assessment of joint effusion, synovial hypertrophy, and cartilage erosions by ultrasound can provide information about the severity of the disease.

Erosions and focal or diffuse thinning of the articular cartilage also can be detected, but only peripherally in the joint. Color Doppler ultrasound enables the detection of perisynovial hyperemia. Studies in children[85,86] have demonstrated the ability of color and power Doppler sonography, with or without intravenous injection of contrast agents, to estimate synovial activity in JIA. Resistive indices and fraction of color pixels may be used as quantitative measurements of the blood flow.[87,88] Contrast-enhanced sonography holds potential for detection of active synovial inflammatory disease in persons with subclinical JIA and may help guide early treatment.[85]

Very limited information is available about the diagnostic performance of ultrasound compared with MRI or clinical examination (in knees, sensitivity for joint effusion is 62%,[89] ranging between 60% and 90% for clinically active joints and approximately 70% for clinically inactive joints[90-92]; for superficial cartilage destruction, overall sensitivity is 60%).[89] Ultrasound-determined synovial thickness of the knee seems to correlate with clinical and laboratory (sedimentation rate

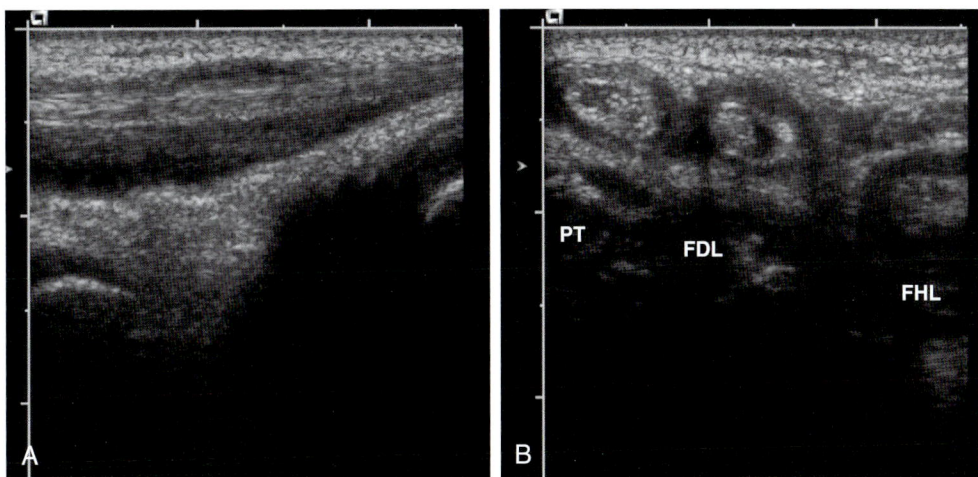

Figure 137-10   A 10-year-old girl with polyarticular juvenile idiopathic arthritis. The longitudinal gray-scale ultrasound scan along the medial aspect of the patient's left ankle shows an increased amount of fluid within the posterior tibialis tendon (**A**). Corresponding transverse (**B**) sonograms demonstrate tenosynovitis involving the posterior tibialis (*PT*), flexor digitorum longus (*FDL*), and flexor hallucis longus (*FHL*) tendons of this ankle.

and C-reactive protein levels) disease activity scores and with biomarkers of disease activity.[92] In ankles, however, very poor agreement was observed comparing clinical and ultrasound scores.[93]

TREATMENT AND FOLLOW-UP

A recent systematic review on the best evidence for treatment of JIA[94] showed that nonsteroidal antiinflammatory drugs are effective only for a minority of patients, mainly those with oligoarthritis. Intraarticular corticosteroid injections are very effective for persons with oligoarthritis. Methotrexate is effective for the treatment of persons with extended oligoarthritis and polyarthritis and less effective for persons with

systemic arthritis. Sulfasalazine and leflunomide may be alternatives to methotrexate. Antitumor necrosis factor medications are highly effective for polyarticular JIA that is not responsive to methotrexate but are less effective in persons with systemic arthritis. Therefore despite many advances in the treatment of persons with JIA, evidence is still lacking for treatment of several disease subtypes.

With regard to the use of intraarticular corticosteroids, studies have shown that as many as 70% of patients with oligoarthritis do not have reactivation of disease in the injected joint for at least 1 year, and 40% do not have reactivation for more than 2 years.[95-97] Radiographic and MRI studies have shown a marked decrease in synovial volume after injection without deleterious effects on the cartilage.[98]

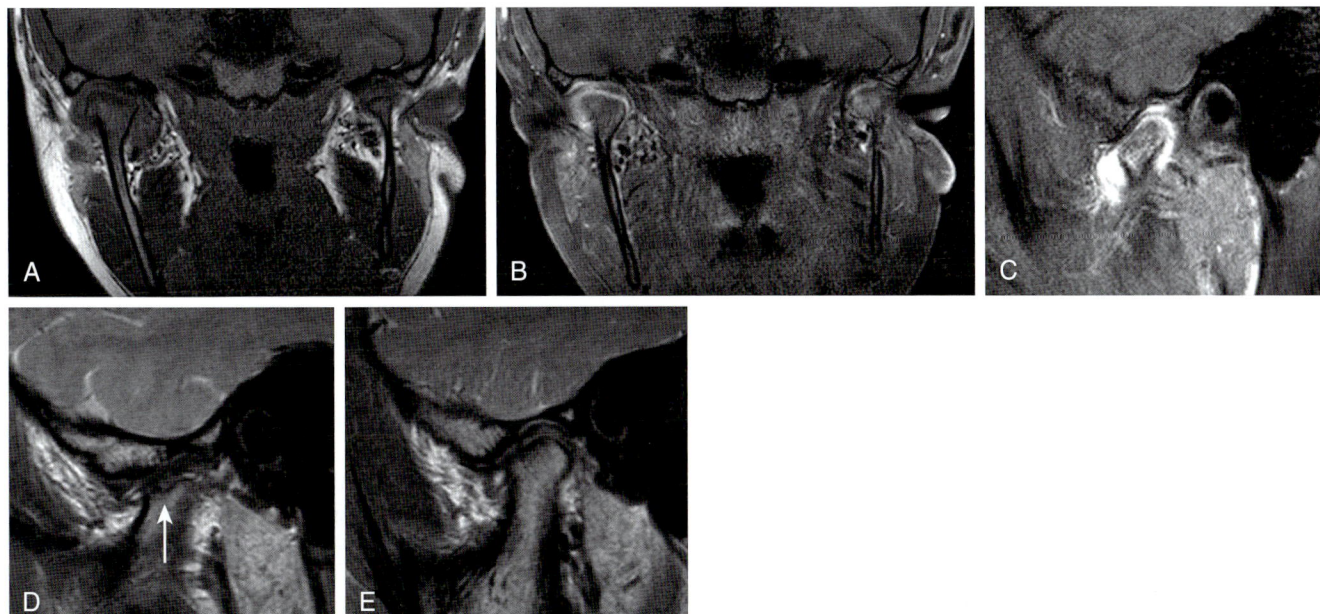

Figure 137-12   A 12-year-old girl with longstanding juvenile idiopathic arthritis and symptomatic and asymmetrically involved temporomandibular (TMJ) joints clinically. A coronal T1 image (**A**), a contrast-enhanced coronal T1 spectral presaturation inversion recovery (SPIR) image (**B**), a contrast-enhanced T1 SPIR image (**C,** right TMJ), a sagittal proton density image (**D,** left TMJ), and a sagittal PD image (**E,** right TMJ) show moderate right acute TMJ synovitis and mild left acute synovitis. Established chronic arthropathic changes are seen in the left TMJ joint with definite erosive changes. Incipient evidence of chronic arthropathy is noted in the right TMJ. Note a hypoplastic left mandibular ramus in **A** and **B**.

Imaging in the Assessment of Response to Therapy

Once therapy has begun for patients with JIA, imaging can be a helpful adjunct to assess disease activity and response to therapy. To date, several studies have examined radiographic changes before and after initiation of therapy, whereas more recent studies have used CT and/or MRI to describe joint changes and also have begun to use more quantitative measures of disease activity, including measurement of synovial volume.

Radiography

Radiography is able to demonstrate epiphyseal overgrowth and osteopenia after the injection of intraarticular triamcinolone hexacetonide.[99] Carpal length, defined as the radiometacarpal length plotted against the length of the second metacarpal bone on a chart with normal growth carpal scores, as described by Poznanski et al.,[100] is another parameter that has been used in follow-up with an interval increase in carpal length (a positive change) indicating improvement.

Sonography

Eich et al.[99] used ultrasound to determine the presence of effusion, pannus, popliteal cysts, and lymphadenopathy in 10 children with JIA affecting 15 joints (11 knee and 4 hip joints) before and after intraarticular therapy and concluded that ultrasound was as sensitive as MRI in demonstrating joint effusion and/or pannus but that differentiation between the two was difficult, particularly in the hip joint. Sureda et al.[90] reported that 2 out of 16 patients (12.5%) had marked clinical improvement with a corresponding decrease in cartilage thickness (insufficient evidence).

Magnetic Resonance Imaging

Although CT is able to demonstrate joint space narrowing, erosions, and condylar flattening,[101] MRI is currently the modality of choice to document changes before and after therapy. MRI can be used to monitor cartilage and bone erosions, effusion, pannus, and synovial volumes.[39] In studies of children with arthritis who received intraarticular steroid injections, MRI has shown that intraarticular steroid therapy has a long-lasting beneficial effect, with suppression of synovial inflammation and reversion of pannus formation.[98,99,103]

Quantitative dynamic contrast-enhanced MRI based on pharmacokinetic modeling can be used to evaluate disease activity in the knee. A study of pharmacokinetic parameters and synovial volumes showed significant decreases at 12 months after intraarticular steroid therapy; however, improvement in synovial volume appeared to lag behind dynamic parameters, reflecting delay or subclinical synovitis.[62] Of all the imaging modalities, MRI has been shown to be the most sensitive modality in the assessment of temporomandibular joint arthritis in children and has been used as a reference standard measure for comparison of clinical examination and ultrasound in clinical studies.[45] Ultrasound has been shown to be less useful than clinical examination to exclude active temporomandibular joint arthritis in patients with JIA.[45]

Complications and Adverse Effects of Joint Injections

It is difficult to determine whether other postinjection changes in JIA patients reflect the underlying severity of the disease or the effects of the local treatment.[104] The most common radiographic finding after injection is intraarticular calcification (e-Fig. 137-13). This calcification can resolve or persist for some time. It typically does not impair joint function. Damage to cartilage during the procedure is a potential complication.[98] Additional complications of intraarticular steroid injections include skin depigmentation, overlying skin atrophy, and iatrogenic infection.

Enthesitis-Related Arthritis

ETIOLOGY, PATHOPHYSIOLOGY, AND CLINICAL PRESENTATION

Enthesitis-related arthritis (ERA) affects 1% to 7% of patients with JIA and includes patients with arthritis *and* enthesitis, or with arthritis *or* enthesitis, as well as two of five defined criteria, including a history of sacroiliac joint tenderness and/or lumbosacral pain, the presence of the HLA-B27 antigen, the onset of arthritis in a male patient older than 6 years, uveitis, or a history of ankylosing spondylitis, inflammatory bowel disease, or uveitis in a first-degree relative.[1] The term "ERA" was introduced in lieu of the term "pediatric spondyloarthropathies" to emphasize that (1) axial skeletal involvement in children is rare and large joint appendicular involvement is more common at presentation, and (2) the disease commonly involves tendon/ligamentous insertions and origins in children.

IMAGING

Radiography

Radiographic findings of ERA and other spondyloarthropathies are similar to those encountered in other forms of JIA with the exception of sacroiliitis and enthesitis, which are more specific for spondyloarthropathy (Box 137-4).[105,106] In the appendicular skeleton, radiography typically shows asymmetrical involvement of the large joints of the lower limb, that is, the hip, ankle, knee, and tarsal joints. The interphalangeal joint of the hallux is also frequently involved. Radiographs may be normal initially or can demonstrate soft tissue swelling, effusion, ossification and epiphyseal overgrowth, erosions (Fig. 137-14), osteopenia, joint space narrowing, or, rarely, fusion. Bone erosions may be associated with irregular bone apposition at joint margins, referred to as "whiskering." With hip involvement, these proliferative changes are noted at the junction of the femoral head and neck. Dactylitis may be seen with soft tissue swelling and periosteal reaction along the shaft of metacarpals, metatarsals, or phalanges.

Enthesitis can involve the calcaneal and tibial tuberosities with soft tissue swelling at tendon insertions, localized osteopenia, and bone erosion and/or spur formation. Common sites include Achilles tendon insertion, plantar aponeurosis origin, or at the patella. Periostitis also may be seen.

In ERA, changes in the spine and sacroiliac joints generally are not seen until the latter part of the second decade or

Box 137-4 Radiographic Features of Enthesitis-Related Arthritis and Spondyloarthropathies

Peripheral Joints
- Asymmetrical involvement of large lower limb joints
- Involvement of interphalanged joint of the hallux
- New bone at the margins of erosions
- Affected joints show swelling, effusion, epiphyseal overgrowth, erosions, osteopenia, cartilage space narrowing, and rarely fusion
- Dactylitis-swelling and periosteal new bone of gingers or toes
- Periosteal new bone—for example, metatarsals, proximal femur

Entheses
- Especially tibial tubercle and posterior aspect of calcaneus
- Swelling, erosion, new bone formation

Sacroiliitis
- Radiographic changes generally delayed until late teens
- Asymmetrical involvement may occur early, then become symmetrical
- Erosions occur first on the iliac side of the sacroiliac joint
- "Pseudowidening" occurs as a result of erosion
- Sclerosis and finally ankylosis develop

From Jacobs JC, Berdon WE, Johnston AD. HLA-B27-associated spondylarthritis and enthesopathy in childhood: clinical, pathologic, and radiographic observations in 58 patients. *J Pediatr.* 1982;100:521-528.

even adulthood. It is unusual for ERA to present initially with spinal involvement in children. Spinal involvement includes localized osteitis, erosions, and sclerosis, particularly at vertebral margins. Syndesmophytes and atlantoaxial subluxation are rarely seen in children. Radiographs may demonstrate unilateral or bilateral sacroiliitis (Fig. 137-14) with indistinct articular margins (also known as pseudowidening), erosions, and sclerosis, particularly on the iliac side of the joint. Radiography shows asymmetrical sacroiliac joint space widening initially, but eventually the classic bilateral, symmetrical joint involvement can be seen, with joint space narrowing and ankylosis. Radiographic evaluation of the sacroiliac joints is often especially difficult in teenagers. Diffuse osteopenia of the pelvic bones is also seen as a late change.

Sonography

On sonography, enthesitis may show loss of the normal fibrillar echotexture of the tendon and irregular fusiform thickening.[107] Doppler sonography can be used to assess low-velocity flow in small synovial vessels.[108] Using Doppler sonography, Tse et al.[80] demonstrated the ability of color Doppler sonography to show decreased hyperemia at the cortical bone insertion of enthesis and along the adjacent synovium in children undergoing treatment, suggesting that this technique may add valuable information to gray-scale sonography.

Magnetic Resonance Imaging

Bone marrow edema, tenosynovitis, granulation tissue, or cortical erosion at the site of enthesitis in the appendicular skeleton may be seen with MRI.[38] MRI can demonstrate early inflammatory changes in the sacroiliac joints and spine and is especially sensitive for evaluation of subchondral bone marrow edema not shown on other types of imaging.[109]

The administration of contrast material improves the detection of early sacroiliitis and enthesitis-related arthritis (Fig. 137-15). On MRI, a periarticular low signal may be seen on T1-weighted images, with a high signal on T2-weighted images from inflammatory changes in bone marrow, whereas a low signal on both sequences will be seen with bone sclerosis. MRI also may demonstrate erosions in articular cartilage.[38] Evaluation of more widespread anatomic assessment, including whole body MRI, is currently under way and appears useful at least in demonstrating the presence of multiple sites of enthesitis-related disease.

Computed Tomography

Sacroiliitis may be demonstrated on either computed tomography (CT) or MRI at an earlier stage compared with radiography. A CT scan of the sacroiliac joints is useful in demonstrating sclerosis or erosive disease that is not evident on radiographs. Although MRI is preferable, if CT is used, angled scans through the sacroiliac joint should be used to lower the gonadal radiation dose.

TREATMENT AND FOLLOW-UP

Evidence for the optimal treatment of enthesitis-related arthritis is lacking.[94] Conventional treatments frequently offer limited efficacy. Treatment with nonsteroidal antiinflammatory drugs and corticosteroids may provide symptomatic improvement but do not alter disease progression. It was found that sulfasalazine is not significantly better than placebo.[110] Methotrexate has an uncertain effect and has not been demonstrated to modify disease course.[111] Treatment directed against tumor necrosis factor-α seems to significantly improve the arthritis and enthesis.[111,112] Infliximab treatment yielded responses in young adults presenting with peripheral enthesitis inflammatory heel pain.[113]

Psoriatic Arthritis

ETIOLOGY, PATHOPHYSIOLOGY, AND CLINICAL PRESENTATION

Psoriatic arthritis involves 2% to 15% of patients with JIA and may involve either larger joints such as the knees and ankles or interphalangeal joints of hands and feet, resulting in the characteristic "sausage digits."[20] Unlike in adults, in children, arthritis actually may precede skin manifestations.

IMAGING

Radiography

Radiographs obtained in the initial phase of the disease may be normal or show juxtaarticular osteoporosis. Characteristic radiographic features of psoriatic arthritis include asymmetric involvement, sausage digits (Fig. 137-16), joint erosions, joint space narrowing, bony proliferation including periarticular and shaft periostitis, enthesitis, osteolysis including "pencil-in-cup" deformity (Fig. 137-17), acro-osteolysis, spur formation, and ankylosis.[35] The bone erosions tend to

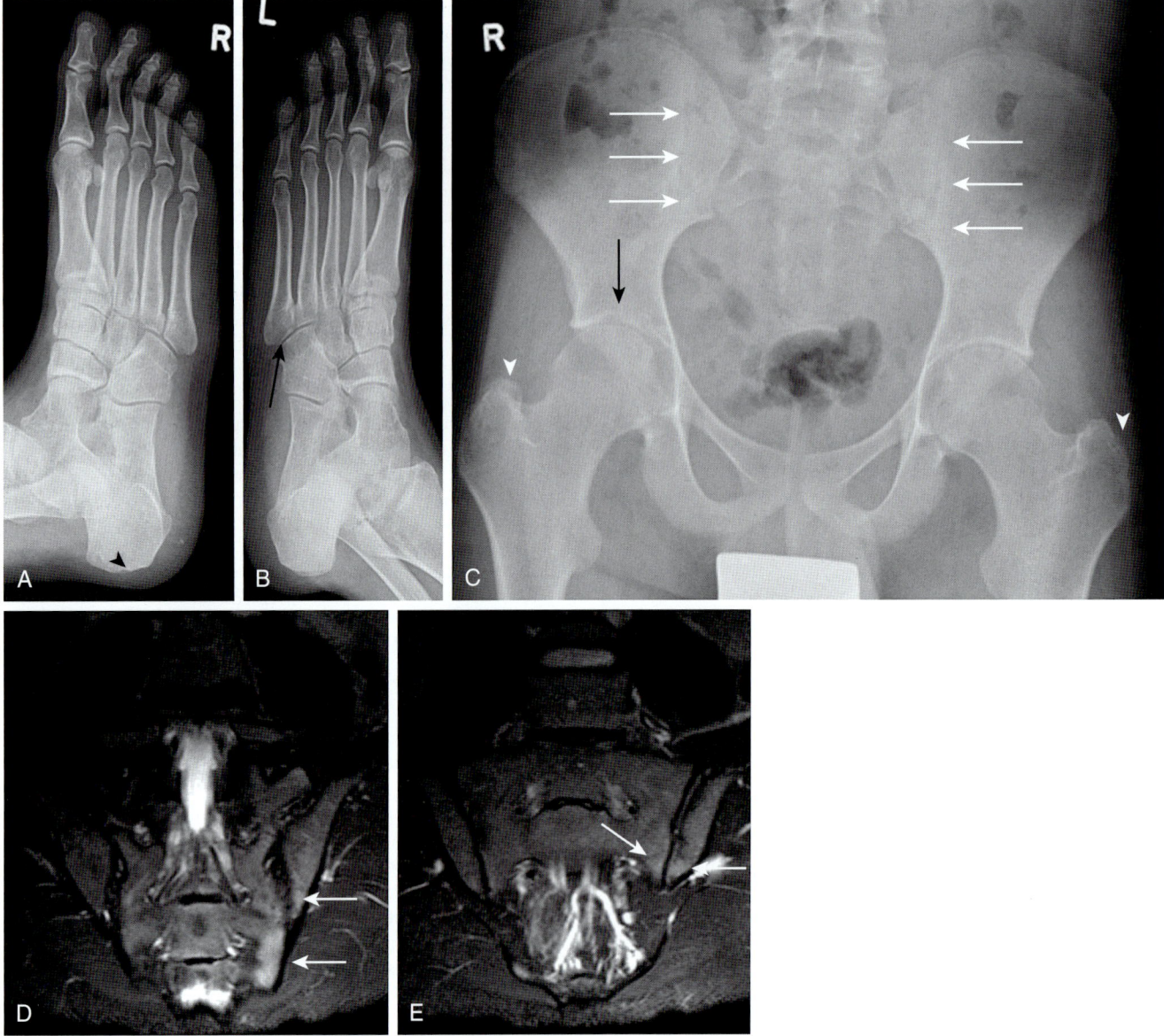

Figure 137-14   Oblique radiographs of the feet in a 16-year-old boy newly diagnosed with enthesitis-related B27 negative arthritis. **A,** An erosion is seen at the Achilles tendon insertion of the right calcaneal tuberosity (*arrowhead*). **B,** Mild narrowing is noted at the left fifth tarsometatarsal joint (*arrow*). **C,** On the frontal radiograph of the pelvis, slight irregularity and sclerosis is seen along both sacroiliac joints (*white arrows*) suggestive of bilateral sacroiliitis. Uniform narrowing is noted in both hip joints in association with erosions and a subchondral cyst (*black arrow*) along the superior acetabulum and erosive changes at both greater trochanters (*arrowheads*), representing signs of enthesitis. **D** and **E,** Coronal T2-weighted magnetic resonance images with fat saturation obtained 2 months after the aforementioned radiographs show heterogeneous high bone marrow signal involving the iliac and sacral aspect of the left sacroiliac joint (*arrows*) confirming the presence of sacroiliitis.

be larger and more asymmetrical than those seen in persons with JIA, but the radiographic features may be indistinguishable from other forms of JIA. The characteristic adult changes seen at the distal interphalangeal joints are uncommon in children.

Sacroiliitis and vertebral involvement typically manifest later during the progression of the disease. The sacroiliitis of juvenile psoriasis is usually asymmetric and resembles that of reactive arthritis. Syndesmophytes, paraspinal calcification, and atlantoaxial subluxation are rare in children.[35]

Sonography

Sonography with Doppler evaluation is more sensitive than clinical examination for detection of abnormalities in the hands and wrists, along with calcaneal enthesitis of adults with psoriatic arthritis, and it is a reliable tool for assessment of joint response to therapy with biological agents.

Magnetic Resonance Imaging

In persons with psoriatic arthritis, MRI demonstrates erosive changes, joint space narrowing, ligament disruption, and tenosynovitis. Sausage digits are seen in patients with psoriatic arthritis and reactive arthritis. These swollen fingers or toes result from tenosynovitis, soft tissue edema, and synovial proliferation.[114] MRI may also be used to evaluate the responsiveness of therapy as noted by a significant reduction in gadolinium uptake after treatment with infliximab.[115] In the axial skeleton, contrast-enhanced MRI can demonstrate

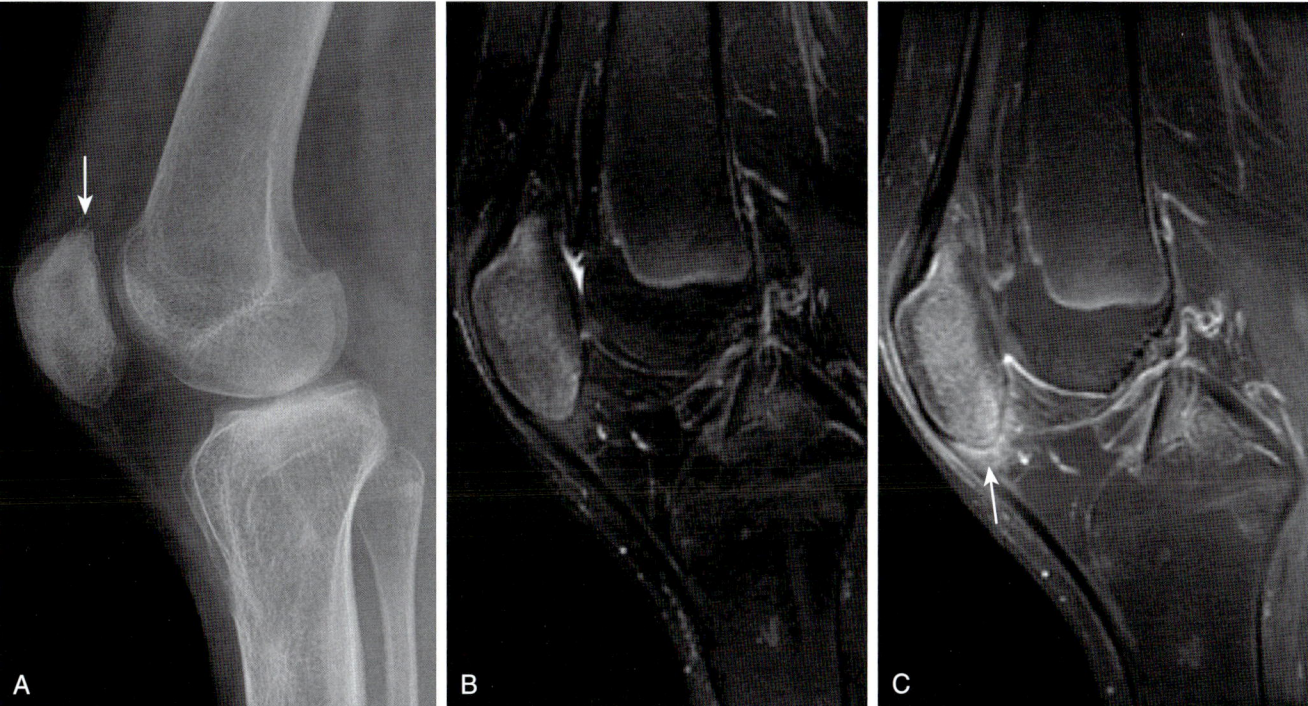

Figure 137-15 A 13-year-old boy with enthesitis-related arthritis. **A,** A lateral radiograph shows spurring at the upper aspect of the patella (*arrow*). Corresponding sagittal T2 fast spin echo fat-saturated (**B**) and contrast-enhanced sagittal T1-weighted fat-saturated (**C**) magnetic resonance images reveal increased signal intensity in the patellar and postcontrast enhancement at the origin of the patellar tendon and adjacent Hoffa's fat pad (*arrow*).

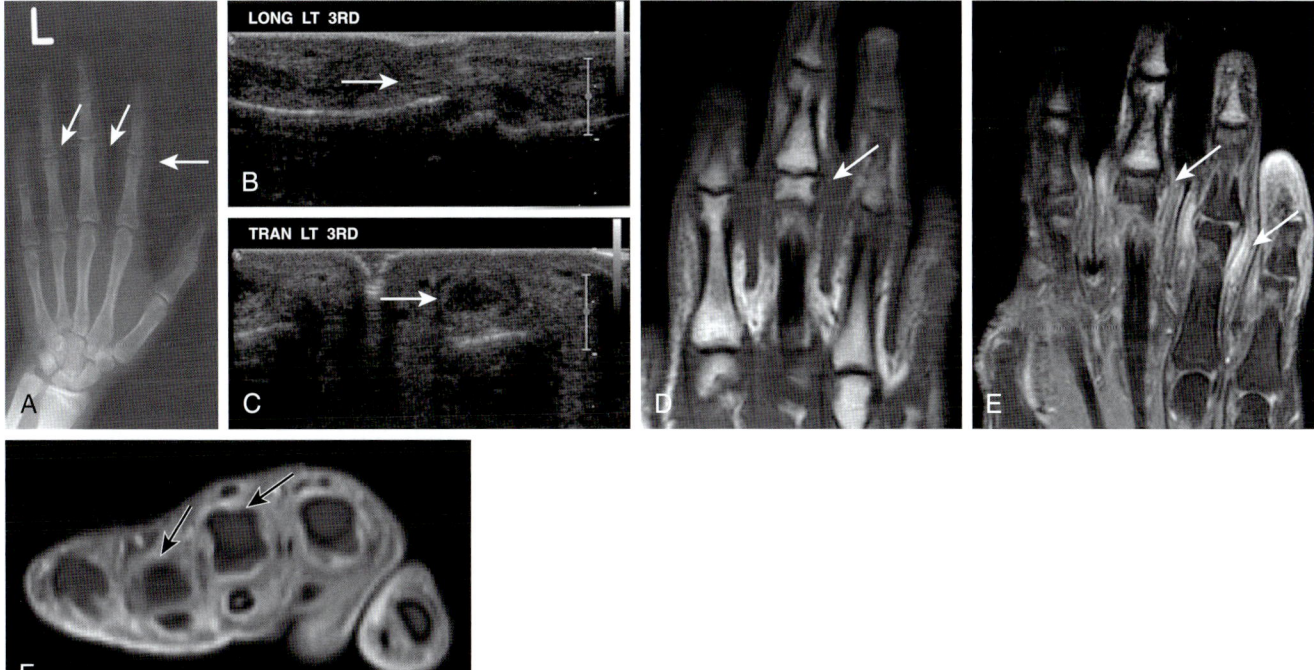

Figure 137-16 A 16-year-old boy with psoriatic arthritis. **A,** A frontal radiograph of the patient's left hand shows soft tissue swelling at the proximal interphalangeal joint level at the right second, third, and fourth digits. Corresponding longitudinal (**B**) and transverse (**C**) ultrasound images demonstrate fusiform swelling surrounding the proximal interphalangeal joints of the right hand. Localized echogenic thickened tissue compatible with synovial hypertrophy is seen (*arrows*) within the left third interphalangeal joint. Corresponding unenhanced coronal non–fat-saturated (**D**) and contrast-enhanced fat-saturated coronal (**E**) and axial T1-weighted images (**F**) of the left hand show prominent synovial hypertrophy and soft tissue enhancement (*arrows*) of the left third and fourth proximal interphalangeal joints.

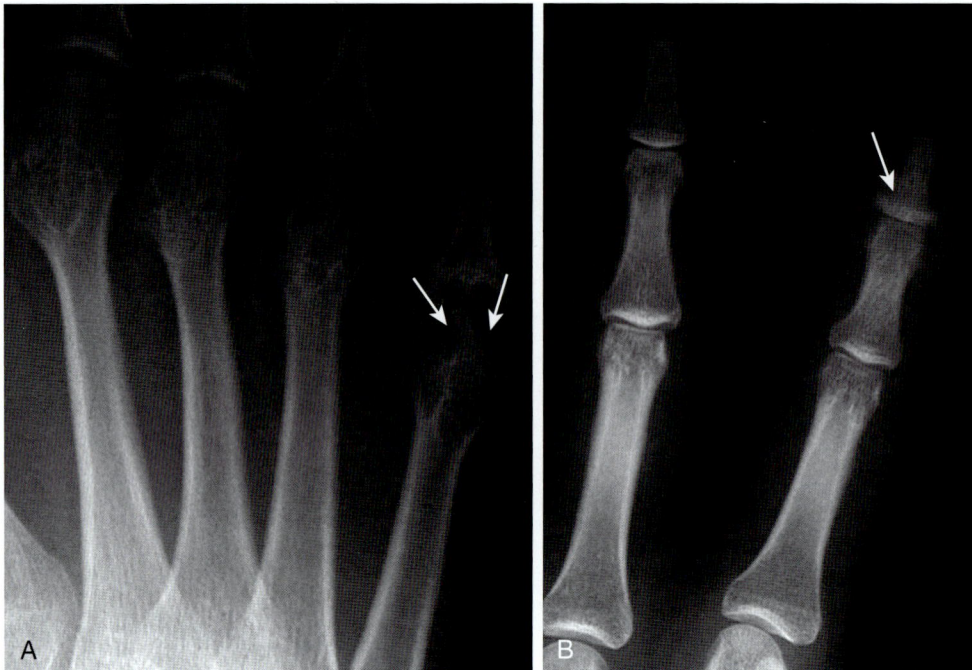

Figure 137-17 **A patient with advanced psoriatic arthritis.** Radiographs of the digits reveal extensive erosive changes at the distal end of the fifth metacarpal, resulting in a "pencil-in-cup" appearance at the proximal interphalangeal joint (**A,** *arrows*), and bony proliferation at the base of the distal phalanx (**B,** *arrow*).

synovitis (e-Fig. 137-18) and may be a useful tool for follow-up of response to therapy.

Computed Tomography

CT may be useful in assessing spine disease, but it has little role in the assessment of peripheral joints. Previous studies have shown that CT is as accurate as MRI for assessment of erosions in the sacroiliac joints but is not as affective for identifying synovial inflammation.[114a] CT can be used to guide sacroiliac joint injection.[115]

Hemophilic Arthritis

ETIOLOGY, PATHOPHYSIOLOGY, AND CLINICAL PRESENTATION

Hemophilia, an X-linked recessive disorder characterized by abnormality of the coagulation mechanism, affects 20 in every 100,000 males in North America.[116] It may be a result of a deficiency in factor VIII as in classic hemophilia (hemophilia A), or it may result from a deficiency of factor IX in persons with Christmas disease (hemophilia B).[116]

Hemarthrosis occurs in 75% to 90% of patients with hemophilia[117,118] and starts in the first and second decades of life. The most commonly affected joints include the knee, elbow, and ankle. Recurrent joint bleeding leads to secondary inflammation and hypertrophy of the synovium in response to blood products, and the cartilage degeneration and development of erosions and subchondral cysts[119] are similar to a primary inflammatory arthritis. Hemophilic pseudotumors, which are often intramuscular in location, may develop in these patients.

IMAGING

Radiography

The radiographic changes may be identical to those in children with JIA, but clinical findings and typical joint involvement help distinguish these entities.[120] Radiodense joint effusions and subchondral cystic changes are more common in persons with hemophilic arthropathy. In the knee, the classic radiographic findings include squaring of the femoral condyles (Fig. 137-19), multiple erosions, a widened intercondylar notch, and squaring of the patella.[25]

Magnetic Resonance Imaging

MRI can detect acute and subclinical prior hemarthrosis.[117] In a cohort study evaluating ankles, elbows, and knees of 24 boys with severe hemophilia examined by MRI at a median age of 8.8 years (range, 6.2 to 11.5 years), hemosiderin deposition was detected by MRI in 26% of joints (ankles, 63%; elbows, 16%; and knees, 12%) with no history of clinically evident bleeding.[120]

Acute hemarthrosis and chronic joint effusion may be indistinguishable with a low signal on T1-weighted images and a high signal on T2-weighted images.[121] Subacute hemarthrosis usually has a high signal on both T1- and T2-weighted images, which is related to the presence of extracellular methemoglobin.[121] Hemosiderin deposition can occur in persons with JIA but is more frequently seen in persons with other disorders, including hemophilic arthropathy, pigmented villonodular synovitis, synovial venous malformation, and posttraumatic synovitis.[122-124]

On MRI, gradient echo sequences are most sensitive in detecting synovial hemosiderin deposition, with signal loss

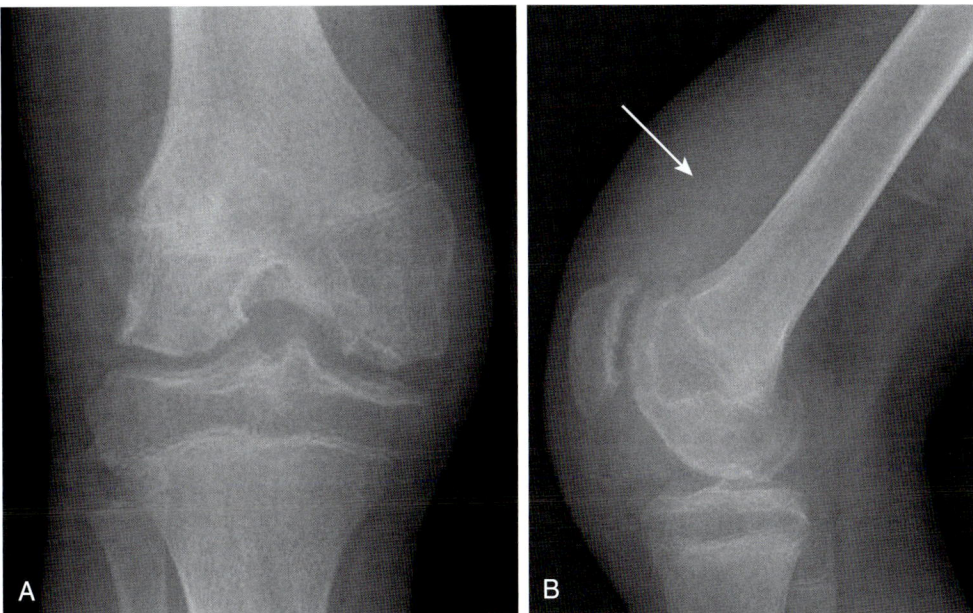

Figure 137-19 An adolescent boy with hemophilic arthritis. Frontal (**A**) and lateral (**B**) radiographs demonstrate widening of the intercondylar notch, epiphyseal cortical angular deformities related to innumerable erosions, and a large radiodense suprapatellar soft tissue density related to hemarthrosis (*arrow*).

occurring because of increased magnetic susceptibility (Fig. 137-20). Synovitis that contains hemosiderin appears very low in signal on all MRI sequences, and this finding is accentuated on gradient echo sequences.[125,126] The synovial thickening often has areas of low signal on T1- and T2-weighted imaging related to fibrosis or hemosiderin deposition.[121] Although gadolinium can better delineate the extent of synovial thickening, which shows less enhancement compared with rheumatoid arthritis, previous studies[127] have shown that dynamic MRI is not useful for evaluating hemophilic arthropathy, and gadolinium contrast agents are not routinely indicated.

Sonography

A major advantage of ultrasound over MRI in the assessment of hemophilic joints is the lack of interference of susceptibility artifacts, which are seen commonly on gradient-echo MRI sequences[128] and may obscure the synovium in the joint. In a patient with intraarticular bleeding with significant hemosiderin deposition, gradient-echo MRI sequences cannot tell whether the patient has mild, moderate, or large synovial hypertrophy. Ultrasound, on the other hand, is able to quantify the amount of synovial hypertrophy regardless of the amount of the hemosiderin deposition (e-Fig. 137-21). This advantage of ultrasound is particularly important for evaluating patients who may be candidates for radiosynovectomy.

Recently, a few systematic protocols for ultrasound imaging of hemophilic joints have been developed,[129-131] which enable systematization of imaging protocols and future comparative clinical trials. Although a prior study found a very close relationship between ultrasound and MRI in the assessment of the synovium and a good correlation between the degree of cartilage damage in ultrasound and the progression of bone changes in radiographs,[132] further investigation is required to determine the value of ultrasound

for assessment of cartilage changes. Ultrasound has limitations in the assessment of deeper cartilage surface abnormalities that are expected to occur in early stages of hemophilic arthropathy, given the centrifugal progression of cartilage degeneration.[133,134]

TREATMENT AND FOLLOW-UP

Treatments for hemarthrosis include injection of the deficient coagulation factor, cryotherapy, arthrocentesis of intraarticular blood (guided by ultrasound), and arterial embolization (in cases in which an arteriogram has identified a bleeding vessel).[135] Radioactive injections into joints (radionuclide synovectomy) initially were used in cases of JIA but have been shown to be effective in reducing bleeding and effusion in selected cases of hemophilic arthropathy. Radionuclide synovectomy has a good record for low complication rates; however, concern remains that the radiation exposure in young children could lead to radiation necrosis or tumor induction.[136]

Prophylaxis is the first therapeutic option in noninhibitor hemophilic patients.[137] This therapy reduces the joint symptoms and avoids further degeneration of the joints and should be started prior to the development of cartilage lesions. MRI is used to detect early hemophilic disease and to help direct the appropriate therapy. The role of ultrasound for detecting early cartilage lesions is still under investigation.[138]

Transient Synovitis

ETIOLOGY, PATHOPHYSIOLOGY, AND CLINICAL PRESENTATION

Transient synovitis is the most common cause of childhood hip pain and can be mimicked by a number of more serious

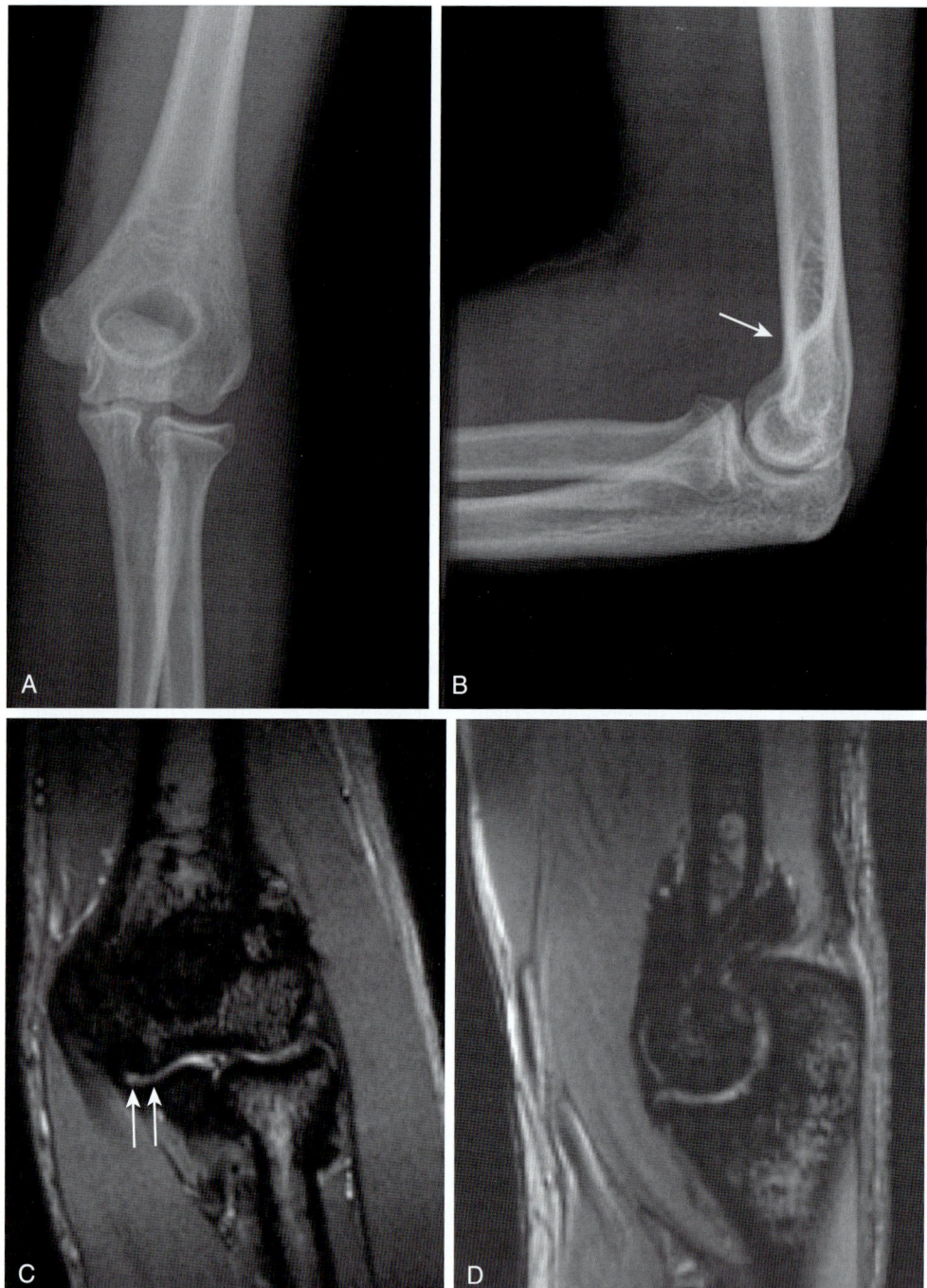

Figure 137-20 Hemophilia. Frontal (**A**) and lateral (**B**) radiographs of the left elbow of a 16-year-old hemophilic boy. A subtle anterior fat pad is visible as a sign of joint effusion/synovial thickening (*arrow*). Note is made of slight overgrowth of the radial head. Coronal (**C**) and sagittal (**D**) multiplanar gradient-recalled acquisition magnetic resonance images of this elbow show severe synovial hypertrophy and hemosiderin deposition, as well as surface erosions and cartilage loss (*arrows*).

hip disorders, including Legg-Calvé-Perthes disease, slipped capital femoral epiphysis, JIA, septic arthritis, and malignancy.[139] Transient synovitis is an acute, self-limiting disorder of unknown origin.[139]

IMAGING

Imaging is usually performed with conventional radiography or ultrasound. It has been proposed that radiography should

not be used in the primary evaluation of most children with hip pain because the results are generally normal or show only subtle findings of joint effusion. Exceptions should be made in infants younger than 1 year of age and in children older than 8 years because of the lower incidence of transient synovitis in these age groups, with the higher risk of child abuse and septic arthritis in infancy, and the occurrence of slipped capital femoral epiphysis in the older age group.[139] Although sonography is a sensitive and noninvasive method

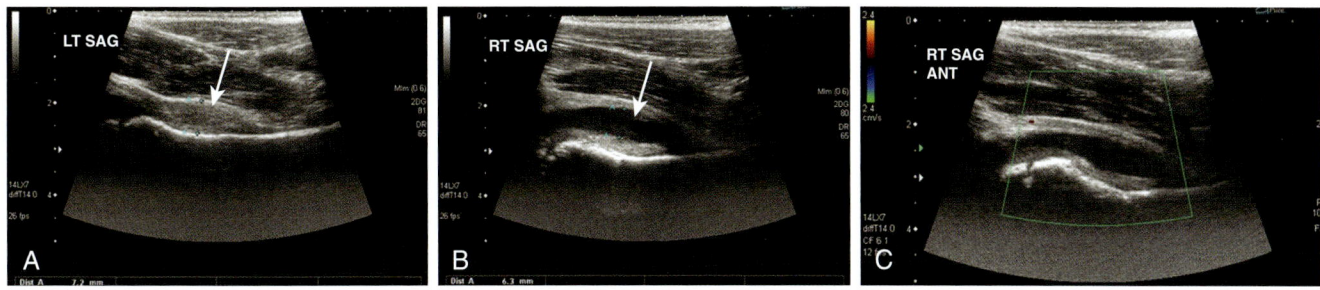

Figure 137-22 A 7-year-old girl with transient synovitis. Longitudinal gray-scale ultrasound images of the right hip show marked synovial hypertrophy (**A**, *arrow*) and joint effusion (**B**, *arrow*). No significant synovial hyperemia is noted on color Doppler (**C**). *ANT*, Anterior; *LT*, left; *RT*, right; *SAG*, sagittal.

of detecting hip joint effusion in persons with transient synovitis (Fig. 137-22),[140] it is unable to distinguish between different types of synovitis. Thus the combination of the patient's age, history of fever, and laboratory studies is useful to distinguish transient synovitis and septic arthritis.[141]

Nevertheless, the major contribution of ultrasound is to confirm the presence of joint effusion.[141] An ultrasound joint space thickness difference >2.0 mm between asymptomatic and symptomatic hips has been considered valid for the presence of effusion.[142] Other modalities such as bone scans, CT, and MRI are not used initially in the evaluation of irritable hips because of their higher cost and limited benefit.[25]

TREATMENT AND FOLLOW-UP

Aspiration is required if infection is a consideration and is readily accomplished with ultrasound guidance.[143] Treatment for hip pain related to transient synovitis can include traction of the hip in 45° of flexion, which may minimize intracapsular pressure. Treatment with ibuprofen may shorten the duration of symptoms.[144]

Malignancies

ETIOLOGY, PATHOPHYSIOLOGY, AND CLINICAL PRESENTATION

Any of the childhood malignancies, especially the leukemias and neuroblastoma, can mimic rheumatic disease. These malignancies may (Fig. 137-23) or may not involve the joint itself. Leukemic arthritis typically presents with transient arthralgias and joint pain, often involving the knees, shoulders, and ankles.[30] Joint effusion is postulated to occur in relation to either synovial infiltration with leukemic cells and/or an autoimmune response related to the leukemia. However, differentiating leukemic arthritis from infection is not possible, and aspiration may be necessary.

IMAGING

Although radiologic findings often are normal, they can include joint effusion, osteopenia, periostitis, lytic or sclerotic bone lesions, and metaphyseal radiolucent bands.[145,146] Diffuse abnormal signal intensity of bone marrow, which is low on T1-weighted sequences and high on T2-weighted sequences, can be seen on MRI (Fig. 137-23).

Pigmented Villonodular Synovitis

ETIOLOGY, PATHOPHYSIOLOGY, AND CLINICAL PRESENTATION

Pigmented villonodular synovitis (PVNS) is a benign proliferative disorder of uncertain etiology that affects synovial lined joints, bursae, and tendon sheaths (where it is sometimes termed "cell tumor of tendon sheath"). PVNS mostly occurs in the third and fourth decades of life[147] but can affect persons of any age.[148]

Gross pathologic features include a thickened synovium with a combination of villous and nodular proliferation, depending on the site of involvement. PVNS can either be focal or diffuse (i.e., involving nearly the entire synovial lining). On microscopy, PVNS is characterized by the presence of hemosiderin–laden, multinucleated giant cells. In addition, lipid-laden macrophages, fibroblasts, and other large, mononuclear cells are present. Hemosiderin also is found within the surrounding tissues. The ubiquitous presence of hemosiderin lends the tissue a characteristic pigmented appearance. The lesions tend to be hypervascular and demonstrate synovial hyperplasia.[148] PVNS typically invades local tissues and has the potential for extensive local destruction, even though it rarely metastasizes.[149]

IMAGING

Radiographs show soft tissue swelling without calcification; in advanced stages, findings are of degenerative arthritis, including bony erosions and subchondral cysts. The invasion of the subchondral bone, with resultant cyst formation, is a characteristic finding.[150] When PVNS involves relatively constricted joint spaces such as the hip, erosions related to intraarticular mass effect may be seen earlier compared with more capacious joints such as the knee.

On MRI, diffuse or nodular synovial thickening is noted, with low to intermediate T1 signal. Thick frondlike synovial excrescences often are identified extending into a joint effusion. Hemosiderin deposition results in linear low T2 signal, particularly at the periphery of the thickened synovium, which is more prominent on gradient-echo sequences; anecdotally, this finding is less likely to be seen in younger children. On postcontrast imaging, homogeneous enhancement is seen (Fig. 137-24).[20,151] Focal PVNS usually is a well-defined solitary masslike lesion that superficially may not appear to arise from synovium (Fig. 137-25), whereas masses

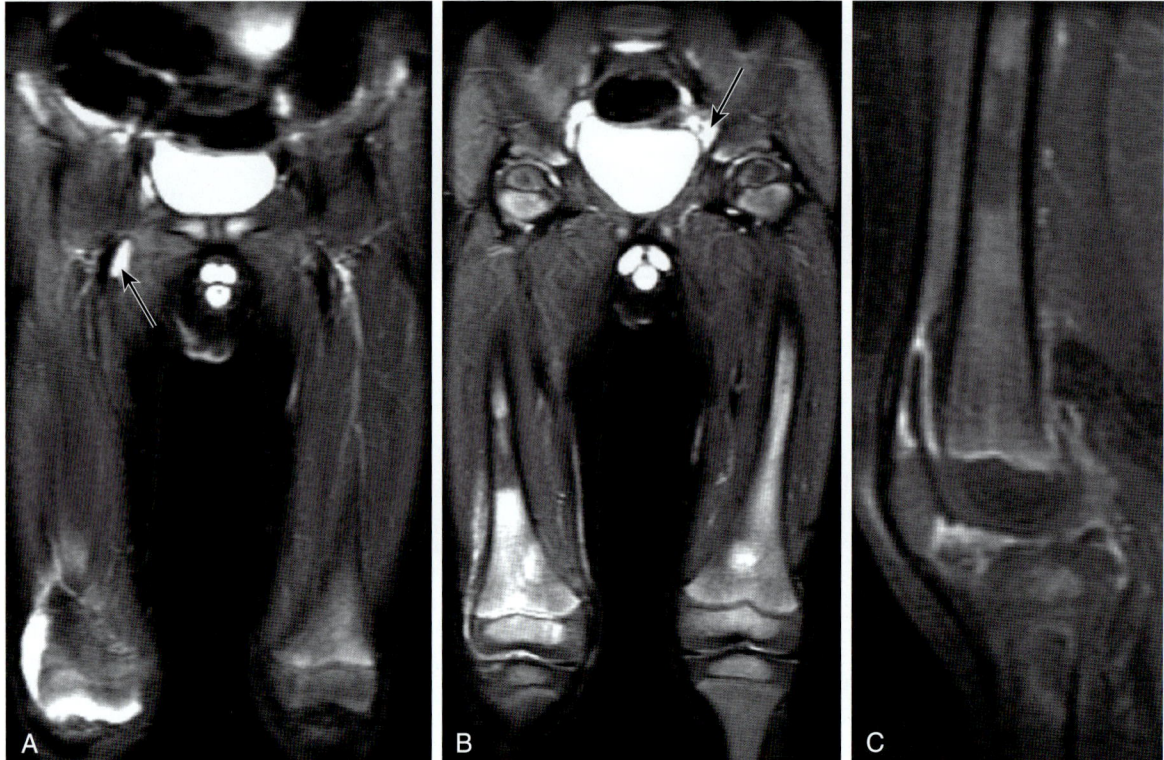

Figure 137-23 . **A patient with leukemia.** Coronal inversion-recovery (**A** and **B**) and contrast-enhanced sagittal T1-weighted fat-saturated (**C**) magnetic resonance images of the lower extremities show a large right joint effusion (**A**) with synovial enhancement representing synovitis (**C**). Diffuse heterogeneous signal abnormality is seen within the bone marrow of the femora and right proximal tibia, along with generalized adenopathy (**A**). Note is made of patchy metaphyseal enhancement in the proximal right tibia likely reflecting early bone marrow ischemia. This patient was diagnosed with acute lymphocytic leukemia.

related to diffuse PVNS originate from the synovium (see Fig. 137-24).

TREATMENT AND FOLLOW-UP

Definitive treatment requires synovectomy, but there is a high (up to 50%) incidence of local recurrence.[151]

Synovial Chondromatosis/ Osteochondromatosis

ETIOLOGY, PATHOPHYSIOLOGY, AND CLINICAL PRESENTATION

Synovial chondromatosis/osteochondromatosis is a benign condition of unknown etiology characterized by synovial membrane proliferation and metaplasia. It is rare in children,[152,153] and mostly occurs in the third to fifth decades of life.[154] The synovium undergoes neoplastic nodular proliferation, and fragments may break off into the joint. There, nourished by synovial fluid, the fragments may grow, calcify, or ossify. The fragments may be found free within the joint cavity, or they may be embedded within the proliferating synovium, which may extend into the surrounding soft tissues.[154] The natural history of synovial osteochondromatosis is gradual progression of disease, joint deterioration, and secondary osteoarthritis.

IMAGING

Imaging findings depend on the degree of mineralization of the chondro-osseous bodies. Ossification (synovial osteochondromatosis) is seen in 70% of patients.[20] Unlike with adults, children rarely present with radiographically detectable ossified loose bodies. Therefore the initial diagnosis often is suggested from MRI, where these particles may mimic pannus, rice bodies, and PVNS. On MRI, a non-calcified lesion is seen as an isointense T1-weighted and high T2-weighted signal mass. In a calcified lesion, focal areas of bone marrow signal are noted on all sequences (Fig. 137-26) but appear most conspicuous on gradient–echo sequences.[20]

When intraarticular particles are relatively uniform in size, the term *primary synovial osteochondromatosis* may be used. When the intraarticular particles are nonuniform and are heterogeneous in size and shape, secondary synovial osteochondromatosis should be considered. Secondary causes include trauma, infection, and nonpyogenic inflammatory arthritis.

TREATMENT AND FOLLOW-UP

Synovial osteochondromatosis is usually treated by surgical resection of the proliferative synovium and removal of the loose bodies, but the local recurrence rate is up to 23%.[154]

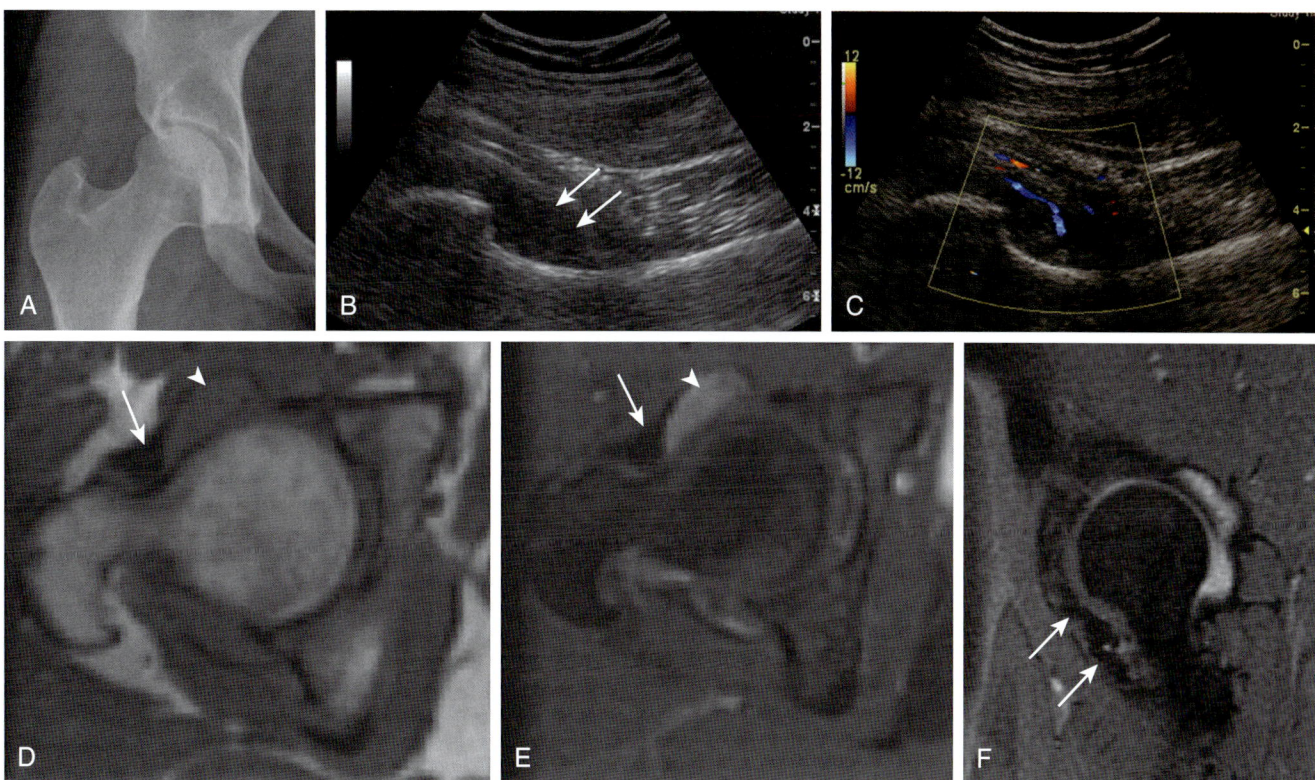

Figure 137-24 Pigmented villonodular synovitis (PVNS). A 17-year-old girl with a history of right hip pain for 3 years has a biopsy-proven diagnosis of PVNS. A frontal radiograph of the pelvis (**A**) shows a slight increase in the right femoroacetabular joint space medially. A subsequent longitudinal ultrasound of the right hip (**B** and **C**) demonstrates an area of synovial thickening within the anteroinferior aspect of the right hip with fine internal solid echogenicity (**B,** *arrows*) and internal vascularity on color Doppler (**C**). Mild right hip effusion was confirmed on the corresponding magnetic resonance imaging (MRI) examination. Unenhanced (**D**) and contrast-enhanced (**E**) axial T1-weighted MR images of the right hip reveal moderate thickening and enhancement of the synovium (*arrowheads*). A sagittal multiplanar gradient-recalled acquisition (**F**) MR image shows low signal intensity within the anteroinferior aspect of the right hip with mild blooming artifact consistent with extracellular hemosiderin (*arrows*). No invasion of the adjacent bone is noted.

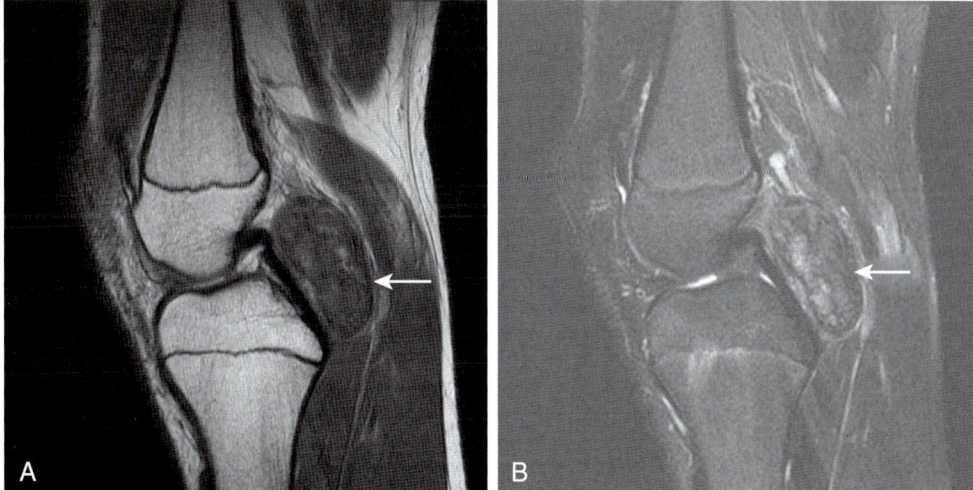

Figure 137-25   A 15-year-old girl with focal pigmented villonodular synovitis (PVNS). Sagittal proton density (**A**) and T2-weighted fat saturated sagittal (**B**) images of the knee demonstrate a well-circumscribed mass with heterogeneous signal on fluid sensitive sequences in the posterior knee joint space (*arrow*), with a biopsy confirming PVNS.

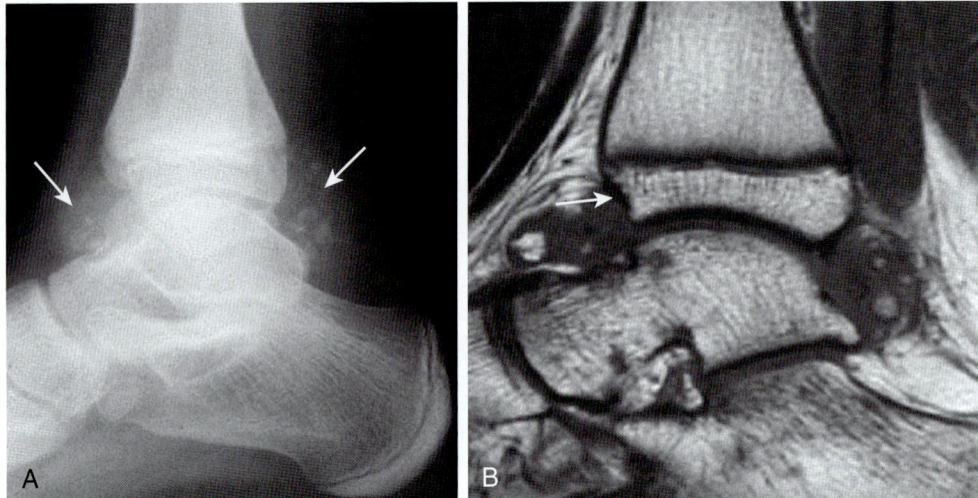

Figure 137-26 *Synovial osteochondromatosis.* An adolescent had a history of pain in the right ankle for years. A lateral radiograph (**A**) shows soft tissue swelling with multifocal calcific concretions within the anterior and posterior synovial recesses of the ankle (*arrows*). The corresponding sagittal T1-weighted image (**B**) of this ankle demonstrates large nodular synovial proliferation within the anterior and posterior synovial recesses with bony fragments seen within the synovial tissue. Associated incipient erosive changes at the anterior distal tibial epiphysis are best demonstrated by magnetic resonance imaging (*arrow*).

Lipoma Arborescens

ETIOLOGY, PATHOPHYSIOLOGY, AND CLINICAL PRESENTATION

Lipoma arborescens is a rare intraarticular lesion of unknown etiology characterized by replacement of synovial cells by fat cells, producing villous transformation of the synovium. It is not a true neoplasm and most commonly affects the suprapatellar bursa of the knee in patients between the fifth and seventh decades of life.[155,156] Patients present with painless joint swelling and effusions.[155]

Lipoma arborescens associated with degenerative joint disease and chronic inflammatory arthritis (secondary lipoma arborescens) is more common in the adult population, whereas primary lipoma arborescens (without a primary etiology) is seen predominantly in a younger population.[157]

IMAGING

The characteristic MRI appearance is frondlike synovial proliferation with fat signal intensity on all pulse sequences (Fig. 137-27), but it is best seen on T1-weighted and fat-suppressed T2-weighted sequences.[155,156]

TREATMENT AND FOLLOW-UP

Although the recommended treatment for lipoma arborescens is arthrotomy and synovectomy, arthroscopic[158] and yttrium-90 radiosynovectomy[159] treatments have been described.

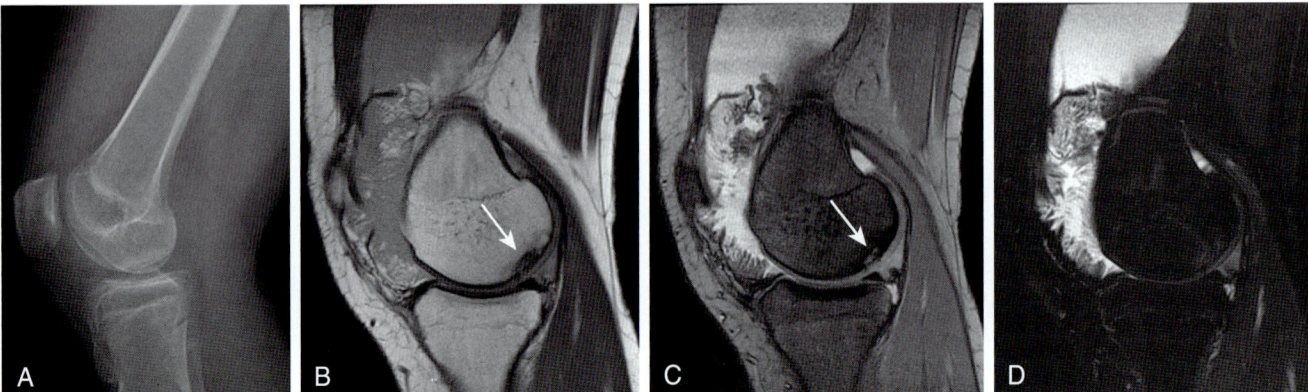

Figure 137-27 A 15-year-old girl with a diagnosis of psoriatic arthritis, lipoma arborescens, and osteochondritis dissecans. A lateral view of the radiograph of the right knee (**A**) shows a large joint effusion and an osteochondral defect (in the medial right femoral condyle; *arrow*). Corresponding sagittal proton-density (**B**), multiplanar gradient-recalled acquisition (**C**), and T2-weighted fat-saturated fast spin echo (**D**) magnetic resonance images of the patient's right knee demonstrate, in addition to the known osteochondral defect, a large effusion with fat signal frondlike synovial proliferation in keeping with lipoma arborescens.

Vascular Malformations

ETIOLOGY, PATHOPHYSIOLOGY, AND CLINICAL PRESENTATION

Vascular malformations are benign lesions that usually are diagnosed in childhood or young adulthood. The Mulliken and Glowacki classification for these lesions separates these lesions as high flow (arteriovenous malformations and fistulas) and low flow (venous, lymphatic, capillary) lesions and reserves the term *hemangioma* for vascular tumors that present during infancy.[160] The most frequent vascular malformation that may present with arthropathic changes is a venous malformation with synovial involvement,[161] although in the literature, these lesions often are erroneously referred to as "synovial hemangiomas."[162] Clinically, they mimic chronic arthritis because of recurrent bleeding of the involved synovium, and not uncommonly, diagnosis is delayed. They may have associated cutaneous lesions, recurrent hemarthrosis, and arthropathy (Fig. 137-28). The knee is the most commonly affected joint, but other joints such as the elbow, wrist, and ankle also can be affected, along with tendon sheaths. These lesions often have both a synovial component and a large extrasynovial component.[161]

IMAGING

Radiography can demonstrate phleboliths in the setting of synovial venous malformations, a soft tissue mass, joint effusion, osteoporosis, advanced epiphyseal maturation, leg length discrepancy, arthropathy simulating hemophilia, and periosteal reaction.[161]

The MRI appearance varies from slightly lobulated, nonencapsulated masses to infiltrating serpentine vascular masses to a combination of these morphologies. They are usually isointense to hypointense to muscle on T1-weighted images and hyperintense on T2-weighted images, with variable contrast enhancement.[161,162] Venous components tend to enhance and may demonstrate hematocrit levels within their tubular channels related to sluggish flow and microthrombi. Phleboliths are characteristic of venous malformations and typically present with low signal intensity on all sequences. Intraarticular fluid-fluid levels, synovial blooming artifact on gradient-echo images because of the presence of hemosiderin, or bone erosions due to a reactive arthritis as a result of the presence of intraarticular blood may be present (e-Fig. 137-29).

TREATMENT AND FOLLOW-UP

Intraarticular vascular malformations, particularly venous malformations, have a propensity to bleed. When these lesions bleed, the blood products cause an inflammatory response, and the presentation in a child may be that of inflammatory arthritis. Therefore treatment may be necessary to decrease bleeding incidence, including malformation resection, synovectomy, and palliative sclerotherapy.

Juvenile Dermatomyositis

ETIOLOGY, PATHOPHYSIOLOGY, AND CLINICAL PRESENTATION

Juvenile dermatomyositis (JDM) is an autoimmune inflammatory myopathy characterized by diffuse nonsuppurative inflammation of muscle fibers and skin.[163] The inflammatory infiltrates are predominantly perivascular, in the interfascicular septa, or around the fascicles.[164] The incidence of JDM in the United States is 3.2 per million children per year.[165] The ratio of girls to boys is 2.3 to 1.[166] JDM most commonly presents between the ages of 5 and 14 years.[167] Clinical findings

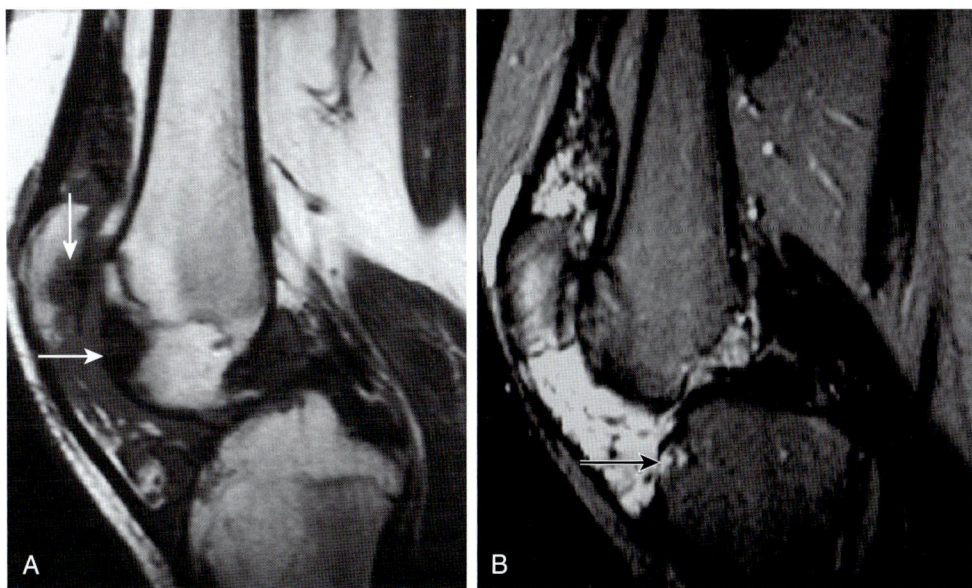

Figure 137-28 Venous malformation. An adolescent presented with chronic pain in the left knee. Sagittal T1-weighted (**A**) and T2-weighted fat-saturated (**B**) magnetic resonance images show an extensive soft tissue mass with predominant low signal intensity on a T1-weighted image (**A**) and high signal intensity on a T2-weighted image (**B**) involving the suprapatellar bursa and Hoffa's fat pad of this knee. Focal areas of low signal intensity on both T1- and T2-weighted images suggest the presence of hemosiderin deposition from previous hemarthrosis. Erosive and subchondral abnormalities are noted along the articular surface of the tibial plateau, patella, and anterior aspect of the femoral condyle (*arrows*) as a result of inflammatory arthropathy generated by the presence of intraarticular blood products.

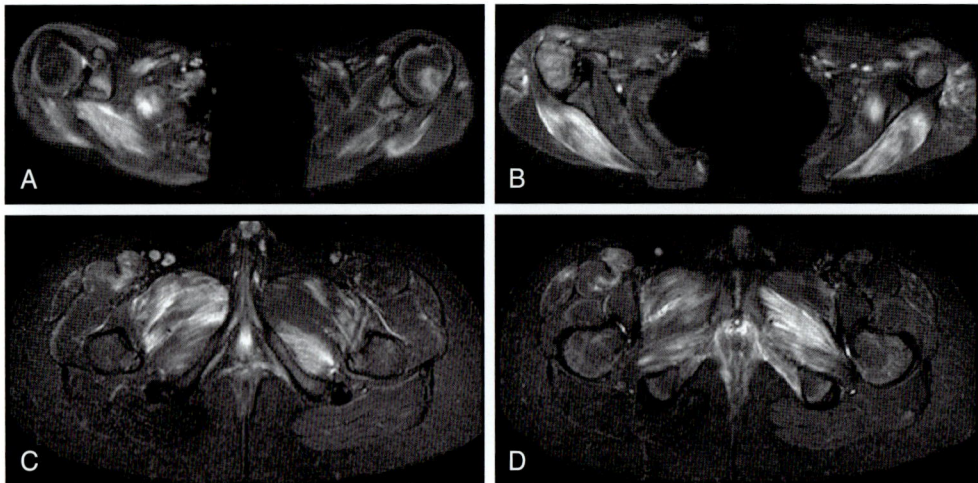

Figure 137-30 An 11-year-old boy with juvenile dermatomyositis. Axial inversion-recovery images of the upper extremities (**A** and **B**) show patchy asymmetric involvement of bilateral deltoid muscles, pectoralis minor muscle, triceps, supraspinatus, infraspinatus, teres minor, teres major, paraspinal and subscapularis muscles. Within the lower extremities (**C** and **D**), patchy asymmetric signal abnormality was noted in the adductor compartment, internal obturator, tensor fascia lata, quadriceps, hamstring, iliopsoas, gluteus maximum, and gluteus medius and minimum muscles.

include severe proximal muscle weakness, fatigue, heliotrope rash (a pink or purple rash on the face and knuckles), and underlying vasculitic pathology.[167,168]

IMAGING

Radiography

In the acute stage of JDM, radiologic changes are minimal. However, incipient soft tissue swelling and subcutaneous edema represented by blurring of fat planes can be noted in the proximal appendicular skeleton in some cases. The muscles of the scapular and pelvic girdles are most frequently affected, and their involvement is typically symmetrical (Figs. 137-29 and 137-30).[169,170] In chronic disease, radiographs demonstrate soft tissue loss and muscle atrophy. Marked osteoporosis of the long bones and vertebral bodies also may be present. The most characteristic finding of chronic disease, however, is the deposition of calcium in the soft tissues (Fig. 137-31), which is identified in 25% to 50% of cases.[171] The calcium deposits may present as subcutaneous plaques, nodules, periarticular calcific foci, and large clumps or sheets of calcium within muscle or subcutaneous tissue.[172] The arthritis associated with JDM is usually transient and nondeforming in nature.[172]

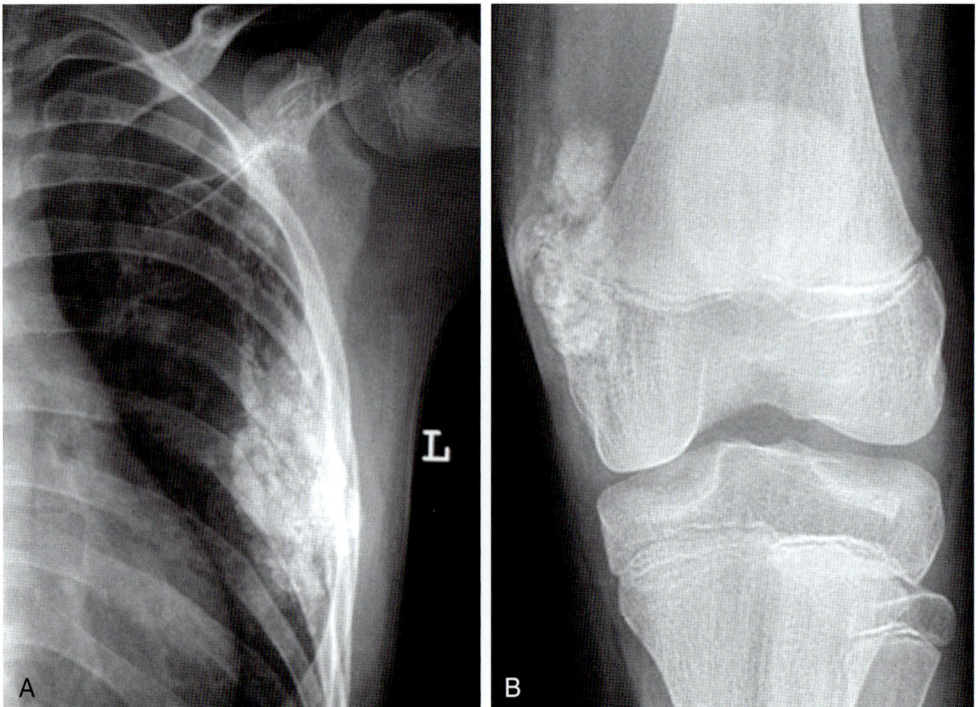

Figure 137-31 Juvenile dermatomyositis in a 15-year-old boy with juvenile dermatomyositis and severe heterotopic calcifications. Frontal radiographs of the left lateral chest wall (**A**) and left knee (**B**) show extensive soft tissue calcium deposits.

Ultrasonography

Ultrasound scanning of the involved musculature shows diffusely increased echogenicity of the soft tissues and acoustic shadowing within the musculature in regions of calcium deposits. Histopathologically, muscle lipomatosis significantly correlates to muscle echogenicity.[164] Other sonographic findings include atrophy and decreased muscular bulk, soft tissue fasciculation, tenosynovitis, and soft tissue nodularities.[173]

Magnetic Resonance Imaging

Ultrasound and MRI have a similar capacity to demonstrate the features of inflammatory muscle disease, but MRI is more sensitive for the detection of edema, representing inflammation, in the acute phase of the disease. Both MRI and ultrasound allow guided biopsy and aspiration of muscle abnormalities.[174-177] MRI reveals increased water content (edema) as increased signal intensity on T2-weighted and short tau inversion recovery MR images (Figs. 137-29 and 137-30) within infarcted muscles as a result of vasculitis.[178] In fact, T2 relaxation time can be used as a quantitative measure of muscle inflammation and correlates well with other measures of disease activity.[179] Because physical exercise can induce changes that mimic inflammation of muscle, children with JDM should be at rest for at least 30 minutes before MR imaging to assess disease activity.[180]

In chronic disease, focal areas of low signal intensity usually are seen on all MRI sequences, which represent calcific and fibrotic foci. Focal areas of increased signal intensity on T1-weighted images representing partial fatty replacement of muscles and tenosynovitis-related changes also may be identified.[178]

Computed Tomography

Although CT does not detect inflammatory changes in muscle tissue, it is the modality of choice for identifying soft tissue calcifications in soft tissues associated with JDM.[181] It also allows quantification of muscle atrophy and fatty replacement in deep muscles.

Scintigraphy

Whole-body thallium-201 chloride and technetium-99m-methylene diphosphonate (^{99m}technetium-MDP) muscle scintigraphy a potentially useful tool to investigate occult muscle groups affected by dermatomyositis; however, further investigation in the pediatric population is required.[182,183] Furthermore, bone scans with ^{99m}technetium-MDP can function as auxiliary tools to evaluate calcinosis in patients with JDM.[181-183]

TREATMENT AND FOLLOW-UP

Since the 1970s, standard treatment for JDM has been high-dose daily oral corticosteroids, which is continued until clinical and laboratory improvement are evident, and then slowly reduced over at least a 2-year period.[184] Methotrexate is an important ancillary treatment. Early studies suggested that methotrexate improves strength and reduces other signs of disease activity in steroid-resistant patients[185] with acceptable adverse effects.[186,187] Other treatments, including cyclosporine, hydroxychloroquine, tacrolimus, azathioprine, mycophenolate mofetil, and cyclophosphamide for severe disease, have shown some benefit in cases of refractory disease.[188]

Biological agents, which are used widely in persons with other rheumatic diseases, are being developed for the treatment of childhood myositis. The few studies[189,190] of rituximab in persons with JDM suggest a favorable response; however, biologic agents currently are reserved for patients with recalcitrant disease.[191]

Physical disability from muscle weakness or contractures represents a significant problem. Physiotherapy plays an important role in the rehabilitation of patients with JDM.[192] Studies using MRI T2-weighted relaxation time suggest that moderate exercise does not increase muscle inflammation.[193] In another study,[194] aerobic exercise limitation in JDM was shown to correlate best with measures of disease damage (e.g., global damage assessment, T1-weighted MRI, and disease duration).

Chronic Recurrent Multifocal Osteomyelitis

ETIOLOGY, PATHOPHYSIOLOGY, AND CLINICAL PRESENTATION

Chronic recurrent multifocal osteomyelitis (CRMO) is a skeletal disorder of unknown origin mainly occurring in children and adolescents.[195] It is characterized by multifocal non-pyogenic inflammatory bone lesions, a course of exacerbations and remissions, and an association with other inflammatory disorders.[196] The association of CRMO with dermatologic disorders (such as psoriasis) and inflammatory bowel disease and its response to steroids has led to the suggestion of an autoimmune cause.[197-199] More recently, a genetic origin for CRMO has been suggested as a result of observation of disease in siblings and monozygotic twins.[200-202]

SAPHO (synovitis, acne, pustulosis, hyperostosis, osteitis) syndrome is the adult equivalent of CRMO.[203] Whereas CRMO typically manifests in the first decade of life, the mean age of onset for SAPHO syndrome is 28 years.[204] CRMO is a diagnosis of exclusion, distinct from bacterial osteomyelitis, based on the following criteria:

1. Bone lesions with a radiographic picture suggesting subacute or chronic osteomyelitis
2. An unusual location of lesions when compared with infectious osteomyelitis and frequent multifocality
3. No abscess formation, fistula, or sequestra
4. Lack of a causative organism
5. Nonspecific histopathologic and laboratory findings compatible with subacute or chronic osteomyelitis
6. A characteristic prolonged, fluctuating course with recurrent episodes of pain
7. Occasional accompanying skin disease[195]

IMAGING

The imaging evaluation of CRMO should start with radiographic evaluation of the symptomatic sites. If the radiographs have negative findings in the presence of significant clinical symptoms, further evaluation with MRI should be considered to evaluate for bone marrow edema. Whole-body evaluation traditionally has been performed with [99m]technetium bone scintigraphy,[205] although whole-body MRI is being used increasingly for evaluation of multifocal bone lesions in persons with CRMO.[206] The diagnosis of CRMO typically is confirmed by means of a bone biopsy; with MRI guidance, a biopsy of CRMO bone lesions that are visible on MRI but are occult on radiography and CT can be performed.[207]

The three most common sites of disease at initial presentation are the lower extremities (39.7%) (Fig. 137-32 and e-Fig. 137-33), spine (25.9%), and pelvis (20.7%),[203] followed by the clavicle, the spine, the mandible (see Fig. 137-34), and pelvic bones.[208,209] In tubular bones, metaphyseal lesions are the most common, accounting for 49% of all long bone lesions.[203] When the shoulder girdle is involved, the term *sternocostoclavicular hyperostosis* is used.

The differential diagnosis of CRMO includes subacute and chronic infectious osteomyelitis, histiocytosis, hypophosphatasia, and malignancies such as leukemia, lymphoma, and Ewing sarcoma.[210] The imaging features may mimic pyogenic, chronic osteomyelitis, and ultimately, it may be necessary to perform a biopsy in clinically equivocal cases. Multifocal metaphyseal-based lesions favor a diagnosis of CRMO after pyogenic infection has been excluded. Langerhans cell histiocytosis is a less likely consideration when multifocal lesions involve the metaphysis because Langerhans cell histiocytosis tends to affect the axial skeleton or diaphysis.

CRMO of long bones can result in orthopedic complications such as bony overgrowth, angular deformities, and limb-length discrepancy.[211] Because of its tendency to occur near the physes, CRMO can cause premature physeal closure, resulting in growth arrest. The hyperemia caused by chronic inflammation may result in diffuse demineralization, predisposing to fractures.[212]

TREATMENT AND FOLLOW-UP

Suggestion of the diagnosis by a radiologist could help avoid unnecessary diagnostic procedures and antibiotic therapy and initiate an appropriate therapy.[203] Many different treatments have been used in persons with CRMO, including nonsteroidal antiinflammatory agents, corticosteroids,[213] azithromycin, tumor necrosis factor-blocker (infliximab),[214,215] and interferon.[216] Bisphosphonates have been used in persons with CRMO for pain relief, control of disease progression,[217] and when simple therapies fail to control symptoms or disease progression.[217]

ACKNOWLEDGEMENT

We would like to acknowledge the contributions of Sarah Teich, a summer student at The Hospital for Sick Children, and Nasir A. Khan, a medical student at the University of Toronto.

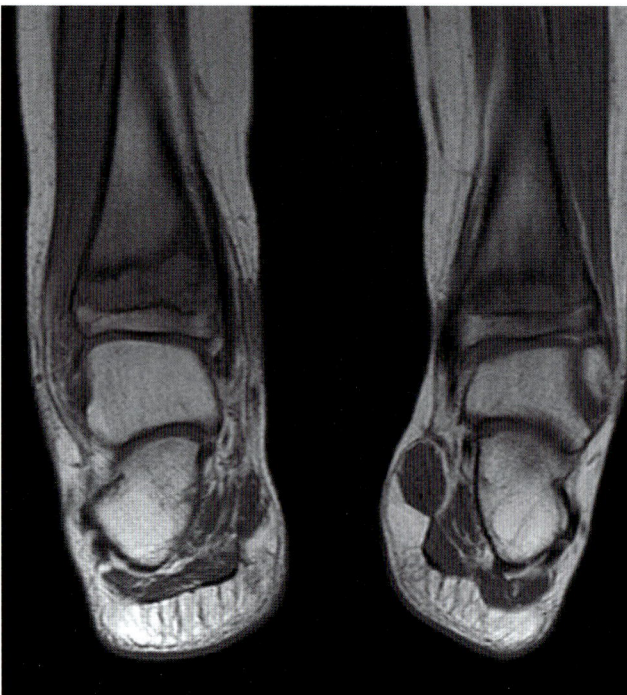

Figure 137-32 An adolescent girl with bilateral distal tibial juxtaphyseal metaphyseal widening seen on T1-weighted coronal sequences. After infection was excluded, the diagnosis of chronic recurrent multifocal osteomyelitis was established.

Key Points

Because the clinical and laboratory diagnosis of early joint changes in children with JIA is suboptimal, imaging becomes an ideal noninvasive outcome measure for early diagnosis and follow-up of joint changes. Imaging plays a key role in establishing the presence, severity, and extent of joint disease and also can help monitor for disease complications, exclude other diagnoses, and assess treatment response.

Both MRI and ultrasound can detect JIA synovial hypertrophy, cartilage erosions, and joint effusion in peripheral joints and monitor clinically meaningful response to treatment. Ultrasound is less sensitive than MRI for assessment of both soft tissue findings and superficial cartilage loss.

Radiographic findings of ERA and other spondyloarthropathies are similar to those encountered in other forms of JIA, with the exception of sacroiliitis and enthesitis, which are more specific for spondyloarthropathy.

The radiographic changes in hemophilic arthropathy may be identical to JIA, but clinical findings related to hemarthrosis and typical large joint involvement help distinguish these entities.

Pigmented villonodular synovitis is a benign proliferative disorder of uncertain etiology characterized by synovial hyperplasia that affects synovial lined joints, bursae, and tendon sheaths, having potential for extensive local destruction. The presence of hemosiderin may lend the tissue a characteristic pigmented appearance.

In juvenile dermatomyositis, the muscles of the scapular and pelvic girdles are most frequently affected, and their involvement typically is symmetrical. MRI is more sensitive than ultrasound for the detection of edema, representing inflammation, within infarcted muscles as a result of the vasculitis in the acute phase of the disease.

Chronic recurrent multifocal osteomyelitis is characterized by multifocal nonpyogenic inflammatory bone lesions, a course of exacerbations and remissions, and an association with other inflammatory disorders. If the radiographs are negative in the presence of significant clinical symptoms, further evaluation with MRI should be considered to evaluate for marrow edema.

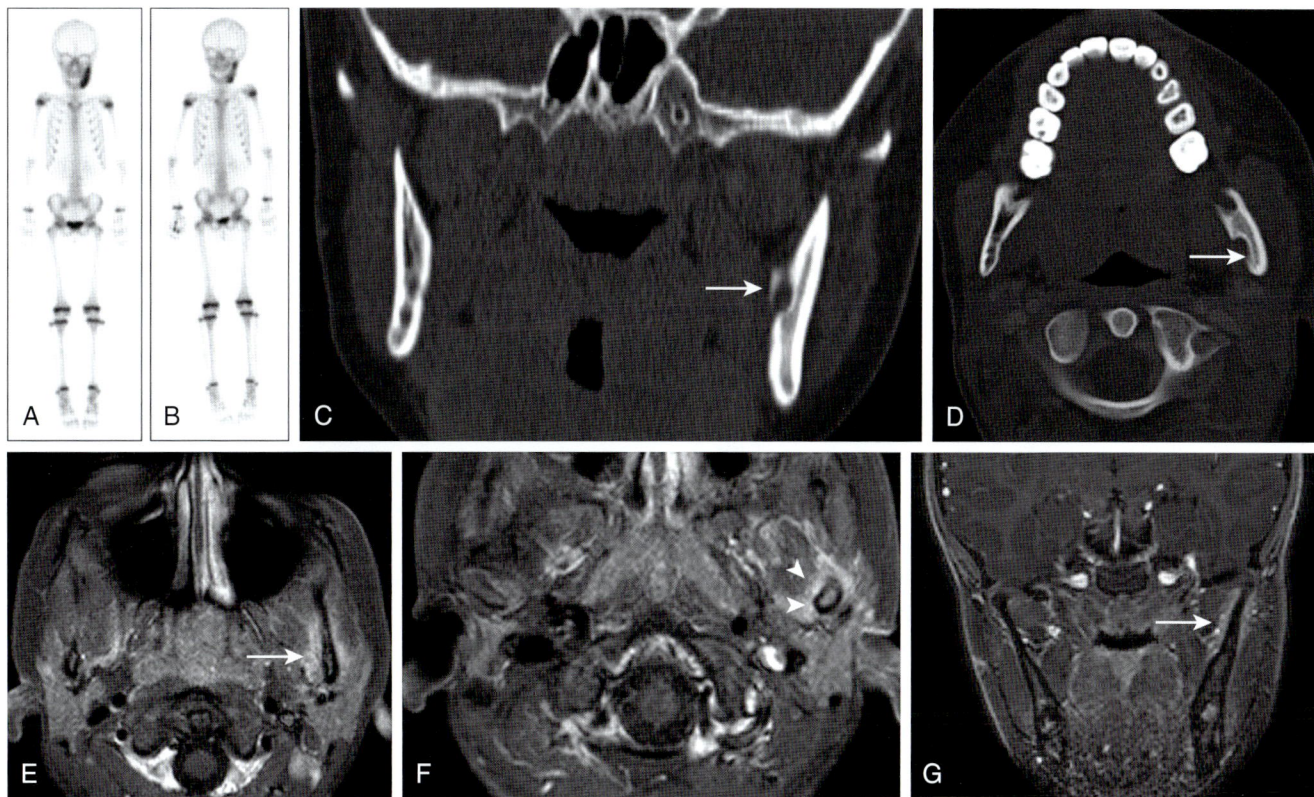

Figure 137-34 Chronic recurrent multifocal osteomyelitis. At the age of 6 years, this girl started to present with pain in the left mandible. At that time the bone scan (**A**) showed a very hyperemic focus in the left mandibular ramus. Eight months later, diffuse increased activity was still noted in the left mandible on a bone scan (**B**); however, it was less intense than in the previous study. Subsequently, the patient started treatment with pamidronate. Three years later, coronal (**C**) and axial (**D**) computed tomography (CT) scans of the mandibles showed a lytic left mandibular lesion (9 × 6 mm) posterior to an unerupted molar (*arrows*). Magnetic resonance imaging (MRI) (postcontrast axial T1-weighted turbo spin echo spectral presaturation inversion recovery (SPIR), **E** and **F**; coronal T1-weighted three-dimensional fast field echo postcontrast, **G**) performed 2 months after the CT scan confirmed the cysticlike lesion noted within the inferior aspect of the left mandibular ramus, which likely represented previous sequela from the local inflammatory process. The MRI also showed the interval development of an inflammatory process involving the bone and adjacent soft tissues in the mid and superior aspects of the left mandibular ramus (*arrows*) with associated mild reactive synovitis (*arrowheads*). Three years after the performance of the CT and MRI scans, pain started to develop in the right knee. *Continued*

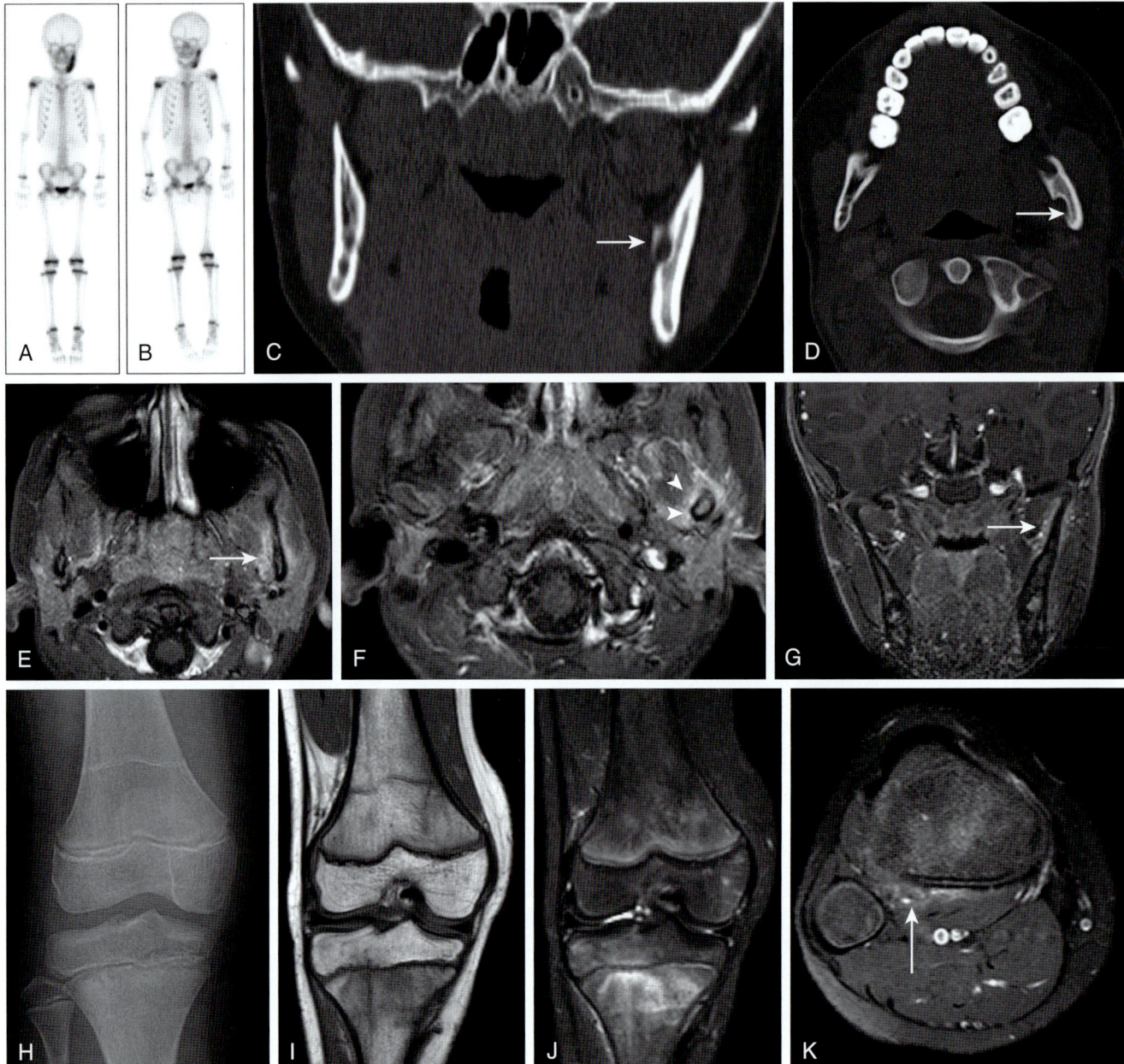

Figure 137-34, cont'd. The frontal radiograph (**H**) and MRI of the right knee (coronal T1-weighted, **I**; coronal short tau inversion recovery, **J**; and postcontrast axial T1-weighted SPIR, **K**) showed patchy bone marrow signal changes involving the right distal femoral and proximal tibial metaphysis and epiphysis with mild associated soft tissue changes adjacent to the right proximal tibia (*arrow*).

Suggested Readings

Chan WP, Liu GC. MR imaging of primary skeletal muscle diseases in children. *AJR Am J Roentgenol.* 2002;179:989-997.

Doria A, Lundin B. Imaging modalities for assessment of hemophilic arthropathy. In: Lee C, Berntorp E, Hoots K, eds. *Textbook of hemophilia.* West Sussex, UK: Wiley-Blackwell; 2009:191-199.

Khanna G, Sato TS, Ferguson P. Imaging of chronic recurrent multifocal osteomyelitis. *Radiographics.* 2009;29:1159-1177.

Miller E, Doria AS. Imaging for early assessment of peripheral joints in juvenile idiopathic arthritis. In: Santiago Medina L, Applegate K, Blackmore C, eds. *Evidence-based imaging in pediatrics: optimizing imaging in pediatric patient care.* New York, NY: Springer; 2010:219-273.

References

Full references for this chapter can be found on www.expertconsult.com.

Chapter 138

Musculoskeletal Infections

J. HERMAN KAN and E. MICHEL AZOUZ

Overview of Musculoskeletal Infections

Musculoskeletal infections remain a diagnostic and therapeutic medical challenge. Historically, the workup and treatment of such infections has been based on clinical grounds supplemented by diagnostic aspiration and subsequent surgical incision and drainage. Today, imaging plays a critical role in the diagnosis and management of musculoskeletal infections as a result of increased utilization of cross-sectional imaging.

This chapter will review the clinical presentation, pathophysiology, imaging, and treatment spectrum of osteomyelitis, septic arthritis, and soft tissue infections of the appendicular skeleton.

ACUTE PYOGENIC OSTEOMYELITIS

Etiology, Pathophysiology, and Clinical Presentation Osteomyelitis may occur from direct or hematogenous inoculation; it may be iatrogenic, related to orthopedic implants; or it may be from secondary extension from primary septic arthritis or pyomyositis. Hematogenous osteomyelitis is preponderantly a disease of children; however, infantile and even neonatal cases are not uncommon. Bacteria are the most common inflammatory agents, but growing bones may also be invaded by other pathogens, including viruses, spirochetes, and fungi.

The incidence of pediatric osteomyelitis in the United States is 1 in 5150 and has increased 2.8-fold in 20 years.[1] This increased incidence is confounded, however, because of differences in access to health care and advances in imaging diagnosis. *Staphylococcus aureus* remains the most common causative organism of acute osteomyelitis in children. Unfortunately, community-acquired methicillin-resistant *S. aureus* (MRSA) strains are increasing in prevalence.[2] *Haemophilus influenzae* osteomyelitis and septic arthritis have become less common since the availability of effective vaccination (*H. influenzae* type B vaccine).[3]

In sickle cell disease, bone complications include osteonecrosis and osteomyelitis. Osteonecrosis is approximately 50 times more frequent than osteomyelitis.[4] The proposed mechanism of osteomyelitis is hematogenous, with bacteria gaining entrance to blood vessels through ischemic bowel and finding suitable culture material in foci of infarcted bone marrow. Both *S. aureus* and *Salmonella* commonly occur in sickle cell patients.[2]

In chronic granulomatous disease of childhood, an X-linked recessive disorder of leukocyte function, repeated infections occur in solid organs, skin, and bone. Approximately one third of patients develop osteomyelitis. Phagocytes are unable to kill catalase-positive organisms such as *Staphylococcus* and *Aspergillus*.[5]

Hematogenous osteomyelitis usually involves the highly vascularized metaphysis of the fastest growing bones, such as the distal femur and radius and the proximal tibia and humerus. The most common location for hematogenous osteomyelitis is about the knee (distal femur, proximal tibia).[2] Pain, localized signs, fever, reduced range of motion, and reduced weightbearing are the most common initial clinical features. A history of trauma is seen in approximately 30% of cases,[2] and the male-to-female ratio is approximately 1.8:1.

Organisms lodge most frequently in the terminal capillary sinusoids of the metaphyses.[6] Rarely, they may locate initially in the epiphyses related to the terminal capillary sinusoids of the metaphyseal equivalent region immediately next to the spherical growth plate (Fig. 138-1). A small abscess forms in the marrow of the metaphysis, followed by local decalcification and destruction of the adjacent bone. When focal abscesses are generated, multiple small foci of bone destruction develop and later coalesce. Inflammatory swelling increases the intraosseous pressure because of the rigid bony walls of the marrow cavity; this can force extension of the infected exudate into several sites, as indicated in Figure 138-2. The most common route is via the haversian canals of the cortex to the subperiosteal space, where a subperiosteal abscess is formed. Simultaneously, spread also occurs farther within the medullary cavity. Rupture of the periosteal abscess is responsible for extension of infection into the adjacent soft tissues. Inflammation and rapidly increased intraosseous pressure may cause thrombosis of the vascular channels.

The most common location for direct inoculation osteomyelitis is the foot. Plantar puncture wounds secondary to walking on broken glass, metal (nail), or vegetable matter (thorn, toothpick) may result in infectious cellulitis, plantar fasciitis, and osteomyelitis, whether the foreign body is removed or retained. The calcaneus is often involved, and *Pseudomonas aeruginosa* is often found related to direct inoculation, usually with a history of a puncture through a shoe.[5]

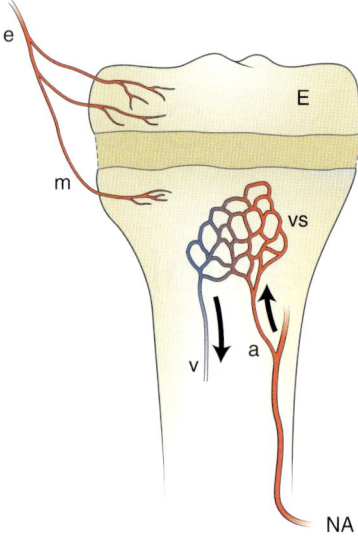

Figure 138-1 The blood supply to the metaphysis and epiphysis of a child and the arterial channels through which invading organisms enter the growing bone. An epiphyseal artery (e) supplies the epiphysis (E) and may branch to give (minor) metaphyseal vessels (m). The major blood supply of the metaphysis comes from the nutrient artery. a, arteriole; NA, nutrient artery; v. venule; vs, venous sinuses in the metaphysis.

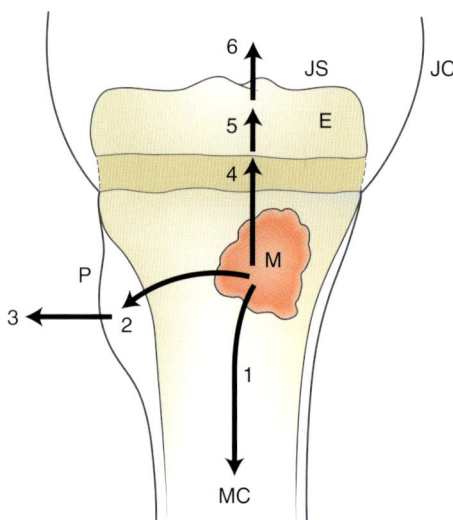

Figure 138-2 Pathways of infection after hematogeneous implantation in the metaphysis and formation of a metaphyseal focus (M) of bone infection (bone abscess). 1, spread to the medullary canal (MC); 2, formation of a subperiosteal abscess; 3, penetration of the periosteum (P) and spread to the adjacent soft tissues; 4, 5, and 6, spread across the growth plate to the epiphysis (E), and eventually to the joint space (JS). JC, joint capsule.

Imaging Imaging guidelines for the evaluation of suspected osteomyelitis include radiographs first to exclude alternative etiologies, such as a fracture or neoplasm, as an explanation for symptoms. If radiographs are normal, ultrasound (US) is recommended if the symptoms are localized to an osteoarticular region. If US is negative, scintigraphy is the next study of choice, if symptoms are nonlocalizable.[7] If symptoms can be localized, targeted magnetic resonance imaging (MRI) of the affected region should be performed both for diagnostic purposes and for planning surgical treatment.[8,9]

Radiography With acute osteomyelitis, the earliest change on radiographs is soft tissue swelling; osseous changes are seldom present until the second week of disease (Fig. 138-3).[10] The earliest bone changes seen on conventional images are one or more small radiolucencies, usually in the

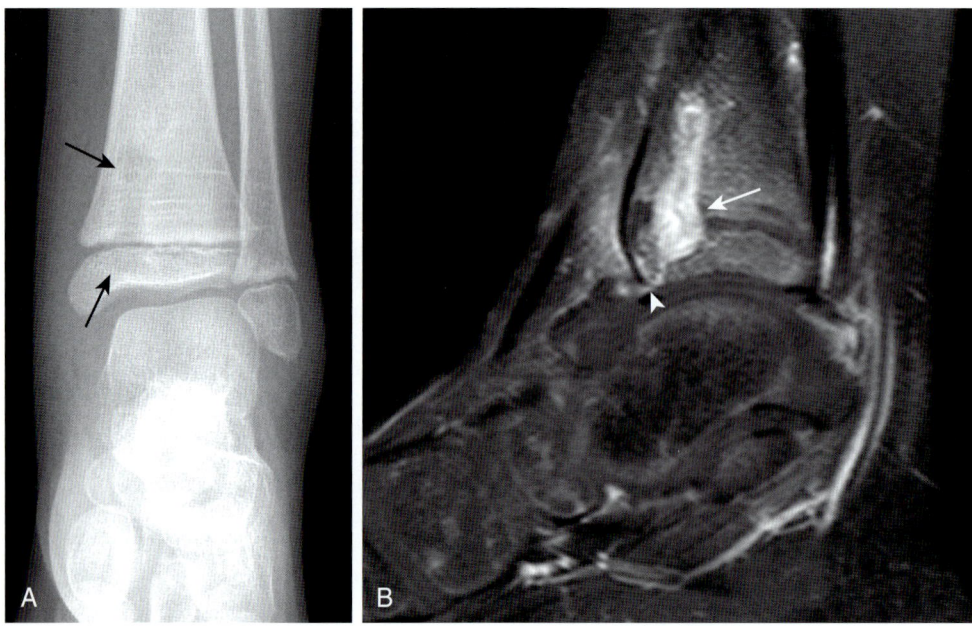

Figure 138-3 Osteomyelitis in a 6-year-old girl. **A,** Frontal radiograph demonstrates a lytic lesion in the distal tibia metaphysis extending into the epiphysis (*arrows*). **B,** T1-weighted fat-saturated post-gadolinium sagittal view demonstrates a thick, rim-enhancing lesion with a small amount of non-enhancing fluid consistent with early abscess formation with epiphyseal extension (*arrow*) and a small cloaca (*arrowhead*) extending to the tibiotalar joint.

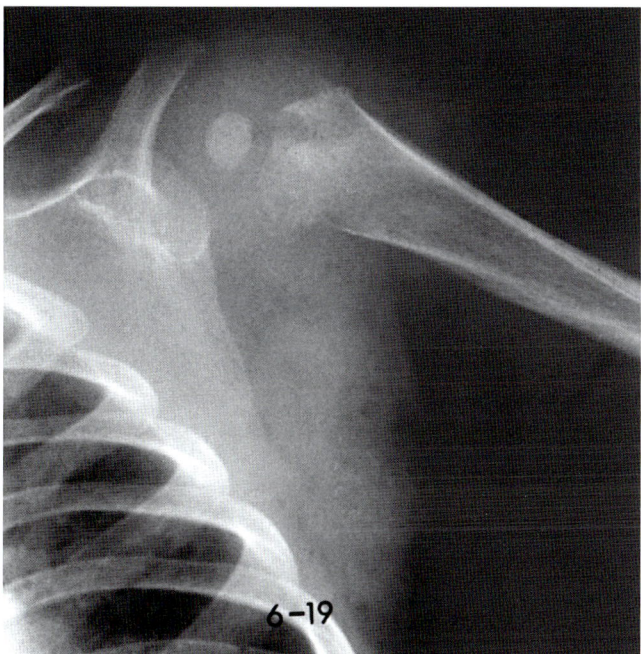

Figure 138-4 Early radiographic changes of osteomyelitis in the proximal left humeral metaphysis. This 9-month-old boy had fever and local signs and symptoms for 12 days. Metaphyseal areas of bone destruction are visualized as irregular, ill-defined lucencies.

metaphyseal region, where necrosis and destruction of bone has occurred (Fig. 138-4). On serial examinations, these areas of bone destruction enlarge and become confluent.

With continuing appropriate antibiotic therapy, periostitis is visible when the periosteum begins to produce new bone on its undersurface after the second or third week (Fig. 138-5). Osteogenic function by the periosteum suggests that infection has been at least partly locally controlled. Subsequent healing may involve remodeling of the cortical new

bone and reconstitution of the underlying bone or, if damage has been extensive, it may involve an increase in the amount of periosteal reaction to form an involucrum (Fig. 138-6), a living bone sheath around the fragments of the old devitalized bone (sequestrum).

Scintigraphy Early bone scans may demonstrate a "cold" metaphyseal lesion as a result of compression or occlusion of the metaphyseal vessels. In these cases, increased activity is observed toward the diaphysis, beyond the cold metaphyseal area, which subsequently becomes "hot" and merges with the adjacent increased activity. The multiphase bone scan is very sensitive and is usually positive 24 to 48 hours after the onset of symptoms.[7] It can detect extension of metaphyseal osteomyelitis into the epiphysis through the growth plate (Fig. 138-7).

In the early detection of acute bone infection, radionuclide imaging is more sensitive than radiographs and can identify additional foci of disease not clinically apparent. Vascular phase images done within the first 5 minutes following injection, delayed images with pinhole collimators, and special attention to the affected area have proven of great value. Osteomyelitis appears as an area of increased tracer activity that reflects the hyperemia and bone turnover induced by the infectious process. In a study of 100 children with acute limb pain, the sensitivity and specificity of three–phase bone scans for acute osteomyelitis were 84% and 97%, respectively.[11] Errors arise from simulation of infection by fracture or sickle cell disease, obscuration of osteomyelitis by septic arthritis, prior antibiotic treatment, and "cold" defects that result from ischemia. It is difficult to detect infection close to the growth plate, because both the growing physis and the nearby area of infection show increased activity.

Computed Tomography Computed tomography (CT) is of limited clinical value in acute osteomyelitis.[12] It is more useful in advanced or chronic disease to help determine the quality

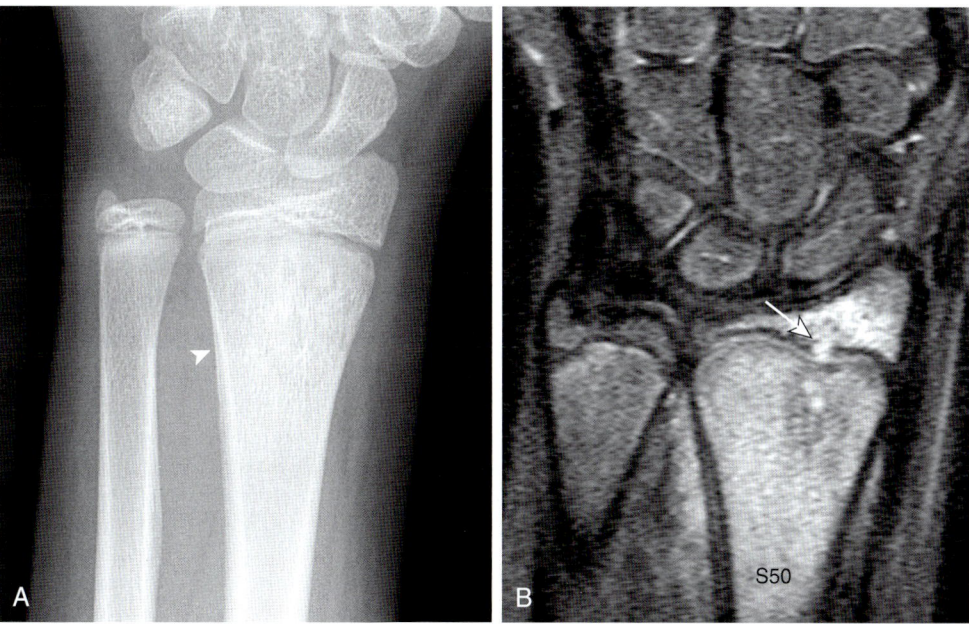

Figure 138-5 Osteomyelitis in a 12-year-old boy. **A,** Frontal radiograph demonstrates distal radial moth-eaten bone destruction with periostitis (*arrowhead*). **B,** Short tau inversion recovery coronal image demonstrates diffuse marrow edema with transphyseal extension (*arrow*) into the epiphysis.

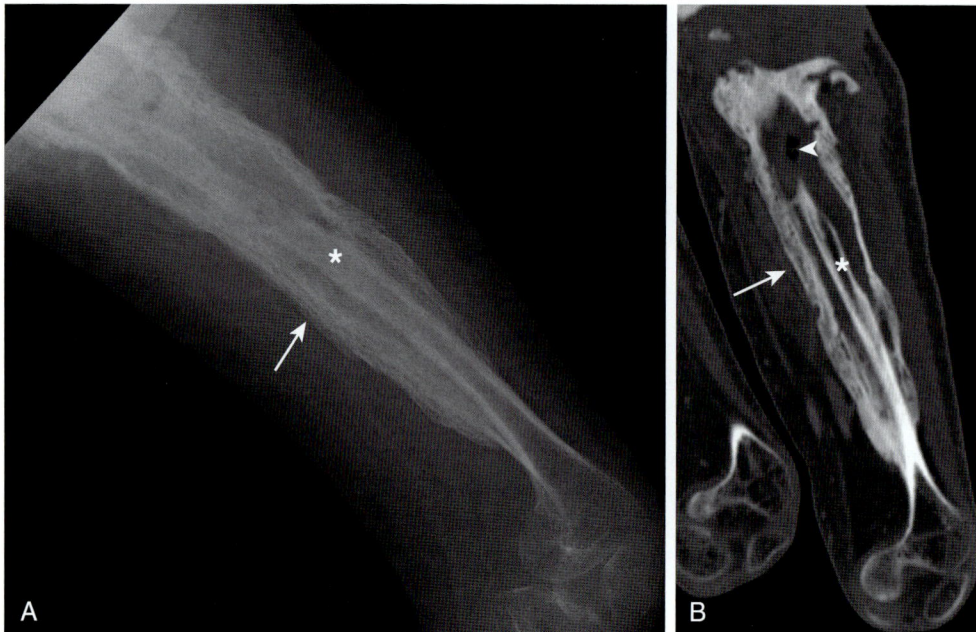

Figure 138-6 Chronic osteomyelitis of the left femur in a 17-year-old boy. Radiograph (**A**) and computed tomography scan (**B**) demonstrate involucrum (*arrow*) that surrounds sequestrum (*asterisk*). Note air within the proximal femoral diaphysis related to abscess (*arrowhead*).

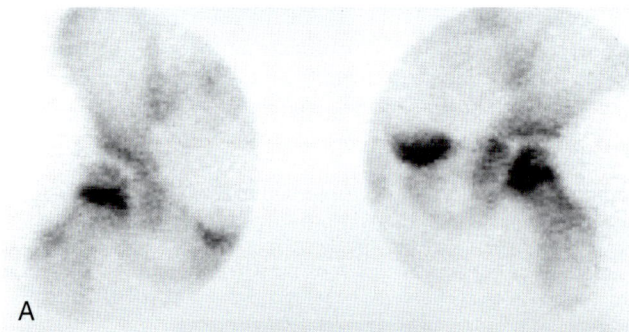

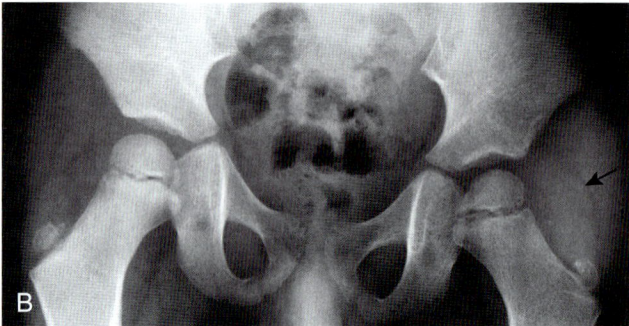

Figure 138-7 A 4-year-old boy with fever and inability to walk or move the left lower extremity for 6 days. **A,** Bone scan shows increased uptake in the femoral neck and head on the left side, likely resulting from extension of an initial metaphyseal focus of infection into the epiphysis. The right hip shows normal increased uptake in the region of the growth plate. **B,** Radiograph of the hips 2 weeks after the beginning of symptoms shows osteopenia on the left side, ill-defined medial metaphyseal and epiphyseal bone lucencies on each side of the growth plate, and indirect evidence of left hip joint effusion. Fat line (*arrow*) is displaced laterally by the joint fluid. Adjacent deep soft tissues also appear swollen and edematous compared with the normal right side.

of bone stock, including determinations of cortical destruction, involucrum, and sequestra (see Fig. 138-6).

Magnetic Resonance Imaging MRI is the optimal study to evaluate for infection and alternative etiologies for symptoms, particularly when radiographs are normal. MRI can identify early bone changes, and it delineates the anatomy and extent of marrow involvement; for this reason, it has become an important tool for imaging of suspected osseous infection. However, MRI does carry additional cost, and depending on the availability of scanner time and the need for sedation or anesthesia, delays in definitive diagnosis and treatment are possible. Imaging should aim at guiding or modifying treatment if necessary.

When precontrast MRI exams are entirely normal and show no evidence to suggest osteomyelitis, routine postgadolinium images may not be necessary.[13,14] When abnormal, MRI can reveal marrow alterations and extent of disease in bone, soft tissues, or adjacent joints (Fig. 138-8).[15] Early MRI findings of osteomyelitis may have a tumefactive appearance and may be paradoxically hypointense on fluid-sensitive sequences (e-Fig. 138-9). Over time, the lesion may remain masslike and demonstrates the expected, more homogeneous hyperintense signal on fluid-sensitive sequences, indicative of its inflammatory nature (Fig. 138-10). Eventually, periostitis and adjacent soft tissue involvement may be seen in the early phase of osteomyelitis (e-Fig. 138-11). Subperiosteal abscess formation may be seen by sonography (Fig. 138-12) or MRI (Fig. 138-13), preceding radiographic bony changes. A salt-and-pepper appearance to the marrow may be seen in the late acute phase of osteomyelitis and is presumed to represent small areas of noncoalescent microabscess formation and early bone destruction (Fig. 138-14).

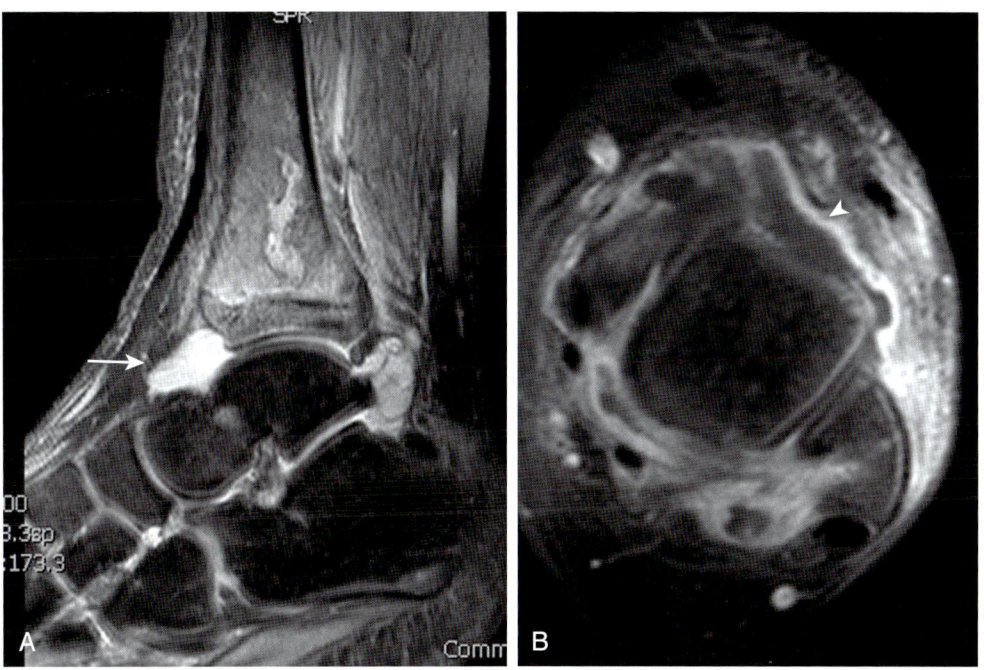

Figure 138-8 Distal tibial osteomyelitis and tibiotalar septic arthritis in an 11-year-old boy. **A,** T2-weighted fat-saturated sagittal magnetic resonance image demonstrates diffuse marrow edema that includes transphyseal extension to the epiphysis and juxtacortical soft tissue edema. A large joint effusion is present (*arrow*) with T1-weighted fat-saturated post-gadolinium axial images (**B**) that demonstrate thick synovial enhancement (*arrowhead*).

SUBACUTE AND CHRONIC OSTEOMYELITIS

Subacute or chronic osteomyelitis may develop as a result of partial host response to contain the infection. Distinguishing between subacute and chronic osteomyelitis is arbitrary.[16] The initial purulent exudate is replaced by granulation tissue, and the clinical manifestations are mild and consist mainly of local pain. A Brodie abscess may then develop, typically in the metaphysis and less commonly in the epiphysis, because the growth plate is only a partial barrier against the spread of infection. A Brodie abscess is characterized radiographically by a central or eccentric round or oval radiolucency.[17] The

cavity may contain a small, dense sequestrum. On MRI, lesions have a characteristic layered appearance with a high-signal periphery as a result of edema (penumbra sign)[18] and a double-line sign (rim sign), which on fluid-sensitive sequences is delineated as a low-signal outer rim because of sclerosis; an inner rind of intermediate signal because of granulation tissue; and a central, hyperintense region related to abscess (Fig. 138-15).[19] With contrast–enhanced imaging, the inner granulation layer will show enhancement around the nonenhancing central abscess.

Adjacent soft tissue swelling and edema and periosteal new bone formation may be present. In spite of occasional growth

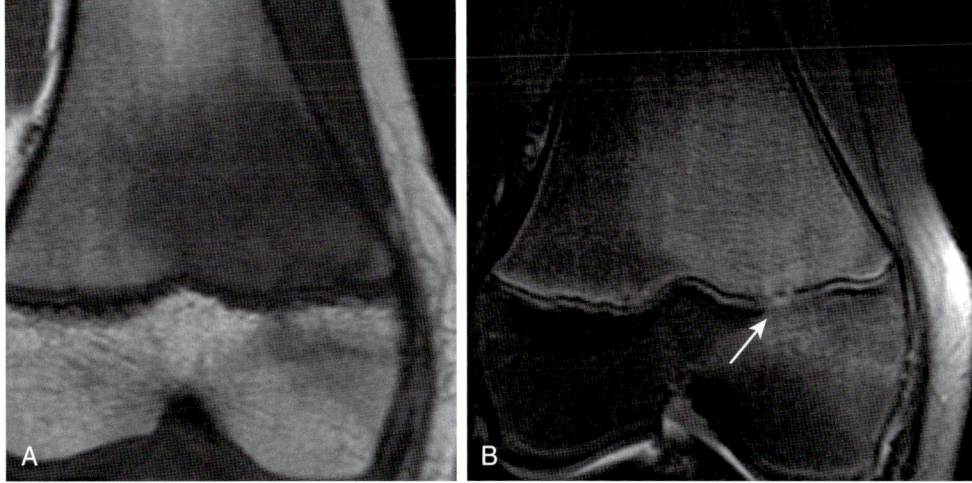

Figure 138-10 Child with biopsy-confirmed osteomyelitis of the distal femur. **A,** T1-weighted coronal magnetic resonance imaging (MRI) demonstrates tumefactive marrow replacement in the distal femur. **B,** Short tau inversion recovery coronal MRI demonstrates diffuse homogeneous hyperintensity in the same distribution with early physeal extension of infection (*arrow*).

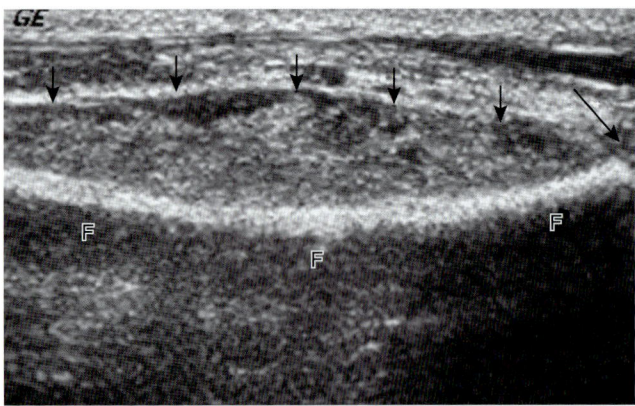

Figure 138-12 Acute osteomyelitis of the distal fibula in a 12-year-old boy. Ultrasound shows a large subperiosteal abscess (*small arrows*) and distal fibular growth plate (*long arrow*). F, fibula.

plate involvement, the incidence of premature growth plate fusion after subacute osteomyelitis is rare.[20]

Cortical and trabecular bone sclerosis, cavities, involucra, and sequestra are characteristic of advanced osteomyelitis.[21] The affected bone is thickened, and its outline may be wavy, with or without periosteal cloaking of new bone. An involucrum of reactive, viable bone may cloak an area of infection (Fig. 138-16). The involucrum may be perforated by a cloaca, which is a tract or communication between bone and the surrounding soft tissues (e-Fig. 138-17). If the cloaca extends to the skin surface, it is termed a *sinus tract* (see Fig. 138-16).[22] The necrotic, devitalized bone of a sequestrum is surrounded by inflammatory granulation tissue and may be located within a bone abscess cavity. The dead bone of a sequestrum is relatively sclerotic. Sequestra may be demonstrated on radiography, CT, or MRI, but it is best seen with CT (see Figs. 138-6 and 138-16). Sequestration is now relatively rare owing

to earlier diagnosis, largely because of advances in imaging, and more effective antibiotic therapies.

Radiographs will suggest the diagnosis of subacute or chronic osteomyelitis and may be used to follow up for gross changes. Although CT is of limited clinical value in acute osteomyelitis, it is very useful in imaging chronic disease to evaluate bone stock quality and to detect cortical metaphyseal tracts and channels, sequestra, and bone destruction. MRI will detect any reactivation or persistence of infection by showing focal active disease in the bone marrow and also showing juxtacortical soft tissue hyperemia and edema. Serial MRI after an established diagnosis of osteomyelitis has been made, and after medical or surgical treatment, has limited utility.[23]

Not all marrow edema and granulation tissue identified on MRI represents a diagnosis of osteomyelitis, therefore a combination of imaging features and clinical history should be used in concert to arrive at such a diagnosis. Stress reaction may superficially mimic early osteomyelitis, and Ewing sarcoma may superficially mimic subacute or chronic osteomyelitis, with the mass related to Ewing sarcoma mimicking granulation tissue.

Treatment Although the mortality and morbidity of bone infection have decreased significantly, permanent sequelae do occur, largely as a result of delay in diagnosis or inadequate treatment with complications related to generalized bacterial sepsis.[24] Complications of bone infection include pathologic fracture through regions of bone destruction,[25] venous thrombosis,[26] and adjacent infectious arthritis and destruction of joints (Fig. 138-18).

Identification of a bacterial pathogen for underlying osteomyelitis ranges from 9% to 22% by blood culture and 40% to 50% by bone or joint aspiration.[24] MRI is useful for confirming or excluding the diagnosis of osteomyelitis, identifying fluid for culture, and preoperative planning for

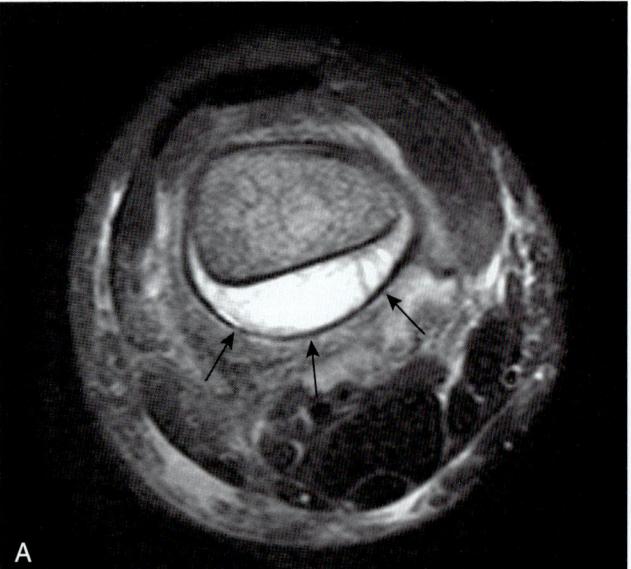
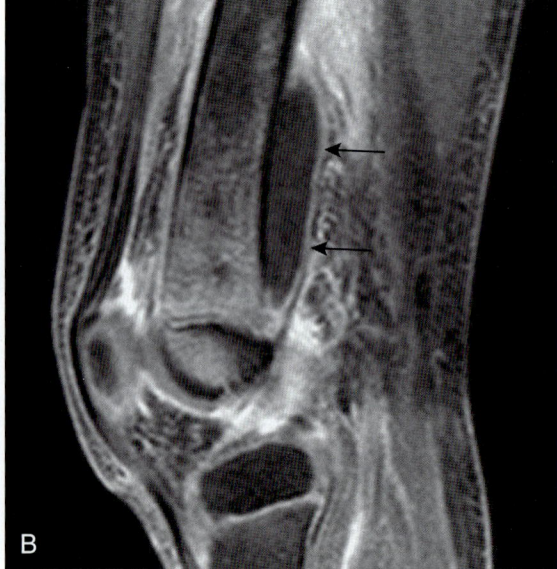

Figure 138-13 Acute osteomyelitis of the distal femur in a 5-year-old boy. **A,** T2-weighted fat-saturated axial magnetic resonance imaging (MRI) shows a large subperiosteal abscess (*arrows*) at the posterior aspect of the femur. Increased signal is seen within the bone, and there is adjacent soft tissue edema. **B,** T1-weighted fat-saturated post-gadolinium sagittal MRI shows the longitudinal extent of the subperiosteal abscess with enhancing wall (*arrows*).

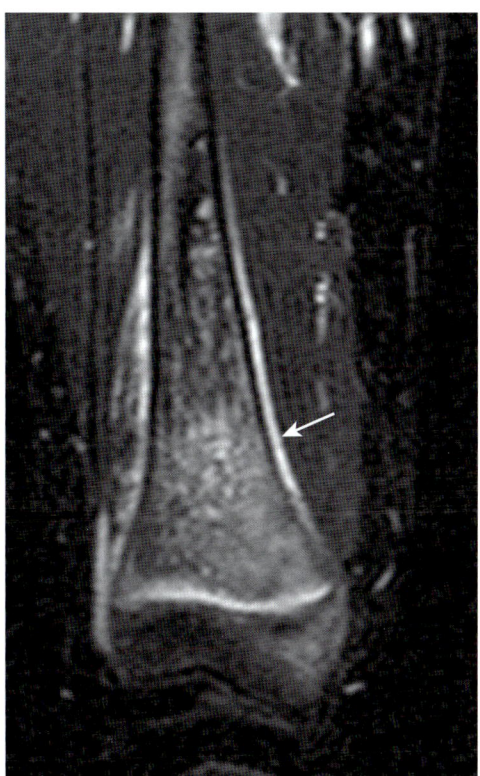

Figure 138-14 Femoral osteomyelitis in a 13-year-old girl. Short tau inversion recovery coronal magnetic resonance image demonstrates a salt-and-pepper appearance to marrow edema and periosteal reaction (*arrow*).

incision and drainage of potential intraosseous and extraosseous abscesses.[8]

To decrease the chance of complications, empiric antibiotic therapy is often initiated even before bacterial culture is isolated.[27] Treatment includes parenteral antibiotics followed by a long course of oral antibiotics, provided the child is not immunocompromised.[28]

Surgical drainage is recommended if the child has not responded to antibiotics after 48 to 72 hours, or if a substantial abscess is identified by MRI.[24] If adjacent septic arthritis is present, the joint will need to be débrided as well. Aseptic reactive effusions may occur, so not all adjacent joint effusions near an area of osteomyelitis should be categorically diagnosed as secondary septic arthritis. Sequestrae are foci for continued infection, and their detection and localization are crucial in view of surgical excision.[24]

NEONATAL OSTEOMYELITIS

Etiology, Pathophysiology, and Clinical Presentation In the neonatal period, the incidence of epiphyseal and joint involvement is higher, and multifocal disease may be seen.[29] This is because of the persistence of metaphyseal vessels that cross the physis and extend into the intraarticularly located epiphysis. Also, osteomyelitis is often indolent in onset or is masked by other medical conditions. Risk factors include prematurity and vascular catheter-related sepsis.[30] The most common causative organism is *S. aureus*. Other isolated organisms include *Escherichia coli*, group B streptococci, Gram-negative rods, and *Candida albicans*.[29] The hip is frequently involved,[31] and neonatal calcaneal osteomyelitis may develop after heel pad puncture for blood drawing.[32]

Imaging Bone scan is very helpful for early diagnosis, particularly if symptoms and clinical findings are nonlocalizable.[7] The bone scan will be positive several days before radiographic findings become manifest (~ 2 weeks). The initial radiographic findings may be soft tissue swelling with bone rarefaction and destruction seen later. Because of the high incidence of coexisting septic arthritis related to neonatal osteomyelitis, US of the adjacent joint may be performed to identify effusion. MRI may better delineate early epiphyseal cartilage involvement (Fig. 138-19).[33] Complications related to neonatal osteomyelitis include premature physeal fusion, epiphyseal osteonecrosis, joint dislocation, and joint arthrodesis.[29]

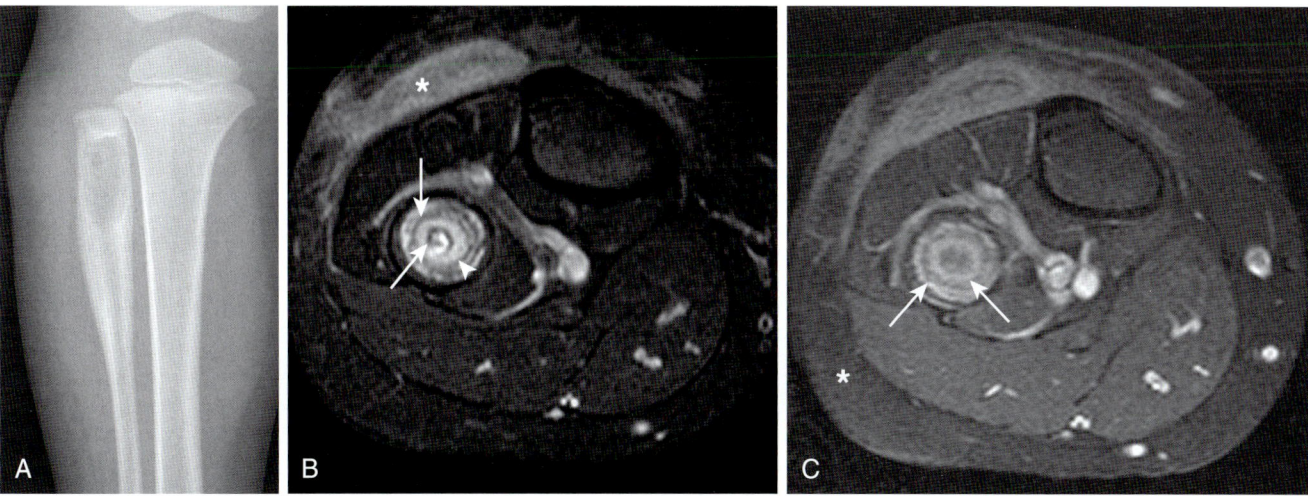

Figure 138-15 Brodie abscess in a 3-year-old boy. **A,** Radiograph demonstrates a lytic lesion in the proximal fibula with laminated thick periostitis. T2-weighted fat-saturated axial (**B**) and T1-weighted fat-saturated post-gadolinium axial (**C**) magnetic resonance images demonstrate a Brodie abscess with sclerotic outer rim (*asterisk*) and inner granulation tissue with enhancement (*arrowhead*). Note the nonenhancing central abscess, which contains a small sequestrum (*arrows*) that is only seen on the T2-weighted fat-saturated sequence.

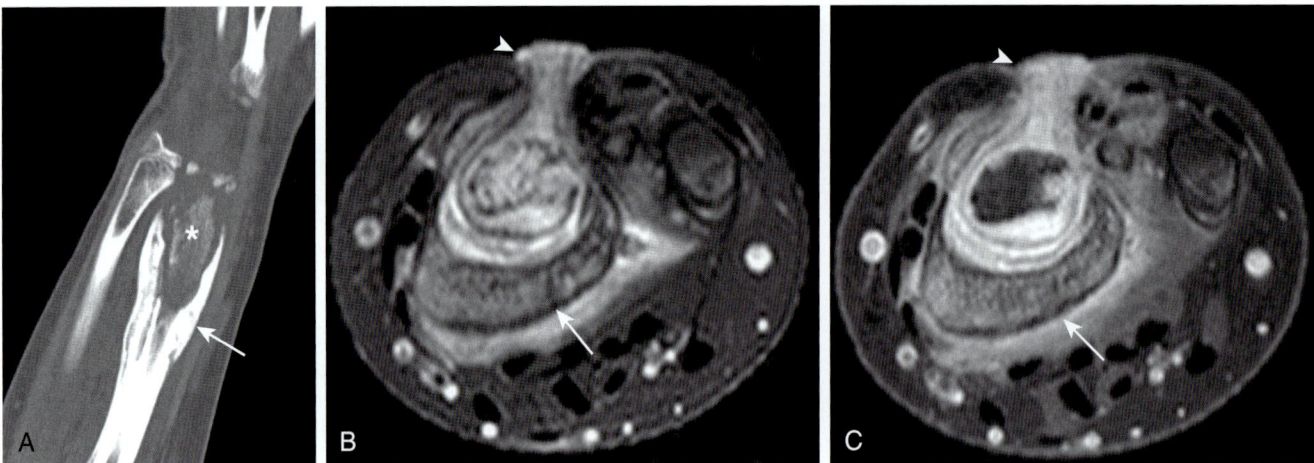

Figure 138-16 Chronic osteomyelitis of the distal radius in a 13-year-old girl. **A,** Computed tomographic coronal reformat shows involucrum (*arrow*) surrounding sequestrum (*asterisk*). T2-weighted fat-saturated axial (**B**) and T1-weighted fat-saturated axial (**C**) post-gadolinium magnetic resonance image shows involucrum (*arrow*) that surrounds the nonenhancing sequestrum. Note granulation along the sinus tract that extends from the radial metaphysis sequestrum and abscess to the skin surface (*arrowhead*).

EPIPHYSEAL OSTEOMYELITIS

Etiology, Pathophysiology, and Clinical Presentation In tubular bones, the early changes of pyogenic hematogenous osteomyelitis are usually localized to the metaphysis, where capillary vascularization is very rich, and blood flow is slow on the venous side of the sinusoidal loops. Infection may spread from the metaphysis through the growth plate to the epiphysis (see Fig. 138-2).[12] Epiphyseal osteomyelitis and septic arthritis occur more commonly in infants younger than 15 months of age, because metaphyseal vessels penetrate the growth plate and enter the epiphysis.[34]

Imaging Radiography usually demonstrates a focus of epiphyseal bone destruction (Fig. 138-20, *A*). In subacute and chronic cases, a small round or oval epiphyseal abscess cavity with well-defined borders is seen. CT is useful for imaging of the bone cavity and detection of a sequestrum. MRI reveals the epiphyseal focus of infection as low signal on T1-weighted images and high signal on T2-weighted images (Fig. 138-20, *B*). Imaging after gadolinium injection may show rim enhancement outlining the abscess cavity of the epiphyseal ossification center. Browne et al showed epiphyseal cartilage involvement was seen in 52% of cases of *S. aureus* infections in children under 18 months of age.[33] Enhancement defects in the epiphyseal cartilage are commonly seen in the setting of osteomyelitis, but they do not routinely reflect true epiphyseal cartilage abscesses (see Fig. 138-19); only one fifth to one third represent true epiphyseal cartilage abscesses.[34] The importance of identifying epiphyseal cartilage involvement is both to determine underlying epiphyseal abscess formation and to provide prognostic information related to growth disturbance of the spherical growth plate of the epiphysis.

The differential diagnosis of an epiphyseal (or apophyseal) lucent lesion in a child is infection and chondroblastoma.

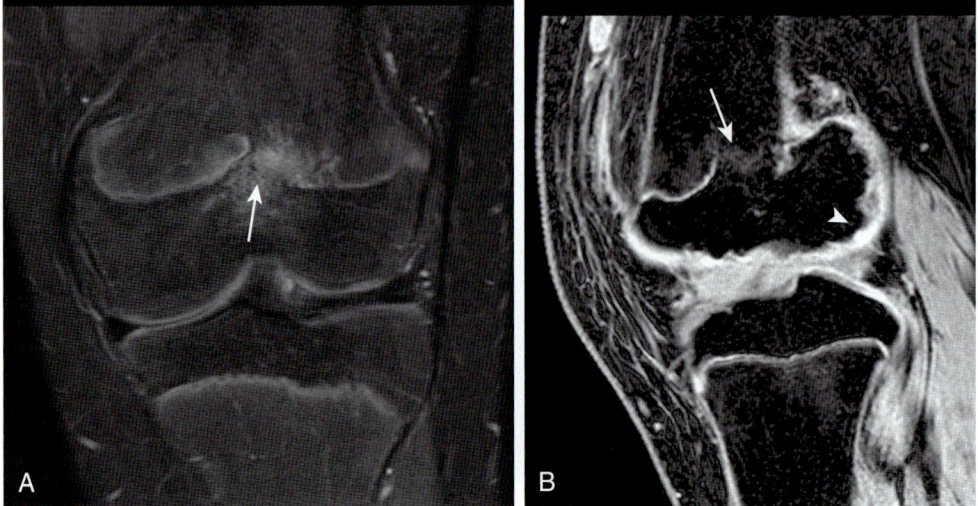

Figure 138-18 A 14-year-old boy with a remote history of distal femoral osteomyelitis and septic arthritis. Physeal bar (*arrows*) and femoral condylar epiphyseal irregularity (*arrowhead*) are seen on T2-weighted fat-saturated coronal (**A**) and gradient recalled echo sagittal (**B**) magnetic resonance image.

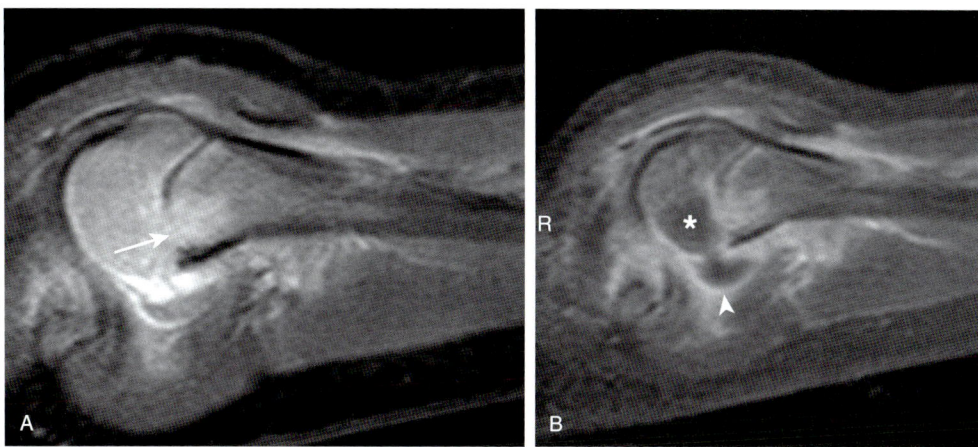

Figure 138-19 Acute proximal humeral osteomyelitis and septic arthritis in a 3-year-old boy. **A,** Short tau inversion recovery sagittal magnetic resonance imaging (MRI) demonstrates proximal metaphyseal edema with physeal involvement (*arrow*). **B,** T1-weighted post-gadolinium sagittal MRI demonstrates glenohumeral effusion with synovial enhancement (*arrowhead*) and nonenhancing humeral epiphyseal cartilage, consistent with chondral involvement (*asterisk*).

Treatment Epiphyseal osteomyelitis may lead to growth disturbance of the epiphyseal ossification center and physis.[33] Early osteoarthritis may also occur with epiphyseal and articular cartilage destruction. Because the epiphysis is an intraarticular structure, coexisting septic arthritis may often be present. Surgically, these children will require exploration and débridement of both the epiphyseal bone and joint space, when those are involved, based on preoperative MRI. Care should be made to differentiate epiphyseal cartilage enhancement defects from true epiphyseal abscesses.[34]

FUNGAL OSTEOMYELITIS

Fungal infections of bone are becoming more common as the immunosuppressed population increases. *Aspergillus,* *Candida, Histoplasma, Blastomyces,* and other pathogens have been implicated. The radiographic changes are similar to those of chronic pyogenic osteomyelitis or tuberculosis (TB): destruction of bone and periosteal reaction with areas of cortical thickening and trabecular sclerosis. Fungal osteomyelitis may be multicencentric, masslike, and may superficially mimic osteonecrosis.[31,35,36]

TUBERCULOUS OSTEOMYELITIS

Etiology, Pathophysiology, and Clinical Presentation Although osseous TB is a relatively rare condition today, cases are still encountered that are not diagnosed until an extensive, and expensive, workup has been completed. Hematogenous metastases of tubercle bacilli to the skeleton may take place

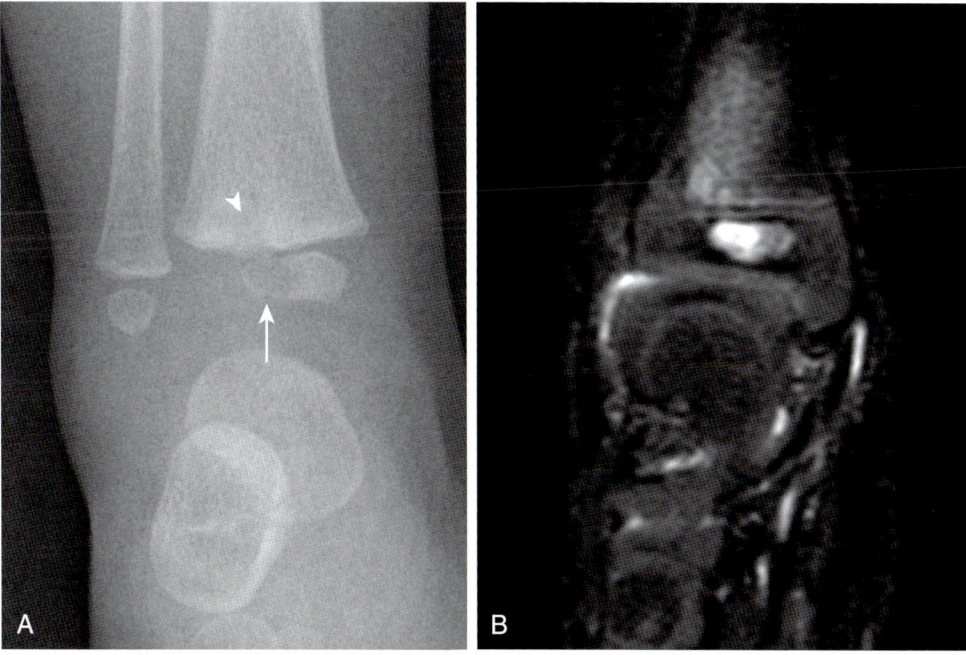

Figure 138-20 Epiphyseal osteomyelitis in a 1-year-old girl. **A,** Radiograph demonstrates epiphyseolysis (*arrow*) and metaphyseal destruction (*arrowhead*). **B,** Short tau inversion recovery coronal magnetic resonance image demonstrates epiphyseal bone abscess and metaphyseal edema.

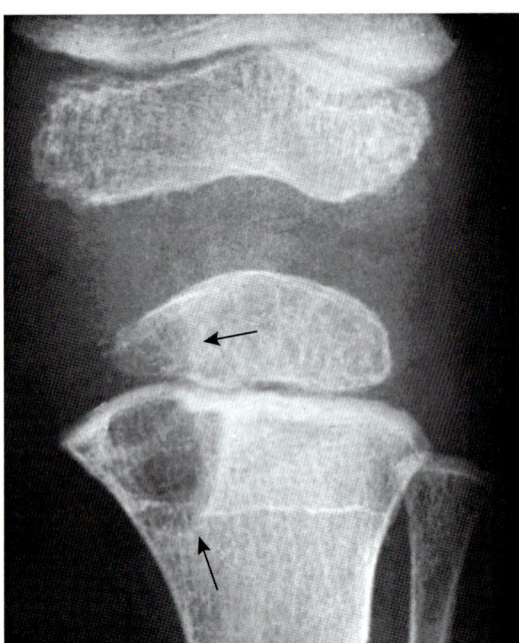

Figure 138-21 Tuberculous metaphysitis and epiphysitis of the tibia and arthritis of the knee in a 3-year-old boy. Large areas of destruction are present in the medial aspects of the metaphysis and the epiphyseal ossification center (*arrows*).

early during the active phase of the primary complex in the thorax or later from postprimary tuberculous foci. Musculoskeletal involvement of TB is seen in approximately 10% to 15% of all TB cases.[37] After implantation in the bone, an immediate active inflammatory reaction may develop, or the bacilli may be dormant for years until activated by local factors, such as trauma to the bone or joint. The synovial surface may be infected before the bones are involved; the infection may then spread from the joint into the contiguous epiphysis and metaphysis. In a large South African experience, the distribution of childhood skeletal TB is 60% to 70% vertebral, 20% to 25% large joints, and 10% to 15% tubular and flat bones.[38]

Imaging   TB produces a chronic inflammatory reaction in the bones that is similar in its macroscopic aspects to chronic pyogenic osteomyelitis. Local necrosis of the intraosseous tissues develops at the site of implantation and is then followed by regional decalcification and bone destruction. Spread of infection takes place through the same pathways as those described in the pathogenesis of pyogenic osteomyelitis. During infancy and early childhood, when the epiphyseal cartilages are relatively thick, direct transfer of the infection from the joint to the bone, or infection across joints, is uncommon. The articular cartilages are preserved longer in tuberculous osteomyelitis and arthritis than in pyogenic arthritis because of the lack of a destructive proteolytic enzyme in tuberculous exudates.[39] Sinus formation and cold abscesses are common; involucrum formation and sequestration are rare.

The radiographic findings also are similar to those of chronic pyogenic osteomyelitis, so that TB should be added regularly to the differential diagnosis of focal bone disease. Unlike pyogenic osteomyelitis, radiographs are usually

abnormal at the initial clinical presentation of tuberculous osteomyelitis.[37]

Certain imaging features can suggest the diagnosis of TB. In the metaphyses and epiphyses, destruction of bone is more prominent than production of bone (Fig. 138-21).[39] The joint space is characteristically preserved in the early phases of tuberculous arthritis. The epiphysis is a site of predilection in primary skeletal TB. In the diaphyses of tubular bones, long segments may exhibit destructive and productive changes, whereas metaphyseal regions are unaffected (e-Fig. 138-22). Sometimes, sharply defined rarefactions are present that gave rise to the term *cystic TB* of bone. In the short bones of the hands and feet, tuberculous lesions may cause bone expansion, so-called spina ventosa (Fig. 138-23). Skeletal TB may affect multiple sites, and a bone scan is recommended to detect the presence of quiescent lesions. MRI is useful in certain cases and clearly demonstrates the full extent of the bone marrow, subperiosteal, and soft tissue involvement as well as any extension into the adjacent joint.

Growth disturbances of bones infected with TB are common and may result from partial destruction and premature fusion of growth plates. Disuse osteopenia is a constant feature of the bones when movement has been limited for more than a few weeks. Limitation of movement may contribute to the occasional premature fusion of the growth plates on both sides of a joint with subsequent limb shortening.

When multifocal at presentation, TB (osteitis cystica tuberculosa multiplex) and fungal infections may superficially mimic metastatic disease.

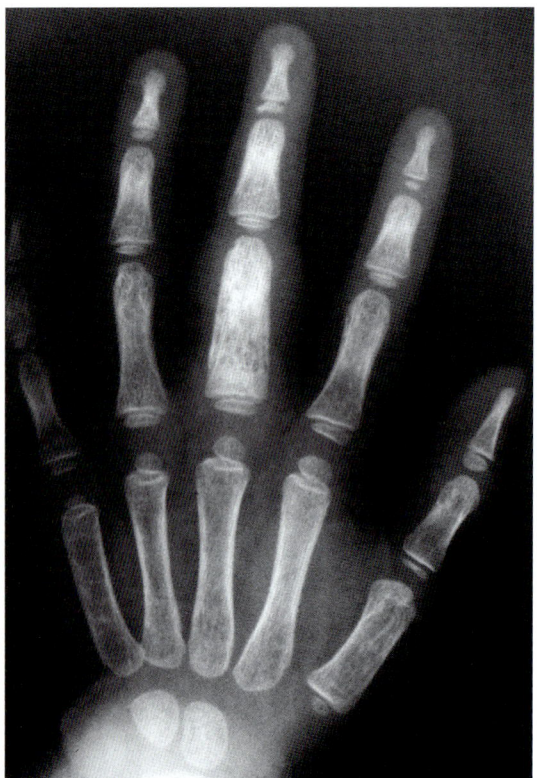

Figure 138-23 Tuberculous dactylitis (spina ventosa) in the proximal phalanx of the third finger in a 2-year-old girl. The whole diaphysis is involved, but the epiphysis is spared. Expansion of the rest of the phalanx shows mixed areas of bone destruction and sclerosis.

Treatment The standard treatment for TB is multidrug therapy inclusive of isoniazid, rifampin, pyrazinamide, and ethambutol for a minimum of 6 to 9 months.[37] Extrapulmonary TB treatment is longer (12 to 18 months) because of relatively poor osseous and fibrous tissue penetration.

CONGENITAL SYPHILIS

Etiology, Pathophysiology, and Clinical Presentation Congenital syphilis (*Treponema pallidum*) causes hepatosplenomegaly, lymphadenopathy, skin rash, and anemia.[40] Bones are often involved, but this may not become clinically or radiologically manifest in the first weeks of life. Bone pain in one or more extremities may be severe and may result in lack of movement of those extremities, a condition termed *Parrot pseudoparalysis*. Syphilis of bone can be suggested on the basis of radiologic signs, when it has not been considered on clinical grounds. The diagnosis, however, still rests on appropriate serologic tests. Two main forms are observed, infantile and juvenile, and their radiographic features are different.

Imaging The unique imaging characteristic of *infantile syphilis* is multiple bone involvement with almost selective localization in the metaphyses. Broad bands of metaphyseal radiolucency were considered evidence of "metaphysitis" but are now known to be nonspecific responses to the stress of disseminated infection.[41] Syphilitic granulation tissue can, however, occur in these regions (e-Fig. 138-24). Radiographically, the two causes cannot be distinguished, but when associated with metaphyseal serration, the so-called sawtooth metaphysis (Fig. 138-25), the diagnosis of congenital syphilis is practically assured. Similar diagnostic

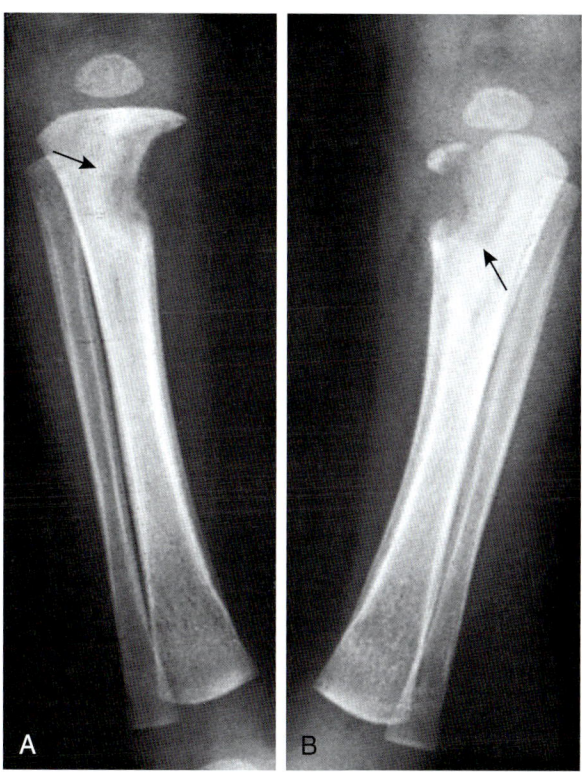

Figure 138-26 Bilateral, symmetric, destructive syphilitic metaphysitis of the proximal ends of the tibias (Wimberger sign) in a 2-month-old infant. Large areas of destruction of the spongiosa and overlying cortex are seen at the medial aspects of the tibias (*arrows*). In the left tibia, the medial segment of the epiphyseal plate is partially destroyed. Note also diffuse periosteal thickening of the diaphyses.

"specificity" is provided by the Wimberger sign after the newborn period, when destructive foci are found in the metaphyseal regions of tubular bones, particularly the medial tibial metaphyses at the knee (Fig. 138-26). Metaphyseal destructive lytic lesions may lead to pathologic fractures, and child abuse is in the differential diagnosis.[42] Although metaphyseal lesions are characteristic of congenital syphilis, they are not pathognomonic and may be seen with ordinary osteomyelitis, hyperparathyroidism, skeletal infantile myofibromatosis, and metastases. Diaphyseal involvement, especially with periosteal new bone formation, also tends to occur after the first month and may be associated with some destructive foci and even scattered focal cortical destruction and expansion of the medullary cavity (e-Fig. 138-27). The epiphyses are generally spared. Healing of the bone lesions in the infantile form of the disease occurs with or without therapy, usually without deformity.

Juvenile syphilis is observed radiographically in childhood and is manifested by diffuse or localized subperiosteal thickening of the cortex (Fig. 138-28). Associated focal destructive lesions, resembling cystic TB, occasionally are present. Thickening of the anterior cortex of the tibia is responsible for the "saber shin" deformity of congenital syphilis that appears in late childhood.[43]

SEPTIC ARTHRITIS

Etiology, Pathophysiology, and Clinical Presentation The annual per capita incidence of septic arthritis in a study based

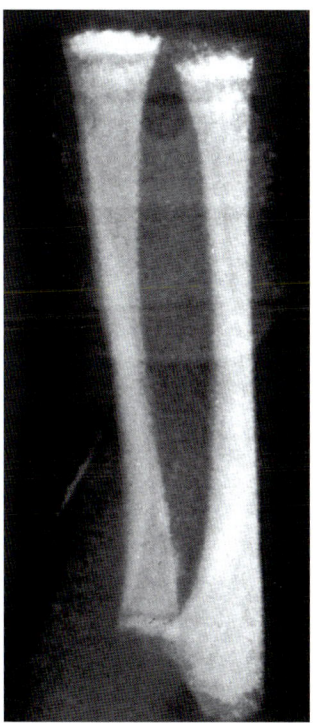

Figure 138-25 Newborn infant with congenital syphilis and sawtooth metaphysis. This patient had a rash and mucocutaneous lesions characteristic of the disease.

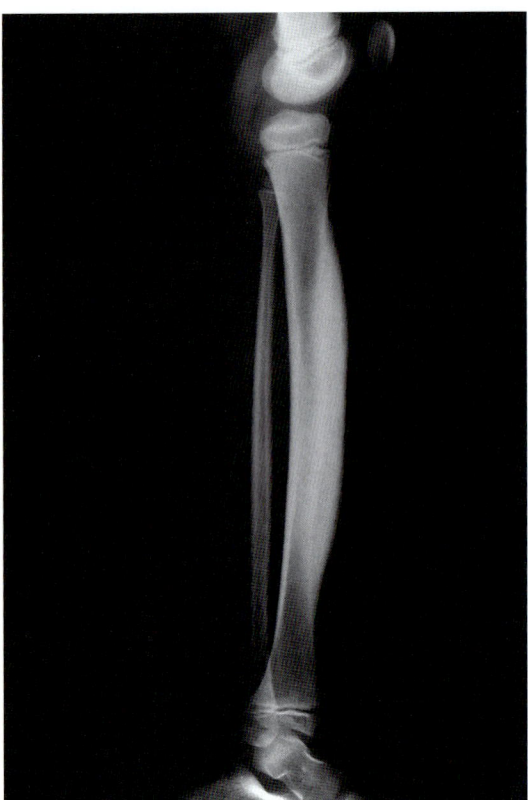

Figure 138-28 An 8-year-old boy with saber shin as a result of congenital syphilis. Lateral view of the leg shows extensive anterior cortical and periosteal thickening of the tibial diaphysis.

rule out an obvious alternative cause for symptoms, such as an underlying fracture. The initial findings may be nonspecific soft tissue swelling about a joint. In certain joints—such as the elbow, knee, and ankle—a joint effusion may be seen and is best delineated on a lateral radiograph.

The role of US is to identify the presence or absence of an underlying joint effusion or to determine whether pathology is intraarticular or extraarticular, such as adjacent tenosynovitis.[46,47] When a joint effusion is present, no sonographic features are evident that predict the presence or absence of septic arthritis.[48-50] Capsular distension with anechoic or hypoechoic fluid is usually seen. Debris and septations within the joint, as well as hyperemic flow in the synovium, can be seen on power Doppler; but this can also be seen in JIA, transient synovitis,[50] and posttraumatic arthritis (Fig. 138-29).

The MRI findings of isolated septic arthritis are also nonspecific.[51,52] Synovial thickening, enhancement, effusions, and juxtasynovial soft tissue edema may be seen, but this is indistinguishable from transient synovitis and JIA. The role of MRI is not to diagnose septic arthritis but to identify the presence or absence of coexisting osteomyelitis (see Fig. 138-8), epiphyseal cartilage involvement (e-Fig. 138-30), and juxtasynovial muscle inflammation (Fig. 138-31) or abscesses, because this will affect medical and surgical management.

in the United States is approximately 1 in 93,500.[1] *S. aureus* is the most commonly isolated organism, the majority of which are MRSA. The knee is most commonly affected (41.4%) followed by the hip (22.6%) and ankle (13.6%).

Bacterial entry into the joint can occur by two mechanisms: direct inoculation from a penetrating injury and hematogenous inoculation. The vascular synovium may be hematogenously inoculated.[12] Alternatively, inoculation may occur secondarily by way of osteomyelitis. This may occur with higher frequency in infants when transphyseal vessels extend from the metaphysis to the intraarticular epiphysis.[44]

Septic arthritis causes rapid cartilage loss and joint destruction and therefore is a medical and surgical emergency. Diagnosis is based on clinical grounds and laboratory data. A history of fever, non-weightbearing, an erythrocyte sedimentation rate above 40 mm/hour, and a white blood cell count greater than 12,000 cells/mm^3 are four consistent variables that occur frequently in the setting of septic arthritis as extensively studied in the hip.[45] When present in isolation, each of these individual variables has low accuracy for the diagnosis of septic arthritis, but when three or more of these variables are present at the same time, the chance of a positive diagnosis of septic arthritis of the hip is greater than 93%.[45]

Many nonbacterial entities may mimic septic arthritis; these include transient synovitis, juvenile idiopathic arthritis (JIA), Lyme arthritis, posttraumatic arthritis, and epiphyseal osteonecrosis.

Imaging Radiography is the first line of imaging in the setting of suspected septic arthritis. Radiographs are used to

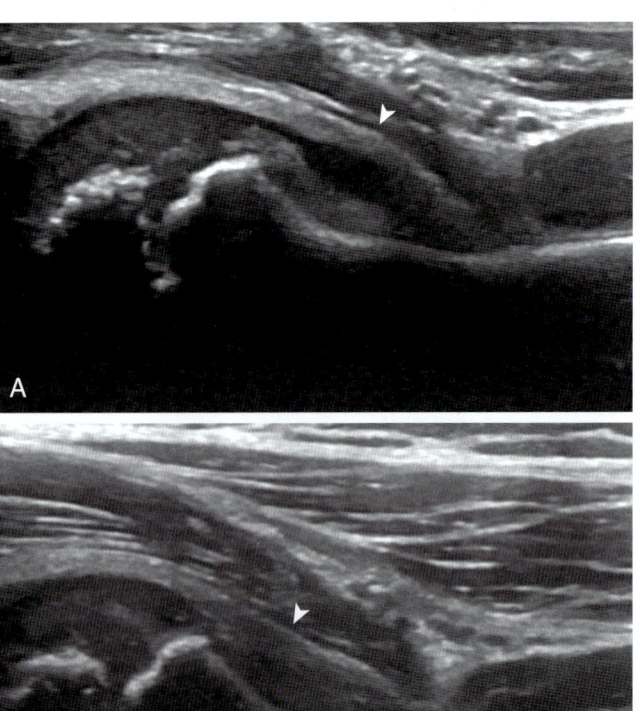

Figure 138-29 Transient synovitis of the hip in a 1-year-old girl. **A,** Longitudinal imaging of the symptomatic right hip shows capsular distension (*arrowhead*) because of a large effusion. **B,** Imaging of the asymptomatic left hip shows a normal amount of hip fluid; note the capsule (*arrowhead*).

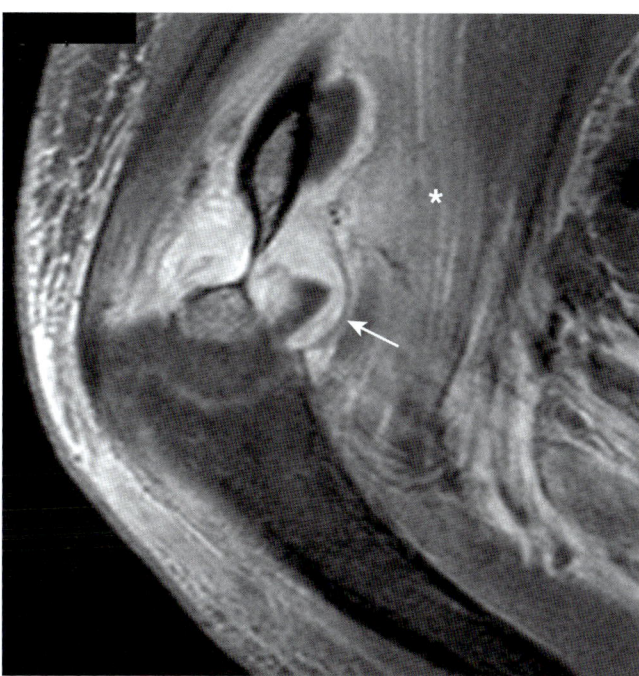

Figure 138-31 Elbow septic arthritis and distal humeral osteomyelitis in an 11-year-old boy. T1-weighted fat-saturated post-gadolinium sagittal magnetic resonance image demonstrates thick synovial enhancement (*arrow*) and juxtasynovial myositis (*asterisk*). Marrow edema is also seen in the distal humerus.

Treatment US may be used to both identify the presence or absence of a joint effusion and to provide needle guidance for diagnostic joint aspiration.[47] Emergent arthrotomy and washout is recommended to prevent complications of septic arthritis. If septic arthritis is a complicating feature of osteomyelitis, the underlying bone should also be débrided. Complications of septic arthritis include sepsis, chondrolysis, and osteonecrosis.[53] Antibiotic treatment is similar to the treatment of osteomyelitis at all ages: a total of 4 to 6 weeks of therapy.[51]

PYOMYOSITIS

Etiology, Pathophysiology, and Clinical Presentation Pyomyositis is a localized primary infection of muscle characterized by progression to abscess formation that can mimic tumor, trauma (hematoma), osteomyelitis, septic arthritis, cellulitis, or thrombophlebitis. This disorder is endemic in Africa, South America, southeastern Asia, and the South Pacific; it is increasingly reported in temperate climates, including the northern United States. Pyomyositis occurs in otherwise healthy children and in those predisposed to infection by debilitating diseases, including human immunodeficiency virus infection. *S. aureus* is the most commonly identified organism; it is isolated in 45% of cases in a U.S.-based study, followed by group A β-hemolytic streptococci (GABHS; 10%).[1] GABHS infections may occur in the setting of *Varicella* infection,[55] and multifocal pyomyositis may be seen as a complication of bacterial endocarditis. Secondary pyomyositis may also occur as the result of extension from adjacent osteomyelitis, particularly in the pelvis. Damaged muscle with some degree of underlying immune suppression and a source of bacteremia are the key predisposing elements.

Clinically, the gluteal muscles, thighs, and calves are more commonly affected than the upper extremities, trunk, and chest wall.[56] Approximately 25% of patients have a history of antecedent trauma. Usually, only a single muscle is involved. Early in the course of illness, patients experience low-grade fevers, general malaise, and dull, cramping pain.[57] The involved area lacks the cutaneous erythema usually evident with cellulitis, and it has a "woody" nonfluctuant feel. Fever usually occurs as infection advances. Infections of the pelvic musculature may clinically mimic osteomyelitis or septic arthritis by producing hip or groin pain. Infection of the piriformis muscle may irritate the adjacent sciatic nerve and produce pain that extends into the ipsilateral lower extremity.[58] Pyomyositis is usually accompanied by elevations in white blood cell count, erythrocyte sedimentation rate, and C-reactive protein level.

Imaging Early in the development of pyomyositis, the affected muscle is enlarged and edematous without a frank abscess. Without treatment, the process progresses to form an intramuscular abscess. US may be helpful in localizing relatively superficial sites of pyomyositis (Fig. 138-32).[59] Infections at deeper sites and infections that have not yet formed an intramuscular abscess are less readily detected with US. Although CT is not the imaging modality of choice, most intramuscular abscesses are readily seen at all locations. CT findings indicative of abscess include enlargement of the involved muscle, central low-attenuation fluid collection, and a peripheral rim that enhances with contrast (e-Fig. 138-33).[60]

MRI is the preferred modality for imaging of suspected pyomyositis in children, and it is particularly valuable in cases of pelvic involvement.[61] On MRI, the involved muscle appears enlarged and edematous with increased signal on T2-weighted and inversion recovery sequences. On T1-weighted images, the signal intensity of some abscesses is homogeneously greater than that of the involved muscle. On T2-weighted images, the abscess is seen as high signal with a hypointense rim and less well-defined hyperintensity of the adjacent muscle (Fig. 138-34). Post-gadolinium T1-weighted images best reveal the abscess, and the abscess wall densely enhances (see Fig. 138-32). Changes may result from associated cellulitis and include skin thickening, stranding of subcutaneous fat, and swelling of fascial planes; these findings are best seen on fat-saturated T2-weighted and inversion recovery images. A sympathetic effusion may be present if infection is near a joint. Often, the chief clinical differential diagnosis is osteomyelitis. In pyomyositis, underlying bones usually appear normal, and the process is displaced or eccentric to underlying bone, whereas in osteomyelitis, signal abnormality is seen within the medullary space, and the process is centered on involved bone.

Muscle abscesses show avidity for gallium-67– and indium-labeled leukocytes; however, these techniques are usually reserved for patients in whom the site of infection is not localized or in whom multifocal disease is suspected.

Treatment Appropriate antibiotic therapy is usually curative for pyomyositis. More aggressive abscesses may require abscess drainage and débridement of muscle.[62]

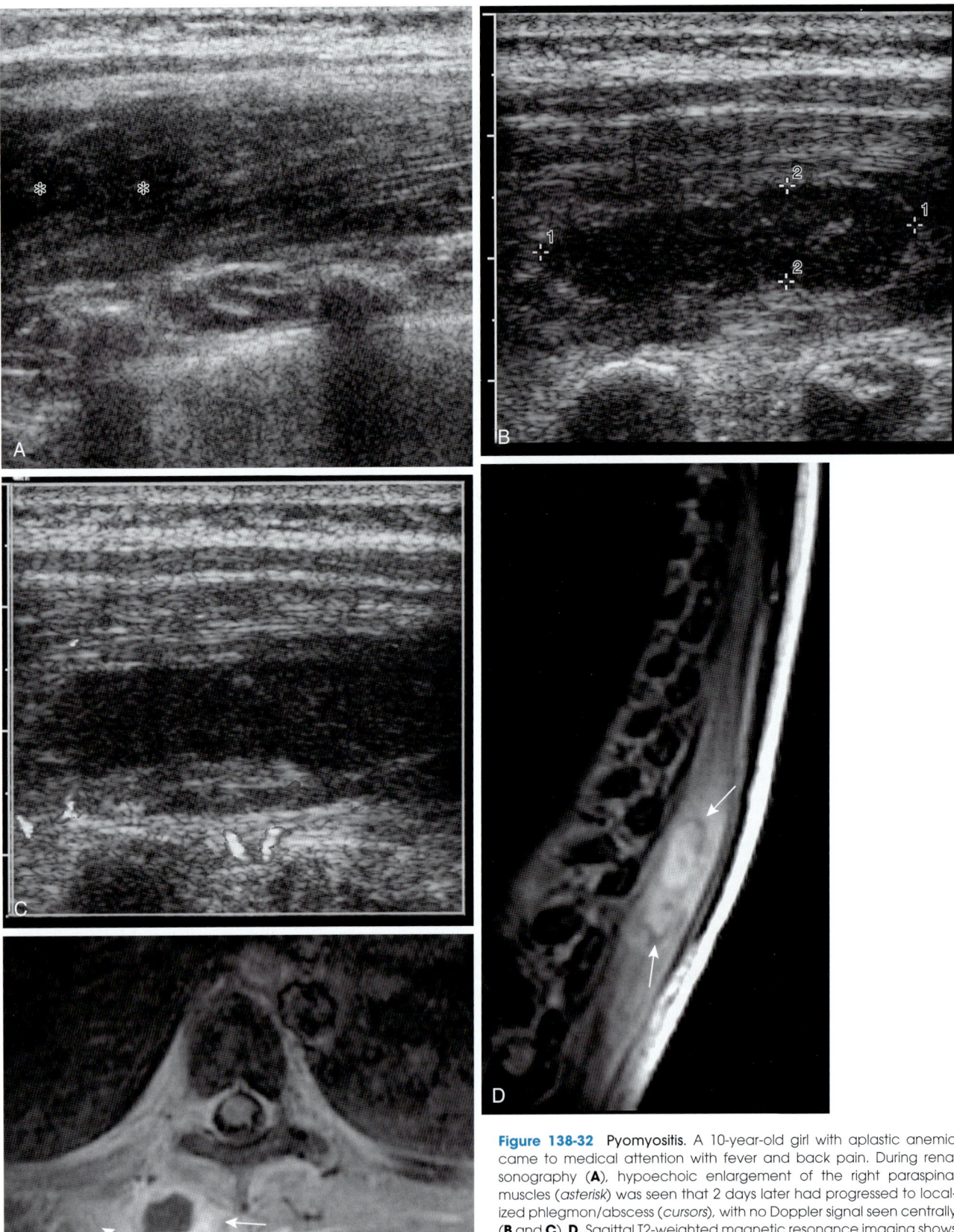

Figure 138-32 Pyomyositis. A 10-year-old girl with aplastic anemia came to medical attention with fever and back pain. During renal sonography (**A**), hypoechoic enlargement of the right paraspinal muscles (*asterisk*) was seen that 2 days later had progressed to localized phlegmon/abscess (*cursors*), with no Doppler signal seen centrally (**B** and **C**). **D,** Sagittal T2-weighted magnetic resonance imaging shows right paraspinal muscle edema with a central higher signal intensity collection surrounded by a lower signal intensity rim (*arrows*). **E,** On axial fat-suppressed post-gadolinium T1-weighted images, the collection (*arrows*) is characterized by an irregular rim of enhancement and lack of contrast enhancement centrally. Note low signal intensity marrow, likely the result of iron deposition from multiple transfusions.

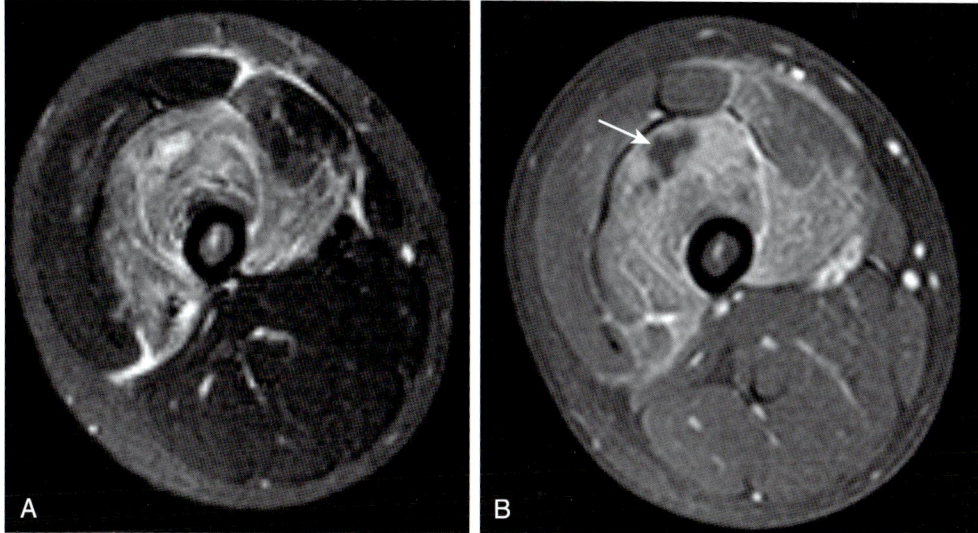

Figure 138-34 A 6-year-old girl with pyomyositis and early abscess formation (*arrow*) in the quadriceps mechanism seen on short tau inversion recovery axial (**A**) and post-gadolinium T1 fat-saturated axial (**B**) magnetic resonance image.

NECROTIZING FASCIITIS/CELLULITIS

Etiology, Pathophysiology, and Clinical Presentation Necrotizing fasciitis is a rapidly progressive, sometimes fatal soft tissue infection that characteristically involves the deep fascia of the extremities and trunk.[57] The disease tends to affect the elderly and those with impaired immunity, but it can occur in immune-competent patients of any age. Underlying skin infection related to lesions such as furuncles, insect bites, and even minor trauma or surgery has been associated. Necrotizing fasciitis is most commonly a polymicrobial infection with both aerobic and anaerobic organisms. In children with chicken pox, secondary infection of vesicular skin lesions with *S. aureus* or GABHS has been linked to development of cellulitis and, less frequently, necrotizing fasciitis.[63]

The early clinical presentation of necrotizing fasciitis is nonspecific and may be accompanied by vague complaints of fever and malaise with rapid progression to sepsis and acute renal failure. Initial soft tissue findings are those of warmth and induration. A high index of suspicion is paramount for early diagnosis.

Imaging Imaging can facilitate the diagnosis. Radiographs are insensitive to changes of necrotizing fasciitis until they are advanced, at which time gas can be seen in the soft tissues. Characteristic CT findings include soft tissue air, deep fascial fluid collections, and fascial enhancement, although these findings are not consistently seen (e-Fig. 138-35). Ultrasonography may depict deep soft tissue changes and fluid collections and offers the benefits of portability along with the ability to guide diagnostic aspiration.

Pathologic changes and extent of necrotizing fasciitis and cellulitis are detected most sensitively on MRI with fat-suppressed T2-weighted, short tau inversion recovery sequences, and post-gadolinium fat-suppressed T1-weighted imaging (Fig. 138-36). Cellulitis is characterized by high T2 signal thickening and gadolinium enhancement with or without fluid collection in the subcutaneous tissue and superficial fascia (e-Fig. 138-37). Necrotizing fasciitis should be considered when these changes extend to the deep fascia. Patients with necrotizing fasciitis may have thick (> 3 mm) fascial signal intensity or low signal intensity in the deep fascia on T2-weighted images, along with focal or diffuse nonenhancing portions of deep fascia and involvement of three or more compartments in one extremity.[64] Soft tissue gas appears as areas of signal absence with susceptibility artifact. To help guide therapy, it is important to distinguish by MRI whether necrotizing fasciitis is related to underlying osteomyelitis and/or septic arthritis versus infection confined to the muscles and fascia.

Edema of fascia and muscles is nonspecific on MRI and overlaps with that of other pathologic conditions, including dermatomyositis, pyomyositis, and lymphedema. Additionally, in the very early stages of necrotizing fasciitis, deep fascial involvement may be minimal or lacking. Therefore even though exclusion of deep fascial involvement on MRI is fairly reliable for exclusion of necrotizing fasciitis, ultimate patient management relies on a combination of imaging and clinical findings.

Treatment Cellulitis is amenable to medical therapy with intravenous antibiotics; necrotizing fasciitis is a life-threatening emergency that requires additional urgent surgical débridement of necrotic tissue.[65] Therefore distinction between these two entities is critical for patient management.

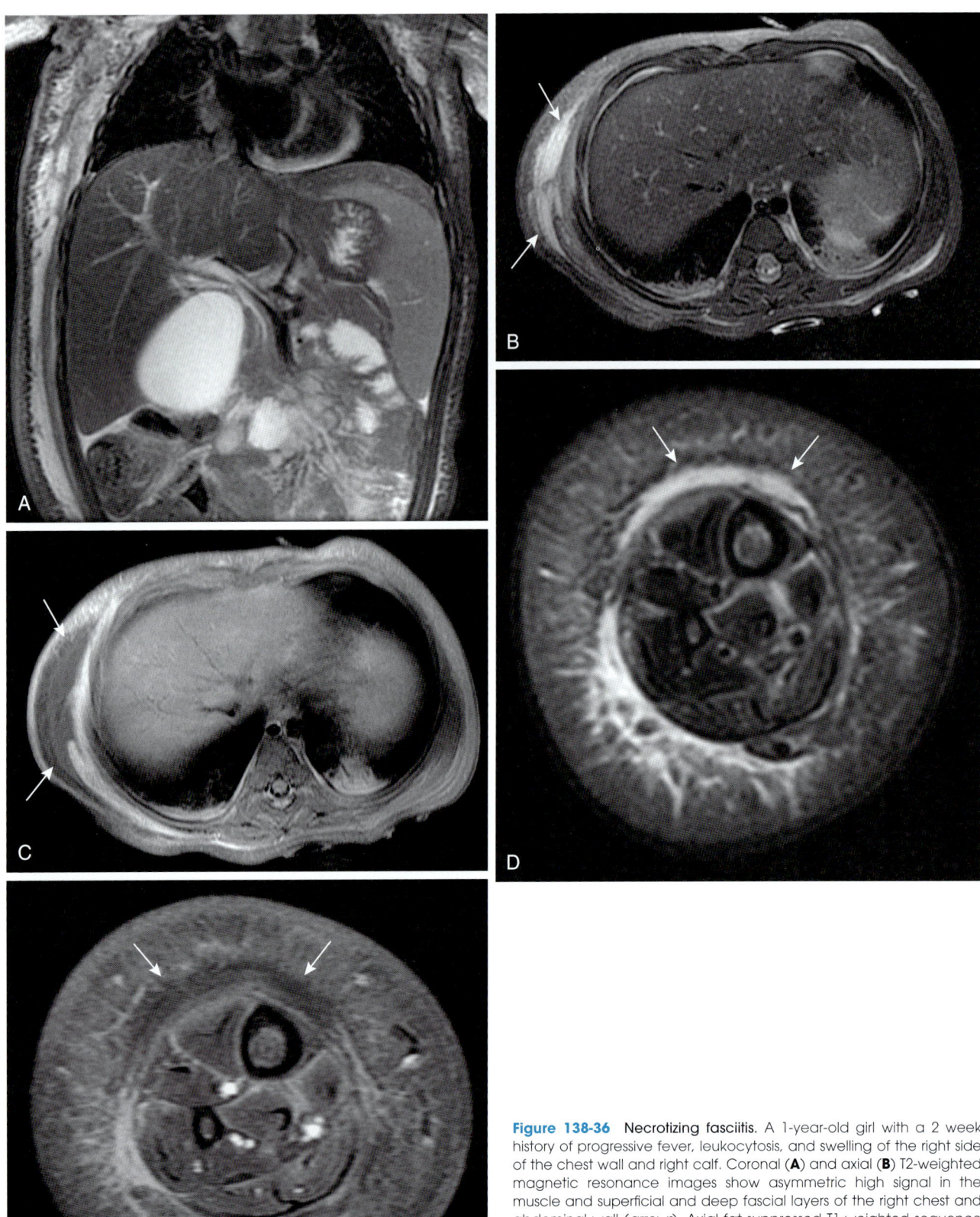

Figure 138-36 Necrotizing fasciitis. A 1-year-old girl with a 2 week history of progressive fever, leukocytosis, and swelling of the right side of the chest wall and right calf. Coronal (**A**) and axial (**B**) T2-weighted magnetic resonance images show asymmetric high signal in the muscle and superficial and deep fascial layers of the right chest and abdominal wall (*arrows*). Axial fat-suppressed T1-weighted sequence (**C**) after intravenous gadolinium administration shows enhancement of these areas with more superficial nonenhancing fluid lacking rim enhancement (*arrows*). Similar changes (*arrows*) are seen in the right lower leg on axial T2-weighted (**D**) and post-contrast fat-suppressed T1-weighted images (**E**). Biopsy of both sites showed acute inflammation with coagulative necrosis. Cultures were negative, but dramatic clinical improvement was noted with intravenous antibiotic therapy.

Key Points

Distinguish alternative causes for marrow edema. Not all marrow edema is osteomyelitis.

Radiographs should always be obtained prior to advanced imaging to rule out obvious alternative causes for symptoms, such as a fracture.

When infection is a concern and symptoms are nonlocalizing, bone scan is recommended. If symptoms are localizing, MRI is recommended.

When osteomyelitis is present, identify and measure all abscesses, their location, and whether there is secondary involvement of a nearby joint.

US and MRI are not able to distinguish pyogenic and nonpyogenic joint effusions. Therefore when a joint effusion is present without additional findings, such as nearby osteomyelitis, do not attribute an infectious cause for the effusion.

ACKNOWLEDGEMENT

This chapter includes material from Chapter 159, "The Soft Tissues," in the previous edition of this text, originally written by Kathleen H. Emery, MD.

Suggested Readings

Jaramillo D. Infection: musculoskeletal. *Pediatr Radiol.* 2011;41(Suppl 1):S127-S134.

Kocher MS, Zurakowski D, Kasser JR. Differentiating between septic arthritis and transient synovitis of the hip in children: an evidence-based clinical prediction algorithm. *J Bone Joint Surg.* 1999;81-A(12):1662-1670.

Tureck MB, Taljanovic MS, Stubbs AY, et al. Imaging of musculoskeletal soft tissue infections. *Skeletal Radiol.* 2010;39(10):957-971.

References

Full references for this chapter can be found on www.expertconsult.com.

Chapter 139

Soft Tissue and Bone Tumors

MAHESH M. THAPA, SUE CREVISTON KASTE, and JAMES S. MEYER

Soft Tissue Tumors

OVERVIEW

In general, clinical presentation and findings guide diagnostic imaging in the assessment of soft tissue neoplasms. In children with subtle masses, the primary objective of imaging is to confirm or exclude the presence of a mass. In children with obvious masses, imaging is performed to assess the local extent of the tumor, to provide a differential diagnosis, and to guide potential biopsy.

Most soft tissue tumors in children are benign.[1] When the mass is hard and fixed, conventional radiographs are often performed to determine whether an underlying bone lesion is present that is simulating, or is associated with, a soft tissue mass. Conventional radiographs may show secondary changes in the configuration of adjacent bones and may also reveal the presence of cortical bone erosion, periosteal reaction, and soft tissue calcifications. Occasionally, radiolucency indicates the presence of a fat-containing tumor.[1]

Superficial masses are often assessed by ultrasonography (US), a modality that is easily accessible, lacks ionizing radiation, and rarely requires sedation.[2] In addition, color and spectral Doppler analysis can assess and characterize vascularity.

Nuclear medicine also plays a significant role in the assessment of soft tissue tumors. Many soft tissue sarcomas are detected by gallium-67 and thallium-201 scintigraphy.[3,4] Technetium-99m–methylene diphosphonate (99mTc-MDP) bone scintigraphy may be performed to identify local bone involvement and distant skeletal metastases. In addition, positron emission tomography (PET) and PET computed tomography (CT) are playing an increasing role in initial tumor assessment and evaluation of tumor response and recurrence.

With continuing advances in magnetic resonance imaging (MRI), the role of CT has become limited. CT offers similar but more detailed information than that provided by conventional radiographs. Two areas in which CT has a clear advantage over MRI are in the detection of calcification, such as in myositis ossificans, and when lesions are present along the anterior abdominal wall or chest, where artifact may significantly degrade MRI quality.[1] Also, CT of the lungs is usually performed to assess for metastatic disease.

MRI is the imaging study of choice for assessment of most soft tissue tumors. The superb soft tissue contrast and multiplanar images provide details on the tumor's extent and relationship to underlying anatomic structures.

Although MRI technology continues to evolve, the basic tenets of the MRI examination of a child with a soft tissue tumor have remained constant. First, images should cover the entire tumor, including its margins, and they should include any needle biopsy tracts that may have to be excised at the time of surgical resection. Care must be taken to ensure quality images and coverage of the entire lesion and important adjacent structures. The area that contains the tumor should be imaged in at least two orthogonal planes. T1- and T2-weighted images should be obtained. Fat saturation is often added to confirm the presence of fat in a lesion and/or to highlight the presence of enhancement after intravenous gadolinium administration. Short tau inversion recovery (STIR) sequences are also useful, because they inherently suppress signal from fat and do not require a homogeneous magnetic field. Gadolinium-enhanced T1-weighted images add information about tumor vascularity and are helpful in guiding percutaneous biopsy in that viable tumor can be differentiated from areas of necrosis.[5] Cystic lesions may be identified by their lack of central enhancement.[6] MR angiography (MRA) is useful for detecting the presence of blood flow within the tumor and for planning the optimal surgical approach when large vessels may be involved. Most soft tissue tumors have prolonged T1 and T2 signal characteristics.[7] The MRI signal characteristics of most soft tissue tumors are nonspecific and usually cannot predict histology, nor can they differentiate between benign and malignant neoplasms. Biopsy is necessary for histologic diagnosis.

BENIGN SOFT TISSUE TUMORS

Desmoid Tumors

Overview Desmoid tumors, representing deep or aggressive fibromatosis, are rare mesenchymal neoplasms with a fibrotic texture.[8,9] Although distant metastases do not occur, these tumors are locally aggressive and can lead to significant morbidity and mortality. Desmoid tumors are slightly more common in females, with an incidence of 2 to 4 cases per million per year. The peak incidence is in the third and fourth decades of life.[10] When these tumors occur in younger patients, they tend to be more aggressive, with recurrence rates up to 87%.[11]

Etiology Desmoid tumors are classified into superficial and deep groups. Superficial tumors are usually small and slow growing, and deep lesions may occur in the abdomen or extraabdominally. In children, extraabdominal desmoid tumors are more common than the abdominal type. Most desmoid tumors in patients with Gardner syndrome are found in the abdomen. Extraabdominal desmoid tumors, also referred to as *aggressive fibromatosis,* are usually solitary and arise from the fascial sheaths and aponeuroses of striated muscle. In a series of tumors studied at St. Jude Children's Research Hospital, head and neck, trunk, and extremity involvement was seen with approximately equal frequency.[12] Histologically, desmoid tumors consist of benign fibrous tissues that contain spindle cells and abundant collagen. Although they do not metastasize, desmoid tumors can infiltrate contiguous structures, including bone.

Imaging Desmoid tumors are variably echogenic on US, and their borders may be smooth or irregular. On contrast-enhanced CT, most appear more attenuated than striated muscle (Fig. 139-1). On MRI, these tumors may be nodular with infiltrative or well-defined margins. Tumors may be homogeneous or heterogeneous with varying signal characteristics. Some lesions are low signal on T1- and T2-weighted images, but more often tumors are heterogeneous and contain areas that are hyperintense to "fat" on T2-weighted images. On T1-weighted images, these masses contain areas that are hypointense, isointense, or slightly hyperintense when compared with muscle. This variability in signal reflects differences in the relative proportions of collagen, spindle cells, and mucopolysaccharides within the lesion (e-Fig. 139-2). On T2-weighted images, low signal generally reflects collagen, and high signal reflects a greater quantity of cellular tissue.[13] Tumors with high signal on T1-weighted images have been found to contain fat or myxoid material. Contrast enhancement may be homogeneous, heterogeneous, or absent and does not correlate with clinical outcome.[14]

A desmoid tumor may be prospectively suggested by the presence of areas of T2 hypointensity suggestive of collagen stroma within the mass, but biopsy is ultimately required for definitive diagnosis.

Treatment Stable asymptomatic desmoid tumors are often treated conservatively and observed for changes.[15] Symptomatic desmoids must be treated, and therapy often depends on anatomic location. If possible, surgical resection with wide margins is the treatment of choice.[10] However, recurrence is common (19% to 77%) and is more frequent with extraabdominal desmoids (30% to 50%) than with intraabdominal desmoids (15% to 30%).[8,9,16] If surgery is not possible, systemic therapy should be considered. This is often the case when desmoids are associated with familial adenomatous polyposis or Gardner syndrome. These conditions increase the likelihood of postoperative complications such as hemorrhage, short-bowel syndrome, intestinal ischemia, obstruction, or fistula formation.[9,15] Nonsurgical treatment options that include radiation and systemic therapy are also available. Patients treated with chemotherapy have a lower incidence of tumor recurrence compared with those treated with radiation.[13]

Infantile Myofibromatosis

Infantile myofibromatosis is the most common fibrous tumor of infancy. Tumors may involve skin, muscle, bone, or viscera and may be solitary (myofibroma) or multiple (myofibromatosis). Myofibromatosis occurs in children younger than 2 years of age. The prognosis of musculoskeletal lesions is excellent, and spontaneous resolution usually occurs, although visceral involvement may portend a poorer prognosis. Lesions have a variable appearance on US and range from solid to anechoic centrally with a thick wall. On CT, myofibromas enhance to a lesser degree or similarly to muscle and often exhibit a peripheral rim of enhancement. On MRI, lesions are low signal on T1 weighting and usually high signal on T2 weighting. Some masses show decreased central signal on T2 weighting, because these masses are composed of collagen and have cellular elements. Enhancement of the fibrous and cellular components is seen with gadolinium administration (Fig. 139-3).[12,17-21] Osseous lesions tend to occur in the metaphysis and have a lytic appearance (Fig. 139-4).[20]

Benign Peripheral Nerve Sheath Tumors

Overview Benign peripheral nerve sheath tumors are divided into schwannomas, also known as *neurinomas* and *neurilemomas,* and neurofibromas. Benign neurofibromas and, less commonly, schwannomas are frequently multiple and are associated with neurofibromatosis type 1 (NF1). However, both tumors may be solitary and may occur sporadically.

Etiologies and Clinical Presentation Schwannomas account for approximately 5% of all benign soft tissue neoplasms, and they are usually found as a solitary lesion in individuals between 20 and 50 years of age. Although they may occur virtually anywhere in the body, the head and neck, flexor surfaces of extremities (notably the ulnar and peroneal nerves), mediastinum, and retroperitoneum are the most commonly involved sites.[22] If the lesion is large, pain and neurologic symptoms may be clinical manifestations; otherwise, patients are usually asymptomatic.[23,24]

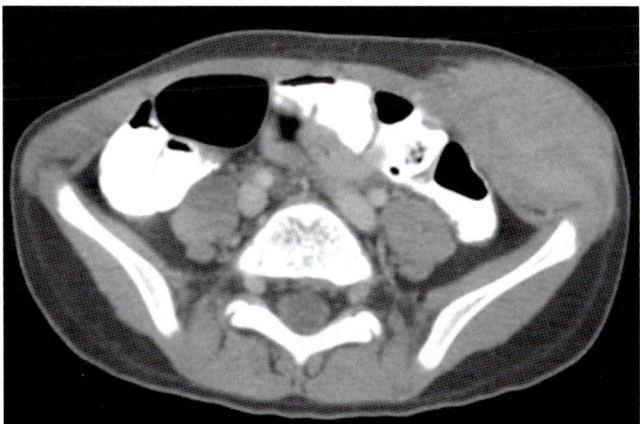

Figure 139-1 Extraabdominal desmoid tumor (Gardner fibroma) in a 5-year-old girl. Axial contrast-enhanced computed tomographic image shows a large lenticular-shaped mass originating in the anterior abdominal wall musculature.

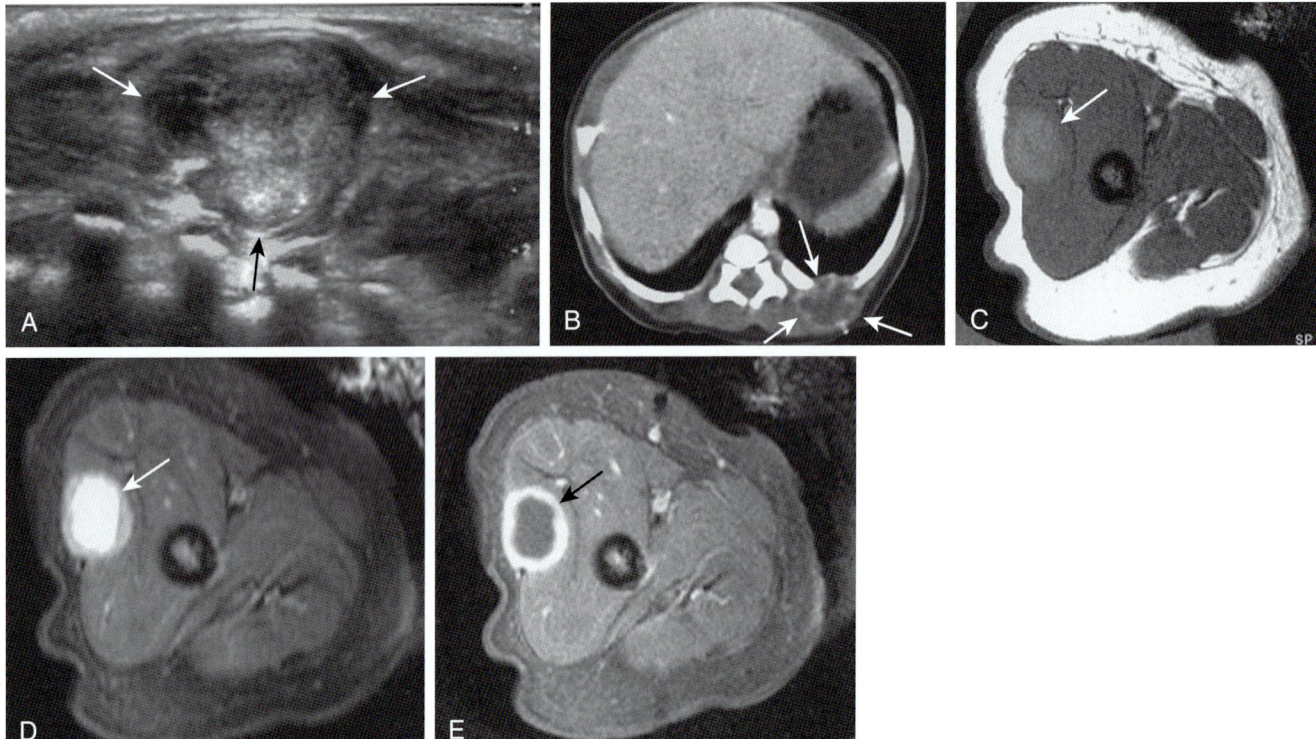

Figure 139-3 Infantile myofibromatosis in a neonate. **A,** Ultrasound shows a solid, intramuscular subscapular mass (*arrows*). **B,** Axial contrast-enhanced computed tomographic image shows peripheral enhancement within the mass (*arrows*). **C,** Thigh lesion in the same patient shows hyperintense signal on T1-weighted magnetic resonance imaging. **D,** T2-weighted image with fat saturation demonstrates cystic changes with a thick, irregular rind of soft tissue. **E,** Post-gadolinium T1-weighted fat-saturated images demonstrate enhancement of the rind of soft tissue and central areas of nonenhancement.

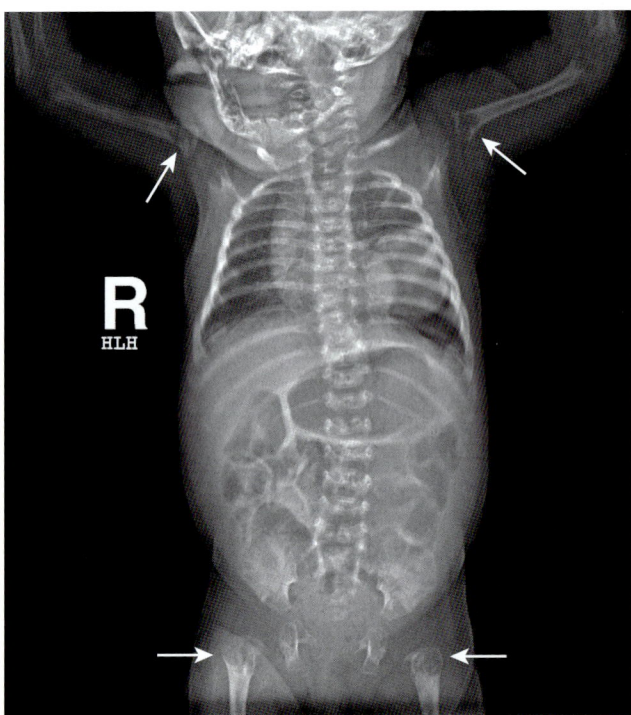

Figure 139-4 Newborn girl with multifocal myofibromatosis with preferential involvement of metaphyses (*arrows*).

Neurofibromas may be localized, plexiform, or diffuse, and the localized form accounts for 90% of cases and is not usually associated with NF1, unlike the diffuse and plexiform subtypes.[22] *Localized neurofibromas* account for approximately 5% of all benign soft tissue tumors and are typically seen in younger patients between 20 and 30 years of age.[22] They often come to medical attention as a painless, slowly growing mass.[23]

Schwannomas and localized neurofibromas are similar histologically and are composed primarily of Schwann cells, therefore they exhibit similar imaging characteristics. Microscopic examination reveals a dense central core of Schwann cells surrounded by a peripheral zone of myxoid tissue. Peripheral nerve sheath tumors have a low incidence of malignant degeneration.[22]

Imaging A tumor can be suspected to have a neurogenic origin if it is located along the distribution of a peripheral nerve. Calcification in degenerating ("ancient") schwannomas may be visible radiographically; on bone scintigrams, these tumors have been observed to take up 99mTc-MDP.[25] Peripheral nerve sheath tumors may be accompanied by subtle atrophy of surrounding or distally innervated muscle. Most of these tumors are well-defined spherical or fusiform masses. On CT images, they tend to be hypoattenuated, possibly because of lipids in their Schwann cells, adipocytes, and perineural tissues.[26] On MRI, the bulk of the tumor shows low intensity on T1-weighted sequences and high intensity on T2-weighted sequences. Typically, the central zone consists of collagen and neurofibroma cells and is hypointense on T2-weighted images, lending a "target" appearance to the lesion that can also be seen on contrast-enhanced T1-weighted images; it is more easily appreciated when wide window settings are used to view the images. The presence of a target sign helps to distinguish these benign tumors from their less well-organized malignant counterparts (Fig. 139-5).[27-30]

On MRI, differentiating a schwannoma from a neurofibroma can be difficult; however, schwannomas may contain more prominent areas of hemorrhage, cystic change, and necrosis with resultant heterogeneous signal intensities. In addition, neurofibromas intimately involve and are inseparable from the normal nerve. Schwannomas are eccentric to the nerve, and this may be apparent on MRI in tumors that involve larger nerves. When smaller nerves are involved, schwannomas may obliterate the nerve of origin, and

the MRI appearance is indistinguishable from that of a neurofibroma.[31]

Plexiform neurofibromas arise from the axis of a primary nerve and form tortuous, cordlike tumors along its axis. They are regarded as indicators of neurofibromatosis, even when they are the sole manifestation of the disease. Tumors tend to appear as lobulated, amorphous masses with ill-defined borders. Similar to solitary neurofibromas, these tumors are usually hyperintense on T2-weighted imaging and often have well-defined, central, tubular, hypointense structures, or they may form large masses that resemble a "bag of worms" on transverse images.[32]

Diffuse neurofibromas are particularly uncommon and are often associated with NF1 (7 of 10 patients in one series).[33] These lesions occur primarily in children and young adults and most commonly involve the head and neck regions. These ill-defined, infiltrative lesions tend to be located in the skin and subcutaneous tissues. They appear as linear or reticular strands of intermediate signal on T1-weighted images and are of high signal intensity on T2-weighted images, with linear areas of enhancement after gadolinium administration.

Benign Fatty Tumors

Overview The 2002 World Health Organization (WHO) Soft Tissue Tumor Classification includes nine types of benign fatty tumor: lipoma, lipomatosis, lipomatosis of nerve, lipoblastoma/lipoblastomatosis, angiolipoma, myolipoma of soft tissue, chondroid lipoma, spindle cell/pleomorphic lipoma, and hibernoma. Except for lipoblastoma, all of these tumors are more common in adults than in children.[24]

Lipoblastoma and lipoblastomatosis are benign mesenchymal tumors of immature fat that occur primarily in infants and young children, most often in boys younger than 8 years of age. The average age of patients at the time of presentation is 3.6 years.[34] Lipoblastomas are usually painless superficial tumors most commonly located in the extremities and the head and neck region, but they may also involve the trunk and deeper structures, such as the mediastinum and retroperitoneum. The tumor consists of lobules of immature adipose tissue with a variable amount of myxoid stroma separated by richly vascularized septa composed of connective tissue. The discrete form, *lipoblastoma,* is a well-circumscribed lesion that occurs in approximately 70% of cases and involves the superficial soft tissues. Lipoblastomas eventually evolve into mature lipomas. The term *lipoblastomatosis* refers to the diffuse type that often infiltrates adjacent deeper tissues, such as muscle, and has a tendency to recur locally[35]; spontaneous resolution has also been reported.[36,37]

Imaging Imaging features reflect the amount of fatty tissue present. On US images, hyperechoic fat can be clearly delineated from the myxoid component, and CT images show a similar combination of hypoattenuated fat and denser myxoid tissue. On MRI, the signal is often heterogeneous (e-Fig. 139-6), and lipomatous elements appear hyperintense to muscle on T1-weighted images and isointense to subcutaneous fat on T2-weighted images; nonfatty tissues produce lower signal intensity than fat on T1-weighted images and are more intense than fat on T2-weighted images. In addition to low-signal myxoid components on T1 imaging, the fatty

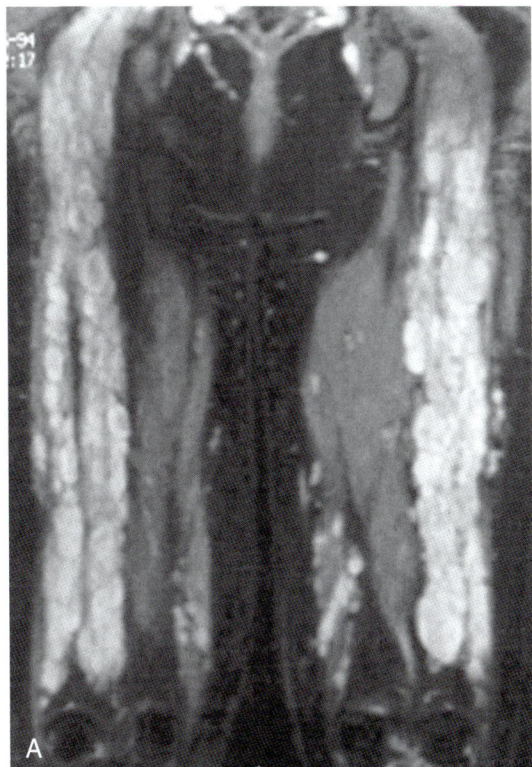

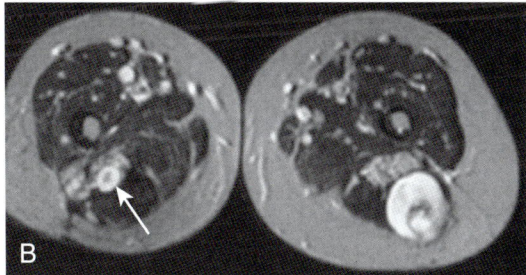

Figure 139-5 A young woman first seen at the age of 16 with a malignant peripheral nerve sheath tumor. **A,** Coronal short tau inversion recovery magnetic resonance image of the thighs shows multiple plexiform neurofibromas distributed along the sciatic nerves. **B,** Transverse T2-weighted images show multiple, discrete, high-intensity neurofibromas. A characteristic target sign is evident (*arrow*). The larger lesion in the posterior left thigh, which had shown recent growth, was a low-grade malignant peripheral nerve sheath tumor.

mass may contain low-signal fibrous septa that show contrast enhancement.[38-40]

The differential diagnosis includes lipoma, which is much more prevalent in adults than in children; hibernoma, a rare tumor analogous to brown fat; and myxoid liposarcoma. Liposarcoma is rare in children younger than 5 years of age.[41] Thus, a fat-containing tumor that occurs in a child younger than 2 years of age, even with nonlipomatous components, is almost invariably a lipoblastoma.

Treatment   The majority of fat-containing masses in children are benign. Although complete surgical resection is the treatment of choice for focal lesions,[34] subtotal resection may therefore be considered, particularly when surgical resection may involve critical neurovascular structures, or when it may lead to significant cosmetic deformity.

MALIGNANT SOFT TISSUE TUMORS

Rhabdomyosarcoma

Overview   The head and neck and genitourinary tract are the most frequent locations of rhabdomyosarcoma (RMS). About 20% of these tumors occur in the extremities. Most extremity RMS is of the alveolar or undifferentiated histologic types, not the embryonal or botryoid types found in the face and neck and in the genitourinary system.[42] Prognosis is less favorable for patients with RMS of the extremities than for those with tumors that arise from the genitourinary system or the head and neck region.[43] In the extremities, tumors tend to be deep and tend to spread along fascial planes, and RMS may cause erosion of adjacent bone.

Etiologies, Pathophysiology, and Clinical Presentation   RMS contains a mixture of rhabdomyoblasts, which are recognized by their typical cross striations, and undifferentiated cells. These tumors are thought to arise from progenitor cells for striated muscle and can occur anywhere in the body, even in areas with no striated muscle. RMS accounts for more than 60% of soft tissue sarcoma (STS) in children younger

than 5 years of age but only 25% of STS in those aged 15 to 19 years.[44]

Imaging   Imaging is usually nonspecific but is essential for staging and surgical management. MRI has superseded CT and US in this clinical setting, because it can define the anatomic location of the tumor (unicompartmental vs. multicompartmental), indicate its relationship to important nerves and blood vessels, and reveal local involvement of bone or lymph nodes. MRI characteristics are nonspecific, and most tumors are predominantly low signal on T1-weighted images, high signal on T2-weighted images, and demonstrate central tumoral enhancement (Fig. 139-7). Only 15% to 20% of patients with RMS have clinically detectable metastases at presentation. The lungs, bone marrow, and bone are the most common sites of distant metastases. Lymph nodes may also be involved. Bone metastases resemble those that occur with neuroblastoma; they have been reported even in the absence of detectable primary tumor.

Treatment   Even if not clinically detectable, all patients are considered to have micrometastatic disease; this has resulted in the universal use of chemotherapy. The 5-year survival rate for children with RMS has improved from 55% in the 1970s to more than 70% in modern times.[45]

Primitive Peripheral Neuroectodermal Tumor and Extraosseous Ewing Sarcoma

Overview   Primitive peripheral neuroectodermal tumor (PPNET) and extraosseous Ewing sarcoma (EOES) are small round cell neoplasms that belong to the Ewing sarcoma family of tumors; they can arise in both soft tissue and bone. These neoplasms are related histogenically and share a common cytogenetic characteristic, the translocation of bands 24 and 12 of the short arms of chromosomes 11 and 22, but they are often indistinguishable histologically. Also known as *peripheral neuroepithelioma,* PPNETs have a higher degree of neural differentiation than is seen with Ewing sarcoma; thus

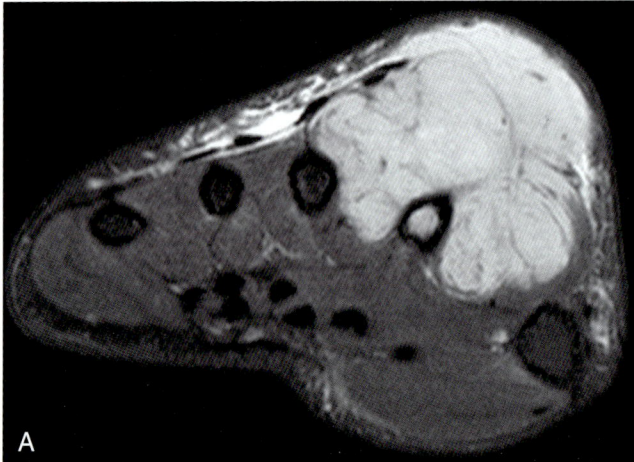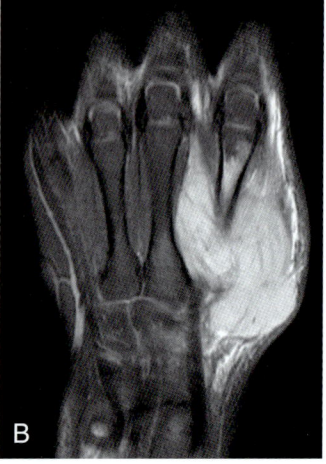

Figure 139-7   Rhabdomyosarcoma of the hand in an 11-year-old boy. **A,** T2-weighted fat-saturated magnetic resonance imaging (MRI) demonstrates a multilobulated, multicompartment mass with secondary involvement of the second metacarpal bone. Note that the mass has a sharp interface with the second metacarpal cortex, an indication that the mass abuts and secondarily involves the bone rather than arising primarily from the bone. **B,** Post-gadolinium T1-weighted fat-saturated coronal MRI demonstrates diffuse tumoral enhancement of the mass.

these two tumors can be distinguished on the basis of immunohistochemical markers. This distinction is important, because disease-free survival is poorer for patients with PPNETs than for those with EOES.[46,47]

Etiologies, Pathophysiology, and Clinical Presentation Both tumors occur most commonly in truncal and paravertebral soft tissues (50% to 60% of cases) and in the extremities (25% of cases), although PPNET occurs less commonly in the extremities than does EOES, and patients with EOES are generally younger. Askin tumors are thoracic PPNETs that involve the chest wall.[48] These tumors can be very large at the time of presentation and tend to be poorly circumscribed. The soft tissue mass does not calcify but may erode adjacent bone.

Imaging On MRI, these tumors have a nonspecific imaging appearance. PPNET and EOES are typically isointense to muscle on T1-weighted images and inhomogeneously hyperintense on T2-weighted and STIR images; they show variable contrast enhancement. When these lesions outgrow their blood supply or, alternatively, when masses hemorrhage spontaneously or after minor trauma, cystic components may be seen; these lesions may superficially mimic a hematoma (Fig. 139-8). Postcontrast imaging is helpful in these circumstances to help identify solid soft tissue components and guide biopsy of viable tumor cells. Distant spread occurs to bone, lung, liver, and brain.[49,50]

Treatment Treatment is dictated by location and extent of disease and may involve surgery for localized disease with or without adjuvant/neoadjuvant chemoradiotherapy.[51]

Synovial Sarcoma

Overview, Etiologies, Pathophysiology, and Clinical Presentation Synovial sarcomas predominantly occur in adults younger than 50 years of age, but they account for about 10% of pediatric STS. These tumors arise from undifferentiated mesenchymal cells, not from true synovial cells. A monophasic variety comprises spindle cells, and a biphasic variety consists of spindle cells and epithelial elements. Although synovial sarcomas often occur close to joints, tendons, and bursae, they are rarely intraarticular.[52] About 80% of synovial sarcomas occur in the extremities, and considerably more lower than upper extremity involvement has been noted. Synovial sarcomas may spread to regional lymph nodes, and the lungs are the most common sites of distant metastasis.[53]

Imaging Radiographically visible calcifications are present in 30% of cases. On MRI, synovial sarcomas are often lobulated, well-defined, deep-seated lesions, although they may be infiltrative and can encase major blood vessels. Femoral vein invasion has been described, and erosion of the cortex of adjacent bones is present in up to 20% of patients.

MRI signal characteristics are nonspecific. Synovial sarcomas are usually isointense to muscle on T1-weighted images. Foci of high T1-weighted signal may be present, and fluid-fluid levels are caused by hemorrhage; tumors generally have heterogeneous signal with areas of high intensity on T2-weighted images (Fig. 139-9). In one large series, 35% of tumors showed a triple-signal pattern on T2-weighted images; these findings are consistent with high (fluid) signal intensity, intermediate signal intensity similar to that of fat, and low

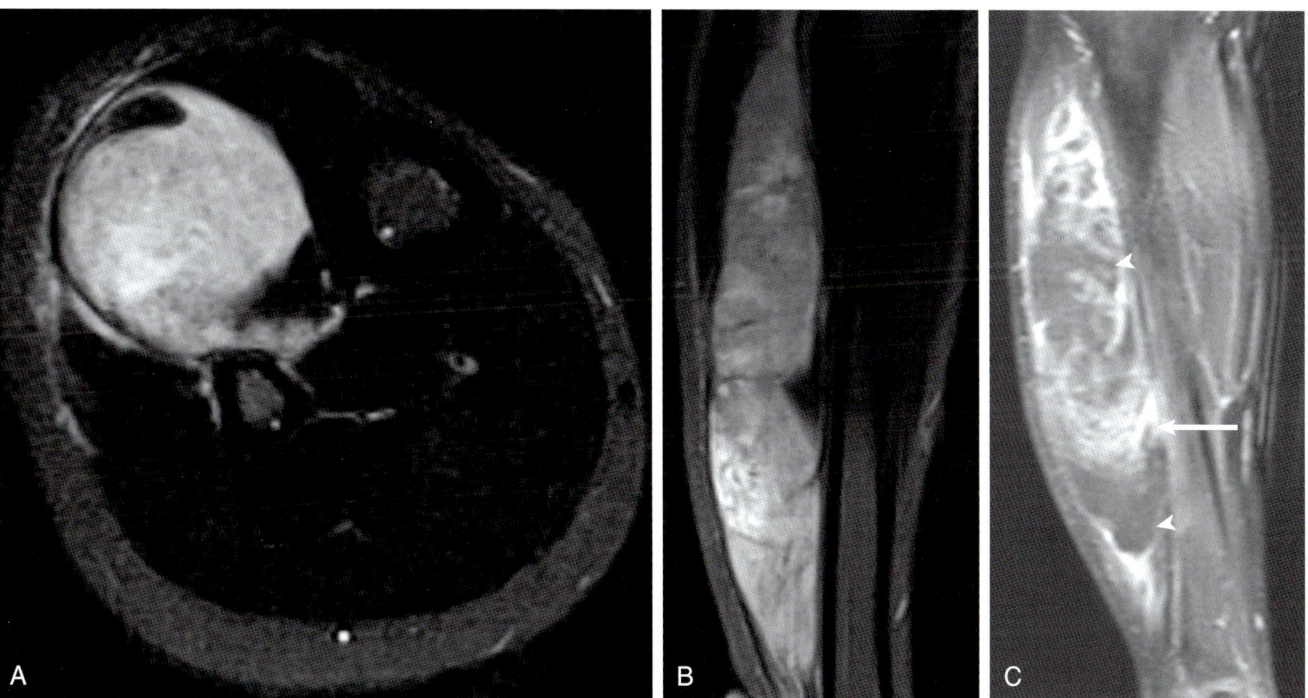

Figure 139-8 Anterior leg primitive neuroectodermal tumor in a 12-year-old boy. Short tau inversion recovery axial (**A**) and coronal (**B**) images demonstrate an extraosseous mass with extensive peritumoral edema. **C,** Post-gadolinium T1-weighted fat-saturated coronal magnetic resonance image demonstrates cystic nonenhancing components of the tumor (*arrowheads*) and solid enhancing components (*arrow*).

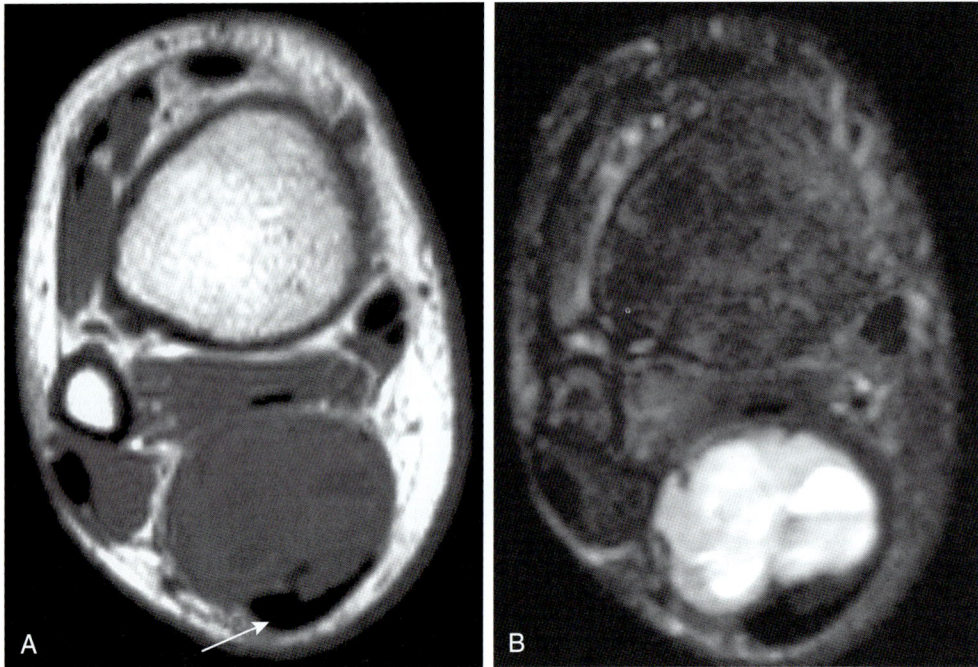

Figure 139-9 Synovial sarcoma adjacent to the Achilles tendon. **A,** Transverse T1-weighted magnetic resonance imaging (MRI) shows mixed intermediate and low signal in the mass. The Achilles tendon (*arrow*) is shown. **B,** A transverse fat-saturated T2-weighted MRI at the same level shows a fluid-fluid level typical of hemorrhage.

signal intensity resembling that of fibrous tissue (see Fig. 139-9, *B*).[54] Some synovial sarcomas superficially mimic ganglion cysts (e-Fig. 139-10). A multilocular appearance with fluid-fluid levels may be seen in 18% to 25% of these tumors. As a rule of thumb, a diagnosis of ganglion cyst should only be considered when a fluid-filled neck can be seen extending from the cyst to a joint or tendon sheath, and no solid components lie within the cystlike lesion. Otherwise, a diagnosis of neoplasm should be favored, with biopsy recommended.[54-57]

Treatment The treatment of choice is surgery with or without adjuvant and neoadjuvant chemotherapy. A recent multicenter study of patients under 20 years of age with a minimum of 10 years of follow-up found that wide surgical resection is the most efficacious method of treatment. Presence of tumor in the trunk and high histologic grade were negative factors for recurrence-free and metastasis-free survival.[58]

Malignant Peripheral Nerve Sheath Tumor

Overview *Malignant peripheral nerve sheath tumor* (MPNST) is the accepted name for a spindle cell sarcoma that arises from a nerve or a neurofibroma. In contrast to other STS that is of mesenchymal cell origin, MPNSTs are of neuroectodermal origin. The MPNST designation has replaced many formerly used terms, including *malignant schwannoma, neurofibrosarcoma, neurogenic sarcoma,* and *malignant neural neoplasm.* A variant of MPNST is the so-called triton tumor (named after a salamander) that contains neural and rhabdomyosarcomatous elements.[22]

Etiologies, Pathophysiology, and Clinical Presentation MPNST accounts for about 4% to 10% of STS, and they are the most common malignancy associated with NF1. Half of these tumors occur in patients with NF1; conversely, 2% to 29% of patients with NF1 develop MPNSTs—a much higher incidence than is seen in the general population. MPNST patients with NF1 are usually younger than those without associated NF1. Furthermore, in patients with NF1, MPNSTs tend to arise in preexisting benign neurofibromas; they are high-grade tumors that have a tendency to recur locally and metastasize. MPNSTs may also arise at previously irradiated sites.[31]

Imaging Similar to benign neurofibromas, MPNSTs are deep soft tissue lesions that are often associated with primary nerves, especially those of the thigh and lower extremities. CT and MRI appearance is nonspecific. Tumors may be well or poorly defined, homogeneous or inhomogeneous, and they occasionally erode bone. Malignant transformation of benign neurofibromas should be considered in patients in whom the mass is painful or enlarging, or when the typical target appearance of a benign neurofibroma is absent (Fig. 139-11). Tumor uptake on gallium scintigraphy may indicate malignant transformation or progressive growth of neurofibromas; however, biopsy is usually necessary to confirm malignancy.[23,24,26,28-30]

Treatment Surgical resection with or without adjuvant and neoadjuvant chemoradiotherapy is used for treatment, depending on the tumor's location.

Infantile Fibrosarcoma

Overview, Etiologies, Pathophysiology, and Clinical Presentation Infantile fibrosarcoma is an uncommon tumor that contains fibroblasts and myoblasts and occurs in young children,

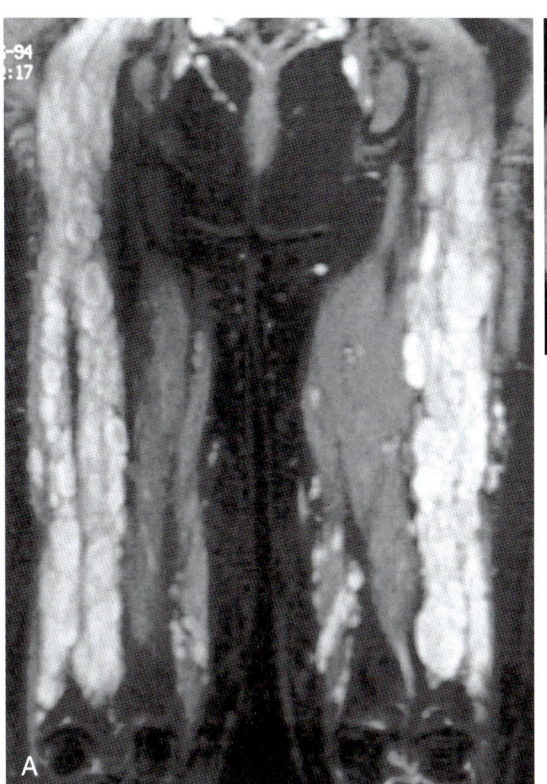
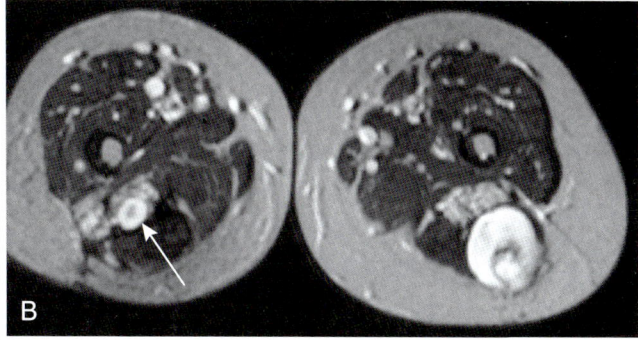

Figure 139-11 Multiple neurofibromas. **A,** Coronal short tau inversion recovery magnetic resonance image of the thighs shows multiple neurofibromas distributed along the sciatic nerves of a young woman first seen at the age of 16 with a malignant peripheral nerve sheath tumor. **B,** Transverse T2-weighted images show multiple, discrete, high-intensity neurofibromas. A characteristic target sign is present (*arrow*). The larger lesion in the posterior left thigh, which had shown recent growth, was a low-grade malignant peripheral nerve sheath tumor.

especially in the first 3 months of life.[59] This tumor is now considered a low-grade malignancy, in distinction from an adult-type fibrosarcoma that occurs in older children (10 to 15 years of age) and is more aggressive. Clinically, infantile fibrosarcomas present as enlarging, sometimes painful masses. Tumors often occur in the distal ends of the extremities and occasionally in the head, neck, and trunk. Because of their high degree of vascularization, they may be confused with hemangiomas on physical and imaging examinations.[60] These tumors may rarely erode adjacent bone, and angiographic studies may reveal tumor vasculature.[61,62]

Imaging Because these masses are often present during fetal life, extensive remodeling of adjacent bones may occur (e-Fig. 139-12). MRI characteristics are nonspecific. Fibrosarcomas are usually isointense to muscle on T1-weighted images and are hyperintense on T2-weighted images. They may contain hypointense foci, which correlate with fibrosis.[63]

Treatment These tumors recur in up to 30% of cases, and metastases occur in about 5%.[64,65] Unlike congenital RMS, infantile fibrosarcoma has an excellent prognosis, with 5-year survival up to 84%.[66]

Dermatofibrosarcoma Protuberans

Overview, Etiologies, Pathophysiology, and Clinical Presentation *Dermatofibrosarcoma protuberans* is an intermediate-grade malignancy that involves the dermis. This tumor is most

often seen in adults; it occurs rarely in children but may be seen at birth. The tumor most commonly appears as a red-blue or pink plaque that grows slowly and may become nodular. A less common atrophic variant occurs as a depressed plaque. Lesions are typically fixed to the dermis but may extend into the underlying tissues. Lesions frequently recur locally, and metastasis occurs in 1% to 6% of patients; 75% of metastases occur in the lungs.[67,68]

Imaging MRI is useful for determining the extent of disease, especially with deep tumor invasion. MRI characteristics are nonspecific. On T1-weighted images, lesions are hypointense to fat and may be isointense, hyperintense, or slightly hypointense to muscle. On T2-weighted images, lesions are isointense or hyperintense to fat. Lesions can enhance after gadolinium administration. On MRI, these tumors may be confused with subcutaneous granuloma annulare, a benign localized inflammatory dermatosis that occurs in children.[69]

Therapy Treatment involves surgical resection with or without adjuvant and neoadjuvant chemoradiotherapy. One review found that only the presence of metastasis had an overall decreased patient survival rate, and those with fibrosarcomatous change or acral location had a decreased disease-free interval despite wide local resection.[70]

Malignant Fibrous Histiocytoma

The 2002 WHO Soft Tissue Tumor Classification has changed the designation of *malignant fibrous histiocytoma*

(MFH). *Pleomorphic MFH* is no longer considered a definable or reproducible entity. As a result, many lesions that had been regarded as MFH will be classified as other entities. The term *pleomorphic MFH* is now synonymous with *undifferentiated pleomorphic sarcoma,* which is essentially a diagnosis of exclusion that accounts for approximately 5% of adult STS.[71-73]

DISSEMINATED DISEASE OF SOFT TISSUES

Lymphoma

Overview, Etiologies, Pathophysiology, and Clinical Presentation Muscle involvement by non-Hodgkin lymphoma (NHL) is usually due to metastatic spread via lymphatic and hematogeneous routes; however, it may be the result of direct extension from primary bone lymphoma. Much less commonly, muscle lymphoma occurs as a primary extranodal tumor. The disease can cross compartmental boundaries, or it may invade subcutaneous tissues. Involvement of adjacent bone and bone marrow may also be noted. Primary T-cell lymphoma of the skin is referred to as *mycosis fungoides.* Typical findings include focal thickening caused by dermal and epidural infiltrates and lymphadenopathy in advanced-stage disease.[74]

Imaging Muscle involvement results in solitary or multiple masses detectable on CT and MRI and with the use of gallium-67 scintigraphy and fluorodeoxyglucose (FDG)-PET. On CT, muscles affected by lymphoma appear diffusely enlarged with or without obliteration of normal fat planes. The tumor may be poorly defined, and its attenuation is equal to or slightly less than that of normal muscle on contrast-enhanced and noncontrast CT images. On MRI, masses are isointense or slightly hypointense to normal muscle on T1-weighted images; they are hyperintense on T2-weighted images and markedly hyperintense on STIR images, and they enhance homogeneously with gadolinium (e-Fig. 139-13). Abnormal activity on gallium-67 and FDG-PET scans correlates well with MRI findings.[75-77]

Granulocytic Sarcoma

Overview, Etiologies, Pathophysiology, and Clinical Presentation *Granulocytic sarcoma* is a rare solid tumor of primitive precursors of white blood cells and is also known as *chloroma* and *extramedullary myeloblastoma.* It occurs in patients with acute and chronic myelogenous leukemia and other myeloproliferative diseases. Children are more often affected than adults, and 60% of these tumors occur in children younger than 15 years of age.[78]

Imaging Chloromas may be solitary or multiple, and they can involve any part of the body, including the brain and muscles. Orbits and subcutaneous tissues, however, are the most common sites (see Chapter 7). These tumors are typically isoattenuating to slightly hyperattenuating to muscle on noncontrast CT and hyperattenuating to muscle on contrast CT. On MRI, lesions are typically isointense to muscle on T1-weighted images and hyperintense to muscle on T2-weighted images. Tumors usually enhance after gadolinium administration.[79-81]

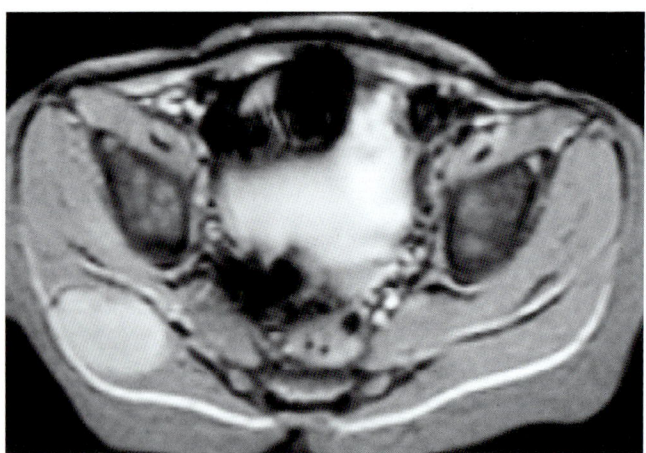

Figure 139-14 Neuroblastoma. A transverse T2-weighted magnetic resonance image of the pelvis of a 2-year-old girl with stage IV neuroblastoma shows a large metastasis in the right gluteal muscle.

Metastases

Subcutaneous tissues and muscles may be involved in metastatic lesions. Neuroblastoma, in particular, may metastasize to the skin, subcutaneous tissue, or muscle (Fig. 139-14). Despite its large volume, muscle is not a frequent site for metastatic disease. On CT, muscle metastases produce low-attenuation masses with loss of normal muscle planes. On MRI, metastases are similar in intensity to muscle on T1-weighted images and are hyperintense on T2-weighted images. Contrast-enhanced T1-weighted images show masses of high signal intensity. Focal necrosis may also occur.[82,83]

Bone Tumors

RADIOGRAPHIC EVALUATION OF BONE TUMORS

Regardless of the site and aggressiveness of a bone lesion, the initial mode of imaging of bone tumors is radiography. Radiographs serve to confirm the presence and site of a tumor, assist in the formulation of differential diagnoses, characterize the tumor, and guide in the selection of further imaging.[84,85] The decision to obtain radiographs is a clinical one, based on presentation, history, physical examination, and occasionally on laboratory tests. The differential diagnosis of a pediatric bone tumor can be narrowed down by asking a few simple questions.

How Old Is the Child?

Most bone tumors have a proclivity to occur within a certain age range. The differential diagnosis of a bone tumor in a 1-year-old infant is much different than that of a 16-year-old teenager or a 5-year-old child. Box 139-1 lists common pediatric bone tumors in accordance with the peak age at which they most commonly occur.[86-88]

What Is the Location of the Lesion? What Bone? What Part of the Bone?

Many bone tumors have a proclivity to affect certain bones within the skeleton or to occur at certain locations within

---

Box 139-1 Pediatric Bone Tumors: Peak Age of Occurrence

Infant and Toddler (≤5 Years)
Infantile myofibromatosis
Leukemia
Langerhans cell histiocytosis (multifocal)
Metastatic neuroblastoma
Osteofibrous dysplasia

Child (5-10 Years)
Ewing sarcoma of long bone
Langerhans cell histiocytosis (unifocal)

Adolescent (10-20 Years)
Aneurysmal bone cyst
Chondroblastoma
Chondromyxoid fibroma
Ewing sarcoma of axial skeleton
Fibrous dysplasia
Osteochondroma
Leukemia (second peak)
Nonossifying fibroma/fibrous cortical defect
Osteoblastoma
Osteoid osteoma
Osteosarcoma
Periosteal chondroma
Primary lymphoma of bone
Simple bone cyst

Adult
Adamantinoma
Enchondroma
Giant cell tumor (rare until physes fuse)
Parosteal osteosarcoma
Periosteal osteosarcoma

Box 139-2 Pediatric Bone Tumors: Location in Long Bones

Epiphysis
Chondroblastoma
Giant cell tumor (after physeal fusion)
Langerhans cell histiocytosis

Metaphysis
Aneurysmal bone cyst
Chondromyxoid fibroma
Enchondroma
Leukemia
Metastases
Nonossifying fibroma/fibrous cortical defect*
Osteochondroma*
Osteoid osteoma
Osteosarcoma
Parosteal osteosarcoma
Simple bone cyst*

Diaphysis
Adamantinoma
Ewing sarcoma/primitive neuroectodermal tumor
Fibrous dysplasia
Nonossifying fibroma/fibrous cortical defect (in older patients)*
Osteochondroma (in older patients)*
Osteofibrous dysplasia
Osteoid osteoma
Periosteal osteosarcoma
Simple bone cyst (in older patients)*

*Osteochondromas, nonossifying fibromas/fibrous cortical defects, and simple bone cysts begin in the metaphyses. With maturation, these lesions may "migrate" into metadiaphysis and diaphysis.

---

a bone. Box 139-2 lists common pediatric bone tumors according to their preferred location in growing long bones. Lesions also vary in their centricity relative to the involved bone. Some tumors, such as a simple bone cyst, are central, whereas others are eccentric within bone (nonossifying fibroma) or juxtacortical (osteochondroma, periosteal osteosarcoma).[86,87,89]

Is the Lesion Unifocal or Multifocal?

Some lesions are always solitary, and others are usually multifocal. Some may be solitary or multifocal, although multifocal disease often implies a systemic disease or an underlying syndrome predisposing the patient to the development of a particular type of bone tumor. Box 139-3 lists common pediatric bone tumors that are multifocal.

Is the Lesion Aggressive or Nonaggressive in Appearance?

In general, unlike malignant lesions, benign lesions have a nonaggressive radiographic appearance. Exceptions are common, and some lesions may have both aggressive and nonaggressive features. Box 139-4 lists lesions covered in this chapter by their characteristic radiographic appearance—aggressive, nonaggressive, or indeterminate.

Radiographic features of a nonaggressive and usually benign bone tumor are well-defined margins with a narrow zone of transition, particularly with sclerosis; expansion of bone contour from slow growth; smooth, single-layered periosteal new bone; and absence of an associated soft tissue mass. Radiographic features of an aggressive and usually malignant

---

Box 139-3 Pediatric Bone Tumors: Multifocal Lesions

Brown tumors (hyperparathyroidism)
Cystic angiomatosis/lymphangiomatosis
Enchondroma (Ollier disease, Maffucci syndrome)
Fibrous dysplasia (McCune-Albright syndrome)
Infantile myofibromatosis
Langerhans cell histiocytosis
Leukemia
Metastases (i.e., from neuroblastoma)
Multifocal osteosarcoma
Nonossifying fibromas/fibrous cortical defects
Osteochondroma (osteochondromatosis)

bone tumor are poorly defined margins with a wide zone of transition, permeative or "moth-eaten" bone destruction, frank destruction of bone without remodeling, aggressive forms of periosteal new bone, interrupted periosteal new bone, and the presence of an associated soft tissue mass. Aggressive forms of periosteal reaction include layering, or "onionskin," and "hair-on-end" periosteal new bone. Interrupted periosteal new bone may take the form of a Codman triangle, a sign of an aggressive process.[90]

By answering the aforementioned four questions, the radiologist can often arrive at a single diagnosis or can at least narrow the differential to a few lesions. Most significant is the distinction between an aggressive and nonaggressive lesion; this is of major importance in guiding further imaging and initial therapy.

Some benign bone tumors are adequately defined by radiography and do not require any further imaging for diagnosis or treatment. Most bone tumors, however, do require additional imaging; this may take the form of CT, MRI, scintigraphy, PET scanning, and rarely even US. The choice of imaging for a given tumor depends on the differential diagnostic considerations, possible treatment options, and whether the lesion is aggressive or nonaggressive. MRI is usually the preferred modality in the delineation of aggressive and suspected malignant lesions, and radiographs followed by MRI adequately define most bone lesions. As opposed to radiography, on MRI an aggressive lesion may have a well-defined margin, particularly with T1 weighting. Although MR is also very good at delineating nonaggressive and likely benign lesions, CT is better able to delineate ossified bone and thus occasionally may better define the characteristics and anatomy of many benign lesions. Image-guided biopsy has become a viable option to determine or confirm the diagnosis of many bone lesions. CT, US, fluoroscopy, and even MRI may be used for guidance.[91-95]

BENIGN BONE TUMORS

The vast majority of pediatric bone tumors are benign. It is important that radiologists recognize the typical benign tumors to avoid unnecessary diagnostic procedures. The differentiation of a nonaggressive lesion from an aggressive lesion will significantly affect the course of subsequent imaging evaluations, the approach to biopsy, and the preliminary choice of definitive treatment.

Cartilaginous Tumors

Osteochondroma (Exostosis)

Overview, Etiologies, Pathophysiology, and Clinical Presentation In pathologic series, osteochondroma is the most common pediatric bone tumor. Rather than a true tumor, osteochondromas are thought to be a developmental defect of growing bone in which an injury to the perichondrium causes bone growth in an aberrant direction. It is theorized that islets of cartilage from the physis are displaced along the metaphyseal surface and then grow. Osteochondromas occur in approximately 1% of the general population. Solitary osteochondroma is slightly more common in boys than girls. Growth ceases at skeletal maturity, and lesions are usually detected in the second decade of life as they grow. Most osteochondromas are asymptomatic and are discovered incidentally. However, a host of complications can occur (Box 139-5). When one of a pair of adjacent bones is affected, the osteochondroma can cause pressure deformity of the other bone. Symptomatic presentations of osteochondroma are usually due to irritation of adjacent muscles, tendons, nerves, or rarely blood vessels.[96,97] Pseudoaneurysm is a rare complication. A bursa may develop over an osteochondroma as a result of inflammation, and a pedunculated osteochondroma may fracture. Presentation with pain as a result of malignant transformation of a solitary osteochondroma in a child is extraordinarily rare.[98,99]

Osteochondromas develop in 6% to 12% of patients who received radiation at a young age. Latent periods vary from 3 to 16 years. Osteochondromas can occur even after low doses of radiation therapy and often occur in bones that were in the periphery of the radiation field. Multiple osteochondromas have been found in patients who received total-body irradiation as preparation for bone marrow transplantation at a young age. Sarcomatous degeneration of radiation-induced osteochondroma is very rare and of no greater incidence than with other osteochondromas.[100]

Patients with hereditary osteochondromatosis (multiple exostoses, diaphyseal aclasis) develop multiple osteochondromas throughout the skeleton. The disorder is autosomal dominant, and 10% of cases arise spontaneously. Patients have a mutation of the *EXT1* gene family that results in an error in regulation of normal chondrocyte proliferation and

Box 139-5 Complications of Osteochondroma

Musculoskeletal Complications

Cosmetic and functional deformity

Pseudo-Madelung deformity

Radial head subluxation/dislocation

Coxa valga

Genu valga

Tibiotalar tilt

Leg-length discrepancy

Decreased range of motion

Impingement syndrome

Muscle/tendon irritation

Tenosynovitis

Snapping tendon

Tendon dislocation

Bursa formation

Synovial (osteo)chondromatosis

Synostosis

Pseudarthrosis

Short stature

Fracture

Vascular Complications

Displacement

Stenosis/occlusion

Claudication

Pseudoaneurysm

Venous compression/deep venous thrombosis/pulmonary embolism

Neurologic Complications

Peripheral nerve compression/entrapment

Cranial neuropathy

Spinal stenosis

Thoracic Complications

Hemothorax

Pneumothorax

Ruptured pericardium

Thoracic outlet syndrome

Dysphagia

Malignant transformation

---

maturation.[101,102] In most patients, the disorder becomes manifest by 10 years of age. The multiplicity of lesions in these patients may lead to substantial deformity. Axial osteochondromas are frequently seen and may cause complications. Small lesions are common on tubular the bones of the hand. Most notable is a pseudo-Madelung deformity of the wrist because of forearm exostoses that cause ulnar shortening and angular deformity of the distal radius. Multiple metaphyseal lesions may interfere with normal modeling of the metaphyses.[103]

Malignant transformation of solitary osteochondromas, even those that are radiation induced, is exceedingly rare and probably occurs in fewer than 1% of patients.[100,104] However, the reported incidence of transformation to chondrosarcoma in patients with hereditary osteochondromatosis is 0.5% to 25%. Wide variation reflects patient selection biases; the actual incidence is probably less than 5%. Malignant transformation does not occur until well after skeletal maturity. Clinical and imaging findings suggestive of malignant transformation include an osteochondroma that grows or begins to produce symptoms after physeal closure, a cartilaginous cap greater than 1.5 to 2 cm thick, indistinct lesion margins, new lucency within an osteochondroma, and an associated soft tissue mass. Chondrosarcomas tend to arise at the periphery of an osteochondroma and are usually of low histologic grade. If a diagnosis of chondrosarcoma is suggested based on pathology in someone in the first or second decade of life, it usually is misdiagnosed as chondroblastic conventional osteosarcoma or periosteal osteosarcoma, which are invariably chondroblastic.[105,106]

Dysplasia epiphysealis hemimelica (DEH), also known as *Trevor disease,* may be a manifestation of epiphyseal osteochondroma. Patients come to medical attention before 15 years of age, and 75% of patients are boys. Patients are seen initially with deformity, swelling, and pain. These patients form osteochondroma-like protuberances from the epiphyses. The lesions are usually confined to one side of the joint (medial more than lateral) and may occasionally involve contiguous joints in one extremity. The lower extremity (femur, tibia, talus) is usually affected, and the most commonly affected region is the ankle and hindfoot.[107] Radiographs show deformity with irregular enlargement of one side of the epiphysis, and MRI is necessary to define the abnormality in younger children, because the lesions may be predominantly cartilaginous. With further ossification in older children, CT is preferred.

Subungual exostosis is a broad-based irregular osteochondroma of the tuft of the finger under the nail bed. The lesion is most common in males in the second decade of life and most commonly affects the great toe. Unlike conventional osteochondroma, there is no medullary continuity of the exostosis with the underlying bone.[108,109]

Imaging On radiography, CT, and MRI, a hallmark of osteochondroma is continuity of the cortex and medullary space from the underlying bone into the lesion. On radiography, osteochondromas are most often found on the long-bone metaphyses, and 35% occur at the knee. Lesions in younger patients tend to be closer to the growth plates. Osteochondromas may also form on the pelvis, ribs, and scapulae; spinal lesions are rare. Underlying metaphyses are broadened as a result of disturbance of normal modeling. The shape of osteochondromas varies from sessile, plaquelike lesions (Fig. 139-15) to pedunculated lesions (Fig. 139-16) with a long stalk. The stalk of a pedunculated lesion is directed away from the adjacent joint. En face, osteochondromas may be mistaken for sclerotic intramedullary lesions.

CT nicely demonstrates the morphology of the lesions and usually confirms the diagnosis; however, MRI much better demonstrates the cartilaginous cap characteristic of the lesion (Fig. 139-17). On T2-weighted images and with other cartilage-sensitive sequences, the cartilaginous cap is seen as a well-defined, thin, high-signal crescent that caps the osteochondroma. The role of MRI is not to define the presence or absence of malignancy but to identify pathologic fractures or overlying soft tissue impingement. Pedunculated osteochondromas tend to fracture and cause soft tissue impingement, whereas sessile osteochondromas tend to only cause soft tissue impingement.[110]

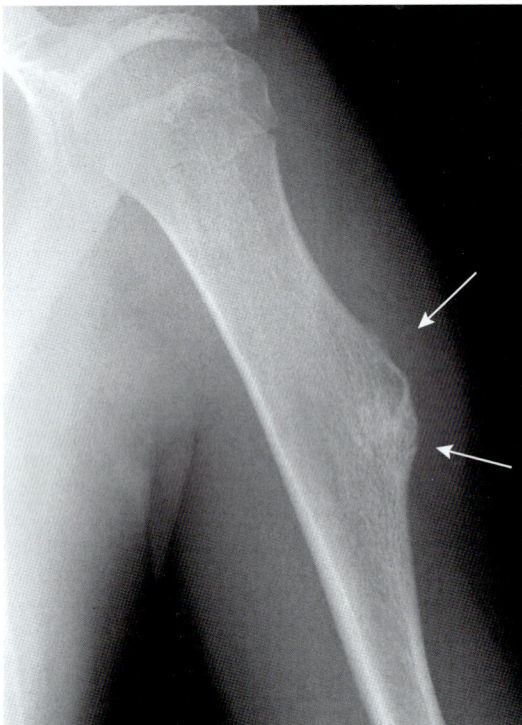

Figure 139-15 Sessile osteochondroma (*arrows*) of the proximal humeral diaphysis in a 16-year-old girl.

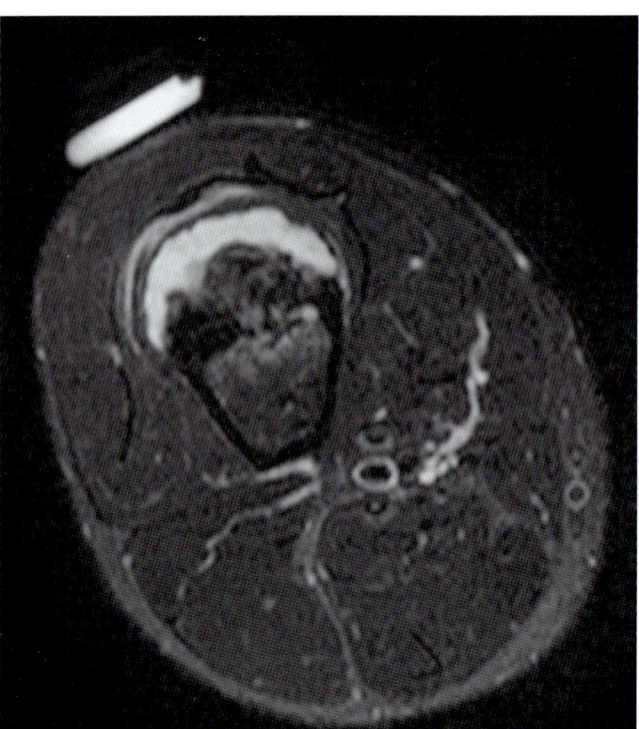

Figure 139-17 Sessile osteochondroma in a 14-year-old boy. T2-weighted magnetic resonance image with fat saturation shows a broad, high-signal cartilaginous cap that covers the osteochondroma. Note the developing, overlying pseudobursa. The anterior cortex under the cartilaginous cap is thickened. An external vitamin E marker was placed anteriorly over the palpable abnormality for localization.

In DEH, radiographs show deformity with irregular enlargement of one side of the epiphysis (Fig. 139-18). MRI is necessary to define the abnormality in younger children, because the lesions may be predominantly cartilaginous. With further ossification in older children, CT is preferred.

Treatment Osteochondromas are treated nonoperatively, unless soft tissue impingement is significant, or the lesion causes biomechanical alignment disorders. Treatment of epiphyseal osteochondromas are problematic, but nonarticular components may be resected. The articular components of epiphyseal osteochondromas usually are smooth, and the affected joint typically adapts over time.[111]

Enchondroma

Overview, Etiologies, Pathophysiology, and Clinical Presentation Enchondromas form owing to a failure of normal endochondral ossification adjacent to a physis. Tumors are composed of cartilage cells derived from the neighboring physis. Enchondromas are most frequently located in the small tubular bones of the hands and feet and in the metaphyses and metadiaphyses of the long bones. Enchondromas represent 80% of primary hand tumors in children and can form in any bone that forms in cartilage. Rib and vertebral lesions are uncommon. Enchondromas become more common with age, with a peak age for diagnosis in the third decade.

Enchondroma protuberans is an enchondroma variant that can resemble either a periosteal chondroma or a sessile osteochondroma (e-Fig. 139-19).[112] It has been described as an exophytic, exaggerated, eccentric from of enchondroma. This tumor arises in the medulla and expands eccentrically through the cortex so that the tumor eventually protrudes beyond it.[113] Rather than a cartilaginous cap, the tumor is covered by a thin layer of cortex and periosteum. This enchondroma

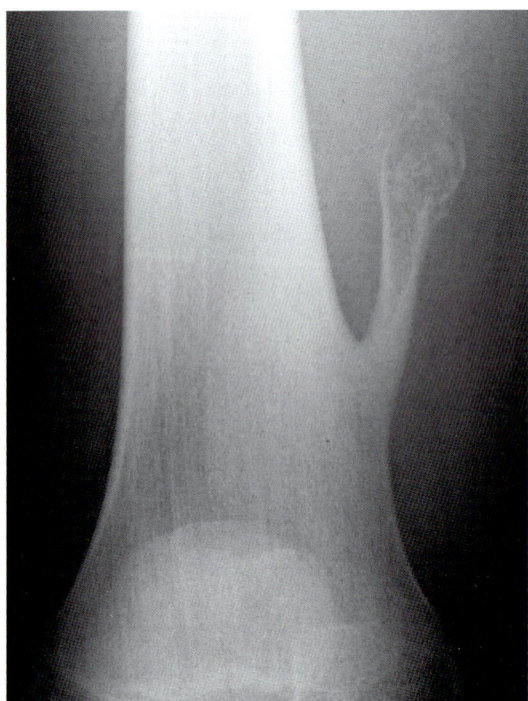

Figure 139-16 Pedunculated osteochondroma of the distal femoral metaphysis in a 14-year-old boy.

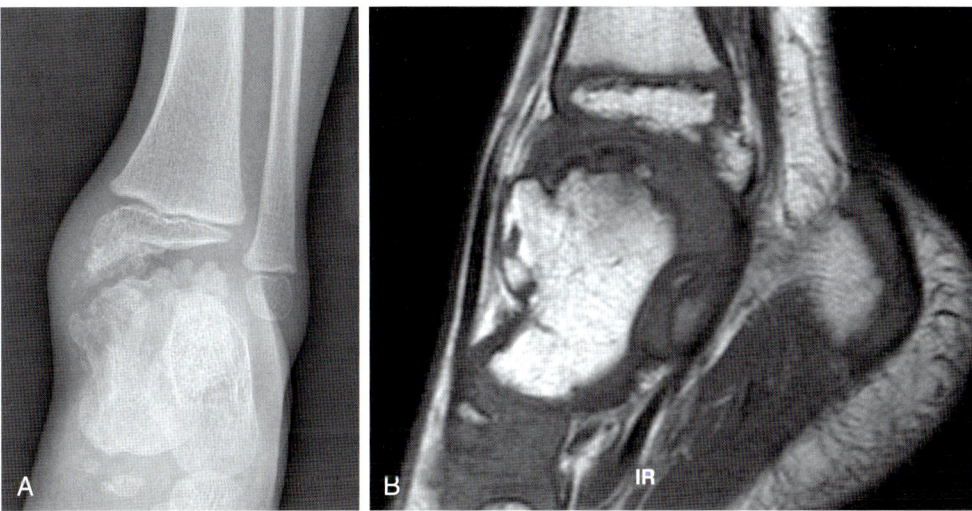

Figure 139-18 Trevor disease (dysplasia epiphysealis hemimelica) in a 3-year-old boy. **A,** Radiography demonstrates "kissing" epiphyseal osteochondromas at the level of the tibiotalar joint. **B,** T1-weighted sagittal magnetic resonance image shows talar marrow continuity with the epiphyseal osteochondromas.

variant most commonly occurs in the proximal humerus and in the hand.[114]

Ollier disease (enchondromatosis) is a nonheritable disorder of cartilage proliferation in which enchondromas involve multiple bones. It is a mesodermal dysplasia and broader dyschondrogenesis that can affect any part of endochondrally formed bones, and it is more common in boys. Enchondromas form in any bone with a physis, although the hands may be disparately affected and may be grotesquely deformed. Enchondromas are bilateral but usually asymmetric in severity. Onset during infancy or early childhood may result in severe skeletal deformity. Enchondromas may interfere with growth plate function and may lead to limb shortening. The lesions of Ollier disease are expansile and lucent or trabeculated, usually with a shell of thin cortex. In the long bones, longitudinal lucent columns or streaks are characteristic.

Enchondromatosis accompanied by vascular malformations is known as *Maffucci syndrome,* which is also nonhereditary and a form of mesodermal dysplasia. The vascular malformations are predominantly venous but may be capillary and occasionally lymphatic. Calcified phleboliths may be demonstrated radiographically in the vascular soft tissue masses.

Malignant transformation is extremely rare with a solitary enchondroma, particularly in childhood. Unlike in adults, chondrosarcoma is very rare in children. Approximately 5% of patients with chondrosarcoma have Ollier disease. Patients with Maffucci syndrome also have an increased risk of central nervous system and intraabdominal malignancy.

Metachondromatosis is a very rare disorder that is a combination of enchondromatosis and osteochondromatosis.[115]

Imaging On radiography, as with other cartilaginous tumors, enchondromas exhibit a lobulated growth pattern that results in asymmetric expansion of the medullary cavity and endosteal scalloping (e-Fig. 139-20). The lesions may have characteristic channel-lytic lucencies that are perpendicular to the physis. Lesions are oval, well-circumscribed, and lucent with thin eggshell-like margins (Fig. 139-21). Focal, punctate calcifications may be evident on radiographs but are better appreciated with CT. The cartilaginous "ring and arc" pattern may be seen on CT. Margins of the lesion are sclerotic. The lesion may scallop the endosteum, erode cortex, and expand or distort the bone. Periosteal reaction is absent. The tumor is isointense with muscle on T1-weighted MRI and exhibits a heterogeneous, predominantly high T2-weighted signal. Signal intensity of the lesion parallels cartilage on all sequences. Enhancement with gadolinium varies; some lesions enhance peripherally, whereas others enhance more homogeneously. Adjacent bone marrow edema and enhancement are typically absent, but bone scans typically show increased activity.[116]

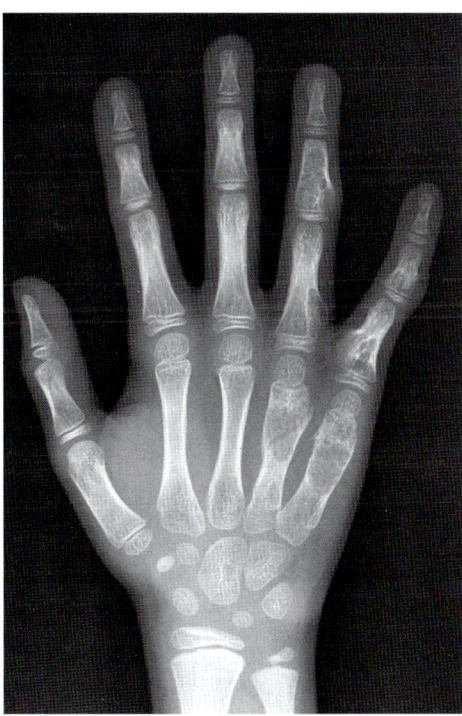

Figure 139-21 Enchondromatosis in a 13-year-old girl. Multiple, well-defined, lucent, expansile lesions are present in the metacarpals and phalanges of the ring and little fingers. A pathologic fracture is seen through an enchondroma in the distal fourth metacarpal.

Treatment Enchondromas are managed nonoperatively and do not need to be longitudinally followed by imaging, unless new symptoms of pain or a pathologic fracture occur. These lesions do not need to be biopsied to confirm diagnosis.

Periosteal (Juxtacortical) Chondroma

Overview, Etiologies, Pathophysiology, and Clinical Presentation This rare tumor is a surface variant of an enchondroma that arises from the periosteal surface of the cortex of the large and small tubular bones. One theory holds that the tumor is posttraumatic in origin, located under the periosteum and external to the cortex. Some tumors, such as within the femoral neck, are not covered with periosteum and are better labeled "juxtacortical." Periosteal chondroma most commonly occurs in the proximal humerus metaphysis, phalanges of the hands and feet, femur, and proximal tibia. Patients are usually 10 to 30 years of age, and peak incidence is in the second decade of life; most come to medical attention with mild pain and swelling.[117] The lesion is more frequent in boys, and periosteal chondromas may be seen in patients with Ollier disease.

Periosteal chondroma does not have malignant potential, but biopsy may be advisable to distinguish it from periosteal osteosarcoma.

Imaging Radiographically, although periosteal chondroma may bear superficial similarity to a sessile osteochondroma, it is associated with sclerosis and external cortical scalloping, forming a periosteal shelf (e-Fig. 139-22). Focal calcifications of matrix within the lesion may be seen. Cross-sectional imaging delineates the underlying cortex and clearly distinguishes the lesion from a sessile osteochondroma. CT may show chondroid calcification (Fig. 139-23). MRI shows chondroid composition of the lesion, and peripheral enhancement is usually seen with gadolinium.[118] The tumor is usually 1 to 3 cm in size. A shell of reactive bone may be seen around the lesion, adjacent cortex is eroded or saucerized, and reactive bone sclerosis and buttressing is seen.

Treatment These benign lesions require biopsy to distinguish them from periosteal osteosarcomas. Lesions do not need to be longitudinally followed by imaging after histologic diagnosis, because they are benign.

Chondroblastoma

Overview, Etiologies, Pathophysiology, and Clinical Presentation Chondroblastoma, an uncommon tumor composed of primitive cartilage cells, usually occurs in the second decade of life. Roughly half occur before the physes close. The most specific feature of chondroblastoma is its location in the epiphysis of a long bone, most often the proximal humerus, distal femur, or proximal tibia. Chondroblastoma may also occur in epiphyseal equivalent regions such as apophyses, the patella, and carpal and tarsal bones. Larger lesions often may extend into an adjacent metaphysis.[119] Up to 15% of chondroblastomas have a component of aneurysmal bone cyst (ABC). Larger lesions may extend into an adjacent metaphysis, particularly in skeletally mature patients. The tumor evokes a striking inflammatory response, which may help to distinguish it from other lesions.[120,121]

Included in the differential diagnoses for a lucent epiphyseal lesion in a child are chondroblastoma, osteomyelitis, and, after physeal closure, giant cell tumor (GCT).

Imaging Radiographically, a chondroblastoma is seen as an eccentric, lucent, well-defined smooth or lobulated lesion with sclerotic borders within an epiphysis or epiphyseal equivalent (Fig. 139-24). The lesion may expand the bone, but the cortex is usually intact. Periosteal reaction distant from the lesion is another common feature suggestive of an accompanying inflammatory process.[122] Periosteal reaction on an adjacent metaphysis is seen in 30% to 50% of cases.

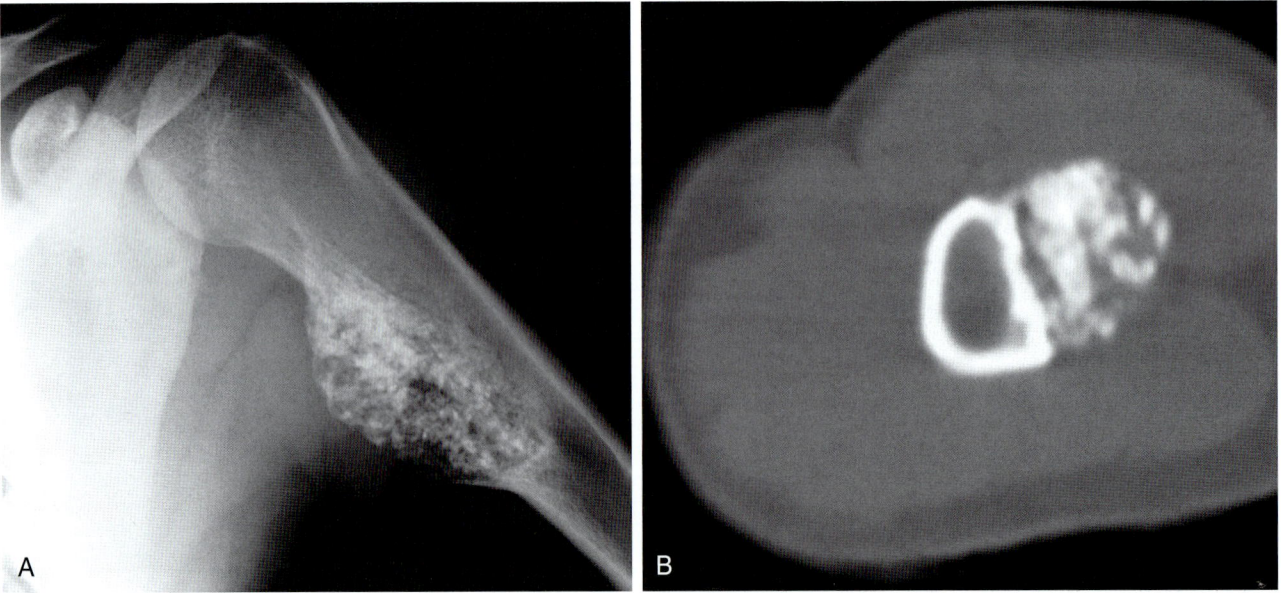

Figure 139-23 Periosteal chondroma in a 19-year-old girl. **A,** Anteroposterior view of the humerus shows a broad-based tumor with a lobular mineralized matrix. **B,** Computed tomography shows the superficial nature of the lesion, which is separated from the medulla by cortical bone.

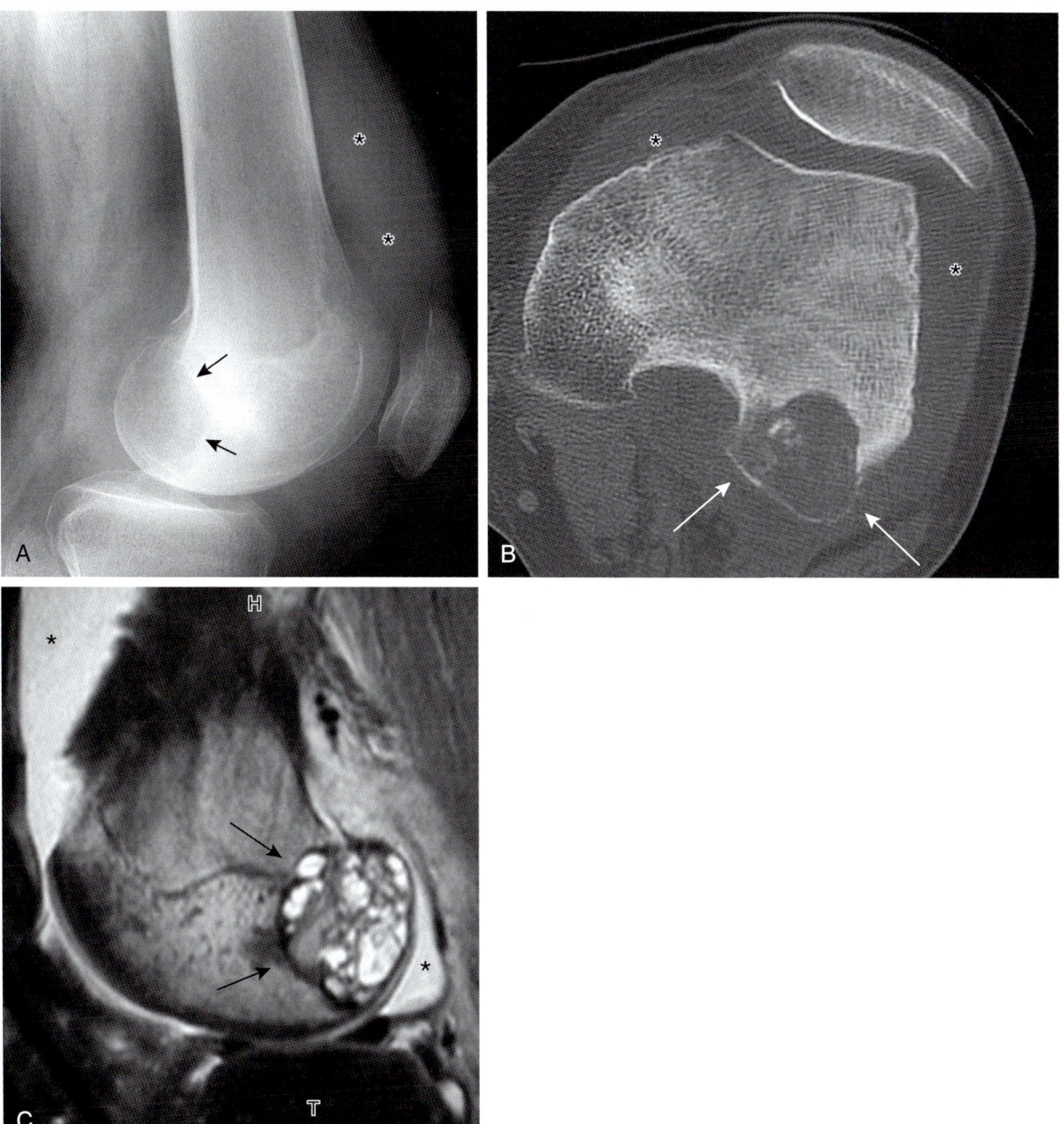

Figure 139-24 Chondroblastoma in a 17-year-old boy. **A,** Radiograph shows a lucent lesion within the posterior aspect of the lateral femoral condyle (*arrows*). An effusion distends the suprapatellar pouch (*asterisks*). **B,** Computed tomography image shows a well-defined lesion (*arrows*) with some calcified cartilaginous matrix and effusion (*asterisks*). **C,** Sagittal T2-weighted magnetic resonance image with fat saturation shows the lesion to be of mixed high-signal intensity with multiple cysts consistent with secondary aneurysmal bone cyst formation (*arrows*). Note internal regions of low signal intensity consistent with chondroid matrix. Bone marrow edema is seen in the femur (compare with the tibia (T)). Knee-joint effusion (*asterisk*) and adjacent soft tissue edema are noted.

Approximately one third of chondroblastomas have a calcified chondroid matrix. This is better demonstrated by CT, which may also show cortical destruction (see Fig. 139-24). On MRI, chondroblastoma typically parallels cartilage signal intensity on all sequences. Signal intensity varies with the degree of calcification in the lesion. The rim of the tumor may have a lower intensity, and some foci give no signal because of calcification. Adjacent inflammatory changes consist of bone marrow and soft tissue edema and joint effusion and are usually prominent (see Fig. 139-24).[123,124]

Chondroblastomas superficially will mimic an epiphyseal Brodie abscess. MRI is useful in this circumstance. Both chondroblastomas and epiphyseal Brodie abscesses may demonstrate exuberant adjacent marrow and soft tissue edema, effusions, and reactive bone proliferation. However, on post-contrast imaging, chondroblastomas will demonstrate central enhancement, whereas Brodie abscesses will not.[125]

Treatment Chondroblastomas are treated with curettage and bone grafting. Approximately 20% of lesions recur. Otherwise, the prognosis is good. There are rare reports of metastatic chondroblastoma.

Chondromyxoid Fibroma

Overview, Etiologies, Pathophysiology, and Clinical Presentation Chondromyxoid fibroma (CMF) is a benign rare tumor that predominantly affects males in the second or third decade of life. Patients come to medical attention with pain. The lesion is a rubbery mix of fibrous, myxoid, and chondroid tissue. CMF most frequently arises within ilium, long bones at the knee, and tubular bones of the foot, although the proximal tibia is the most common site. The tumor is metaphyseal and often extends into metadiaphysis, but very rarely does it extend past a physis.[126,127]

Imaging On radiography, CMF has a characteristic but nonspecific appearance of a solitary, eccentric, lucent, well-defined lesion with sclerotic margins, and septations may be evident within the lesion. In the short bones of the hands and feet, the lesion appears more central. The underlying cortex may be expanded, thinned, and occasionally absent. The lesion may appear bubbly, similar to an ABC.[128] Most lesions are elongated and oriented parallel to the long axis of the involved bone (Fig. 139-25). Matrix calcification and periosteal new bone formation usually do not occur. On MRI, CMF produces variable and often heterogeneous signal intensity depending on the composition of the lesion. In general, the lesion is of low signal on T1- and intermediate to high signal on T2-weighted imaging.[126]

Treatment Treatment of CMF is excision, and 25% of lesions recur. Multiple recurrences are common.

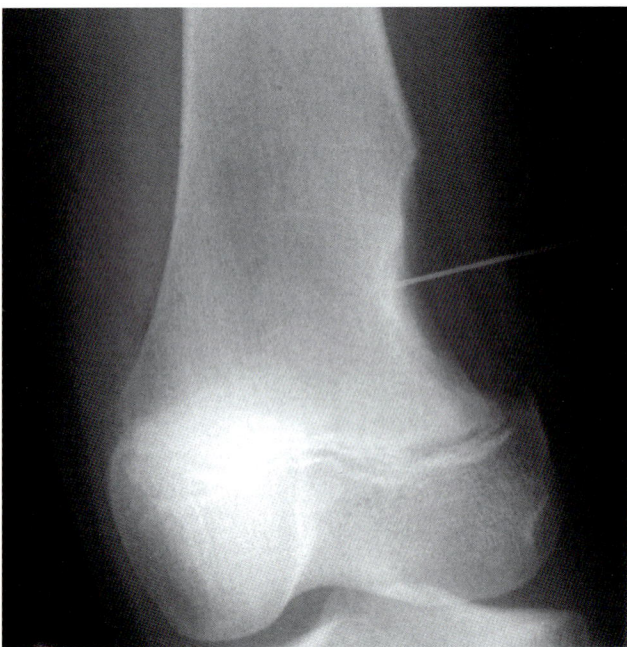

Figure 139-25 Chondromyxoid fibroma in a 14-year-old boy. The lesion has produced a well-defined scalloped defect in the distal tibial metaphysis. A biopsy needle is shown.

Cysts

Simple Bone Cyst

Overview, Etiologies, Pathophysiology, and Clinical Presentation A simple bone cyst is also referred to as a *solitary cyst* or *unicameral bone cyst* (UBC), although the latter term is a misnomer, because these cysts may be septated. One theory holds that bone cysts arise because of a defect in endochondral bone formation or altered hemodynamics with venous occlusion that elevates intraosseous pressure and leads to cyst formation. Bone cysts have a membrane of loose vascular connective tissue and contain osteoclast-like giant cells and accumulations of fibrinoid material. The cyst space is usually filled with yellow, sometimes bloody fluid.

Cysts are more common in boys than girls by threefold, and 75% are seen in patients younger than 25 years of age; 25% are found incidentally. Bone cysts typically occur centrally in the metaphyses of the long bones and most commonly involve the proximal humerus (50%) and proximal femur (20%). Cysts have an "active phase," during which they increase in size and remain in close proximity to the physis. "Latent phase" cysts are found farther from the physis and usually do not continue to grow. Cysts may appear to "migrate" into the diaphysis, but actually it is the growth plate that migrates away from the cyst. In older patients, pelvic and calcaneal bone cysts become more common.[129]

Solitary UBCs are occasionally found in the calcanei of pediatric patients.[130] Often, these cysts are painless and are first detected by radiography of acute injuries to the feet. Calcaneal bone cysts are nearly always located near the base of the neck of the calcaneus. The thin, overlying lateral cortical wall of the calcaneus forms a well-defined bony border that allows differentiation from the "physiologic" pseudocystic radiolucent areas observed in the same region of normal bones.

Bone cysts are asymptomatic unless complicated by fracture; however, 75% of patients come in with a pathologic fracture. Bone cysts are the most common cause of pathologic fracture in children.

Imaging On radiography, bone cysts have a central, medullary location within the metaphysis. Most cysts are less than 3 cm in diameter but may be much larger in long axis. The cyst wall is well defined and sclerotic; the overlying cortex is thinned, and the lesion may be mildly expansile.[131] With fracture, a fragment of bone may be seen dependently within the cyst. This "fallen fragment" sign is considered pathognomonic for a simple bone cyst (Fig. 139-26). CT delineates the cyst and confirms a fallen fragment, but the study is rarely necessary. In atypical cases, MRI is performed and confirms the cystic nature of the lesion. The fluid contents are low signal on T1- and high signal on T2-weighted imaging. With contrast, the cyst lining enhances, but the contents do not (Fig. 139-27).[132]

Occasionally, with preceding intralesional hemorrhage from fracture, fluid-fluid levels may be seen that represent settled, degraded blood products. When UBCs heal after pathologic fracture, they may have multiple septations and fluid-fluid levels within them, and they may superficially mimic an ABC. As a general rule, if the lesion diameter is smaller than the thickest diameter of the affected bone, the lesion should be considered a complicated UBC. If the lesion

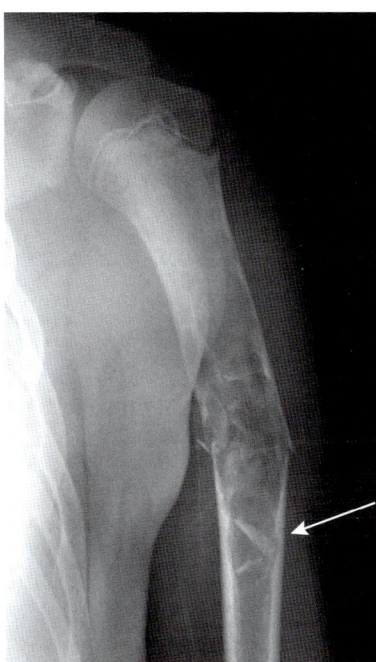

Figure 139-26 Simple bone cyst with pathologic fracture in a 12-year-old boy. The cyst has thinned and scalloped the overlying cortex. A fallen fragment is noted (*arrow*).

diameter is greater than the thickest diameter of the affected bone, an ABC should be considered.

Treatment Fractured cysts tend to heal spontaneously; however, larger cysts with or without fracture are usually treated with curettage and bone grafting. The prognosis is excellent, although 35% to 50% of bone cysts recur, in some cases multiple times. Treated cysts often have a complex appearance with mixed sclerosis and lucency, septations, and mild expansion and deformity of the involved bone. Premature growth plate closure may occur as a complication of treatment or pathologic fracture but not as a result of the cyst itself. Cyst aspiration with corticosteroid injection or sclerotherapy has also been used for treatment.

Aneurysmal Bone Cyst

Overview, Etiologies, Pathophysiology, and Clinical Presentation ABC is a pseudolesion that occurs as a result of intraosseous or subperiosteal hemorrhage, or it occurs as a transitional lesion secondary to an underlying primary bone tumor. Histologically an ABC is composed of anastomosing channels that contain blood and are variably lined with fibrous walls that contain red blood cells, hemosiderin granules, foreign body giant cells, and spicules of reactive bone. The etiology of an ABC is poorly understood and may be primary or, more commonly, secondary and/or reactive. A wide variety of lesions may act as the nidus for ABC development, and underlying lesions are pathologically identified in one third of cases. A large ABC may obscure the underlying lesion, or it may represent only a small component of a larger tumor. In lesions without an underlying tumor, the role of antecedent trauma acting as a nidus has been proposed. ABC is slightly more common in girls. Whether primary or

secondary, the lesion is most common in the first three decades of life, and it is rare in patients younger than 5 years. Patients usually come to medical attention with nonspecific pain and swelling, and 10% come in with pathologic fracture.[133] ABC is most common in the metaphyses of long bones, the craniofacial bones, and the spine; spinal lesions occur in the posterior elements. Long-bone lesions can be subclassified as either *intramedullary* or *juxtacortical* (cortical or subperiosteal). A subperiosteal ABC is rare and mimics other subperiosteal tumors and pathologies.[134-136]

An unusual solid variant of ABC has radiographic features similar to those of the typical ABC.[137,138] The solid variant lacks cavernous, blood-containing spaces and is characterized histologically by the solid elements—proliferating fibrous tissue, benign giant cells, and newly formed osteoid matrix—found in typical ABCs. A third of these tumors are not "aneurysmal." The solid variant of ABCs is histologically indistinguishable from extragnathic giant cell (reparative) granuloma. It is most common in the second and third decade. The lesion favors the axial skeleton over appendicular locations, and the most common locations are in the craniofacial bones, small tubular bones of the hands and feet, and the femur.

Imaging On radiography, ABC appears as a lucent, expansile, "blowout" or "soap-bubble" lesion with thin, smooth, bony walls (e-Figs. 139-28 and 139-29). As a general rule, if the lesion diameter is greater than the widest part of the affected normal bone, an ABC should be considered (see e-Fig. 28). If the diameter is less than the widest part of the

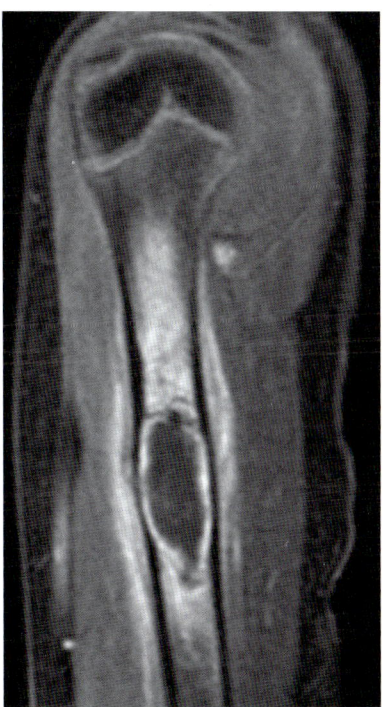

Figure 139-27 Simple bone cyst in an 8-year-old boy. Sagittal T1-weighted magnetic resonance image with fat saturation post gadolinium shows a lesion that contains fluid with an enhancing rim. Enhancement is also seen in the adjacent marrow and soft tissues. The degree of enhancement is increased in this patient owing to a healing pathologic fracture through the lesion.

affected normal bone, a UBC should be considered. Lesions are multiloculated, and the cortex is usually intact but may be markedly thinned to the point of being invisible, and periosteal new bone may be present. Both CT and MRI demonstrate fluid-fluid levels (see e-Fig. 139-28, *B*), which are characteristic of the lesion.[139,140] This finding is due to sedimentation of degraded blood products, especially methemoglobin, which has a much shorter T1 relaxation time than that of hemoglobin. Fluid-fluid levels may be single or multiple and may be seen as varying horizontal levels within separate loculations (see e-Figs. 139-28 and 139-29). If the loculations are very small, fluid-fluid levels may be less apparent. The signal characteristics of the cyst contents are variable and are probably dependent on the relative age and concentration of the blood components. Abundant hemosiderin may produce foci of low signal, which may be diffuse throughout the lesion. Cyst contents do not enhance, but the septations do.

It may not be possible to differentiate primary and secondary ABCs. Secondary ABCs can occur with numerous benign and malignant bone lesions, including fibrous dysplasia, chondroblastoma, GCT, nonossifying fibroma, simple bone cyst, and osteosarcoma, particularly the telangiectatic variant.[141,142] Any solid component suggests an underlying tumor. Lesions composed of a greater percentage composition of fluid-fluid levels are more likely benign in origin. Differentiation of ABC from telangiectatic osteosarcoma is particularly difficult and at times cannot be achieved by imaging. Greater bone destruction may be evident with telangiectatic osteosarcoma. It should be noted that ABC may also develop within a conventional osteosarcoma

On MRI, solid ABCs demonstrate low signal on both T1 and T2 images because of fibrosis. The lesion enhances with gadolinium. The solid variant of ABC may occasionally produce osteoid that may be evident on radiographs or CT.

Treatment ABC is treated with curettage and bone grafting, although 20% of ABCs recur after grafting. Vascular embolization and percutaneous sclerotherapy have also been used. The utility of MRI is to identify any solid components to direct the surgeon for biopsy.

Giant Cell Tumor

Overview, Etiologies, Pathophysiology, and Clinical Presentation GCT, also known as *osteoclastoma,* is an uncommon neoplasm that rarely occurs before skeletal maturity. Approximately 5% of cases are reported before skeletal maturity,[143] most in the second decade, and rarely in the first decade of life.[144] The lesion is most common in the long bones, particularly the distal femur and proximal tibia; it is less common in the short bones of the hands and feet, and in children, it rarely occurs elsewhere.[145] In skeletally mature individuals, the lesion is uniformly within the epiphysis with variable extension into the adjacent metaphysis. Epiphyseal lesions abut the articular surface. In skeletally immature patients, the lesion is almost uniformly metaphyseal and usually abuts the physis. Epiphyseal involvement is very rare before physeal closure, and multifocal GCT is very rare in children. Patients with GCT come to medical attention with pain and tenderness, swelling, and limited range of motion of the adjacent joint.[146]

Imaging On radiographs, GCT appears as a geographic, lytic lesion (Fig. 139-30). Margins vary from sclerotic to ill defined. Frequently, a relatively sharp but nonsclerotic margin is apparent. Periosteal new bone, expansion of bone, and pathologic fracture are common. The metaphyseal end of the lesion tends to be less well defined, although CT delineates the lesion and its margins. No calcified or ossified matrix is seen.

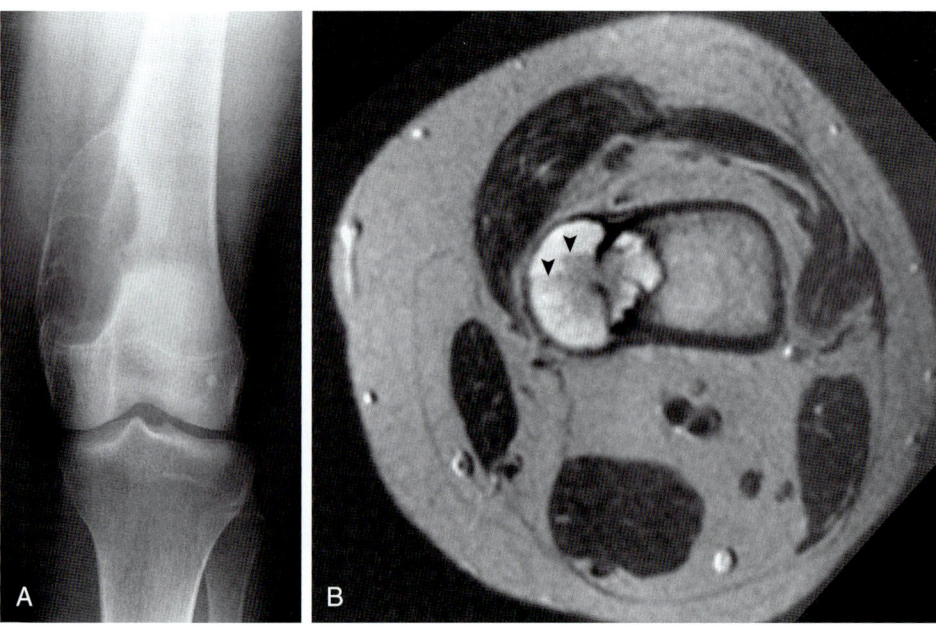

Figure 139-29 Aneurysmal bone cyst in a 13-year-old. **A,** Radiograph of the knee shows an eccentric, expansile, lucent lesion with a thin, bony shell that involves the medial aspect of the distal femur. **B,** On a transverse T2-weighted magnetic resonance image, the lesion is seen to penetrate the cortex of the femur and extend into the adjacent soft tissues. Several fluid-fluid levels are demonstrated (*arrowheads*).

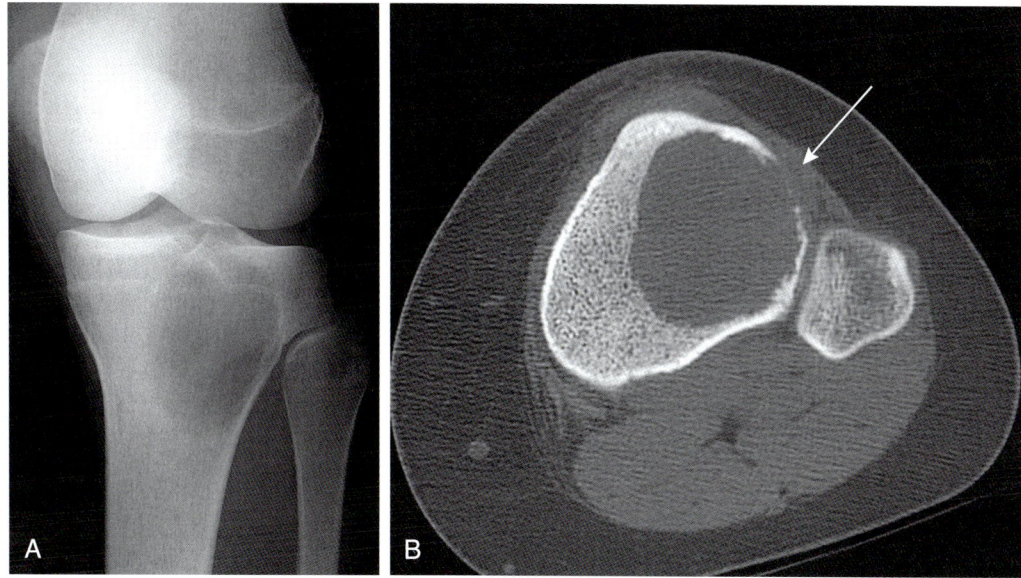

Figure 139-30   Giant cell tumor in a 14-year-old girl. **A,** Radiograph shows a relatively well-defined lucent lesion in the proximal tibial metaphysis and epiphysis. The lesion does not have sclerotic margins and is near the articular surface but does not abut it. **B,** Axial computed tomography shows a large lucent lesion of the tibia. The lesion margins are well-defined but not sclerotic. The anterolateral cortex is destroyed (*arrow*).

MRI findings vary. In one large series, 56% of tumors were solid or solid with cystic change, and 44% were cystic.[143] Solid areas tend to have intermediate T1 and T2 signal. Hemosiderin from intratumoral hemorrhage may produce foci of low signal. Occasionally, a GCT may have a more aggressive appearance, with cortical penetration and soft tissue extension. Approximately 15% of GCTs have an associated component of ABC and appear more expansile.[147] The prognosis of GCT is excellent, although up to 25% of tumors recur locally. Malignant GCT and metastasizing GCT have rarely been reported in children. The pulmonary "implants" from GCT are usually of self-limiting growth potential, but recurrence and disease progression is possible.[148]

Treatment   For resectable GCTs, en bloc excision has a lower recurrence rate compared with intralesional curettage.[149] The local recurrence rate with en bloc resection is approximately 20%, compared with 50% for intralesional curettage.

Fibrous Tumors

Fibrous Cortical Defect and Nonossifying Fibroma (Fibroxanthoma)

Overview, Etiologies, Pathophysiology, and Clinical Presentation   Fibrous cortical defect (FCD) and nonossifying fibroma (NOF) are extremely common tumors that occur in the metaphyses of the long bones of children. FCDs are essentially a normal variant and are found in up to 40% of children during development. FCD and NOF are histologically identical and are composed of highly cellular stroma with spindle-shaped fibroblasts, osteoclast-like multinucleated giant cells, and foam or xanthoma cells. Arbitrarily, lesions smaller than 2 cm are considered an FCD, and those larger than 2 cm are called NOFs. Lesions probably represent a developmental defect in the periosteum of cortical bone and are seen in the latter part of the first decade until shortly after skeletal maturation. The average time from diagnosis to spontaneous regression is 29 to 52 months; lesions become inactive after skeletal maturity, although rarely, an NOF may persist into adulthood.[150,151]

FCD and NOF are usually detected incidentally. The lesions are asymptomatic, with the exception of very large lesions, which may cause dull pain. Uncommonly, an NOF may be large enough to cause a pathologic fracture or lead to a stress fracture. FCD and NOF are most common in the metaphyses of the long bones of the lower extremity, especially at the knee. Lesions are more commonly posterior. FCDs and cortical desmoids of the posteromedial distal femoral metaphysis are histologically similar.[152]

Multiple NOFs may be seen with neurofibromatosis. In Jaffe-Campanacci syndrome, disseminated NOFs are associated with cystic lesions of the jaw, café-au-lait skin lesions, mental retardation, ocular anomalies, hypogonadism, and cardiovascular anomalies in the absence of other signs of neurofibromatosis. There is debate that Jaffe-Campanacci syndrome is a *forme fruste* of neurofibromatosis.[153-156]

Imaging   On radiography, FCDs are seen as small, well-defined, ovoid, cortically based lesions. NOFs appear to be similar but are larger (Fig. 139-31), more lobular, and multilocular with a characteristic "soap bubble" appearance. Usually, the lesions extend inward; however, the outer cortex may be thinned and bulging. In thinner bones, such as the fibula, the lesion may occupy the entire width of the bone. FCDs and NOFs originate in metaphysis near the growth plate and migrate into metadiaphysis and diaphysis with maturation, and their radiographic appearance is sufficiently specific that neither additional imaging nor biopsy is indicated.

The radiographic features of FCD and NOF are also manifest on CT. On MRI, lesions are well defined, lobular, and cortically based. Low signal is seen on T1, and T2 signal and enhancement with gadolinium varies with the stage of

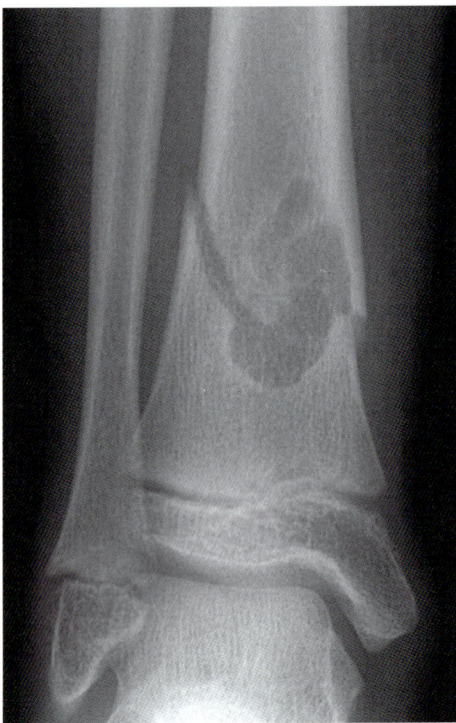

Figure 139-31 Pathologic fracture through a nonossifying fibroma in a 10-year-old boy. The lesion has well-defined, minimally sclerotic margins.

lesion development. Active, early lesions are high signal on T2-weighted imaging, and they enhance. Involuting lesions are low signal on T2 and do not enhance, and no peritumoral edema is seen.[157] Active, early lesions may also show uptake on bone scans and PET scans.[158]

Treatment The natural history of the lesions is for involution to occur with progressive sclerosis of the lesion.

Fibrous Dysplasia

Overview, Etiologies, Pathophysiology, and Clinical Presentation Although it is not a true neoplasm, fibrous dysplasia that involves a long bone may mimic a bone tumor or cyst, especially when it causes localized expansion of the bone and is monostotic.[159] Pathologically, fibro-osseous tissue replaces the normal medullary space. Fibrous dysplasia can be monostotic or polyostotic and monomelic or polymelic, although 70% to 80% of cases are monostotic. Fibrous dysplasia is more common in girls than in boys, and most patients with focal disease are adolescents or young adults, but patients are occasionally seen in the first decade of life. Any bone may be affected. The most common presentation is monostotic disease that affects craniofacial bones, especially the skull base; a long bone, most commonly the femur; or a rib. Lesions may involve metaphysis and diaphysis but spare the epiphysis before physeal fusion. Patients with solitary lesions come to medical attention with pain, edema, deformity, or pathologic or fatigue fracture. Patients with polyostotic disease are seen with similar signs and symptoms, but often at a younger age (i.e., first decade). Polyostotic disease predominates on one side, is often syndrome related, and may be suspected based on other clinical findings.[160,161]

In 2% to 3% of patients, fibrous dysplasia is associated with endocrine disorders, mostly of hypothalamic dysfunction. In McCune-Albright syndrome, female patients are seen with precocious puberty, cutaneous café-au-lait spots, and unilateral polyostotic fibrous dysplasia. Mazabraud syndrome, characterized by polyostotic fibrous dysplasia and intramuscular myxoma, is rare in children.[162]

Imaging Fibrous dysplasia in the long bones causes expansion of the medullary cavity, endosteal scalloping, coarse trabeculation, and sclerotic margins that form a "rind." Bowing of the affected bone may occur. In the femur, the resulting deformity is called a *shepherd's crook* (Fig. 139-32).

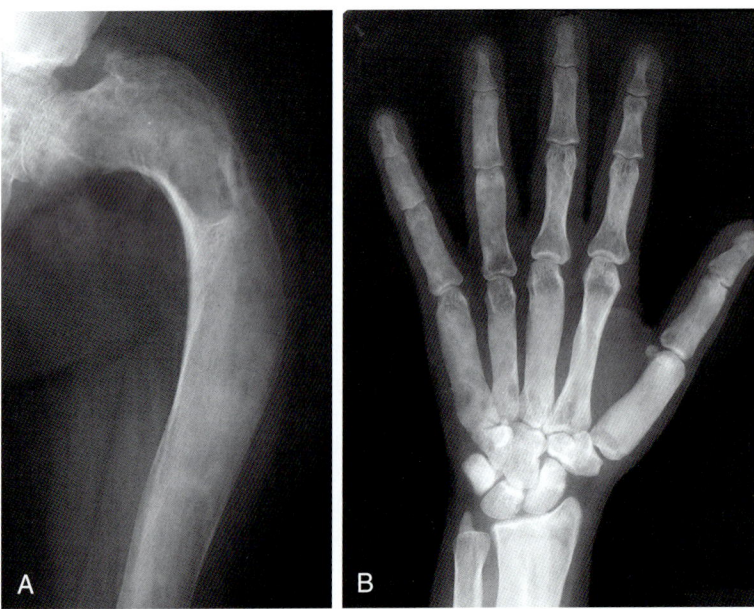

Figure 139-32 Polyostotic fibrous dysplasia in a 22-year-old woman. **A,** The femur is expanded and bowed with a "shepherd's crook" deformity. The femoral trabeculae are replaced by "ground glass" matrix. **B,** Diffuse sclerosis is seen in the hand and wrist with mild expansion and indistinct transition from cortex to medullary space.

Lesions may be central or eccentric. Because the radiographic opacity of a fibrous dysplasia lesion depends on the relative amount of dysplastic bone and fibrous material within the lesion, the appearance varies, from having the look of ground glass to appearing radiolucent. The ground-glass appearance is due to matrix that contains a fine meshlike pattern of delicate bone spicules (Fig. 139-33; see also Fig. 132). It is relatively specific for fibrous dysplasia but may be simulated by other lesions that replace the medullary trabeculae. Lucent lesions usually have a sclerotic margin, and small cartilaginous foci within the lesion may develop chondroid calcification (osteocartilaginous fibrous dysplasia). In addition, a single lesion or involved bone may demonstrate varying appearances within different areas. Active, early lesions tend to be radiolucent, whereas older lesions may be more sclerotic. No periosteal reaction is present unless there is a fracture. Similar findings are visible with CT.

On MRI, lesions are similar in signal intensity to muscle on T1-weighted imaging. On T2, lesion signal intensity varies depending on the composition of the lesion; pure fibrous tissue is hypointense on T2. However, lesions of fibrous dysplasia are often hyperintense[163] because of the inhomogeneous nature of the lesion, which consists of spindle cells, trabeculae of immature woven bone with osteoid seams, and small cysts. Fluid-fluid levels have been reported,[164] but soft tissue extension is rare. Central or, less frequently, peripheral enhancement may occur with gadolinium, and lesion uptake on bone scans is variable and may even be normal. Fibrous dysplasia lesions of the face or skull may be quite debilitating and clinically challenging.

Treatment Treatment is supportive for this benign lesion. Imaging findings are diagnostic, and biopsy is rarely necessary. Surgical treatment is predicated on the presence or absence of pathologic fracture or impending biomechanical failure.

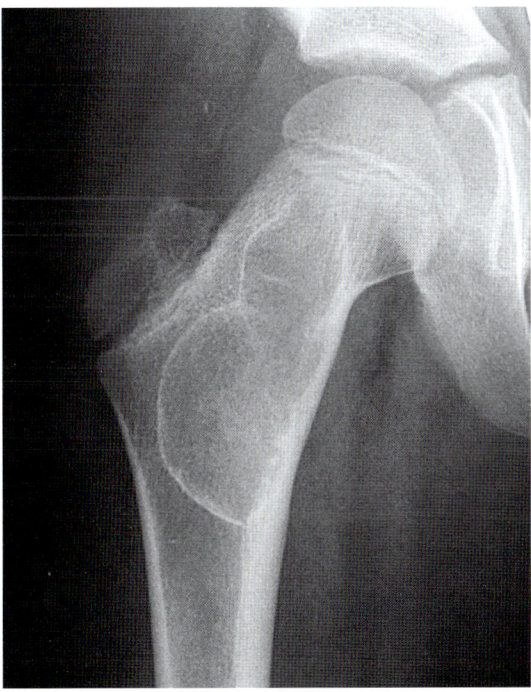

Figure 139-33 Focal fibrous dysplasia in an 11-year-old boy. The lesion has well-defined, sclerotic margins and a ground-glass matrix.

Orthopedic implants are used to reinforce and stabilize affected bones.

Osteofibrous Dysplasia

Overview, Etiologies, Pathophysiology, and Clinical Presentation Osteofibrous dysplasia (OFD), also known as *extragnathic ossifying fibroma* or *intracortical fibrous dysplasia,* is a proliferation of fibro-osseous tissue. OFD is usually sporadic, although a kindred with six affected members by autosomal-dominant inheritance has been reported.[165] Most cases occur during the first decade of life, and some tumors have been found in newborns.[166,167] OFD is a rare lesion that is usually confined to the diaphysis and metadiaphysis of the tibia but can also involve the fibula, sometimes synchronously in the same patient. Rarely, lesions may be multiple and bilateral. OFD is usually painless and is characterized by deformity that can progress until physeal fusion occurs. Patients may come to medical attention with anterior bowing, and fracture or pseudoarthrosis may complicate the disease's course.

OFD is histologically similar to fibrous dysplasia in that it contains well-differentiated fibroblasts, collagen, and bony trabeculae. The main differentiating feature is the presence of active osteoblasts in OFD. Differentiated adamantinoma and adamantinoma are closely related to OFD, because they share similar histochemical properties.[168] Especially in the second decade, radiologic and even pathologic distinction between OFD, differentiated adamantinoma, and adamantinoma is difficult, although OFD tends to occur at a younger age than adamantinoma. This differentiation is discussed later in this chapter.

Imaging By radiography, OFD is an eccentric, lucent, solitary or multiloculated lesion that involves the anterior cortex of the tibia (Fig. 139-34). The lesion may be rounded in appearance or ovoid and may be longitudinally oriented with the tibial shaft; it may be purely intraosseous, or it may have a minor extraosseous component. Involvement of the tibia is more commonly proximal, but distal lesions occur and may be complicated by pseudarthrosis. The cortex is expanded, and larger lesions will expand posteriorly and may replace the medullary cavity. Lesions appear lucent or similar to ground glass and are associated with cortical thickening and anterior bowing of the bone. Cross-sectional imaging is very helpful in determining the lesion's intracortical location, an important feature in distinguishing OFD from fibrous dysplasia, which is intramedullary.

Long-Bone Adamantinoma

Overview, Etiologies, Pathophysiology, and Clinical Presentation Long-bone adamantinomas are rare tumors in children, and patients are often seen initially with pain and anterior tibial bowing.[169] As opposed to OFD, adamantinoma is potentially progressive and malignant acting. Up to 15% of affected patients die of metastatic disease. On the basis of clinical, radiologic, histologic, and histochemical characteristics, long-bone adamantinomas (unrelated to the jaw lesion of the same name) have recently been divided into two groups: *classic* and *differentiated* (OFD-like). Both types involve the tibia, the fibula, or both bones. The classic form occurs almost exclusively in adults and is found in either the cortex

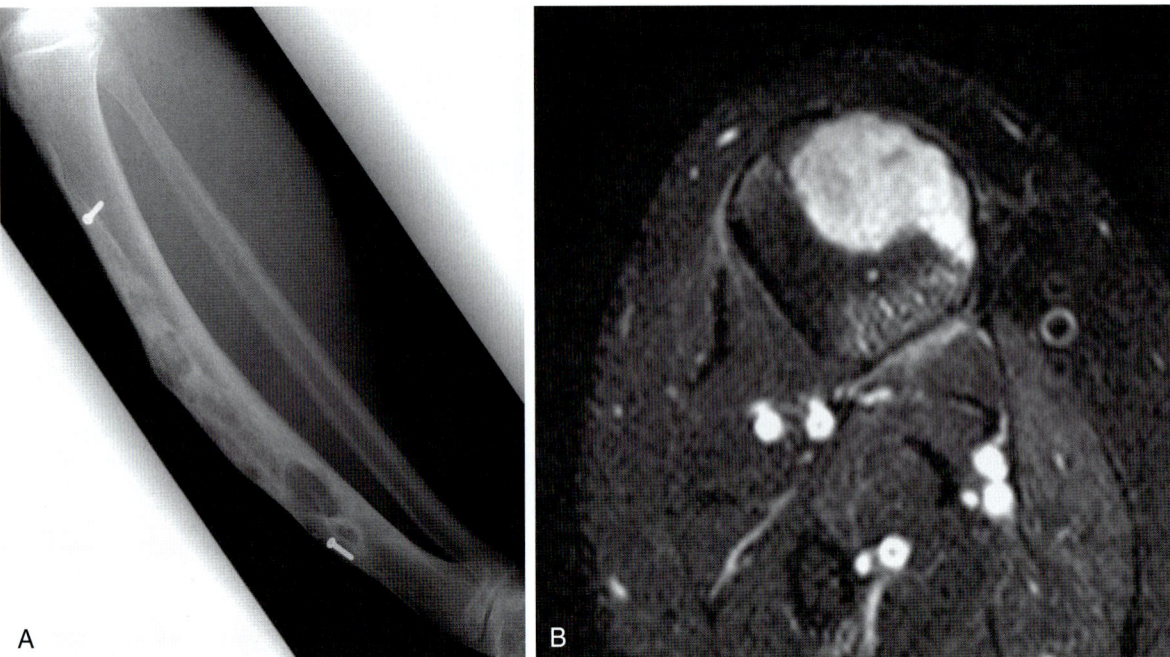

Figure 139-34   Osteofibrous dysplasia in a 15-year-old boy. Biopsies obtained several years prior had led to a diagnosis of adamantinoma, for which surgical excision with grafting had been performed (screws are related to the prior graft). Symptoms recurred. **A,** Lateral radiograph shows anterior tibial bowing with mixed sclerosis and cystic lucencies centered anteriorly within the tibia. **B,** Axial T2-weighted magnetic resonance image with fat saturation shows homogeneous, high-signal soft tissue within the lesion. Percutaneous and excisional biopsies both showed osteofibrous dysplasia.

or the medulla, but it can expand through the cortex and periosteum. The differentiated form is seen in children and young adults up to 20 years of age and has been reported in newborn infants. The tumor is limited to the bony cortex and has a radiographic appearance identical to that of OFD. However, adamantinoma are OFD pathologically distinct: epithelial and mesenchymal cells, which express immunoreactive cytokeratin and vimentin, are present in adamantinomas. Epithelial elements are absent in classic OFD and are minimal in differentiated adamantinoma.[170]

Clinical, radiologic, and pathologic distinction of adamantinoma from OFD is challenging. The concept of a differentiated form implies a continuum between OFD and adamantinoma and suggests that OFD may be a regressive phase of adamantinoma. Some well-documented cases in the literature support this contention. Czerniak and colleagues[171,172] suggested that patients with the differentiated type have a more favorable prognosis than those with classic adamantinoma—no differentiated tumors have been known to metastasize—and that long-bone adamantinoma could be included among the few neoplasms capable of spontaneous regression.

Imaging   Radiographic findings of long-bone adamantinoma are analogous to those of OFD. Variable features that might raise suspicion for adamantinoma are periosteal reaction, moth-eaten destruction, and soft tissue extension. MRI of adamantinoma is nonspecific. The T1- and T2-weighted signal characteristics are similar to those of other tumors. Soft tissue extension may also be evident.[168,173,174]

Treatment   Treatment of adamantinoma is usually en bloc resection. Treatment for OFD and differentiated adamantinoma is much more conservative. If surgery is to be

performed for OFD or differentiated adamantinoma, it should be performed after the child reaches puberty, and only if the disease is extensive and has caused deformity.[168]

Langerhans Cell Histiocytosis

Overview, Etiologies, Pathophysiology, and Clinical Presentation   The cause of Langerhans cell histiocytosis (LCH) is unknown. An infectious etiology was postulated in the past, but recent evidence of clonal proliferation of Langerhans cells suggests a neoplastic etiology. The unifying pathologic feature of LCH is in an inappropriate proliferation of Langerhans cells. Like the cells of monocyte-macrophage lineage, the Langerhans cell originates from CD34+ stem cells of the bone marrow. Histologically, the tumors are composed of Langerhans histiocytes that contain characteristic cleaved nuclei, and on electron microscopy, racquet-shaped Birbeck granules are seen in the cytoplasm adjacent to the cell membrane; lesions also contain ordinary histocytes and eosinophils. Immunohistochemical staining for S100 protein and CD1a antigen are used in making the diagnosis.[175,176]

Focal LCH is a relatively common pediatric bone tumor and represents a continuum of disease that ranges from a single, indolent, self-limiting osseous lesion to a fulminant disseminated disorder that involves multiple organs systems. Approximately 80% of patients with LCH have osseous involvement. In the past, patients with LCH pathology were divided into three diagnoses: *eosinophilic granuloma* referred to localized skeletal disease, usually a single lesion, and 70% of patients fall into this category; children with *Hand-Schüller-Christian disease* had the triad of geographic bone lesions, proptosis, and diabetes insipidus—a triad rarely seen in an individual patient; and *Letterer-Siwe disease* referred to the fulminant, disseminated, often fatal multisystem form. Fewer than 10% of patients fall into this category. It is now recognized that LCH is a spectrum of disease rather than these three distinct entities.[177,178]

LCH is more common in whites, is twice as common in boys, and is seen from the neonatal period into adulthood. Most patients are younger than 15 years at presentation, with a peak incidence from 1 to 5 years of age. Focal lesions tend to be found in children who are slightly older, with an average age of 10 to 12 years. Multifocal and systemic disease is most common in infants and younger children. Fulminant life-threatening LCH is usually seen in the first two decades of life and is rare beyond 3 years of age. Disseminated disease may cause lymphadenopathy, hepatosplenomegaly, skin lesions (purpuric rash), diabetes insipidus, exophthalmos, thrombocytopenia, and anemia. Pulmonary involvement of LCH in children is seen almost always in the setting of disseminated disease, in which osseous lesions vary from relatively few to a diffuse, confluent involvement.[179,180]

Solitary LCH lesions usually come to attention with local pain, tenderness, and an occasional palpable mass. Symptoms also relate to the involved bone: mastoid lesions may manifest as ear disease, and spinal lesions may show up as painful scoliosis or kyphosis. In addition, patients may have a low-grade fever, and erythrocyte sedimentation rate and C-reactive protein levels may be elevated.

The skull is the most frequent site of LCH, followed by the femur, mandible, pelvis, ribs, and spine; in addition, 70% of lesions occur in flat bones, and 30% occur in tubular bones (long bones, clavicle, hands, and feet). Lesions are usually located in the medulla. Primary lesions of the cortex are rare; however, the cortex is often secondarily affected by expansion of an intramedullary lesion. Long-bone lesions occur in the diaphysis or metaphysis, with rare involvement of the epiphysis. Rarely, lesions may cross an open growth plate. Multiple bone lesions occur in approximately 25% of patients.[181,182]

Imaging In the extremities, most LCH lesions are purely osteolytic with well-defined, minimally sclerotic borders. Many lesions are mildly expansile. Endosteal scalloping may be prominent and may progress to cortical disruption. Some lesions are permeative, and periosteal new bone formation may occur, giving them an aggressive appearance. Periosteal new bone may be in single or multiple layers. Although it is often said that LCH can have any radiographic appearance, lesions often have both aggressive and nonaggressive features. When such an indeterminate lesion is identified, LCH is high on the list of differential diagnoses.

Radiographically, LCH of the calvaria typically appears as a lytic bone lesion with a well-defined "punched out" appearance. Skull lesions appear geographic with beveled borders as a result of differential destruction of the inner and outer tables (Fig. 139-35; see also Chapter 21). A so-called button sequestrum may be seen, and lesions of the maxilla and mandible produce "floating teeth" (e-Fig. 139-36). Vertebral lesions produce compression deformities, most commonly in the thoracic spine, followed by the lumbar and cervical regions. LCH often produces vertebra plana with marked loss of height of a single vertebral body (Fig. 139-37). With vertebral involvement, soft tissue extension into the spinal canal may be apparent and is best assessed by MRI. The height of affected vertebral segments tends to

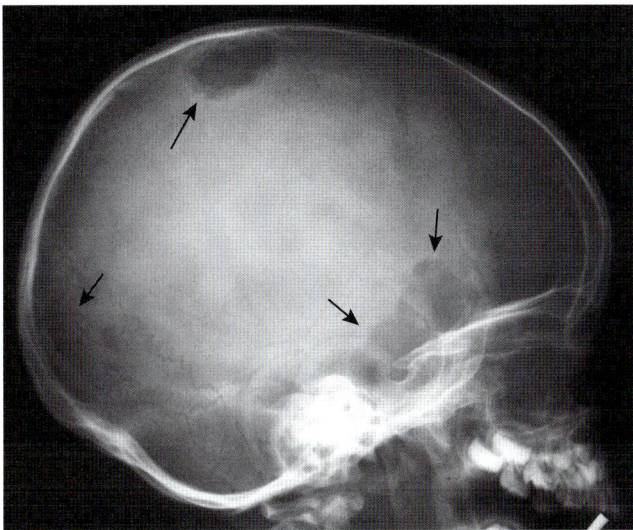

Figure 139-35 Langerhans cell histiocytosis in a 2-year-old girl. Lateral skull radiograph shows three lytic lesions in the skull. The lesion at the vertex has beveled edges.

reconstitute after therapy. Involvement of the posterior element may occur but is less common than vertebral body involvement.[183-185]

The imaging appearance of LCH depends on the stage and activity of the lesions. The natural history is for spontaneous involution of some lesions to occur. Even at the time of diagnosis, some lesions may be present that are already in a state of involution or quiescence. Involuting lesions will be

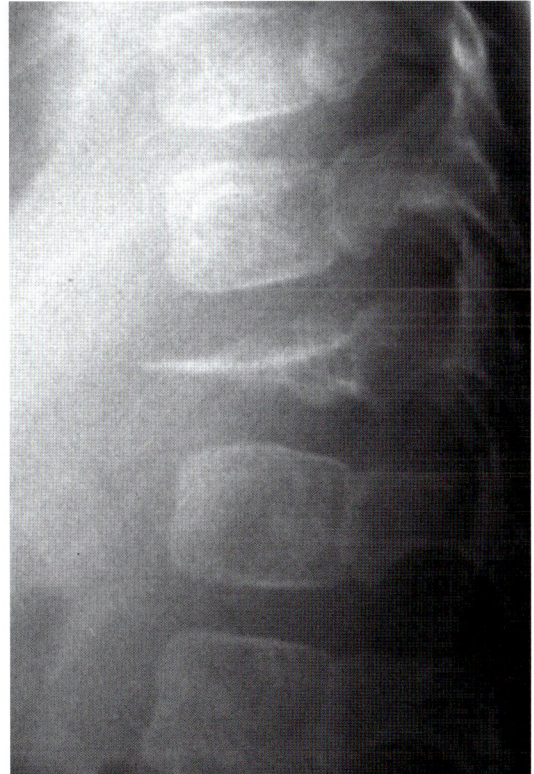

Figure 139-37 Vertebra plana as a sequela of Langerhans cell histiocytosis in a 20-month-old girl.

less well defined and will show sclerosis. Both CT and MRI can be used for further delineation of osseous lesions. On CT, active lesions usually have a well-defined, nonsclerotic margin. A cortical break and soft tissue mass may be seen. MRI is preferred to CT, owing to the lack of ionizing radiation and superior tissue contrast. On MRI, active lesions are composed of soft tissue, which is low signal on T1- and high signal on T2-wieghted imaging, and it enhances relatively homogeneously (see e-Fig. 139-36). About half of the lesions will be hyperintense to muscle on T1-weighted images, and extensive bone marrow and soft tissue edema produces high signal on T2-weighted images and enhances (Fig. 139-38). This prominent inflammatory reaction produces an aggressive appearance suggestive of a malignant process. LCH lesions that disrupt the cortex may also produce a sizable soft tissue mass (seen in 30% of cases on MRI) and may simulate malignancy. Older, involuted, or involuting lesions appear as low signal on T1- and T2-weighted images. Also, a multiplicity of lesions is very suggestive of LCH, as opposed to many other entities that are usually unifocal. If LCH is a consideration, a radiographic skeletal survey may be beneficial in identifying other lesions. Often, the presenting lesion is not at the best site for biopsy, and other unsuspected sites may prove more suitable for tissue diagnosis. Because multiple skeletal lesions may coexist, skeletal imaging is necessary at the time of diagnosis and for purposes of follow-up. Some controversy exists about the relative accuracy of radiographic skeletal surveys and radionuclide bone scintigraphy, because up to 35% of lesions may be missed by bone scans.

Whole-body MRI may become an alternative method for identifying and following multifocal disease. PET scans have also shown utility in identifying sites of active disease and for following response to therapy.[186-188]

Treatment   LCH localized to the skeleton carries a favorable prognosis. Recurrences are not uncommon. Solitary lesions are watched and usually involute spontaneously. More aggressive therapy may be occasionally warranted, depending on symptoms and lesion characteristics. Curettage and ablative techniques have been used, and children with multiple lesions and/or associated systemic disease are treated more aggressively with steroids and chemotherapy.[189] The disease is thus treated in a manner similar to that for a malignant process. The morbidity in children with systemic disease varies depending on the organs involved and the histologic pattern of disease. Children in whom organ function is unaffected and who respond well to initial therapy show a better long-term prognosis. Mortality of disseminated disease is approximately 10%.

Osseous Tumors

Osteoid Osteoma

Overview, Etiologies, Pathophysiology, and Clinical Presentation   Osteoid osteoma is a common, benign tumor of bone that has a characteristic presentation and radiologic appearance. These tumors occur predominantly in boys, usually those in the second decade of life; however, it is not uncommon in both sexes from the first decade until the mid fourth decade, with a strong prevalence in whites. Pathologically, osteoid osteoma consists of a nidus that is usually surrounded by dense sclerotic bone. The nidus contains interlacing

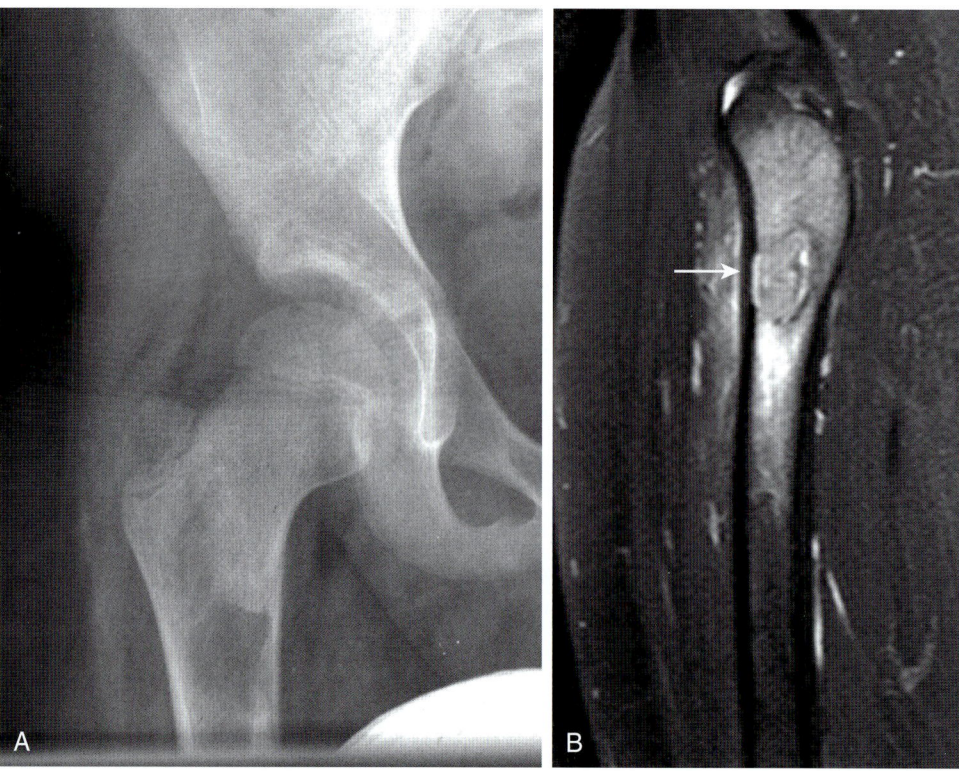

Figure 139-38   Biopsy-proven Langerhans cell histiocytosis in an 8-year-old boy. **A,** Radiograph demonstrates a lytic lesion in the right subtrochanteric femur. **B,** Short tau inversion recovery sagittal magnetic resonance image of the right femur demonstrates the primary mass (*arrow*) with extensive adjacent bone and soft tissue edema.

trabeculae at various stages of ossification within a stroma of loose, vascular connective tissue. Three types of osteoid osteoma are recognized: cortical (most common), cancellous or medullary, and subperiosteal (least common). The latter two types produce less sclerotic bone than cortical lesions, making radiologic diagnosis difficult. Osteoid osteomas can also be subdivided into *extraarticular* and *intraarticular* types. The incidence of medullary and subperiosteal types is higher at juxtaarticular and intraarticular locations.

Osteoid osteomas may develop in any bone. The single most common location of osteoid osteoma is the femur, and specifically, the femoral neck. The tibia is the next most frequent site. Osteoid osteomas occur less frequently in the upper extremities than in the lower extremities but frequently affect the tubular bones of the hands and feet. Osteoid osteomas most commonly affect the metaphysis or metadiaphysis, less commonly the diaphysis, and rarely the epiphysis. They are less common in flat bones and the spine, where they tend to affect the vertebral posterior arches. In such cases, patients usually are seen initially with painful scoliosis.[190] The classic presentation of osteoid osteoma is well-localized pain that is especially severe at night and relieved by aspirin or another nonsteroidal antiinflammatory drugs (NSAIDs); aspirin relieves the pain in 75% of patients. Lesions near a joint may mimic arthritis.

Imaging   Radiographically, the nidus may be purely radiolucent or may contain a dense center. The lucent nidus ranges from a few millimeters to 15 mm in diameter. With cortical osteoid osteomas the nidus is encased by a broad zone of dense bone (Fig. 139-39).[191] Intraarticular osteoid osteomas tend to have little reactive bone or periosteal new bone formation. This type most frequently affects the hip, where it causes osteopenia and joint effusion.[192] Regardless of location, the nidus of an osteoma may be difficult to see on radiography.

CT is valuable in showing the lesion, confirming the diagnosis, and determining the anatomic location of the lesion before percutaneous therapy or surgical excision. The CT appearance of a lucent nidus with central sequestrum opacity and surrounding sclerosis is usually diagnostic of osteoid osteoma, particularly if the clinical presentation is classic (see Fig. 139-39). Intramedullary and subperiosteal lesions show less sclerosis. Subperiosteal osteoid osteomas lie on top of the cortex and may erode it,[193] and they may or may not have ossification within the nidus. Without the ossification, findings are less specific. CT shows the nidus of an osteoid osteoma better than MRI. On MRI, low intensity may be seen on both T1 and T2 images, depending on the relative amount of ossification and fibrovascular tissue. Although there is no signal from the sclerotic bone, the inherent contrast resolution of MRI provides precise definition of potentially extensive reactive changes in the bone marrow and adjacent soft tissues. Osteoid osteoma may produce an intense inflammatory response within adjacent bone, joint, and soft tissues. If the nidus is not identified, a more aggressive process can be suggested.[194] Both the nidus and the adjacent inflamed tissues enhance with gadolinium.[195] Intraarticular osteoid osteomas produce joint effusions and synovial proliferation that also appear of high intensity on T2-weighted images and enhance after gadolinium.

The chief imaging-based differential diagnoses for osteoid osteoma are stress fracture and osteomyelitis. Usually, clinical presentation and laboratory results point toward the correct diagnosis. Imaging findings of osteoid osteoma tend to be specific.

Treatment   The traditional treatment for osteoid osteoma has been surgical excision, however, localization of the lesion and confirmation of excision may be challenging in the operating room. Recently, percutaneous methods of treatment have been developed. Other percutaneous methods include

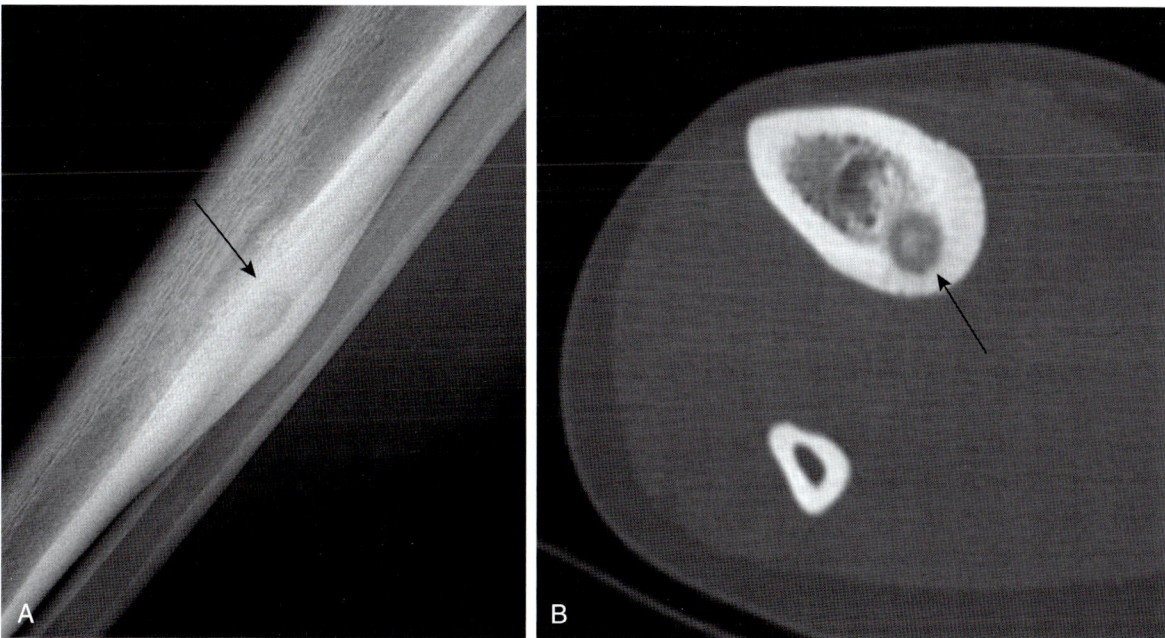

Figure 139-39   Osteoid osteoma of the tibia in a 15-year-old girl. **A,** Radiograph shows cortical thickening posteriorly. The lucent nidus is faintly seen (*arrow*). **B,** Computed tomography better shows the nidus (*arrow*). A small radiopaque sequestrum is present within the nidus.

excision with a large-bore needle or drill and cryoablation,[196] but percutaneous radio frequency ablation is now the preferred method of treatment of osteoid osteoma.[197] Complex lesions or lesions located where percutaneous methods are contraindicated may still require surgical excision. Surgical or percutaneous methods are successful in approximately 90% of patients on the initial attempt.

Osteoblastoma

Overview, Etiologies, Pathophysiology, and Clinical Presentation Osteoblastomas are closely related to osteoid osteomas and have in the past been considered a larger version of that tumor (giant osteoid osteoma). The two lesions are nearly identical histologically.[198] Osteoblastoma consists of numerous osteoblast-lined trabeculae that contain osteoid.[199] However, these trabeculae are less organized than those in osteoid osteoma. Size is an important consideration in distinguishing between the two types of tumors: those less than 1.5 cm in diameter are considered to be osteoid osteomas, whereas tumors larger than 1.5 cm are usually osteoblastomas.[200] The two types of tumors can also be distinguished by differences in clinical presentation, anatomic location, and imaging features. Osteoblastoma most commonly occurs in patients in the second and third decades of life,[201] and it is more common in boys. Osteoblastomas are not associated with a typical pattern of pain, and if painful, they do not typically respond to NSAIDs. Many osteoblastomas are found in the posterior elements of the vertebrae, where they can cause scoliosis and neurologic deficits. Nearly half of these tumors occur in the appendicular skeleton, primarily in the proximal femoral diaphysis and metaphysis. Tibial lesions are next most common. Long-bone lesions may be cortical or medullary in location. Another characteristic location for osteoblastoma is the neck of the talus, usually at its dorsal margin.

Imaging Osteoblastoma appears as three distinct radiologic variants: 1) an osteoid osteoma–like appearance, but larger; 2) an ABC-like appearance, most commonly in the spine; and 3) an aggressive appearance that mimics a malignancy, which is uncommon.[202] Osteoblastomas vary from 1 to 10 cm in size. Most are lytic with a well-defined sclerotic margin, but the tumor usually lacks the wide, dense rim of sclerosis typical of osteoid osteoma. Lesions in the spine are often expansile (Fig. 139-40). Adjacent sclerosis with spinal lesions may be minimal or absent. In the long bones, osteoblastomas appear radiologically as round or oval lucent tumors, eccentric within the medulla or cortex. Some sclerosis is seen adjacent to the lesion, and mineralization of the matrix is frequently present. Periosteal reaction is common and is solid or layered. Talar lesions may expand into the soft tissues, and osteoporosis of the talus and other bones of the foot may be an associated finding. The calcified or ossified matrix of an osteoblastoma and the tumor's thin, bony outer shell are especially well visualized on CT images. Edema in the soft tissues or marrow may give high signal on T2-weighted MRI, but signal characteristics are not specific; osteoid within the lesion may cause areas of decreased signal, and bone scans may help in determining the location of a lesion. In addition, osteoblastomas are relatively vascular, hence angiography may reveal a dense capillary blush.

Treatment Treatment of osteoblastoma is by surgical excision or curettage, but there is a moderate recurrence rate.

MALIGNANT BONE TUMORS

Approximately 50% of all bone tumors in the pediatric age group are malignant; nearly two thirds of these are osteosarcomas. Ewing sarcomas of bone comprise most of the remainder. Other types of osseous malignancies, such as chondrosarcoma, are extremely rare in children, although non-Hodgkin lymphoma occasionally occurs as a primary bone neoplasm. Osteosarcoma and Ewing sarcoma differ sufficiently, both in their clinical and imaging presentation, such that they can usually be distinguished from one another. Their characteristic features, discussed in this chapter, are summarized in Table 139-1.

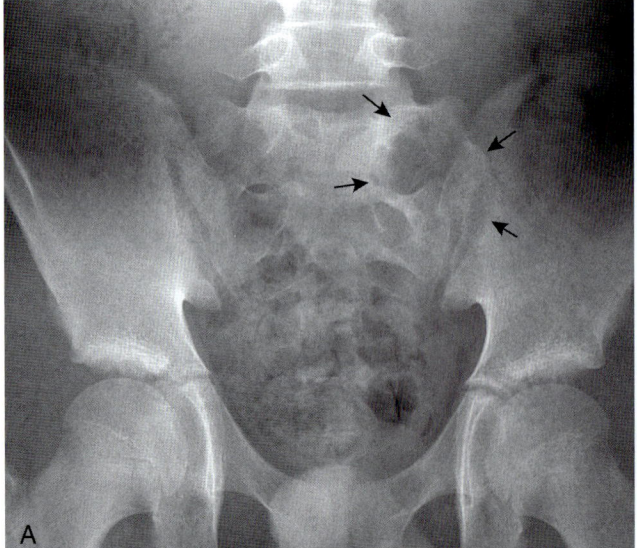
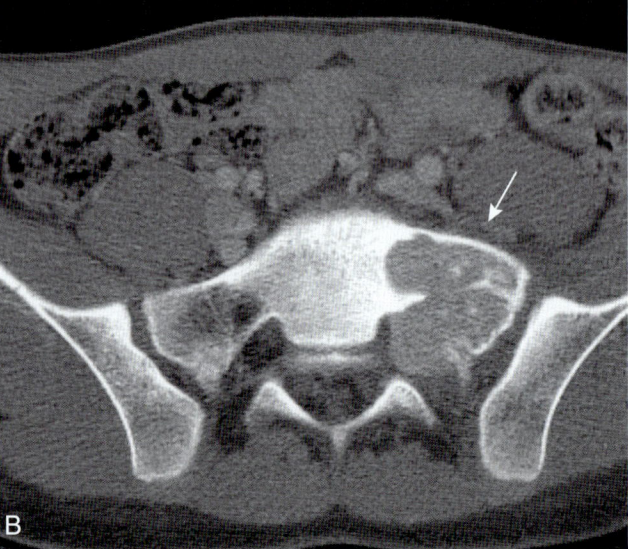

Figure 139-40 Osteoblastoma of the sacrum in a 12-year-old boy. A well-defined, lucent, expansile lesion (*arrows*) is seen within the left sacrum on radiography (**A**) and computed tomography (**B**).

Table 139-1

Differentiating Features of Osteosarcoma and Ewing Sarcoma

Feature	Osteosarcoma	Ewing Sarcoma
Age range	15 to 25 years	0 to 25 years
Incidence	More common	Less common
		Rare in nonwhites
Location	Metaphyses of long bones	Metadiaphysis of long bones
		Axial, flat-bone involvement more common than osteosarcoma
Matrix	Usually "cloudlike" mineralization	Not mineralized or sclerotic
Periosteal reaction	"Sunburst"	"Onionskin"
	Codman triangles	
Metastases	Lung (80%)	Lung, rarely bone, marrow, lymph nodes
	Bone (20%)	
Other	Occasional multifocal disease	11:22 translocation
	Association with retinoblastoma	Radiation sensitive

Osteosarcoma

Overview, Etiologies, Pathophysiology, and Clinical Presentation Osteosarcoma is the most common malignant primary bone tumor in the pediatric population. The peak incidence of osteosarcoma is in patients 15 to 25 years of age, but the youngest patient described to date with osteosarcoma was a 19-month-old girl.[203] The tumors are slightly more common in males, and the long bones are affected in approximately 70% of cases; more than half of osteosarcomas are distributed about the bones of the knee, and the face, mandible, cranium, and axial skeleton are among the less commonly affected sites (Fig. 139-41). Most osteosarcomas are single, primary neoplasms that arise from the medullary cavity of the metaphyses of the long bones. The diaphyses alone are less commonly involved, which occurs in 2% to 11% of cases; an epiphyseal origin of osteosarcoma is extremely rare. Osteosarcomas can involve multiple skeletal sites synchronously, a condition known as *osteosarcomatosis*.[204,205] Extremely rare in children, extraskeletal osteosarcomas are found in various organs or in the soft tissues of the extremities of adults.[206,207]

Often referred to as *conventional osteosarcomas,* most are considered to be high grade because of their degree of cellular atypia and anaplasia. Other much less common categories of this tumor include well-differentiated medullary osteosarcoma, telangiectatic osteosarcoma, and surface osteosarcomas, including intracortical osteosarcoma and parosteal, periosteal, and high-grade surface osteosarcomas. Secondary osteosarcomas, which are rare in children, are usually associated with previous radiation therapy. Osteosarcoma can also arise in patients with inherited (usually bilateral) retinoblastoma who have a defect in a specific gene, or it can arise in patients who have undergone a spontaneous mutation of that gene. Although radiation therapy increases the incidence of osteosarcoma in these patients, secondary osteosarcoma may develop in sites remote from radiation fields. Osteosarcoma unassociated with other malignancies is occasionally familial and has been identified in siblings.

Intramedullary Osteosarcoma

Conventional Osteosarcoma

Overview, Etiologies, Pathophysiology, and Clinical Presentation Approximately 75% of osteosarcomas are the high-grade variant, and 75% of cases occur in patients between the ages of 15 and 25 years. The histologic hallmark of osteosarcoma is the presence of an osteoid matrix produced by sarcoma cells. In most cases, there is extensive immature bone formation. However, other tissues may predominate in the tumor matrix. The three main types of osteosarcoma, based on matrix type, are *osteoblastic, chondroblastic,* and *fibroblastic.* These tumors have differing mineral content.[207]

Imaging Radiography remains the primary method of diagnosis for conventional osteosarcoma. Other imaging methods are used mainly for staging purposes and to assist with surgical planning. Osteosarcoma typically manifests as a large, mixed sclerotic–lytic mass with a cloudlike matrix that involves the long-bone metaphyses. The tumors cause cortical erosion and destruction rather than expansion. Resultant periosteal new bone formation, often of the spiculated "sunburst" variety (Fig. 139-42), and periosteal elevation are often observed, frequently with Codman triangles (Fig. 139-43). However, conventional osteosarcomas are occasionally purely lytic and exhibit no periosteal reaction. Osteosarcomas with chondroblastic elements tend to be more lytic on radiography (see Fig. 139-43), and osteoblastic dominant osteosarcomas will demonstrate increased osteoid matrix (see Fig. 139-42).

CT is superior to radiographs for delineating osteoid matrix. Like radiographs, CT often underestimates the true extent of bone involvement (Fig. 139-44).

MRI is used extensively to evaluate osteosarcoma. The longitudinal extent of marrow involvement, an important determinant of surgical therapy, is accurately shown as well-defined hypointense signal within hyperintense fatty marrow on T1-weighted images obtained in either coronal or sagittal planes. It is important to obtain a longitudinal T1-weighted image of the entire bone to measure intramedullary tumor length, to assess possible epiphyseal involvement (seen in as many as 80% of metaphyseal tumors), and to detect skip metastases that occur in a small percentage of cases. On T2-weighted images, the tumor-containing marrow can be either hyperintense or, if there is sufficient bone formation, hypointense to normal fat (see Fig. 139-42). The soft tissue component is usually of heterogeneous, mainly high-intensity signals that contrast greatly with surrounding structures. STIR

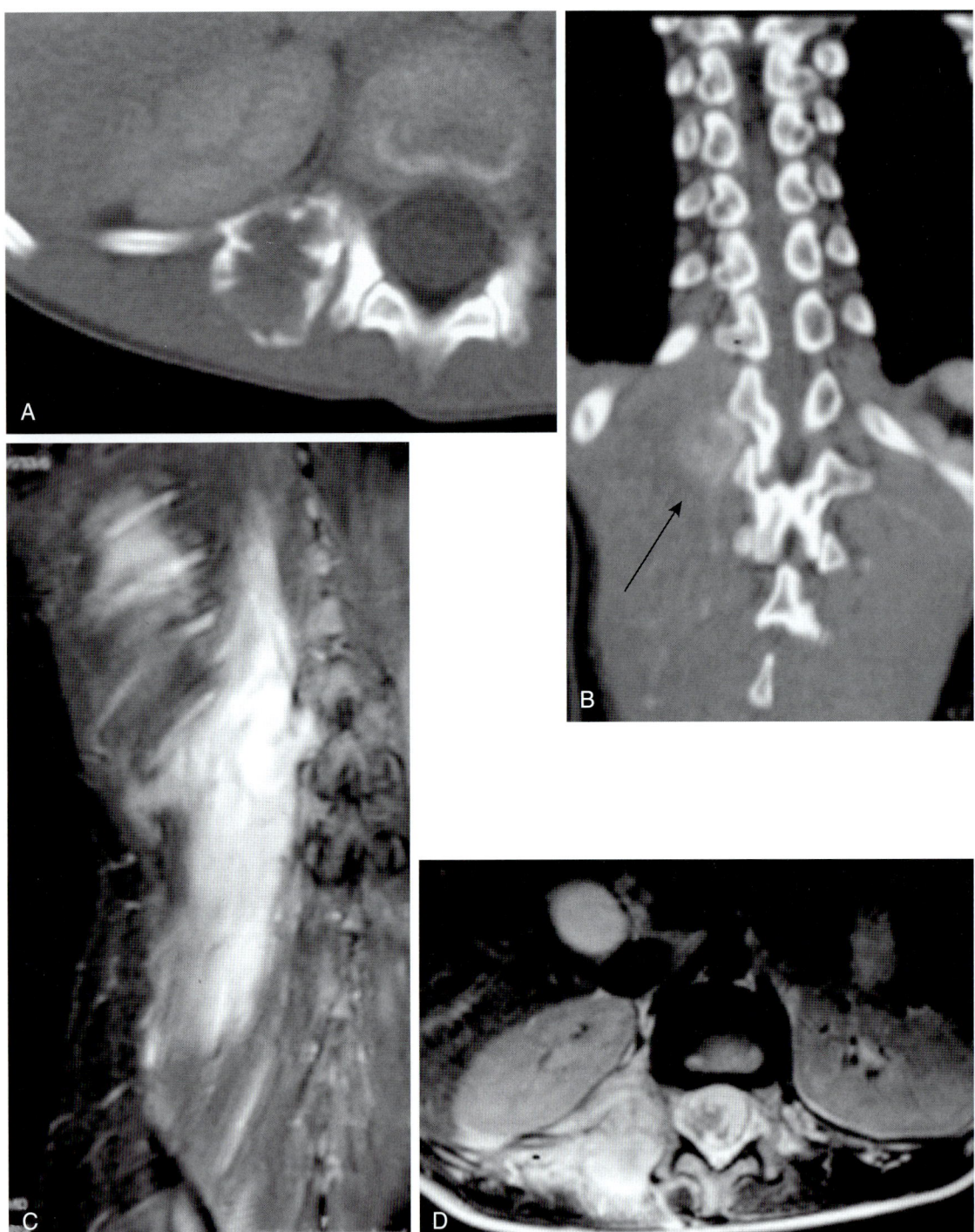

Figure 139-41 Osteosarcoma of the spine in an 8-year-old girl. **A,** Axial contrast-enhanced computed tomography through T12 after 10 weeks of chemotherapy shows a peripherally sclerotic expansile mass arising from the right costovertebral junction. Note disruption of the cortex posteriorly. **B,** Coronal reconstruction shows the relationship of the mass (*arrow*) to the apex of the scoliosis. **C,** Coronal short tau inversion recovery magnetic resonance imaging (MRI) demonstrates massive edema in the paraspinal muscles in response to the osteosarcoma. **D,** Axial contrast-enhanced T1-weighted MRI with fat saturation demonstrates intense tumor enhancement and moderate enhancement of the surrounding paraspinous musculature.

images are very sensitive to the water content of tumors, thus they markedly increase the conspicuity of most osteosarcomas; the intramedullary length of tumor extension may be overestimated on STIR sequences.[208] Contrast-enhanced T1-weighted images, preferably obtained with fat saturation, provide similar contrast and better signal-to-noise ratios than T2-weighted images. Furthermore, contrast-enhanced

T1-weighted images are especially useful in determining the relationship between the tumor and the major blood vessels, in detecting joint involvement in the presence of effusion,[209] and in estimating the amount of necrosis within the tumor. Osteosarcoma is frequently accompanied by edema of the adjacent soft tissues that is hyperintense to muscle on T2-weighted STIR images and contrast-enhanced

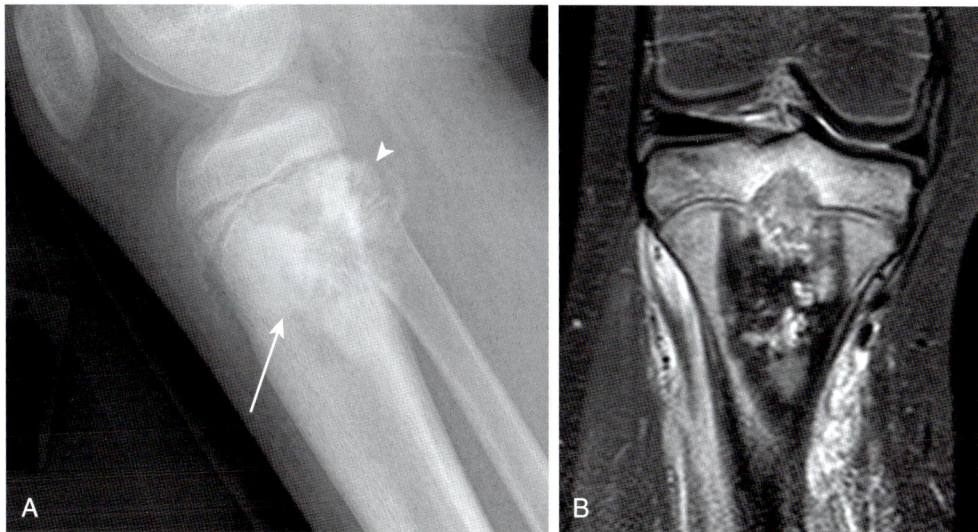

Figure 139-42 Proximal tibial osteosarcoma in an 11-year-old boy. **A,** Radiograph demonstrates osteoblastic osteosarcoma with osteoid matrix (*arrow*) and "sunburst" periostitis (*arrowhead*). **B,** Corresponding short tau inversion recovery coronal magnetic resonance image shows low signal intensity throughout the majority of the mass, indicative of osteoid matrix. Note the presence also of transphyseal transgression through the central physis.

T1-weighted images. This edema can be localized to the tumor periphery, or it can involve whole muscle groups, as in the case of larger tumors. The latter finding has been associated with a poor prognosis.[210]

Between 10% and 20% of patients with osteosarcoma have metastases at the time of diagnosis, mainly to the lungs; therefore chest CT is essential in the search for pulmonary lesions at presentation. Like the primary tumor, these metastases can be calcified and therefore difficult to distinguish from calcified granulomas. Pleural-based lung metastases can also produce pneumothorax, hemothorax, or malignant pleural effusion. Such findings may be the first sign of pulmonary metastases at the time of diagnosis or at follow-up. Bone metastases are much less frequent, but radionuclide

bone scans are justified to detect these lesions and to assess the extent of the primary tumor.

Telangiectatic Osteosarcoma

Overview, Etiologies, Pathophysiology, and Clinical Presentation Telangiectatic osteosarcoma comprises about 2% of all osteosarcomas. Like conventional osteosarcomas, telangiectatic osteosarcoma tends to occur in the long bones adjacent to the knee and is seen more frequently in boys than in girls. These tumors contain little osteoid and do not form bone but rather are composed of single or multiple cavities that contain blood or necrotic tumor with septa of anaplastic cells.[211,212] Telangiectatic osteosarcomas by definition are

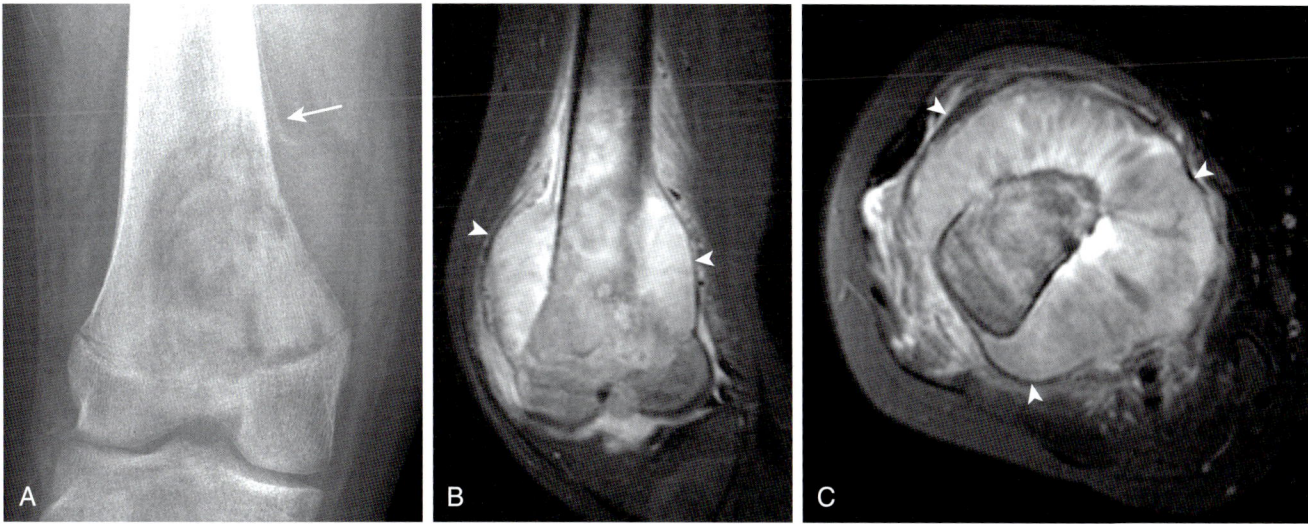

Figure 139-43 Osteosarcoma in a 13-year-old girl. **A,** Radiograph demonstrates permeative lytic destruction in the distal femur metaphysis with aggressive periosteal reaction with a Codman triangle (*arrow*). Short tau inversion recovery coronal (**B**) and axial (**C**) magnetic resonance image demonstrates distal femoral metaphyseal mass with transphyseal transgression into the epiphysis with a large extraosseous tumor component with intermediate signal intensity, consistent with osteoid matrix. Note the displaced periosteal envelope (*arrowheads*).

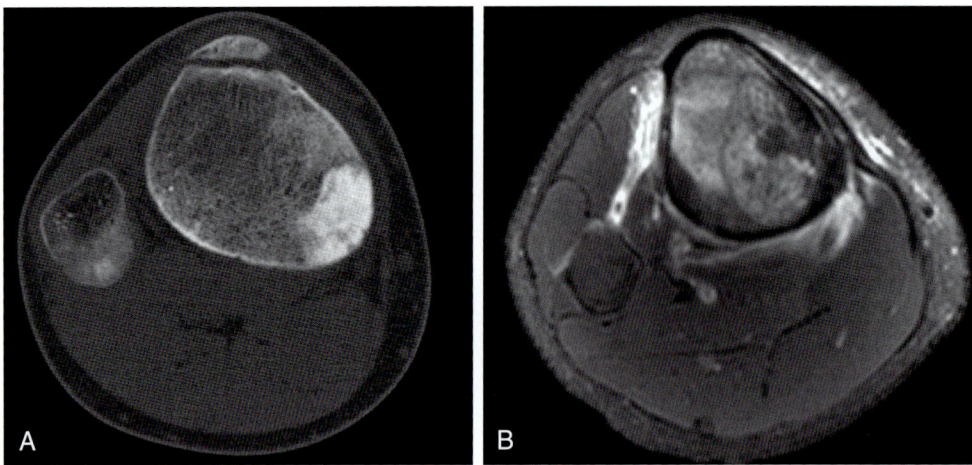

Figure 139-44 Tibial osteosarcoma in a 14-year-old boy. **A,** Axial computed tomography demonstrates intraosseous osteoblastic matrix replacing a portion of the medullary cavity. **B,** Short tau inversion recovery axial magnetic resonance image through the same level demonstrates near complete intramedullary involvement.

composed of approximately 90% cystic components prior to treatment.[213]

Imaging Radiographically, telangiectactic osteosarcomas tend to be lytic, and they tend to expand, rather than destroy, the cortex; they may also be associated with a soft tissue mass. Except for the presence of malignant cells that are often at the periphery of the cavity, the pathologic appearance of telangiectatic osteosarcoma mimics that of an ABC. Indeed, on MRI, the appearance of telangiectatic osteosarcoma and ABC may be identical; both may have single or multiple fluid-fluid levels produced by blood products of differing ages that are best demonstrated on T2-weighted images.[214] Telangiectatic osteosarcomas are characterized by enhancing soft tissue in the periphery and septations of the tumor, features absent in ABCs.[215] Biopsy is necessary to differentiate telangiectatic osteosarcoma from an ABC. The prognosis of patients with telangiectatic osteosarcoma is similar to that of patients with conventional osteosarcoma.

Surface Osteosarcomas

Overview, Etiologies, Pathophysiology, and Clinical Presentation Surface osteosarcomas are classified by histologic grade as low-, intermediate-, and high-grade lesions.[216] *Parosteal osteosarcoma* is more common in girls than in boys, tends to occur after skeletal maturity has been achieved, and is of low histologic grade. *Periosteal osteosarcoma* probably arises from the deep layers of periosteum or the outer cortex and is classified as an intermediate-grade osteosarcoma; most periosteal osteosarcomas are chondroblastic,[217] and they may be mistaken for a chondrosarcoma by pathologists unfamiliar with pediatric orthopedic oncology. *High-grade surface osteosarcomas* comprise dedifferentiated parosteal osteosarcoma and high-grade surface osteosarcoma. The origin of high-grade surface osteosarcoma is controversial; histologically, it is difficult to differentiate from the much more common, conventional, intramedullary high-grade osteosarcomas.

Patients with parosteal osteosarcoma generally have an excellent prognosis, although this may be affected adversely by ingrowth into the medullary cavity. Parosteal osteosarcomas are composed of extensive osteoid tissue with a fibrous stroma and form a lobulated, ossified, juxtacortical mass. Early lesions may have a radiologic cleavage plane between the cortex and the tumor. Patients with periosteal and high-grade surface osteosarcomas have similar prognoses compared with those with conventional, intramedullary high-grade osteosarcomas.

Imaging Parosteal osteosarcomas are very osteoblastic and are slow growing. They demonstrate mature periosteal ossification and most commonly occur in the posterior aspect of the distal femur (Fig. 139-45). Superficially, parosteal osteosarcoma may mimic a sessile osteochondroma. MRI is used to define the degree of intramedullary extension, if present, and adjacent neurovascular and muscle involvement.

Periosteal osteosarcomas also arise from the surface and may have adjacent intramedullary marrow edema, but true invasion is rare.[217] Because these lesions are invariably chondroblastic, they often have little to no matrix on radiography and are hyperintense on fluid-sensitive sequences (Fig. 139-46). Superficially, these lesions may mimic a juxtacortical chondroma.

Treatment Osteosarcomas are not radiosensitive. Thus, treatment consists of preoperative chemotherapy; extirpation of resectable lesions, usually by limb-sparing surgery; and postoperative chemotherapy. MRI serves as a surgical road map to define the presence or absence of neurovascular involvement, physeal and epiphyseal extension, and joint involvement. If the physis is spared, physeal-sparing surgery can be attempted with an intercalary graft. When the epiphysis is involved, morbidity is higher, and a joint prosthesis is necessary.

Prognosis is influenced by response to initial chemotherapy, which is evaluated postoperatively by histologic estimation of necrosis within the treated tumor. Little change in tumor size is expected, even in tumors that respond well to chemotherapy. Imaging methods of assessing the effects of therapy include thallium-201 scintigraphy and dynamic contrast-enhanced MRI. Although PET and PET-CT appear

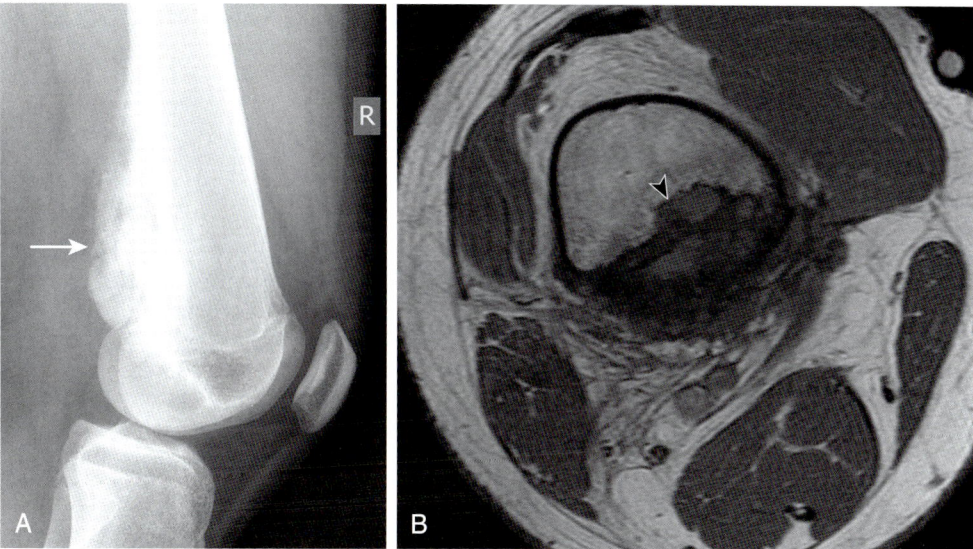

Figure 139-45 Parosteal osteosarcoma in a 14-year-old boy. **A,** Lateral radiograph demonstrates a surface-based osteoblastic mass in the distal femur (*arrow*). **B,** T1-weighted axial magnetic resonance image through the distal femur demonstrates the surface-based mass with intramedullary extension (*arrowhead*).

to be useful in both staging and monitoring response, experience is currently limited in its use for osteosarcoma and other bone tumors. Long-term follow-up of osteosarcoma and other malignant bone tumors in children is essential and extends over many months.[218,219]

Bone scintigraphy and chest CT should be performed periodically after treatment, especially within the 2 years following therapy: 80% of relapses occur in the lung only, and 20% occur in the skeleton. Local or distant lymph node involvement is extremely rare.

Ewing Sarcoma

Overview, Etiologies, Pathophysiology, and Clinical Presentation In 1921, James Ewing described a radium-sensitive bone tumor, which he called an *endothelioma,* that consisted of sheets of small polyhedral cells of probable endothelial origin.[220] Although the origin of this undifferentiated tumor has been debated since its initial description, what we now know as *Ewing sarcoma* has proved to be a distinct entity with characteristic histologic, radiologic, and cytogenetic features. The Ewing family of tumors includes Ewing sarcoma of bone, extraosseous Ewing sarcoma (EOES), and primitive neuroectodermal tumor (PNET), also known as *peripheral neuroepithelioma.* PNETs exhibit neural differentiation and may arise from either bone or soft tissues. The Ewing family of tumors shares a distinctive cytogenetic feature: reciprocal translocation of chromosome bands q24 and q12 of chromosomes 11 and 22. This same translocation is also found in Askin tumor of the thorax.[221-223]

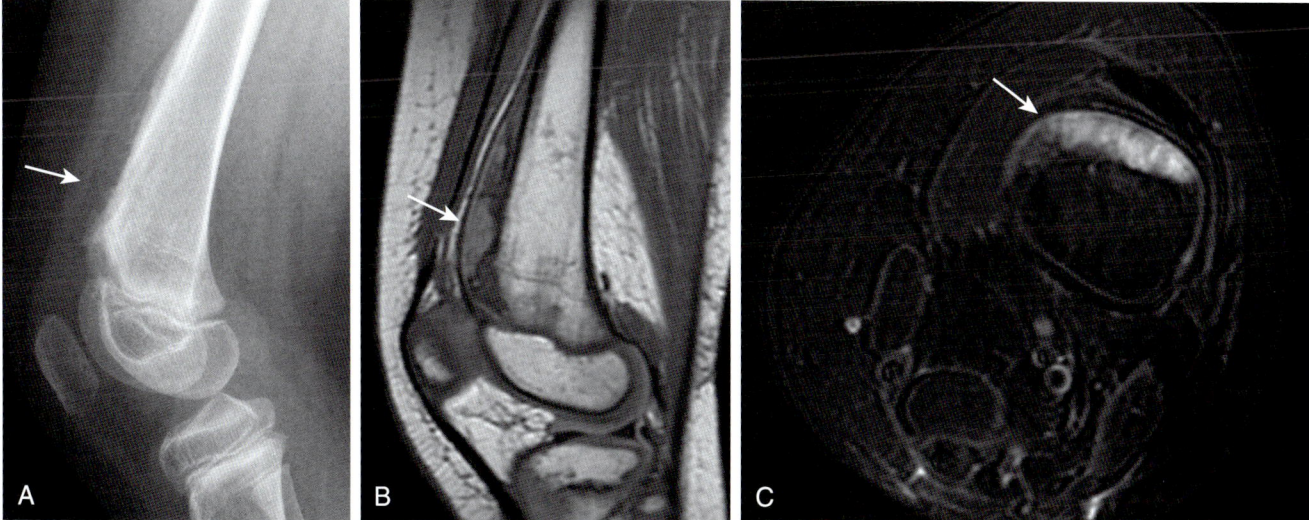

Figure 139-46 Periosteal osteosarcoma in an 11-year-old boy. **A,** Lateral radiograph demonstrates aggressive, perpendicularly oriented periosteal reaction with little to no matrix (*arrow*). **B,** Sagittal proton-density magnetic resonance imaging (MRI) demonstrates an intermediate signal lesion. **C,** On T2-weighted fat-saturated axial MRI, it is hyperintense and surface based, indicative of its chondroblastic composition (*arrow*).

In younger patients, Ewing sarcoma of bone occurs less frequently than osteosarcoma, with 2.9 cases per million diagnosed in patients younger than 20 years of age. Most cases are detected in patients between 10 and 25 years of age (median 15 years). Like osteosarcoma, Ewing sarcoma occurs slightly more often in boys and is much more common in whites. Fever, leukocytosis, and elevation of the erythrocyte sedimentation rate may accompany these neoplasms. More than 50% of Ewing sarcomas involve a single long bone; Ewing sarcoma involving the bones of the hands and feet, often initially diagnosed as an infection, is rare. Within the long bones, the metaphysis and diaphysis are the usual locations. The flat bones, especially the ribs and pelvis, are also commonly involved. Most Ewing sarcomas appear to arise from the medullary cavity. Multifocal osseous involvement at the time of diagnosis is rare.[223-225]

Imaging The typical radiographic appearance of Ewing sarcoma in the long bones is that of a permeative lesion with a lamellar "onionskin" periosteal reaction (see Fig. 139-47). However, nearly 40% of these tumors display diffuse sclerosis, sometimes with a mixed lytic–sclerotic pattern. The sclerosis correlates histologically with the presence of dead bone.[226] Because Ewing sarcomas do not ossify, soft tissue extension is often poorly detected by radiographs but is almost always apparent on CT or MRI (see Fig. 139-48). Indeed, the soft tissue masses tend to be disproportionately large in comparison to the amount of bone destruction, and they are especially extensive in Ewing sarcoma of the pelvis (Fig. 139-49). Cortical permeation and destruction may be visible on CT or MRI. However, these tumors can permeate haversian canals and can grow into the soft tissues without causing large areas of cortical loss. Extensive marrow involvement is particularly well shown as nonspecific low signal, isointense to muscle on T1-weighted images. It has been observed that most Ewing sarcomas found in the medullary cavity display intermediate signal that is isointense to that of fat on T2-weighted images. Rarely, Ewing sarcoma can arise from the surface of the bone rather than from the medullary cavity. In this periosteal or subperiosteal location, Ewing sarcoma resembles other surface malignancies, such as periosteal osteosarcoma with periosteal elevation and Codman triangles.[227] The affected cortex is typically excavated or saucerized,[228] and cross-sectional imaging is required to exclude medullary involvement. Patients with this form of Ewing sarcoma are thought to have a relatively favorable prognosis.

Treatment With appropriate multimodal therapy, the long-term survival rate of patients with nonmetastatic medullary Ewing sarcoma approaches that of patients with osteosarcoma (about 65%). In some series, tumor volume has been shown to influence prognosis. Survival of patients with pelvic tumors may be somewhat shortened and is much reduced in patients with metastatic disease. As many as 25% of patients with Ewing sarcoma have detectable metastases at the time of diagnosis; most of these are found in the lung, therefore chest CT is necessary for disease staging. Local and regional lymph node involvement may rarely occur, and metastases in bone or bone marrow are less frequent, although skip metastases have been reported.[229]

In addition to MRI of the primary tumor, bone scintigraphy, thoracic CT scanning, and bone marrow examination should be performed to detect possible disseminated disease. Early experience indicates that PET and PET-CT are useful for detection of metastatic sites of disease and for monitoring therapeutic response. Most Ewing sarcomas respond well to initial chemotherapy; increased bony sclerosis develops, and the soft tissue mass disappears.

Percentage change in size of the soft tissue mass appears to be an important prognostic indicator.[230] T2-weighted MRI shows an increase in intensity of the treated medullary component because of serous atrophy, with increased interstitial fluid of the yellow marrow and replacement of cytoplasmic lipid with serous material. High T2-weighted signal intensity caused by radiation-induced inflammatory reactions may also be observed in those patients treated with radiation therapy.[231-234]

The surgical approach to resection of Ewing sarcoma is similar to osteosarcoma.

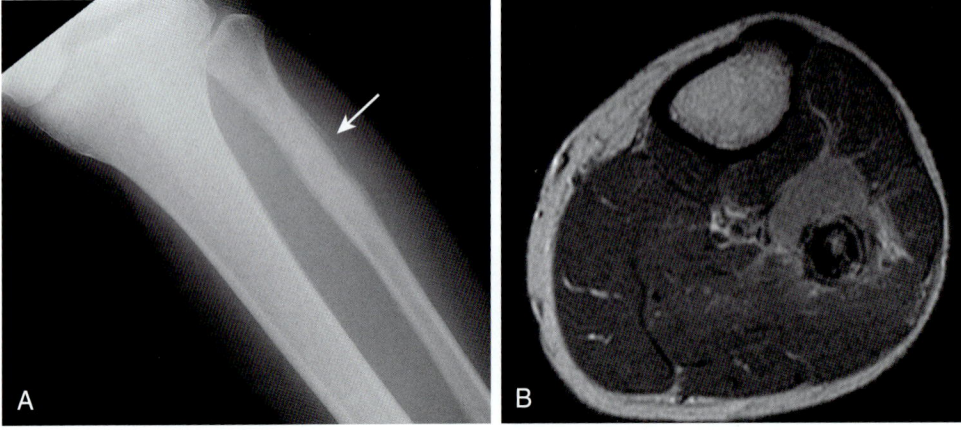

Figure 139-47 Ewing sarcoma of the fibula in a 17-year-old. **A,** Anteroposterior radiograph of the leg demonstrates aggressive "onionskin" periostitis of the proximal fibula (*arrow*). **B,** T1-weighted axial postcontrast magnetic resonance image demonstrates a large extraosseous mass that arises from the fibula with cortical destruction.

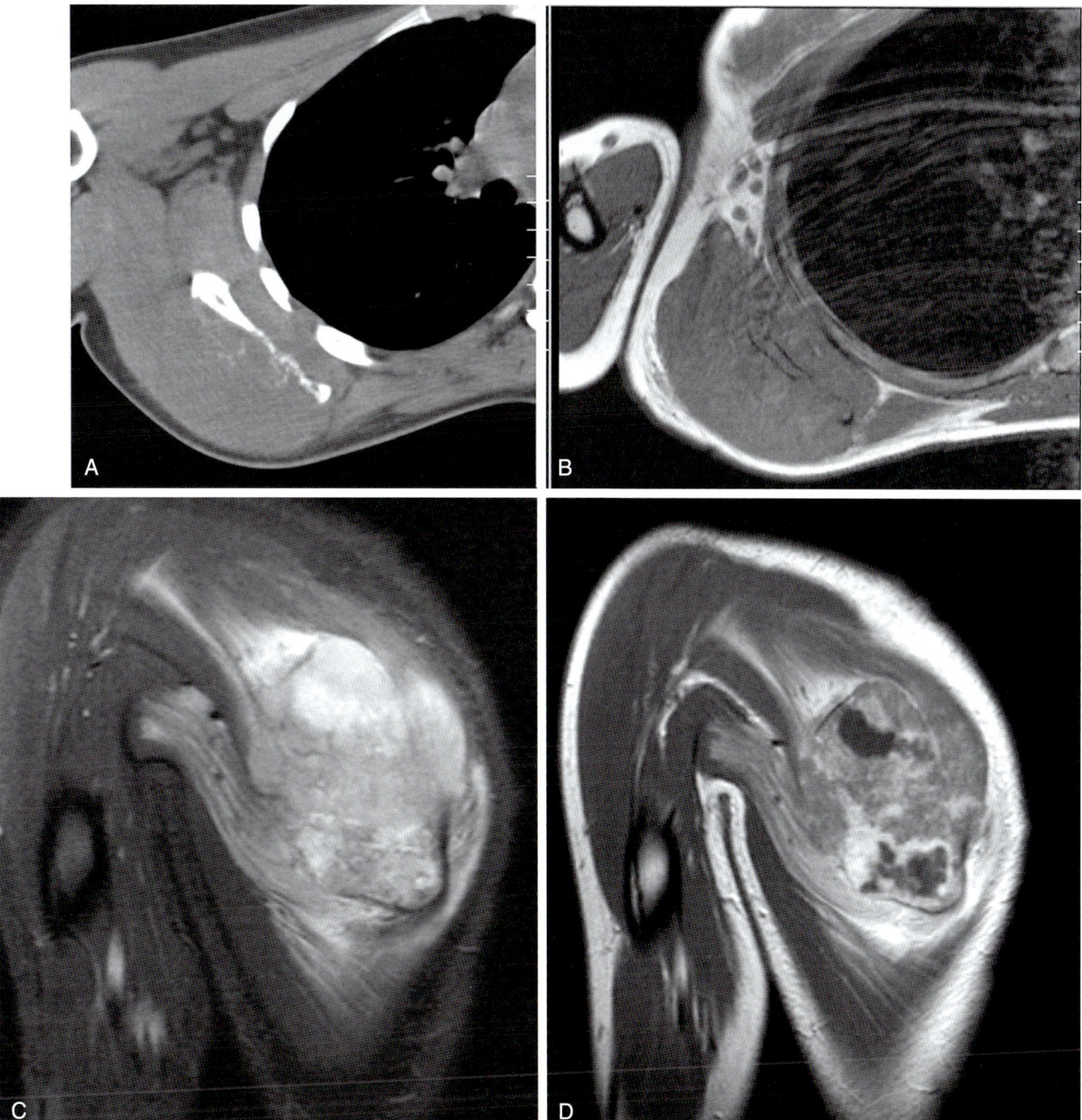

Figure 139-48 Ewing sarcoma of the right scapula in a 16-year-old girl. **A,** Axial computed tomographic image shows a permeative pattern to the scapula with subtle dystrophic calcifications within the soft tissue mass. **B,** T1 axial magnetic resonance imaging (MRI) shows marrow replacement and cortical destruction by the mass. **C,** Short tau inversion recovery sagittal MRI demonstrates a large heterogeneous mass with cortical destruction and intramuscular invasion. **D,** T1 postcontrast MRI demonstrates heterogeneous central tumoral enhancement with areas of nonenhancement consistent with tumoral necrosis.

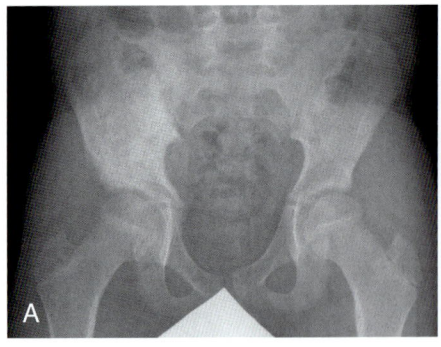 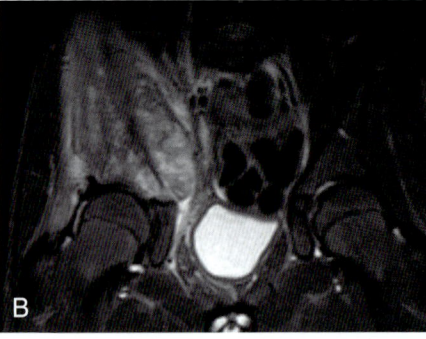 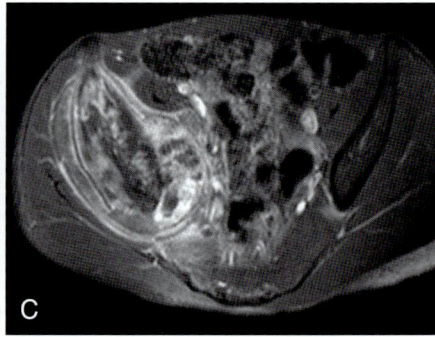

Figure 139-49 Ewing sarcoma of the right iliac bone in an 11-year-old girl. **A,** Frontal radiograph of the pelvis demonstrates a mixed lytic and blastic lesion of the right iliac bone. **B,** Short tau inversion recovery coronal magnetic resonance imaging (MRI) demonstrates a right iliac mass with extraosseous extension. **C,** Postcontrast T1-weighted axial MRI demonstrates heterogeneous enhancement of the mass, as it better delineates both extraperitoneal extension and posterior extension into the pelvic abductor muscles.

WHAT THE CLINICIAN NEEDS TO KNOW

- What are the location, size, and extent of the tumor?
- Is the soft tissue or bony lesion benign, malignant, or indeterminate?
- Is follow-up or additional imaging necessary?
- Are neurovascular structures involved?
- Does the lesion cross the joint space?

Key Points

MRI features highly suggestive of soft-tissue malignancy are neurovascular encasement, adjacent bone or joint involvement, and marrow abnormality.

Any fat-containing soft tissue mass in a child younger than 3 years of age is likely benign.

In general, osteosarcoma has a predilection for the metaphysis, and Ewing sarcoma, for the diaphysis. The matrix in osteosarcoma may be cloudlike.

ABCs may be primary or secondary. In addition, they may be associated with another benign or malignant lesion. Telangiectatic osteosarcoma can have a similar appearance.

Suggested Readings

Laor T. MR imaging of soft tissue tumors and tumor-like lesions. *Pediatr Radiol.* 2004;34(1):24-37.

Levine SM, Lambiase RE, Petchprapa CN. Cortical lesions of the tibia: characteristic appearances at conventional radiography. *Radiographics.* 23:157-177, 2003.

Murphey MD, Robbin MR, McRae GA, et al. The many faces of osteosarcoma. *Radiographics.* 1997;17:1205-1231.

Navarro OM, Laffan EE, Ngan B-Y. Pediatric soft-tissue tumors and pseudo-tumors: MR imaging features with pathologic correlation: part 1. Imaging approach, pseudotumors, vascular lesions, and adipocytic tumors. *Radiographics.* 2009;29(3):887-906.

O'Donnell P, Saifuddin A. The prevalence and diagnostic significance of fluid-fluid levels in focal lesions of bone. *Skeletal Radiol.* 2004;33:330-336.

References

Full references for this chapter can be found on www.expertconsult.com.

Chapter 140

Metabolic Bone Disease

RICHARD M. SHORE

Skeletal ossification and mineralization are influenced by many metabolic factors, with sometimes arbitrary distinctions between metabolic bone disorders, endocrine bone disorders, and inherited skeletal dysplasias. Accurate diagnosis is essential because many of these disorders require specific therapy for both their skeletal and extraskeletal effects.

Abnormalities of Mineralization

BONE MINERAL PHYSIOLOGY

In the process of bone formation, osteoblasts produce organic bone matrix (osteoid), which then must be mineralized with deposition of hydroxyapatite crystals.[1-4] Mineralization of cartilage and osteoid requires sufficient levels of circulating calcium and phosphate as reflected in an adequate calcium x phosphate product. Mineralization also requires alkaline phosphatase to hydrolyze pyrophosphate, which otherwise would inhibit crystal formation.[5] Hence deficient mineralization of cartilage and osteoid may be due to either an insufficient calcium x phosphate product as in rickets and osteomalacia or alkaline phosphatase deficiency as in hypophosphatasia. Rickets is a complex disorder of the growth plate that involves not only deficient mineralization of cartilage and osteoid but also disruption of endochondral ossification, leading to the accumulation of excessive cartilage. This phenomenon results from failure of hypertrophic chondrocytes to undergo normal apoptosis, which is now believed to be caused by hypophosphatemia as the common metabolic pathway of all forms of rickets (in calcipenic rickets, hypophosphatemia results from secondary hyperparathyroidism).[6] Osteomalacia is a pure disorder of insufficient mineralization of osteoid at sites other than the physes, hence at either sites of bone turnover or intramembranous bone formation. Forms of rickets due to insufficient calcium are mostly a result of abnormalities of vitamin D, whose major function is maintenance of a sufficient calcium x phosphate product. Vitamin D may be synthesized in the skin from 7-dehydrocholesterol upon exposure to sunlight containing ultraviolet B radiation (290 to 315 nm) or it may be provided in the diet, although natural dietary sources of vitamin D are quite limited. Vitamin D then undergoes 25-hydroxylation in the liver followed by highly regulated 1-α-hydroxylation in the kidney to produce 1,25(OH)$_2$-vitamin D, which is the active form of vitamin D (calcitriol). The most important biological function of calcitriol is facilitation of gastrointestinal absorption of calcium by inducing transcription of the gene for calcium-binding protein. Calcitriol synthesis by 1-α-hydroxylase is promoted by parathyroid hormone (PTH) in response to hypocalcemia.

Rickets also may result from a variety of disorders that cause hypophosphatemia, in most instances from renal tubular phosphate wasting. Renal tubular phosphate wasting or retention is regulated by PTH and by a variety of other factors, most of which are produced in bone by osteocytes.[7-12] The most important of these is fibroblast growth factor 23 (FGF23), which causes renal tubular phosphate wasting by downregulating the sodium-phosphate cotransporter that facilitates phosphate reabsorption. Additionally, FGF23 downregulates 1-α-hydroxylase, leading to diminished calcitriol with excessive FGF23 signaling. Similarly, insufficient FGF23 signaling increases calcitriol.

Nutritional (Vitamin D–Deficiency) Rickets

Etiology Both inadequate exposure to sunlight and insufficient dietary intake of vitamin D must be present for rickets to occur.[1-3,13-16] The first and most severe epidemic of rickets occurred during the industrial revolution as a result of urbanization and diminished exposure to sunlight from smog and the practice of staying indoors. This epidemic largely ended with food fortification after the discovery of vitamin D synthesis. However, rickets then became more prevalent in the United States during the mid 1990s with increased breast feeding in the African American and Hispanic populations, because breast milk provides relatively little vitamin D. Less commonly, nutritional rickets may result from insufficient calcium intake.[17]

Because 25(OH)D readily crosses the placenta, infants born to vitamin D–replete mothers have sufficient stores, and thus nutritional rickets usually is not apparent before 3 to 6 months. However, if the mother is deficient in vitamin D, nutritional rickets may be seen earlier.

Clinical manifestations of rickets include failure to thrive, short stature, bowing deformities, and predisposition to fractures. In addition, prominence of anterior rib ends causing a "rachitic rosary" and craniotabes (i.e., a ping-pong ball deformity of the skull) may be seen. Weakness is a clinical feature of rickets, correlating with the presence of vitamin D receptors in skeletal muscle.[18]

Imaging The manifestations of rickets are most pronounced with rapid bone growth with mineralization that is unable to keep pace with new bone formation. As a result the features of rickets are most pronounced in regions of greatest bone growth, particularly the distal radius and ulna, distal femur, proximal tibia, proximal humerus, and anterior rib ends. An insufficient calcium x phosphate product causes decreased mineralization of the zone of provisional calcification and lack of normal chondrocytic terminal differentiation. As a result the initial radiographic finding is rarefaction of the normally sharply defined zone of provisional calcification on the metaphyseal side of the growth plate so that metaphyseal bone fades gradually into the lucent physeal and epiphyseal cartilage (Fig. 140-1 and e-Fig. 140-2). Also seen is loss of definition of the Laval-Jeantet collar, a short cylindrical segment of the metaphysis adjacent to the growth plate that is an indicator of the most recently formed bone in young infants.[19] Deficient chondrocyte terminal differentiation and apoptosis causes accumulation of disorganized cartilage in the metaphysis in addition to nonmineralized osteoid, leading to widening of the distance between the epiphysis and metaphysis, metaphyseal fraying, and metaphyseal concavity (cupping). Metaphyseal concavity varies by site, being most pronounced in the distal forearm bones (see Fig. 140-1). However, distal ulnar metaphyseal concavity with no other abnormality should be recognized as a normal finding. Metaphyseal findings that may be recognized on chest radiographs include involvement of the proximal humeral metaphyses and rib ends, producing the rachitic rosary (Fig. 140-3), although this term more properly refers to the bulbous rib ends on physical examination. The classic metaphyseal findings of rickets are best illustrated by comparison of active and healed or healing phases (see Fig. 140-1 and e-Fig 140-2). Similar but less pronounced findings may be seen in the slower growing

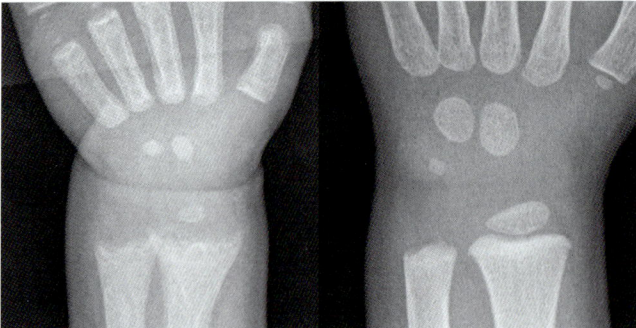

Figure 140-1 Vitamin D deficiency rickets. A 14-month-old child with growth failure and severe rickets who responded well to vitamin D therapy. The initial image (*left*) shows loss of definition of the zones of provisional calcification for the distal radial and ulnar metaphyses along with metaphyseal fraying and concavity ("cupping") and physeal widening with an increased distance between the epiphysis and visualized portion of the metaphysis. Periosteal new bone also is present that is seen best along the metacarpals but also is present along the distal radius. With healing (*right*), the zone of provisional calcification is well mineralized and the other findings have resolved.

epiphyses and small bones with loss of definition of the zone of provisional calcification surrounding the ossification centers.[19]

Long bone shaft findings lag behind those in the metaphysis. In rickets due to vitamin D abnormality, PTH rises in an attempt to restore a normal serum calcium concentration, producing secondary hyperparathyroidism (HPTH) with subperiosteal bone resorption, intracortical tunneling, and overall demineralization (Fig. 140-4). With ongoing bone remodeling, as nonmineralized osteoid replaces mineralized bone (osteomalacia), cortical demineralization and coarsening of the trabecular pattern in the shafts occurs, predisposing a person to insufficiency fractures. Paradoxically, periosteal new bone formation also may be seen in rickets even before

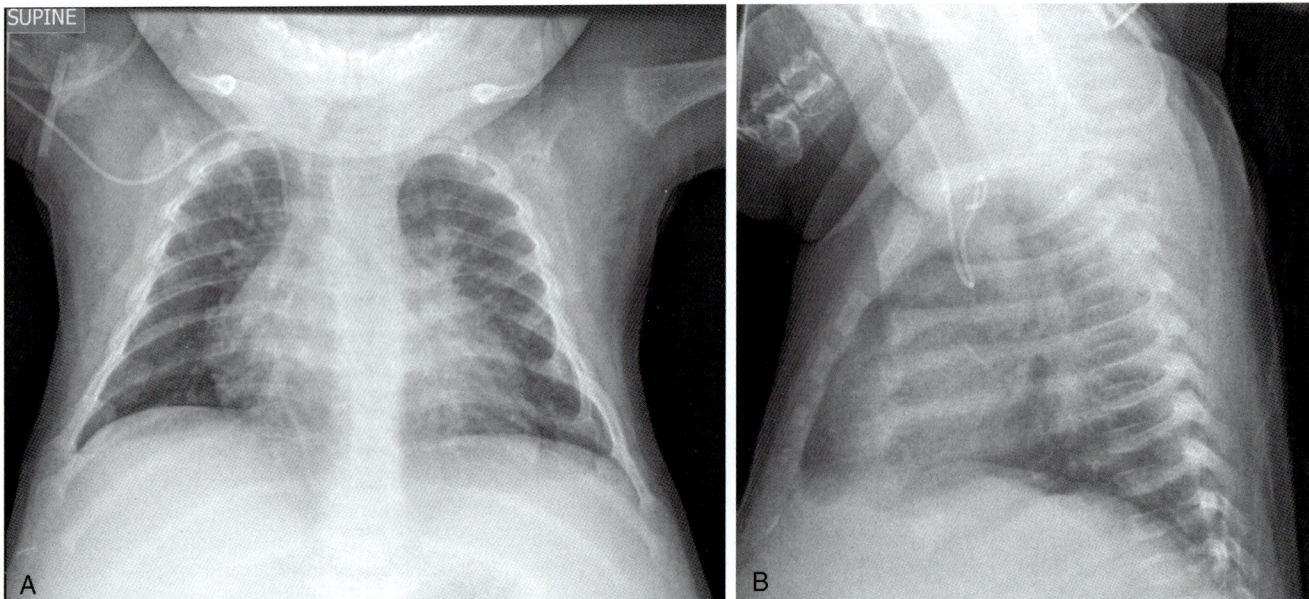

Figure 140-3 Anteroposterior (A) and lateral (B) chest radiograph views in a 5-month-old child with rickets from biliary atresia. Note rickets in the proximal humeral metaphyses and anterior rib ends. The rib findings are best seen on the lateral view.

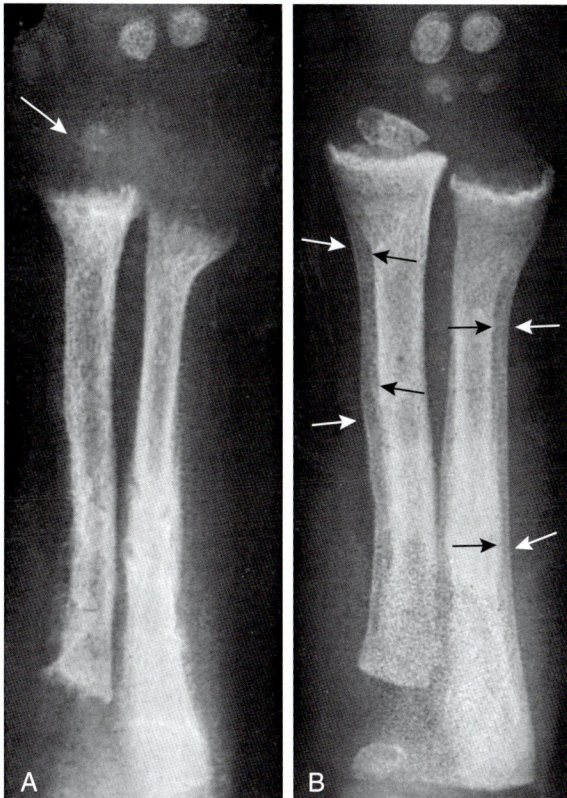

Figure 140-4 Diaphyseal findings in a patient with severe vitamin D deficiency rickets. During the active phase (**A**), coarse demineralization and subperiosteal bone resorption are present, which are indicative of hyperparathyroidism as a result of rickets. Also note the severe rachitic findings in the metaphysis and poor mineralization of the distal radial epiphysis with loss of the zones of provisional calcification (*arrow*). With healing 3 months later (**B**), extensive periosteal new bone is seen (*white arrows*) with calcification of previously nonmineralized osteoid (*black arrows*) produced by periosteal osteoblasts.

healing, which likely is an anabolic effect of PTH (see Fig. 140-1).

Bowing in rickets is most pronounced in the tibias and is due to loss of normal bone rigidity in the metaphyses and shafts. The large zone of nonmineralized cartilage and osteoid in the rachitic metaphyses is particularly deformable and subject to bending.

With healing (see Fig. 140-1, e-Fig. 140-2, and Fig. 140-4), mineral deposition in the zone of provisional calcification and restoration of chondrocyte terminal differentiation occurs. The initial radiographic finding of healing is reidentification of the zone of provisional calcification as a thin opaque line that is separated from the identifiable shaft by the intervening lucent nonmineralized cartilage and osteoid. With further healing, this metaphyseal region calcifies, which may give the false impression of rapid bone growth. Less often, newly mineralized osteoid also may be seen in the metaphyseal equivalent region of the epiphysis (e-Fig. 140-5). With healing of cortical bone, the subperiosteal osteoid becomes calcified, producing either a uniform or lamellated layer.

Additional imaging features of rickets include chest wall (Harrison) grooves related to diaphragmatic insertions. Scoliosis and kyphosis also may be seen.

Treatment and Follow-up   Prevention of vitamin D deficiency is a controversial issue because of lack of consensus regarding the level of vitamin D that is considered sufficient. The 2011 Institute of Medicine report[20] concluded that a serum level of 25-hydroxy-vitamin D of at least 20 ng/mL is normal, although many experts in vitamin D research argue that higher levels are needed. Accordingly, the Institute of Medicine recommends 400 IU of vitamin D daily during the first year of life and 600 IU daily thereafter, with higher amounts suggested by researchers who believe that higher serum levels are needed.

Treatment guidelines for vitamin D deficiency are those of the Lawson Wilkins Pediatric Endocrine Society.[21] Treatment is recommended for clinical manifestations of vitamin D deficiency or 25-hydroxy-vitamin D levels less than 15 ng/mL, beginning with higher doses than those used for prevention. With treatment, if radiographic evidence of healing is seen by 3 months, vitamin D dosage can be reduced to preventive levels. Because a major cause of treatment failure is noncompliance, intermittent high-dose vitamin D therapy also has been suggested.

Other Forms of Rickets

Many other conditions may result in an insufficient calcium x phosphate product, causing rickets. The radiographic manifestations described for vitamin D insufficiency rickets are etiologically nonspecific and are similar in the other forms of rickets unless otherwise indicated.

Malabsorption and Hepatobiliary Disease

Vitamin D malabsorption may cause rickets in disorders such as celiac disease and cystic fibrosis. Rickets with hepatobiliary disease is mostly a result of decreased intake and intestinal absorption of fat-soluble vitamins (A, D, E, and K); decreased hepatic 25-hydroxylation of vitamin D usually is not significant. Associated vitamin K deficiency in hepatobiliary disease may lead to recurrent hemarthrosis, most frequently involving the knee.

Vitamin D–Dependent Rickets, Types I and II

In autosomal-recessive vitamin D–dependent rickets (VDDR) type I, a defect in the renal 1-α-hydroxylase leads to undetectable or very low calcitriol levels.[22,23] Rickets in VDDR I is severe, presents in the first few months of life, and has more secondary HPTH than do other forms of rickets. VDDR I responds to physiologic doses of calcitriol. Rickets also can result from a defect in the receptor for calcitriol, causing vitamin D nonresponsiveness.[23,24] The designation of VDDR type II for this disorder is inappropriate because it is resistant to all forms of vitamin D, and hence the term "calcitriol-resistant rickets" is preferred. In addition to severe rickets, approximately half of the patients have manifestations of ectodermal dysplasia.

Hypophosphatemic Rickets

Hypophosphatemic forms of rickets are seen in hereditary hypophosphatemia, tumor-induced rickets and osteomalacia, and intrinsic renal tubular disease. Additionally, a major component of rickets of prematurity (i.e., metabolic bone disease of prematurity) is likely phosphate deficiency.

Hereditary Hypophosphatemic Disorders

Etiology X-linked hypophosphatemia (XLH), also known as familial vitamin D–resistant rickets, is the most common hereditary cause of hypophosphatemia, with rare autosomal-dominant and recessive variants.[7,9,11,16] The discovery that the autosomal-dominant variant was due to a gain of function for FGF23 led to the recognition of FGF23 as a major phosphaturic factor. In XLH, FGF23 also is increased, although it is not clearly understood how this increase is caused by a mutation in the *PHEX* gene.

XLH is characterized clinically by short stature and prominent bowing deformities of the lower extremities. Although X-linked dominant, it often is less severe in female heterozygotes than in male hemizygotes. Biochemically, serum phosphate is low and phosphate excretion is elevated. Calcium and PTH are normal and calcitriol is either low or inappropriately normal.

Imaging Lower extremity bowing usually is quite prominent in XLH (Fig. 140-6), whereas the rachitic findings of XLH are often (but not always) relatively mild. Because no hypocalcemia is present, secondary HPTH is not seen in hypophosphatemic rickets. Looser zones (a feature of osteomalacia) are present more often in XLH than in nutritional rickets, likely because of the chronicity of the mineralization disorder. Looser zones, or pseudofractures, are radiolucent lines oriented perpendicular to the cortex as a result of poor mineralization of osteoid at sites of stress, which lead to increased

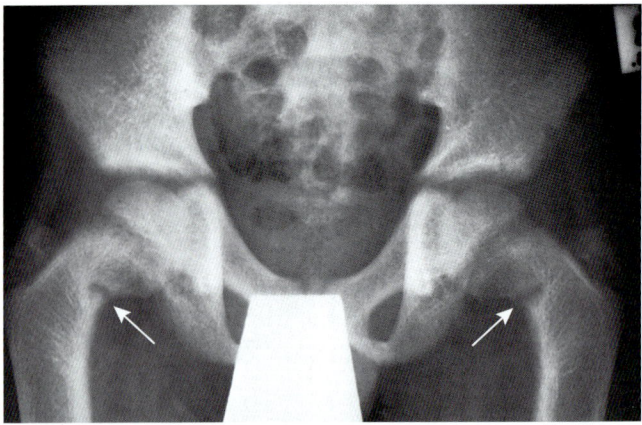

Figure 140-7 Looser zones in a child with X-linked hypophosphatemia. Symmetric transverse lucent areas in the medial aspect of the femoral necks (*arrows*) are a manifestation of osteomalacia. Also note the patchy increased density, coarse trabeculations, and rachitic irregularity of the metaphyses.

bone remodeling. Characteristic sites include the medial aspect of the femoral neck (Fig. 140-7), the extensor surface of the ulna, the axillary border of the scapula, and the pubic ramus, with these findings often being bilateral. In infants, craniosynostosis may complicate XLH.[25,26] In older patients, XLH may be associated with enthesopathy and paravertebral ossification, similar to diffuse idiopathic skeletal hyperostosis.

Treatment and Follow-up Treatment of XLH includes oral phosphate replacement and calcitriol because phosphate replacement alone often leads to secondary HPTH. However, excessive calcitriol may lead to hypercalcemia, nephrocalcinosis, and nephrolithiasis; renal ultrasonography often is used to screen for this complication.[27]

Tumor-Induced Rickets and Osteomalacia (Oncologic Osteomalacia)

Etiology Hypophosphatemic rickets and osteomalacia may be caused by certain tumors and tumorlike conditions that are capable of producing FGF23, with healing of rickets after removal of the tumor.[28,29] TIRO may occur at any age but is quite uncommon in children. Although a large variety of benign and malignant mesenchymal neoplasms initially were described, many of these neoplasms more recently have been recategorized pathologically as "phosphaturic mesenchymal tumor, mixed connective tissue variant."[30] Other conditions causing rickets that are considered to be within the spectrum of TIRO include neurofibromatosis, polyostotic fibrous dysplasia (with or without other features of McCune-Albright syndrome), epidermal nevus syndrome, and Gorham massive osteolysis syndrome (Fig. 140-8).

Patients with TIRO may present with chronic vague symptoms, including generalized pain and muscle weakness. TIRO should be suspected in cases of hypophosphatemic rickets with no family history or evidence of renal tubular disease.

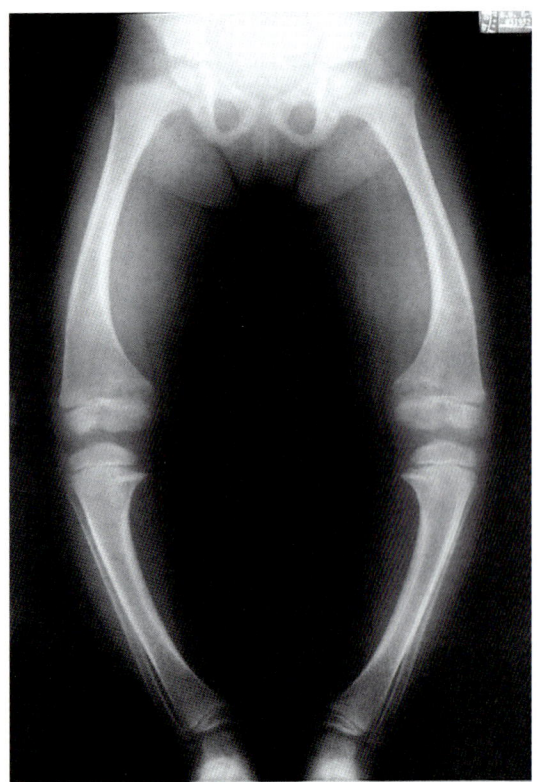

Figure 140-6 X-linked hypophosphatemia in a 3½-year-old girl. Prominent convex lateral bowing of the femurs and tibias is present, along with rachitic findings in the metaphyses.

Imaging The radiographic findings of TIRO are similar to those of other forms of chronic rickets such as XLH. Imaging also plays a role in the search for the causative tumor, which

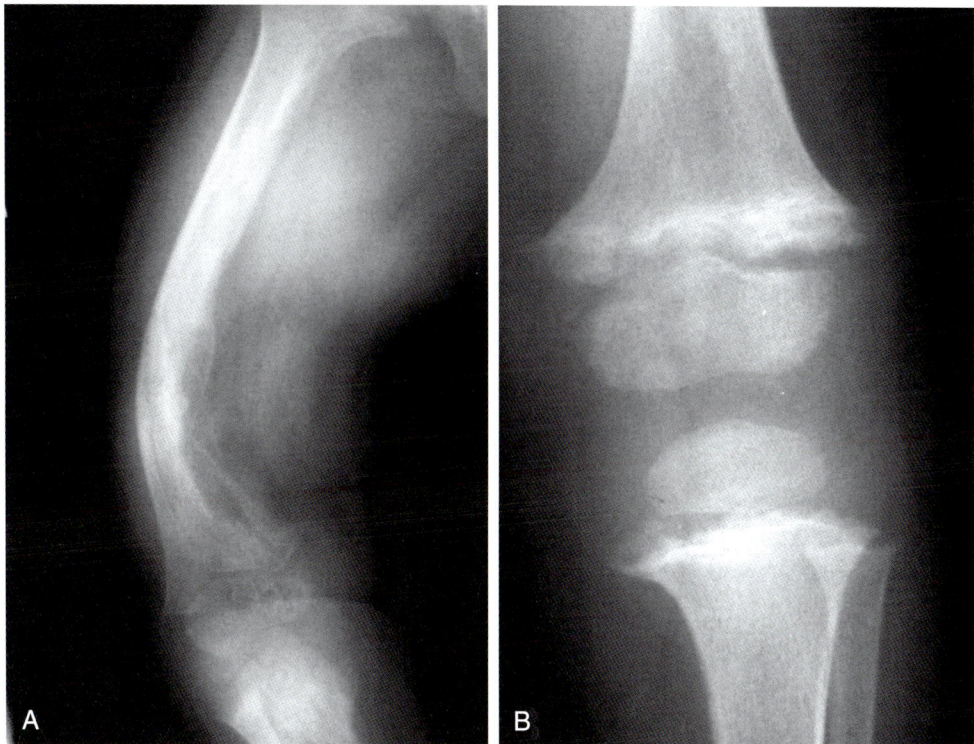

Figure 140-8 "Tumor-induced" hypophosphatemic rickets in a girl aged 2 years and 4 months with Gorham massive osteolysis syndrome. The right femur (**A**) shows extensive osteolysis. The left hemiskeleton was unaffected by osteolysis, but the left knee (**B**) shows typical features of rickets.

usually is small and grows slowly. Because phosphaturic mesenchymal tumors often express somatostatin receptors, In-111 octreotide scintigraphy has been used.[31] Reports also indicate that fluorine-18-deoxyglucose positron emission tomography/computed tomography may be helpful.[32]

Renal Tubular Disease Many disorders including cystinosis, tyrosinemia, galactosemia, Lowe syndrome, Wilson disease, and toxins may cause global renal tubular dysfunction, hyperphosphaturia, renal tubular acidosis, and wasting of other substances.

Rickets of Prematurity

Etiology Rickets of prematurity, also known as metabolic bone disease of prematurity, is most common in infants with a birth weight below 1 kg or gestational age younger than 28 weeks.[33,34] Normally, 80% of gestational bone mineral accretion occurs during the third trimester,[34] and thus infants born prematurely must accumulate mineral at a high rate to make up for this deficit. Although dietary mineral deficiency is rare in term infants and older children, inadequate intake of calcium and especially phosphorus is a major cause of metabolic bone disease of prematurity. Breast milk and infant formulas do not supply sufficient calcium and phosphorus for premature infants, and this deficiency becomes most pronounced during the period of "catch-up" growth, often near the time of hospital discharge.

Imaging Radiographic features include generalized osteopenia, fractures, and rachitic changes in the metaphyses (Fig. 140-9). However, the rachitic findings may be masked when the infant is not growing. The fractures often are not recognized acutely and, if first discovered after discharge, may be confused with nonaccidental trauma. Extremity fractures are common and usually do not lead to long-term morbidity because ample opportunity exists for remodeling.

Hypophosphatasia

Etiology Hypophosphatasia is a rare inherited condition in which deficient mineralization of cartilage and osteoid are attributed to alkaline phosphatase deficiency rather than an insufficient calcium x phosphate product (which characterizes rickets).[5,16,35,36] In hypophosphatasia, a defect in the gene encoding alkaline phosphatase results in accumulation of pyrophosphate, which interferes with the formation of hydroxyapatite crystals. The severe perinatal and infantile forms are autosomal recessive, with autosomal-recessive and dominant inheritance for the milder forms.

Hypophosphatasia is divided clinically into perinatal, infantile, childhood, and adult forms, with decreasing severity as the age of presentation increases. The perinatal form features severe lack of mineralization of the skeleton and short and deformed limbs. Absence of structural support for the thorax leads to respiratory insufficiency, predisposition to pneumonia, and early death. The infantile form has a less severe mineralization defect. Patients present before 6 months of age with lethargy, leading to poor feeding and failure to thrive. Rachitic-appearing ribs and multiple rib fractures may be seen. Craniosynostosis often is present and may be associated with increased intracranial pressure despite a wide appearance of the sutures radiographically. Prognosis for the infantile form is quite variable; approximately half die from respiratory causes and others improve spontaneously. Progression of skeletal findings suggests a poor and likely fatal

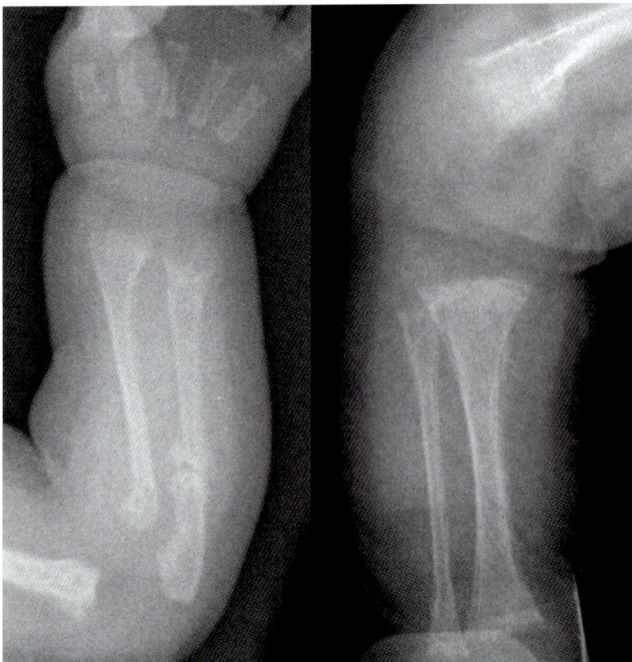

Figure 140-9 Metabolic bone disease of prematurity in a former premature infant who is now 3 months of age. Findings include severe diffuse demineralization, rachitic findings in major long bone metaphyses, and healing fractures of the ulnar diaphysis and distal femur.

outcome. The childhood and adult forms are milder with extremity pain, gait disturbance, weakness, and premature loss of deciduous teeth. The skeletal manifestations of childhood hypophosphatasia improve during adolescence, but symptoms of the "adult" form recur later in life. The adult form often presents in middle age with features simulating osteomalacia, including recurrent metatarsal stress fractures, femoral pseudofractures, arthropathy, and other recurrent orthopedic symptoms.

Imaging The perinatal form (Fig. 140-10) is characterized by severe failure of mineralization of much of the skeleton. Although the skull base usually is mineralized, the calvarium may be nearly completely nonmineralized. The remainder of the axial skeleton has varying mineralization. The extremities are short and incompletely mineralized. The overall skeletal deficiency in perinatal hypophosphatasia is worse than that in the severe in utero form of osteogenesis imperfecta. In infantile and childhood hypophosphatasia, the diaphyses appear normal and the metaphyses are poorly mineralized, suggesting a process similar to rickets. However, the "rachitic" changes of hypophosphatasia are not as uniformly distributed across the growth plate. Rather, it involves a more localized portion of the growth plate with deficient mineralization extending into the metaphysis, creating a "chewed out" appearance of the metaphyses (Fig. 140-11). Because of poor calvarial mineralization, the sutures may appear widened despite actual premature closure. The adult form simulates osteomalacia with a coarse trabecular pattern, Looser zones, and metatarsal fractures.

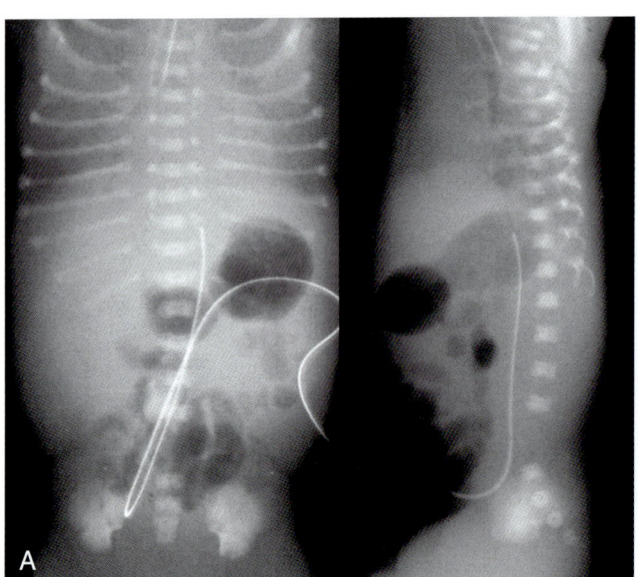

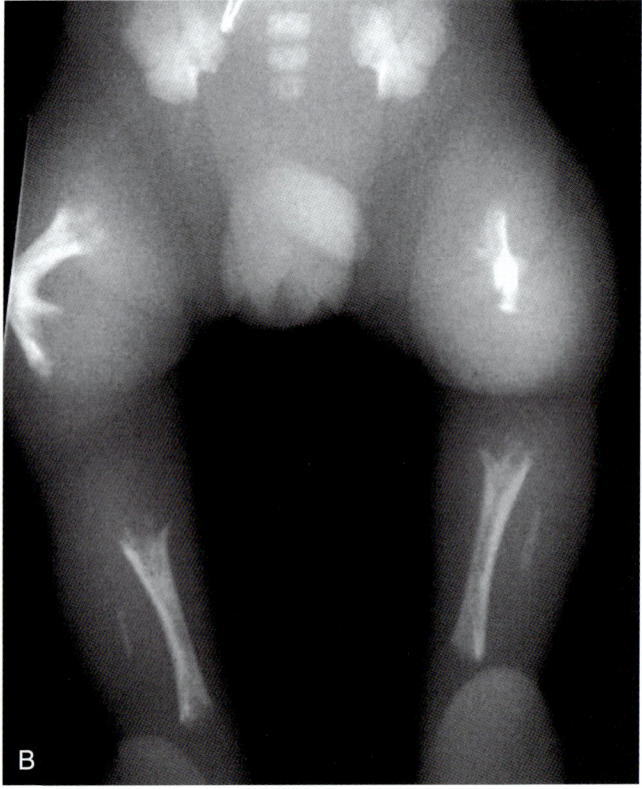

Figure 140-10 Perinatal hypophosphatasia. **A,** The skull is nonmineralized except for part of the base, a portion of the occipital bone. **B,** The posterior elements of the entire spine and the lower lumbar vertebral bodies are nonmineralized. (Courtesy Ellen Benya, MD, Chicago, IL.)

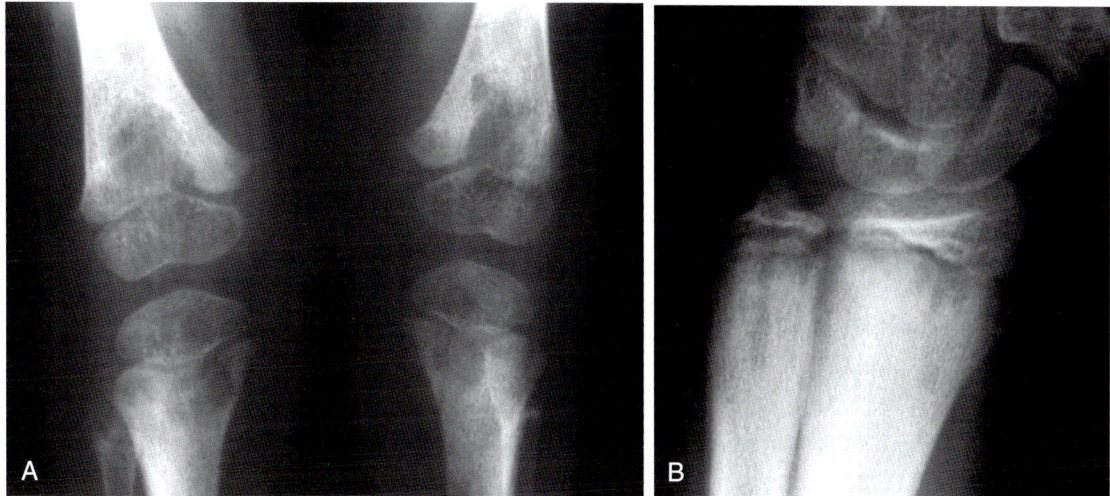

Figure 140-11 Childhood hypophosphatasia. Prominent lucent defects extend into the metaphyses from the growth plates with a more focal and "chewed out" appearance than the uniform mineralization defect of rickets.

Treatment and Follow-up Initial attempts to treat severe forms of hypophosphatasia with alkaline phosphatase infusion were ineffective, although more recent work with a bone-targeted human recombinant enzyme is encouraging.[37] Bone marrow transplantation also has been used in the treatment of infantile hypophosphatasia.[38] The milder forms are treated symptomatically.

Hyperphosphatemic Disorders

Etiology The major conditions causing hyperphosphatemia include renal insufficiency, tumoral calcinosis (TC), and hyperostosis hyperphosphatemia syndrome (HHS). TC and HHS are now considered to be different manifestations of the same disorder, with some patients showing features of each.[39] TC is an autosomal-recessive disorder characterized by prominent calcific deposits and hyperphosphatemia. It usually is seen in adolescents and young adults but may present earlier. In the United States, TC is most common in African Americans. HHS is most common in the Middle East and usually presents in childhood with extremity pain and swelling along with imaging findings that mimic osteomyelitis. Recognition of hyperphosphatemia and knowledge of this condition are essential in offering an alternative diagnosis. TC and HHS biochemically mirror image hypophosphatemic rickets with hyperphosphatemia and elevated or inappropriately normal calcitriol levels. These effects are secondary to decreased FGF23 signaling, which in turn is caused by mutations affecting either FGF23 an enzyme that stabilizes it, or its receptor.[40-43]

TC should be distinguished from secondary causes of heterotopic bone formation, such as is seen in chronic renal insufficiency and posttraumatic myositis ossificans.

Imaging The major finding in TC is the deposition of large calcific masses in the paraarticular soft tissues (Fig. 140-12, A).[44-46] In descending order, the hips, elbows, shoulders, and feet are most frequently involved. These masses often are cystic and may show layering of chalky fluid on cross-sectional imaging or even horizontal beam radiography. Some patients with TC may also have manifestations of HHS, including medullary sclerosis, extensive periosteal new bone, abnormalities on skeletal scintigraphy, and bone marrow edema on magnetic resonance imaging (Fig. 140-12, B). These features are related to bone marrow involvement and may mimic osteomyelitis or other infiltrative disorders.

Treatment and Follow-up The calcified masses of TC are amenable to surgical excision if they become painful or cause deformity or functional impairment. Many forms of therapy have been used to diminish or prevent these deposits, although they all have limited supporting data. Most often used is dietary phosphate restriction, which often is combined with aluminum-based phosphate binders. No forms of therapy have been found to be useful in patients with hyperostosis HHS, a disorder that usually shows spontaneous subsidence, often followed by recurrence.

Abnormalities of Bone Matrix Formation

Bone matrix (osteoid) is the organic framework upon which mineral, in the form of hydroxyapatite, is deposited. The most common cause of insufficient matrix formation is osteogenesis imperfecta with defects in the genes encoding type I collagen. Normal collagen synthesis also depends on ascorbic acid (vitamin C) and ascorbic acid oxidase, a copper-dependent enzyme. Hence matrix synthesis is impaired in vitamin C deficiency (scurvy), copper deficiency, and some abnormalities of copper metabolism.

SCURVY

Etiology Scurvy is caused by dietary deficiency of vitamin C.[47-49] Although infantile scurvy is now quite rare, it may be underdiagnosed. Adult scurvy remains a significant problem, particularly in elderly persons.[50] Historically, infantile scurvy occurred almost exclusively in babies fed pasteurized or boiled milk, because of heat destruction of vitamin C. Scurvy nearly always presents after 6 months of age; when similar

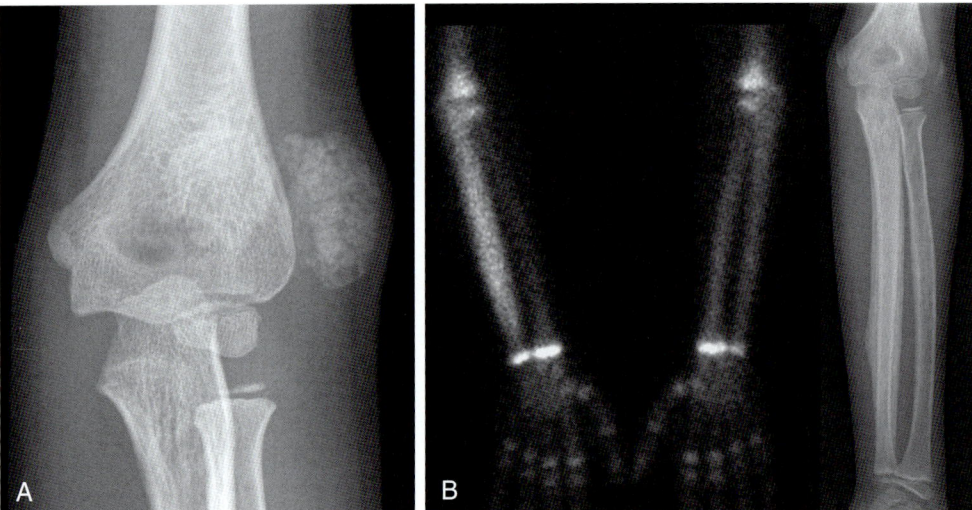

Figure 140-12 Tumoral calcinosis/hyperostosis hyperphosphatemia syndrome. **A,** A left elbow radiograph at age 7 years shows a multiloculated calcified mass lateral to the left elbow. A similar mass also was present lateral to the right hip (not shown). These masses were excised with confirmation of tumoral calcinosis. **B,** At age 9 years, evaluation for left forearm and mandibular pain included a bone scan showing increased localization of technicium-99m diphosphonate throughout the left ulna with extensive periosteal new bone on the corresponding radiograph. The mandible and maxilla also were abnormal on the bone scan (not shown).

findings are seen earlier, alternative diagnoses such as congenital syphilis should be considered.

Imaging Decreased osteoid formation in scurvy causes an imbalance between bone production and resorption, leading to generalized atrophy of the cortex and spongiosa. However, chondrocyte terminal differentiation and cartilage calcification are normal, forming a well-mineralized zone of provisional calcification. On the diaphyseal side of the physis, resorption of calcified cartilage is diminished, leading to a thickened zone of provisional calcification. Radiographically, this thickened zone is seen as a prominent opaque line (Fig. 140-13), designated as the white line of scurvy (white line of Fränkel). Despite its thickness, this zone is brittle and may fracture. The bone just beneath the thickened provisional zone is demineralized and also brittle with a sparse trabecular pattern, producing a lucent zone adjacent to the zone of provisional calcification (see Fig. 140-13) known as the scurvy zone (the Trümmerfeld zone). Later, transverse fractures may develop through the brittle zone of provisional calcification and the demineralized metaphyseal scurvy zone. If this fracture is limited to a peripheral portion of the scurvy zone, a subphyseal lucent cleft will be seen (Fig. 140-14). With transverse displacement of the epiphysis and zone of provisional calcification from the rest of the shaft, the heavily mineralized zone of provisional calcification projects peripherally, forming a metaphyseal spur (Pelkan spur), another characteristic radiographic feature of scurvy. These changes should not be confused with metaphyseal fractures of child abuse. Similar changes in the epiphyses lead to a thickened peripheral shell of calcified cartilage surrounding rarefied trabecular bone within the epiphysis, producing the Wimberger ring (see Fig. 140-13), one of the most characteristic findings of scurvy. This appearance is opposite that of rickets, in which the peripheral ring is lost with relative sparing of the central trabecular bone. In the shaft, the findings are those of generalized osteopenia with cortical thinning, although diaphyseal fractures are uncommon compared with those through

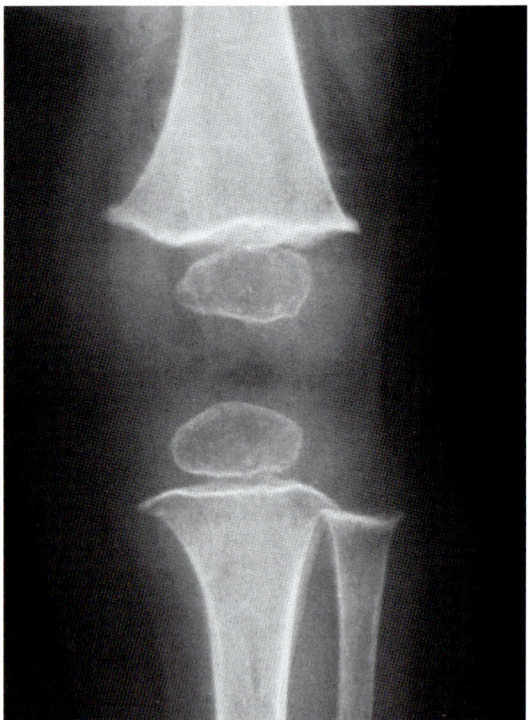

Figure 140-13 Scurvy. The zones of provisional calcification are prominent and form the white line of scurvy. These zones stand out in high contrast compared with the subjacent demineralized scurvy zone, which is better seen for the proximal tibia than for the distal femur. Similar findings also are present at the margins of the epiphyses where the epiphyseal zone of provisional calcification forms the Wimberger ring surrounding the centrally lucent epiphysis. A small spur is present at the lateral aspect of the distal femoral metaphysis, and a proximal tibial spur is partially obscured by the fibula.

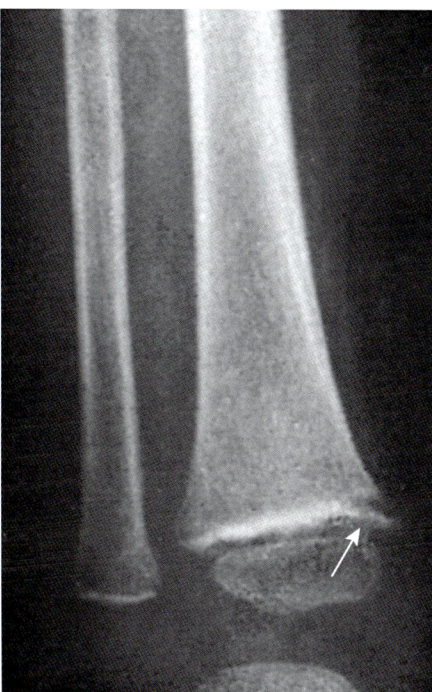

Figure 140-14 A peripheral metaphyseal cleft in a 14-month-old child with scurvy. An eccentric lucent cortical and trabecular defect produces a cleft (*arrow*) just beneath the zone of provisional calcification, with the peripheral aspect of the zone of provisional calcification separated from the shaft and tilted off the shaft toward the epiphysis.

the scurvy and provisional calcification zones. Subperiosteal hemorrhage due to capillary fragility is a frequent manifestation of scurvy and is most common in the larger tubular bones such as the femur, tibia, and humerus. Initially, subperiosteal hemorrhage is seen as increased soft tissue opacity. Subsequently, the periosteum produces a cloak of new bone surrounding the shaft, which eventually will become the new cortex (Fig. 140-15).

Treatment and Follow-up   The diagnosis of scurvy usually is based on a combination of the clinical and radiographic findings; an appropriate dietary history also may be helpful. Laboratory testing usually is not helpful. Although orange juice or tomato juice may be used, treatment with ascorbic acid usually is provided. The clinical response is usually rapid, confirming the diagnosis.

COPPER DEFICIENCY AND MENKES DISEASE

Ascorbic acid oxidase is a copper-dependent enzyme, and hence copper deficiency results in deficient matrix formation and osteopenia. These findings are nonspecific, and copper deficiency has been confused with metabolic bone disease of prematurity, although neutropenia and anemia serve as other markers of copper deficiency. Menkes disease is an X-linked condition that is characterized by kinky hair, osteopenia and bone fragility, mental retardation, seizures, and intracranial hemorrhage as a result of widespread arterial abnormalities.[36,51] Menkes disease is a result of deficiency of a cation-transporting enzyme needed for transport of copper from the gut and its intracellular delivery to copper-dependent enzymes, including lysyl oxidase, which is needed for proper

cross-linking of collagen and elastin. This deficiency results in abnormal collagen and elastin, leading to osteopenia and increased bone fragility. Fractures in Menkes disease may follow minor trauma; in addition, metaphyseal fractures with spurring may appear similar to the metaphyseal fractures of nonaccidental trauma,[52] which in some cases erroneously has led to that diagnosis (e-Fig. 140-16).

Hypervitaminosis A

Etiology   Vitamin A is a fat-soluble vitamin needed for vision and many other essential processes. In addition to its role in light reception, it is essential for normal epithelial differentiation of mucous membranes, and hence vitamin A deficiency causes xerophthalmia (dry ulcerating eye), the leading cause of blindness worldwide. Historically, fish liver oil and other preparations used for prevention and treatment xerophthalmia had been the major cause of vitamin A toxicity in young children, with cases often blamed on overly diligent caregivers. With discontinuation of these preparations, infantile hypervitaminosis A has become quite rare. More recently, toxicity has been from high-potency vitamin A analogs used for their pharmacologic rather than physiologic effects in dermatologic disorders.

Chronic vitamin A toxicity usually presents at least 6 months after the beginning of excessive vitamin A intake. Initial symptoms are nonspecific, with anorexia and irritability. Dry, pruritic skin with desquamation, lip fissuring, and hepatomegaly may be present. The extremities demonstrate focal regions of swelling and pain that overlie the skeletal findings. Acute vitamin A poisoning is rare and usually presents with central nervous system signs and symptoms from increased intracranial pressure.

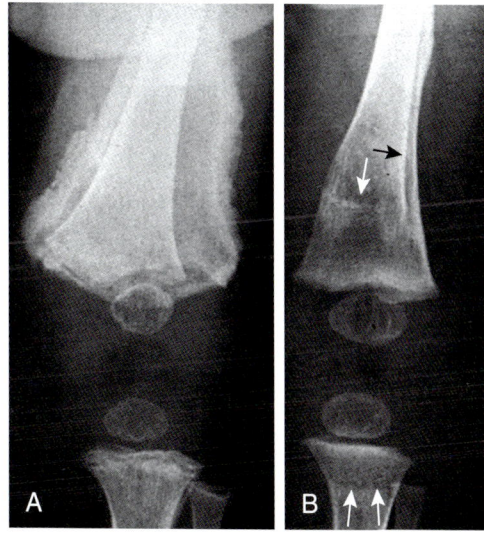

Figure 140-15 Scurvy with displaced fracture and a subperiosteal hematoma. **A,** The left distal femoral epiphysis is displaced laterally relative to the metaphysis with a fracture through the brittle zone of provisional calcification. A large subperiosteal hematoma is present with periosteal calcification. Also note a nondisplaced fracture through the proximal tibial zone of provisional calcification and Wimberger rings for the distal femur and proximal tibia. **B,** Four months later the periosteal new bone is producing a new cortex with remodeling and eventual anatomic alignment of the prior epiphyseal displacement. Arrows indicate the initial cortex and zone of provisional calcification.

Imaging The skeletal manifestation of hypervitaminosis A may be extremely helpful in establishing this diagnosis in a child with a confusing clinical picture.[53,54] Long bone hyperostosis is the most frequent and most well-recognized finding, with periosteal new bone formation leading to undulating diaphyseal cortical thickening, most frequently involving the ulnae (Fig. 140-17) and metatarsals. Radiographically, these findings have been confused with infantile cortical hyperostosis (Caffey disease). However, age and distribution usually differentiate these, with presentation after 11 months and metatarsal involvement suggesting hypervitaminosis A, whereas presentation before 5 months and mandibular involvement suggests infantile cortical hyperostosis.[53] Premature central growth plate closure also may be seen in hypervitaminosis A,[55,56] likely because of an effect of retinoic acid on promoting chondrocyte terminal differentiation, thus accelerating endochondral ossification.[57] This effect may lead to cone-shaped epiphyses that are invaginated into the metaphyses, mimicking the appearance of prior meningococcemia (Fig. 140-18). High-potency synthetic vitamin A analogs (e.g., isotretinoin) that are used for prolonged treatment of keratinizing disorders such as ichthyosis also may cause hyperostosis, although the pattern is different with involvement of the axial skeleton, resembling diffuse idiopathic skeletal hyperostosis.[58] Beaklike ossifications also occur at the calcaneus and near the ends of the long bones compared with the diaphyseal involvement from vitamin A toxicity.

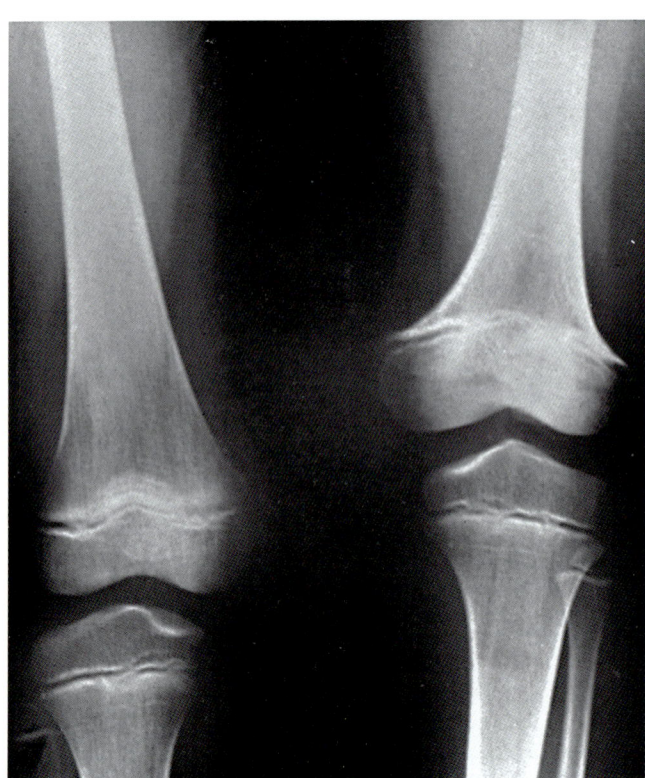

Figure 140-18 Premature central growth plate closure from vitamin A causing a short left femur and a cone-shaped physis. In other cases involvement can be more generalized. (Courtesy Charles N. Pease, Chicago, IL.)

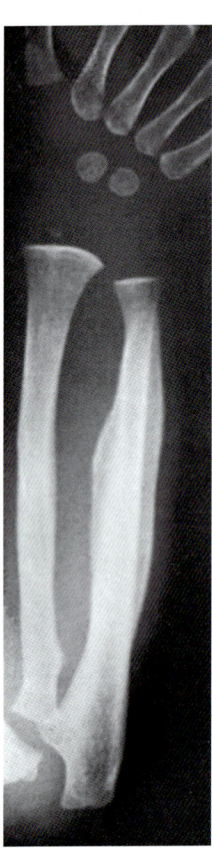

Figure 140-17 Mature periosteal new bone producing cortical hyperostosis in the right ulna from vitamin A toxicity. The finding was symmetrical with an identical appearance of the left ulna (not shown).

Hypervitaminosis D

Etiology Production of calcitriol, the most active vitamin D metabolite, is a highly regulated process that provides inherent protection against vitamin D toxicity, which would require either excessive calcitriol ingestion or massive doses of less potent forms of vitamin D. Iatrogenic vitamin D poisoning has occurred in patients with physiologic bowlegs who mistakenly were thought to have XLH (vitamin D–resistant rickets) and were given escalating doses of vitamin D. The Schmid type of metaphyseal chondrodysplasia also can mimic XLH, and large doses of vitamin D will not "cure" the bowing or metaphyseal irregularity.

Vitamin D poisoning may be acute or chronic. Most symptoms and signs are associated with manifestations of hypercalcemia. Massive overdosage (4 to 18 million U/day) may cause severe illness or even death. Manifestations may include vomiting, dehydration, fever, coma, convulsions, abdominal cramps, and "bone pain." In cases of chronic poisoning, the common early symptoms are lethargy, thirst, anorexia, vomiting, diarrhea, and abdominal discomfort. Excessive calcium excretion leads to renal damage.

Imaging Skeletal findings include cortical thickening, osteoporosis, and alternating bands of increased and decreased opacity (Fig. 140-19). Metastatic calcifications also may be present in blood vessels, the flax cerebri, and many organs, including the kidneys, stomach, lungs, bronchi, and adrenal gland.[59]

Heavy Metal Poisoning

Etiology Lead poisoning is the most common form of heavy metal poisoning. In children, lead poisoning usually occurs as a result of the ingestion of lead that is contained in paint chips in older housing; in the United States, the sale of house paint containing lead was discontinued in 1978. Although the incidence of lead poisoning has declined with public health and education efforts, it remains a significant problem, particularly in older neighborhoods. Other environmental sources of lead are less common. Lead bullets result in toxicity only if they are within a serous space such as a synovium-lined joint, where lead will cause both systemic toxicity and synovitis, resulting in lead arthropathy.

Lead poisoning is characterized by abdominal pain, encephalopathy, peripheral neuropathy, and anemia with basophilic stippling.

Imaging Chronic lead toxicity causes bands of increased opacity (lead lines) in the metaphyses. The amount of lead in these regions is far below the amount that would be needed to produce opaque bands. Rather, lead toxicity causes defective resorption of calcified cartilage in the primary spongiosa, which builds up, producing the opaque bands. When they are first formed, these bands are located along the zone of provisional calcification of long bone metaphyses and other metaphyseal equivalent regions, such as the iliac crests. The major differential diagnostic consideration is normal–variant opaque metaphyseal bands, and correlation with lead levels often is needed. Usually, the more opaque the metaphyseal band, the more likely it is to be pathologic. However, lead lines can be clearly distinguished from normal opaque metaphyseal bands once interval bone growth separates the abnormally sclerotic bone from the zone of provisional calcification. Normal opaque metaphyseal bands are always contiguous with the zone of provisional calcification, with the sclerotic bone being resorbed by the time that it "migrates away" from the physis (Fig. 140-20).

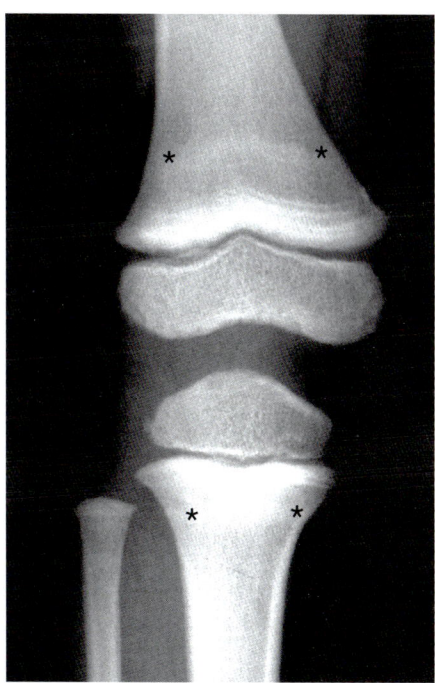

Figure 140-20 **Lead toxicity.** In addition to the opaque bands at the zones of provisional calcification, faint opaque bands also are present (between *asterisks*) that have "migrated away," clearly establishing that they are abnormal rather than normal-variant opaque metaphyseal bands, which are always in continuity with the zone of provisional calcification.

Treatment and Follow-up Steps to prevent further exposure to lead are mandatory. Removal of radiographically identified lead chips from the stomach by gastric lavage has been performed to prevent subsequent absorption. However, use of this technique is controversial because the lead chips usually are poorly absorbed, and the American Academy of Clinical Toxicology does not support its use. In addition, no evidence exists to support the use of charcoal as a gastrointestinal binder to prevent absorption. For patients with particularly high lead levels, chelation therapy is indicated and is best managed by an expert in clinical toxicology who is familiar with the criteria for treatment, the agents used, and potential complications.

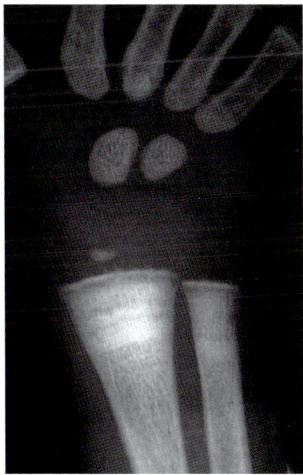

Figure 140-19 **Iatrogenic vitamin D intoxication in a child with physiological bowlegs who mistakenly was thought to have X-linked hypophosphatemia.** Multiple opaque bands are present in the distal radial metaphysis.

Key Points

The initial radiographic finding in rickets is loss of mineralization of the zone of provisional calcification.

Isolated distal ulnar metaphyseal cupping is a normal variant in an infant and should not be confused with rickets.

In scurvy, maintenance of the zone of provisional calcification with subjacent demineralization occurs and gives an opposite appearance to rickets in both the metaphyses and epiphyses.

Metaphyseal skeletal changes with scurvy may superficially mimic classic metaphyseal fractures of child abuse.

Suggested Readings

Alizadeh Naderi AS, Reilly RF. Hereditary disorders of renal phosphate wasting. *Nat Rev Nephrol.* 2010;6:657-665.

Holick MF. Vitamin D deficiency. *N Engl J Med.* 2007;357:266-281.

Pettifor JM. Rickets and vitamin D deficiency in children and adolescents. *Endocrinol Metab Clin North Am.* 2005;34:537-553.

Rajakumar K, Thomas SB. Reemerging nutritional rickets: a historical perspective. *Arch Pediatr Adolesc Med.* 2005;159:335-341.

Whyte MP. Physiological role of alkaline phosphatase explored in hypophosphatasia. *Ann N Y Acad Sci.* 2010;1192:190-200.

References

Full references for this chapter can be found on www.expertconsult.com.

Chapter 141

Endocrine Disorders

RICHARD M. SHORE

Several endocrine glands have significant effects on skeletal growth, maturation, and modeling, and understanding these effects facilitates correct radiographic interpretation, allowing for optimal therapy. The parathyroid glands are also intimately involved in mineral homeostasis and have major effects on bone mineralization and resorption.[1,2] Because of the importance of hyperparathyroidism (HPTH) in its pathophysiology, renal osteodystrophy is also included in this chapter as are other related conditions such as those causing neonatal hypercalcemia and disorders of bone resorption.

Hyperparathyroidism and Renal Osteodystrophy

Etiology   The parathyroid glands act to maintain a normal circulating calcium concentration. Synthesis and secretion of parathyroid hormone (PTH) are regulated by the parathyroid calcium sensing receptor, which increases PTH in response to hypocalcemia. PTH then has many effects that function to restore the serum calcium concentration. PTH promotes bone resorption to mobilize calcium. In the kidney, PTH upregulates renal 1-α-hydroxylase to produce calcitriol (1,25[OH]$_2$-vitamin D) which then acts on the gut to absorb calcium. PTH also decreases renal calcium excretion and increases phosphate excretion.

Bone resorption is mediated by multinucleated osteoclasts, which are derived from the monocyte–macrophage lineage. Their development is stimulated by osteoclast differentiation factor that is produced by osteoblasts. Osteoclast differentiation factor (RANK-ligand or RANKL) binds to a cell surface receptor called *RANK*. PTH has a major role in stimulating osteoclastic bone resorption, probably acting both directly and indirectly through stimulation of *RANKL*. Calcitriol also stimulates osteoclastic differentiation and function through RANKL, whereas calcitonin transiently inhibits osteoclastic resorption. Activated osteoclasts then form a sealed-off compartment along the resorption surface. Within this localized compartment, bone is dissolved by highly concentrated enzymes in acidified extracellular fluid.

Primary HPTH may be caused by diffuse parathyroid hyperplasia or parathyroid adenoma. Parathyroid adenomas are infrequent in children and are usually associated with multiple endocrine neoplasia (MEN) I. Parathyroid hyperplasia may be seen with MEN II and MEN III.

In secondary HPTH, PTH secretion is increased in response to hypocalcemia. Secondary HPTH is more frequent than primary HPTH in children and most often caused by chronic renal failure. Rickets and some other disorders of calcium metabolism may also cause secondary HPTH. HPTH in children is most often caused by chronic renal failure.

RENAL OSTEODYSTROPHY

Renal osteodystrophy (ROD)[3-5] comprises a variety of skeletal manifestations of chronic renal failure, the most important of which is secondary HPTH. In chronic renal failure, as the glomerular filtration rate falls, less phosphate is filtered. Phosphate retention and the slight decrease in the ionized calcium concentration caused by it, each stimulates PTH which then acts to promote phosphaturia and increase calcium. Although this initially normalizes calcium and phosphate concentrations, it does so at the expense of elevating PTH and mobilizing calcium and phosphate from bone. With advancing renal failure, decreased renal mass also reduces calcitriol synthesis, leading to rickets and osteomalacia. However, this effect on the skeleton is less pronounced than is HPTH, and many of the manifestations of "renal rickets" are actually those of HPTH.

Imaging   PTH stimulation of osteoclasts leads to bone resorption at multiple sites.[3-6] The most specific radiographic manifestation of HPTH is subperiosteal resorption, initially seen along the radial aspects of the index and the middle finger middle phalanges (Fig. 141-1). The distal phalangeal terminal tufts are also involved relatively early. With progression, subperiosteal resorption is noted along the ulnar aspects of the phalanges and other bones including the medial aspects of the humeral and femoral necks and the medial aspects of the proximal tibial metaphyses. Although less specific than subperiosteal resorption, HPTH may lead to intracortical resorption, or "tunneling," causing a striated appearance of the cortex, as well as endosteal, subchondral, and subligamentous resorption (Fig. 141-2). Subphyseal resorption (a form of subchondral resorption) leads to resorption of the zone of provisional calcification and metaphyseal bone beneath the physis, simulating the appearance of rickets. Additional findings of HPTH include resorption of the lamina dura, which forms the thin opaque line surrounding tooth roots (Figs. 141-3 and 141-4), cystic-appearing "brown tumors"

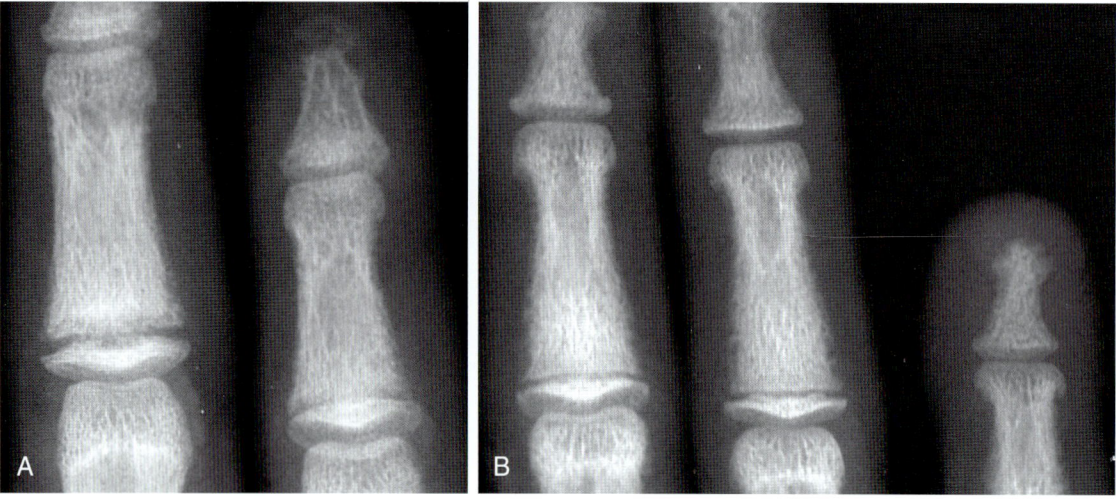

Figure 141-1 Subperiosteal bone resorption involving the radial aspects of the middle phalanges from secondary hyperparathyroidism in renal osteodystrophy.

(osteoclastomas), and bone sclerosis. Although brown tumors are more characteristic of primary HPTH, overall, they are seen more often in secondary HPTH because it is much more common than primary HPTH in children. Osteosclerosis, most often seen with renal osteodystrophy, may be generalized or most pronounced subjacent to the vertebral end plates, resulting in a "rugger jersey" appearance (Fig. 141-5).

Slipped epiphyses (e-Fig. 141-6) are an important complication of renal osteodystrophy in children, accounting for more cases than other predisposing conditions such as hypothyroidism, hypogonadism, and growth hormone deficiency. Although subphyseal resorption can mimic the radiographic appearance of rickets, the radiolucent material beneath the growth plate is fibrous tissue of osteitis fibrosa cystica, which is weaker than the nonmineralized cartilage and osteoid in true rickets, accounting for slipped epiphyses in renal osteodystrophy but not true rickets. Radiographic findings indicating a particularly high risk of slippage include coxa vara with reorientation of the physis from horizontal toward vertical, increased width of the growth plate, and subperiosteal resorption of the adjacent metaphysis. The risk of epiphyseal slippage is particularly high when growth hormone is used to treat short stature, a major clinical problem in children with chronic renal failure. Although slipped epiphyses are seen

most frequently in the proximal femur, many other sites may also be involved.

True rickets and osteomalacia may also be seen from decreased production of calcitriol. It is often not possible to distinguish true rickets from the rachitic appearance of osteitis fibrosa cystica. Looser zones, if present, indicate osteomalacia. Renal osteodystrophy usually manifests a "high turnover" state from HPTH. Less often, an adynamic "low turnover" state may also be seen. Previously, adynamic bone disease was often due to aluminum toxicity, which occurred as a complication of dialysis or aluminum-based phosphate binders. Presently, causes of adynamic bone disease include calcitriol therapy (which suppresses PTH), malnutrition, immobilization, corticosteroid therapy, and prior parathyroidectomy.

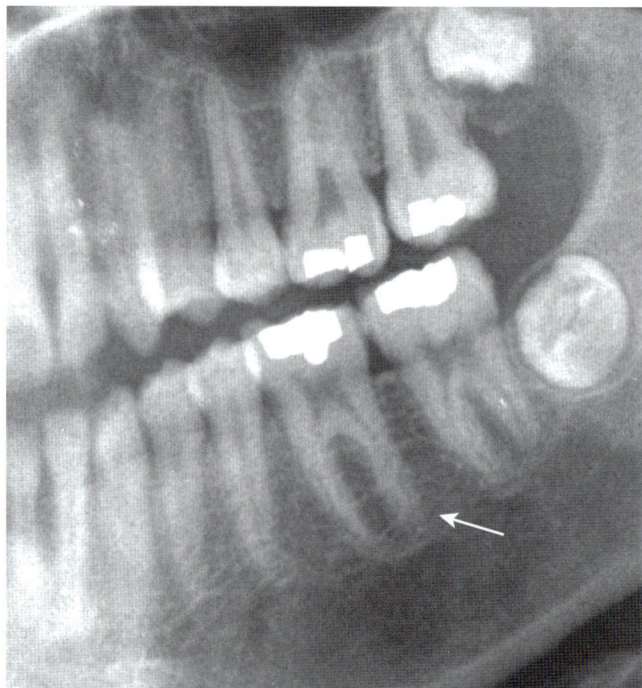

Figure 141-2 Subligamentous resorption at coracoclavicular ligament (*arrows*) in secondary hyperparathyroidism of renal osteodystrophy.

Figure 141-3 A 16-year-old girl with loss of normal lamina dura (*arrow*) and a history of hyperparathyroidism caused by chronic renal failure.

Fractures may occur in renal osteodystrophy with HPTH predisposing to metaphyseal fractures (e-Fig. 141-7).

Treatment and Follow-up Treatment of secondary HPTH in children with chronic renal disease is directed toward normalization of mineral metabolism to improve growth, decrease skeletal deformity and fragility, and prevent extraskeletal calcification, most importantly vascular calcification.[4,7] Treatment is often initiated at stage 3 chronic renal disease (GFR <60 mL/min/1.73 m^2) when positive phosphate balance and calcitriol deficiency appear. Dietary phosphate restriction is often difficult to achieve while maintaining adequate protein intake. Hence, intestinal phosphate binders are used. Although calcium-containing phosphate binders such as calcium carbonate have been used extensively, they pose a risk of hypercalcemia and vascular calcification, particular when used along with calcitriol. Aluminum-containing phosphate binders may cause aluminum bone disease and should be avoided. Sevelamer is a newer phosphate binder that does not contain calcium and has been shown to lower phosphate and control the skeletal lesions of HPTH without the adverse effects on vascular calcification that are seen with calcium-containing binders.

Vitamin D analogs are also important in control of second-degree HPTH, beginning with vitamin D repletion, as many patients are deficient. Additionally, active vitamin D metabolites, most often calcitriol, act to lower PTH both indirectly by increasing intestinal calcium absorption and directly by inhibiting transcription for the gene encoding PTH. The use of calcitriol requires monitoring for hypercalcemia. Hypercalcemia can be managed by decreasing or discontinuing calcium-containing phosphate binders or reducing calcitriol. Specific vitamin D analogs, which lower PTH mostly by inhibiting its gene transcription with relatively little effect on intestinal calcium absorption, are also available. Calcimimetics are allosteric modulators of the parathyroid calcium sensing receptor, which increase the sensitivity of the receptor to calcium. This effectively lowers the level at which the circulating calcium concentration suppresses PTH synthesis and secretion, thereby lowering both calcium and PTH.

Despite medical therapy, parathyroidectomy may still be needed in some patients with renal osteodystrophy and severe HPTH. Documentation of severe HPTH and absence of aluminum accumulation by bone biopsy prior to parathyroidectomy has been suggested. Postoperative hypocalcemia should be expected and managed accordingly.

Other Disorders of Hyperparathyroidism and Causes of Bone Resorption

NEONATAL HYPERPARATHYROIDISM

Primary HPTH in neonates is quite rare and is usually caused by hyperplasia rather than parathyroid adenoma.[8] Some cases, neonatal HPTH may result from homozygosity of the gene for familial hypocalciuric hypercalcemia, which usually causes asymptomatic hypercalcemia in adults.[9] Additional causes of HPTH in neonates include Jansen metaphyseal chondrodysplasia and I-cell disease. Although Williams syndrome may also cause neonatal hypercalcemia, PTH is not elevated.

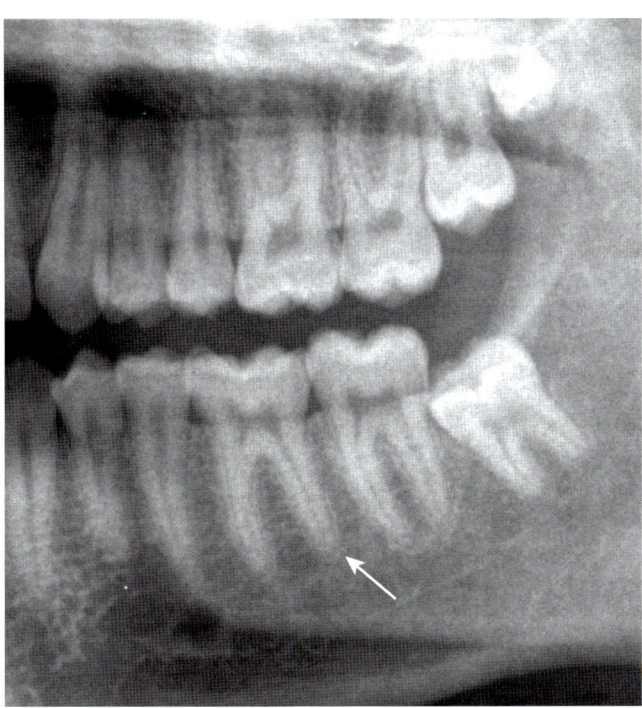

Figure 141-4 A 16-year-old boy with intact lamina dura (*arrow*) for comparison.

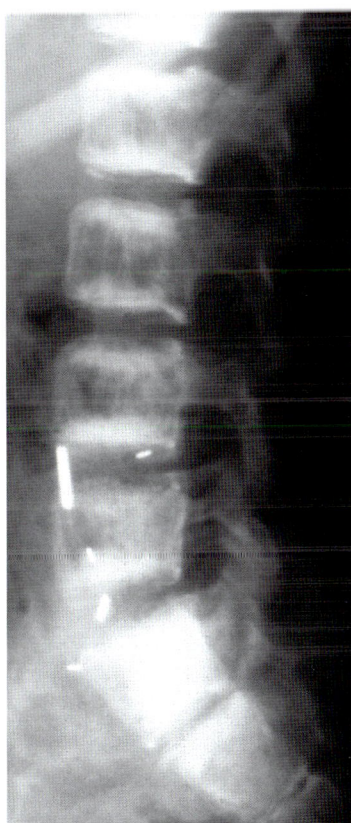

Figure 141-5 Rugger jersey spine. The lateral view of the lumbar spine shows vertebral end plate sclerosis producing rugger jersey appearance.

JANSEN METAPHYSEAL CHONDRODYSPLASIA

Jansen metaphyseal chondrodysplasia is an autosomal dominant condition with hypercalcemia and other findings suggestive of severe HPTH during the neonatal period and short-limbed dwarfism later in life. It is caused by a mutation of the receptor for PTH and PTH–related peptide (PTHrP) that causes the receptor to be constantly activated.[10,11] Hence, even though no PTH or PTHrP are detectable, PTH signaling is increased, producing effective HPTH with hypercalcemia and bone resorption, which are most prominent early in life (Fig. 141-8). Similarly, constitutive activation of the PTH/PTHrP receptor also leads to excessive PTHrP signaling, which inhibits endochondral ossification by preventing proliferating chondrocytes from entering hypertrophic differentiation.[12] This causes an ossification defect leading to buildup of a large amount nonossified cartilage and creating a lucent gap between the epiphysis and the ossified portion of the shaft (see Fig. 141-8). Subsequently, bizarre chondroid calcifications develop within these regions, which become widened and dysplastic. Eventually, the skeleton becomes fully ossified with residual shortening and deformity. The opposite effects are seen in Blomstrand lethal chondrodysplasia with an inactivating mutation of the PTH/PTHrP receptor.[13] The lack of PTHrP signaling leads to accelerated endochondral ossification, causing severe growth failure from loss of proliferating chondrocytes and markedly premature physeal closure.

MUCOLIPIDOSIS II

Mucolipidosis II (I-cell disease) is an autosomal recessive storage disorder with clinical and radiographic features similar to those of the mucopolysaccharidosis Hurler syndrome. In addition, some infants with mucolipidosis II have skeletal features of HPTH, including generalized demineralization and subperiosteal bone resorption.[14] Although PTH is elevated, calcium is not, indicating that this is a form of second-degree HPTH. It is speculated that placental involvement by this storage disorder impairs calcium transport leading to fetal and neonatal calcium deficiency causing second-degree HPTH.

OTHER DISORDERS OF BONE RESORPTION

Abnormal bone resorption may also be seen in conditions other than HTPH. Decreased resorption, usually caused by a defect in osteoclastic acidification, leads to osteopetrosis. Increased resorption is seen in hyperphosphatasia and some endocrine disorders such as glucocorticoid excess. Hyperphosphatasia, also known as *juvenile Paget disease*, is a rare autosomal recessive condition with increased bone turnover caused by deficiency of osteoprotegerin.[15,16] Osteoprotegerin normally suppresses bone turnover by acting as a "decoy receptor" for the osteoclast differentiation factor RANKL. In the absence of this decoy receptor, excessive RANKL signaling stimulates osteoclast differentiation and activity, causing

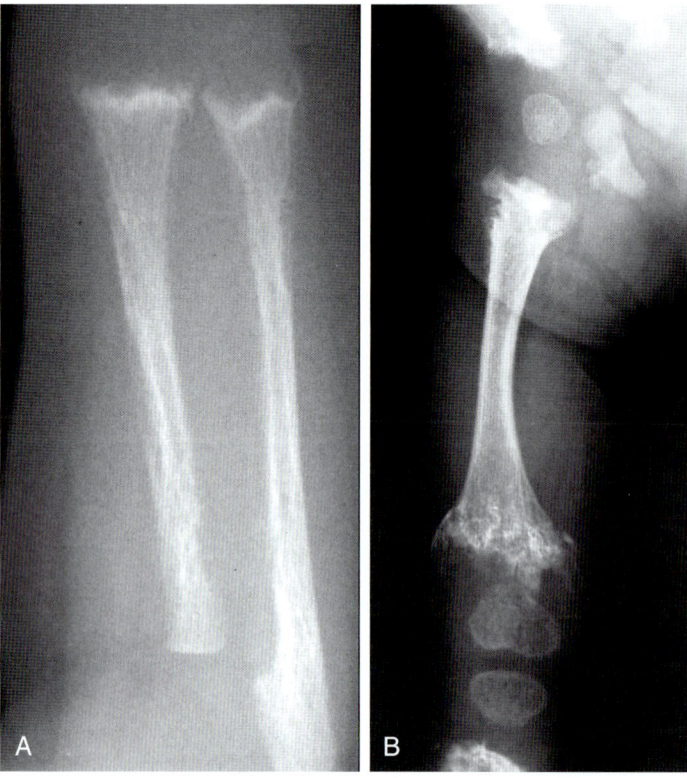

Figure 141-8 Jansen metaphyseal chondrodysplasia, with manifestations of parathyroid hormone/parathyroid hormone–related peptide (PTH/PTHrP) receptor activation. At 5 days of age, the forearm shows severe demineralization and subperiosteal resorption indicative of a hyperparathyroid state from increased PTH signaling. Also prominent are rachitic findings in the metaphyses. Impaired endochondral ossification from excessive PTHrP signaling is demonstrated in the right femur at 15 months with a large lucent zone between the shaft and epiphyses, comprising nonossified cartilage. These lucent zones are beginning to fill in with disorganized chondroid calcifications, which are most apparent distally. This disorganized pattern of ossification leads to the marked metaphyseal dysplasia of this condition.

accelerated bone resorption and hence bone turnover. Hyperphosphatasia often presents at 2 to 3 years of age with short stature, bone fragility, and deformity, including long bone bowing, kyphoscoliosis, and pectus carinatum. Unlike adult Paget disease, which involves limited portions of the skeleton, hyperphosphatasia is more generalized. The radiographic features may be striking, with overall demineralization, coarse trabecular pattern, cortical thickening, widened cylindrical long bones with decreased tubulation, and markedly variable bone texture with osteosclerosis intermixed with regions of cystic-appearing lucency (Fig. 141-9). Bowing and pathologic fractures are common. The skull shows thickening and regions of lucency combined with "cottonwool" sclerosis, similar to adult Paget disease. Familial expansile osteolysis is a related condition with deafness, loss of teeth, expansion of bones, painful phalanges, and episodic hypercalcemia caused by duplication of the gene for the osteoclast membrane-bound receptor that is activated by RANKL.[17]

HYPOPARATHYROIDISM

Etiology Idiopathic hypoparathyroidism in children is most commonly part of polyglandular autoimmune disease type I.[18] This autosomal recessive condition targets multiple endocrine glands, most frequently the parathyroids and adrenals. Other causes of hypoparathyroidism in children include congenital absence of the parathyroids, which may accompany thymic absence in DiGeorge syndrome, surgical removal during thyroidectomy, and transient suppression of fetal parathyroids by maternal HPTH.[19]

Imaging Skeletal manifestations of hypoparathyroidism include osteosclerosis, dense metaphyseal bands, cranial vault

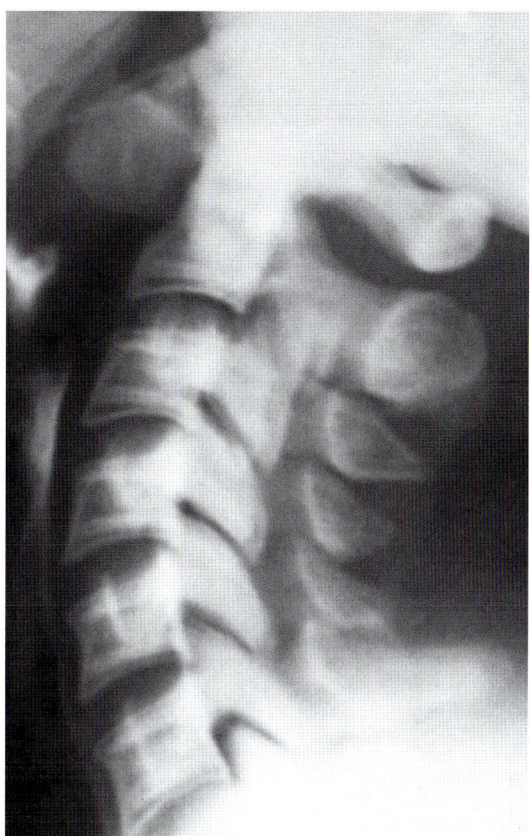

Figure 141-10 Idiopathic hypoparathyroidism. Bone-within-bone appearance and patchy osteosclerosis of cervical vertebrae are observed in a patient with idiopathic hypoparathyroidism.

thickening, intracranial calcifications such as basal ganglia and choroid plexus, and dental abnormalities. Vertebral findings include marginal sclerosis, "bone within bone" appearance (Fig. 141-10), and paravertebral ossification.

PSEUDOHYPOPARATHYROIDISM

Etiology Pseudohypoparathyroidism is characterized by variable resistance to PTH and, less often, other hormones, as well as typical somatic features known as *Albright hereditary osteodystrophy (AHO)*.[18,20] The hormone resistance results from an inactivating mutation of the *GNAS1* gene, which is involved in G-protein biosignaling. In pseudopseudohypoparathyroidism, the somatic features of AHO are seen without hormone resistance.

Imaging The somatic features of AHO include short stature, obesity, a round face, variable degrees of subnormal intelligence, subcutaneous calcification and ossification, small exostoses, and brachydactyly of hands and feet (Fig. 141-11). The brachydactyly is often associated with premature growth plate closure that results from impaired PTHrP signaling leading to accelerated endochondral ossification. Brachydactyly E, Turner syndrome, and acrodysostosis are differential considerations. Resistance to PTH leads to manifestations of hypoparathyroidism including hypocalcemia and soft tissue and basal ganglia calcifications despite elevated PTH levels. Although hormone resistance often involves both kidney and bone, skeletal resistance is variable. With skeletal

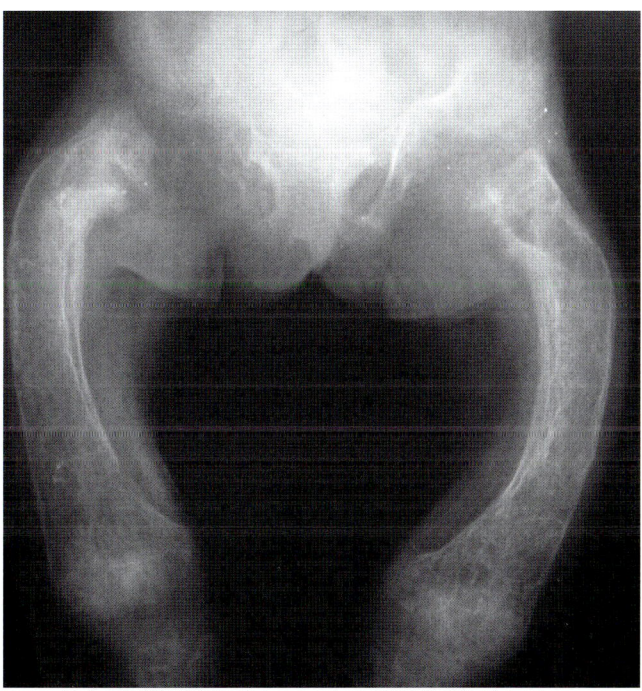

Figure 141-9 Hyperphosphatasia. The diaphyses are expanded and bowed. Demineralization is marked and has a highly heterogeneous pattern. The findings are symmetric, unlike the more focal appearance of adult Paget disease.

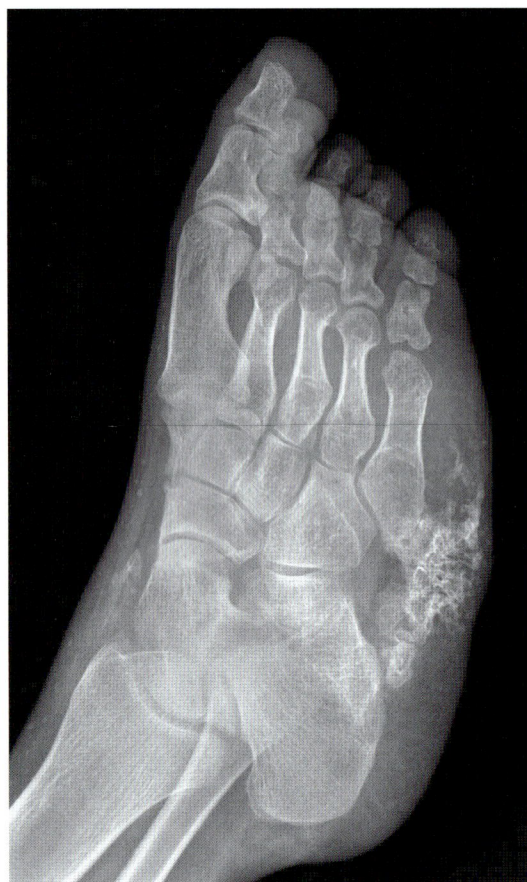

Figure 141-11   Pseudohypoparathyroidism in a 14-year-old with extensive heterotopic ossification along the lateral aspect of foot. Also note brachydactyly involving some of the metatarsals.

responsiveness to PTH, manifestations of HPTH such as subperiosteal bone resorption and brown tumors (Fig. 141-12) may be seen.[21,22]

Nonparathyroid Endocrine Disorders

Several other endocrine disorders have important skeletal effects. These primarily influence skeletal growth and maturation often by their effects on endochondral bone formation at the growth plates.

GROWTH HORMONE DISORDERS

Etiology   Growth hormone (GH) is an important positive regulator of postnatal longitudinal growth, acting directly as well as indirectly through insulin-like growth factor (IGF), to stimulate proliferation of physeal chondrocytes.[23-25] Prenatal growth depends mostly on IGF, accounting for the relative preservation of prenatal growth in GH deficiency. In GH deficiency, skeletal growth and maturation are retarded to a similar degree, resulting in a similar height age and bone age. Maturation of the carpal bones is often more delayed compared with the phalanges. The retarded growth and maturation of GH deficiency may be mimicked by deprivational dwarfism ("psychosocial dwarfism") although the presence of multiple growth restart lines favors deprivational dwarfism

(e-Fig. 141-13).[26] Slipped capital femoral epiphysis (SCFE) may be seen with growth hormone deficiency either prior to or following growth hormone therapy.

Imaging   The effects of growth hormone excess are different in children than in adults. Prior to skeletal maturity, GH excess causes gigantism with increased linear growth, a relatively rare condition and usually caused by an isolated pituitary adenoma. Approximately 20% of cases are associated with McCune-Albright syndrome with growth hormone excess caused by either adenoma or hyperplasia. In most cases, skeletal maturation is normal. With increased linear growth and advanced skeletal maturation, other endocrinopathies such as excessive gonadal or adrenal androgens should be considered. After skeletal maturity has been attained, increased GH leads to increased periosteal bone formation, reactivation of endochondral bone formation at chondro-osseous junctions, and cartilage and soft tissue hypertrophy. These processes lead to acromegaly, which is predominantly an adult disorder.

HYPOTHYROIDISM

Etiology   Thyroid hormone (TH) is essential for normal brain development during the first 3 years of life, as well for normal skeletal growth and maturation.[23,24,27-29] Although TH does not directly affect chondrocyte proliferation, the positive effects of GH and IGF on proliferation require the presence of TH. Additionally, TH has a major effect on skeletal maturation by inhibiting PTHrP signaling which ordinarily retards endochondral ossification. Hence increased PTHrP signaling in hypothyroidism causes impaired endochondral ossification.

Imaging   Skeletal maturation is delayed to an even greater degree than linear growth, whereas in GH deficiency, growth and maturation are proportionately diminished. Impaired ossification not only delays the appearance of epiphyses but also leads to an abnormal pattern with multiple fragmented ossification centers, which is known as *epiphyseal dysgenesis*. Although these eventually coalesce, the epiphysis often has uneven opacity and irregular margins (Fig. 141-14). Although the term *stippled* is often used for these epiphyses, the appearance is distinct from chondrodysplasia punctata and associated

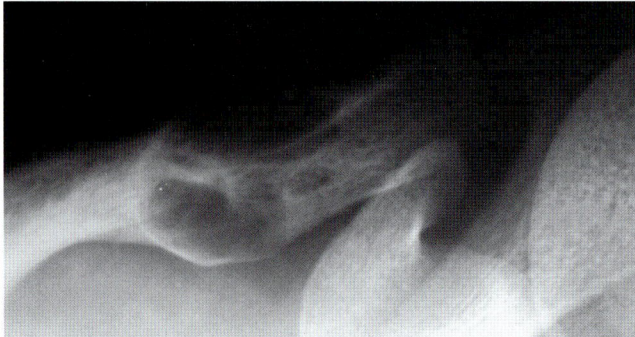

Figure 141-12   Pseudohypoparathyroidism with skeletal responsiveness to parathyroid hormone leading to a distal clavicular brown tumor. Other manifestations of hyperparathyroidism in this patient included subperiosteal bone resorption and bilateral slipped capital femoral epiphyses (*not shown*).

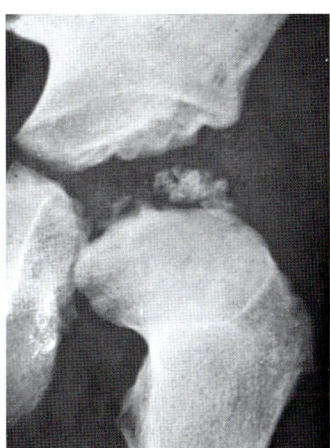

Figure 141-14 Epiphyseal dysgenesis in a 9-year-old hypothyroid girl who had started treatment 1 year earlier. The femoral head is small, flattened, and contains multiple small fragmented ossification centers. At the beginning of treatment 1 year earlier, no ossification of the femoral heads was seen. With follow-up, these ossification centers were observed to be coalesced, but the femoral heads remained flattened. Similar finding were also present in several major epiphyses.

disorders. Epiphyseal dysgenesis is particularly common in the hips. With treatment, the findings of epiphyseal dysgenesis resolve. SCFE may be a presenting manifestation of hypothyroidism, often bilateral and occurring at a younger age than idiopathic SCFE.[30,31] In the skull, hypothyroidism may cause multiple wormian bones, enlargement of the sella from pituitary hyperplasia, and brachycephaly from decreased growth at the spheno-occipital synchondrosis. Radiographs of hands may show small projections of bone extending from the distal phalangeal metaphyses into the growth plates (Fig. 141-15).[32]

HYPERTHYROIDISM

Etiology As discussed for hypothyroidism, TH inhibits PTHrP and hence promotes hypertrophic differentiation of proliferating chondrocytes leading to accelerated skeletal maturation. Hyperthyroidism in the pediatric age range is most frequent in adolescent girls. Hyperthyroidism may also occur as a manifestation of McCune-Albright syndrome, although precocious puberty is most common.

Imaging Skeletal maturation in hyperthyroidism may be normal or mildly advanced. Accelerated maturation may be seen in infants born to mothers with uncontrolled hyperthyroidism during the last trimester of pregnancy. Although hyperthyroidism is uncommon in infancy, acceleration of skeletal maturation is greatest in this group and may include premature craniosynostosis.[33] Other skeletal manifestations of hyperthyroidism include calcification of costal cartilage and tracheal rings, diffuse osteopenia, and cortical striations, which are indicative of increased bone turnover. Hyperthyroidism may mimic osteomalacia, including the presence of Looser transformation zones, although excessive nonmineralized osteoid is the result of overproduction of osteoid rather than impairment of its mineralization. Although it is predominantly an adult disorder, thyroid acropachy may be seen in adolescents with spiculated or feathery appearing

periosteal new bone involving the metacarpals, metatarsals, and phalanges.

GLUCOCORTICOID EXCESS

Etiology Cushing syndrome refers to the systemic effects of glucocorticoid excess. Most cases of Cushing syndrome in children are iatrogenic and result from pharmacologic dosages of glucocorticoids used for treatment of chronic inflammatory or autoimmune disorders. Endogenous Cushing syndrome in children is uncommon and usually caused by primary adrenal lesions in those below 5 years of age and pituitary lesions in those above 5 years. Glucocorticoids decrease linear growth and maturation, acting at multiple levels to negatively regulate physeal chondrogenesis by decreasing GH secretion and downregulating GH and IGF receptors in growth plate chondrocytes.[24]

Glucocorticoids also impair skeletal mineralization.[34,35] Systemically, they negate the positive influence of the sex steroids on mineralization and decrease calcium absorption in the gut. Glucocorticoids also act directly on bone to decrease bone formation and increase osteoclastic resorption by increasing RANKL and decreasing osteoprotegerin expression. Osteonecrosis is an additional complication of endogenous or exogenous glucocorticoid excess. Its pathogenesis is not well understood; potential mechanisms include compromise of intraosseous perfusion caused by increased intraosseous pressure from fat deposition in marrow and fat embolization resulting from fatty liver.

Imaging The skeletal findings of endogenous or exogenous corticosteroid excess are mostly nonspecific generalized osteopenia with cortical thinning, trabecular rarefaction, and vertebral compression fracture. In addition, more specific findings include vertebral end plate sclerosis, abundant callus formation at fracture sites, and osteonecrosis. Excessive callus formation associated with compression fractures of vertebral bodies probably accounts for end plate sclerosis, which may be a clue in the diagnosis of Cushing syndrome in a patient with osteopenia. Glucocorticoid induced osteonecrosis most frequently involves the femoral head, with the humeral head and femoral condyles being next in frequency. Radiographic

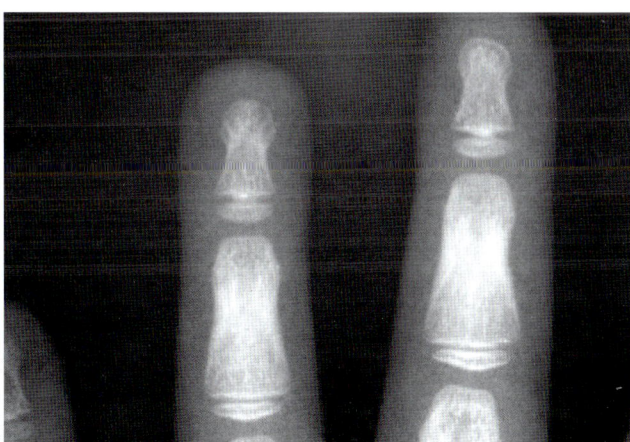

Figure 141-15 Hypothyroidism in an 11-year-old boy. Small spikelike projections of bone extend into the growth plates from the distal phalangeal metaphyses.

findings include subcortical fracture, bone collapse, fragmentation, and patchy osteosclerosis.

ADRENAL ANDROGEN EXCESS

Etiology   Adrenogenital syndrome, the most frequent cause of excessive adrenal androgens excess, results from a biosynthetic defect in the production of cortisol with compensatorily increased adrenocorticotropic hormone driving excessive production of adrenal androgens.[35] Excessive amounts of adrenal androgens may also be secreted by adrenal cortical neoplasms. Although they are weaker than testosterone, adrenal androgens promote virilization and accelerate skeletal maturation.

Imaging   Although growth is initially accelerated, this effect is less pronounced than is advancement of maturation. Hence, physeal closure occurs prematurely, and final height is decreased rather than increased. Advancement of skeletal maturation caused by excessive androgens is more pronounced than that caused by hyperthyroidism.

GONADAL DISORDERS

Etiology   Although previously thought that normal skeletal maturation was mediated by estrogens in females and androgens in males, the effects of sex steroids on physeal fusion and bone mineral accretion are currently believed to be caused by estrogen, with these processes mediated in males by estrogens formed from peripheral conversion of androgens.[36-38]

Imaging   Increased production of androgens and estrogens by gonadal tumors may accelerate skeletal maturation, whereas gonadal insufficiency delays maturation.[24]

Key Points

The most common cause of HPTH in children is chronic renal insufficiency and the major manifestations of renal osteodystrophy are those of HPTH.

In renal osteodystrophy, the lucent material adjacent to the growth plates is fibrous tissue of osteitis fibrosa cystica. This simulates the appearance of rickets but is weaker than osteoid, leading to slipped epiphyses.

PTHrP signaling inhibits endochondral ossification by retarding hypertrophic differentiation.

In GH deficiency, skeletal growth and maturation are proportionally decreased.

TH promotes hypertrophic differentiation. Hence, in hypothyroidism, skeletal maturation is impaired to a greater degree than is growth.

Suggested Readings

Bastepe M. The GNAS locus and pseudohypoparathyroidism. *Adv Exp Med Biol.* 2008;626:27-40.

Dabbagh S. Renal osteodystrophy. *Curr Opin Pediatr.* 1998;10:190-196.

Loder RT, Wittenberg B, DeSilva G. Slipped capital femoral epiphysis associated with endocrine disorders. *J Pediatr Orthop.* 1995;15:349-356.

Sanchez CP. Mineral metabolism and bone abnormalities in children with chronic renal failure. *Rev Endocr Metab Disord.* 2008;9:131-137.

Weinstein LS, Liu J, Sakamoto A, et al. Mini-review: GNAS: normal and abnormal functions. *Endocrinology.* 2004;145:5459-5464.

References

Full references for this chapter can be found on www.expertconsult.com.

Chapter 142

Skeletal Manifestations of Systemic Disease

ROBERT C. ORTH and R. PAUL GUILLERMAN

Normal Bone Marrow

OVERVIEW

Bone marrow is one of the largest and most dynamic tissues in the body. Its functions include the production of red and white blood cells and platelets for tissue oxygenation, cellular immunity, and blood coagulation, respectively. Bone marrow occupies approximately 85% of the medullary cavity and is supported by a network of trabecular bone.[1] In addition to hematopoietic elements, it contains stromal cells, collagen, nerves, and a variable amount of fat.

FUNCTION AND COMPOSITION

Physiology On gross examination, bone marrow may be red because of hemoglobin in the erythrocytes and their precursors, indicating active hematopoietic marrow, or it may be yellow as a result of the presence of carotenoid derivatives dissolved in fat droplets within adipocytes.[1] Hematopoietic marrow is rich in vascular sinusoids, whereas fatty marrow is considerably less vascular. During periods of decreased hematopoiesis, the fat cells increase in size and number. During periods of increased hematopoiesis, the fat cells atrophy.

The cellularity of bone marrow diminishes most rapidly in the first two decades of life. The cellularity of hematopoietic marrow is near 100% at birth and decreases to 50% to 75% by 15 years of age. By adulthood, the hematopoietic marrow is composed of approximately 40% fat, 40% water, and 20% protein, with 60% of cells being hematopoietic and 40% being adipocytes.[1] In contrast, the fatty marrow is composed of 80% fat, 15% water, and 5% protein, with 95% of cells being adipocytes (e-Fig. 142-1).[1,2]

Imaging Conventional radiography, computed tomography, and ultrasonography are of limited value in the assessment of bone marrow.[3] Since the first reports of magnetic resonance imaging (MRI) of the marrow in children were published in 1984, MRI has emerged as the primary imaging modality to evaluate the bone marrow. It provides a noninvasive method for visualizing the gross anatomic structure of a large sample of the bone marrow and for inferring alterations in its chemical and cellular composition related to a variety of physiologic and pathologic processes. Furthermore, MRI can provide valuable information about regions of the bone marrow that may be inaccessible or difficult to biopsy.

The constituents of bone marrow that contribute to the signal characteristics on MRI are fat, water, and, to a lesser extent, mineralized matrix.[3] Fat is the dominant contributor to both hematopoietic and fatty marrow signal intensity patterns. Most fat protons are in hydrophobic methylene ($-CH_2-$) groups of relatively heavy molecular complexes, conferring very efficient spin-lattice relaxation; this results in a short T1 relaxation time, which results in high signal intensity on T1-weighted sequences.[1] The T2 relaxation time of fat is much shorter than that of free water protons, and water contributes much more to the signal intensity of hematopoietic marrow than fatty marrow.[1] The mineralized matrix of bone has a low density of hydrogen protons that lack mobility within the crystalline structure of bone, accounting for very long T1 and short T2 relaxation times and low signal intensity of mineralized matrix on T1- and T2-weighted sequences. In addition, local field gradients at the trabecular surface are generated by the fixed dipole from the immobile protons and cause magnetic field inhomogeneity. This magnetic susceptibility effect, as well as that resulting from iron deposition, can play a large role in the signal characteristics of hematopoietic and fatty marrow on gradient echo (GRE) images.[1]

The normal intervertebral disks, skeletal muscle, and subcutaneous fat have little interindividual and intraindividual variation in signal intensity on T1-weighted sequences during childhood and consequently serve as convenient internal reference standards for comparison with the signal intensity of the marrow.[1,4] Fatty marrow has high signal intensity on conventional spin echo T1-weighted sequences. The relative amounts of fat, water, and protein contribute in a complex fashion to produce a longer T1 relaxation time in hematopoietic marrow, with signal intensity that ranges from intermediate to low (less than that of muscle or intervertebral disks) in fat-poor hematopoietic marrow to intermediate to high (greater than that of muscle or the intervertebral disks but less than that of subcutaneous fat) in hematopoietic marrow with larger proportions of fat.[1,5] In neonates, hematopoietic marrow contains minimal fat and has low signal intensity on T1-weighted sequences. With aging, hematopoietic marrow signal intensity progressively increases on T1-weighted sequences, reflecting a progressive increase in fat content. After the neonatal period, hematopoietic marrow has signal intensity equal to or slightly greater than muscle and the intervertebral disks but much less than subcutaneous fat on T1-weighted sequences, whereas fatty marrow approaches the signal intensity of subcutaneous fat on T1-weighted sequences.[5] Because of the similar proton densities of hematopoietic and fatty marrow, proton density sequences without fat suppression are less useful than T1-weighted sequences.[6]

On fat-suppressed fast spin echo (FSE) T2-weighted and short tau inversion recovery (STIR) sequences, normal hematopoietic marrow in childhood shows higher signal intensity than fatty marrow and higher signal intensity than muscle; the signal intensity of hematopoietic marrow decreases with age and approaches that of muscle by adolescence.

The signal characteristics of marrow are highly variable on GRE sequences, with which images that exploit chemical shift can be obtained by choosing an echo time in which the phases of relaxing water and fat protons are either opposed 180° (out-of-phase or opposed-phase sequences) or coincide (in-phase sequences) related to differences in their resonance frequencies.[1] When hematopoietic marrow contains approximately equivalent amounts of water and fat, as in normal adults, the signal intensity is markedly diminished on opposed-phase T1-weighted sequences, compared with in-phase T1-weighted sequences, as a result of intravoxel chemical shift effect.[1] When the amount of fat and water is no longer balanced, for example, in fatty marrow or in edematous or hypercellular hematopoietic marrow, the marrow signal intensity does not show such a profound difference between the opposed-phase and in-phase T1-weighted images.[1] Magnetic susceptibility effect from trabecular bone and iron leads to a lower signal intensity of the marrow on GRE T2*-weighted sequences than on spin echo sequences.

The degree of contrast enhancement of normal marrow varies with the contrast dose, timing of image acquisition following contrast administration, the age of the patient, and the composition of the marrow. Marrow enhancement peaks within a minute of contrast administration and then slowly declines.[7] Enhancement is greater in children than in adults, greater in the metaphyses than in the epiphyses, and greater in hematopoietic marrow than in fatty marrow. Enhancement can be imperceptible by visual inspection in the marrow of adults and in the marrow of the epiphyses in patients aged more than 2 years. Interindividual variation in the degree of enhancement is also substantial.[7] If gadolinium-enhanced T1-weighted sequences are acquired without fat suppression, contrast between hematopoietic and fatty marrow is decreased, which potentially obscures marrow lesions or age-related marrow conversion changes.[8] Image-subtraction and fat-suppression techniques facilitate the detection of abnormal marrow enhancement on postcontrast T1-weighted sequences.[6]

A combination of T1-weighted and fat-suppressed FSE T2-weighted or STIR sequences is sufficient for the detection and characterization of most marrow lesions.[9] Contrast-enhanced T1-weighted sequences increase the cost and duration of the MRI exam while providing only modest incremental added sensitivity; because of this, they should be reserved for cases with unclear findings on the precontrast sequences. GRE sequences are valuable for the assessment of the iron content of the marrow, and chemical-shift techniques are useful to detect subtle changes in the fat and water fractions of the marrow.

Practical time constraints previously limited MRI scanning of the marrow to only sections of the skeleton. This disadvantage has been mitigated by the development of fast, whole-body MRI scanning techniques that include FSE and single-shot sequences, parallel imaging, rolling table platforms with a large field of view, and global matrix coil concepts.[10-12] Obscuration of lesions by motion artifact may be overcome to some extent by the use of respiratory triggering or other motion-suppression techniques. The lower signal-to-noise ratios in smaller children on whole-body MRI exams can be ameliorated by using MR systems with a higher field strength.[13] Diffusion-weighted whole-body MRI holds particular promise as a technique to globally assess the bone marrow for hematologic disorders and tumor metastases.[14,15]

Molecular diffusion is a stochastic process characterized by brownian motion.[16] Diffusion-weighted imaging (DWI) is based on the MR signal attenuation caused by the brownian motion of water molecules. In biologic tissues, the diffusion of water molecules is influenced by the microstructure of the surrounding environment. Bone marrow is semifluid in consistency and is confined within spaces defined by the bony trabeculae and supported by reticulum cells and adipocytes. DWI is not pure diffusion imaging, and the apparent diffusion coefficient (ADC) reflects both the molecular diffusion of water and the blood perfusion of the microvasculature. At b-values of 30 and 300 seconds/mm^2, the ADC values of marrow are more affected by perfusion effect than by diffusion.[17]

A positive correlation exists between the degree of marrow cellularity and the marrow ADC. Hematopoietic marrow or marrow infiltrated by neoplastic cells has more abundant microvasculature and more intracellular and interstitial free water than fatty marrow, and it exhibits higher ADC values.[18]

Motion and susceptibility artifacts are especially problematic in DWI of the marrow, which is contained by bone and in proximity to physiologic motions, such as cerebrospinal fluid pulsations in the case of the spine.[16] Recent advances have largely overcome these technologic challenges, and diffusion-weighted whole-body MRI is being used to evaluate an increasing number of benign and malignant conditions that include chronic recurrent multifocal osteomyelitis, Langerhans cell histiocytosis, and bony metastases.[19-21]

DISTRIBUTION AND CONVERSION

Physiology Hematopoiesis occurs in the yolk sac in the early stages of fetal development; later in gestation, it shifts to the liver, and to a lesser extent, to the spleen. Bone marrow begins hematopoiesis in the fourth intrauterine month, overtakes the liver in this function by the sixth month, and is entirely responsible for hematopoietic cell production by birth.[22] Shortly before birth, conversion from hematopoietic to fatty marrow begins in the distal phalanges of the hands and feet and proceeds in a centripetal fashion from the distal to the more proximal portions of the appendicular skeleton.[4] Within the long bones, conversion from hematopoietic to fatty marrow proceeds from the mid diaphyses to the distal metaphyses and then to the proximal metaphyses. Conversion also progresses from the central medullary canal to the endosteum. Fatty transformation in the epiphyses and apophyses begins almost as soon as they begin to ossify. In infants, the skull and limbs contain about half of the total amount of hematopoietic marrow.[1,4] By early adulthood, hematopoietic marrow becomes confined to the vertebrae, sternum, ribs, pelvis, skull, proximal humeri, and proximal femurs. Approximately one half of the bone marrow volume is fatty marrow in early adulthood and is located primarily in the appendicular skeleton. The involution of hematopoietic marrow continues throughout adult life, although at a slower pace than during childhood.[1,4,23] Unlike skeletal maturation, there are generally no gender differences in the rate of marrow conversion during childhood.[2] Knowledge of the normal age-related changes in the distribution of hematopoietic and fatty marrow is necessary for the recognition of abnormal conversion and reconversion patterns and for the detection of marrow infiltration by other pathologic processes.

Imaging Conversion from hematopoietic to fatty marrow is readily detected by MRI because of the high sensitivity of T1-weighted spin echo sequences to fat (e-Table 142-1).[1] In fact, marrow conversion is observed earlier by MRI than by gross pathologic inspection because of the capability of MRI to detect microscopic fat present in marrow.[2,4,5,24] Numerous publications detail the temporal and spatial sequence of marrow conversion revealed by MRI. Although there are discrepancies among these publications in the precise ages of transformation, the sequence of conversion is consistent along the long axes of individual bones and in the skeleton as a whole. Conversion occurs at a faster pace in the appendicular skeleton (extremities, shoulders, and pelvic girdle) than in the axial skeleton (skull, spine, ribs, and sternum).[1,4]

Appendicular Skeleton

Marrow conversion follows a similar pattern in both the upper and lower limbs. Within the long bones, conversion initially begins within the diaphysis before spreading to the metaphysis.[24] In general, low signal intensity on T1-weighted images marrow within the long-bone diaphyses is unusual after 10 years of age.[1,5] Long-bone metaphyseal marrow demonstrates high signal intensity on T1-weighted images by 15 to 25 years of age, except for low to intermediate signal intensity hematopoietic marrow that may persist through adulthood in the proximal femoral metaphyses, the metaphyses around the knee, and the proximal humerus, particularly in populations with increased hematopoiesis, such as smokers, endurance athletes, and obese women.[1,4,25]

Under normal circumstances, the epiphyseal ossification centers do not participate in hematopoiesis to any appreciable degree. Soon after the onset of epiphyseal ossification, the low signal intensity bony trabeculae and hematopoietic marrow begin to be replaced by high signal intensity fatty marrow, with near complete conversion within 6 to 8 months from the onset.[26] Fatty marrow appears earlier in the proximal humeral epiphysis, compared with the femur, because of the earlier onset of proximal humeral epiphyseal ossification.[1,27]

The apophyses and sesamoid bones follow a similar pattern to the epiphyses.

Fatty marrow conversion first occurs within the phalanges and is completed in the fingers and toes by 1 year of age.[4] Conversion in the femurs begins in infancy. Fatty marrow is seen in the femoral diaphyses as early as 3 months of age and is commonly observed by 12 months of age.[24] At 1 to 5 years of age, the diaphyseal fat signal becomes homogeneous, and the hematopoietic marrow in the distal femoral metaphyses becomes replaced by fatty marrow at 6 to 15 years of age (Fig. 142-2).[24] However, a mottled pattern of relatively low to intermediate signal intensity in the proximal femoral metaphyses may remain, related to persistent hematopoietic marrow and bony trabeculae extending from the inferolateral aspect of the femoral neck to the superomedial aspect of the femoral head.

Bone marrow conversion in the humerus follows a similar predictable pattern. Conversion to fatty marrow is complete in the proximal humeral epiphyses by 1 year of age, nearly complete in the diaphyses by 5 years of age, and nearly complete in the distal metaphyses by 10 years of age.[27] Conversion occurs less rapidly in the proximal humeral metaphyses and is nearly complete by 15 years of age. However, low to intermediate signal intensity hematopoietic marrow is retained in the proximal humeral metaphyses and subchondral medial aspects of the humeral heads into adulthood, particularly in women.[2,28] The acromion behaves like an epiphysis in regard to marrow distribution and conversion rate.[2]

Conversion of marrow in the forearm and leg bones lags slightly behind the proximal arms and thighs. Conversion to fatty marrow begins in the diaphyses between 1 and 5 years of age and is complete in all portions of the forearm and leg bones by 10 to 15 years of age.[4] Marrow conversion ensues in the tarsal and carpal bones at 2 to 6 months of age and is complete by 6 years of age, with the possible exception of small foci of residual hematopoietic marrow that persists in the tarsal bones up to 15 years of age.[29]

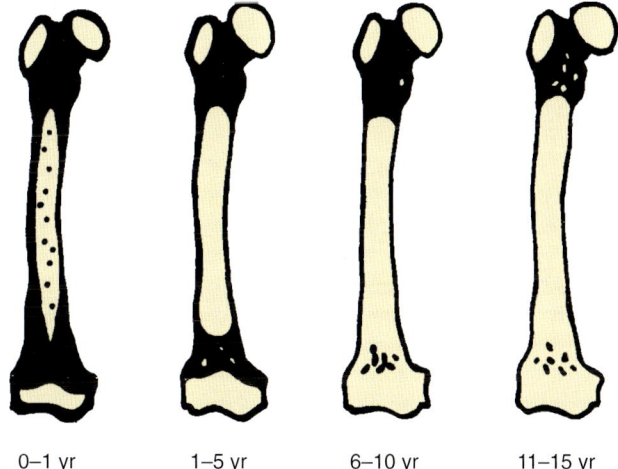

0–1 yr	1–5 yr	6–10 yr	11–15 yr

Figure 142-2 Diagrammatic representation of changes in magnetic resonance imaging appearance of the femoral marrow with increasing age. *Black areas* represent hematopoietic marrow, *black areas* represent fatty marrow or cartilage, and *stippled areas* indicate heterogeneous hematopoietic and fatty marrow. (From Waitches G, Zawin JK, Poznanski AK. Sequence and rate of bone marrow conversion in the femora of children as seen on MR imaging: are accepted standards accurate? *AJR Am J Roentgenol.* 1994;162:1401.)

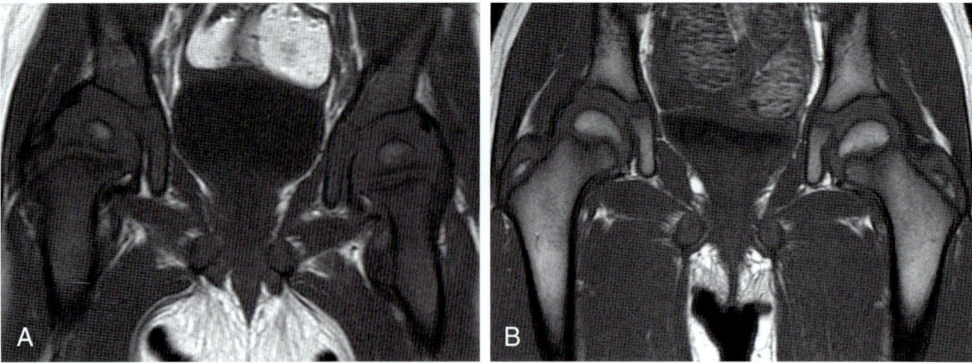

Figure 142-3 Coronal T1-weighted magnetic resonance images of the pelvis showing normal marrow changes. **A,** In an 11-month-old boy, normal low signal intensity hematopoietic marrow is present in the pelvis and proximal femurs. **B,** In a 3-year-old girl, normal conversion to fatty marrow has occurred by this age, manifested by increased signal intensity throughout the pelvis and proximal femurs.

In the first year after birth, hematopoietic marrow is present in the pelvis. Conversion to fatty marrow initially occurs in the anterior ilium and acetabulum, beginning as early as 2 years of age (Fig. 142-3). In the second decade of life, the remainder of the pelvic marrow increases to intermediate signal intensity. Except in infancy, heterogeneous signal intensity of the pelvic marrow is a normal finding and is most prominent in adolescents and adults in the acetabulum and anterior ilium because of macroscopic foci of both hematopoietic and fatty marrow.[30]

Axial Skeleton

During the first month after birth, the vertebral marrow lacks fat and exhibits uniformly lower signal than the adjacent cartilaginous disks on T1-weighted sequences. Later in infancy, as the vertebral ossification center increases in size, and the cartilaginous end plates decrease in prominence, the veterbral body marrow increases in signal intensity on T1-weighted sequences, particularly adjacent to the cartilaginous end plates.[4] Compared with the intervertebral disks and cartilaginous end plates, vertebral body marrow is usually hypointense on T1-weighted images up to the age of 1 year.[31] Vertebral body marrow is commonly isointense or hyperintense on T1-weighted images compared with the intervertebral disks from 1 to 5 years of age. After the age of 5 years, vertebral body marrow signal on T1-weighted images is typically greater than that of the intervertebral disks, and a band of fatty marrow may be conspicuous in the vertebral body centrally or along the basivertebral venous plexus (e-Fig. 142-4).[4,31] The spine continues as a site of hematopoietic marrow throughout life, although the proportion of fatty marrow gradually rises approximately 7% per decade.

The skull is where the bone marrow is most frequently imaged by MRI in childhood, typically incidentally in studies obtained to evaluate the brain.[32] The skull contains 25% of the active hematopoietic marrow at birth, and conversion to fatty marrow begins by 2 years of age within the facial bones and skull base before proceeding to the calvarium.[4] Marrow at the site of the future paranasal sinuses becomes fatty before pneumatization.[32] By 3 to 4 years of age, foci of high signal intensity on T1-weighted sequences are seen in the clivus, and complete conversion is typical by 15 years of age. In the calvarium, conversion begins earlier in the frontal and occipital bones than in the parietal bones.[23] Conversion in the calvarium should be obvious by 7 years of age, and it is complete in the great majority by 15 years of age.[4] The conversion to fatty marrow in the calvarium may occur more slowly in females, an exception to the rule of no gender differences.[3]

Marrow conversion in the sternum precedes that in the ribs. Development of foci of intermediate to high signal intensity on T1-weighted sequences occurs in the sternum after 5 years of age and in the ribs by 10 years of age.[4] The sternum and, to a lesser extent, the ribs remain hematopoietic into adulthood.

Detection of primary or systemic pathology that affects the marrow is usually easier in fatty marrow than in hematopoietic marrow.[33] This includes processes associated with hematopoietic hypercellularity (hemolytic anemia, hematopoietic growth factor treatment, leukemoid reaction, glycogen storage disease type 1b [GSD1b], myelodysplastic syndrome, leukemia), marrow infiltration (metastatic tumor cells, inflammatory cells, Gaucher cells), iron overload, and myelofibrosis.[7] Some of these processes are also associated with an increase in free water in the marrow and manifest as signal intensity higher than that of normal hematopoietic or fatty marrow on fat-suppressed FSE T2-weighted or STIR sequences.

Features that favor normal hematopoietic marrow include signal intensity equal to or only slightly higher than that of muscle on fat-suppressed FSE T2-weighted or STIR sequences, dropout of signal intensity on opposed-phase GRE sequences, a "flame" or "paintbrush" shape (Fig. 142-5), no underlying trabecular disruption, symmetry with the contralateral side, and no associated abnormalities of the cortical bone or extraosseous soft tissues. Residual red marrow may sometimes have a globular appearance on T1-weighted sequences, and this is a normal finding (Fig. 142-6). However, a low-grade infiltrative or edematous process of the marrow can be difficult or impossible to distinguish from hematopoietic marrow on MRI, particularly when the hematopoietic marrow is relatively hypercellular, such as in very young children and in states of marrow reconversion in patients on granulocyte colony-stimulating factor (G-CSF) therapy (Fig 142-7). Normal red marrow should never have a round, well-circumscribed configuration, which suggests a neoplastic process (Fig. 142-8).[34]

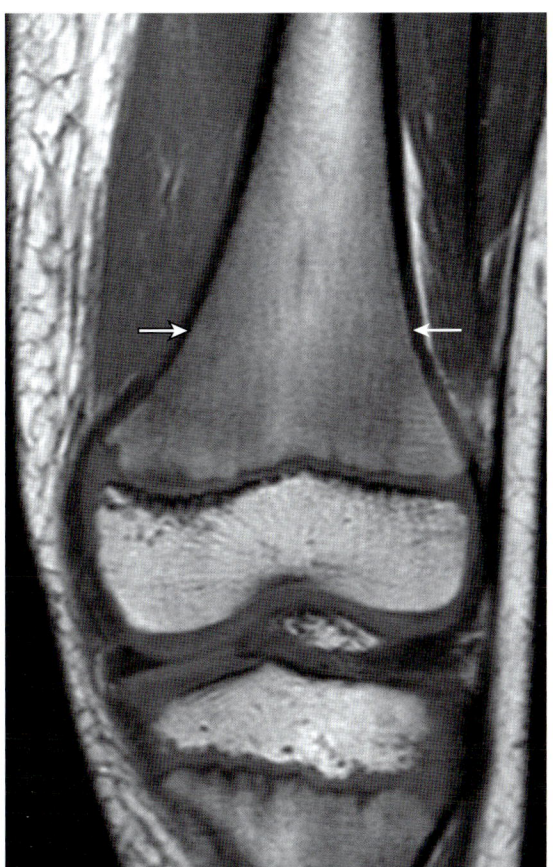

Figure 142-5 An 8-year-old boy with normal marrow. T1-weighted coronal magnetic resonance image demonstrates paintbrush-like pattern of hypointensity (*arrows*) in the femoral metaphysis without underlying trabecular disruption, consistent with normal residual red marrow.

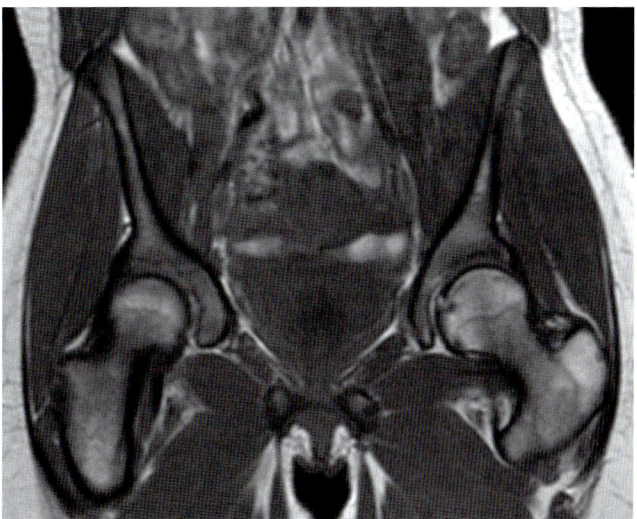

Figure 142-6 A 15-year-old girl with normal marrow. T1-weighted coronal image demonstrates globular areas of decreased signal throughout the proximal femurs and throughout the innominate bones, consistent with normal, residual red marrow.

Processes in which the proportion of fat is increased relative to other components of the bone marrow appear as a focal or diffuse increase in the bone marrow signal intensity on T1-weighted sequences. This occurs physiologically during aging with the conversion from active hematopoietic marrow to hematopoietically quiescent fatty marrow. A pathologic example is the hematopoietic cell depletion associated with aplastic anemia. Some processes are associated with varying degrees of marrow cellularity and fat content, and their MRI appearances vary correspondingly. These include the myelodysplastic syndromes and the responses of marrow to chemotherapy, radiation therapy, and hematopoietic cell transplantation.

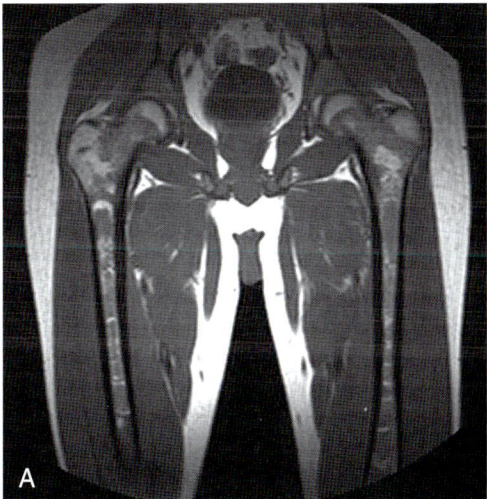
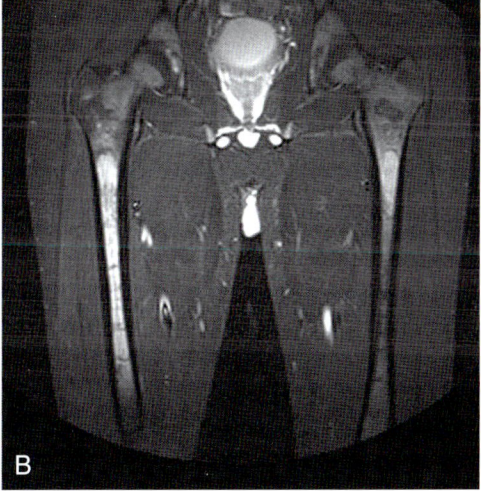

Figure 142-7 Magnetic resonance images of the thighs in a 17-year-old boy on granulocyte colony-stimulating factor (G-CSF) therapy for myelosuppression related to chemotherapy for Hodgkin disease. Coronal T1-weighted image (**A**) and coronal short tau inversion recovery (STIR) magnetic resonance image (**B**) show masslike, patchy, bilateral foci of marrow replacement with low signal intensity on T1-weighted images and high signal intensity on STIR images representing regenerating granulopoeitic marrow in response to G-CSF stimulation. Clinical correlation with the timing of therapy is necessary to distinguish these findings from neoplastic involvement of the marrow.

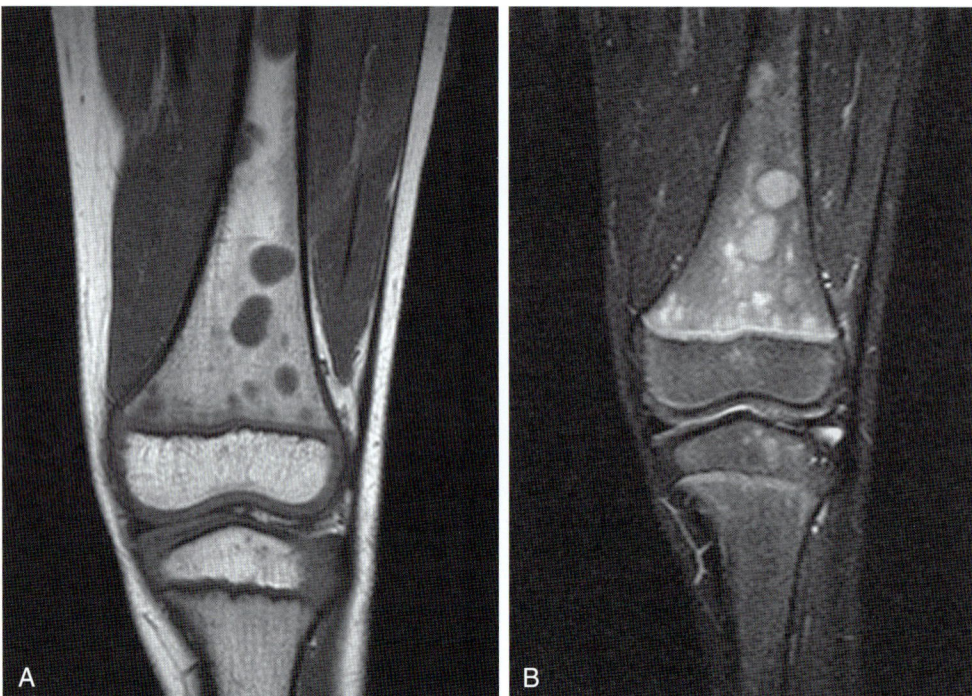

Figure 142-8 Magnetic resonance images of the left knee of a 6-year-old boy with knee pain. **A,** Coronal T1-weighted image. **B,** Short tau inversion recovery (STIR) image. Multiple round, sharply defined masses identified on T1-weighted images are hyperintense on STIR images because of marrow involvement by Burkitt lymphoma.

Marrow Hyperplasia and Reconversion

Overview Reconversion is a process by which established fatty marrow is replaced by hyperplastic hematopoietic marrow in response to conditions that create a demand for increased hematopoiesis. In children, reconversion is commonly encountered in patients with chronic anemia—such as from sickle cell disease, thalassemia, and spherocytosis—and in those administered hematopoietic growth factors, such as G-CSF, granulocyte-macrophage colony-stimulating factor (GM-CSF), and erythropoietin.

Etiology, Pathophysiology, and Clinical Presentation The stimulus for increased oxygen-carrying capacity of the blood in cyanotic congenital heart disease patients, endurance athletes, heavy smokers, and high-altitude dwellers also induces hematopoietic marrow hyperplasia and reconversion. Because marrow conversion is a process that occurs throughout childhood, some of what is construed as reconversion in children actually represents an arrest or delay in conversion from hematopoietic to fatty marrow and is attributable to increased hematopoietic demands (e-Fig. 142-9).[4]

Reconversion occurs in the reverse order of normal marrow conversion, beginning in the axial skeleton and proceeding sequentially to the proximal metaphyses, distal metaphyses, and diaphyses of the long bones of the appendicular skeleton.[4,6] The more distal long bones are the last to undergo this process. The epiphyses are usually spared but can undergo reconversion in response to very high hematopoietic demands.

Imaging Positron-emission tomography (PET) with 18-fluorodeoxyglucose (FDG) may reveal increased FDG uptake in areas of marrow hyperplasia because of the metabolic demands of increased hematopoiesis. The marrow reconversion revealed by MRI is far more extensive than that suggested by technetium-99m (^{99}mTc) phosphonate bone scintigraphy. Marrow reconversion usually begins in the metaphysis. On MRI, reconverted marrow follows the signal intensity of hematopoietic marrow and tends to involve the appendicular skeleton in a symmetric fashion.[1,4] The reconverted hematopoietic marrow may be distributed in either a homogeneous or patchy pattern and may have an appearance overlapping with that of pathologic processes, such as leukemia and storage disorders. Although MRI is very sensitive to changes in marrow fat content, disease specificity is low, and the distinction between reconverted and diseased marrow often requires clinical correlation. Also, some of the conditions that exhibit marrow reconversion have additional superimposed marrow processes that complicate MRI interpretation, such as transfusion hemosiderosis in thalassemia and marrow infarction and fibrosis in sickle cell disease.

THALASSEMIA

Etiology, Pathophysiology, and Clinical Presentation Thalassemia is an inherited hemoglobinopathy characterized by ineffective erythropoiesis, intramedullary hemolysis, and anemia. With effective transfusion therapy, hematopoietic to fatty marrow conversion may proceed in the extremities by puberty. However, hematopoietic marrow hyperplasia in the skull, spine, and pelvis can remain pronounced. The paranasal sinuses often fail to develop, in part as a result of abrogation of the normal fatty conversion of marrow that precedes sinus pneumatization (see Chapter 8).[32]

Thalassemia patients have an increased risk of pathologic fractures because of osteopenia, arthralgias that are believed to be related to iron overload or the use chelation therapy,

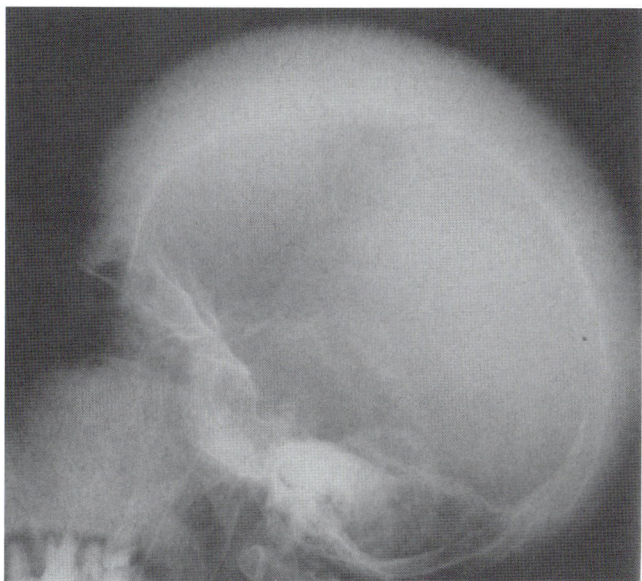

Figure 142-10   Child with thalassemia with diffuse "hair-on-end" appearance of the calvarium. (Courtesy Edward Singleton, MD.)

and back pain as a result of the high incidence of scoliosis and early intervertebral disk degeneration.[35]

Imaging   The radiographic changes of thalassemia are due to chronic hematopoietic marrow hyperplasia. These include diffuse osteopenia, undertubulization of bone, premature physeal fusion, "hair-on-end" appearance of the calvarium with widening of the diploic space (Fig. 142-10), decreased pneumatization of the paranasal sinuses, coarse trabeculation of appendicular bones, expansion of costochondral junctions, scoliosis, and soft tissue masses related to extramedullary hematopoiesis.[36]

The appearance of the bone marrow on MRI is a reflection of the diffuse erythroid marrow hyperplasia, chronic transfusions, and iron chelation therapy.[4] Iron deposition in the marrow results in lowered signal intensity on T1-, T2-, and especially T2*-weighted images because of T2 relaxation-time shortening and magnetic susceptibility effects.[37] However, excess iron deposition can still be identified by MRI in some of those whose chelation is thought to be clinically adequate on the basis of serum ferritin levels. In severe cases of thalassemia, bone marrow transplantation may be pursued as a potentially curative treatment, and MRI can reveal the consequent degree of marrow conversion. FDG-PET in patients with thalassemia shows diffuse increased marrow uptake.[38]

Treatment   Transfusion therapy suppresses the marrow hyperplasia of thalassemia but at the cost of iron overload. The iron deposition occurs preferentially in areas of hematopoietic marrow and is reduced by chelation therapy.[37]

SICKLE CELL DISEASE

Etiology, Pathophysiology, and Clinical Presentation   Sickle cell disease is an inherited hemoglobinopathy characterized by deformation of red blood cells and resultant hemolytic anemia and intravascular sludging of blood. The bone marrow imaging manifestations of sickle cell disease are primarily related to hematopoietic marrow hyperplasia, osteonecrosis,

and perivascular fibrosis.[39] Because the circulation normally passes centrifugally from the medullary cavity to the cortex, sludging of blood flow in the nutrient artery branches places increased demands on the radially arranged periosteal-cortical system of anastomosing blood vessels to supply the marrow, particularly in the peripheral subcortical medullary cavity.[39,40] This, coupled with the increased oxygen needs from increased hematopoietic activity, accounts for the vulnerability of the bone marrow to osteonecrosis.

Imaging   Osseous abnormalities in sickle cell disease are secondary to osteonecrosis and, less often, osteomyelitis. Radiographic findings are similar to osteonecrosis from other causes, with geographic and patchy areas of sclerosis (Fig. 142-11) that most commonly involve the femoral heads. Other common radiographic abnormalities include dactylitis (e-Fig. 142-12), H-shaped, or "Lincoln log" vertebral bodies from central growth plate osteonecrosis (Fig. 142-13), diffuse osteosclerosis, and widespread periostitis.[41]

Findings on MRI include bone marrow changes that reflect red marrow reconversion secondary to chronic anemia, with decreased signal intensity on T1-weighted images and increased signal intensity on fat-suppressed T2-weighted and STIR sequences. Marrow changes secondary to osteonecrosis are more complex and often reflect a combination of acute and chronic processes. Foci of low, serpentine signal intensity on T1-weighted images and abnormal high signal intensity on fat-saturated T2-weighted or STIR images are classic imaging features of osteonecrosis. Chronic osteonecrosis may be suggested when these findings are confined to the

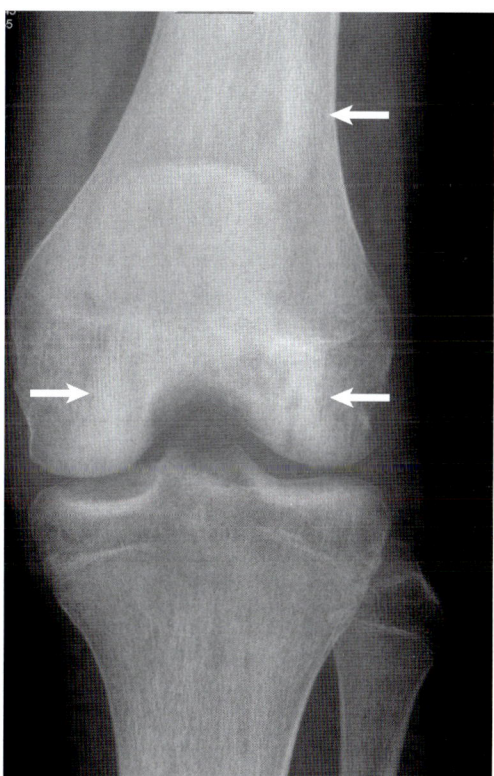

Figure 142-11   Sickle cell disease in a 17-year-old boy. Antereroposterior radiograph of the knee demonstrates multiple areas of sclerosis in the condyles and femoral shaft consistent with areas of osteonecrosis (arrows).

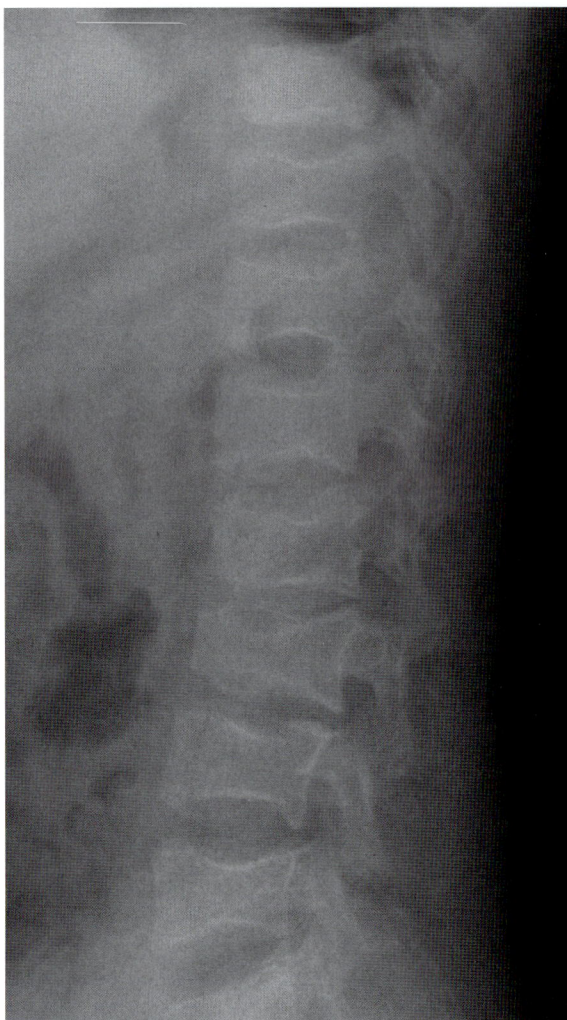

Figure 142-13 Sickle cell disease in an 18-year-old man. Numerous Angulated end-plate depressions ("Lincoln log" vertebrae) are consistent with central growth plate osteonecrosis.

marrow itself with absent joint effusions or juxtacortical soft tissue edema (Fig. 142-14). Acute osteonecrosis may be suggested when there is also infiltrative marrow edema, periostitis, and/or juxtacortical soft tissue edema (Fig. 142-15).

Acute osteomyelitis may be difficult to differentiate by MRI from the more common acute osteonecrosis and vasoocclusive crisis (see Fig. 142-15). Ultimately, aspiration and biopsy may be necessary to distinguish these entities, because both can manifest with marrow signal intensity abnormalities, periosteal reaction, and intraosseous, subperiosteal, or extraosseous soft tissue fluid collections. Gadolinium-enhanced MRI can be useful to distinguish vascularized inflammatory tissue from fluid collections and can guide the aspiration of fluid collections.[42] Some evidence suggests the ability of unenhanced T1-weighted fat-saturated images to differentiate acute osteonecrosis from acute osteomyelitis based on the T1 shortening effects of sequestered red blood cell aggregates in the marrow, but further studies are needed to validate this technique.[43]

Treatment The two most common acute musculoskeletal manifestations of sickle cell disease are vasoocclusive crisis followed by infection. Osteonecrosis is the most frequent presentation of vasoocclusive crisis and is treated with supportive care and pain management.[44] Infections include osteomyelitis and, less commonly, septic arthritis. Unlike the general pediatric population with musculoskeletal infections, *Salmonella* is most commonly identified by culture, followed by *Staphylococcus aureus*[41]; therefore antimicrobial therapy should be tailored accordingly in sickle cell patients.

GLYCOGEN STORAGE DISEASE TYPE 1B

Etiology, Pathophysiology, and Clinical Presentation The musculoskeletal manifestations of GSD1b are related to a defect in myeloid maturation that leads to bone marrow hypercellularity with hyperplasia of the myelopoietic cells and

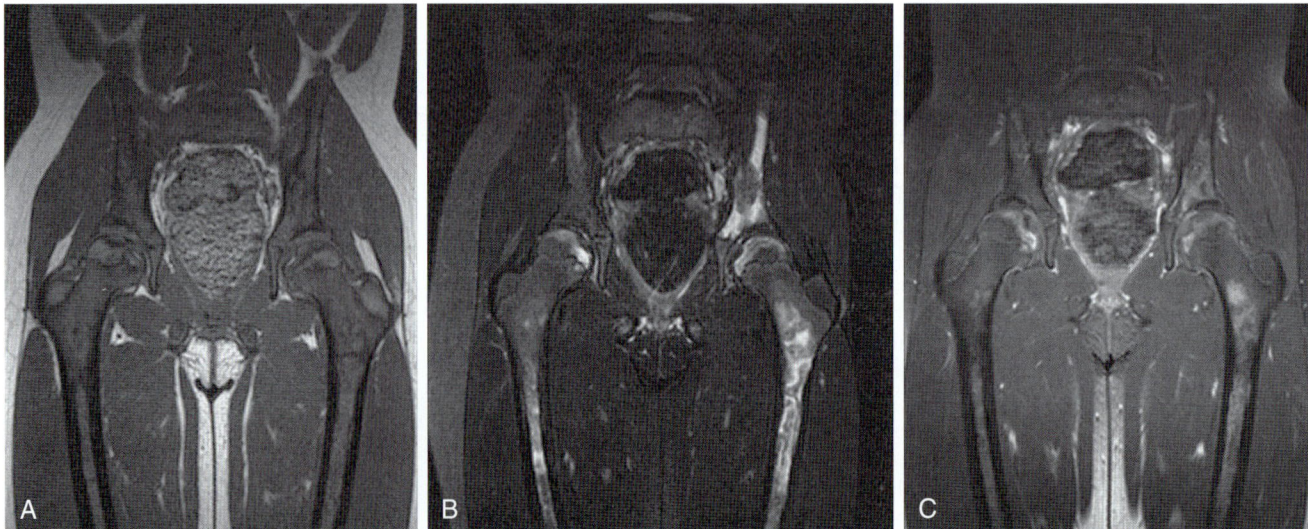

Figure 142-14 Homozygous sickle cell disease in a 10-year-old girl with diffuse changes of osteonecrosis of the pelvic bones and femurs. Coronal T1-weighted (**A**), T2-weighted fat-saturated (**B**), and post-gadolinium T1-weighted fat-saturated (**C**) magnetic resonance images of the pelvis. Note absence of juxtacortical soft tissue edema or hip joint effusions, suggesting that the process is subacute or chronic in nature.

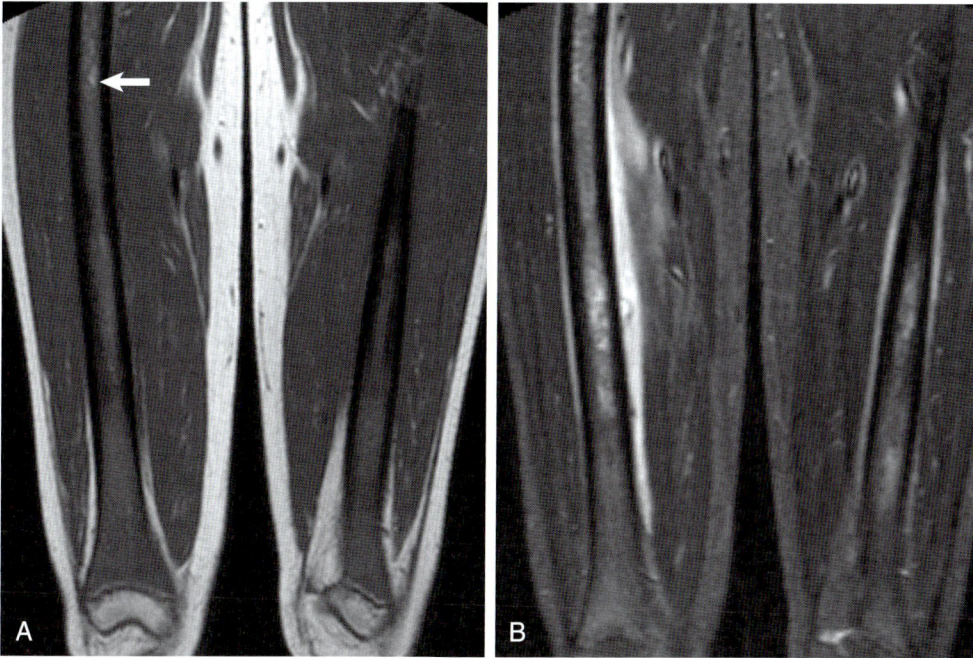

Figure 142-15 Sickle cell disease acute vasoocclusive crisis in a 16-year-old girl. **A,** T1-weighted coronal image demonstrates diffuse red marrow hyperplasia with variegated sclerosis throughout the femoral shafts consistent with prior episodes of osteonecrosis. Note hyperintense T1 focus (*arrow*), which may represent sequestered blood. **B,** Short tau inversion recovery coronal sequence reveals diffuse marrow edema bilaterally, as well as exuberant periostitis bilaterally, and exuberant juxtacortical soft tissue edema on the right.

a leftward shift. Patients with GSD1b have a propensity to develop bacterial infections related to chronic neutropenia.[45]

Imaging   The most common radiographic changes in GSD1b during childhood are osteoporosis, undertubulization of appendicular bones, marked growth retardation, and delayed physeal closure.[46,47] Epiphyseal ossification is often delayed, and open physes may persist into early adulthood. When epiphyseal ossification centers appear, they often have a spiculated and fragmented appearance but eventually normalize in shape as the skeleton matures.

On MRI, the signal intensity of the bone marrow varies and is dependent upon whether G-CSF has been administered for treatment. Without such treatment, patchy areas of low signal intensity on T1-weighted sequences and high signal intensity on T2-weighted FSE and STIR sequences reflect myeloid hyperplasia throughout the axial and appendicular skeleton. MR imaging features of glycogen storage disease may be indistinguishable from marrow hyperplasia related to profound anemia or leukemia. With G-CSF treatment, marrow hyperplasia becomes even more profound, and replacement of yellow marrow at the epiphyses may occur. In addition, G-CSF therapy often creates transverse bands of increased signal intensity on T2-weighted FSE and STIR sequences at the level of the juxtaphyseal metaphysis, likely related to hematopoeitic recruitment.[25,45]

Treatment   Medical nutrition therapy is the primary treatment. Additional therapies include allopurinol to prevent gout, lipid-lowering agents, citrate supplementation to help prevent urinary calculi, angiotensin-converting enzyme inhibitors to treat microalbuminuria, surgery or other treatments for hepatic adenomas, human G-CSF for recurrent infections, and organ transplantation for end-stage kidney and liver disease.[48]

Marrow Infiltration

STORAGE DISORDERS

Gaucher Disease Type 1

Etiology, Pathophysiology, and Clinical Presentation   Gaucher disease is the most prevalent heritable lysosomal storage disorder. Mutations that confer a deficient level of activity of β-glucocerebrosidase lead to accumulation of the lipid glucocerebroside in the lysosomes of macrophage-like Gaucher cells.[49] The symptoms and pathology of the type 1 form of Gaucher disease result from the accumulation of Gaucher cells in various organ systems, including the skeletal system. Those with Gaucher disease are subject to recurrent painful bone crises, like those with sickle cell disease.

Imaging   Skeletal imaging manifestations relate to marrow infiltration by Gaucher cells, leading to osteonecrosis, osteosclerosis, osteomyelitis, and predisposition to fractures.[49,50] The most common radiographic abnormality in untreated Gaucher disease is undertubulation of the distal femoral metaphysis as a result of marrow infiltration, termed the *Erlenmeyer flask deformity*; this is less commonly identified in treated patients.

On MRI, replacement of fatty marrow by Gaucher cells results in low signal intensity of the marrow on T1- and T2-weighted sequences. Initially, marrow replacement is often diffuse and homogeneous and mimics a number of systemic metabolic disorders.[51] Marrow replacement is usually

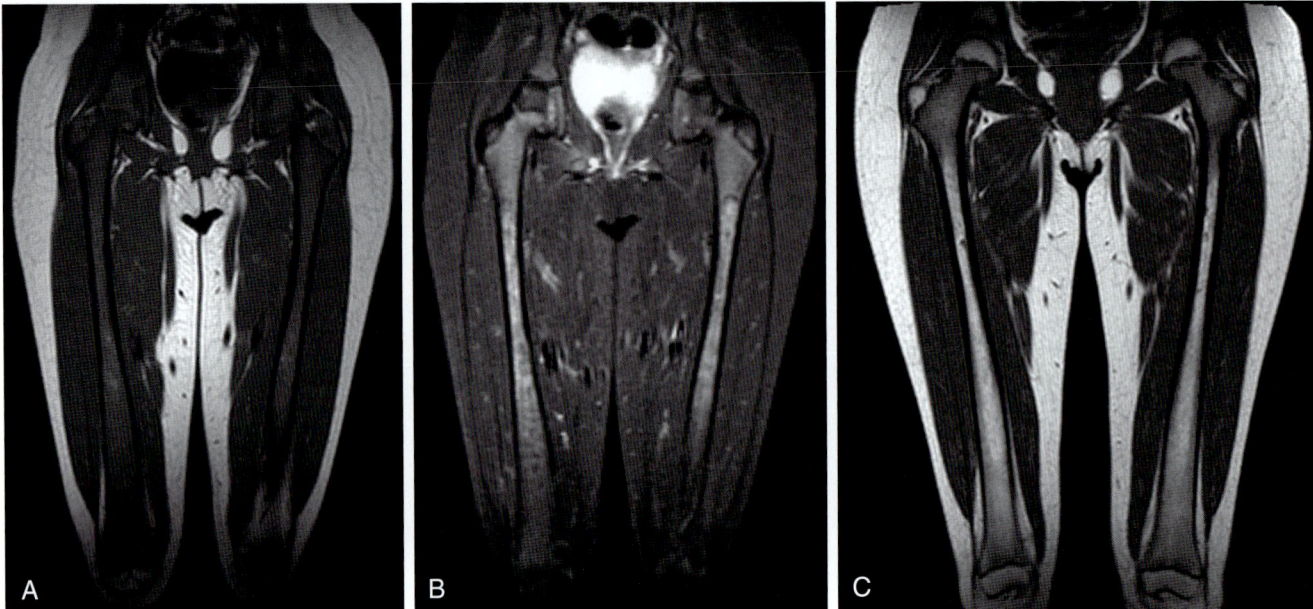

Figure 142-16 Four-year-old girl with Gaucher disease. **A,** T1-weighted coronal image shows diffuse yellow marrow replacement with small diaphyseal islands of yellow marrow. **B,** Short tau inversion recovery coronal image shows lobulated marrow replacement with increased signal with respect to muscle. **C,** T1-weighted coronal image after treatment 7 years later shows yellow marrow conversion in the metaphysis and diaphysis.

confined to the metaphysis and diaphysis, and epiphyseal involvement is unusual except in severe cases.[52] With time and treatment, marrow changes become patchy. Islands of Gaucher cells are separated by intervening fatty marrow throughout the skeleton with relative preservation of the epiphyseal fatty marrow (Fig. 142-16). The intramedullary presence of Gaucher cells is thought to hinder blood flow within the marrow, thereby predisposing these patients to osteonecrosis (e-Fig. 142-17).

Treatment Enzyme-replacement therapy results in degradation of Gaucher cell deposits and reconversion to normal fatty marrow.[52] MRI has been advocated to monitor for an increase in the fat fraction of the marrow as an indicator of response to therapy, and several MRI-based methods of quantifying the bone marrow infiltration in patients with Gaucher disease are under investigation, including Dixon chemical-shift imaging, T1 relaxation-time calculation, and MR spectroscopy.[51]

NEOPLASMS

Leukemia

Etiology, Pathophysiology, and Clinical Presentation Leukemia is the most common childhood malignancy, accounting for up to one third of childhood cancer.[53] Leukemia is classified by the morphology, immunophenotype, and cytogenetics of the leukemic cells. Acute lymphoblastic leukemia (ALL) and acute myeloid leukemia (AML) account for three quarters and one fifth of childhood leukemia cases, respectively. The peak incidence of ALL among children is 2 to 3 years of age, and there is evidence that ALL can initiate in utero.[54] AML rates are highest in the first 2 years of life, decline to a nadir at 6 years of age, and slowly increase during the adolescent years.[55]

An increased risk of leukemia is associated with certain genetic disorders, including trisomy 21, monosomy 7, neurofibromatosis type 1, and DNA repair disorders such as ataxia-telangiectasia.[53] Of special interest to the radiologist, and increasingly the public, is the reported increased risk of leukemia from prenatal or postnatal radiation exposure.[56,57]

Imaging Radiography of the appendicular and axial skeleton is most often normal when the patient is brought to medical attention. When radiographs are abnormal, the most common finding is osteopenia. *Leukemic lines* refers to juxtaphyseal radiolucent metaphyseal bands (Fig. 142-18), and has been attributed to various causes, including disruption of the zone of hypertrophy related to leukemic infiltration, insufficiency fractures of the metaphysis just above the physis, with rarefaction of the juxtaphyseal metaphysis; it has even been proposed to be a visual artifact related to profound osteopenia. Periostitis may also be seen at initial presentation related to the disease process itself or to insufficiency fractures as a result of osteopenia (e-Fig. 142-19).

On MRI, diffuse decreased signal intensity on T1-weighted images[58,59] and increased signal intensity on fat-suppressed T2-weighted and STIR sequences is seen in the setting of leukemic infiltration. The epiphysis is often involved (Fig. 142-20). Marrow involvement may also have a well-defined nodular appearance, especially in the setting of leukemic relapse.[34] The findings are less conspicuous in hematopoietic marrow than in fatty marrow, and consequently these are more difficult to appreciate in younger children, in whom marrow conversion has not yet occurred.[33] The MRI appearance of diffuse cellular infiltration of the marrow in children is not specific for acute leukemia and can also be seen in conditions associated with hematopoietic marrow hyperplasia, in myelodysplastic and myeloproliferative syndromes, and in lymphoma and solid tumor metastases. The findings of periostitis, geographic replacement of fatty marrow by

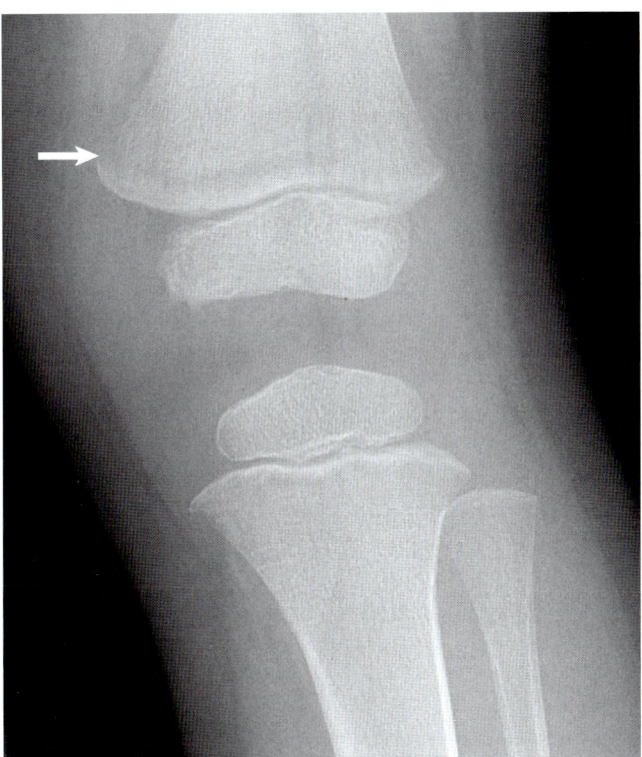

Figure 142-18 One-year-old boy with newly diagnosed acute lymphoblastic leukemia. Leukemic lines manifesting as juxtaphyseal metaphyseal lucency are most pronounced in the distal femur (*arrow*).

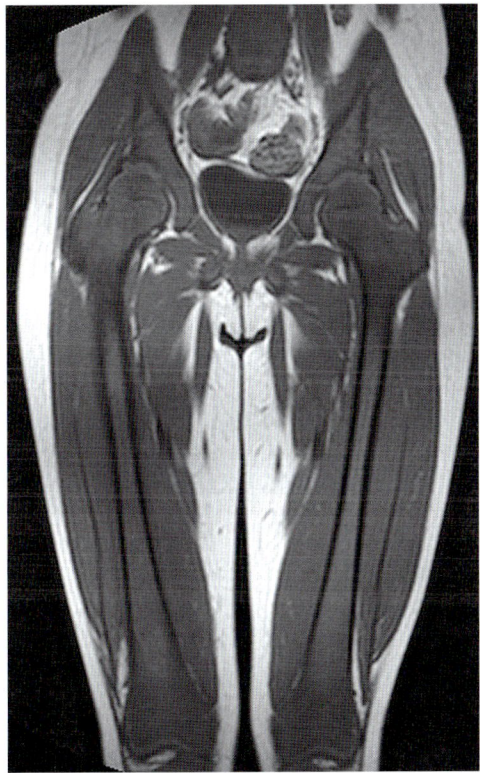

Figure 142-20 Six-year-old girl with newly diagnosed acute lymphoblastic leukemia. Coronal T1-weighted magnetic resonance image of the pelvis and thighs demonstrates diffuse low signal intensity of the bone marrow consistent with leukemic replacement.

hematopoietic marrow throughout the entirety of the long bones and axial skeleton, and juxtacortical soft tissue edema favor a diagnosis of leukemia over hematopoietic marrow hyperplasia.

During chemotherapy for leukemia, the bone marrow becomes hypocellular and edematous. Following chemotherapy, there is progressive regeneration of normal hematopoietic cells and fat (e-Fig. 142-21).[60] A marked increase in the marrow-fat fraction is observed by chemical-shift MRI in patients responding to chemotherapy, whereas a low marrow-fat fraction persists in the setting of unresponsive disease. In children with ALL who enter remission, marrow T1 relaxation time normalizes, whereas it remains prolonged in those who do not enter remission.[59,61] These findings imply that MRI could potentially allow earlier prediction of therapeutic response and identification of residual disease, and it could reduce the need for serial bone marrow biopsies.

Treatment and Follow-up No standard guidelines exist for routine imaging follow-up in children with leukemia. PET imaging, bone densitometry, and whole-body MRI at presentation, treatment, or follow-up may be components of clinical trials or other research investigations but are not part of routine clinical practice.

Imaging is often obtained to evaluate musculoskeletal complications in children treated for leukemia. Musculoskeletal complaints are common at presentation and during follow-up.[62] The most common complications amenable to imaging diagnosis are osteonecrosis and insufficiency fractures. Osteonecrosis is seen in up to 70% of children screened by MRI, and 15% to 20% have symptoms.[63] The reported incidence of fractures in leukemic patients is 18.5% with low lumbar spine bone mineral density and age greater than 10 years as independent predictors of fracture risk.[64]

The most common site of ALL relapse is the marrow, followed by the central nervous system and testes.[55] MRI may be used to evaluate for relapse; however, its specificity is limited by difficulty in differentiating viable neoplasm from effects of therapy, including hematopoietic marrow regeneration (particularly with G-CSF or GM-CSF therapy), hematopoietic marrow reconstitution following stem cell transplantation, marrow iron overload from transfusional hemosiderosis, and marrow infarction and fibrosis.[65-67] Because of these limitations, MR imaging has not replaced marrow aspirate or biopsy for assessment of therapeutic response in leukemia.[68]

Lymphoma

Etiology, Pathophysiology, and Clinical Presentation Marrow involvement by lymphoma in children usually occurs with Burkitt and lymphoblastic lymphomas and with lymphocyte-depleted Hodgkin disease. The pattern of involvement is usually multifocal, and there is a predilection for sites of predominantly hematopoietic marrow. When involvement is diffuse, an arbitrary threshold of neoplastic lymphoid cells constituting 25% or greater of the marrow cellularity differentiates the diagnosis of lymphoblastic leukemia from lymphoma.[69]

Primary lymphoma of bone should be distinguished from Hodgkin and non-Hodgkin lymphoma with bone involvement. When isolated disease is confined to marrow without disease elsewhere for at least 6 months, a diagnosis of primary bone lymphoma can be made.[70]

Imaging Disseminated lymphoma with marrow involvement may be indistinguishable from leukemia by imaging. However, primary lymphoma of bone may be seen initially as isolated focal bone involvement that may mimic other primary bone neoplasms. The most common radiographic pattern is lytic-destructive (Fig. 142-22).[71] The lytic pattern may be permeative, consisting of many uniform small lucencies or "moth-eaten" areas made of larger, poorly marginated lucencies.[70] Primary bone lymphoma often involves the flat bones of the pelvis and shoulder girdle as well as the diaphyses of long bones, similar to Ewing sarcoma.

Unlike leukemia, primary bone lymphoma usually presents as a well-defined intramedullary mass with variable cortical destruction and soft tissue extension. The involved sites typically show low signal intensity on T1-weighted sequences and high signal intensity on fat-suppressed T2-weighted and STIR sequences (see Fig. 142-8). When primary bone lymphoma is unifocal on MRI with masslike features, it cannot be distinguished from other aggressive lesions, such as Ewing sarcoma and Langerhans cell histiocytosis. When diffuse, involvement is often patchy, and up to one third of lymphoma patients with negative bone marrow biopsies have lymphoma involvement visible by MRI distant from the standard iliac crest biopsy sites.[67,72]

Although MRI is a sensitive modality for detecting marrow infiltration, it is not routinely used for the staging of lymphoma. FDG-PET detects lymphoma on the basis of the increased glucose transporter activity and glycolysis in lymphoma, and it is emerging as the functional imaging study of choice for the evaluation of lymphoma. Like MRI, FDG-PET is more sensitive than standard bone scintigraphy for the detection of bone marrow involvement.[72] However, assessment of lymphoma in the marrow after therapy may be limited, with false-positive findings as a result of hematopoietic growth factor effects.[72]

Treatment and Follow-up Systemic lymphoma with marrow involvement portends a worse prognosis and is considered stage IV disease.[53] Imaging follow-up is based on nonosseous disease, including nodal involvement. Patients with primary bone lymphoma have an excellent prognosis, and treatment is usually tailored to the site of involvement.[73]

Osteonecrosis

Etiology, Pathophysiology, and Clinical Presentation Although often asymptomatic and rarely extensive enough to impair hematopoietic function, osteonecrosis can cause pain and disability. It can be separated into *epiphyseal* and *nonepiphyseal* osteonecrosis. The terms *aseptic* and *avascular necrosis* are alternative terms for *epiphyseal osteonecrosis,* and *bone infarction* is an alternative term for *nonepiphyseal osteonecrosis.*

Epiphyseal osteonecrosis portends a worse prognosis compared with nonepiphyseal osteonecrosis. This is because epiphyseal osteonecrosis and its complications—including cartilage injury, subchondral collapse, and subsequent early osteoarthritis—may compromise joint function.

Conditions associated with an increased risk of osteonecrosis include repetitive trauma, sickle cell disease, Gaucher disease, chronic renal failure, bone marrow transplantation, steroid therapy, pancreatitis, and highly active antiretroviral therapy for HIV infection.[74] Putative pathophysiologic mechanisms related to nontraumatic spontaneous osteonecrosis include vascular occlusion, elevated medullary cavity pressure, coagulopathy, and altered lipid metabolism. Osteonecrosis most commonly occurs in regions of fatty marrow and is unusual in hematopoietic marrow, except in patients with a hemoglobinopathy.[74]

Legg-Calvé-Perthes (LCP) disease, also called *idiopathic osteonecrosis of the capital femoral epiphysis,* is one of the most common forms of epiphyseal osteonecrosis. LCP is a classic illustrative example of the clinical course and prognosis related to epiphyseal osteonecrosis at the femoral head and

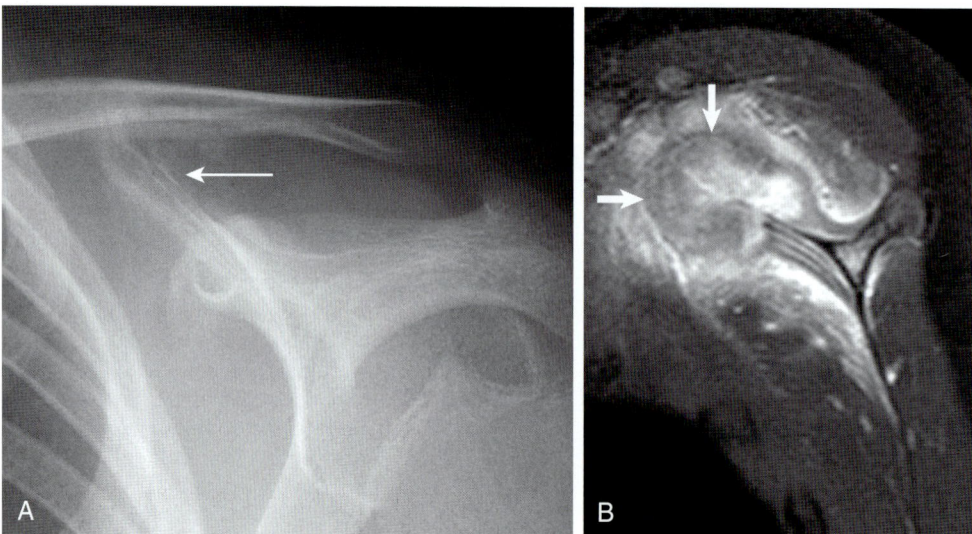

Figure 142-22 Fourteen-year-old boy with left shoulder pain. **A,** Frontal radiograph of the left scapula at initial presentation shows periosteal reaction and irregularity (*arrow*) at the superomedial scapula. **B,** T1-weighted image with fat saturation shows cortical destruction, bone marrow edema, and a large heterogeneously enhancing soft tissue mass arising from the superior scapula (*arrows*) with adjacent soft tissue edema. Open surgical biopsy revealed large cell anaplastic lymphoma.

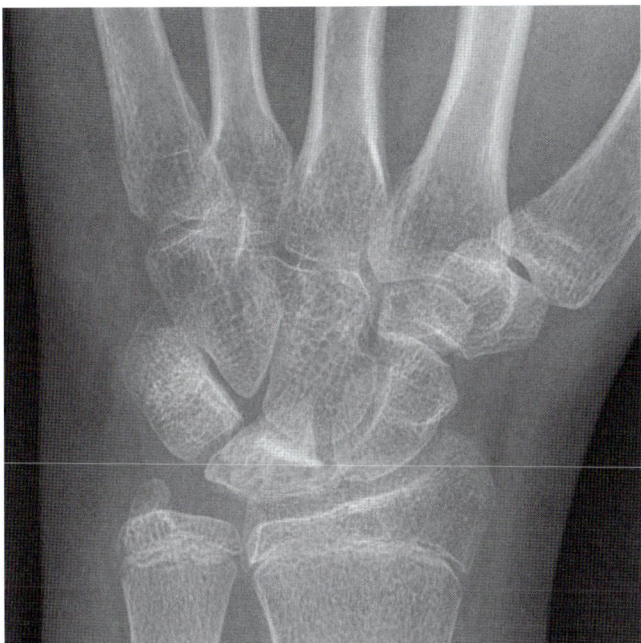

Figure 142-23 Fourteen-year-old girl with Keinboch disease with flattening and sclerosis of the lunate bone.

elsewhere. LCP affects boys between 2 and 14 years of age with peak incidence around 5 to 6 years (male/female ratio, 5:1). Bilateral involvement is seen in about 10% to 15% of cases, although it is almost always asynchronous.[75] Forms of idiopathic osteonecrosis that affect other bones include but are not limited to Kienböck disease (lunate; Fig. 142-23), Köhler disease (navicular; Fig. 142-24), and Freiberg infraction (second or third metatarsal head; Fig. 142-25).

For LCP, deformity of the femoral head, neck, and acetabulum results is a common cause of degenerative disease of the hip, particularly in men. Children who come to medical attention before 6 years of age generally have a benign course, whereas those who seek care after 8 years of age fare less well and often require surgery.[76]

Children with LCP are typically seen after having had several weeks or months of limping, often without pain. Physical findings include spasm, limitation of abduction and internal rotation, and atrophy of the thigh and buttocks in a child who is otherwise normal.

Imaging In acute osteonecrosis, radiographs are usually normal. With subacute and chronic osteonecrosis, radiographs will show geographic and patchy areas of sclerosis (see Fig. 142-11).

In the acute phase of osteonecrosis, marrow hemorrhage, edema, and liquefactive necrosis are evident. On MRI, this may be difficult to distinguish from infection and/or superimposed stress reaction. Acute-on-chronic osteonecrosis may occur, and the presence of edema and periostitis are helpful clues to identify the acute component (Fig. 142-26). Rarely, this may superficially mimic a neoplastic process. Unfortunately, early infection and superimposed stress reaction may be indistinguishable. During the reparative phase, central fatty marrow replacement usually occurs (Fig. 142-27). Osteonecrosis often has a geographic shape with a serpentine margin of low signal intensity on T1-weighted sequences and often does not respect epiphyseal, metaphyseal, and diaphyseal boundaries of the long bones (see Fig. 142-27). T2-weighted sequences may demonstrate a characteristic "double-line sign" consisting of an outer rim of low signal intensity corresponding to sclerotic bone and an inner rim of high signal intensity corresponding to vascularized granulation tissue (Fig. 142-28). Areas of low signal intensity on both T1- and T2-weighted sequences related to osteonecrosis represent fibrosis or calcification. Fatty marrow infiltration manifested by increased signal intensity on T1-weighted sequences within the area of osteonecrosis is believed to indicate central revascularization (see Fig. 142-27). Intense contrast enhancement is common at the periphery of evolving areas of osteonecrosis, and dynamic contrast-enhanced MRI has been advocated for early diagnosis but probably is not necessary in children with established osteonecrosis. The diagnosis can usually confidently be made on conventional MRI sequences without intravenous contrast.[74]

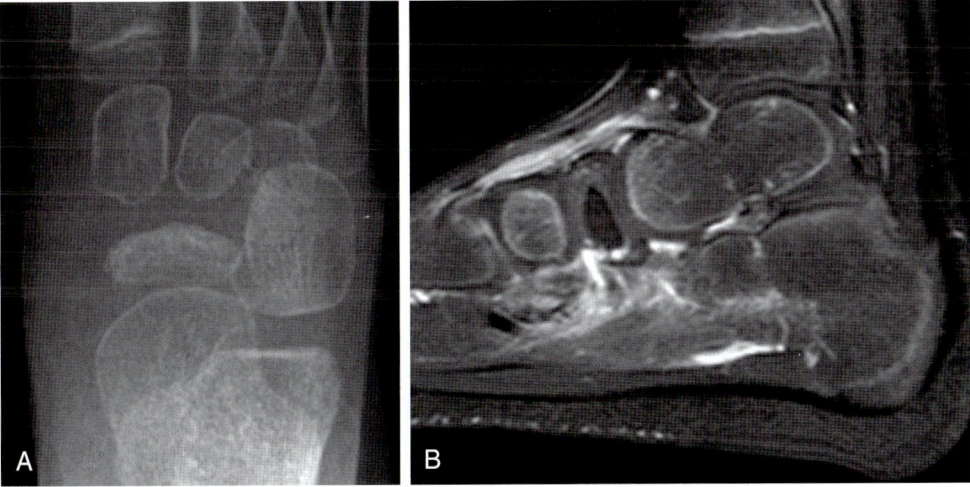

Figure 142-24 Fifteen-year-old girl with Kohler disease. **A,** Anteroposterior view of the foot shows sclerosis and mild flattening of the navicular bone. **B,** Postcontrast T1-weighted fat-saturated sagittal image shows nonenhancement of the navicular bone and soft tissue edema about the dorsal and plantar surface of the midfoot.

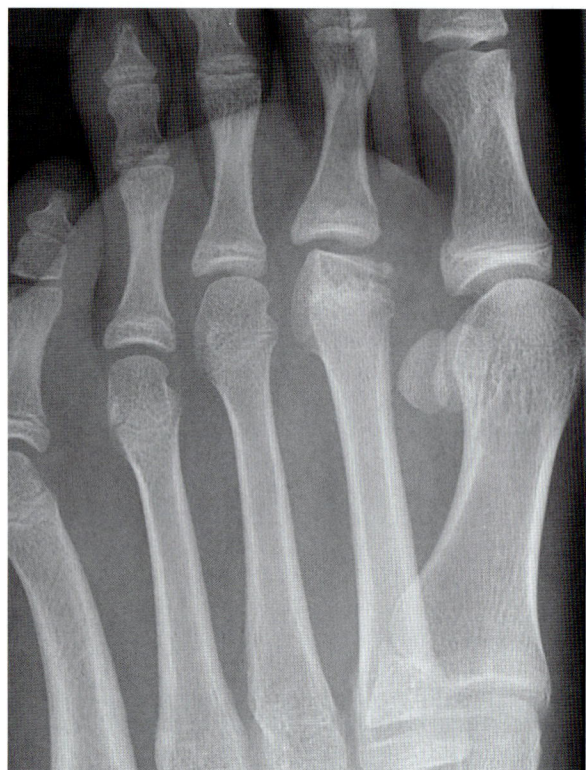

Figure 142-25 Freiberg infraction in an 11-year-old girl. Oblique view of the forefoot shows flattening and collapse of the second metatarsal head.

Imaging findings of epiphyseal osteonecrosis related to other causes are indistinguishable from those of LCP, which progresses through four main stages: 1) avascularity, 2) revascularization, 3) healing, and 4) residual deformity (e-Fig. 142-29). Early radiographic diagnosis is based on the detection of periarticular osteoporosis, medial joint space widening and lateral displacement of the femoral head, and eventually a relatively smaller and denser appearance of the femoral head.[77,78]

During the revascularization stage, which lasts from 1 to 4 years, surrounding tissues react to the dead bone. In this stage, the child experiences pain, and the most dramatic radiographic changes occur.[79] The ossific nucleus appears even denser because of new bone formation that occurs within the dead trabeculae; it is easily flattened and deformed. A pathologic subchondral fracture in the anterosuperior ossific nucleus creates the radiographic "crescent sign." The epiphyseal ossification center undergoes varying degrees of fragmentation, primarily in its central portion (e-Fig. 142-30). The adjacent metaphysis sometimes develops cystic changes and broadens. Disturbed endochondral ossification from ischemia probably results in residual cartilage in the metaphysis.[80]

During the healing phase, new bone slowly replaces granulation tissue in the ossific nucleus, and the epiphysis regains its height. The better the femoral head is contained by the acetabulum, the more spherically the femoral head will remodel. On MRI performed during the healing phase, the physeal cartilage may exhibit irregularity or bridging. Epiphyseal deformity is more pronounced anteriorly; hence, sagittal images are more useful for evaluation.

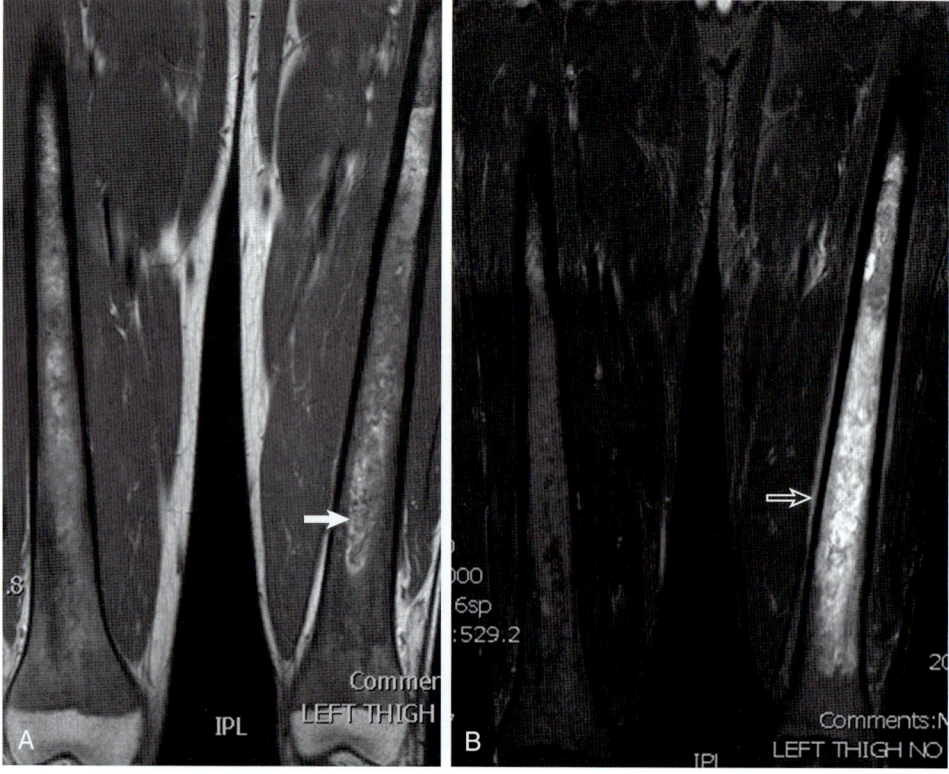

Figure 142-26 20-year-old man with sickle cell disease with acute bone infarction. **A,** T1-weighted coronal image shows diffuse red marrow of the metaphyses and diaphyses. Hyperintense foci are apparent within the medullary cavity (*arrow*), presumably representing sequestered blood. **B,** Short tau inversion recovery coronal image shows diffuse marrow edema and periostitis (*open arrow*), consistent with acute bone infarction.

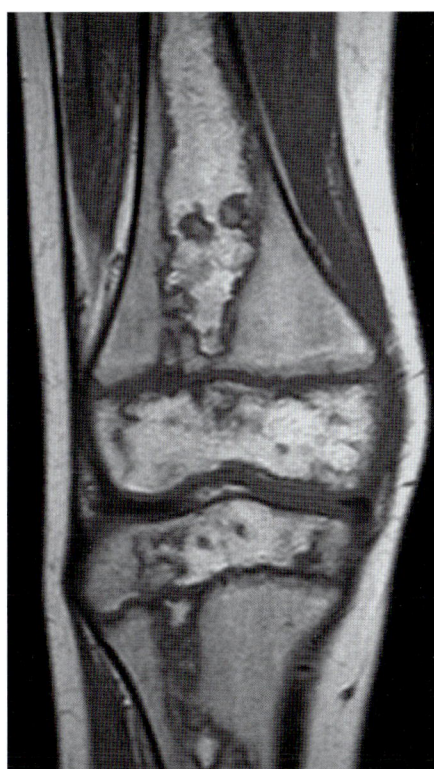

Figure 142-27 Diffuse osteonecrosis in an 11-year-old boy. T1-weighted coronal image shows diaphyseal, metaphyseal, and epiphyseal involvement of osteonecrosis. Note central areas of increased signal intensity within the areas of osteonecrosis, believed to represent fatty marrow conversion.

Residual deformity persists after healing, although the articular cartilage is reasonably preserved. As a result, joint function may be satisfactory for several years. Abnormal shape of the healed epiphysis is characterized by *coxa magna,* a residual enlargement of the femoral head and neck, and *coxa breva,* a short femoral neck as a result of premature physeal

arrest. Subsequent varus or valgus hip deformity may occur, depending on the location of the physeal fusion. A deformed femoral head, especially with a large anterolateral segment that is uncovered, can impinge on the lateral acetabular lip and cause clinical symptoms of decreased range of motion, pain, and a "clunking" sensation. Joint incongruity leads to degenerative joint disease later in life.

Treatment Treatment is aimed at managing the underlying condition or modifying administration of the causative agent, such as decreasing corticosteroid dosage. Resting the affected joint may help slow disease progression and may prevent complications, including pathologic fractures. Children with osteonecrosis are predisposed to pathologic fractures, and subchondral collapse occurs with epiphyseal osteonecrosis and pathologic long-bone fractures with nonepiphyseal involvement. For epiphyseal osteonecrosis, the most important predictors of patient outcome, aside from age of onset, are joint congruency and motion.

Treatment of LCP is individualized on the basis of clinical and radiographic findings, including age of onset, range of motion in the hip joint, extent of femoral head involvement, presence or absence of femoral deformity, and lateral subluxation of the femoral head. For many patients, a combination of traction treatment with an abduction cast, nonsteroidal antiinflammatory agents, and gentle range-of-motion exercises are used to enhance molding of the femoral head by the acetabulum. Surgery is indicated in children younger than 8 years who have femoral head deformity and in those older than 8 years even in the absence of deformity. Because LCP often affects the proximal femoral physeal vertex while preserving normal medial physeal physiology, a relative coxa valga may develop related to vertex physeal growth disturbance. As a consequence, surgical reduction to contain the femoral head is often indicated, including subtrochanteric varus osteotomies with or without congruent periacetabular shelf osteotomies, particularly in older patients (second decade). The main goals of surgical therapy are to preserve joint congruity during the active phase of the disease and to

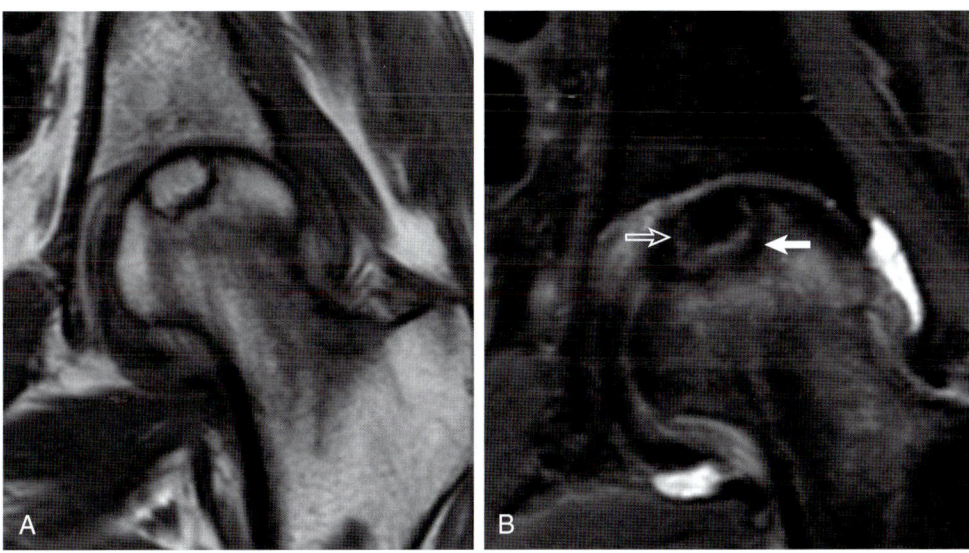

Figure 142-28 Epiphyseal osteonecrosis of the femoral head in an 18-year-old woman. T1-weighted (**A**) and short tau inversion recovery coronal images (**B**) demonstrate a "double-line sign" with inner white line (*open arrow*) and outer dark line (*solid arrow*). Note central area of increased T1 signal consistent with fatty marrow replacement.

contain the femoral head within the acetabulum, preventing extrusion and subluxation. A femoral head that is contained by the acetabulum tends to heal more spherically than one that is partially subluxed. In severe cases, a vicious cycle ensues in which decreased containment leads to increased deformity that in turn leads to further subluxation. Surgery can prevent this progression and can be used to maintain a full range of motion at the hip joint.[81]

Effects of Therapy

HEMATOPOIETIC GROWTH FACTORS

Etiology, Pathophysiology, and Clinical Presentation Hematopoietic growth factors such as G-CSF, GM-CSF, and erythropoietin are cytokines that regulate the proliferation and differentiation of hematopoietic progenitor cells in the bone marrow.[82,83] Recombinant human hematopoietic growth factors are commonly used to hasten the recovery of hematopoietic marrow from myelosuppressive chemotherapy or bone marrow failure syndromes and to stimulate more effective myelopoiesis in GSD1b.[45]

Imaging In those treated with G-CSF or GM-CSF, MRI will show signal intensity changes associated with reconversion of fatty marrow to hypercellular hematopoietic marrow that coincide temporally with increases in the absolute neutrophil count. These changes may be observed incidentally on routine imaging studies or on imaging studies prompted by bone pain accompanying G-CSF administration.[25] As in other instances of marrow hyperplasia, the imaging changes

follow a signal intensity similar to that of red marrow. GRE out-of-phase sequences designed to detect altered proportions of fat and water may be the most sensitive for the effects of G-CSF therapy. The peak of hematopoietic marrow hyperplasia observed by MRI occurs about 2 weeks after discontinuation of G-CSF administration, and the bone marrow alterations normalize in most patients within 6 weeks after treatment. The marrow changes may be diffuse, patchy, or have a masslike appearance, and they can be asymmetric and simulate bone marrow involvement by leukemia, metastatic disease, or other infiltrative process.[66] The masslike appearance of red marrow on T1-weighted images may have well-defined margins rather than the wisplike, feathery appearance of residual red marrow (see Fig. 142-5). Marrow changes as a result of G-CSF may not follow the typical red marrow pattern of reconversion seen in patients who are anemic. For instance, diaphyseal red marrow islands may appear before metaphyseal red marrow changes are seen. The changes can also obscure underlying marrow lesions.[84] Masslike marrow replacement owing to G-CSF usually is not associated with juxtacortical soft tissue edema at the same level of the lesion that is more likely with metastatic marrow replacement. Consideration of the timing of the therapy and imaging is necessary to avoid misinterpretation of the marrow changes (see Fig. 142-7).

Similarly, FDG-PET, ^{99m}Tc sulfur colloid scintigraphy, gallium-67 scintigraphy, and thallium-201 scintigraphy can show elevated radiopharmaceutical uptake by the stimulated hematopoietic marrow (Fig. 142-31). Large interindividual variability is seen in marrow FDG uptake induced by hematopoietic growth factors. FDG marrow uptake returns to

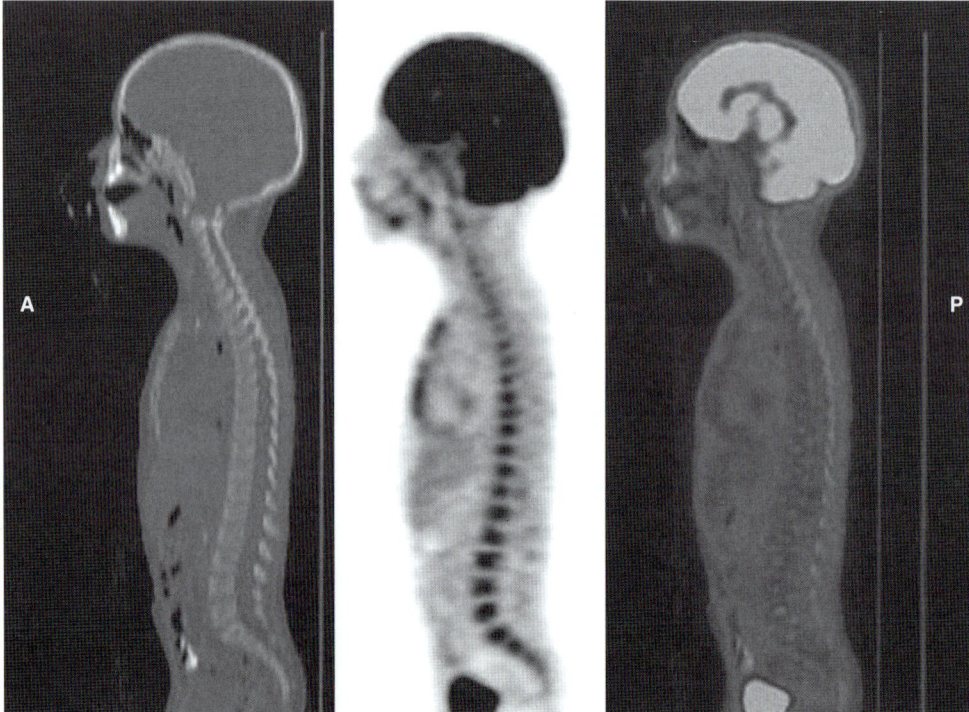

Figure 142-31 Fluorodeoxyglucose positron-emission tomography (FDG-PET) computed tomographic images of a 4-year-old boy on granulocyte-colony stimulating factor therapy to mitigate the myelosuppressive effects of Wilms tumor treatment. Diffuse increased uptake of FDG by the bone marrow of the spine and sternum reflects the increased metabolic demand from stimulation of granulopoiesis in the marrow. (Courtesy Dr. Barry Shulkin, St. Jude Children's Research Hospital, Memphis, TN.)

normal within 1 month after the discontinuation of G-CSF treatment in most individuals.[84]

The anemia of end-stage renal disease can be treated with recombinant human erythropoietin, which induces an increase in the erythropoeitic marrow that manifests as decreased signal intensity on T1-weighted sequences. Erythropoietin also increases the bone marrow uptake of FDG.

RADIATION THERAPY

Etiology, Pathophysiology, and Clinical Presentation In the acute phase, radiation therapy causes depression of the marrow cellularity and vascular sinusoid injury with edema and hemorrhage.[85] In the chronic phase, the vascular sinusoids are obliterated, and hematopoietic marrow is replaced by fat and fibrosis.[86]

The process of fatty replacement of the marrow is largely irreversible for doses higher than 30 to 40 Gy, because destruction of the vascular sinusoids prevents migration of hematopoietic cells into the irradiated marrow.[6] For doses less than 30 to 40 Gy, the fatty replacement of the marrow is less complete, because regeneration of the hematopoietic marrow may occur. This regeneration of hematopoietic marrow manifests as a mottled or band pattern in the vertebrae of children between 11 and 30 months after spinal irradiation of doses no greater than 40 Gy, and similar findings have been observed in the marrow of the long bones after irradiation.[87] Marrow regeneration is more likely to occur with larger volumes of irradiated marrow, suggesting that partial spinal irradiation may not provide enough stimuli for regeneration, because the nonirradiated marrow is sufficient to meet hematopoietic demands.[87]

Imaging STIR sequences are the most sensitive conventional MRI technique for depicting early postradiation changes in the marrow, and they can detect the effects of radiation therapy within a few days after initiation of treatment.[6] Areas of increased signal intensity in the marrow on STIR sequences peak 9 days after therapy and reflect edema, hemorrhage, and early influx of nonirradiated cells.[4,25,84] T1-weighted sequences in the acute phase show a corresponding decrease in the signal intensity of the bone marrow and a corresponding increased signal intensity on STIR sequences indicative of marrow edema. From 2 to 6 weeks after irradiation, the signal intensity of the bone marrow begins to increase on T1-weighted sequences and decrease on STIR sequences (Fig. 142-32).[84] After 6 weeks, the marrow pattern either becomes more homogeneous, with high signal intensity on T1-weighted sequences and low signal intensity on STIR sequences, or it develops a band pattern of peripheral intermediate signal intensity surrounding central high signal intensity on T1-weighted sequences and produces reciprocal changes on STIR sequences.[84,87] In the chronic phase, the marrow also shows a marked decrease in contrast enhancement, reflecting vascular obliteration.[25,85]

Marrow regeneration after radiation usually occurs when less than 40 Gy is administered.[87] Marrow fibrosis is more likely to occur when more than 40 Gy is administered.

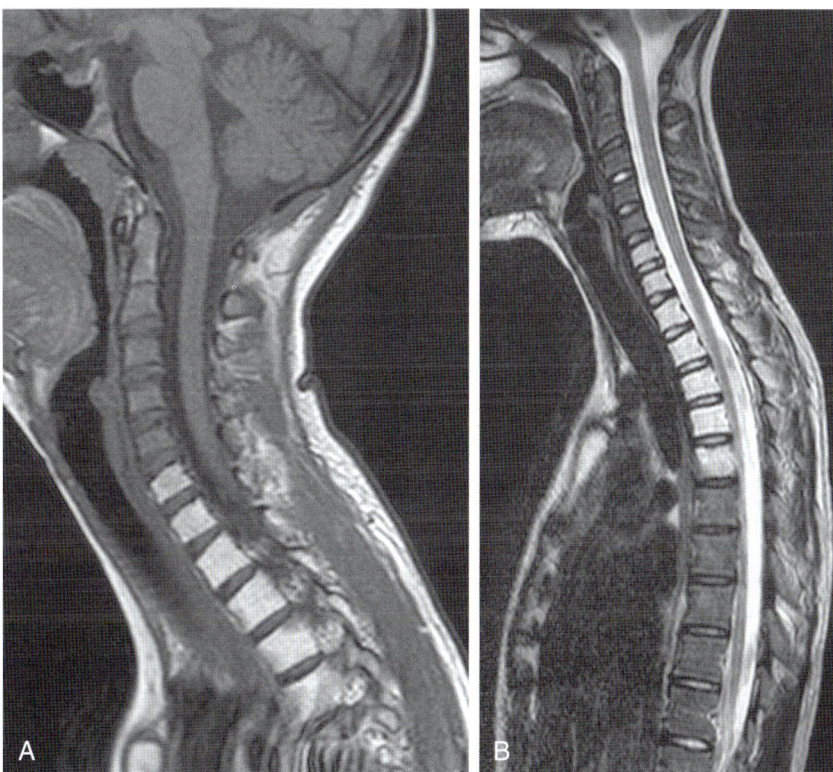

Figure 142-32 Fifteen-year-old girl with a history of local radiation therapy for an extraosseous Ewing sarcoma of the left supraclavicular region. Sagittal T1-weighted (**A**) and turbo spin echo T2-weighted (**B**) magnetic resonance imaging of the upper spine reveals sharply demarcated, homogeneous high signal intensity of the marrow of the lower cervical spine, upper thoracic spine, and upper sternum that corresponds to fatty transformation of the marrow within the irradiated field.

Additional late changes after radiation therapy include osteo-necrosis and radiation-induced osteochondromas.[25]

BONE MARROW TRANSPLANTATION

Etiology, Pathophysiology, and Clinical Presentation Bone marrow transplantation is used in the treatment of numerous pediatric malignancies, as well as severe aplastic anemia, hereditary hemoglobinopathies, inborn errors of metabolism, and certain immunodeficiency and autoimmune syndromes. In preparation for bone marrow transplantation, the host marrow is ablated and conditioned by chemotherapy and possibly also by fractionated total-body irradiation to induce immune suppression and eliminate residual malignant cells, if applicable. Stem cells are then infused intravenously and engraft in the marrow within 2 to 4 weeks. Typical fatty and hematopoietic bone marrow is usually seen within 90 days after transplantation.[4]

Imaging In the interval following bone marrow transplantation, until the recovery of hematopoiesis, hematopoietic growth factors and multiple blood transfusions may be given, and the appearance of the marrow on MRI during this time will reflect the combined effects of marrow necrosis, early hematopoietic reconstitution, and possibly iron overload.[88,89]

Within 40 to 90 days after transplantation, a band pattern in the vertebral bodies may develop, consisting of a peripheral zone of intermediate signal intensity and a central zone of high signal intensity on T1-weighted sequences with recipro-cal signal intensities on STIR sequences.[88] This pattern cor-responds to regenerating hematopoietic marrow peripherally and fatty marrow centrally. The band pattern may gradually evolve into a homogeneous appearance of the marrow.[6] However, the hematopoietic marrow recovery after bone marrow transplantation may not achieve full reconstitution, corroborated by the observation that the fat fraction in the vertebral and pelvic marrow determined by chemical-shift MRI is higher in transplanted patients for several years after transplantation.[25]

WHAT THE CLINICIAN NEEDS TO KNOW

Alterations from age-appropriate bone marrow signal

Extent of abnormal marrow, focal or diffuse

Whether complications such as fractures are present

If changes are potentially treatment related

Whether a mass or other features suspicious for neoplasm are present

Any significant change from prior examinations

Key Points

MRI is the primary imaging modality for evaluating bone marrow. A combination of T1-weighted and fat-saturated T2-weighted or STIR sequences is sufficient for the detection and characterization of most marrow lesions. Contrast-enhanced MRI is reserved for when findings are unclear on precontrast images.

Conversion from hematopoietic to fatty marrow in the axial skeleton occurs in a distal-to-proximal direction and from diaphyses to metaphyses in the long bones. Fatty conversion in the epiphyses and apophyses begins soon after ossification, and marrow reconversion occurs in the reverse order of marrow conversion.

The MRI appearance of marrow in thalassemia and sickle cell disease reflects the combined effects of red marrow hyperplasia, iron deposition, iron chelation therapy, and in the case of sickle cell disease, medullary infarcts. Acute medullary infarcts are often indistinguishable from acute osteomyelitis on MRI.

Treatment-related marrow changes, particularly with hematopoietic growth factors, cause bone marrow changes that can simulate involvement by leukemia, metastatic disease, and other infiltrative processes. Knowledge of the timing of therapy and imaging is necessary for accurate image interpretation.

ACKNOWLEDGMENT

We acknowledge the contributions of Jennifer D. Smith, MD, and Diego Jaramillo, MD, MPH, from prior editions of this book.

Suggested Reading

Burdiles A, Babyn PS. Pediatric bone marrow MR imaging. *Magn Reson Imaging Clin N Am.* 2009;17(3):391-409.

Fletcher BD. Effects of pediatric cancer therapy on the musculoskeletal system. *Pediatr Radiol.* 1997;27(8):623-636.

Foster K, Chapman S, Johnson K. MRI of the marrow in the paediatric skeleton. *Clin Radiol.* 2004;59(8):651-673.

Jaramillo D, Kasser JR, Villegas-Medina OL, et al. Cartilaginous abnormali-ties and growth disturbances in Legg-Calvé-Perthes disease: evaluation with MR imaging. *Radiology.* 1995;197(3):767-773.

Saini A, Saifuddin A. MRI of osteonecrosis. *Clin Radiol.* 2004; 59(12):1079-1093.

Vande Berg BC, Malghem J, Lecouvet FE, et al. Magnetic resonance imaging of normal bone marrow. *Eur Radiol.* 1998;8(8):1327-1334.

References

Full references for this chapter can be found on www.expertconsult.com.

Chapter 143

Skeletal Trauma

DEEPA R. PAI and PETER J. STROUSE

General Overview

In this chapter, traumatic injuries to the pediatric appendicular skeleton and pelvis are discussed. Injuries to the axial skeleton, including the skull, spine, and bony thorax, are covered in separate chapters dedicated to those portions of the body. This chapter will concentrate on fractures in children; however, other forms of trauma to the pediatric skeleton are briefly covered.

The dictum "Children are not small adults" holds more weight than in any other situation with regard to skeletal trauma. Fracture patterns and fracture healing are different processes in children than in adults.[1,2] Unfortunately, a fracture may interfere with subsequent normal growth of a bone.[1,2] Fortunately, such complications are relatively uncommon. In healthy children, the process of fracture healing and remodeling is rapid, particularly in the vascularized metaphysis.[3] Most posttraumatic deformities readily correct with healing and remodeling.[1,2] The composition of a child's bones and the presence of the growth process both predispose children to types and complications of fractures that are different from those seen in adults.[1,2,4]

General Etiologies, Pathophysiology, and Clinical Presentation (Mechanism, Healing, Complications)

Mechanism Many mechanisms may play a role in pediatric trauma. Falls, injuries at play, and motor vehicle accidents account for a majority of childhood fractures.[5] Unfortunately, younger children may suffer fractures as a consequence of nonaccidental trauma (child abuse). These injuries are often characteristic and are covered in Chapter 144. Children of all ages are increasingly involved in and dedicated to athletics and competitive sports. Certain types of fractures, including stress fractures, are often associated with sporting injury. These fractures are addressed Chapter 145. Pathologic fractures may be seen with bone tumors, and insufficiency fractures may be seen with metabolic bone disease (see Chapter 140).

Fracture Description and Nomenclature Understanding basic fracture nomenclature is important for effective communication with clinicians and other radiologists. Fractures are subdivided into two basic categories: (1) incomplete (plastic) and (2) complete. Incomplete fractures include *greenstick* and *buckle* fractures. Complete fractures should be described based on orientation: *transverse*, *oblique*, *longitudinal*, and *spiral*. Spiral fractures are defined by an approximately 180-degree or greater twist in the fracture plane. For any fracture, angulation, displacement, diastasis, comminution, and impaction must be described. On follow-up radiographs, any change, in addition to the presence or absence of fracture healing, should be described. The term *dislocation* should be reserved for joints only, not fracture sites. In addition, whenever describing fractures, involvement of an open physis and articular surface should be described. For physeal fractures, it is acceptable to describe the fracture using the Salter-Harris classification.

Fracture Healing Fracture healing in children has been described in three phases: (1) inflammatory, (2) reparative, and (3) remodeling (e Fig. 143-1).[6] At the time of fracture, bone and periosteum are disrupted. A hematoma is formed at the site of fracture enveloping the ends of the fractured bone. The hematoma may also contain necrotic fragments of bone, bone marrow, and adjacent tissues. An inflammatory response is initiated (inflammatory phase), and the organization of a hematoma then begins. Osteoclasts and osteoblasts arise from precursor cells of the involved tissues. Bone resorption occurs at areas of necrosis.[7] This peaks 2 to 3 weeks after injury and appears as a poorly defined fracture line.[8] Initial callus (immature woven bone) is formed during the reparative phase.[6] Osteoid and chondroid material (callus) forming within the hematoma envelops the fracture fragments, joining and stabilizing them. Endosteal callus also forms within the fracture fragments and is seen as increased density on radiographs. Devitalized portions of bone at the margin of the fracture fragments may undergo resorption and appear demineralized on radiographs. An injury that is less than 5 to 7 days old will not show any of these described radiographic features.[7] With time, the woven bone of callus is replaced by organized lamellar bone during the remodeling phase. With remodeling, excess thickness from the callus is resorbed and the medullary canal is reestablished. Remodeling lasts months, and occasionally years.[6,7] The healing process is more rapid and complete in children than in adults. Most childhood fractures heal completely and without residual deformity.

Complications   Complications may occur at the time of fracture, during treatment, or as a failure of normal, complete fracture healing. Box 143-1 lists potential complications of pediatric fractures. The incidence of a particular complication varies, depending on many factors, including the site and severity of the fracture, complicating factors (i.e., open fracture), the age and overall health of the patient, associated injuries, and the adequacy of therapy.[9]

In *nonunion*, healing stops before osseous continuity of the fracture fragments occurs. The fracture fragments may form a pseudoarthrosis. Pseudoarthrosis is most common in the clavicle, humerus, and tibia. Nonunion and pseudoarthroses are uncommon in normal children but may be seen with underlying abnormalities such as neurofibromatosis or congenital insensitivity to pain.[10,11] The incidence of nonunion is increased with greater injury, comminution, and distraction and with open fractures complicated by substantial soft tissue injury, infection, or both.[11] *Delayed union* is defined as failure of bone union to occur in the expected time. *Malunion* indicates fusion in a nonanatomic orientation. Mild degrees of malalignment are well tolerated and usually result in

no permanent deformity and resolve overtime because of remodeling. Surgical interruption of the healing process to correct residual malalignment is occasionally necessary. Posttraumatic synostoses are most common in the paired bones of the forearm and leg. Infection may occur due to an open fracture or as a complication of surgery or percutaneous pinning.[11]

Fracture at certain sites may result in neurovascular injury; however, such injuries are rare and usually only seen with substantial displacement and deformity, as may occur with supracondylar fractures of the distal humerus.[9] Compartment syndrome is an uncommon complication of extremity fractures, most commonly in the leg or with supracondylar elbow fractures, and may lead to Volkmann contracture caused by ischemia.[9]

Reflex sympathetic dystrophy syndrome (RSDS; also called "Sudeck atrophy") is a poorly understood dysfunction of the autonomic nervous system after injury. RSDS most commonly affects the lower extremities in children. Patients present with pain, swelling, joint stiffness, and exquisite sensitivity to touch.[12] Onset of symptoms is within 1 week to several months after injury.[9] Radiographs show osteopenia that is difficult to distinguish from disuse osteoporosis. Magnetic resonance imaging (MRI) can show patchy bone marrow edema; however, at times it may be normal.[13] Bone scintigraphy is usually abnormal. Early, increased activity is seen on perfusion, blood pool, and delayed phases. Later, decreased activity may be seen on both perfusion and blood pool phases, with increased activity remaining during the delayed phase for months.[14] The characteristic imaging findings seen in adult patients may not be seen in children.[15] RSDS has been more recently categorized under the more general term *bone marrow edema syndrome*, which includes other transient clinical conditions with an unknown underlying mechanism, such as transient osteoporosis of the hip.[14]

Premature fusion occurs in approximately 15% of physeal fractures.[16] A bony "bridge" or "bar" forms across the physis.[17] Prognosis depends on the involved bone, the extent and location of the physeal bar (central versus eccentric), and the amount of remaining growth.[11,16] Morbidity is greater when the remaining growth potential is higher. The phalanges and distal radius are the most common sites of physeal fracture; however, growth arrest is rare.[16] The distal femur and proximal tibia have high incidence of posttraumatic physeal fusion but are less common sites for physeal fracture.[16] Premature fusion in the distal femur and tibia is also of greater clinical importance because of possible resultant leg length discrepancy or angular deformity.[16] Indirect physeal insult such as burns, frostbite, and electrical injury, which are discussed later in this chapter, and other processes such as infection and secondary ischemic insult related to meningococcemia can also cause premature physeal fusion (Box 143-2).

Central fusions cause loss of growth potential. Central fusions result in a cupped appearance of the physis, with the epiphysis and physis invaginating into the center of the metaphysis.[11,16] Peripheral fusions result in angular deformity.[11,16] Premature physeal fusion usually occurs approximately 3 months after injury.[16] Radiographs may show obliteration of the physeal clear space. Comparison views are often helpful, particularly when evaluating an older child in whom the time of normal physeal closure is near. A secondary sign of premature physeal fusion is tethering of growth

---

Box 143-1 Complications of Fracture

Acute

Neurovascular injury

Hemorrhage

Fat embolism

Compartment syndrome

Subacute or Chronic

Premature growth plate fusion

Delayed union

Nonunion or pseudoarthrosis

Malunion or deformity

Synostosis (cross-union)

Heterotopic ossification or myositis ossificans

Osteomyelitis or septic arthritis

Posttraumatic osteolysis

Avascular necrosis

Posttraumatic cyst

Osteochondroma

Fibrous cortical defect

Aneurysmal bone cyst

Iatrogenic

Soft tissue infection

Hardware misplacement, migration, or infection

Casting complications

Hypocalcemia of immobilization

Superior mesenteric artery syndrome

Deep Venous Thrombosis or Pulmonary Embolism

Overgrowth

Refracture

Reflex sympathetic dystrophy syndrome

Premature degenerative joint disease (osteoarthritis)

Box 143-2 Causes of Physeal Arrest

Trauma
Fracture (Salter-Harris I–IV)
Crush or compression (Salter-Harris V)
Stress fracture
Neuropathic (i.e., myelodysplasia)
Infection
Osteomyelitis
Meningococcemia
Ischemia
Thalassemia
Sickle cell anemia
Radiation therapy
Electrical injury
Burn
Frostbite
Iatrogenic (epiphysiodesis)
Disuse
Tumor
Developmental
Blount disease
Madelung deformity
Metabolic
Chronic vitamin A intoxication
Scurvy

lines.[16] Growth lines normally form during the healing process. Normal growth lines parallel the physis, whereas with premature fusion, growth lines are angled toward a bony bar.[16]

Both computed tomography (CT) and MRI have been used to diagnose and map areas of premature fusion. With CT, a limited scan with narrow collimation is obtained through the physis. A standard protocol obtains 1.25-mm images overlapping at 0.625-mm intervals. Sagittal and coronal reformats will show the area of fusion. Small bars may be seen as a sclerotic band across the physis, whereas with larger areas of fusion, continuity of the marrow space across the fusion is seen.[11,16,18] Cartilage-sensitive sequences (proton density with fat saturation, three-dimensional spoiled gradient recalled echo with fat saturation) can be employed on MRI to delineate the physis (Fig. 143-2). Areas of fusion will be seen as defects within the bright signal of the cartilaginous physis.[16,19] These sequences can also be helpful to detect the potential fracture complication of trapped periosteum within the physis.[20] With either CT or MRI, maps can be created showing the degree and site of fusion.

When a child is less than 2 years old or has 2 cm of growth remaining or when the bar involves less than 50% of the physis, resection of the bar can be considered.[11,21] A plug of fatty tissue can be placed in the void.[21] Premature fusion may recur. If greater than 50% of the physis is fused, resection of the bar may be impractical. Depending on the deformity and growth potential of the patient, other orthopedic techniques may be utilized to minimize morbidity from the premature fusion, including osteotomy and contralateral epiphysiodesis (surgical physeal fusion).[11]

Imaging Radiographs are the mainstay of imaging of traumatic injuries to the pediatric skeleton. As a general rule, two orthogonal views are obtained to assess for fracture at non-osteoarticular locations and an additional oblique view at osteoarticular locations. At some locations, normal anatomy limits the value of orthogonal projections (i.e., the pelvis). At other locations, unique projections are helpful for delineation of anatomy (i.e., an axillary view of the shoulder, and a sunrise view of the knee). When imaging a long bone, both the proximal and distal joints must be included.

Contralateral comparison views are not routinely obtained, but frequently aid in differentiating normal developmental variation from pathology.[22] Comparison views are most helpful in areas of complex anatomy such as the elbow. Normal variants are common and may mimic fracture.

At certain sites and with complex patterns of injury, CT is very helpful in diagnosing fractures and delineating the anatomy of fracture planes and resultant deformity. Occasionally, MRI or ultrasonography can be used to diagnose fractures in children; however, these modalities excel in delineating associated soft tissue injury rather than osseous injury. Ultrasonography, however, may be particularly helpful in infants whose epiphyses are not yet ossified. It also can be used to detect lipohemarthrosis as an indirect sign of fracture or to aid in diagnosis of an occult fracture.[23] The cartilaginous epiphysis is well seen with ultrasonography, and its relationship and continuity with an adjacent metaphysis can be readily assessed. With the increasing capabilities of cross-sectional imaging, nuclear scintigraphy is less utilized than in the past. Nonetheless, scintigraphy can be a valuable tool to identify an occult fracture. Bone scans typically become positive 24 to 48 hours after a fracture.

Plastic Fractures

Etiology, Pathophysiology, and Clinical Presentation The composition of bones in a child is different from that of bones in an adult.[24] The most apparent anatomic difference in the pediatric skeleton is the presence of the physis and a thick periosteum.[25] The plasticity of a child's bones allows for substantial deformity prior to fracture (e-Fig. 143-3).[2] Bone may give way and may become permanently deformed prior to a complete break. The result is an "incomplete fracture" or a "plastic fracture."

A *greenstick fracture* occurs when a cortical fracture occurs on the tension side of bone with intact cortex on the loading side of bone. A torus or buckle fracture is a cortical fracture occurring on the loading side of bone with intact cortex on the tension side. A bowing deformity does not have a radiographically identifiable fracture line on either the tension or loading side of bone.

Greenstick fractures most commonly occur in long bones, particularly the radius and ulna.[2] These fractures are most common in the first decade of life, are uncommon in the second decade of life, and are not seen in normally developed and mineralized bones of adults.[2] *Buckle fractures* most commonly affect the distal radius and ulna, tibia, and proximal first metatarsal bone.

Imaging Radiographs are the standard method of evaluation and advanced imaging is usually not indicated. Subtypes of

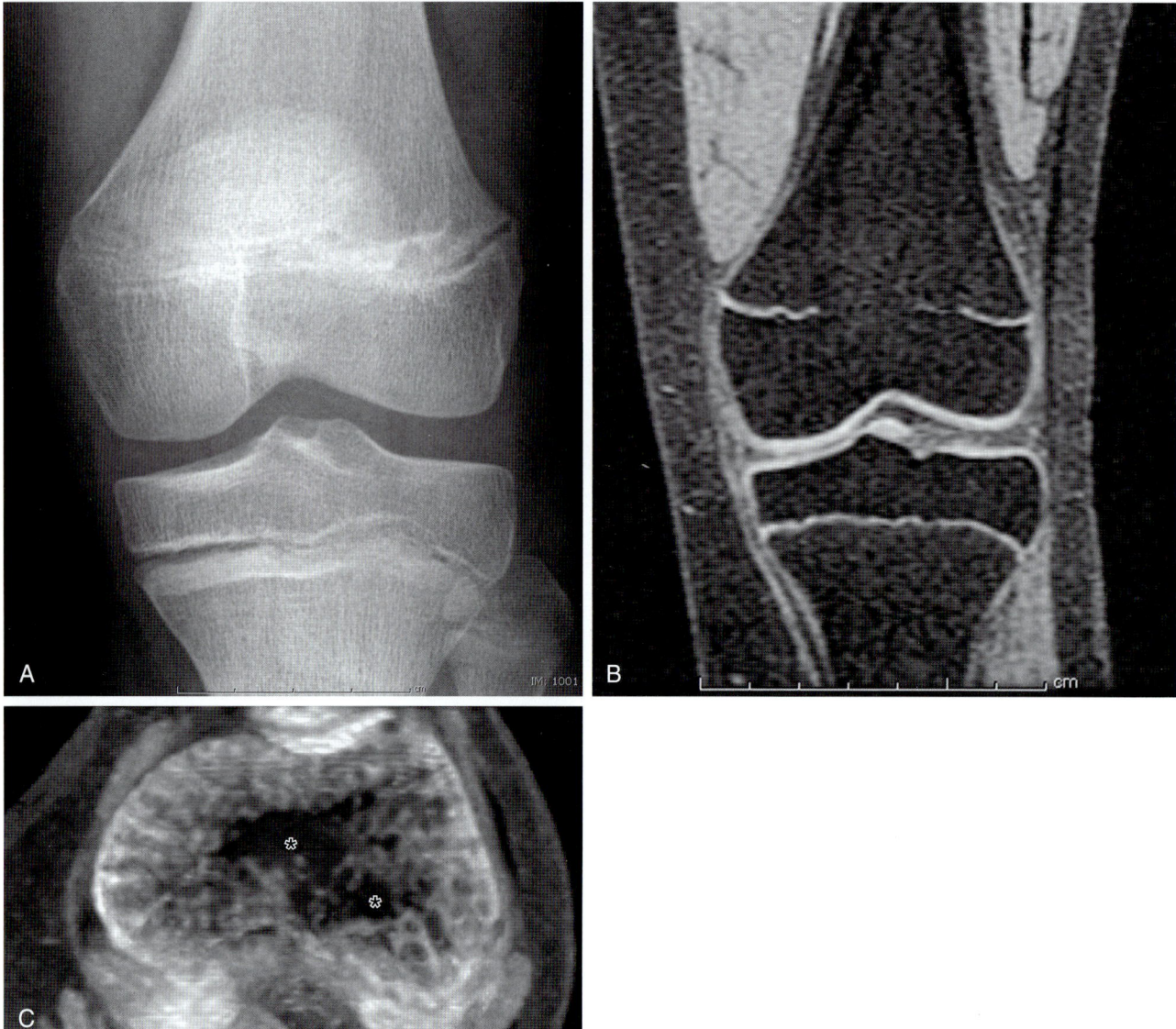

Figure 143-2   Premature growth plate fusion. A, On radiography, the central portion of the distal femoral growth plate is poorly defined; however, the extent of fusion is poorly delineated. **B,** Coronal spoiled gradient recalled echo magnetic resonance image with fat saturation. The central growth plate is fused. **C,** Axial maximum intensity projection image constructed from the stack of coronal spoiled gradient recalled echo with fat saturation images. The area of growth plate fusion is mapped (*asterisks*). (Courtesy of Dr. K. Ecklund, Boston, MA.)

incomplete fractures are buckle or torus fractures (Fig. 143-4), lead pipe fractures (part transverse fracture or part buckle fracture), greenstick fractures (Fig. 143-5), and bowing deformities (e-Fig. 143-6). With incomplete fractures, the periosteum is intact wherever the cortex is intact.[2]

Treatment Cast and splinting is usually performed for pain control since most of these fractures are stable. Plastic fractures usually heal completely and have a good prognosis. Rarely, it may be necessary to operatively "complete" the fracture for reduction of severe angular deformity. Mild angular deformities (<15 degrees) usually do not need to be reduced and will remodel nicely without permanent sequelae.

Physeal (Salter-Harris) Fractures

Etiology, Pathophysiology, and Clinical Presentation For the musculoskeletal unit of the child, the physis and physeal equivalent regions are points of relative weakness and are thus predisposed to mechanical failure leading to fractures.[26] The physis usually fails before ligamentous or tendinous soft tissue structures fail after biomechanical stress. This occurs more frequently during growth spurts, and affects the lower extremities more frequently than the upper extremities. Once the physis fuses, ligamentous and tendon soft tissue injuries become more frequent, as do metadiaphyseal fractures. Fracture patterns in older children are similar to fracture patterns seen in adults.

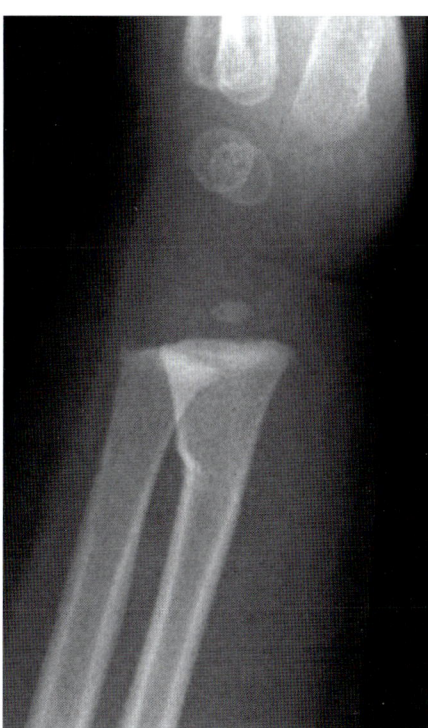

Figure 143-4 Buckle fracture of the distal radius in a 19-month-old boy. The distal radius is slightly angulated posteriorly.

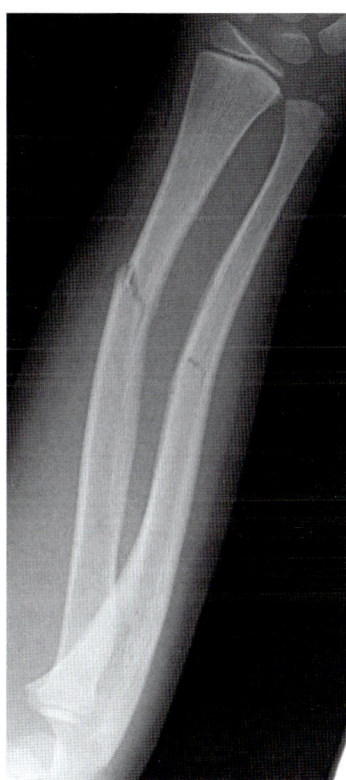

Figure 143-5 Greenstick fractures of the radial and ulnar diaphyses in an 8-year-old boy. The fracture lines only extend through part of the cortex.

Approximately 18% of pediatric fractures involve the physes.[27] Physeal fractures are classified by the system of Salter and Harris (Fig. 143-7). The Salter-Harris classification is a well-accepted classification scheme for describing physeal fractures and therefore facilitates efficient communication between clinicians and radiologists.

Imaging Most physeal fractures are adequately delineated by radiography. Since these fractures are at the ends of bones, potential epiphyseal and intraarticular extent of fracture may be present and therefore, three views are necessary (frontal, lateral, oblique). The Salter-Harris classification of fractures, the degree of diastasis and angulation, if present, loose bodies, and any intraarticular involvement should be considered.

Fractures through the physis may pass solely and directly through the physis (Salter-Harris I; e-Fig. 143-8), involve the physis and a portion of the metaphysis (Salter-Harris II; Fig. 143-9), involve the physis and a portion of the epiphysis (Salter-Harris III; e-Fig. 143-10), or cross the physis in single plane involving both epiphysis and metaphysis (Salter-Harris IV; e-Fig. 143-11). Crush injury of the physis (Salter-Harris V) is rare as an isolated injury to the bone and is rarely, if ever, diagnosed prospectively. Although not in common use, additional fracture types are included in an expanded Salter-Harris classification. A Salter-Harris VI fracture occurs at the perichondral ring at the edge of the physis. A Salter-Harris VII fracture is confined to the epiphyses.[2,26,28]

Many lesser grades of Salter-Harris fractures that proceed to premature physeal fusion probably have a component of Salter-Harris V injury. The Salter-Harris classification serves to assign prognosis. Higher grade Salter-Harris fractures have a higher incidence of premature physeal fusion. Most physeal fractures, however, are either Salter-Harris I (approximately 10%) or Salter-Harris II (approximately 75%). Thus, although premature physeal fusion is more likely to occur with a higher grade Salter-Harris fracture, this complication is probably more commonly the result of a lower grade Salter-Harris fracture.

Fracture planes within the physis pass through the zone of calcified cartilage and adjacent newly formed bone, which represent the point of least resistance to fracture forces. Fracture lines that extend into the epiphysis (Salter-Harris III and IV) cross the zone of proliferating cartilage, which is more susceptible to damage leading to premature physeal fusion. The zone of proliferating cartilage is thought to be damaged by Salter-Harris V fractures. Malalignment of Salter-Harris IV fracture fragments may promote formation of a bridge across the healing fracture from metaphysis to epiphysis.[28]

At certain locations, CT or MRI may be used to confirm or further delineate fractures, especially for defining exact measurements of fracture diastasis and whether involvement of an articular surface exists. Defining exact measurements of fracture diastasis is important especially when an articular cartilage is involved, especially at weightbearing zones (e.g., tibial plafond). On MRI, physeal fractures are diagnosed by widening and increased T2-weighted signal within the fractured portion of the physis, adjacent bone marrow edema, associated metaphyseal (Salter-Harris II) or epiphyseal (Salter-Harris III) fracture lines, and periosteal disruption.[29] The most significant complication of physeal injuries is growth arrest (see Fig. 143-2), which can lead to deformity and limb length discrepancies.[30] A rare complication of physeal fracture

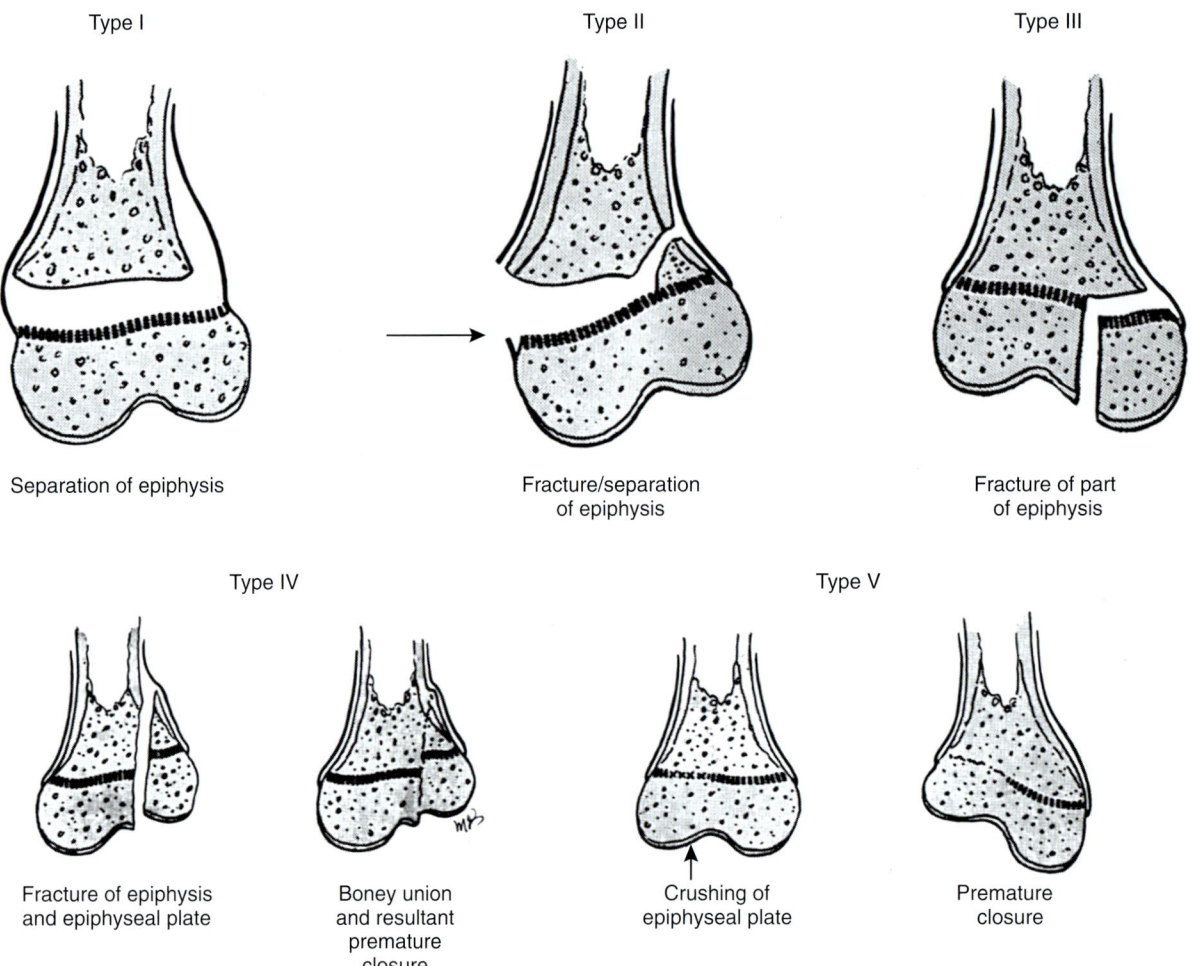

Type I

Separation of epiphysis

Type II

Fracture/separation
of epiphysis

Type III

Fracture of part
of epiphysis

Type IV

Fracture of epiphysis
and epiphyseal plate

Boney union
and resultant
premature
closure

Type V

Crushing of
epiphyseal plate

Premature
closure

Figure 143-7 Injuries to the cartilage plate classified according to Salter and Harris. *Type I,* Complete transverse laceration of the physis with longitudinal distraction and some transverse displacement of the epiphysis. The bone itself is not broken. *Type II,* Incomplete transverse laceration of the physis through a variable distance is associated with an oblique fracture of the contiguous metaphysis with a triangular fragment of metaphysis attached to the displaced epiphysis. The prognosis is good. *Type III,* Short incomplete transverse laceration of the physis with longitudinal fracture extending through the epiphyseal ossification center toward the joint. The prognosis is poor if the epiphyseal fracture is not reduced with smooth joint surfaces. *Type IV,* Oblique longitudinal fracture extending from the articular cartilage through the epiphyseal ossification center, across the physis, and through a short segment of the metaphysis through the cortical wall. This type is most frequently seen at the lateral condyle of the humerus. Perfect reduction is essential for a good prognosis. *Type V,* Segmental crushing of the physis, often followed by closure of the plate prematurely and stoppage of growth. (From Salter RE, Harris WR. Injuries involving the epiphyseal plate. *J Bone Joint Surg Am.* 1963;45:587-622.)

diagnosed by MRI is entrapment of periosteum within the fracture (e-Fig. 143-12). The entrapped periosteum will prevent complete reduction of the fracture. MRI can also be used to evaluate physeal fractures that have a significant risk of complications.[31]

Treatment Salter-Harris I and II fractures are usually treated by closed manipulation followed by casting. Salter-Harris type III and IV fractures usually require open reduction and internal fixation, as often, these types of fractures are displaced and extend to the joint. To prevent posttraumatic osteoarthritis, it is important to create a smooth articular surface; therefore, Salter-Harris fractures with epiphyseal involvement and greater than 2 mm of diastasis or significant angulation usually need the epiphyseal component surgically reduced with orthopedic fixation.

Most (85%) of growth plate injuries heal without complication; however, in a subset of patients angulation and growth arrest may occur, and this depends on the location of the physeal insult.[28,32] Angular deformities tend to occur when the physeal insult is eccentric, and limb shortening without angulation may occur when the physeal insult is central. Sometimes, paradoxic overgrowth may result after a Salter-Harris fracture. This is related to regional trophic effects associated with fracture healing.

Traumatic Injuries of the Humerus

Etiology, Pathophysiology, and Clinical Presentation Injury to the proximal humerus varies with the age of the child. Infants and toddlers are likely to have a Salter-Harris I fracture of the proximal humeral physis. From 5 to 10 years of age, buckle fractures of the proximal humeral metaphysis are most prevalent (e-Fig. 143-13). These fractures may have considerable angulation. In older children, Salter-Harris II fractures predominate (e-Fig. 143-14). Fractures of the humeral diaphysis are also common.[33]

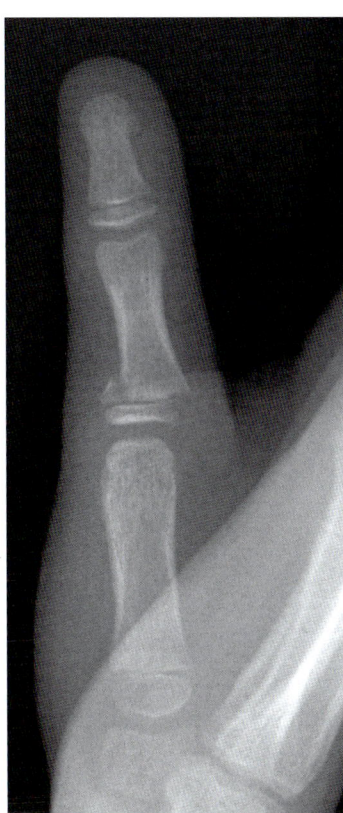

Figure 143-9 Salter-Harris II fracture of the proximal phalanx of the thumb in a 10-year-old boy. The distal fragment is slightly displaced medially.

Glenohumeral dislocation and instability is uncommon in younger children.[34] This is because the physis and metaphysis are less resilient to biomechanical stress compared with the glenohumeral capsule and ligaments. Glenohumeral dislocation is common in older teens and patterns of injury are similar to those in young adults.

The proximal humeral physis can be a site of birth trauma with the middle third of the humerus most commonly fractured.[35] Similar injuries can also be seen with child abuse.

Imaging Anteroposterior and lateral radiographs of the humerus should be obtained to initially evaluate a fracture. If the fracture is near or involves the glenohumeral joint, an additional axillary view is recommended. If a Salter-Harris type I fracture is suspected in the neonate, evaluation with ultrasonography is preferable, as the proximal humeral epiphysis is cartilaginous and therefore better assessed with ultrasonography. For older patients or those with complex proximal humeral fractures, CT or MRI may be useful to evaluate for intraarticular extension and for involvement of the greater and lesser tuberosities.

Radiographically, since the humeral head is usually not ossified or only slightly ossified at birth, fracture through the physis mimics dislocation of the shoulder (e-Fig. 143-15). The humeral metaphysis may appear to align inferior to the glenoid. In the newborn, Salter-Harris I fracture of the proximal humerus is much more common than glenohumeral dislocation.[36] Ultrasound may be used to diagnose the fracture by showing malalignment of the cartilaginous humeral head

with the proximal humeral metaphysis and showing motion at the physis (e-Fig. 143-16).[36,37]

Salter-Harris fractures of the proximal humerus in older children are usually Salter-Harris II fractures, although the metaphyseal fragment is often very small. Occasionally, no metaphyseal fragment exists. Such Salter-Harris I fractures are sometimes called "slipped capital humeral epiphysis." Typically, with a Salter-Harris I or II fracture of the proximal humerus, the epiphyseal fragment rotates medially because of unopposed pull by the rotator cuff.[35] Salter-Harris III and IV fractures of the proximal humerus are extraordinarily rare. Avulsion of the greater tuberosity is a Salter-Harris III fracture. Avulsions of the lesser tuberosity caused by hyperextension with avulsion of the subscapularis tendon are rare and often delayed in diagnosis and are best delineated by an axillary view.[38,39] Chronic avulsive injury of the deltoid insertion site has been reported.[40]

In very young children, fractures of the humeral diaphysis may be incomplete fractures; however, beyond the toddler years, most fractures of the humeral diaphysis are complete fractures. The humerus is one of the more common sites for a pathologic fracture because of its propensity to develop bone cysts.[41] The positioning and alignment of the fragments of a humeral fracture are dependent on the site of fracture and its relationship to the deltoid and pectoral muscular insertions.

Management Treatment is variable. Proximal humeral fractures are usually treated nonsurgically, including those with significant angulation and displacement. Fractures will heal and remodel without long-term orthopedic sequelae. However, some advocate operative management in certain situations.[42,43] Reduction may be necessary in patients near skeletal maturity if the fracture has more than 50 to 70 degrees of angulation in the coronal or sagittal plane.[44] Operative intervention also is indicated in those patients with associated neurovascular injury or who have intraarticular or open fractures.

Traumatic Injuries of the Elbow

OVERVIEW

Fractures of the elbow are one of the most common types of injuries in the pediatric population.[45] The complex articulation of the elbow joint and the immaturity of the pediatric skeleton make this joint particularly susceptible to injury.[46] Frequently, these fractures can be subtle. Familiarity with developmental anatomy of elbow ossification centers and assessment of fat pads and alignment aids in interpreting elbow radiography. Knowledge of common fracture patterns also assists in arriving at a correct diagnosis. Complications, although uncommon, include neurovascular injury, malunion, and compartment syndrome.[47]

OSSIFICATION CENTERS

The normal, orderly progression of the appearance of the ossification of the six major ossifications centers of the elbow (Fig. 143-17) is as follows: capitellum (~1 to 2 years), radial head (~2 to 4 years), medial (internal) epicondyle (~4 to 6 years), trochlea (~9 to 10 years), olecranon (~9 to 11 years), and lateral (external) epicondyle (~9.5 to 11.5 years).[48] This

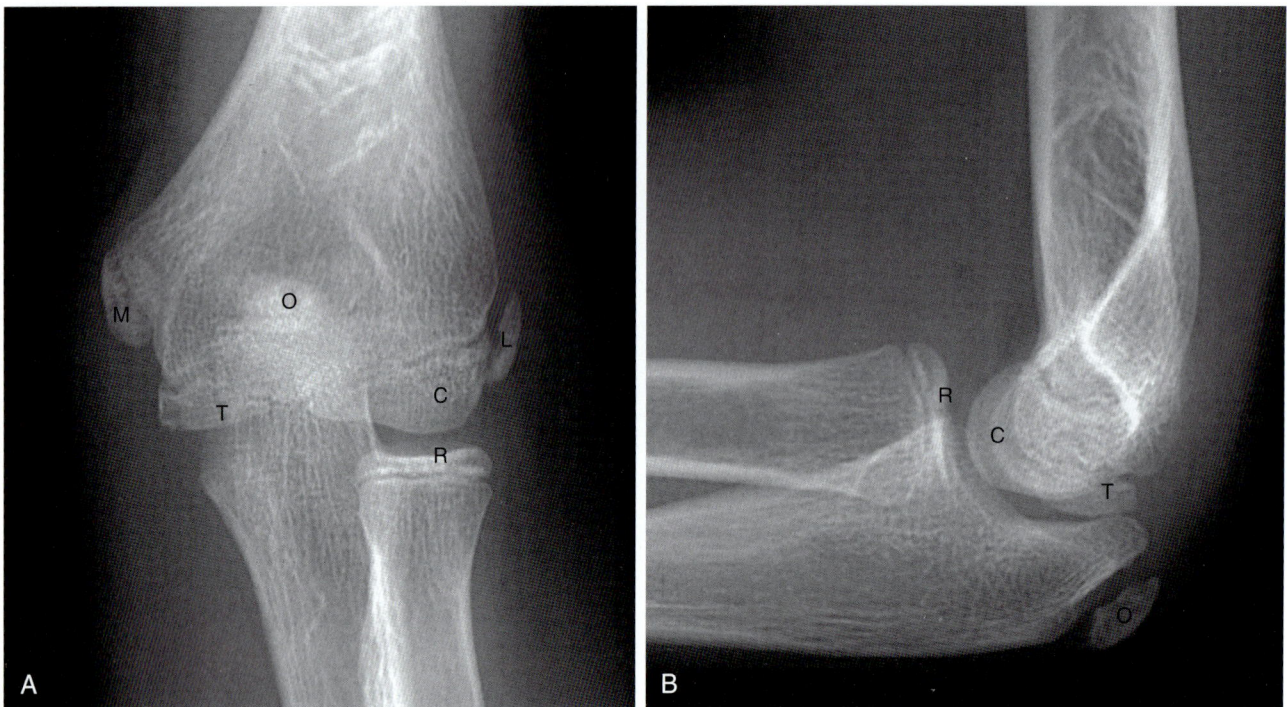

Figure 143-17 Radiographs of a normal elbow in a 14-year-old boy. Anteroposterior (**A**) and lateral (**B**) views. *C*, capitellum; *L*, lateral epicondyle; *M*, medial epicondyle; *O*, olecranon; *R*, radial head; *T*, trochlea.

can be remembered by using the acronyms CRMTOL or CRITOE. With very rare exceptions, the medial epicondyle ossifies prior to the trochlea. If the trochlea is ossified, so should be the medial epicondyle. Fusion of the elbow ossification centers is less orderly, occurring after puberty. Although appearance and fusion of the elbow ossification centers are related to a range in age, they appear and fuse earlier in females compared with males.[49]

JOINT EFFUSION

Acute intraarticular fractures of the elbow will usually have an elbow joint effusion.[50,51] The effusion causes displacement of the anterior and posterior fat pads of the elbow (Fig. 143-18). Although the anterior fat pad is seen normally, it may appear elevated by an effusion ("sail sign") and have an abnormal concave shape inferiorly. The normal anterior fat pad is usually convex in shape or sliverlike. The posterior fat pad normally resides within the olecranon fossa and is not seen on radiographs unless a large joint effusion is present. Ultrasonography may be useful to evaluate for the presence of effusions.[52] Multidetector array computed tomography (MDCT) is a sensitive modality for evaluating radiographically occult fractures with posttraumatic elbow effusions and has a high negative predictive value.[53]

The presence of an elbow joint effusion is strong evidence for the presence of a fracture.[54,55] Usually, the fracture is obvious. In younger children, a subtle buckle or greenstick fracture of the supracondylar distal humerus may occur. In older children, a subtle fracture of the radial head or radial neck may occur. The presence of an effusion is not unequivocal evidence for a fracture.[56] The prevalence of elbow fractures with a joint effusion and no other radiographic findings of a fracture range from 6% to 76%, depending on the

study.[55,57] A normal anterior fat pad is highly associated with absence of a fracture.[58] However, as fractures are often subtle or occult, the presence of an effusion without an identifiable fracture usually prompts splinting of the arm with follow-up radiographs to assess for healing of an occult fracture. Alternatively, MRI has been used by some centers to evaluate for fracture.[59-61] However, MRI may identify some subtle fractures that are probably of little clinical importance.[62]

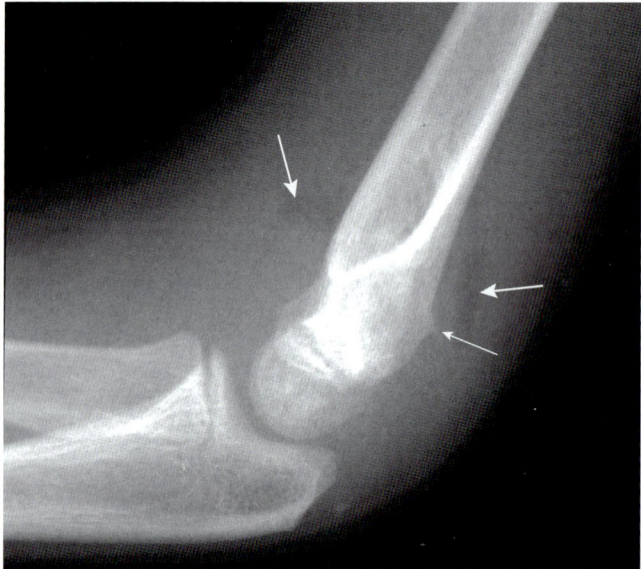

Figure 143-18 Buckle-type supracondylar fracture (*small arrow*) in a 6-year-old boy. The anterior and posterior fat pads (*large arrows*) are displaced by an elbow joint effusion. Note that the anterior humeral cortical line passes along the anterior margin of the capitellum, indicating posterior angulation of the distal fragment.

ALIGNMENT LINES

On a properly positioned lateral view, the anterior humeral cortical line is drawn along the anterior cortex of the humerus. This line should pass through the middle third of the capitellum in the majority of normal elbows; however, in children under 4 years of age, the anterior humeral line passes equally through the anterior or middle third of the capitellum.[63] Disruption of this relationship aids in the detection of supracondylar fractures, which are usually posteriorly angulated and displaced. The radiocapitellar line is drawn along the axis of the radius. Regardless of patient positioning or projection, this line should pass through the capitellum (Fig. 143-19). Disruption of this relationship aids in detection of radiocapitellar dislocation.[64] Other reasons for disruption of this line include lateral condylar, radial neck, and Monteggia fractures.[65]

Supracondylar Fractures

Etiology, Pathophysiology, and Clinical Presentation Supracondylar fractures of the distal humerus account for 60% of pediatric elbow fractures.[66] The usual mechanism of injury is hyperextension with impingement of the olecranon on the posterior distal humerus.[67] Fractures vary widely in severity from a faintly perceptible buckle fracture to a complete fracture with marked displacement and angulation. A significant percentage of patients with a supracondylar fracture will have an ipsilateral forearm fracture.[68]

Imaging Anteroposterior, oblique, and lateral radiographs are required not only for diagnosis but also to guide

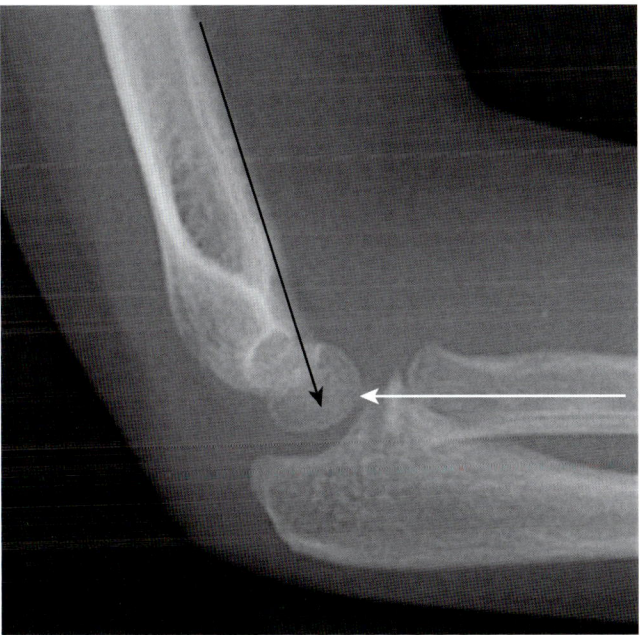

Figure 143-19 *Lateral radiograph of a normal elbow demonstrating normal elbow alignment.* The anterior humeral line is drawn along the anterior cortex of the humerus and should intersect the middle third of the capitellum. The radiocapitellar line is drawn along the axis of the radius. Regardless of patient positioning or projection, this line should pass through the capitellum.

appropriate management.[47] Comparison with the contralateral elbow may be helpful in some instances but is not routinely necessary.[69] The distal fragment of a supracondylar fracture is often displaced or angulated posteriorly. As a result, the anterior humeral cortical line will not bisect the capitellum. In a normal elbow, anterior angulation of the distal humeral condyles causes the anterior humeral cortical line to pass through the center of the capitellar ossification center. If this line passes through the anterior third of the capitellar ossification center or anterior to it, then a supracondylar fracture is likely present.[65] It is important to assess for this finding on a properly positioned lateral view of the distal humerus. Obliquity of the distal humerus may cause the capitellar ossification center to appear falsely posterior relative to the anterior humeral cortical line.[65] Supracondylar fractures invariably involve the distal humeral metaphysis but physeal involvement is unusual.

The modified Gartland classification system of supracondylar fractures is the most commonly used to succinctly describe the fracture and for treatment planning.[70] Type I supracondylar fractures are nondisplaced or minimally displaced less than 2 mm and have an intact anterior humeral line (see Fig. 143-18). Type II fractures are displaced greater than 2 mm with angulation and disruption of the anterior humeral line, but with an intact posterior cortex. Type III fractures are displaced with no cortical continuity (e-Fig. 143-20). Type III fractures are subdivided into posteromedial and posterolateral fractures on the basis of displacement. Most type II and all type III fractures are treated surgically.[67] The risk of developing epiphyseal osteonecrosis of the trochlea should be considered if surgery is delayed.[71] Neurovascular injury may occur with displaced supracondylar fractures.

Underreduced supracondylar fractures may cause clinically significant limitations in elbow flexion.[72] After reduction, supracondylar fractures often demonstrate a mild degree of posterior displacement or angulation. This will not adversely affect functional outcome; however, fusion with loss of normal cubitus valgus will potentially inhibit the range of motion of the elbow. Normally, slight lateral angulation of the radius exists relative to the humerus (cubitus valgus) and is greater in females. The Baumann angle is created by the intersection of the humeral axis with a line tangent to the physis of the lateral condyle (e-Fig. 143-21). The normal angle is approximately 75 degrees. With posttraumatic cubitus varus, the Baumann angle is greater than 83 degrees.[73] Unfortunately, the Baumann angle is somewhat dependent on positioning. Cubitus varus deformity is thought to occur secondary to medial angulation of the distal fracture fragment.[74] Severe deformity of the distal humerus with cubitus varus has been called "gun stock deformity."

Treatment Conservative versus operative management generally depends on the degree of displacement, age of the patient, location of the fracture, stability of the fracture, and associated injuries. A nondisplaced or acceptably displaced fracture will be treated conservatively; an *acceptable displacement* is defined as one that will be corrected by expected growth and thickness of the injured bone.[75] For example, most type I or nondisplaced supracondylar fractures can be treated conservatively in a long arm cast for 3 to 4 weeks with the elbow held in 90 to 110 degrees of flexion. Most type II and III supracondylar fractures are treated operatively with closed reduction and percutaneous pinning.[76,77] Most supracondylar fractures can be electively treated (i.e., next morning for a fracture identified afterhours), including type III fractures. Patients exhibiting neurovascular compromise, however, require immediate treatment.

Lateral Condylar Fractures

Etiology, Pathophysiology, and Clinical Presentation Lateral condylar fractures are the second most common type of fracture of the pediatric elbow, accounting for 12% to 20% of pediatric elbow fractures.[78] The mechanism is hyperextension with varus stress.[66] Lateral condylar fractures are considered Salter-Harris IV fractures until proven otherwise.

Imaging In addition to the standard anteroposterior and lateral radiographs, some advocate obtaining an internal oblique view to better delineate the lateral condylar fracture gap.[79] External oblique views tend to obscure the lateral condylar fracture but are better for delineating the radial head and neck. MDCT may be useful in certain cases to decide between surgical and nonsurgical management.[80] The severity of lateral condylar fractures varies considerably. The fracture may or may not extend through the unossified portion of the distal humeral epiphysis (e-Fig. 143-22). "Stable" lateral condylar fractures (type I) do not traverse the cartilaginous epiphysis and are incomplete and thus nondisplaced or minimally displaced (Fig. 143-23). Type II lateral condylar fractures are complete and thus "unstable" but with little or no displacement. The lateral condylar fracture line may be quite subtle, often paralleling the adjacent metaphyseal margin.

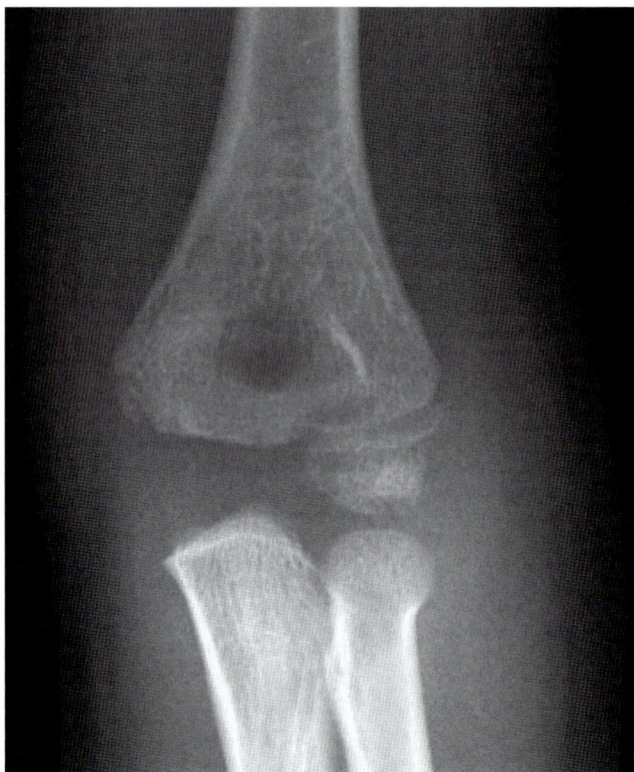

Figure 143-23 Nondisplaced lateral condylar fracture in a 6-year-old boy.

In the past, arthrography (with or without CT) was occasionally used to assess for the epiphyseal fracture line.[81] Both MRI and ultrasonography have proven capable of demonstrating the fracture through epiphyseal cartilage indicating a Salter-Harris IV fracture.[82] With complete or "unstable" fractures, the lateral condylar fragment is displaced and rotated (type III; e-Fig. 143-24).

Treatment Lateral condylar fractures that are nondisplaced (stable) or are displaced 2 mm or less are managed with cast immobilization. Those that are displaced greater than 2 mm (unstable) are treated with surgical fixation with lateral entry pins.[78] A lower threshold exists for surgical intervention of lateral condylar fractures compared with supracondylar fractures because these fractures involve the physis and may have an intraarticular component. Physeal growth arrest and post-traumatic osteoarthritis are more common complications of lateral condylar fractures compared with supracondylar fractures. The most common long-term deformity is relative lateral overgrowth with subsequent cubitus varus.[83]

Medial Epicondyle Avulsion

Etiology, Pathophysiology, and Clinical Presentation The medial epicondyle ossifies by age 7 years and fuses by age 16 years.[84] The medial epicondyle is the origin of the forearm flexor mechanism and ulnar collateral ligaments. Avulsions thus occur within this age range, although rare avulsions of the unossified medial epicondyle have been reported.[85] The two chief mechanisms of acute avulsion fracture of the medial epicondyle are (1) throwing injury and (2) elbow dislocation.[84,86] Acute avulsion of the medial epicondyle is but one of several injuries that can occur in the elbow of a skeletally immature throwing athlete.[87] The avulsion occurs because of hyperextension, with valgus stress producing traction on the apophysis by the flexor tendons and pronators. In the setting of an acute avulsion, the child will experience sudden-onset medial elbow pain while throwing and have point tenderness over the medial epicondyle.[87] Rarely, the medial epicondyle may displace into the joint mimicking a trochlear ossification center. This occurs because the valgus stress of throwing temporarily widens the joint.

Imaging Initial assessment should include anteroposterior, oblique, and lateral radiographs of the elbow (Fig. 143-25). With elbow dislocation in the skeletally immature patient, the medial epicondyle is often avulsed from its normal location. When assessing the images of a dislocated elbow, the status of the medial epicondyle should be specifically addressed (e-Fig. 143-26). In addition, radiographs should address the type of avulsion fracture when present at the level of the medial epicondyle chondro-osseous junction, physeal equivalent, or at the juxtaphyseal metaphyseal equivalent region with displaced and fragmented bone.

Some cases of medial epicondyle avulsion fracture occur with a transient, unrecognized dislocation. When an elbow dislocation is reduced, the medial epicondyle may be trapped in the elbow joint (Fig. 143-27). A trapped medial epicondyle may superficially mimic a trochlear ossification center in the first decade of life. However, absence of the medial epicondyle at its normal location should prompt a search for it

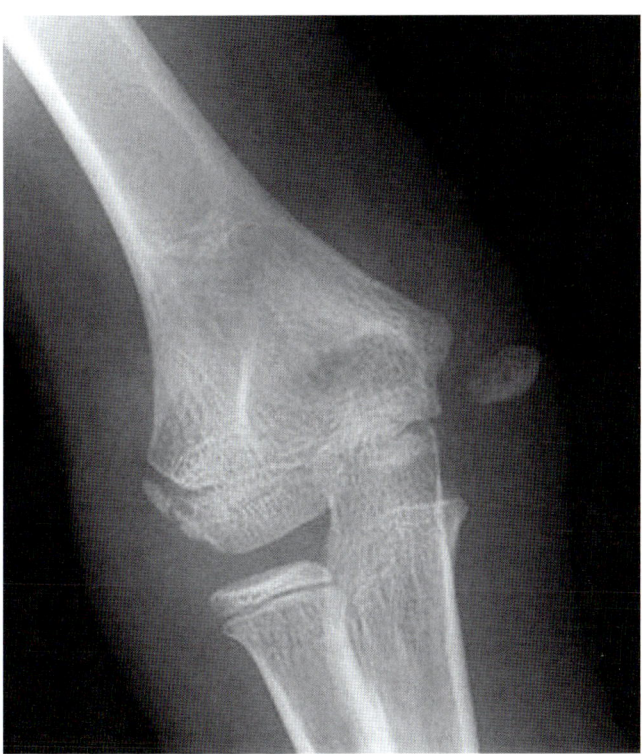

Figure 143-25 Avulsed medial epicondyle in an adolescent boy.

the medial epicondyle physeal equivalent region; however, they are usually not necessary. MRI and CT will often demonstrate associated findings such as injury to the ulnar collateral ligament and the sublime tubercle of the ulna, as well as compression-type injuries in the lateral compartment, such as radiocapitellar osteochondral injuries and bone contusions. However, these additional findings often will not change clinical management.[88,89] MRI and CT are useful when radiographs do not demonstrate a clear fracture and an alternative etiology for the child's symptoms are sought. Avulsion of the medial epicondyle prior to its ossification is distinctly rare but has been reported. Ultrasonography as well as CT or MRI can be used for fracture delineation.[90]

Treatment Both surgical and nonsurgical management has been supported in the literature.[65] Indication for operative treatment include entrapment of the medial epicondyle in the joint and the uncommon occurrence of an open fracture.[65] Medial epicondyle avulsion fractures can be treated conservatively if the avulsed fragment is not intraarticular, if the child is less than 5 years of age or the degree of displacement is less than 4 mm. Generally, the need for intervention increases with the age of the child, degree of dislocation, and athletic activity.[91]

within the joint. If the trochlea is ossified, the medial epicondyle should be as well. Visualization of the trochlea without the medial epicondyle may be caused by displacement of the medial epicondyle or by a displaced medial epicondyle being mistaken for the trochlea.

Comparison views may be helpful in confirming mildly displaced medial epicondylar avulsion injuries at the level of

Medial Condylar Fractures

Etiology, Pathophysiology, and Clinical Presentation Medial condylar fracture, not to be confused with medial epicondylar avulsion (see above), has an appearance similar to the more common lateral condylar fracture. Medial condylar fractures are uncommon and account for 1% to 2% of pediatric elbow fractures.[66] These are typically Salter-Harris type IV fractures.

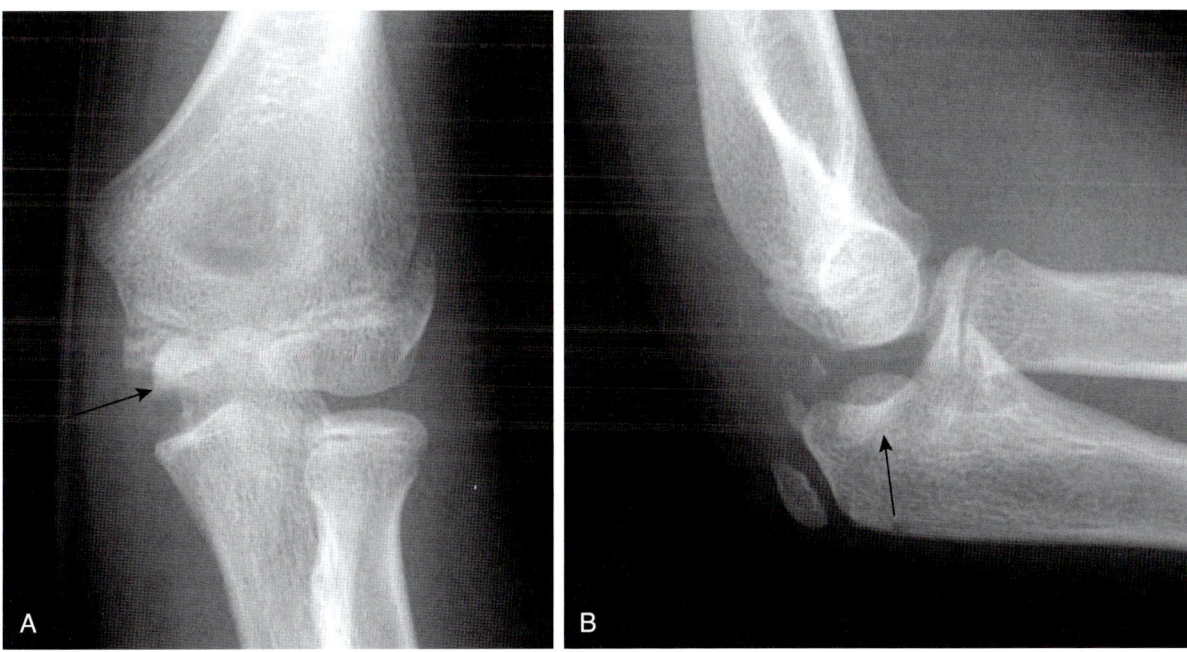

Figure 143-27 Anteroposterior (A) and lateral (B) radiographs after reduction of a dislocated elbow in a 10-year-old girl. The avulsed medial epicondyle (*arrows*) is trapped in the elbow joint.

Imaging   Initial assessment should include anteroposterior, external oblique, and lateral radiographs of the elbow. The fracture line extends through the medial metaphysis separating the metaphysis and medial epicondyle from the remainder of the humerus; the fracture line extends to the trochlear articular surface. MRI can also be useful to evaluate these fractures particularly in young children in whom the diagnosis can be difficult.[92]

Treatment   Most minimally displaced fractures can be treated conservatively with immobilization. Surgical treatment is usually performed if displacement at the fracture site is greater than 2 mm.[92]

Distal Humeral Salter-Harris I Fracture (Transcondylar)

Etiology, Pathophysiology, and Clinical Presentation   Distal humeral Salter-Harris I fracture is an uncommon fracture that occurs from birth to approximately age 7 years, peaking at age 2.5 years. It is typically an injury of infants and young toddlers and is caused by child abuse in half of the cases, or by a rare birth injury.[66,93]

Imaging   Radiographically, the fracture may be mistaken for a dislocation of the elbow, as the bones do not appear to align. The radial axis will be normally aligned with the capitellum, but the capitellum itself will be abnormally related to the distal humeral metaphysis (e-Figs. 143-28 through 143-30). The radius, ulna and humeral epiphysis will be medially displaced. Fractures may occur prior to capitellar ossification.[94]

Treatment   Nondisplaced fractures will be treated with splinting or percutaneous pinning. Displaced fractures usually are treated with open reduction and internal fixation.

Radial Head and Neck Fractures

Etiology, Pathophysiology, and Clinical Presentation   Fractures of the radial head and neck account for 5% of pediatric elbow fractures.[66] Mechanism of injury is falling on an outstretched hand. Fractures in children often occur at or just distal to the physis; this is unlike the adult population where fractures typically involve the radial head.[66] Associated injuries include fracture of the olecranon, avulsion of the medial epicondyle, or medial collateral ligament injury.[66]

Imaging   Radiographs are usually sufficient for diagnosis and follow-up. External oblique views best delineate the radial head and neck morphology, whereas internal oblique views are better for delineating the lateral condylar region. Radial neck fractures are usually buckle fractures followed by Salter-Harris fractures. Isolated radial neck fractures as well as fractures with extension to the radial head are unusual. The radiocapitellar joint is often preserved even when radial neck fractures are displaced and angulated (e-Fig. 143-31).

Treatment   Most pediatric radial head and neck fractures can be treated nonoperatively with closed reduction and immobilization. If there is greater than 30 degrees of residual angulation, greater than 3 to 4 mm of displacement at the fracture site or less than 45 degrees of pronation or supination, then operative intervention is suggested.[95]

Olecranon Fractures

Etiology, Pathophysiology, and Clinical Presentation   Olecranon fractures are relatively uncommon accounting for approximately 4% to 6% of elbow fractures in children.[66] Common mechanisms include falling on an outstretched hand, twisting injury, or direct trauma.[66] The olecranon is the insertion site of the triceps muscle and prone to avulsion fractures. Although most are nondisplaced, olecranon fractures commonly have associated injuries, including radial neck fractures, medial epicondylar fractures, coronoid fractures, and osteochondral injuries.[66]

Imaging   Radiography is usually sufficient for defining olecranon fractures. Fractures should describe the degree of displacement, if any, intraarticular involvement, involvement of the olecranon physeal equivalent zone, and distinguish any additional fractures from normal olecranon ossification centers. Olecranon fractures may be transverse, oblique, or longitudinal. Buckle, bowing, or greenstick fractures are common in younger patients.

CT or MRI is reserved for those olecranon fractures that may have additional injuries elsewhere, to define the degree of intraarticular involvement of the fracture, or to search for loose bodies.

The olecranon physis and apophyseal ossification centers vary considerably in size, location, and degree of fragmentation.[96] The juxtaphyseal fragmentary appearance of the olecranon ossification center may be mistaken for fracture, and vice versa. Comparison views are helpful. Olecranon ossifications are well corticated and appear oval or round. Olecranon fractures have a thin, sliverlike appearance, are usually not corticated, and are located near and parallel the olecranon metaphyseal equivalent zone (e-Fig. 143-32). Other olecranon injuries include stress fractures and sleeve fractures. An olecranon sleeve fracture is an avulsion of the triceps tendon from the olecranon process (e-Fig. 143-33). Stress fractures of the olecranon physis occur in adolescent baseball pitchers.[97] Nondisplaced stress fractures of the olecranon most commonly occur in adolescence and may only be visible on CT or MRI scans.

Treatment   Nondisplaced or minimally displaced fractures are treated conservatively with immobilization and splinting.[96] Displaced fractures are treated with tension wiring across the apophysis rather than screw fixation.[95]

Nursemaid's Elbow

Etiology, Pathophysiology, and Clinical Presentation   *Nursemaid's elbow* occurs due to an upward pull on an extended elbow in pronation. The annular ligament of the proximal radius is disrupted or displaced, allowing the radial head to sublux or dislocate anteriorly relative to the capitellum.

(e-Fig. 143-34).[98] This injury most commonly occurs in the toddler years, up to age 5 years.[99]

Imaging An astute pediatrician will make the diagnosis clinically and reduce the radius without imaging. Often, when imaging is requested, the dislocation is reduced in the course of properly positioning the hand in supination for the anteroposterior view of the elbow. Ultrasonography may also play a role in detecting dislocation of the radial head with respect to the annular ligament.[100] The utility of radiography is not to make the diagnosis of nursemaid's elbow, but to exclude an underlying fracture. After nursemaid's elbow is successfully reduced, the only radiographic sequelae may be a joint effusion without underlying fracture.

When radiographs demonstrate a persistent anterior dislocation despite attempts at reduction, a congenital radial head dislocation should be considered, which has characteristic findings including a convex radial head, small capitellum, and concave shaped posterior margin of the olecranon (e-Fig. 143-35).

MRI may be indicated when radiographs show persistent radial head dislocation despite attempted reduction to look for intrinsic obstacles to reduction such as an entrapped annular ligament.

Treatment Supinating the child's forearm with the elbow in flexion will usually reduce the dislocation. Often, the dislocation is reduced at the time of imaging as described above. A small percentage of children may have recurrent dislocations, with a higher risk the younger the first dislocation occurs.

Traumatic Injuries of the Forearm

Etiology, Pathophysiology, and Clinical Presentation Fractures of the distal radius and ulna are very common. The distal radius is the most common site of buckle fractures in children and usually occurs after a fall on an outstretched arm. Salter-Harris fractures of the distal radius and transverse fractures of the distal radial metaphysis are also very common.[101] Physeal fractures of the distal radius are usually Salter-Harris II fractures. Stress injury to the distal radial physis is frequently seen in gymnasts. Fractures of the radial and ulnar shafts usually occur together. Often, the fracture in one bone is complete, whereas the other bone has an incomplete fracture.

Forearm fractures may also be associated with dislocations. *Monteggia injury* is defined as a fracture of the proximal third of the ulna with dislocation of the radiocapitellar joint.

Galeazzi injury is a fracture of the distal radial shaft with a dislocation of the distal radioulnar joint. These injuries seem to be rarely diagnosed in children, as distal radioulnar joint disruption is uncommon, perhaps because of underrecognition. The distal ulna is most commonly subluxed or dislocated in the direction opposite that of distal radial displacement.

Imaging At least anteroposterior and lateral radiographs of the injured extremity should be obtained. Dedicated osteoarticular radiographic imaging should be performed of the elbow in the presence of a Monteggia fracture, and dedicated osteoarticular radiographic imaging of the wrist should be performed for Galeazzi fractures. CT is usually reserved for injuries that are complex and are accompanied by an associated injury of an osteoarticular joint or for defining the articular surface displacement, which is necessary for surgical planning.

In radial buckle fractures, the cortex tends to buckle dorsally. A fracture line may be present volarly. Distal radial buckle fractures may be extremely subtle and are commonly missed by inexperienced readers. It is important to look at all views for a subtle disruption of the normal smooth flared curve of the metaphyseal margin. Any extra angulation or "bump" is likely a fracture. An associated distal ulnar fracture may or may not be present. With a subtle distal radial fracture, the accompanying distal ulnar buckle fracture may be even more occult, often not identified until signs of healing are seen on follow-up radiographs. Distal radial buckle fractures may also be associated with triangular fibrocartilage injuries and fractures of the ulnar styloid process. Associated carpal injuries are uncommon.[102]

As with buckle fractures, Salter-Harris fractures of the distal radius and transverse fractures of the distal radial metaphysis often occur from falling on an outstretched arm. The distal fragment is usually dorsally displaced or angulated, or both.

Several subtypes of Monteggia fractures are determined on the basis of the anatomy of the ulnar fracture and the direction of radial head dislocation.[103-105] The most common direction of radial head dislocation is anterior with respect to the capitellum (Fig. 143-36). The ulnar fracture may be complete or incomplete.

Treatment Buckle fractures, including those with mild angulation, are usually treated with a splint. Nondisplaced,

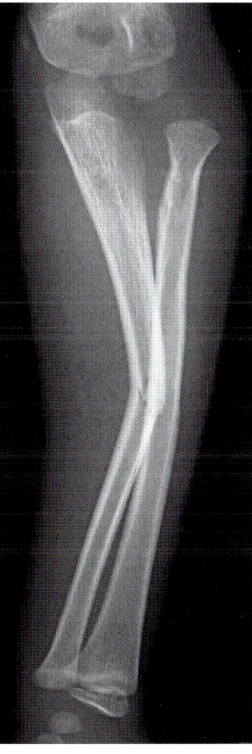

Figure 143-36 Monteggia fracture-dislocation in a 6-year-old boy. A greenstick fracture of the ulna is present with medial angulation of the distal ulna. The radial head is anteriorly dislocated.

complete, nonphyseal fractures are casted. Fractures that involve the distal radial physis usually require closed reduction if displaced. The amount of accepted displacement depends on the type and location of the fracture, age of the child, and direction of angular deformity. In children older than age 10 years, fractures involving the proximal one third of the radius and those with angulation appear to be at higher risk for failure when treated nonoperatively.[106] Surgical reduction is performed with pin fixation across the fracture. With Monteggia fractures, it is the nature of the ulnar fracture rather than the direction of radial head dislocation that is useful in determining optimal treatment for these injuries. Stable anatomic reduction of the ulnar fractures results in stable anatomic reduction of the radial head.[107] Nonsurgical management of Galeazzi fractures with anatomic reduction and immobilization in a long-arm cast has been successful in children.[108]

Traumatic Injuries of the Wrist

Etiology, Pathophysiology, and Clinical Presentation Carpal bone fractures and intercarpal ligament injuries usually occur during the second decade, when children are near skeletal maturity, and follow an adult pattern of injury. Carpal fractures in the first decade are exceedingly rare because of two reasons: (1) the carpal bones have significant epiphyseal equivalent cartilage cushioning the primary carpal ossification centers from injury; and (2) the point of maximal weakness of the forearm and wrist is at the level of the radial and ulnar physis, leading to Salter-Harris fractures, as well as the level of metadiaphyseal cortex where buckle fractures occur. Therefore, in the first decade, Salter-Harris fractures and buckle fractures are far more common compared with carpal bone fractures and ligamentous injuries.

The scaphoid is the most frequently fractured carpal bone. Scaphoid fractures most commonly are transverse and extend through the scaphoid waist. Fractures of the triquetrum are the next most reported carpal bone fracture, followed by the trapezium.[2]

Imaging Scaphoid views with ulnar deviation will better profile the scaphoid and can be added as a supplement to the standard three view wrist series. CT or MRI (e-Fig. 143-37) can be used to confirm the diagnosis and assess for alternative etiologies for wrist pain.[109] Alternatively, if clinical suspicion persists because of mechanism or physical examination findings (snuffbox tenderness), then splints may be applied, with follow-up radiographs obtained after 10 to 14 days to reassess for fracture.

The scaphoid artery enters from the distal pole and extends proximally to supply the proximal pole. As a result, proximal pole osteonecrosis may occur after midpole scaphoid fractures. Osteonecrosis is less frequent in the pediatric population compared with the adult population.[2] The affected proximal pole of the scaphoid will appear dense relative to the other bones of the wrist (Fig. 143-38). Nonunion of the scaphoid can occur with or without epiphyseal osteonecrosis. The incidence of nonunion is increased with delay in diagnosis, although it is generally uncommon.[110,111]

Fractures of the triquetrum (Fig. 143-39) are seen as a small bony fragment projecting dorsally. Fractures of the hook of the hamate may occur in athletes. Carpal dislocations are rare in children. As in adults, these dislocations may involve a fracture of the scaphoid. Carpal instability rarely manifests in childhood.[110]

Treatment Scaphoid fractures usually heal with closed treatment and immobilization. Displaced fractures may require either open or closed reduction with internal fixation to minimize the risk of nonunion.[110] Triquetral fractures are usually treated nonoperatively.

Traumatic Injuries of the Hands

Etiology, Pathophysiology, and Clinical Presentation Fractures of the hand are common in children. The incidence peak is bimodal, the first peak being at age 1 to 2 years and the second at age 12 years. At age 1 to 2 years, the most common hand injury is a distal phalanx fracture with soft tissue

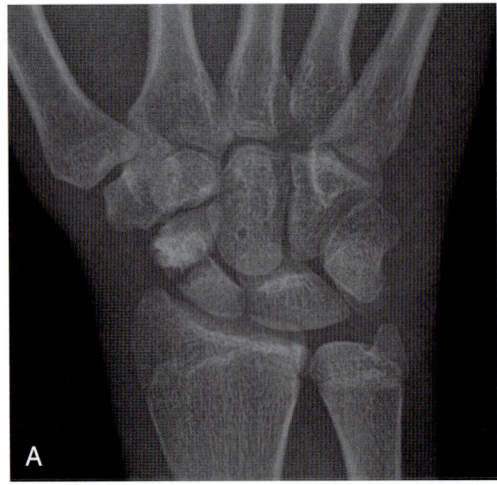 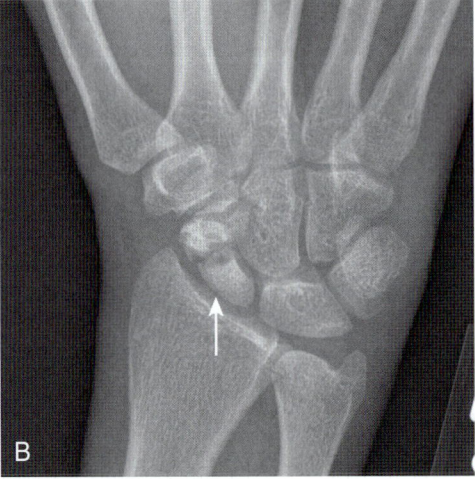

Figure 143-38 A 16-year-old boy with scaphoid waist fracture. **A,** Radiograph at presentation demonstrates a mildly displaced scaphoid waist fracture. **B,** Repeat radiograph 6 months later shows no appreciable callus formation at the fracture site, and subtle increased proximal pole radiodensity (*arrow*) without collapse, suggestive of early osteonecrosis.

The most common metacarpal fracture in adolescents is that of the fifth metacarpal ("boxer's fracture") in adolescents.[112] The fracture plane is transverse or oblique through the metaphysis at the distal aspect of the fifth metacarpal. The distal fragment is angulated toward the palm (e-Fig. 143-44).

Salter-Harris III fractures of the first metacarpal bone are analogous to a Bennett fracture occurring after skeletal maturity (e-Fig. 143-45). A Bennett fracture is an intraarticular fracture at the base of the first metacarpal with first carpometacarpal subluxation. A Rolando fracture is a comminuted version of the Bennett fracture. These injuries are rare in children.

"Gamekeeper's thumb" (e-Fig. 143-46) is a traumatic avulsion fracture at the proximal phalangeal insertion of the ulnar collateral ligament. Historically described in Scottish gamekeepers, this injury most commonly occurs in children from ski pole injury or breakdancing.[114] An avulsion may be seen at the ulnar volar base of the proximal phalanx of the thumb, or a Salter-Harris III fracture if the physis is not yet fused. Radial subluxation of the proximal phalanx may be evident, but stress views may be required to show instability in the absence of fracture. Ulnar collateral ligament avulsion may also cause a Stener lesion with the adductor aponeurosis interposed between the torn ulnar collateral ligament and its insertion, preventing approximation.

Treatment   Nearly all metacarpal and phalangeal fractures are treated nonsurgically with 3 to 4 weeks of immobilization.[2] Surgical pinning is required for intraarticular fractures, particularly those involving the interphalangeal and metacarpophalangeal joints.

Fractures should probably not be immobilized greater than 6 weeks in children unless a significant delay occurs in healing or if a change in treatment is required (i.e., open reduction internal fixation).[2] Nondisplaced avulsion fractures are typically treated by brace taping, or buddy taping, the injured digit to its neighbor. Stener lesions are managed operatively.[113]

Traumatic Injuries of the Pelvis and Hip

PELVIC FRACTURES

Overview   Pelvic fractures are not common in children.[115] Pedestrian–motor vehicle collisions account for the majority of cases, followed by falls, and the majority of victims are boys.[115,116] The presence of a pelvic injury in a child is a marker of severe injury and should alert the clinician to search for additional injury.[116,117] Apophyseal avulsion injuries of the pelvis are covered in Chapter 145.

Etiology, Pathophysiology, and Clinical Presentation   Once a patient has reached skeletal maturity, pelvic ring fracture patterns follow the adult fracture pattern and classification.[118] Several classifications schemes have been applied to pediatric pelvic fractures. In the classification scheme of Torode and Zieg (e-Fig. 143-47), type I fractures are avulsions, type II are iliac wing fractures, type III are simple ring fractures

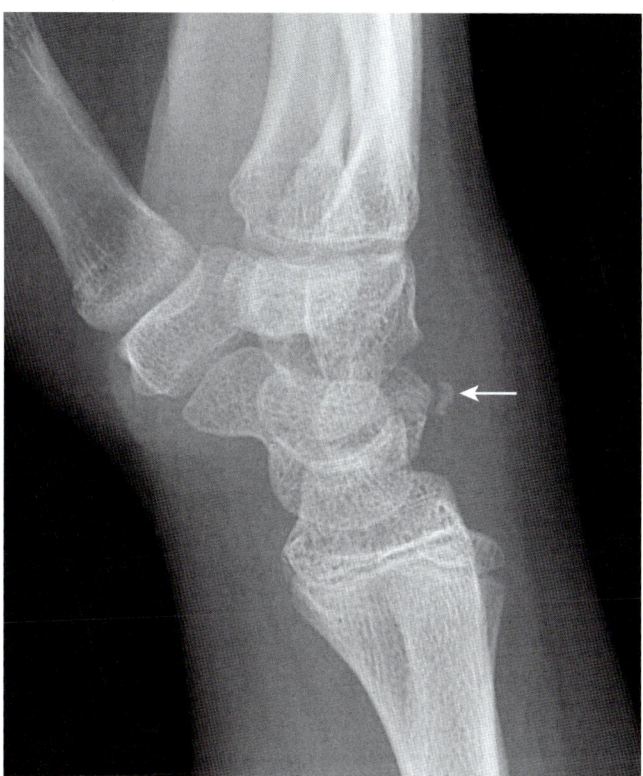

Figure 143-39   An 11-year-old girl with minimally displaced triquetral fracture seen on lateral view (*arrow*).

laceration. At age 12 years, the most common hand injury is fracture of the proximal phalanx of the little finger, followed by metacarpal fractures.[112] In general, phalangeal fractures and interphalangeal dislocations are relatively common injuries. Fractures of the hand often involve the physis[113] and Salter-Harris fractures are common. Growth disturbances in this region are relatively uncommon.[2]

Imaging   Radiography with at least anteroposterior, oblique, and lateral views should be obtained tailored to the specific injured digit rather than imaging the entirety of the hand. Advanced cross-sectional imaging is rarely necessary.

Avulsion injuries usually occur from hyperextension, hyperflexion, or "jamming" of the finger into an object. "Mallet finger" is the result of forced flexion of a distal interphalangeal joint leading to Salter-Harris III fracture–avulsion of the dorsal aspect of the terminal phalanx (e-Fig. 143-40).[113] Volar plate Salter-Harris III avulsion fractures occur along the volar side and may occur at either the terminal phalanx or middle phalanx insertion of the flexor digitorum tendons (e-Fig. 143-41). Salter-Harris type fractures may also be related to terminal phalangeal crush injuries (e-Fig. 143-42).

Salter-Harris II fractures are common and frequently involve the proximal phalanx of the thumb.[113] Displacement is variable. The fractures may be very subtle with minimal physeal widening or a tiny metaphyseal fragment (e-Fig. 143-43). It may be difficult to distinguish between a Salter-Harris II fracture of the proximal phalanx and a bifid epiphysis, an uncommon normal variant. Salter-Harris I and III fractures occur occasionally.

with no clinical instability, and type IV are pelvic ring disruptions with instability. Type IV fractures include straddle injuries with bilateral pubic rami fractures and Malgaigne fractures with anterior and posterior disruption on the same side.[119] Disruption of the sacroiliac joints or pubic symphysis may accompany pelvic fractures. Plastic or incomplete fractures may be seen in children. Usually, if a break in the obturator ring or pelvic ring is present, another break is also present. Younger children, however, may not follow this rule because of the plasticity of their bones.[120,121]

Fractures involving the acetabulum of young children are fortunately rare. Acetabular fractures become more common in the later teen years because of motor vehicle accidents.[120] Fractures of the acetabulum in older children follow patterns similar to those in adults. Most occur in association with hip dislocations.[121]

Imaging CT is the preferred modality for delineation of unstable pelvic fractures. Although most fractures are seen on radiography, CT better delineates the full extent of fracture.[122] The utility of radiographs for screening for pelvic fractures has been questioned.[123,124] Radiography probably is not necessary if CT will be performed to evaluate for other injuries.[123]

Asymmetric widening of the triradiate cartilage may be noted in acetabular fractures (e-Figs. 143-48 and 143-49). CT is used for delineation of fracture anatomy. In younger children, fractures involving the triradiate cartilage are prone to complications, particularly when displaced fragments are present. Premature fusion of the triradiate cartilage may lead to a shallow acetabulum and progressive hip instability.[120] This complication is more common in children under age 10 years at the time of fracture.

Treatment The majority of pelvic fractures can be treated nonsurgically in children.[116,125,126] Surgical intervention is most often needed for those children who require it for other injuries.[118] However, in unstable or fracture-dislocations, open reduction and stabilization should be performed.[125]

HIP DISLOCATION

Overview Traumatic hip dislocations are more common in adolescence, and the hip usually dislocates posteriorly. Unlike adult patients, these fractures are uncommonly associated with acetabular fractures.[121]

Etiology, Pathophysiology, and Clinical Presentation In adolescents, hip dislocation is usually the sequela of significant trauma such as that sustained in motor vehicle accidents, whereas younger children may dislocate their hips with relatively minor trauma, usually falls.[127] Fractures of the acetabulum and femoral head can occur at the same time. In children who suffer dislocations with minimal trauma, ligamentous laxity should be considered as a possible underlying condition such as that seen with Ehlers-Danlos syndrome, Larsen syndrome, and Down syndrome.

Imaging As with most skeletal trauma, initial imaging evaluation should be radiographs (Fig. 143-50). If asymmetry of the hip joint persists after reduction, then further evaluation with either CT or MRI (e-Fig. 143-51) should be considered

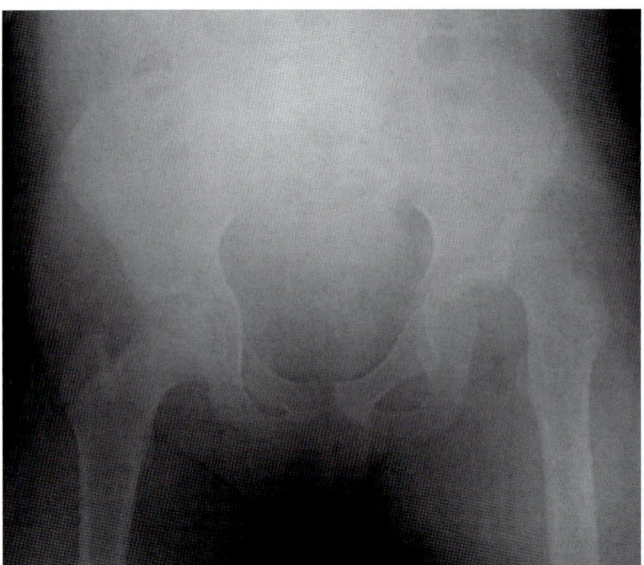

Figure 143-50 A single anteroposterior radiograph of the pelvis in a 9-year-old girl demonstrates superolateral position of the left femoral head compatible with a posterior hip dislocation.

to evaluate for labral entrapment or interposed osteochondral fragments. Most hip dislocations are posterior related to dashboard impact in motor vehicle accidents. With a fracture of the acetabular wall or femoral head, cross-sectional imaging should also be obtained, as it could lead to alterations in patient management. Some have advocated performing a bone scan or MRI 2 weeks after reduction to look for abnormal uptake or signal in an attempt to predict epiphyseal osteonecrosis.[128,129]

Treatment Most hip dislocations in children are reducible with gentle manipulation; however, closed reduction of the hip in the adolescent population carries a risk of epiphyseal osteonecrosis. Open reduction is necessary when closed reduction fails or when interposition of soft tissue or bone exists. Additional complications of hip dislocations include premature osteoarthritis and sciatic nerve injury. If the delay in reduction is greater than 6 hours, the risk of osteonecrosis is significantly increased.[130,131]

SLIPPED CAPITAL FEMORAL EPIPHYSIS

Etiology, Pathophysiology, and Clinical Presentation Slipped capital femoral epiphysis (SCFE) is the most common hip disorder affecting the adolescent population.[132] The physis is the weakest component of the proximal femur, and therefore, SCFE injuries are more common than isolated femoral neck fractures. SCFE is essentially a Salter-Harris I fracture of the proximal femoral physis. SCFE occurs more frequently in boys than in girls, tends to occur earlier in age in girls compared with boys, and occurs more commonly in African Americans. SCFE is usually idiopathic with a higher incidence in children who are clinically obese.[132,133] Risk factors for SCFE include hypothyroidism, pituitary dysfunction, hypogonadism, and renal osteodystrophy.[134,135] Hips within a radiation treatment field are at increased risk. When a child presents with bilateral symmetric SCFE or outside of the typical age range, an underlying disorder should be suspected.[136]

Approximately 25% of patients will have bilateral SCFEs, but the reported prevalence of bilateral SCFEs ranges from 20% to 80%.[134,135] Approximately half of patients with bilateral SCFE present synchronously. Risk for contralateral SCFE is greatest in the first 2 years after initial diagnosis of SCFE.[134]

Children with SCFE usually present with hip, groin, or thigh pain. Symptoms may first occur after minor trauma. Up to one quarter of patients present with referred knee pain.[136] Hip radiographs are therefore recommended in the adolescent with unexplained knee pain.

By definition, children with "acute" SCFE have had symptoms for less than 3 weeks and children with "chronic" SCFE (approximately 85% of cases) have had symptoms for greater than 3 weeks.[137-139] Acute or subacute persistent hip pain in an adolescent should immediately raise suspicion for SCFE.

SCFE patients presenting with hip pain with an inability to walk are considered to have an unstable SCFE.[140] SCFE patients who are able to walk are considered to have stable SCFE. This is an important clinical differentiation, since it affects timing of surgical intervention and prognosis.

Imaging Radiography for suspected SCFE should include a pelvic anteroposterior and "frogleg" lateral view. Both hips should be included. Epiphyseal slips may occur in the medial direction, posterior direction, or both. The frogleg lateral view is helpful, since most epiphyseal slips occur in the posterior direction, which can be subtle on the anteroposterior view (Fig. 143-52). The anteroposterior view best assesses the degree of medial displacement, which is often subtle. Klein's line is drawn parallel to the lateral margin of the femoral neck on the anteroposterior view. Normally, a small portion of the femoral head extends lateral to Klein's line. When the femoral head does not extend lateral to Klein's line, medial displacement should be suspected (see Fig. 143-52).[141] Theoretically, Klein's line can potentially be preserved if the SCFE is directly posterior without a medial component. The smaller the capital femoral epiphysis appears on the anteroposterior view, the greater is the degree of posterior slip.

With chronic slips, sclerosis may be seen in the medial femoral neck with bone remodeling ("buttressing") in response to altered mechanics (e-Fig. 143-53). Physeal widening with juxtaphyseal-, epiphyseal-, and metaphyseal-based lucencies may be seen as well.

CT and MRI may also be used to make the diagnosis of SCFE; however, usually radiographs suffice. Recent uses of MRI include detecting a preslip state, as evidenced by physeal widening with adjacent bone marrow edema and assessing cartilage loss.[142] Joint effusions are invariably present on MRI, presumably due to posttraumatic inflammation related to altered mechanics and hip joint incongruity.

Treatment In situ fixation with transphyseal screw is the treatment for SCFE. Prophylactic pinning of the contralateral hip may be performed in high-risk individuals. Timing of treatment is predicated on symptoms. Stable SCFEs can be electively pinned. Unstable SCFEs usually require urgent or emergent pinning, since they are at higher risk for epiphyseal osteonecrosis. Reduction of the capital femoral epiphysis is performed with extreme caution, since even minimal manipulation may disrupt the epiphyseal blood supply.

Complications after SCFE treatment include epiphyseal osteonecrosis (Fig. 143-54) and chondrolysis (e-Fig. 143-55). Epiphyseal osteonecrosis is more frequent after treatment of unstable SCFE. Chondrolysis used to complicate 5% to 10% of patients with SCFE, but the incidence has substantially

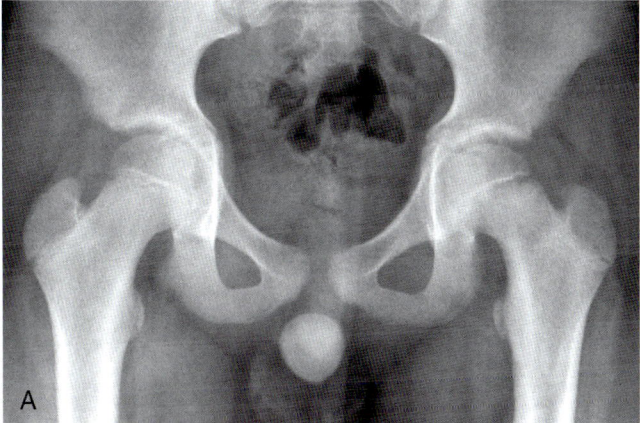
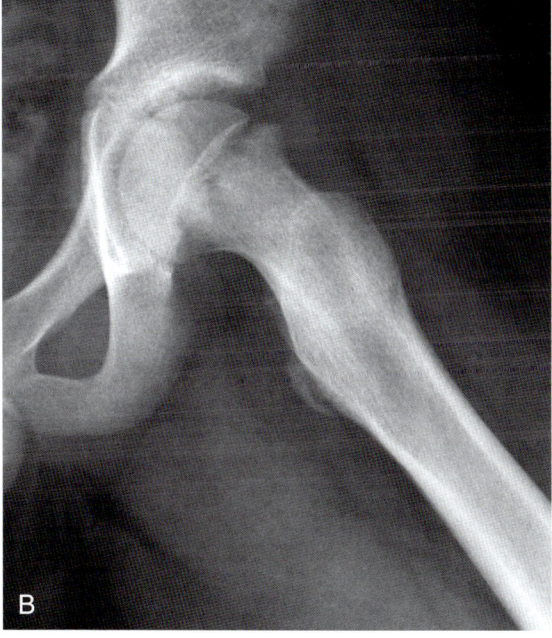

Figure 143-52 Slipped capital femoral epiphysis in an 11-year-old boy with left hip pain. **A,** On the anteroposterior view, the growth plate of the left proximal femur is wide and indistinct. No portion of the left femoral head projects lateral to Klein's line. The right proximal femur is normal. **B,** On the lateral view, malalignment of the femoral head and neck at the growth plate is better seen. The femoral head is displaced posteromedially relative to the femoral neck but is still in continuity.

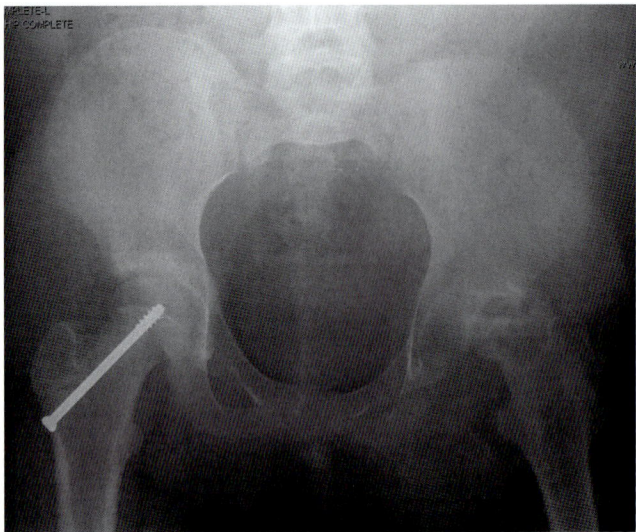

Figure 143-54 Complication of slipped capital femoral epiphysis. Single anteroposterior radiograph of the pelvis in a 14-year-old girl demonstrates left femoral head fragmentation and collapse consistent with osteonecrosis. There are postsurgical changes of the right femur.

lessened with newer fixation techniques.[143] Chondrolysis is now rarely seen without accompanying epiphyseal osteonecrosis. Additional complication of SCFE is cam-type femoroacetabular impingement related to abnormal offset of the femoral head and neck junction (see Chapter 145).

Traumatic Injuries of the Knee

Overview Before physeal fusion, the physes are the usual site of traumatic injury at the knee.[144] Once the physes fuses, cruciate ligament injury becomes much more common.[145] Hemarthrosis of the knee joint which occurs frequently, may be the consequence of major soft tissue injury or fracture.

DISTAL FEMUR

Etiology, Pathophysiology, and Clinical Presentation Two types of distal femoral fractures have been described. Juvenile type injuries (age 2-10 years) are most common secondary to high energy trauma such as a motor vehicle accident, whereas adolescent type injuries are typically sports related.[146] Salter-Harris type II fractures are the most common injury with usual displacement in the coronal plane, medial physeal separation, and associated medial collateral ligament sprain.[146] Salter-Harris type fractures are more common in the distal femur compared with ligamentous injuries of the knee, particularly during periods of rapid growth.

Imaging Initial evaluation begins typically with anteroposterior, lateral, and sunrise views of the knee. Sunrise views are usually not helpful in children under age 5 years, since the patella is undermineralized and patellar fractures are unusual in the first decade. Depending on the mechanism of injury, MRI or CT may be used in certain situations. MRI review of the knee in a child must include specific attention to the unfused physes as part of the search pattern.[145] MRI will also be particularly useful in evaluating tendon and ligamentous

injuries and bone contusions. With intraarticular fracture, lipohemarthrosis may be seen on cross-table lateral radiographs, MRI, or CT.[147] This appearance is secondary to breech of the bone marrow during injury.

Most displaced Salter-Harris fractures of the distal femoral metaphysis are obvious on clinical examination and on radiographs; however, subtle distal femoral Salter-Harris injuries may be occult on radiography and not diagnosed until MRI is performed (e-Fig. 143-56).

Treatment Distal femoral physeal fractures are treated conservatively with immobilization if nondisplaced and stable. Unstable, intraarticular, or displaced fractures are treated operatively with fixation.

PATELLA

Etiology, Pathophysiology, and Clinical Presentation Fractures of the patella in skeletally immature patients are rare.[148] Patellar sleeve fractures are more common and are often related to lateral patellar dislocation (see Chapter 145).[149,150] Direct impaction injury is the most common cause of patellar fractures that are non-sleeve. Like the scaphoid, the patella has a recurrent blood supply. Avascular necrosis of the proximal fragment is a rare complication of transverse patellar fractures.

Imaging Initial evaluation begins typically with anteroposterior and lateral views of the knee. The sunrise view is often challenging to obtain in children with patellar fractures, since this requires the child to flex the knee approximately 115 degrees. A Merchant view may be substituted which requires less knee flexion (45 degree flexion).

Non-sleeve patellar fractures may be simple (e-Fig. 143-57) or comminuted. Intraarticular involvement is important to define for surgical planning, and CT and MRI may be obtained for further evaluation. These fractures should be differentiated from a bipartite patella, which may fracture at the synchondrosis between the patellar body and the smaller superolateral ossification center (e-Fig. 143-58).

Treatment Patellar fractures are treated surgically, depending on several factors, including integrity of the extensor mechanism, degree of displacement, and articular extension. Patellar fractures are particularly difficult to treat conservatively because of issues with nonunion (from chronic traction related to the extensor mechanism), and premature osteoarthritis, since the articular surface is usually involved.

Tibial Tuberosity and Proximal Tibia

Etiology, Pathophysiology, and Clinical Presentation Tibial tuberosity acute and chronic avulsion injuries, physeal equivalent Salter-Harris injuries of the tibial tuberosity, and tibial eminence anterior cruciate ligament avulsion fractures are covered in detail in Chapter 145.

The proximal tibia has an upside-down L–shaped physis and epiphysis. Both the tibial epiphysis and tuberosity are a single entity that fuses to the underlying tibia at approximately age 15 years in girls and age 17 years in boys.[151,152] Therefore, any proximal tibial fracture extending to the tibial physis or tibial tuberosity physeal equivalent region should be considered a Salter-Harris fracture.

Unlike in adult patients, tibial plateau fractures in children are less likely to be depressed because the epiphyseal cartilage is more resilient and acts as a cushion for the tibial epiphyseal bone.

Imaging Initial evaluation begins with anteroposterior and lateral views of the knee. Transverse fractures of the proximal tibia may appear innocuous but are technically Salter-Harris II fractures if they extend to the tibial tuberosity physeal equivalent zone (e-Fig. 143-59). Avulsion fractures that violate the tibial epiphysis or tibial tuberosity are Salter-Harris III fractures (e-Fig. 143-60). CT and MRI are useful to determine the three-dimensional orientation of the fracture and its involvement of the physis. MRI is more useful for fracture delineation when the fracture plane extends to the physeal equivalent region of the tibial tuberosity and may help evaluate if the fracture is a true Salter-Harris type fracture. Involvement of the physis and potential injury to the extensor mechanism can be assessed. MRI is preferred for tibial plateau fractures to evaluate for articular cartilage injury as well as coexisting meniscal and ligamentous injury.

Treatment Salter-Harris fractures involving the proximal tibia weightbearing zone (tibial plateau) and Salter-Harris fractures involving the physeal equivalent region of the tibial tuberosity have different biomechanical challenges related to management. The tibial tuberosity is the insertion of the knee extensor mechanism, and therefore, tibial epiphyseal equivalent fractures in this region may be unstable with knee motion. Tibial plateau fractures are also unstable, but because these are loadbearing surfaces, when the overlying cartilage is violated, it should cause concern about posttraumatic osteoarthritis and coexisting internal derangement and meniscal tears of the knee. For these reasons, a low threshold exists for surgical fixation and immobilization for both tibial tuberosity and tibial epiphyseal Salter-Harris fractures in children.

Toddler Fractures

Etiology, Pathophysiology, and Clinical Presentation Toddler fracture is typically seen between ages 9 months and 3 years and classically involves the distal third of the tibial diaphysis. The toddler fracture spectrum includes any fracture of the leg or foot in the toddler. The tibia is the most commonly fractured, followed by the fibula and cuboid bone.[153]

In the classic clinical toddler fracture history, the child's leg is caught on an object, the leg twists, and the child falls. Some children present with pain and refusal to bear weight without a specific precipitating incident. On physical examination, the child will be point tender over the fracture.[154] Toddler fractures are common once children begin to cruise and walk. The presence of a similar fracture prior to the cruising or ambulatory stage should raise greater concern for abuse.

Imaging Toddler fractures may occur anywhere within the proximal metaphysis, diaphysis, or distal metaphysis of the tibia. The fracture line is oblique or spiral with no distraction or displacement (Fig. 143-61). Acutely, the fracture line may

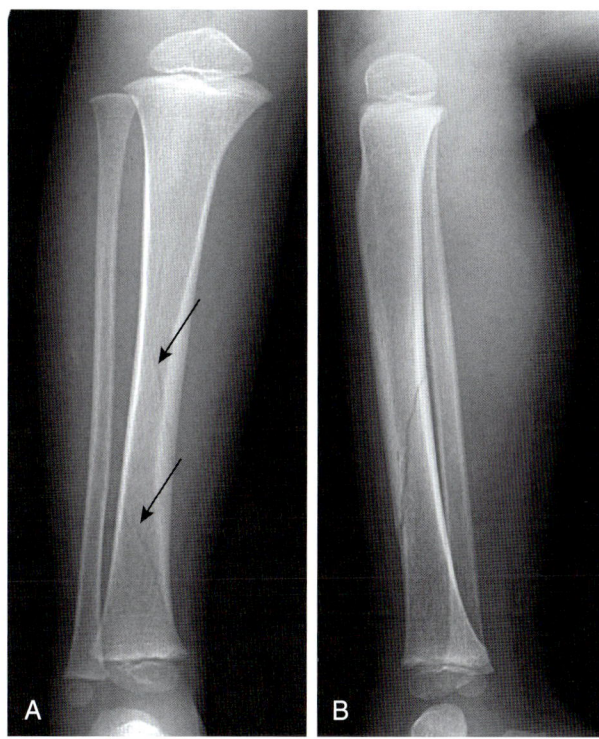

Figure 143-61 Anteroposterior (A) and lateral (B) views of a toddler fracture of the tibia in a 2-year-old girl. The fracture line has a spiral course as shown by two apparent fracture lines on the anteroposterior view (*arrows*) and the intervening single fracture line on the lateral view. Slight soft tissue swelling is seen anterior to the fracture on the lateral view.

be very subtle. In some patients, follow-up radiographs are necessary to confirm the fracture (e-Fig. 143-62). Similarly, acute toddler fractures of the fibula and cuboid (e-Fig. 143-63) may be subtle. The healing process, with sclerosis at the margins of the fracture line and development of periosteal new bone, may increase the conspicuity of the fracture.

Because the fracture line is oblique or spiral and because a particular event may not have led to the fracture, toddler fractures may erroneously be ascribed to child abuse. In the absence of other injury, however, the typical radiographic appearance of a toddler fracture in a child of appropriate age should not in itself raise suspicion for child abuse.

Treatment Treatment is conservative, consisting of immobilization and casting, as well as avoidance of weightbearing.

Other Tibial and Fibular Fractures

Etiology, Pathophysiology, and Clinical Presentation Most tibial fractures occur in the distal metadiaphysis.[155] The distal tibial metaphysis is a common site for buckle fractures in young children. Salter-Harris fractures are also very common at the distal tibia and are covered in detail in the section on ankle fractures (see below). In older children, fractures of the tibial shaft are usually complete with a transverse or oblique fracture plane. The fibula is commonly fractured when a complete fracture of the tibial diaphysis occurs.[156]

Maisonneuve fractures of the proximal fibula may occur with medial ligamentous injury or medial malleolar fracture at the ankle. The mechanism for Maisonneuve fractures is forced ankle valgus injury. These fractures may also occur with juvenile Tillaux or triplane fractures of the distal tibia. With a disruption of medial support at the ankle, the injury force may traverse the interosseous membrane up the leg and pass obliquely through the proximal fibular diaphysis. The presence of a Maisonneuve fracture thus indicates disruption of the interosseous membrane and potential instability if the ligamentous injury is not surgically addressed.

Imaging   Nonphyseal and extraarticular fractures of the leg can be radiographed utilizing anteroposterior and lateral views. Once the physis of either ends of the leg are involved, dedicated osteoarticular imaging is necessary to comprehensively characterize physeal and intraarticular involvement, if present.

Whenever a medially located fracture or ligamentous disruption of the ankle occurs, radiographs of the remainder of the leg should be obtained to rule out a Maisonneuve fracture (e-Fig. 143-64).[157]

Treatment   Treatment of tibial fractures depends on the age of the child, type and location of the fracture, and degree of fracture displacement and angulation. Most tibial fractures can be managed nonoperatively provided that they are purely extraarticular and do not involve a physis. Fibular fractures, including those that have physeal involvement, invariably are treated nonsurgically, since the fibula is a relatively non–load-bearing bone.

Proximal tibial fractures are relatively less common compared with other sites of tibial fractures, but they are more prone to complications, including progressive varus deformity. Type III and IV Salter-Harris type fractures will require operative management. Maisonneuve fractures can be managed nonsurgically if the fracture is stable. With unstable fractures, the syndesmosis needs to be approximated and medial malleolus fixated. The associated proximal fibular fracture is treated conservatively and the deltoid ligament need not be directly repaired.[158]

Distal tibial Salter-Harris III fractures may be seen medially (e-Fig. 143-65) or laterally (juvenile Tillaux fracture; see below). The distal tibial metaphysis is one of the more common locations of Salter-Harris IV fractures (see e-Fig. 143-11 and e-Fig. 143-66).

Traumatic Injuries of the Ankle

TRANSITIONAL ANKLE FRACTURES (JUVENILE TILLAUX AND TRIPLANE)

Etiology, Pathophysiology, and Clinical Presentation   "Transitional" fractures occur in the early teen years when the distal tibial physis is nearing the time of fusion or is already partially fused. The distal tibial physis begins to fuse in the medial central physis. Fusion then proceeds medially and posteriorly (e-Fig. 143-67). The anterolateral portion of the physis is the last portion of the physis to close and thus is the plane of least resistance to fracture.[159,160] The unique pattern of physeal fusion of the distal tibia leads to characteristic fracture patterns in the distal tibia.

Juvenile Tillaux fracture is a Salter-Harris III fracture of the distal tibial physis and epiphysis. Juvenile Tillaux fractures probably represent an anterolateral avulsion of the distal tibial

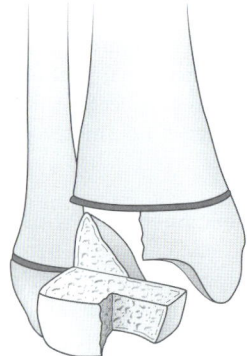

Figure 143-68   Triplane fracture. In a two-part triplane fracture, typically sagittal epiphyseal, transverse physeal, and coronal metaphyseal fracture lines are present. (Modified from Beaty JH, Kasser JR. *Rockwood and Wilkins' fractures in children.* 6th ed. Philadelphia, PA: Lippincott Williams & Wilkins; 2006.)

epiphysis pulled by the anterior tibiofibular ligament and anterior syndesmosis caused by forced external rotation.[161] Triplane fracture is closely related to juvenile Tillaux fracture; however, there is an additional plane of fracture of the distal tibial metaphysis, usually coronal in orientation (Fig. 143-68). The three planes of a triplane fracture are thus: (1) a sagittal fracture through the epiphysis, (2) a transverse fracture through the physis, and (3) a coronal fracture through the metaphysis.[162,163]

Imaging   For juvenile Tillaux fractures, the epiphyseal component of the fracture is usually sagittal or sagittal oblique, with the physeal portion of the fracture coursing through the anterolateral aspect of the distal tibial physis (Fig. 143-69). The vertical fracture line in juvenile Tillaux fractures is invariably located lateral with respect to anteromedial tibial physeal fusion, which is called "Kump's bump" (see Fig. 143-69). This should be distinguished from epiphyseal fractures that are medially located (see e-Figs. 143-65 and 143-66). The concern with juvenile Tillaux fracture of the distal tibia is not possible premature fusion of the physis, since the physis is already fusing, but, rather, involvement of the articular surface. A significant gap or incongruity of the fracture fragments at the articular surface may portend an early progression to degenerative disease in the ankle.

For triplane fractures, the epiphyseal and metaphyseal fracture planes may vary somewhat from true orthogonal orientation. A classic triplane fracture has two parts; however, three-part and four-part variants occasionally occur (Fig. 143-70).[164] Although the triplane fracture involves both the epiphysis and the metaphysis, it is not a true Salter-Harris IV fracture as the epiphyseal and metaphyseal fracture lines are not in continuity within the same plane. More correctly, the triplane fracture is a combination of a Salter-Harris II fracture and a Salter-Harris III fracture.

Superficially, triplane fractures on anteroposterior view may mimic juvenile Tillaux fracture (see Fig. 143-70, *A*). If a Salter-Harris II fracture component is not visualized on the lateral view, CT may be helpful to distinguish these two fractures, since this will alter management.

Radiography is usually sufficient for delineating both juvenile Tillaux and triplane fractures. Sometimes, varus stress maneuvers may be necessary to delineate the epiphyseal fracture component related to juvenille Tillaux fractures. CT

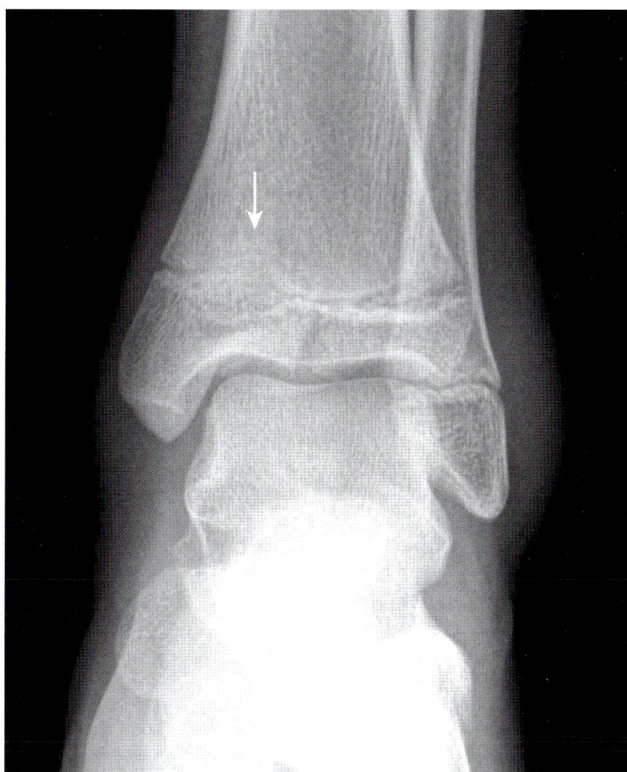

Figure 143-69 A 15-year-old boy with a juvenile Tillaux fracture. Note the Salter-Harris III vertical fracture line is lateral to Kump's bump (*arrow*), the site of initial distal tibia physeal closure.

may be used in preoperative planning to measure displacement at the articular surface and to map the anatomy of the fracture planes (e-Fig. 143-71).[165-169]

Treatment If the fracture line is wider than 2 mm, a transitional fracture will undergo operative fixation.[161] Widening

of the medial joint space may be a sign of fracture displacement.[170] Nondisplaced fractures can be treated with immobilization.[171] Juvenile Tillaux fractures are surgically fixed at the level of the epiphysis. Displaced triplane fractures will require surgical fixation of both the epiphyseal and metaphyseal fracture components.

Traumatic Injuries of the Foot

General Overview Foot fractures account for approximately 5% to 8% of pediatric fractures.[172] These fractures are generally uncommon in infants and toddlers given the significant cartilaginous composition of the foot during this age; the incidence of fractures increases with age as the foot becomes more ossified.[172] The majority of pediatric foot fractures are isolated injuries.[172]

HINDFOOT FRACTURES

Talar Fractures

Etiology, Pathophysiology, and Clinical Presentation Fractures of the talus are uncommon, compromising approximately 2% of pediatric foot fractures.[172] Avulsion fractures are the most common, followed by osteochondral fractures, talar neck, then talar body fractures.[173]

Small avulsion fractures may occur at sites of tendon or ligament attachment. The most common sites are at the medial aspect of the talus and the calcaneus.

The majority of talar neck and body fractures occur with high-energy trauma, usually from a fall or a motor vehicle accident.[172] Complete fractures of the talar neck are seen in older children but are rare.

Younger children may have buckle fractures of the talar neck. The buckle is evident along the dorsal surface of the bone and may be very subtle.[174] The talus is one location of the so-called *tarsal toddler fracture*. These fractures occur from

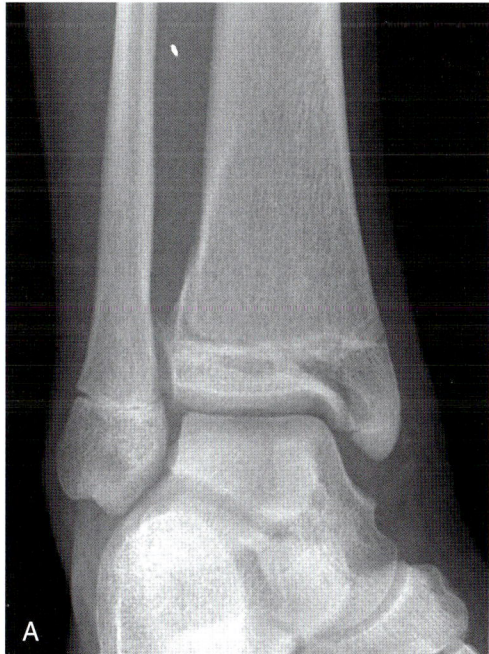
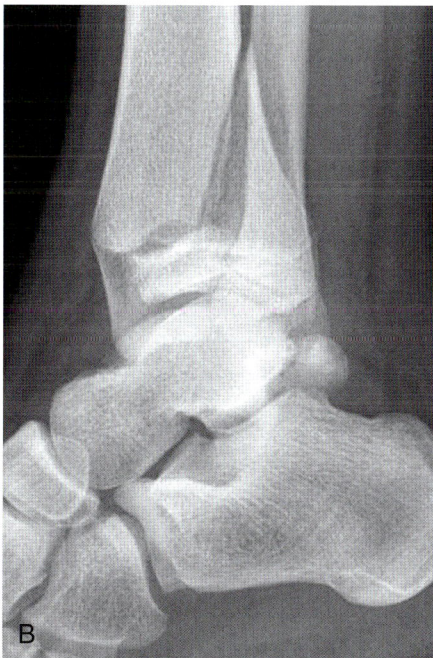

Figure 143-70 Anteroposterior (**A**) and lateral (**B**) views of a triplane fracture in an adolescent. (Courtesy Dr. B. H. Adler, Columbus, OH.)

compression of the talar neck against the anterior margin of the tibia with forced dorsiflexion.[176]

Peritalar dislocations, defined as dislocations of the subtalar and talonavicular joints, are uncommon and are usually the result of high-energy trauma. When a peritalar dislocation is present, additional fractures in the injured foot are common.[175]

Imaging Anteroposterior, oblique, and lateral radiographs of the ankle are initially obtained. Given the complexity of some talar fractures, CT can be used to delineate fracture anatomy and articular involvement (e-Fig. 143-72). Because of the recurrent blood supply of the body of the talus, fractures may be complicated by osteonecrosis of the proximal pole. The dislocated talus is also at risk for subsequent development of osteonecrosis because of disruption of vascular supply. The presence of a subchondral lucency in the talar dome (Hawkins sign) seen approximately 2 months after injury indicates that the talar dome has an adequate blood supply, and therefore, the risk of developing osteonecrosis is low.[172] Other significant complications include posttraumatic arthritis caused by malalignment.[176]

Treatment Treatment of nondisplaced talar fractures includes immobilization and casting, while either closed or open reduction is performed for displaced fractures.

Calcaneal Fractures

Overview Calcaneal fractures are uncommon, comprising only 2% of all pediatric foot fractures. Associated injuries are common.[172] Toddler fractures of the calcaneus, which have been described in the literature, are uncommon.[177]

Etiology, Pathophysiology, and Clinical Presentation Calcaneal fractures most commonly occur with jumps or falls from a large height and from motor vehicle accidents.[172] The mechanism of injury is usually an axial loading force.[178] Prior to apophyseal fusion, the posterior calcaneus may experience fractures involving the apophyseal physis and apophysis that can be classified by the Salter-Harris system.[179]

Imaging Calcaneal fractures may have a variable degree of comminution and of depression of the superior margin of the calcaneus. The Böhler angle can be used to assess for calcaneal depression caused by the fracture. This angle is the posterior angle between two lines, one drawn tangent to the anterior process of the calcaneus and the highest point of the posterior subtalar articular surface, and the other drawn from the latter point to the superior margin of the posterior calcaneus. Normally, the Böhler angle measures 25 to 40 degrees in adults but is less in children.[180] With depressed calcaneal fractures, the Böhler angle is decreased. Although the Essex-Lopresti classification system is widely used, it is important to differentiate between intraarticular and extraarticular fractures with reference to involvement of the subtalar joint.[172] The majority of calcaneal fractures are intraarticular, and the intraarticular component is often best seen on a Harris view (Fig. 143-73).

CT is utilized for full delineation of calcaneal fracture anatomy. Subtle compression fractures of the calcaneal body are not infrequent in younger children. These injuries may be virtually impossible to diagnose acutely from radiographs unless a buckle of the margin of the bone exists. Follow-up radiographs will show an oblique band of sclerosis within the midcalcaneal body (e-Fig. 143-74).

Treatment Displaced, intraarticular fractures of the calcaneus are typically treated surgically with open reduction and internal fixation.[181] Most patients have a good clinical outcome with few complications.[180]

MIDFOOT INJURY

Overview Isolated fractures of the cuneiform bones are rare. "Bunk bed" fractures of the cuboid have been reported (see "Bunk Bed Fracture"). Lisfranc injuries may occur

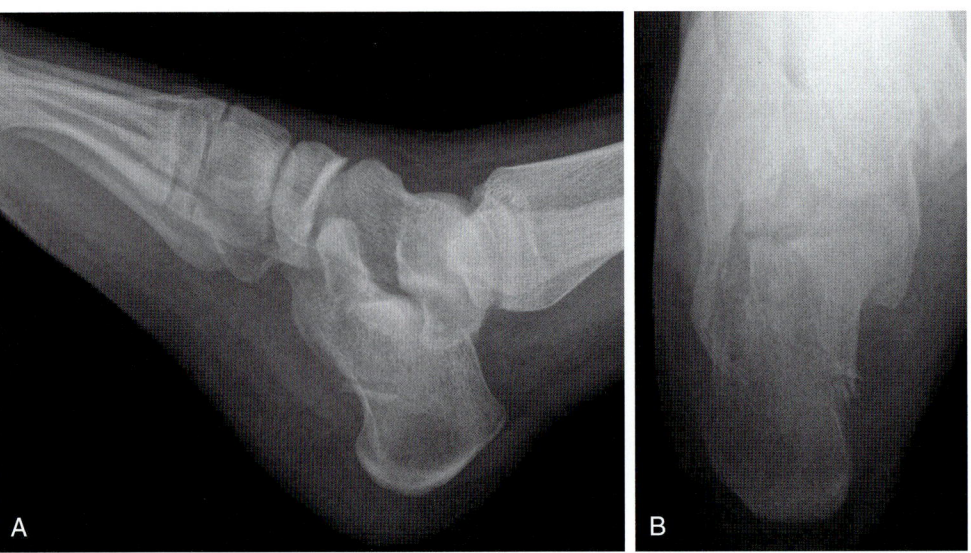

Figure 143-73 A 15-year-old boy with comminuted intra articular fracture of the calcaneus (A). **B,** The subtalar involvement is best seen on the Harris view.

throughout childhood but become more common in older children.

Etiology, Pathophysiology, and Clinical Presentation The mechanism may be direct, from a falling object, or indirect, from forced plantar flexion, abduction, or both.[172] Falls from a height account for the largest number of Lisfranc injuries in children.[172] The Lisfranc joint, which courses between the distal tarsals and the metatarsals, is disrupted. Fractures may be seen within the bases of the metatarsals or within the cuneiforms. Fracture at the base of the second metatarsal is a consistent finding. Multiple metatarsal fractures and midtarsal bone injuries are more likely in children.[2] These fractures may be chondro-osseous separations, which are seen as only as small slivers of bone and often occult with radiographs. Lisfranc injuries can be classified as homolateral, with the first metatarsal displaced in the same direction as the other four metatarsals, or divergent, with the first metatarsal displaced medially and the other metatarsals displaced laterally (e-Figs. 143-75 and 143-76). A fracture of the cuboid with a fracture of the second metatarsal base is compatible with significant tarsometatarsal (TMT) joint injury.

Imaging Radiographic abnormalities may be subtle. Weight-bearing views of the foot are necessary to accurately evaluate alignment of the forefoot and midfoot. Weightbearing will stress the TMT joint and may bring out subtle Lisfranc injuries. Any malalignment between the bases of the metatarsals or with their corresponding tarsal bones on any view should be regarded with suspicion. The midfoot should be closely evaluated for possibility of avulsion fractures. CT is used for confirmation of diagnosis and delineation of comorbid anatomy. Ultrasonography or MRI has been used to evaluate the Lisfranc ligament as well.[183] Ultrasonography and CT are not first line studies for the investigation of TMT injuries. Their role is supplementary when initial radiographs are normal or when it is necessary to identify additional fractures or ligamentous injuries that may affect surgical planning.

Treatment Nondisplaced or minimally displaced TMT dislocations may be treated conservatively. Patients with Lisfranc fracture–dislocations with more than minimal displacement are treated surgically.[172] If closed reduction is not successful, percutaneous pin fixation may be employed for stabilization of the reduction. Stabilizing the fracture of the proximal second metatarsal is important.[2]

FOREFOOT FRACTURES

Overview Metatarsal fractures are one of the most common pediatric foot injuries. Most fractures are nondisplaced or minimally displaced.[178] If the fractures involve the base of the metatarsal, injury to the TMT joint must be considered. Buckle fractures of the phalanges and metatarsals are common in younger children. The most commonly injured metatarsal in younger children is the first metatarsal and in older children the fifth.[184]

Etiology, Pathophysiology, and Clinical Presentation Phalangeal fractures usually occur from objects falling directly on the foot, particularly on the great toe.[178] Salter-Harris fractures may affect the physis of these bones. Salter-Harris III

fractures at the base of the proximal phalanx of the great toe may be mistaken for a bifid epiphysis, and vice versa. Buckle fractures of the phalanges and metatarsals are common in younger children. Often, adjacent bones are fractured together. Oblique or transverse fractures of the metatarsal shafts may be caused by dropped objects, falls, or twisting injuries. In severe twisting injuries in which the foot is caught, multiple adjacent metatarsals may be fractured.

Imaging Dedicated radiographs in three planes of the injured phalanx is preferred rather than imaging the foot in its entirety. Fractures should be defined by its location and extent including: intraarticular or extraarticular extension, location within the phalanx (shaft, neck, or head), and the presence or absence of involvement of an open physes. True lateral radiographs of the isolated symptomatic toe are challenging to obtain because of overlap of adjacent toes but are nevertheless important to obtain for complete fracture assessment, and identifying toe dislocations that may be missed on only anteroposterior and oblique views.

Treatment Displaced fractures need reduction and occasionally need K-wire fixation.[178] Phalangeal fractures heal quickly and usually only buddy taping is required.[178]

Stubbed Great Toe Fracture

Overview Stubbed great toe fractures are considered Salter-Harris I or II fractures of the base of the proximal or distal phalanx of the great toe until proven otherwise.[185] These fractures of the distal phalanx of the great toe are unique given the relationship of the nail bed to the physis and potential for complications (osteomyelitis).

Etiology, Pathophysiology, and Clinical Presentation The nail bed of the great toe is closely apposed to the physis of the distal phalanx of the digit. In fact, the skin is directly attached to the juxtaphyseal periosteum. After an injury, this relationship is thought to allow contamination of the underlying bone and physis.[186] Therefore, any nail bed injury with associated physeal fracture should be considered an open fracture (Fig. 143-77).[187]

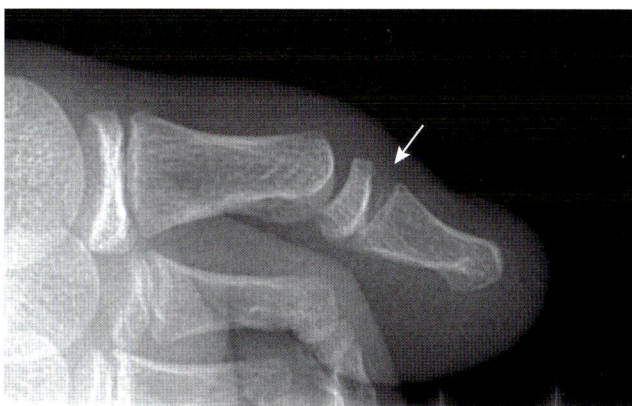

Figure 143-77 *Stubbed great toe fracture in a 12-year-old boy (arrow).* A tiny metaphyseal fragment is present. The patient was prophylactically placed on antibiotics.

Imaging Physeal widening of the terminal phalanx is the most common finding seen with stubbed toe fractures (see Fig. 143-77). Rarefaction and physeal widening can be related to the primary injury, related to superimposed osteomyelitis, or both and usually cannot be distinguished on the basis of radiography alone. If a high clinical concern for superimposed infection exists, MRI is necessary.

Treatment Prophylactic antibiotic therapy is recommended, as these are considered open fractures. The fracture is treated nonsurgically unless complicated by osteomyelitis with abscess formation.

Bunk Bed Fracture

Etiologies, pathophysiology, and clinical presentation A bunk bed fracture is a buckle fracture affecting the metatarsal bone of the first digit. This is most commonly seen in children 3 to 6 years of age.[153,174]

These fractures occur with a fall or a jump from a height onto a hard surface, with the prototypical injury occurring with a jump from the top bunk of a bunk bed onto a hardwood floor, landing in a tiptoe position.[188] The child's entire weight is placed on the first metatarsal (axial loading injury), leading to a buckle fracture. The bunk bed fracture is associated with ligamentous injury of at the TMT junction and is considered a Lisfranc variant.

Imaging Radiography is the primary modality to evaluate these fractures (e-Fig. 143-78). Occasionally, the normal undulation of the physis of the first metatarsal may mimic a bunk bed fracture. This should not cause interruption or buckling of the metaphyseal cortex, however, as is seen with a fracture.

Management Bunk bed fractures are treated conservatively with immobilization and surgical intervention is rarely indicated unless significant displacement or articular involvement has occurred.

Fractures of the Fifth Metatarsal

Overview Fractures at the base of the fifth metatarsal are common. Approximately 40% of all metatarsal fractures involve the fifth metatarsal.[189] The types of fifth metatarsal fractures described in children include tuberosity avulsions, intraarticular, proximal metadiaphyseal, diaphyseal, and neck fractures.

Etiologies, Pathophysiology, and Clinical Presentation The Jones fracture, originally described in the adult population, is a fracture of the proximal fifth metatarsal caused by repetitive inversion.[172] The fracture is transversely oriented and approximately 1.5 cm distal to the tip of the fifth metatarsal tuberosity and extends into the adjacent intermetatarsal facet (e-Fig. 143-79). This should be differentiated from fifth metatarsal stress fractures, which are located greater than 2 cm distal with respect to the fifth metatarsal tuberosity.

Jones and stress fractures of the fifth metatarsal should be differentiated from fifth metatarsal tuberosity avulsion fractures. Fifth metatarsal tuberosity avulsion fractures are fifth digit TMT fractures related to forced flexion and inversion, often due to an unexpected step or falling when on stairs. Tuberosity avulsion fractures were previously thought to be caused by avulsion at the insertion of the peroneus brevis but now appear to be an avulsion from the origin of the abductor digiti minimi.[172] In children, avulsions of the tuberosity are more common than true Jones fractures.

Imaging Initial evaluation should include anteroposterior, lateral, and oblique views. A comparison view of the opposite side obtained in the same position will be confirmatory particularly when apophyseal avulsions are a consideration. The physis of the avulsed apophysis will appear widened. The key is to differentiate base of the fifth metatarsal fractures from the normal fifth metatarsal apophysis. The fifth metatarsal apophysis is longitudinally oriented (e-Fig. 143-80) whereas metatarsal stress and avulsion fractures are horizontally oriented. To add to the confusion of the growing appendicular skeleton, the apophysis of the fifth metatarsal may occasionally avulse (Fig. 143-81).

The transverse fracture line of a tuberosity avulsion may extend through the apophysis and its physis (e-Fig. 143-82). Injuries to the base of the metatarsal can extend into the fifth metatarsal–cuboid joint or into the region between the fourth and fifth metatarsal bases. These fractures should be differentiated from more distally located Jones or stress fractures (e-Fig. 143-83) of the fifth metatarsal shaft.

Treatment Apophyseal avulsions are treated conservatively with immobilization. With Jones fractures, instability can occur at the fracture site. As instability predisposes to delayed union or nonunion, true Jones fractures are usually surgically managed. The fracture site in Jones fracture also has a tenuous blood supply, and therefore, healing may be delayed.[190]

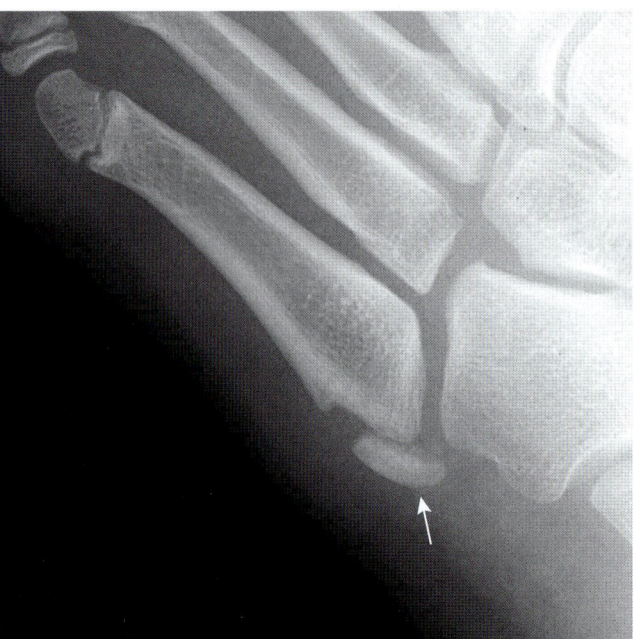

Figure 143-81 Avulsion of the fifth metatarsal apophysis (*arrow*) in a 13-year-old boy. The apophysis is displaced from the underlying bone and retracted proximally.

Neuropathic Injury

Etiologies, Pathophysiology, and Clinical Presentation Causes of neuropathic injury in children include myelomeningocele, syrinx, congenital insensitivity to pain, and familial dysautonomia (Riley-Day syndrome).[191-194] Superimposed infection is common.[191] Neuropathic fractures and joints ("Charcot joints") are much less common in pediatric patients than in adults.

Imaging Neuropathic injury is characterized by the four Ds: (1) dislocation, (2) debris, (3) disorganization (deformity), and (4) density (sclerosis). Injuries fail to heal. Physeal fractures may occur and are often associated with subperiosteal hematoma and exuberant periosteal new bone. Findings may mimic tumor or infection. Repetitive trauma may lead to chronic physeal injury that may lead to premature fusion. Other sequelae include acro-osteolysis, joint deformity, joint dislocation, and epiphyseal osteonecrosis.[191] Neuropathic fractures are most common in the lower extremities in the diaphysis or metaphysis (e-Fig. 143-84). Injury to the fingertips is caused by crush, thermal damage, and chewing (e-Fig. 143-85).

Treatment Treatment is variable and tailored to the underlying problem. Both nonsurgical management and surgical management are used for treating Charcot arthopathy. Nonsurgical treatment includes immobilization and reduction of stress. Examples of surgical management include removal of bony prominences, arthrodesis, plate and screw fixation, bone grafting, and reconstructive surgery.

Physical Agents

FROSTBITE

Etiologies, Pathophysiology, and Clinical Presentation Frostbite injury is most common in children ages 5 to 10 years. The pathophysiologic mechanism of frostbite is not well defined, but a direct injury to chondrocytes may have occurred within the physis.[195] The sequela in children is premature fusion of the physis and shortening of the involved digits. Bone fragmentation may be caused by ischemic damage.[195] Secondary degenerative changes develop from direct articular injury and malapposition of joint surfaces in the affected digits.[196]

Imaging Immediate radiographic findings occurring 1 week after exposure include soft tissue swelling and soft tissue gas, which is a poor prognostic sign.[195] Radiographically identifiable osseous changes manifest weeks to months after injury. Characteristically, the thumb is spared as it is clenched at the time of exposure and covered by the other digits. Findings are most pronounced in the distal phalanges, occasionally affect the middle phalanges, and rarely involve the proximal phalanges or metacarpals (Fig. 143-86).[196]

Treatment Treatment is variable and depends on the degree of injury. Rewarming the extremity, surgical debridement of nonviable tissue, and thrombolytics are potential treatments.

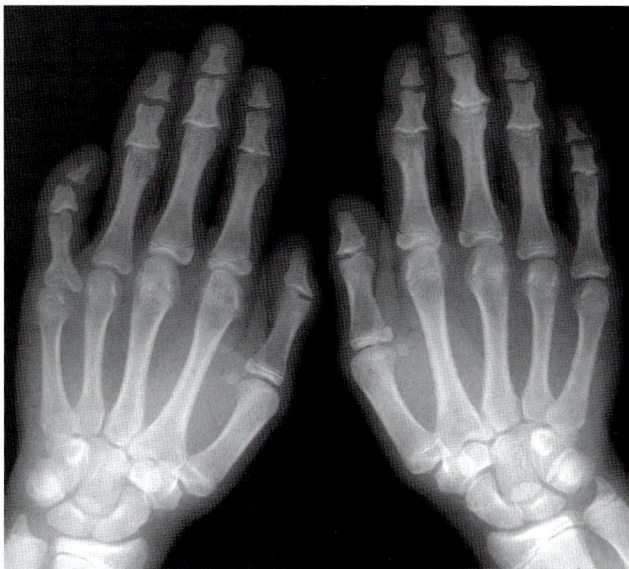

Figure 143-86 Sequelae of frostbite in a 15-year-old girl. Brachydactyly of the distal and middle phalanges was caused by premature growth plate closure. In this patient, the thumbs were not spared. The proximal phalanx of the right fifth finger is also shortened.

Antibiotics are commonly used to prevent or treat superimposed infection.

Thermal and Electrical Injury

Etiologies, Pathophysiology, and Clinical Presentation Thermal injuries are a significant cause of morbidity and mortality in children, most commonly affecting children under age 6 years.[197] The hand is most commonly injured, followed by the face.[197,198]

Imaging Injury from thermal burns is usually to the soft tissues, leading to contractures and ankylosis. Heterotopic bone contributes to ankylosis, as does direct thermal injury of a joint.[199] Direct thermal injury to the physis may lead to premature fusion or growth disturbance (e-Fig. 143-87).[199,200] Electrical injury may lead similar sequelae because of tissue heating. Osteolysis may occur.

Treatment Wound infection and sepsis are common, and surgical intervention may be necessary in some cases.[201,202]

Radiation

Etiologies, Pathophysiology, and Clinical Presentation Irradiation of tissues may cause immediate or delayed injury to tissues.[203] Radiation affects the immature skeleton by interfering with chondrogenesis and causing resorption of bone and cartilage at the physis, therefore affecting younger children who have greater growth potential.[203] Therapeutic radiation doses may be sufficient to cause permanent injury to bone. With regard to growth retardation, microscopic changes are seen with a little as 300 centigrays (cGy) and growth retardation with as low as 400 cGy.[203] Histologic recovery occurs with doses up to 1200 cGy; however, beyond this level, almost uniformly permanent cell damage and premature physeal fusion occur.[203] Radiation-induced sarcomas are uncommon and occur years after therapy.[203]

Imaging Radiation injury includes growth retardation with hypoplasia (e-Fig. 143-88), premature physeal fusion, SCFE, osteonecrosis, osteochondroma formation, and radiation-induced sarcoma.[203-205]

Metaphyseal sclerosis, fraying, and widening can be seen 1 to 2 months following long bone irradiation; this appearance resembles rickets.[203] The affected bone may return to normal after 6 months. A dense metaphyseal band may also be seen shortly after therapy.[203] SCFE can occur anywhere from 1 to 8 years after therapy, and therefore, long-term radiographic follow-up is warranted.[203] Horizontal sclerotic lines parallel to the vertebral body endplates may be seen (bone in bone appearance) 9 to 12 months after irradiation to the spine. With higher doses of radiation (2000 to 3000 cGy), vertebral body scalloping, loss of vertebral body height, and scoliosis from asymmetric vertebral body growth have been reported.[203]

Treatment Initial assessment begins with early diagnosis of radiation injury and determining the amount of radiation exposure. Treatment is variable, depending on the severity of exposure and the location or nature of injury.

Key Points

The composition of a child's bones and the presence of the growth process both predispose the child to different types of fractures and complications of fractures than are seen in the adult.

Higher grade Salter-Harris fractures have a higher incidence of premature physeal fusion.

The medial epicondyle ossifies prior to the trochlea. In an injured elbow, visualization of an ossified trochlea without an ossified medial epicondyle in its normal location should raise suspicion for an avulsed medial epicondyle.

Pelvic fractures in children may be incomplete. Single disruptions in the obturator ring may be caused by the composition of child's bones.

Fractures involving the triradiate cartilage may interfere with subsequent acetabular growth.

When a child presents with bilateral symmetric SCFE or outside of the typical age range, an underlying metabolic disorder should be expected.

Classic toddler fracture of the tibia is one cause of pain and refusal to bear weight. Toddlers may also incur fractures of the fibula and tarsal bones (talus and cuboid) and present similarly.

Because of the proximity of the nail bed, Salter-Harris fractures of the distal phalanx of the great toe are considered open fractures. Children should receive prophylactic antibiotics to prevent osteomyelitis.

✓ WHAT THE CLINICAN NEEDS TO KNOW

- Fracture description, including presence or absence of displacement, angulation, physeal involvement, articular involvement, and fracture orientation (e.g. tranverse, plastic, longitudinal, single, comminuted)
- Differentiation of normal developmental variant from fracture
- Whether an underlying metabolic syndrome predisposes the child to a fracture

Suggested Readings

Ogden JA. *Skeletal injury in the child.* 3rd ed. New York: Springer; 2000.

Ozonoff MG. *Pediatric orthopedic radiology.* 2nd ed. Philadelphia, PA: Saunders; 1992.

Rogers LF, Poznanski AK. Imaging of epiphyseal injuries. *Radiology.* 1994;191:297-308.

Swischuk L, Hernandez JA. Frequently missed fractures in children (value of comparative views). *Emerg Radiol.* 2004;11:22-28.

Wilkins KE. Principles of fracture remodeling in children. *Injury.* 2005;36(suppl 1):A3-A11.

References

Full references for this chapter can be found on www.expertconsult.com.

Chapter 144

Child Abuse

PETER J. STROUSE and DANIELLE K. B. BOAL

Overview

In the decades since the landmark articles by Caffey (1946) and Kempe and Silverman (1962), the medical community, law enforcement, and Child Protective Services (CPS) have developed a much greater awareness and sensitivity to the diagnosis of child abuse; these groups have not only advocated for protection of the child but have also promoted a more aggressive approach to the identification and prosecution of offending individuals.[1,2] Child abuse remains a difficult, emotionally charged topic. The diagnosis of child abuse and the treatment of abused children are intertwined with legal issues of parental rights and family preservation. Because it typically occurs behind closed doors, the abuse is unobserved, and confessions are rare. Presentations are varied, and abuse and neglect may mimic other disease processes.

Etiologies, Pathophysiology, and Clinical Presentation According to the most recent survey from the U.S. Department of Health and Human Services, in the year 2009 an estimated total of 3,043,000 children were the subject of investigations undertaken by CPS agencies as alleged victims of maltreatment, and approximately 702,000 were found to be victims of maltreatment.[3] Thus, in 2009, 40.2 of every 1000 children in the United States were evaluated by CPS for suspected abuse or neglect, and 9.3 of every 1000 children were confirmed by CPS as abused or neglected.[3] Of confirmed cases, children were victims of neglect in 78.3%, physical abuse in 17.8%, sexual abuse in 9.5%, psychological maltreatment in 7.6%, and other forms of maltreatment in 9.6% (>100% as many children are victims of multiple forms).[3] Young children are at greatest risk for fatality; 81% are younger than 4 years of age at the time of death, and 46% are younger than 1 year of age at death.[3] An estimated 1770 children died from abuse or neglect in 2009.[3] More than 90% of all confirmed perpetrators have a parental relationship to the victim (mother, father, step-parent, boyfriend or girlfriend of parent).[3]

Clinical presentations of child abuse are myriad. In some children, abuse is suspected from the start; however, in many, the presentation is cryptic until traumatic findings are made clinically or by imaging.[4] Children commonly present with symptoms related to head, abdominal, or extremity trauma. Children may present with bruising, burns, or evidence of neglect. Not infrequently, manifestations of abuse may be found incidentally on imaging performed to evaluate a nontraumatic process. Therefore, the radiologist is occasionally the first to suggest the possibility of child abuse.

Imaging Initial imaging of the abused child is driven by the clinical presentation.[5,6] Imaging is performed to evaluate for processes that need immediate management or may further threaten the child's well-being if not diagnosed and treated. Once the child's acute medical issues are addressed and their condition is stable, further imaging in the form of a radiographic skeletal survey can be performed to look for occult injuries and evaluate for child abuse as a diagnosis. The role of such imaging is threefold:

1. Recognition of physical abuse, supporting the diagnosis in suspected cases, and recognizing characteristic lesions when the possibility of child abuse has not been suspected.
2. Provision to the prosecution or defense of accused offenders of an understanding of the mechanism, patterns of healing (dating), and likelihood of such injuries with a reasonable degree of medical certainty.
3. Exclusion of the diagnosis of child abuse in cases of true accidental trauma or with variants of normal and disease processes that may mimic abuse.

Computed tomography (CT) and magnetic resonance imaging (MRI) are used to evaluate suspected head trauma. There are no firm indications for CT of the chest in suspected physical abuse or infants with blunt traumatic injury. CT of the abdomen and pelvis is indicated only in children with physical examination, laboratory findings, or both suggesting traumatic intraabdominal injury.[7-9]

In all cases of suspected physical abuse in children younger than 2 years of age, a skeletal survey is mandatory (Box 144-1).[5,6,10] A "babygram" consisting of single or few images of the entire infant is unsatisfactory. If radiographic film is used, high-detail film without a grid is recommended.[10] Digital radiography has replaced film screen skeletal surveys in many centers; however, further evaluation of the technical elements necessary to produce high-detail images is still needed.

Ideally, each skeletal survey is reviewed by a radiologist before the child leaves the radiography suite. Poorly positioned and otherwise suboptimal images should be repeated. Additional views may be obtained to further define

---

Box 144-1 Skeletal Survey*

- Anteroposterior (AP) and lateral of skull (Townes view optional; add if any fracture seen)
- Lateral spine (C-spine may be included on skull radiographs; AP spine is included on AP chest and AP pelvis to include entire spine)
- AP, right posterior oblique, left posterior oblique of chest—rib technique
- AP pelvis
- AP of each femur
- AP of each leg
- AP of each humerus
- AP of each forearm
- Posteroanterior of each hand
- AP (dorsoventral) of each foot

*Images are checked by a radiologist before the patient leaves. Poorly positioned or otherwise suboptimal images should be repeated. Lateral views are added for positive or equivocal findings in the extremities. Coned views of positive or equivocal findings (i.e., at the ends of the long bones, ribs) may be obtained.

---

positive or suspected abnormalities (e-Fig. 144-1). Commonly acquired additional views include lateral views of the extremities, coned views centered at the joints (wrist, ankle, knee), and Townes view of the skull.

A follow-up skeletal survey performed 2 weeks after the initial examination may provide additional information (e-Fig. 144-2).[11,12] As noted by Kleinman, the follow-up survey aids by (1) detecting additional fractures; (2) differentiating fractures from normal developmental variants; and, (3) assisting in dating injuries.[11] Follow-up surveys may be limited or tailored to areas of interest.[13]

In infants and children younger than 2 years, nuclear scintigraphy should be viewed as a complementary modality to radiographic evaluation.[14-16] In general, nuclear medicine bone scans are used for problem solving and in children with a high suspicion for abuse but with negative or equivocal radiography.

The imaging of children between 2 and 5 years of age must be assessed individually. Beyond 2 years of age, the yield of radiographic skeletal survey is low as fractures are less common, fractures are less commonly occult, and the fracture patterns highly specific for abuse are no longer seen. Nevertheless, a skeletal survey may occasionally be warranted on the basis of clinical presentation and high suspicion for abusive trauma, particularly in children who are mentally incapacitated.

In the child older than 5 years, skeletal scintigraphy may be substituted for the radiographic skeletal survey, but neither radiographic nor scintigraphic screening has proved to be useful in the older child.

Whole-body MRI and positron emission tomography have both been studied for the detection of abuse injuries.[17,18] Both modalities lack sensitivity for metaphyseal lesions but do detect many abuse-related lesions.

Radiographic skeletal surveys should be performed in all cases of fatal suspected abuse and unexplained infant death.[19-22] Postmortem surveys follow the same imaging protocol as used in living infants.[20] At present, little experience with postmortem whole body CT exists; however, this technique does show promise for detecting subtle findings to guide the forensic pathologist.[23]

Imaging Findings   No one radiographic finding is pathognomonic of child abuse. Individual radiographic findings vary from high specificity to low specificity.[24,25] High-specificity lesions are seen with abusive trauma but are rarely seen in other forms of trauma. Low-specificity lesions may be commonly seen with abuse-related trauma but are also common with trauma not associated with trauma.

Paul Kleinman has written extensively on the radiography of child abuse and has classified the findings into categories of high, moderate, and low specificities (Box 144-2).[24,25] This categorization is supported by many series in the literature, although a number of reports support slight modifications to the categorization of findings.

Each case must be considered individually with respect to the history provided and the possibility of underlying abnormalities that would predispose to fracture, for example, history of prematurity, metabolic disease, or dysplasia. Certain patterns and types of skeletal injury may occur as a result of abuse. The plausibility of the injury having occurred from accidental non–abuse-related trauma must also be considered. Is the explanation offered for the injury plausible? Is the developmental level of the child consistent with that history?

Infants who are not ambulatory do not normally incur fractures from unintentional injury events. A fall from 3 to 4 feet to a hard surface may result in a linear parietal skull fracture, but rarely do long bone fractures, complex skull fractures, or central nervous system injuries occur in this circumstance. The appropriateness of the history in relation to the mechanism of injury(s) is, thus, often the first and most important clue to the diagnosis of abuse injuries. Inappropriate delay in seeking treatment is also frequent.

The constellation of radiographic findings within the context of the clinical presentation may carry greater

---

Box 144-2 Skeletal Injuries from Child Abuse

High Specificity Findings

- Classic metaphyseal lesions
- Posterior rib fracture
- Scapular fracture
- Sternal fracture
- Spinous process fracture
- First rib fracture

Moderate Specificity Findings

- Multiple fractures
- Fractures of differing age
- Spine fracture
- Complex skull fracture
- Physeal fractures of the long bones
- Digital fractures

Low Specificity Findings

- Diaphyseal fractures of the long bones
- Simple skull fractures
- Clavicle fracture

Modified from Kleinman PK. *Diagnostic imaging of child abuse*. 2nd ed. St Louis, MO: Mosby; 1998.

specificity than any single radiographic finding. Multiple fractures in different stages of healing are highly specific for child abuse, unless an underlying bone dysplasia or metabolic abnormality is diagnosed. Fractures to the rib cage, metaphyseal fractures (classic metaphyseal lesions), and skull fractures predominate in infants younger than age 1 year, whereas diaphyseal long bone fractures are more common in older infants and children.

Rib Fractures

Rib fractures are found in approximately 50% of fatally abused infants.[26] The ribs may be the only site of skeletal trauma in some abused children.[27] In a surviving infant, the astute clinician may palpate callus with healing or, rarely, crepitus, but otherwise, typically, no physical sign of injury is present. Most acute rib fractures are subtle buckle or greenstick type fractures not evident and frequently are not appreciated on radiography until evidence of healing is found (see e-Fig. 144-2).[28] Fracture may occur at any point along the arc of the rib (costovertebral, posterior, lateral, anterior, or costochondral) but frequently involve the posterior rib.[26,29] Posterior rib fractures at the costovertebral junction have a high specificity for abuse.[30-32] Boal and associates reviewed 1463 rib fractures in 141 abused infants and noted that when individual sites along the rib arc were compared, costovertebral junction fractures outnumbered all other individual sites.[30] However, fractures at the costovertebral junction represented only 33% of the total number of rib fractures. Fractures at other sites in the rib arc are very common in abused children, too.[30] Fractures at the costochondral junction appear radiographically similar to classic metaphyseal lesions of the long bones and have a high association with visceral trauma.[33] First rib fractures bear high specificity for child abuse.[34]

A squeezing injury, shaking injury, or a combination of both results in leveraging of the posteromedial rib over the spinal transverse process. Excessive compression and distraction forces are also placed on the lateral and anterior rib arc and at the metaphyseal equivalent region near the costovertebral junction of the rib (Fig. 144-3).[28,35] Multiple fractures may involve a single rib. Oblique views of the ribs increase the sensitivity for rib fractures and aid in their characterization (Fig. 144-4).[36] Nuclear scintigraphy aids in the detection of rib fracture and plays a complementary role to that of radiography (e-Fig. 144-5).[14,15] Follow-up radiographs (see e-Fig. 144-2) and CT also provide increased sensitivity.[37,38] CT may be more sensitive for rib fractures than radiography, but the greater radiation dose of CT limits its use as a screening modality.[37] Nevertheless, focused CT may be helpful in problematic cases. If a CT is performed for evaluation of visceral trauma, reconstruction of images with narrow slice thickness, bone detail algorithm, and multiplanar reformats facilitate identification and delineation of rib fractures (Fig. 144-6).

In contrast to adult ribs, fractures rarely occur in infant ribs because of cardiopulmonary resuscitation.[39-42] Rare fractures caused by infant cardiopulmonary resuscitation are predominantly anterolateral and are usually radiographically occult.[39,40,43] Rib fractures caused by birth trauma are rare.[44] A case report noted posteromedial rib fractures from accidental blunt trauma in an infant.[45] Rib fractures are commonly seen in infants with metabolic bone disease and have been

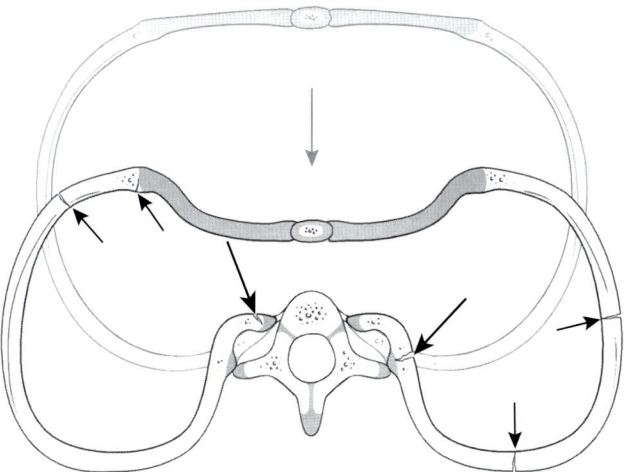

Figure 144-3 Mechanism of rib injury. With anteroposterior compression (*gray arrow*) of the chest, excessive leverage of the posterior ribs occurs over the fulcrum of the transverse processes. This places tension along the inner aspects of the rib head and neck regions, resulting in fractures at these sites (*long black arrows*). This mechanism is consistent with morphologic patterns of injury occurring at other sites along the rib arcs and at the costochondral junctions (*short black arrows*). (From Kleinman PK. *Diagnostic imaging of child abuse.* 2nd ed. St Louis, MO: Mosby; 1998.)

reported after thoracotomy, chest tube placement, and chest physiotherapy.[34,46] However, rib fractures in infants younger than age 12 months without a predisposing condition, for example, instrumentation, prematurity, chronic illness, metabolic bone disease, or all of these, are strongly suspicious for the diagnosis of abuse.[34,47]

Long Bone Fractures

METAPHYSEAL FRACTURES

The classic metaphyseal fracture, first described by Caffey and commonly referred to as a "corner" or "bucket-handle" fracture, was reexamined by Kleinman in 1986 with the use of detailed histopathologic and radiographic studies.[1,48] He determined that the lesions represent a complete shearing or planar fracture that extends through the primary spongiosa of the metaphysis and that it is not an avulsion injury as described by Caffey.[48,49] Depending on size and displacement of the metaphyseal fragment, the positioning of the child and the radiographic projection, this highly specific lesion caused by abuse may appear as a "corner" fracture or as a "bucket-handle" fracture (Fig. 144-7). Metaphyseal fractures of abuse may also be seen on ultrasonography.[50]

The "classic metaphyseal lesion," a term coined by Kleinman, occurs from violent shaking as the infant is held by the trunk or extremities (Figs. 144-8 and 144-9; e-Fig. 144-10; and Fig. 144-11). Some lesions are probably also caused by torsional pulling on a limb. Typically, no bruising or outward sign of injury is evident with a classic metaphyseal lesion. Classic metaphyseal lesions are most commonly seen at the proximal humerus, distal radius, distal femur, proximal tibia, and distal tibia and fibula.[51-54]

Occasionally, classic metaphyseal lesions become more conspicuous on short-term follow-up radiography.[49] With healing, classic metaphyseal lesions typically become indistinct and sclerotic. Kleinman demonstrated subtle extension of

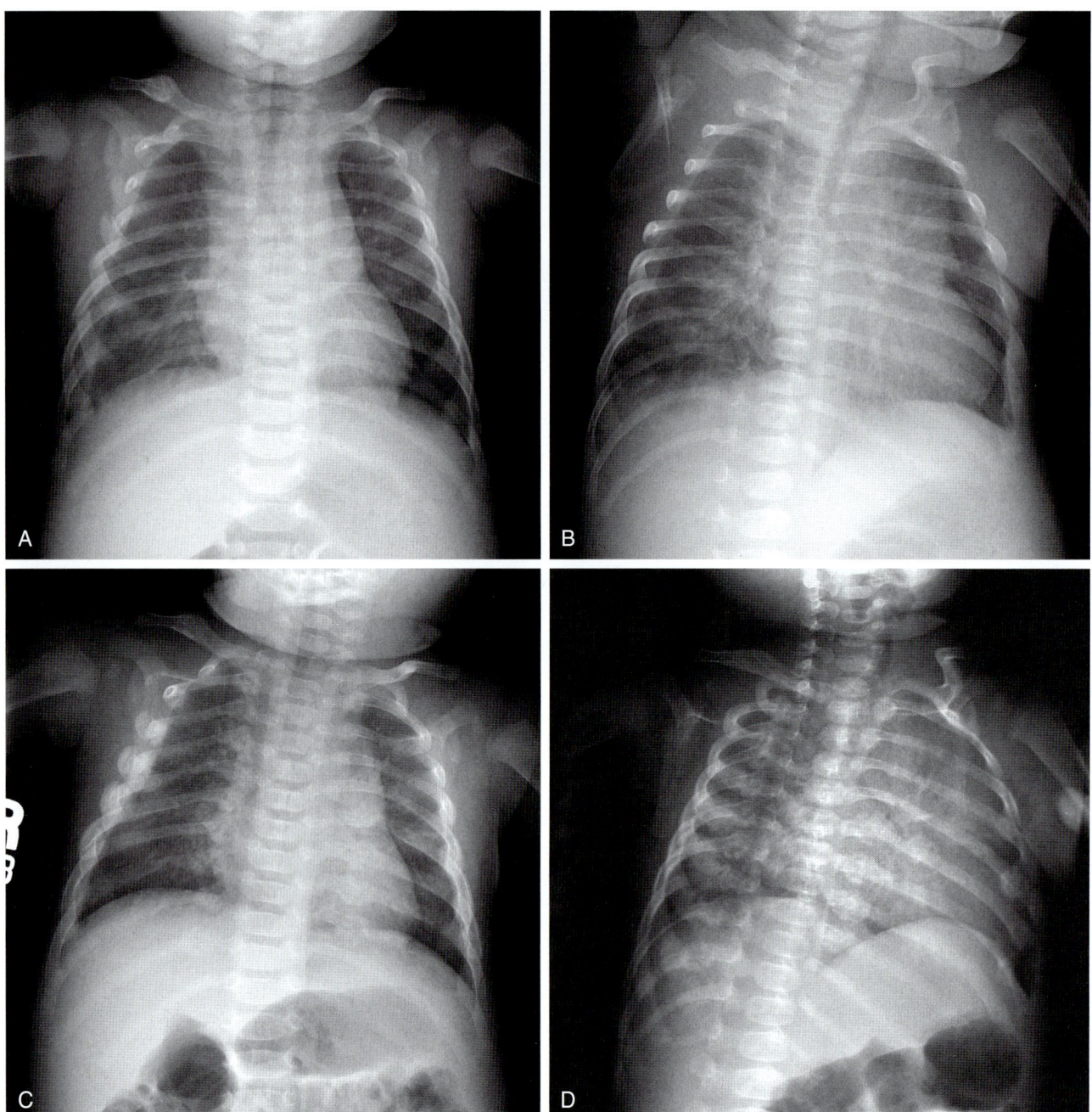

Figure 144-4 A 2-month-old male infant with right pleural effusion. **A,** Anteroposterior radiograph shows healing right clavicular fracture and nine fractures of the right ribs and four fractures of the left ribs on initial survey. **B,** Some fractures are better depicted on the left posterior oblique view. **C** and **D,** Two weeks later, anteroposterior and left posterior oblique radiographs of the chest clearly show 18 right rib fractures and 11 left rib fractures, illustrating the value of a follow-up skeletal survey.

physeal cartilage into the metaphysis as a sign of healing.[55] Subperiosteal new bone is not seen unless there is an associated periosteal injury.

Transverse, greenstick, and buckle fractures of the metaphysis may also be caused by child abuse but do not carry the same specificity as the classic metaphyseal lesions. Such fractures are considered to be of low specificity. Small stepoffs, beaks, and spurs at the metaphyseal margins may mimic abusive injury.[56] Slight fragmentation of metaphyseal margins with physiologic bowing may also mimic abuse.[57] Iatrogenic classic metaphyseal-like lesions have been reported with birth trauma and as a complication of treatment of clubfeet.[50,58,59] Such reports are rare and it is likely that the reported fractures occurred with a similar torsional mechanism as occurs in child abuse.

PHYSEAL FRACTURES

Physeal fractures are uncommon in child abuse. Fractures may be occult or subtle at presentation and some are not recognized until healing occurs.[60] Ultrasonography or MRI may be helpful to image the unossified epiphyses and assess

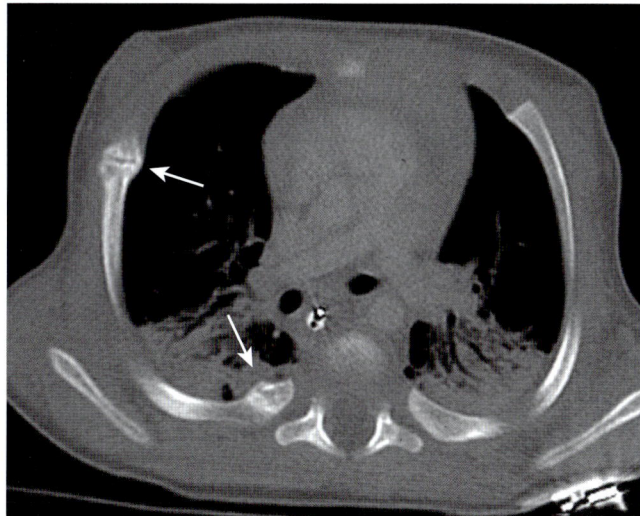

Figure 144-6 A 3-month-old male with multiple rib fractures, multiple metaphyseal fractures (classic metaphyseal lesions), a small subdural hematoma, and disruption of the posterior wall of the hypopharynx. This computed tomography scanning was performed for concern of extension of infection into the chest. Images were also reconstructed with bone algorithm. Arrows indicate healing posterior and anterolateral rib fractures. The fracture lines are indistinct. Callus is present.

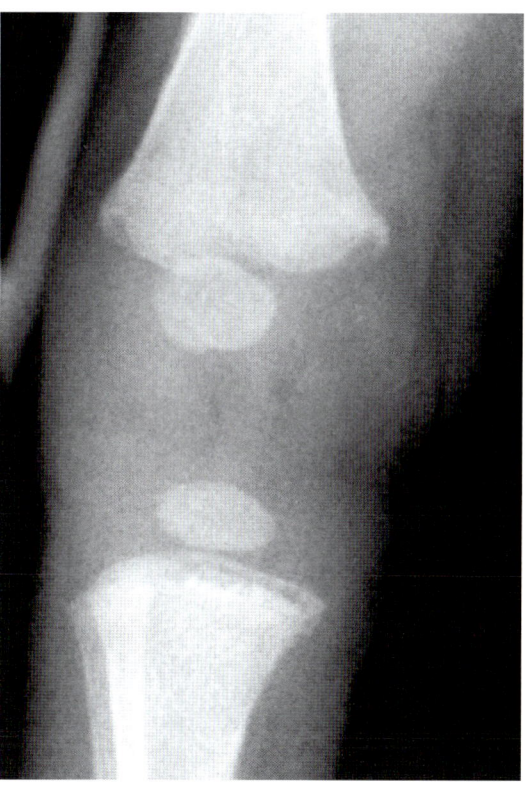

Figure 144-8 A 2½-month-old male infant with acute and chronic subdural hematoma and 18 fractures. Anteroposterior radiograph of the right knee shows classic metaphyseal lesions at the distal femur and the proximal tibia.

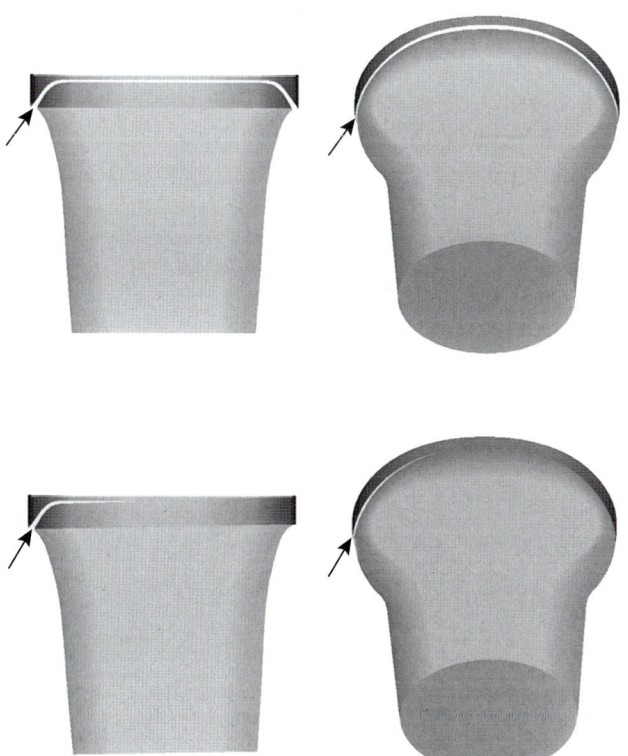

Figure 144-7 Corner and bucket-handle fracture patterns of the classic metaphyseal lesion. Fractures (*arrows*) extend adjacent to the chondroosseous junction and then veer toward the diaphysis to undercut the larger peripheral segment that encompasses the subperiosteal bone collar. When the physis is viewed tangentially, the classic metaphyseal lesion appears as a corner fracture (*left images*). When a view is obtained through beam angulation, a bucket-handle pattern results (*right images*). *Top images,* Diffuse injury; bottom images, localized injury. (From Kleinman PK. *Diagnostic imaging of child abuse.* 2nd ed. St Louis: Mosby; 1998. Originally modified from Kleinman PK, Marks SC, Jr. Relationship of the subperiosteal bone collar to metaphyseal lesions in abused infants. *J Bone Joint Surg Am.* 1995;77:1471-1476.)

the integrity of the physis.[61] Common sites of physeal fracture are the proximal humerus (Fig. 144-12), the distal humerus, and the proximal femur.[60-62] As opposed to classic metaphyseal lesions, which heal without sequelae, physeal fractures may be complicated by malunion and premature physeal fusion.

DIAPHYSEAL FRACTURES

Transverse, oblique and spiral diaphyseal fractures of the long bones in the nonambulatory young infant should raise suspicion for abuse.[63-66] Once ambulatory, true accidental fractures become common.[67] Solitary long bone fractures may occur after accidental trauma in the older infant and child; however, factors that increase the likelihood of an abuse-related injury include association with another fracture and other clinical features that produce a high level of suspicion for abuse, inappropriate clinical history, failure to seek medical attention, and discovery of the fracture in a healing state (Fig. 144-9; also see Fig. 144-13).[66,68,69]

It is risky to assign significance to the pattern of diaphyseal fracture because all patterns occur with unintentional or true accidental trauma as well as with abuse.[65,67,70] Particular note is made of the spiral diaphyseal fracture because this fracture has erroneously become synonymous with abuse.[65] The spiral nature of the fracture indicates only that torque was a component of the stress applied, which resulted in fracture. The fracture is thought to occur when an infant is grabbed or shaken, with the extremity used as a handle. However, spiral

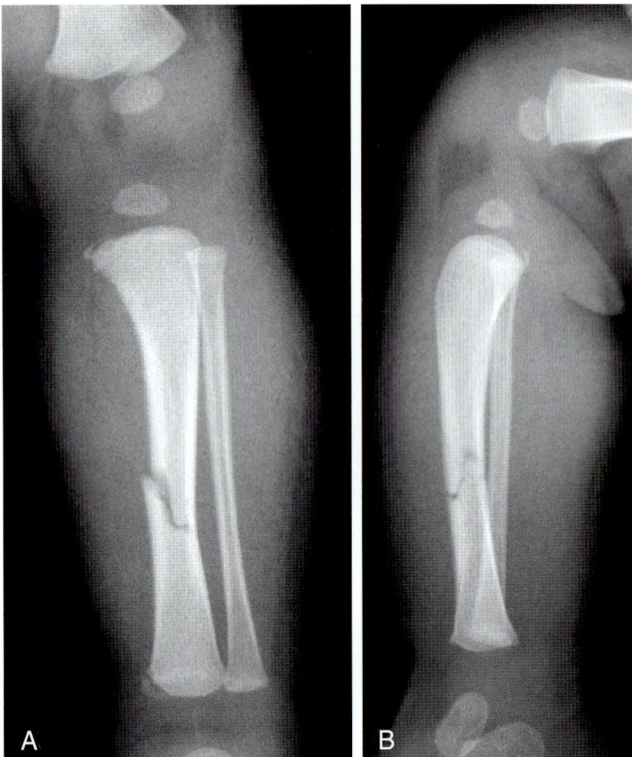

Figure 144-9 A 1-month-old female infant was brought to the emergency department for swelling of the leg without history of trauma. **A,** Anteroposterior view of the left leg. **B,** Lateral view of the left leg shows classic metaphyseal lesions at the proximal and distal tibia, as well as a short oblique mid-diaphyseal fracture. Multiple rib fractures and classic metaphyseal lesions of the right tibia were also discovered.

fractures also occur in a child who is ambulatory, and we now know that they may occur accidentally in younger infants. One mechanism was graphically illustrated and reported by Hymel and Jenny: a 5-month-old infant was being videotaped while lying prone and being rolled to a supine position by his 2-year-old sister; an extended upper extremity was unable to adduct and was pinned under the child as he rolled; an oblique humeral diaphyseal fracture was incurred.[71] It is important to consider whether the explanation offered and the developmental level of the child are appropriate, also considering the apparent age of the fracture at presentation and whether or not other injuries are apparent.

Fractures of the Scapula and Sternum

Any part of the skeleton may be traumatized from abuse. Although uncommon, fracture of the scapula, in particular the acromion, is highly specific for abuse (e-Fig. 144-14).[72] Acromial fracture results from abnormal indirect forces applied during shaking. It is usually accompanied by other bony thoracic trauma. Anatomic variants in the ossification of the acromion may present a diagnostic dilemma.[73,74] Follow-up radiographs taken to assess whether or not healing has occurred allow discrimination between fracture and ossification variant.

Fractures of the sternum are very uncommon in infants, including those who are abused.[72,75] Although Kleinman

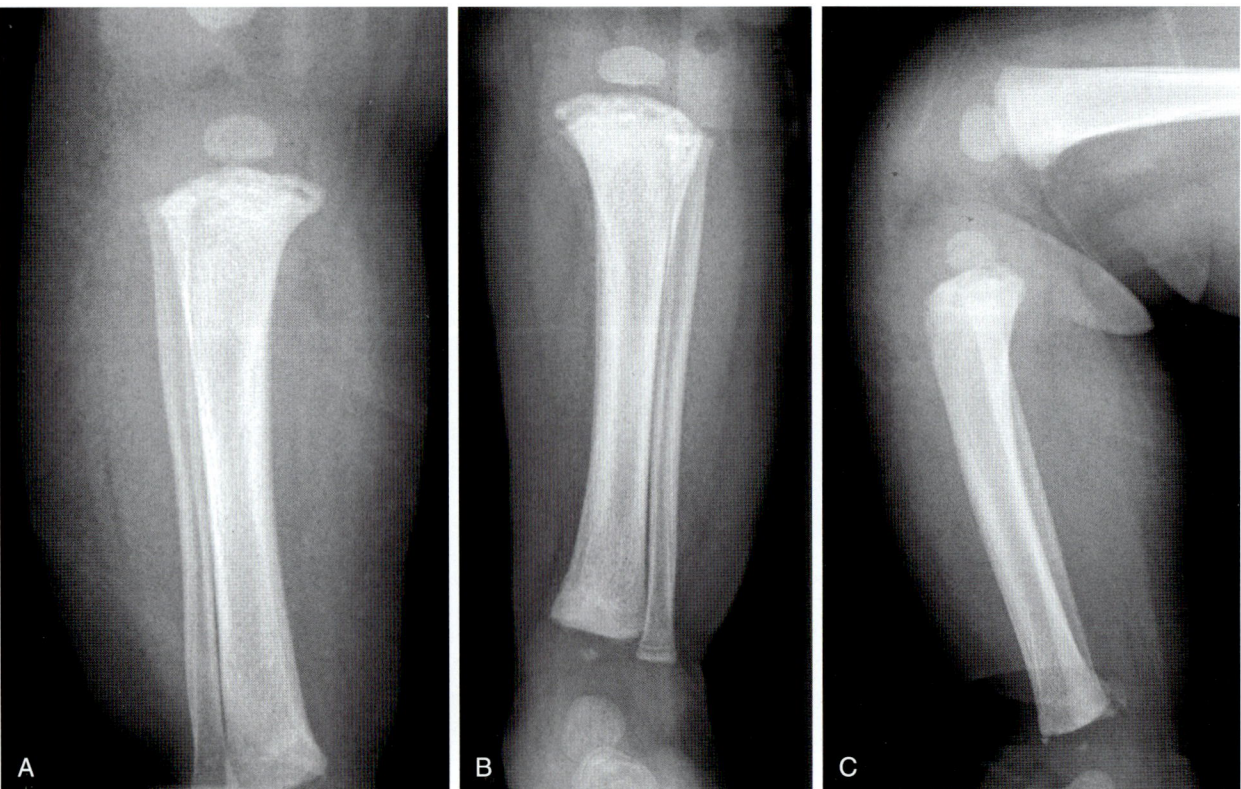

Figure 144-11 Anteroposterior right (**A**) and left (**B**) leg and lateral right (**C**) leg of 3-month-old male infant with an acute occipital skull fracture, classic metaphyseal lesions of the distal femora and proximal and distal tibias, and 23 rib fractures.

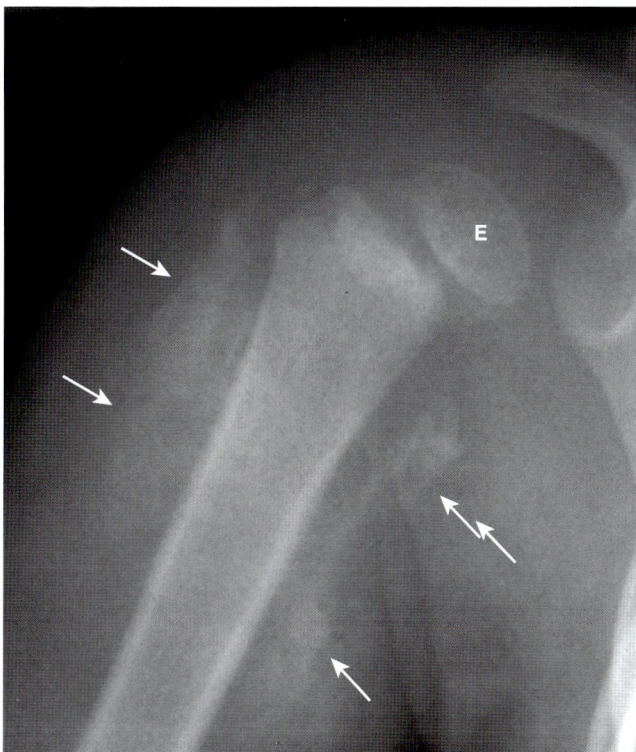

Figure 144-12 A 2-year-old girl with delayed diagnosis of a Salter I fracture of the proximal humerus. The epiphysis (*E*) is displaced medial relative to the proximal humeral metaphysis. A cloak of early callus and subperiosteal new bone is seen around the proximal humerus (*arrows*). The child presented with mental status changes caused by a head injury. This fracture and a subtler fracture of the left proximal humerus were noted on chest radiography after intubation. No other fractures were found on a skeletal survey. Follow-up radiographs demonstrated premature fusion of the right proximal humeral physis with marked shortening of humerus noted at age 6 years.

classifies sternal fractures as highly specific for child abuse, a recent series found these fractures less specific.[75]

Clavicle Fractures

Fractures of the clavicle (Fig. 144-15) are common in child abuse but are also common from accidental and birth trauma. Fractures of the clavicle are therefore considered to be of low specificity for child abuse. Clavicle fractures occur in 0.5% of newborns.[76] Frequently, a history of dystocia exists. It is not uncommon for such fractures to escape detection on the newborn physical examination.[77] Clavicle fractures from birth usually exhibit callus by 10 to 14 days after birth.[77] A fracture which appears acute, without visible callus, in a child older than 10 to 14 days therefore becomes suspicious for having been incurred after birth.

Spinal Fractures

Although rare, spinal fractures in infants and young children are strongly associated with abuse.[72,78-80] The mechanism is thought to be hyperextension, hyperflexion, axial loading, or all. Radiographically, these injuries manifest as compression deformities of the vertebral body, often with associated end plate defects and avulsive injuries of the spinous processes.[79] Fractures may result in listhesis.[80,81] Injuries often involve multiple adjacent vertebral bodies, most often located near the thoracolumbar junction (Fig. 144-16).[78,80]

Cervical spine fractures are fortunately uncommon in child abuse but may be devastating.[80] More severe

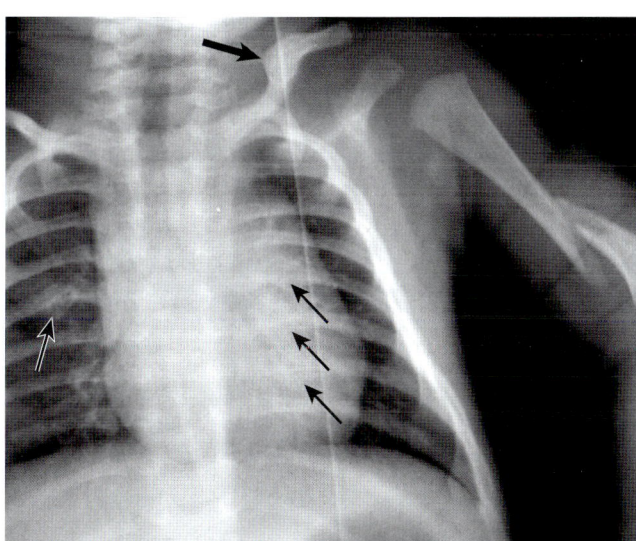

Figure 144-13 A 7-week-old boy with an acute left humeral fracture. The mechanism provided by history was suspect. Additional imaging demonstrated healing clavicular (large arrow) and posterior rib fractures (small arrows). While it is possible that the healing clavicle fracture is due to unrecognized birth trauma, the healing posterior rib fractures are not compatible with birth injury.

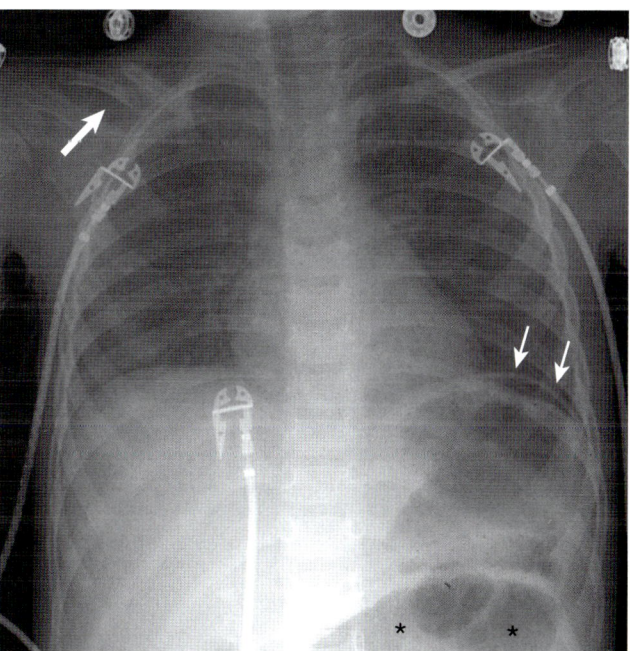

Figure 144-15 A 2-year-old boy with clavicle fracture. The child presented with fever and vomiting. Multiple bruises were noted. This chest radiograph demonstrated a healing, displaced right clavicle fracture with callus (*large arrow*), free air underneath the left hemidiaphragm (*small arrows*), and dilated small bowel in the left abdomen (*asterisks*). At surgery, multiple small bowel perforations were found.

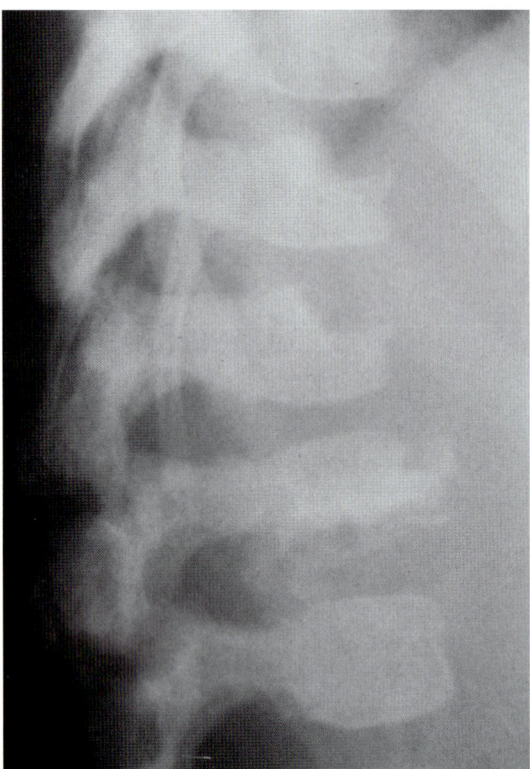

Figure 144-16 A 10-month-old girl with compression fractures of the T12, L1, and L2 vertebral bodies. She presented with paralysis of the lower extremities, and no history of trauma was initially provided. Unfortunately, the child did not recover lower extremity function.

fracture-dislocations have been described, including classic hangman's fracture of the C2 vertebra (e-Fig. 144-17).[82] Although spinal cord injury is uncommon, severe "spinal cord injury without radiographic abnormality" has been described in the shaken infant.[83,84]

Isolated spinous process fractures are considered highly specific for child abuse.[85] Avulsions may be caused by hyperflexion with axial loading or shaking.

Skull Fractures

Skull fractures are frequent in abuse and are indicative of an impact injury. Poor correlation has been shown between the presence of fracture and associated intracranial injury.[86,87] Skull fractures also commonly result from true accidental injury. Several authors have tried to characterize specific patterns of injury that occur in abuse, thereby distinguishing abuse skull fractures from true accidental skull fractures. Some agreement has been expressed that multiple fractures, bilateral fractures, diastasis of fractures and sutures, and fractures that cross suture lines are significantly associated with abuse (Fig. 144-18).[88-90] However, no particular pattern of skull fracture is diagnostic of abuse.[91] Bilateral complex fractures that cross the sagittal suture may result from a single high-impact blow to the midline, and simple linear fractures are seen in abuse and in accidental trauma. One must consider the appropriateness of the history with respect to the type of injury to make the distinction between abuse and

accidental trauma. Simple linear skull fractures are considered to be of low specificity for child abuse.[24] Such fractures are common in short-distance falls onto a hard surface. Other, more complex skull fractures are not expected from short-distance falls in the home environment and are thus considered to be of moderate specificity.[24] Soft tissue swelling is seen with acute fractures; lack of soft tissue swelling suggests that a fracture is not acute.[92] Diastatic fractures or widened skull sutures may indicate a space occupying process within the cranium such as diffuse swelling or large subdural hematoma (Fig. 144-19).

Anteroposterior and lateral skull radiographs are part of the radiographic skeletal survey in suspected abuse, and additional views may be necessary. A Townes view is helpful to evaluate the occipital bone and look for wormian bones in the sutures. Wormian bones are accessory intrasutural bones associated with metabolic bone disease, most notably osteogenesis imperfecta and Menke syndrome.[93] CT alone is inadequate to assess for skull fractures because fractures in the axial plane may be difficult to detect. CT may be indicated to evaluate for suspected intracranial injury; bone window images should be evaluated for signs of skull and other fractures; extracranial soft tissue swelling is also well delineated.

Accessory sutures of the skull may mimic fractures on both radiography and CT. Findings suggesting a fracture are a sharp linear lucency with nonsclerotic edges, widening of the lucency approaching a suture, crossing of a suture, unilaterality or asymmetry, and associated soft tissue swelling.[94] Findings suggesting an accessory suture are a zigzag pattern with sclerotic borders merging with an adjacent suture, bilaterality and symmetry, and lack of associated soft tissue swelling.[94] Accessory sutures tend to occur at characteristic locations.

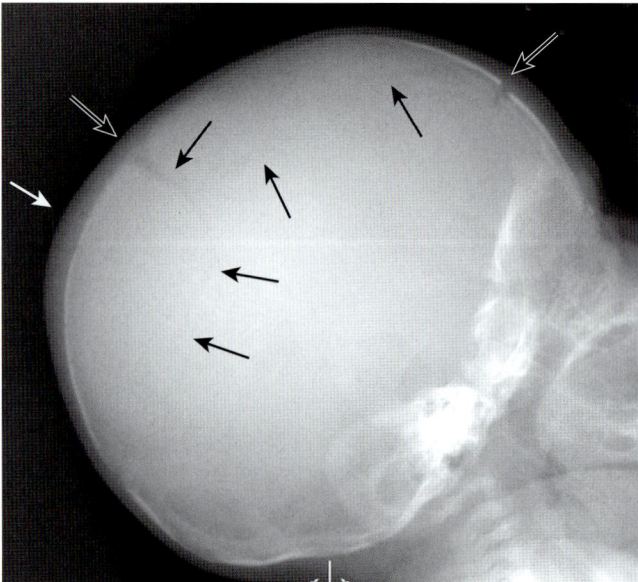

Figure 144-18 A 2-month-old female with complex skull fractures of the involving the right frontal bone and both parietal bones (*open and black arrows*). Extracranial soft tissue swelling is noted (*white arrow*). The child presented to the emergency room with facial bruising. Small bilateral subdural hematomas were found on computed tomography. Multiple healing rib fractures and metaphyseal fractures (classic metaphyseal lesions) were found on skeletal survey.

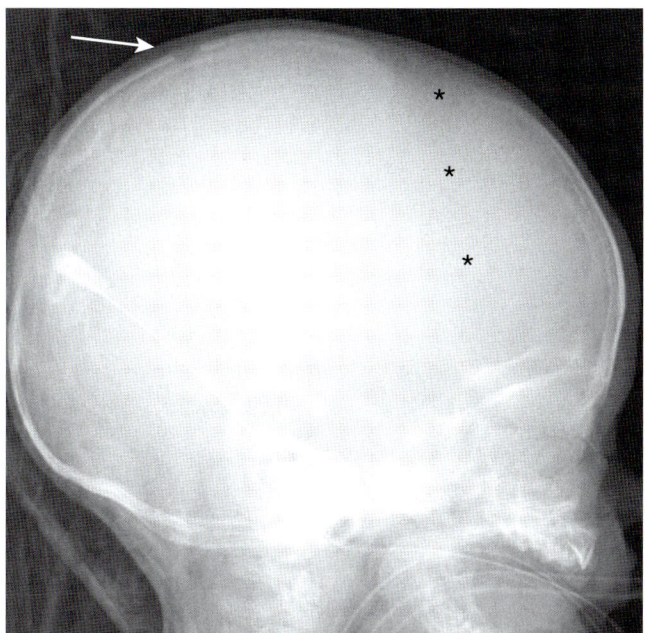

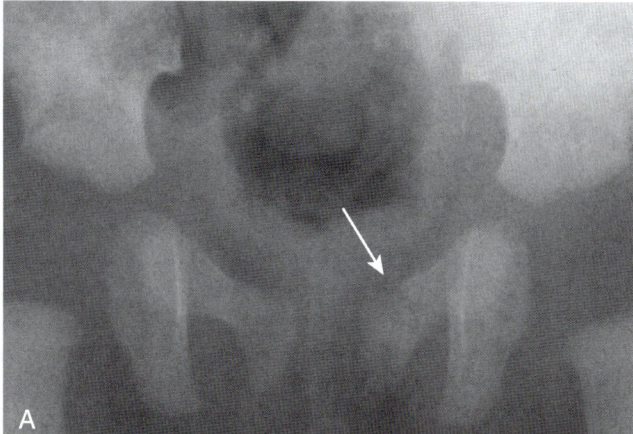

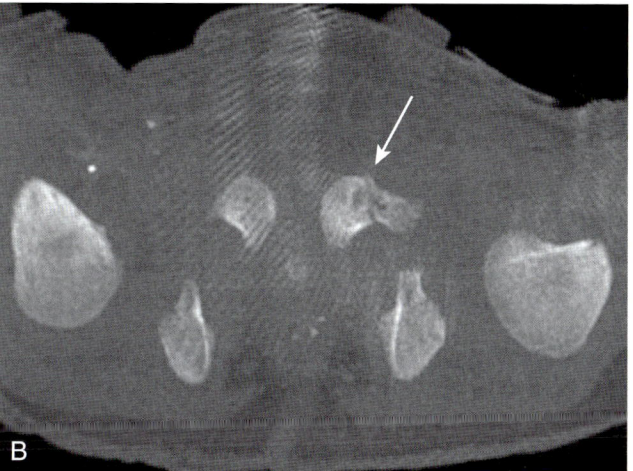

Figure 144-19 A 3-month-old boy with a mildly diastatic parietal skull fracture (*arrow*) and splayed coronal sutures (*asterisks*). Computed tomography showed large bilateral subdural hematomas.

Figure 144-20 A 1-month-old boy presented with failure to thrive and fever. A fracture of the left superior pubic symphysis (*arrows*) is seen on radiography (**A**) and axial bone algorithm computed tomographic (CT) image (**B**), reformatted from a CT scan of the abdomen and pelvis to evaluate for suspected visceral injury. He was also found to have subdural hematomas and healing rib fractures.

Fractures of the Pelvis

Fractures of the pelvic bones are uncommon in child abuse (Fig. 144-20).[95] Fractures of the pubic rami may occur from blunt trauma, particularly in cases of sexual abuse.[96] Variants in pubic ossification may mimic fracture.[97]

Fractures of Hands and Feet

Nonaccidental fractures of the hands and feet occur in abused infants and toddlers (Fig. 144-21).[98] These fractures are often subtle torus fractures and may be better appreciated on oblique views or follow-up radiographs.[98] Fractures of the tubular bones of the hands and feet are probably caused by squeezing by the hands of the abuser.

Dating of Fractures

Dating of fractures is dependent on many variables, including the age of the child, the state of nutrition, immobilization or lack thereof, repetitive injury, and fracture location.[99,100] Fractures of the skull and spine cannot be satisfactorily dated, and the classic metaphyseal lesion is difficult to date with any degree of precision.

In general, a young infant develops subperiosteal new bone much earlier and forms callus more quickly. The range for the appearance of subperiosteal new bone is 4 days to several weeks.[100] Soft tissue swelling resolves during this same period with subsequent loss of fracture line definition and the appearance of soft callus followed by hard callus. Although it is often possible to identify separate fractures as acute or subacute and others as healing, it is very difficult is ascribe different ages to fractures which are healing. Remodeling of

fractures occurs over a span of months to years. Precise dating of fractures is not possible and speculation of fracture age is merely an estimate. Some general guidelines are provided in Table 144-1 (Fig. 144-22).[99,100]

Differential Diagnosis

The differential diagnosis for child abuse is broad and varies considerably, depending on both the clinical presentation and the radiologic findings (Box 144-3).[101,102] True accidental injury is not the only consideration. Unrecognized obstetric trauma may not be noted until days or weeks after birth. Normal processes including metaphyseal variants, physiologic new bone formation, accessory ossification centers, and accessory skull sutures may initially suggest an abuse-related lesion.[103,104] Iatrogenic injury may mimic abuse–related injury.[42,44,46,58,59,105]

Metabolic bone disease of prematurity may result in multiple rib fractures, diaphyseal fractures, and metaphyseal fractures.[106-108] Such fractures are typically buckle or transverse fractures, not classic metaphyseal lesions. Other disease processes, including inherited bone dysplasias, copper deficiency

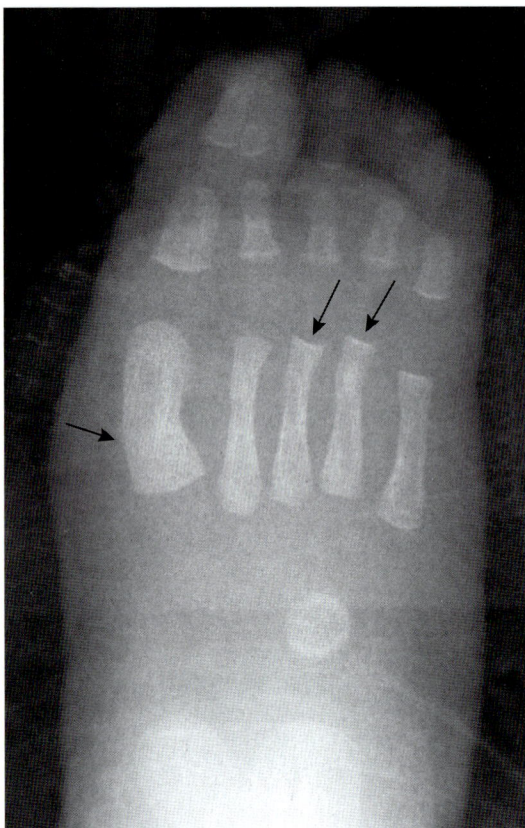

Figure 144-21 A 3-month-old girl with healing fractures of the first, third, and fourth metatarsals (*arrows*). Her twin sister also had metatarsal fractures. Both twins had rib fractures, classic metaphyseal lesions, and skull fractures.

Table 144-1

Timetable of Radiographic Changes in Children's Fractures*			
Finding	**Early**	**Peak**	**Late**
Resolution of soft tissue swelling	2-5 days	4-10 days	10-21 days
Subperiosteal new bone formation	4-10 days	10-14 days	14-21 days
Loss of fracture line definition	10-14 days	14-21 days	
Soft Callus	10-14 days	14-21 days	
Hard Callus	14-21 days	21-42 days	42-90 days
Remodeling	3 months	1 year	2 years to physeal closure

* Repetitive injuries may prolong the presence of findings.
From Kleinman PK. *Diagnostic imaging of child abuse.* 2nd ed. St Louis: Mosby; 1998.

(Menke syndrome), congenital syphilis, Caffey disease, neurologic disorders, and osteogenesis imperfecta may have radiographic features that overlap with those of abuse (see Box 144-3).[101,102,109-113] Most of these disorders are discussed individually in this text. Underlying fragility of the bones may, in turn, predispose some children to iatrogenic injury, which may mimic abuse.

Metaphyseal abnormalities similar to child abuse are seen with some rare skeletal dysplasias, notably spondylometaphyseal dysplasia, Sutcliffe ("corner fracture") type, and metaphyseal dysplasia, Schmid type.[114,115] In such patients, findings may be asymmetric. Clues as to the presence of a dysplasia include family history, short stature, and lack of change of the findings on follow-up radiographs.

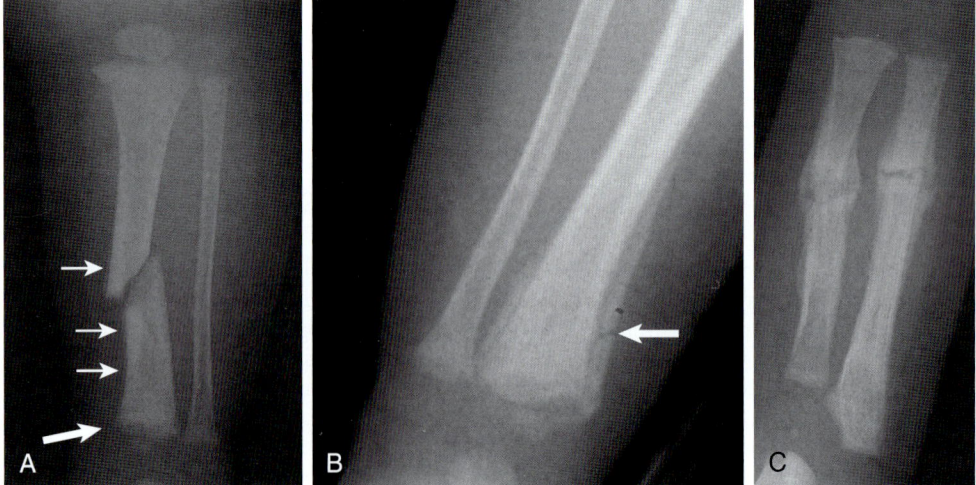

Figure 144-22 A 3-month old boy with multiple fractures of differing age. The child presented with left leg swelling. **A,** Radiograph of the left leg shows an acute or subacute oblique fracture of the left tibia. No ossified callus is seen; however, subperiosteal new bone (*arrows*) is present along the medial margin of the distal tibial, possibly unrelated to the oblique fracture. Irregularity of the distal metaphysis is suggestive of a preceding classic metaphyseal lesion, but not definitive. Soft tissue swelling is noted. **B,** Radiograph of the distal right leg shows a healing bucket handle fracture with associated distal tibial subperiosteal new bone indicative of an injury at least 10 to 14 days old. A fracture through the subperiosteal new bone (*arrow*) indicates injuries of different age. **C,** Transverse fractures of the left radius and ulna show a more advanced state of healing with abundant callus and indistinct, partially obliterated fracture lines. These fractures are clearly older than the oblique left tibial fracture. Images of the ribs showed multiple healing lateral and posterior rib fractures with mature callus.

Box 144-3 Radiographic Differential Diagnostic Considerations for Child Abuse

Trauma
- True accidental trauma
- Birth trauma
- Iatrogenic trauma

Variants of Ossification and Maturation
- Accessory acromial ossification center(s)
- Normal metaphyseal variants of development
- Accessory skull sutures
- Physiologic subperiosteal new bone
- Sternal ossification center (mimicking posterior rib fracture)

Metabolic Bone Disease
- Metabolic bone disease of prematurity
- Copper deficiency (Menke syndrome)
- Rickets
- Vitamin A toxicity

Dysplasia
- Osteogenesis imperfecta
- Metaphyseal and spondylometaphyseal dysplasia

Drug Induced
- Prostaglandin E_1 therapy

Neurogenic
- Spina bifida
- Congenital insensitivity to pain

Miscellaneous
- Caffey disease
- Congenital syphilis
- Neoplastic-metastatic round cell tumors

Kleinman's seminal text *Diagnostic Imaging of Child Abuse* presents an excellent overview of the differential diagnosis and a review of diseases that simulate abuse.[24] Fortunately, it is almost always possible to make an accurate determination as to the presence or absence of genetic disease on the basis of clinical and radiographic examination, along with a review of family and social history. It should be remembered that the presence of an underlying bone disease or dysplasia does not exclude the possibility of physical abuse or neglect.

With regard to the differential diagnosis of the radiographic findings of child abuse, two topics of recent controversy warrant mention—temporary brittle bone disease (TBBD) and vitamin-D deficiency.

TBBD was proposed as a variant of osteogenesis imperfecta by Paterson and colleagues, who identified a group of young infants who were thought to have diminished bone strength, possibly because of temporary deficiency of a metalloenzyme related to copper deficiency.[116] Evidence provided to support the existence of TBBD included denial by caregivers of wrongdoing, absence of episodes of trauma that may explain fractures, lack of bruising, absence of systemic injury, radiographs revealing normal bones, and normal laboratory studies.[116] The purported evidence and the particular diagnosis of TBBD has been refuted by others, including the authors of a critical review of TBBD prepared by the Committee on Child Abuse of the Society for Pediatric Radiology.[113,117,118]

To date, no scientific proof definitively supports the existence of TBBD.

More recently, fractures consistent with abuse have been ascribed to vitamin D deficiency by some authors.[119] While literature supports a high prevalence of infants with low vitamin D levels, the authors did not provide evidence of predisposing low vitamin D levels in their patients or convincing evidence as to the causation of the fractures related to low vitamin D levels.[120] Currently, no evidence exists in the literature to support low levels of vitamin D predisposing children to the high-specificity lesions characteristic of child abuse.[121] It is true, however, that infants and young children with frank rickets caused by vitamin D deficiency are at risk for fracture; however, the pattern of such fractures differs from the high-specificity classic metaphyseal lesions and posterior rib fractures seen with abuse.[122]

Treatment Treatment of the individual patient with abuse-related injuries is dictated by the injuries that are present. Injuries to the brain, spinal cord, and viscera may be life threatening. Brain and spinal cord injuries may cause substantial lifelong morbidity. Treatment is aimed at preserving the life of the child and limiting permanent morbidity. Fortunately, most skeletal injuries heal without permanent sequelae, with fractures of the growth plate being an occasional exception.

Intracranial trauma is the leading cause of death and permanent morbidity in abused infants. It has been nearly 40 years since Caffey proposed his theory on the shaking of infants.[123] In contrast to true accidental head injury, the neurologic deficits that occur in shaken baby syndrome are out of proportion to the degree of physical trauma and to the changes evident on CT and MRI. Debate is ongoing about whether or not shaking alone is sufficient to result in brain injury or whether an impact injury must accompany the shaking event.[124] Apnea and cerebral hypoxia also play a role.

Infants with shaken baby syndrome commonly have subdural hematomas, retinal hemorrhages, and characteristic skeletal injuries (posterior rib fractures and classic metaphyseal lesions). The presence of these osseous lesions is an indication for brain imaging (CT, if emergently indicated; MRI, for more detailed evaluation) and for ophthalmologic evaluation of the eyes for retinal hemorrhage. Retinal hemorrhages are present in 80% to 85% of shaken babies.[125]

Reporting of suspected child abuse is mandated by law. Failure to report suspected child abuse may result in fines, censure, and even prosecution. Radiologists should be aware of the legal requirements and mechanisms for reporting in their state. Fortunately, in nearly every case, responsible treating clinicians or child protection team personnel will take ownership of this task. Nevertheless, the radiologist bears responsibility for reporting if he or she suspects child abuse and no one else reports it.

Imaging findings are just one piece of the clinical, social, and legal investigation of possible child abuse. The radiologist must function as part of the child protection team by providing timely and accurate interpretations that are properly communicated, by providing expertise on the significance of the radiologic findings, and by providing guidance as the utility of additional imaging studies. Radiology reports should be complete, precise, and must appropriately consider the specificity of the findings and the possibility of differential diagnoses. Verbal communications of the report should be properly documented. Proper wording and careful editing of reports avoids embarrassment or confusion in court.

Radiologists are frequently called upon to testify in civil and criminal court proceedings related to cases of suspected child abuse. If called to testify, it is the duty of the radiologist to do so in a professional manner, providing only honest opinions based on personal experience and scientific evidence. Theoretical considerations with no scientific basis have no place in the court room.

WHAT THE CLINICIAN NEEDS TO KNOW

- Presence of injuries requiring emergent management
- Presence or absence or radiographic findings suggesting child abuse
- Specificity of individual findings for child abuse
- Specificity of the constellation of findings for child abuse
- Differentiation of child abuse injury from other processes which may radiographically mimic child abuse, may require treatment, or both
- Recommendations for further imaging

Key Points

The radiologist is occasionally the first to suggest the diagnosis of child abuse.

No one radiographic finding is pathognomonic for child abuse.

Individual radiographic findings may be of low, moderate, or high specificity for child abuse.

The constellation of radiographic findings may bear greater specificity than any one finding.

Many different normal processes, diseases and dysplasias may mimic child abuse radiographically.

Suggested Readings

Carty H. Non-accidental injury: a review of the radiology. *Eur Radiol.* 1997;7:1365-1376.

Dwek JR. The radiographic approach to child abuse. *Clin Orthop Relat Res.* 2011;469:776-789.

Kleinman PK. *Diagnostic imaging of child abuse.* 2nd ed. St. Louis, MO: Mosby; 1998.

Lonergan GJ, Baker AM, Morey MK, et al. From the archives of the AFIP. Child abuse: radiologic-pathologic correlation. *Radiographics.* 2003;23:811-845.

Offiah A, van Rijn RR, Perez-Rossello JM, et al. Skeletal imaging of child abuse (non-accidental injury). *Pediatr Radiol.* 2009;39:461-470.

References

Full references for this chapter can be found on www.expertconsult.com.

Chapter 145

Sports Medicine

J. HERMAN KAN

In the United States, greater than 30 million (approximately one third) of school-aged children participate in organized sports.[1] Sports-related injuries occur more frequently in the lower extremities compared with the upper extremities. This section will review acute and chronic sports injury patterns with an emphasis on entities that are unique in children. This section will cover multimodality imaging and emphasize important magnetic resonance imaging (MRI) features related to pediatric sports injuries. Acute fractures and dislocations are covered in Chapter 143.

Avulsion Injuries and Muscle Injuries

Etiology Avulsion injuries or fractures may occur at muscle attachments to an apophysis or at ligamentous attachments to a chondro-osseous junction.

The musculoskeletal unit of the child is composed of the apophysis, tendon, myotendinous junction, and muscle belly. In the skeletally mature patient, the weakest component of the musculoskeletal unit is the myotendinous junction. In the skeletally immature patient, particularly during periods of rapid growth, the cartilaginous physeal equivalent region of the apophysis is the weakest component of the musculoskeletal unit.[2] As a consequence, apophyseal avulsion injuries (Fig. 145-1), rather than myotendinous tears, may occur when the musculoskeletal unit is stressed.

Apophyseal injuries are more frequent in the lower extremity than in the upper extremity. In the lower extremity, the pelvis and knee are the most common sites for apophyseal avulsion injuries.[3] Ligamentous avulsion injuries similarly are more common in the lower extremity than in the upper extremity.

After the apophysis, the next weakest component of the musculoskeletal unit is the myotendinous junction. Muscle tears most commonly occur at the myotendinous junctions. Myotendinous tears are an acute event during a physical activity in which a child can pinpoint the time (within seconds) in which the injury occurred. This should be differentiated from delayed onset muscle soreness (DOMS). DOMS is not related to a single event but may be caused by an activity with repetitive eccentric and concentric muscle contractions with no acute pain at the time of the activity. Instead, symptoms and pain usually are felt the following day after the activity.[4]

Imaging In the acute setting, the displaced avulsion fracture fragment is present without proliferative callus formation present (see Fig. 145-1). During healing, proliferative callus will be seen, suggesting its subacute or chronic nature.

When radiographs are negative and no displaced fragment exists, an MRI scan may be obtained. MRI may demonstrate subtle edema of the apophysis and metaphyseal equivalent bone, physeal equivalent edema and widening, and adjacent soft tissue edema (e-Fig. 145-2). The term *fracture* should be used only when a linear displaced or nondisplaced fracture is present. When edema alone is present within the apophysis and adjacent soft tissues, the term *avulsion injury* should be used.

MRI may also demonstrate avulsion injuries and fractures at the level of the chondro-osseous junction (Fig. 145-3).

MRI is preferred for delineating the remainder of the musculoskeletal unit. When muscle edema is present related to trauma, three possible etiologies exist: (1) DOMS (Fig. 145-4), (2) direct muscle contusion (e-Fig. 145-5), and (3) myotendinous muscle tear (Fig. 145-6) (Table 145-1). With DOMS, MRI shows diffuse edema on fluid sensitive sequences without discrete fiber disruption. Direct muscle contusions shows similar changes to DOMS but are more focal in nature when injury is mild, with discrete fiber disruption and hematoma formation when the injury is severe. In the setting of muscle hematomas, these may mimic an intramuscular abscess. Gadolinium-enhanced, T1-weighted, fat-saturated imaging may demonstrate rim enhancement for both hematomas and intramuscular abscess. T1-weighted imaging without gadolinium may demonstrate T1-weighted hyperintense foci related to blood products and may suggest muscle hematoma and less likely intramuscular abscess with proteinaceous content. Myotendinous muscle tears may range from partial, with only some fibers disrupted at the level of the aponeurosis, to complete disruption with muscle fiber and aponeurosis retraction.

Treatment and Follow-up Treatment varies, depending on the location of the apophyseal avulsion injury. In the pelvis, the majority of apophyseal avulsion injuries are treated conservatively with rest. Surgical reduction and fixation may be necessary when the avulsed fracture fragment is greater than 2 cm.[3] During the healing phase, radiographs may be helpful to monitor callus formation and healing. Apophyseal avulsion fractures elsewhere are usually treated conservatively, and

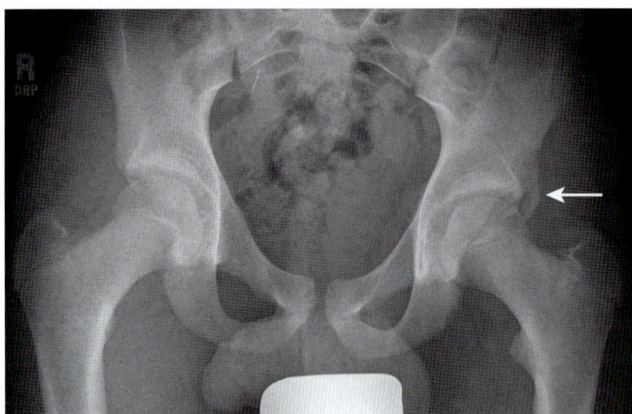

Figure 145-1 A 15-year-old boy with left anteroinferior iliac spine avulsion fracture (*arrow*) related to the rectus femoris origin.

surgical reduction is based on degree of apophyseal displacement. For instance, medial epicondylar avulsion fractures are treated surgically when the displaced fragment is greater than 5 mm.[5]

Myotendinous tears are treated conservatively with 2 to 3 weeks of rest before returning to sport activities.[4] DOMS is also treated conservatively and symptoms usually resolve within a week.

Hyperextension Injuries of the Knee

Etiology The anterior compartment of the knee is composed of the quadriceps tendon, patellar bone, patella tendon, and tibial tuberosity. Patellar bone is a sesamoid equivalent for the quadriceps mechanism. Acute forceful concentric or eccentric contraction of the quadriceps muscle may lead to acute avulsion injuries of the inferior patellar pole (chondro-osseous avulsion injury, patellar sleeve fractures) and tibial tuberosity (apophyseal avulsion injury), as well as tendinopathy of the patella tendon. *Sinding-Larsen-Johansson disease* is the term used for chronic avulsive injuries affecting the inferior patellar pole. *Osgood-Schlatter disease* is the equivalent

Table 145-1

Magnetic Resonance Imaging Appearance and Grading of Myotendinous Tears	
Grade 1	Edema at the myotendinous junction
Grade 2	Partial tearing at the myotendinous junction
Grade 3	Complete tear at the myotendinous junction with tendon retraction

injury affecting the tibial tuberosity.[1] When only a patella tendon tear is present, it is called *jumper's knee* and tends to occur in patients who are skeletally mature. Sinding-Larsen-Johansson and Osgood-Schlatter diseases usually occur during adolescence and often affect both knees. Bone and tendon injuries often may occur in the same knee.

Imaging Although imaging is helpful for the diagnosis of Sinding-Larsen-Johansson and Osgood-Schlatter diseases, the diagnosis for these chronic conditions is made clinically with radiographic confirmation of findings, not by imaging alone. Advanced imaging confirms the diagnosis and excludes alternative etiologies. MRI should not be performed routinely on these patients if radiography and clinical diagnosis confirm the disease.

Patellar sleeve fractures represent an acute avulsion fracture located along the inferior pole of the patella. This occurs at the chondro-osseous junction of the patella tendon origin. On radiography and MRI, a small linear or curvilinear fleck of bone may be identified (Fig. 145-7). On MRI, edema of the patellar bone, edema in the superior aspect of Hoffa's fat pad, and peripatellar edema are often present in the acute setting. This should be differentiated from chronic repetitive avulsive injuries to the inferior patellar pole leading to Sinding-Larsen-Johansson disease. With Sinding-Larsen-Johansson disease, the inferior patellar bone has had time to remodel related to chronic avulsive injury. Therefore, on radiography and MRI, well-formed variable size ossicles may be seen (Fig. 145-8). On MRI, edema within the inferior pole ossicles is related to the acute or chronic nature of the injury.

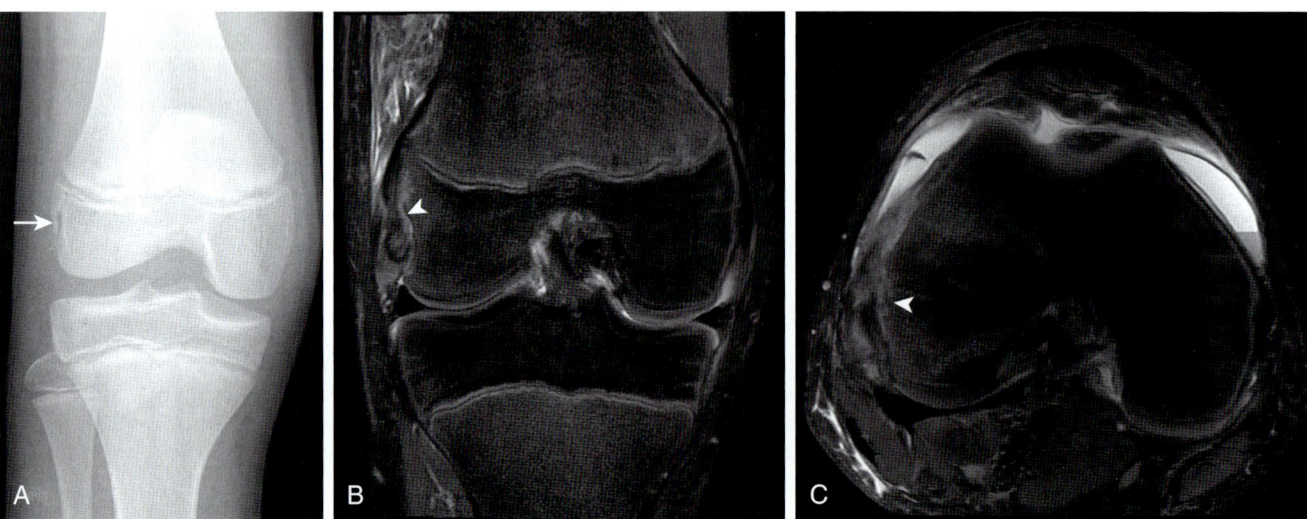

Figure 145-3 A 13-year-old boy with a popliteus origin chondro-osseous avulsion fracture (*arrow*). **A,** An anteroposterior knee radiograph. **B,** Proton density fat-saturated coronal image. **C,** Proton density fat suppression axial image demonstrates chondro-osseous fracture line (*arrowhead*).

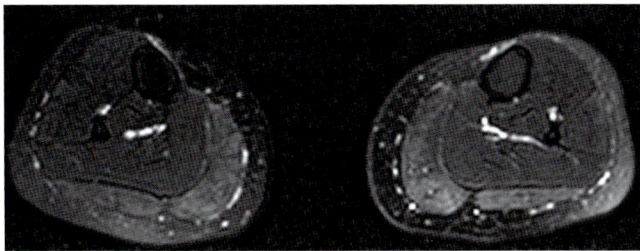

Figure 145-4 A short tau inversion recovery axial image of bilateral calves in an adolescent child with bilateral gastrocnemius myositis consistent with delayed onset muscle soreness.

Acute tibial tuberosity avulsion fractures results from forceful contraction of the patella tendon leading to a tibial tuberosity–sided linear or curvilinear avulsion fracture fragment at the level of the chondro-osseous junction (Fig. 145-9) or to uplifting of the entirety of the tibial tuberosity, with resultant Salter-Harris type injury with physeal equivalent widening (Fig. 145-10). On MRI, often, edema is seen within the tibial tuberosity, and this may extend posteriorly to involve the remainder of the tibial epiphysis. Inferior Hoffa's fat pad and pretibial edema are often present. These changes should be differentiated from chronic repetitive avulsive injury affecting the tibial tuberosity and leading to Osgood-Schlatter disease. With Osgood-Schlatter disease, rather than linear avulsion fracture fragments, the tibial tuberosity and tibial tuberosity avulsion fragments have had time to remodel. Therefore, on radiography and MRI, well-formed variable size well-corticated ossicles may be seen (e-Fig. 145-11). On MRI, edema within the avulsed separate ossicles and tibial tuberosity are present and are related to the acute or chronic nature of the injury. In addition, edema within Hoffa's fat pad and pretibial edema are often present as well.

Patella tendinopathy and patellar tears (e-Fig. 145-12) may be evaluated by ultrasonography or MRI. On MRI, thickening of the tendon with longitudinally or transversely oriented tears may be seen as well as edema within the prepatellar soft tissues and Hoffa's fat pad. MRI diagnosis of jumper's knee should ideally be made on longer echo time sequences to avoid "magic angle artifact."

Treatment and Follow-up Sinding-Larsen-Johansson disease, Osgood-Schlatter disease, and jumper's knee are all treated conservatively with rest. When displaced, acute avulsion fractures of the inferior patellar pole or tibial tuberosity may be treated by open reduction with patellar tendon reconstruction, particularly if patella alta is also present.[6] For avulsion fractures, care should be made to determine if the fracture is complete, incomplete, displaced, or nondisplaced. If the avulsion fracture is incomplete (see Fig. 145-9), affected children may benefit from conservative nonsurgical treatment.

Patellar Dislocation and Patellofemoral Dysplasia

Etiology The patella is a sesamoid equivalent bone of the quadriceps mechanism. Patellar bone has two primary facets: medial and lateral. The lateral facet is usually the dominant and larger facet, and articulates with the lateral aspect of the trochlear fossa. Patellar bone lies within the concave shaped femoral trochlear fossa. With knee flexion, the patella will concentrically locate within the trochlear fossa. With knee extension, patellar bone preferentially subluxes laterally in patients with or without underlying patellofemoral dysplasia because the lateral patellofemoral articulation is shallow compared with the medial articulation and the vastus lateralis activates when the knee is extended.

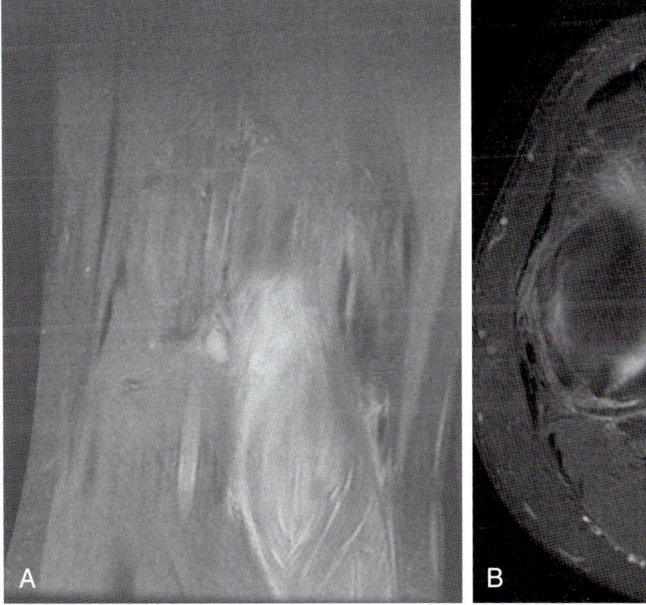
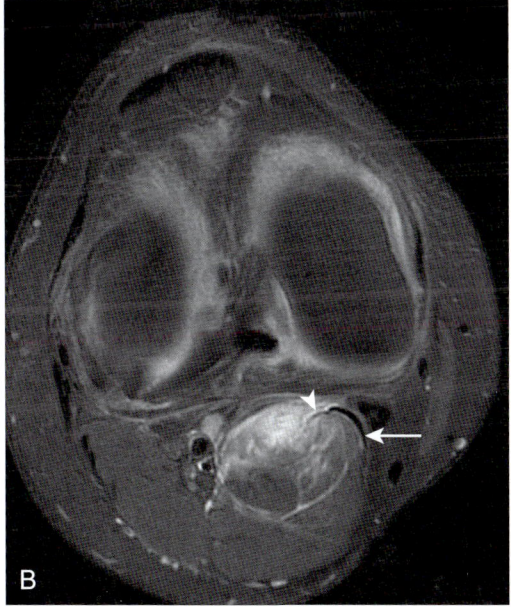

Figure 145-6 **A,** A proton density fat suppression coronal image shows partial myotendinous tear of the medial head of the gastrocnemius muscle. **B,** A proton density fat suppression axial image shows intact aponeurosis (*arrow*) and a partially torn, wavy aponeurosis (*arrowhead*) with infiltrative muscle edema.

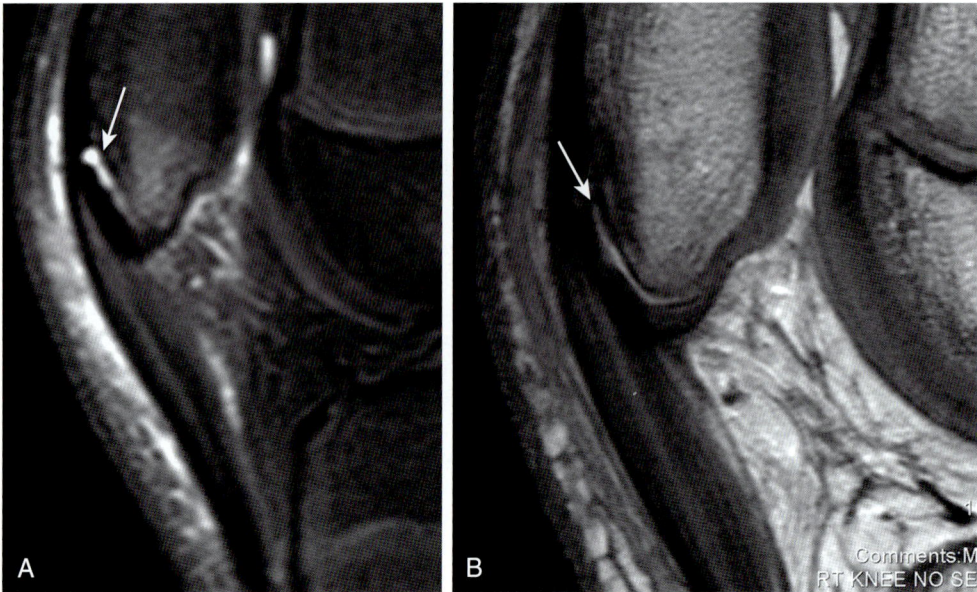

Figure 145-7 **A,** A T2-weighted fat suppression sagittal image. **B,** Proton density sagittal image in a 12-year-old boy with a nondisplaced acute, inferior pole patellar sleeve fracture (*arrows*).

Multiple variables may predispose a patient to patellar dislocation. This includes a large Q-angle, muscle imbalance with dominant vastus lateralis musculature, patella alta, rotational abnormalities of the tibia and femur, and overall ligamentous laxity. The Q-angle is calculated by the angle derived from the intersection of two lines: (1) center of patella and anterosuperior iliac spine and (2) center of patella and tibial tuberosity. The normal Q-angle measures

approximately 15 degrees. The Q-angle is usually larger in females. Larger Q-angles direct the quadriceps muscle vector force on the patella laterally. Patella alta occurs when the ratio of patellar tendon length to patellar bone length is greater than 1:2. Patellar bone captures within the trochlear groove with knee flexion. In the setting of patella alta, it takes

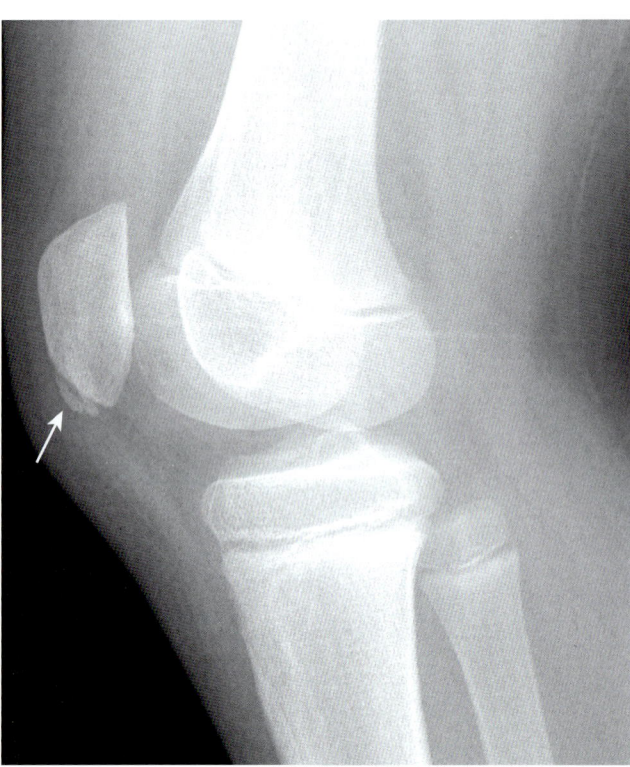

Figure 145-8 A lateral radiograph of the knee demonstrates variable-sized, well-corticated ossicles (*arrow*) consistent with Sinding-Larsen-Johansson disease.

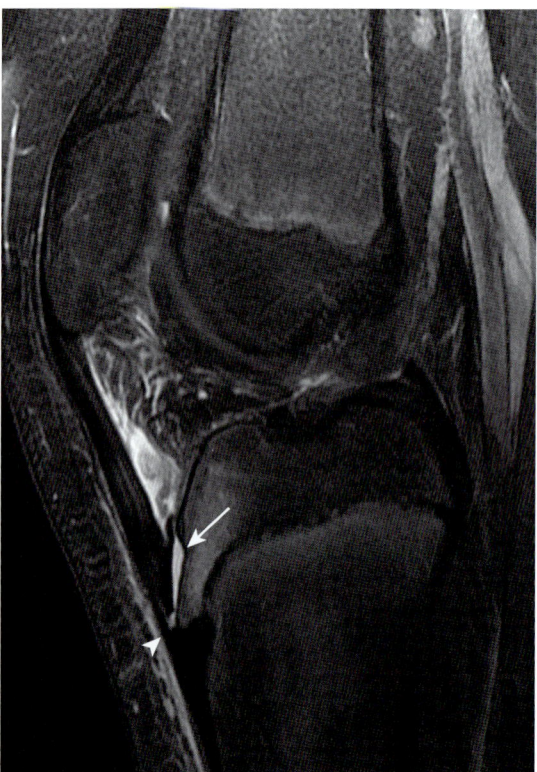

Figure 145-9 A T2-weighted fat suppression sagittal image from a 13-year-old boy demonstrates an acute nondisplaced partial **tibial tuberosity avulsion fracture (*arrow*).** Note that some patella tendon fibers remain intact (*arrowhead*).

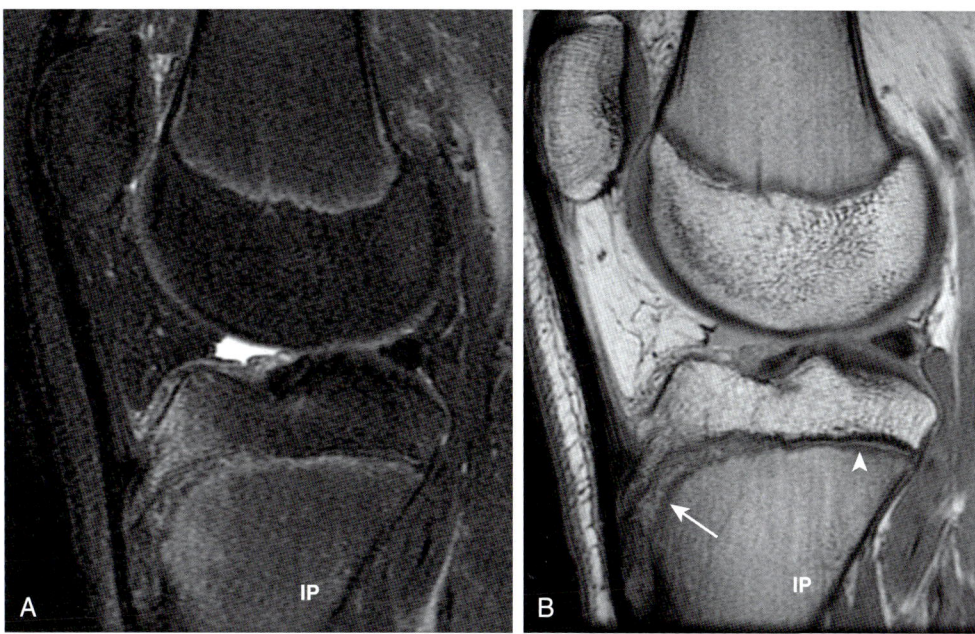

Figure 145-10 A 14-year-old girl with tibial tuberosity equivalent physeal widening. **A,** A T2-weighted fat suppression sagittal image demonstrates diffuse edema of the tibial tuberosity, physis, and deep metaphyseal equivalent region of the tibia. **B,** A proton density sagittal image delineates physeal equivalent widening of the tibial tuberosity (*arrow*). Note the physeal equivalent widening compared with the normal posteriorly located tibial physis (*arrowhead*).

relatively more knee flexion for the patellar bone to capture. Excessive external tibial torsion may also predispose a child to patellar dislocation, as well as increased femoral anteversion.[7,8] The normal degree of external tibial torsion is approximately 28 degrees at age 4 years and increases to approximately 38 degrees at skeletal maturity.[9] The normal degree of femoral anteversion is approximately 40 degrees at birth and approximately 15 degrees at skeletal maturity.

The earlier age first time patellar dislocation occurs, the higher is the incidence of recurrent patellar dislocation. This may be related to remodeling at the level of the patellofemoral joint after initial injury and laxity of the injured medial retinaculum.

Patellofemoral dysplasia may develop as a primary congenital anomaly or may occur as a secondary process. Secondary patellofemoral dysplasia may result from poor articulation at the level of the patellofemoral joint caused by muscle imbalance, as seen in cerebral palsy, or may secondarily develop from remodeling after traumatic patellar dislocation. To form a normal joint, the two opposing bones need to articulate with each other. Patellar bone and the trochlear fossa will not develop normally if they do not properly articulate with each other. Therefore, patients with secondary patellofemoral dysplasia may have had a normally appearing patellofemoral joint at birth, but over time, the joint becomes dysplastic because patellar bone does not properly articulate with the trochlear fossa. The earlier the age at the time of the first traumatic patellar dislocation, the more severe is the associated patellofemoral dysplasia.

Imaging Radiographs should be reviewed to identify loose bodies, subjective determination of patella alta, and patellofemoral dysplasia. The "sunrise view" is helpful to evaluate for patellar sleeve fractures for both acute (Fig. 145-13) and old injuries (e-Fig. 145-14). Acute patellar sleeve fractures are

sliverlike, whereas old injuries are round and corticated. These patellar sleeve fractures occur along the medial pole and are a result of avulsion injury at the medial retinacular attachment to the chondro-osseous junction of the medial patellar pole. The sunrise view is also useful for evaluating for patellofemoral dysplasia. Features suggesting patellofemoral dysplasia include a lateral dominant patellar facet and a flat or even convex appearing trochlear fossa. With progressive patellofemoral dysplasia, the trochlear fossa becomes more

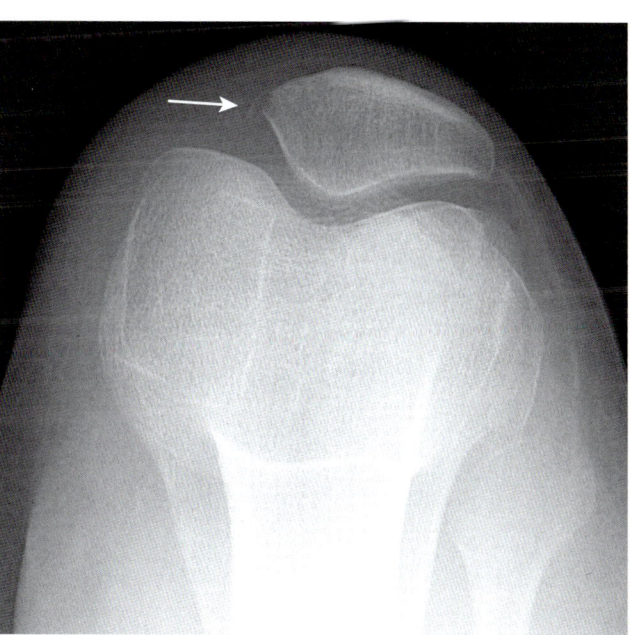

Figure 145-13 An 18-year-old with acute patellar dislocation, with acute, medial patellar sleeve fracture (*arrow*).

convex in appearance and the patellar bone loses its normal angular appearance.

The sunrise view should also be assessed for osteoarthritic changes of the patellofemoral joint. This view may also show lateral patellar tilt, patellar subluxation, or patellar dislocation. With regard to patellar location, the sunrise view may be misleading if not obtained with the knee in 30 degrees flexion. Knee flexion facilitates patella reduction, whereas knee extension may exaggerate patellar tilt and lateral patellar subluxation. When the knee sunrise view is obtained with less knee flexion, the trochlear fossa may appear shallow and should not be mistaken for patellofemoral dysplasia.

Computed tomography (CT) may be obtained in the workup of patellofemoral dysplasia. CT may be used to determine tibial and femoral version. As external tibial torsion and femoral anteversion increases, the child is at higher risk for patellar instability and tilt.[7,8] CT may also be performed with the knees at various degrees of flexion (e-Fig. 145-15). The patella locates with increasing knee flexion and subluxes with increasing knee extension. Three separate CT acquisitions are obtained at different degrees of knee flexion (e.g., 45, 30, and 15 degrees). If the patella dislocates at 15 degrees but is located at 45 and 30 degrees, it is considered a mild degree of patellar dislocation. However, if the patella dislocates at 30 or 45 degrees of knee flexion, it is a more severe degree of patellar dislocation. CT for patellar dislocation should also be used to evaluate the degree of patellofemoral dysplasia and secondary patellofemoral osteoarthritis, with changes similar to what may be seen on sunrise-view radiographs. Lateralization of the tibial tuberosity should also be determined. This represents the distance between the midpoint of the tibial tuberosity and the deepest component of the trochlear groove on axial slices. If the tibial tuberosity is

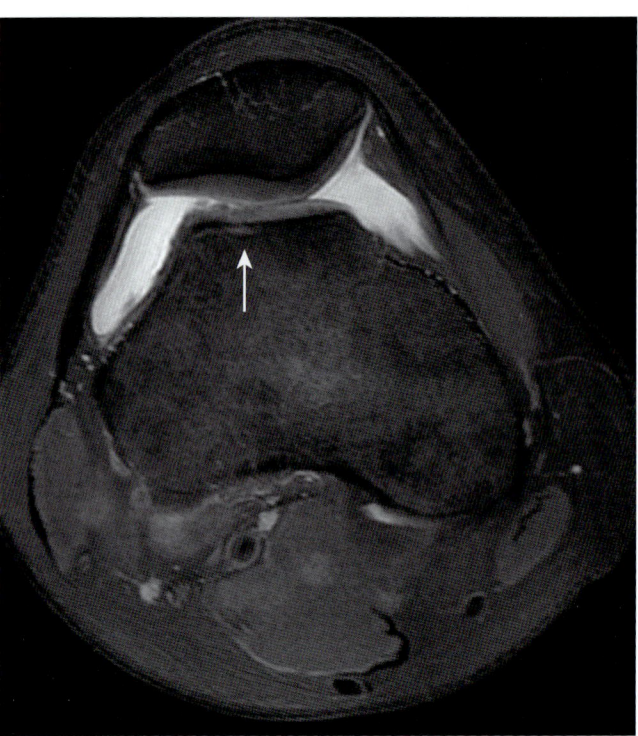

Figure 145-17 A 16-year-old boy with proton density fat suppression axial sequence imaging showing features of patellofemoral dysplasia with a flat (*arrow*) dysplastic trochlear fossa. The normal trochlear fossa has a concave shape.

greater than 2 cm lateral with respect to the trochlear groove, a higher incidence of patellar instability exists.[10]

MRI complements radiography and CT findings. Sometimes, children are referred for knee pain, and the diagnosis of patellar dislocation and patellofemoral dysplasia may be first suspected on MRI. On MRI for acute patellar dislocation, characteristic bone contusions may be seen along the medial patellar pole and anterolateral femoral condyle (Fig. 145-16). The bone contusions occur in relation to relocation of the patella after patellar dislocation. Other findings that may be seen include patellar sleeve fractures, medial retinacular tears, cartilage injuries, and loose bodies. Patellofemoral dysplasia (Fig. 145-17) and secondary degenerative changes should also be assessed by MRI.

Treatment and Follow-up Treatment for patellar dislocation should be approached from two perspectives: (1) treat biomechanical instability, which can be addressed by physical therapy and operative repair, and (2) treat mechanical symptoms related to sequelae from acute dislocation usually from loose bodies or chondral injuries.

Patients with first-time patellar dislocation and those with recurrent patellar dislocation are treated conservatively with physical therapy and bracing. The goal of treatment is to improve gluteal and vastus medialis muscle activity, which facilitates medial location of the patella.[10] Should physical therapy not improve symptoms, surgical repair should be considered, although no one effective surgical technique has been advocated in the literature. Surgical approaches include lateral retinacular release, medial retinacular repair and reconstruction, trochleoplasty (deepen the sulcus), tibial tubercle transfers (medialization of the tibial tubercle), as well as

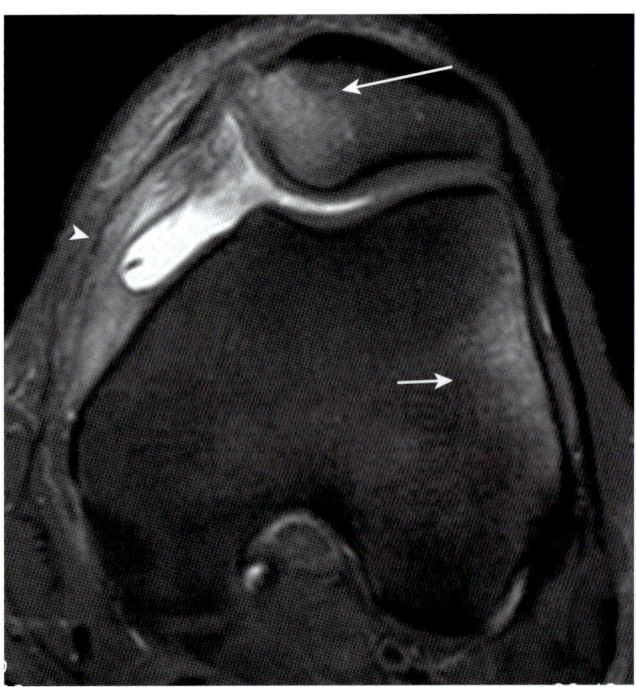

Figure 145-16 A 19-year-old with proton density fat suppression axial sequence imaging showing characteristic kissing contusions related to lateral patellar dislocation (*arrows*). Note partial tearing of the medial retinaculum (*arrowhead*) as well.

rotational osteotomies to treat excessive tibial torsion and femoral version. The surgical goal is to facilitate patellar bone capture by the trochlear fossa and medialization of patellar biomechanical vector forces.

When loose bodies or cartilage injury is identified and the child has mechanical symptoms such as locking, arthroscopy may be performed to remove the loose bodies and perform cartilage debridement to stabilize and smoothen the patello-femoral articulation.[10]

Anterior Cruciate Ligament Complex Injuries

Etiology The anterior cruciate ligament (ACL) complex is composed of the ACL, its femoral origin, and its tibial insertion. The femoral and tibial chondro-osseous attachments of the ACL complex are relatively weak in the skeletally immature, and are predisposed to chondro-osseous avulsion fractures.[11] Chondro-osseous avulsion fractures occur far more commonly at the tibial eminence insertion compared with the femoral origin. The ACL is composed of two fiber bundles: the anteromedial and posterolateral bundles, which extend from the medial aspect of the lateral femoral condyle to the level of the tibial eminence.[12] Coexisting full-thickness ACL tear and complete tibial eminence fractures are unusual since the force of injury usually is dissipated by either the ACL tear or the avulsion fracture. However, in most cases, arthroscopic evidence of ACL incomplete fiber tears is often present in the setting of a complete tibial eminence avulsion fracture. ACL tears are often seen in children with a narrow intercondylar notch, and ACL tibial eminence avulsion fractures tend to occur in children with a wider intercondylar notch.[13,14]

Multiple mechanisms of injury have been attributed as causes for ACL complex injuries in children, including varus or valgus stress, and twisting injuries of the knee. Risk factors include female gender, noncontact indirect injuries, and contact direct injuries (e.g., forceful blow to the lateral knee).

Imaging Radiographic findings that may indicate an ACL complex injury includes Segond (e-Fig. 145-18) and tibial eminence avulsion fractures (Fig. 145-19). A Segond fracture represents an anteromedial capsular avulsion fracture at the chondro-osseous junction of the lateral tibial plateau. Tibial eminence avulsion fractures should be categorized as a single bone avulsion fracture or comminuted, since this may affect treatment strategies. Because of ligamentous instability related to an ACL deficient knee, anterior translation of the tibia may be present on the lateral view.

On MRI, identification of complete disruption of the ACL should be confirmed on all three orthogonal planes (Fig. 145-20). ACL tears should be subcategorized as partial (rare) versus full-thickness tears (more common). Some of the additional features to suggest ACL complex injuries are bone contusions related to anterior translation and twisting of the tibia, including anteromedial or anterolateral femoral condylar bone contusions, with kissing posteromedial or posterolateral tibial plateau contusions (see Fig. 145-20). When bone contusions are evident, a T1-weighted or proton–density sequence is useful for determining is the presence of an underlying

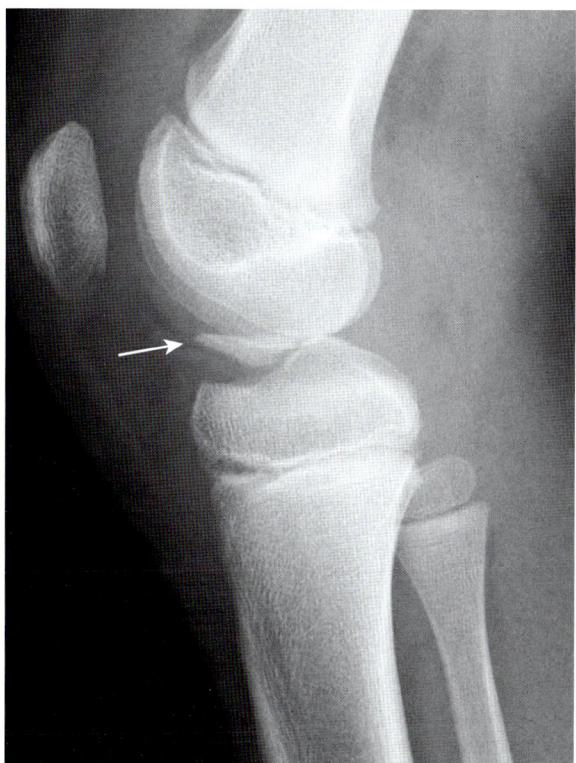

Figure 145-19 A 9-year-old boy with tibial eminence avulsion fracture (*arrow*).

subchondral fracture. When subchondral bone contusions are present, the presence or absence of overlying articular cartilage injury should be identified. Tibial eminence avulsion fractures are also demonstrated by MRI but are more readily identifiable on radiographs (see Fig. 145-19).

Additional findings on MRI include medial collateral ligament tears (e-Fig. 145-21) and meniscal tears. When describing medial collateral ligament tears, its location (femoral or tibial sided) must be identified and the presence of additional involvement of the medial meniscofemoral or medial meniscotibial ligament determined. Meniscal tears can be seen in up to 69% of ACL injuries in children (e-Fig. 145-22).[15] The most common location for meniscal tears is the posterior horn of the lateral meniscus.

Classification of meniscal tears includes vertical (see e-Fig. 145-22), horizontal (e-Fig. 145-23), displaced (Fig. 145-24), and location (red or white zone) types. Vertical tears by definition extend from the superior to inferior articular surface. They are subclassified into radial, longitudinal, or parrot-beak tears. Horizontal tears usually extend to only one articular surface and are usually degenerative in nature. Displaced tears include bucket handle tears (see Fig. 145-24) and displaced free fragment tears. Bucket handle tears by definition are vertical longitudinal tears.

Treatment and Follow-up Treatment for full-thickness ACL tears is surgical. The natural evolution of ACL deficient knees includes early osteoarthritis with cartilage injury and meniscal tears.[16] Diagnosing high-grade partial ACL tears should be approached with extreme caution, since partial ACL tears may heal nonsurgically with appropriate physical therapy and rest. High-grade partial ACL tears are surgically significant if

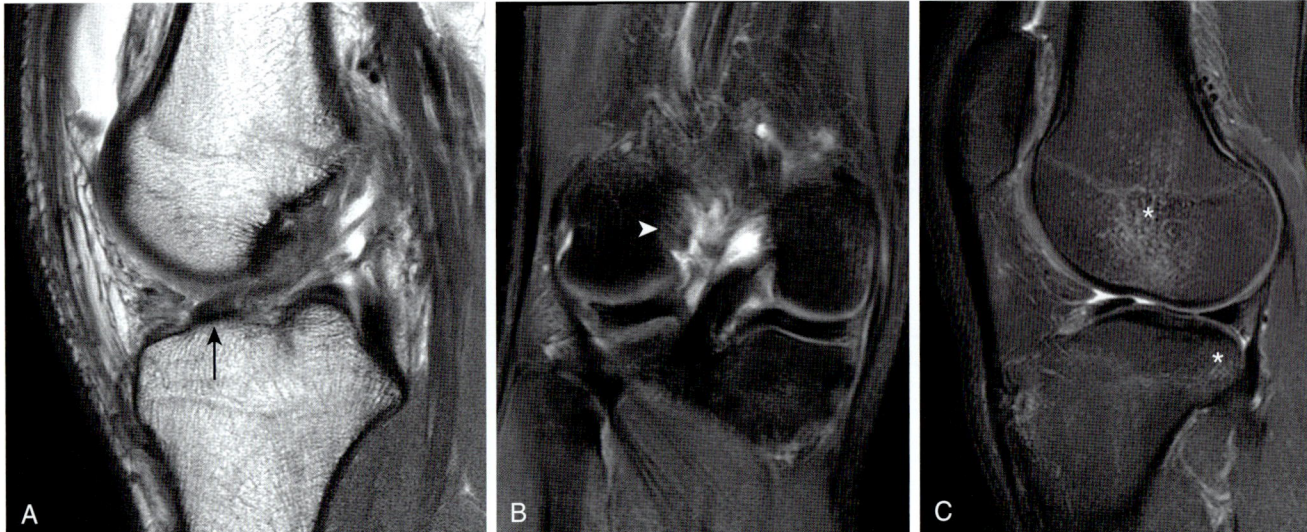

Figure 145-20 A 16-year-old boy with full thickness anterior cruciate ligament (ACL) tear. **A,** Proton density sagittal image demonstrates full-thickness tear of the ACL near its femoral origin with residual tibial insertion fibers (*arrow*). **B,** Proton density fat suppression coronal image demonstrates full-thickness tear with residual femoral origin ACL fibers (*arrowhead*). **C,** A T2-weighted fat suppression sagittal image demonstrates characteristic kissing contusion pattern related to ACL mechanism injury (*asterisk*).

clinical examination suggests an ACL deficient knee or progressive instability of the knee occurs after initial injury. Surgical treatment includes primary ACL or tibial eminence repair, with physeal sparing, transepiphyseal, and transphyseal approaches. Boys over age 16 years, girls age 14 years or older, or those at Tanner stage 5 with closed or near closed physes, can be treated with conventional adult methods for ACL reconstruction.[16] MRI is important presurgically to identify not only the ACL injury but also additional meniscal and cartilage injuries so that these areas can be repaired or débrided during ACL reconstruction.

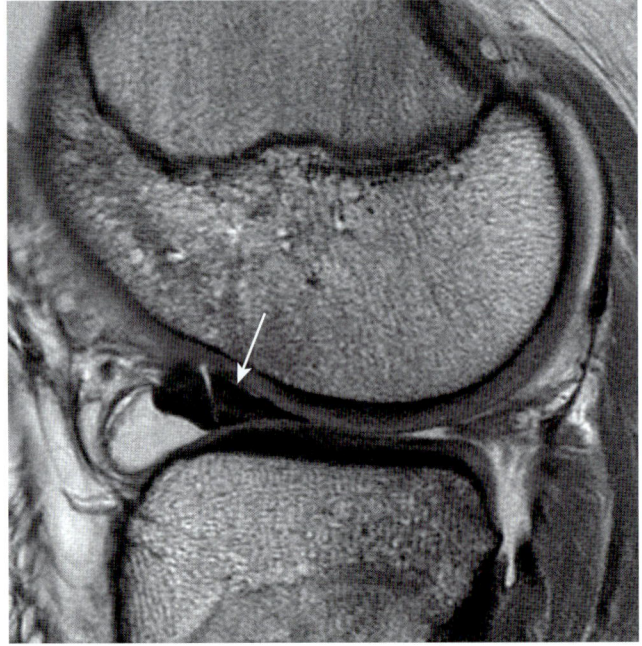

Figure 145-24 A 14-year-old girl with a lateral meniscus bucket handle tear. Proton density sagittal image shows that the posterior horn of the lateral meniscus has flipped anteriorly (*arrow*), leading to a double anterior horn sign.

Discoid Lateral Meniscus

Etiology Discoid menisci most frequently affect the lateral meniscus. This represents a congenital enlargement of the lateral meniscus with respect to the lateral tibiofemoral joint compartment. The relative disproportionate size of the lateral meniscus alters the biomechanics of the lateral tibiofemoral compartment and the meniscus is predisposed to tears and degeneration. The utilization of approximate coverage of the lateral joint space is preferred compared with reference measurement of meniscal size in children. Using the adult reference of 12 mm width for normal meniscal size may be inaccurate in children, particularly in preschoolers who present with suspected lateral discoid menisci.[17]

The Watanabe arthroscopic classification of discoid lateral menisci includes (1) complete, (2) incomplete, and (3) Wrisberg variant.[18] The Wrisberg variant is absence of normal posterior meniscocapsular fascicles and coronary ligaments, with the meniscofemoral ligament being the only attachment.[19] The discoid lateral meniscus subtype of the Wrisberg variant describes the lack of posterior meniscocapsular attachment only and is not predicated on lateral meniscal size. Type 1 and 2 discoid lateral menisci are usually stable, and type 3 is unstable because of its lack of posterolateral meniscocapsular attachment.

Imaging Radiographs may show relative widening of the lateral tibiofemoral joint space in the setting of a discoid lateral meniscus. Radiographs are not adequate to suggest or exclude the diagnosis, since the lateral joint space may be artifactually widened by patient positioning or weightbearing status.

MRI is the optimal method for diagnosing a discoid lateral meniscus. All three orthogonal planes should be used to determine size of the lateral meniscus and degree of coverage of the lateral tibiofemoral joint compartment. When a discoid lateral meniscus is present, it can be partial (e-Fig. 145-25),

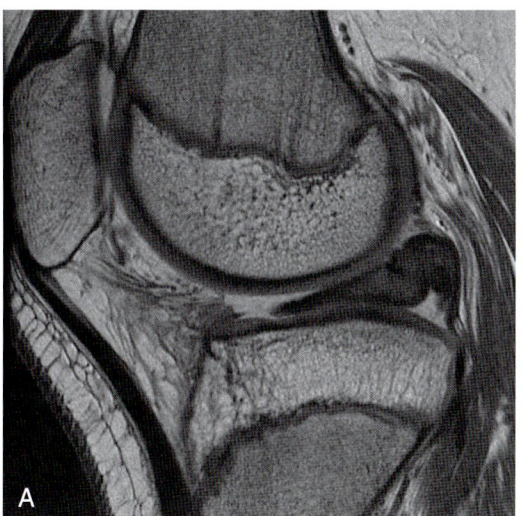 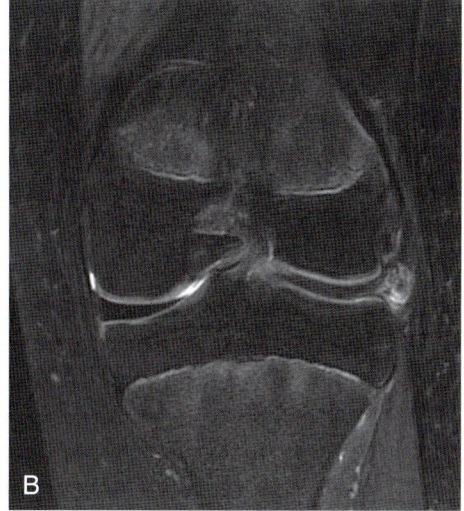

Figure 145-26 14-year-old boy with a complete discoid lateral meniscus seen on (**A**) proton density sagittal and (**B**) proton density fat-saturated coronal images with capsular tear with posterior subluxation of the lateral meniscus.

complete (Fig. 145-26), or a Wrisberg variant. Counting sagittal slices to determine meniscal size is not useful, since no meniscal size references are available for children. The Wrisberg variant may be suggested when normal fascicles connecting the posterior horn of the lateral meniscus with the capsule are absent, independent of the size and shape of the lateral meniscus.

It is important to describe the discoid lateral meniscus morphology, including presence or absence of tears or degeneration, and the nature of the discoid morphology. Discoid lateral meniscus may be uniformly enlarged or may be asymmetrically enlarged with a dominant posterior, midbody, or anterior horn.[19]

Treatment and Follow-up Asymptomatic discoid lateral meniscus is usually observed. Treatment of symptomatic discoid lateral meniscus is surgical. Discoid lateral menisci are usually trimmed and saucerized to conform to the expected normal size and shape of the lateral meniscus and any tears that may also be present are repaired. Tears are débrided and trimmed until a stable margin is created.

Osteochondral Injuries

Etiology Osteochondral lesions represent a broad spectrum of acute or chronic injuries with variable involvement of the articular and epiphyseal cartilage, spherical growth plate, and epiphyseal ossification center. Osteochondral lesions are separated into two basic lesions: (1) acute osteochondral fractures and (2) osteochondritis dissecans. Osteochondritis dissecans results from chronic repetitive injury.

The two types of osteochondritis dissecans are the juvenile and adult types.[20] Juvenile osteochondritis dissecans tends to involve epiphyseal and spherical growth plates with either growth disturbance or injury to the epiphyseal ossification center. These tend to spontaneously heal. Adult osteochondritis dissecans affects articular cartilage and the epiphyseal bone. These lesions occur when the epiphyseal ossification is mature and usually only articular cartilage remains; they less

commonly heal spontaneously and are more likely to be unstable compared with the juvenile variant.

Osteochondritis dissecans most commonly affects the knee but also can occur in the ankle and elbow (Table 145-2). These locations often have different prognostic significance, symptoms, and underlying etiology. For instance, osteochondritis dissecans of the talus tends to be asymptomatic and incidentally noted when the medial talar dome is involved, whereas lateral talar dome lesions tend to be symptomatic. At the level of the elbow, capitellar osteochondritis dissecans often is seen in throwing athletes. Because of repetitive valgus loading of the elbow, capitellar osteochondritis dissecans occurs related to repetitive compressive forces of the radial head abutting the capitellum in the lateral elbow compartment.

Osteochondritis dissecans may also occur as a secondary process when the underlying epiphyseal bone is abnormal, as can be seen in the setting of Perthes disease (e-Fig. 145-27).

Imaging Radiography should be the first line of imaging for osteochondral lesions. Purely cartilaginous lesions are better evaluated by MRI. In osteochondritis dissecans, subchondral fragmentation may be seen (Fig. 145-28). Tunnel views are often ordered in the evaluation of osteochondritis dissecans of the knee, but these are often misleading, since

Table 145-2

Common Locations for Osteochondritis Dissecans

Location of Osteochondritis Dissecans	Most Common Areas	Less Common Areas
Elbow	Capitellum	Radial head
Knee	Lateral aspect of the medial femoral condyle	Lateral femoral condyle, trochlear fossa, patella
Ankle	Medial talar dome	Lateral talar dome, midtalar dome

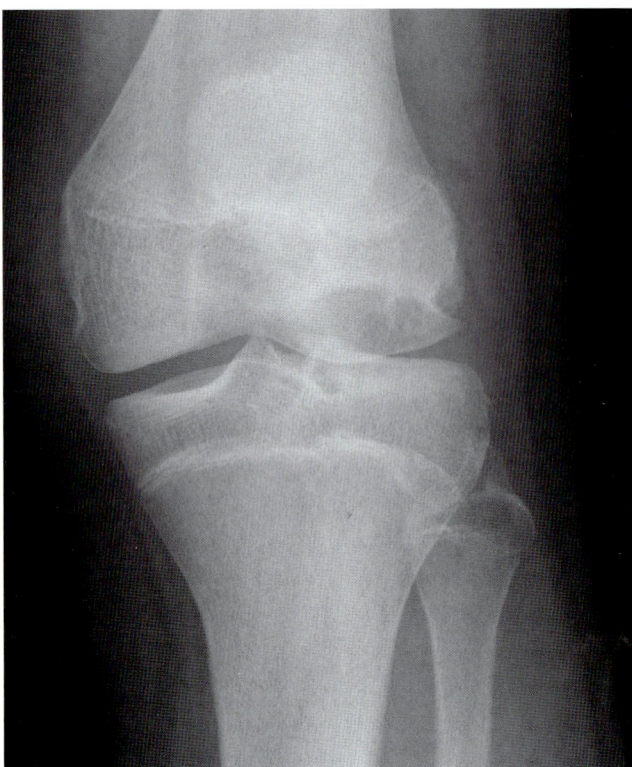

Figure 145-28 An anteroposterior radiograph of the knee in a 16-year-old with large osteochondritis dissecans of the lateral femoral condyle.

they delineate the posterior femoral condylar area in which normal femoral condylar irregularities are usually seen (Fig. 145-29).

MRI is the optimal method for imaging osteochondral injuries. Noncontrast images are usually sufficient, and intraarticularly administered contrast agent is not necessary in most cases when MRI studies are performed using dedicated coils and on a high field magnet.

Acute chondral or osteochondral fractures are classified as partial (Fig. 145-30), full-thickness (Fig. 145-31), or delamination injuries (Fig. 145-32). When only cartilage is involved, these should technically be referred to as *acute chondral fractures* (see Fig. 145-30). The presence or absence of a chondral or osteochondral loose body should be documented when reporting an osteochondral injury.

Osteochondritis dissecans are classified as unstable (Fig. 145-33) or stable (Fig. 145-34). Determining instability is more of an issue related to adult type osteochondritis dissecans, since in most cases, juvenile type osteochondritis dissecans is stable. Instability is suggested when fluid insinuates between the parent bone and osteochondritis dissecans (see Fig. 145-33), junctional cysts are present, the overlying cartilage is deficient, or loose bodies are present. Juvenile osteochondritis dissecans may have features of instability on MRI, but unlike adolescent and adult patients with the same lesion, they are more likely to spontaneously heal without surgical intervention, most likely because their spherical growth plate remains open.

Osteochondritis dissecans should be differentiated from normal condylar fragmentation, which is usually identified along the far posterior, non–weightbearing portion of the femoral condyles (see Fig. 145-29).

Treatment Nonsurgical therapy is recommended when imaging features suggest stability. Juvenile osteochondritis dissecans and osteochondritis dissecans in patients with an open physis are most likely to heal spontaneously, compared with osteochondritis dissecans in older children.[20] Surgical management includes arthroscopic drilling or microfracture methods to improve blood supply and healing, removal of any potential loose bodies, autologous osteochondral plugs,

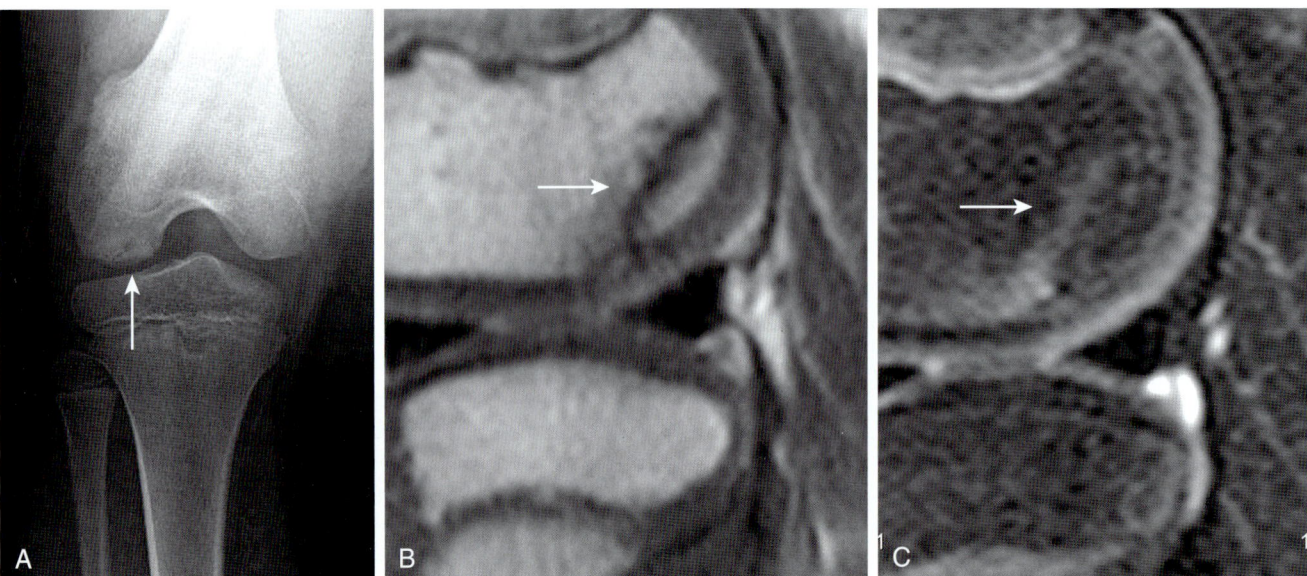

Figure 145-29 **A 10-year-old boy with normal femoral condylar irregularity.** Magnetic resonance imaging of normal femoral condylar irregularities. **A,** Tunnel view demonstrates lateral femoral condylar subchondral irregularities (*arrow*). **B,** Proton density sagittal image. **C,** A T2-weighted fat suppression sagittal image demonstrates subchondral semilunar sharp demarcation between the condylar irregularity and epiphyseal parent bone (*arrow*). Because edema of the subchondral irregularity is not present and because the overlying articular cartilage and spherical growth plate are intact, this is considered a normal finding, not osteochondritis dissecans.

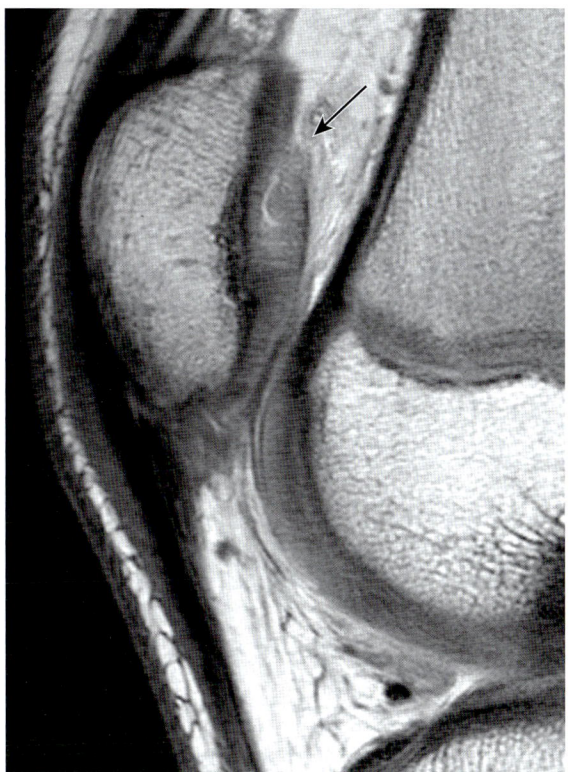

Figure 145-30 A proton density sagittal image demonstrates acute partial thickness cartilage injury (*arrow*) of the patella.

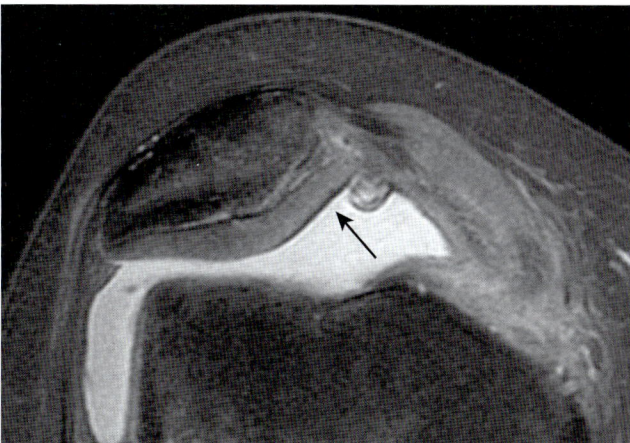

Figure 145-32 A proton density fat suppression axial image demonstrates delamination injury of the medial patella facet (*arrow*) related to lateral patellar dislocation.

and autologous chondrocyte implantation are some methods used to treat unstable osteochondritis dissecans.[20]

Throwing Injuries

Etiology "Little league shoulder" is an overuse injury that may occur with throwing activities, leading to a chronic Salter-Harris I injury of the proximal humerus.[21] The physeal injury occurs related to rotational torque created during throwing.

Little league elbow represents a constellation of medial and lateral compartment soft tissue, cartilage, and bone injuries

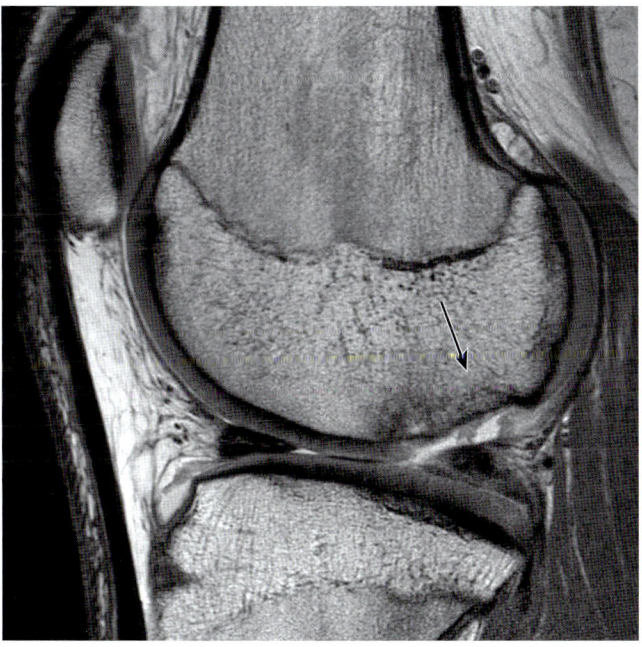

Figure 145-31 A proton density sagittal image of the knee demonstrates full thickness cartilage injury (*arrow*) of the lateral femoral condyle with subchondral bone involvement.

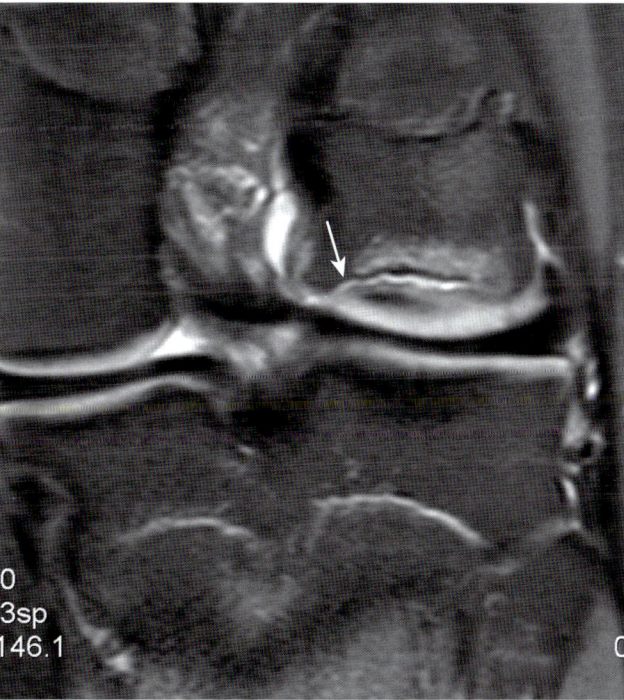

Figure 145-33 A 14-year-old boy with lateral femoral condylar unstable osteochondritis dissecans. A proton density fat suppression coronal image demonstrates fluid signal insinuating between the parent bone and osteochondral fragment (*arrow*).

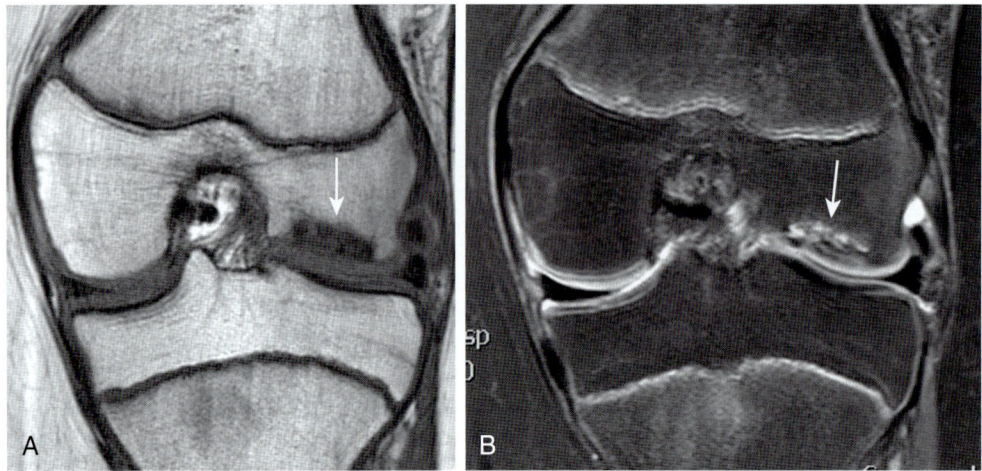

Figure 145-34   A 13-year-old boy with lateral femoral condylar stable osteochondritis dissecans. **A,** A T1-weighted coronal image. **B,** A proton density fat suppression coronal image demonstrates a well-demarcated osteochondritis dissecans with edema and tiny fluid lakes (*arrow*), but without discrete linear fluid signal to suggest instability.

related to throwing. With overhead throwing, repetitive elbow valgus stress occurs and causes tensile forces along the medial joint line and compressive forces along the lateral joint line. Along the medial joint line, this results in medial epi-condylar apophysitis and medial epicondylar avulsion fractures in younger children and anterior band ulnar collateral liga-ment injuries in adolescents who are skeletally mature.[22] Along the lateral joint line, repetitive compressive forces lead to osteochondral lesions of the capitellum, and less frequently osteochondral lesions of the radial head. In younger children, Panner disease may result, rather than discrete osteochondral lesions of the capitellum.

Imaging   Radiographs of little league shoulder manifests with proximal physeal widening, juxtaphyseal metaphyseal fraying (Fig. 145-35), or proximal humeral metaphyseal periostitis. Imaging the contralateral asymptomatic shoulder may be nec-essary when the only finding present is physeal widening. This should be differentiated from physiologic proximal

humeral physeal widening related to growth spurts. Physio-logic proximal humeral physeal widening should be bilateral and symmetric.

Radiographic findings related to throwing injuries of the elbow include medial epicondylar avulsion fractures (Fig. 145-36). The avulsion injury may alternatively occur at the level of the chondro-osseous junction of the medial epicon-dyle with an intact medial epicondylar physeal equivalent region (e-Fig. 145-37). Radiographic features of capitellar osteochondritis dissecans include subchondral lucency (Fig. 145-38), fragmentation, and intraarticular loose bodies.

When radiographs are negative for medial epicondylar avulsion fractures, MRI may be helpful for evaluation of medial epicondylar pain. On MRI, diffuse marrow edema may be seen in the medial epicondyle and adjacent soft tissue. In older adolescents who are skeletally mature, common flexor tendon tears and ulnar collateral ligament tears are more commonly seen. The most common ligament that is torn is the anterior band of the ulnar collateral ligament

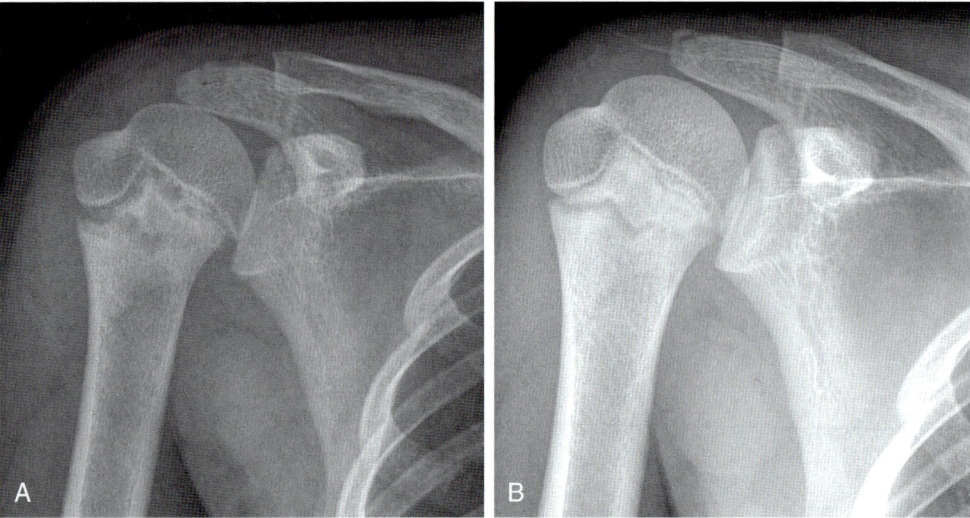

Figure 145-35   A 12-year-old with "Little League" shoulder. **A,** An anteroposterior radiograph at presentation demonstrates proximal humeral physeal widening and metaphyseal fraying. **B,** An anteroposterior radiograph 3 months later shows resolution with rest.

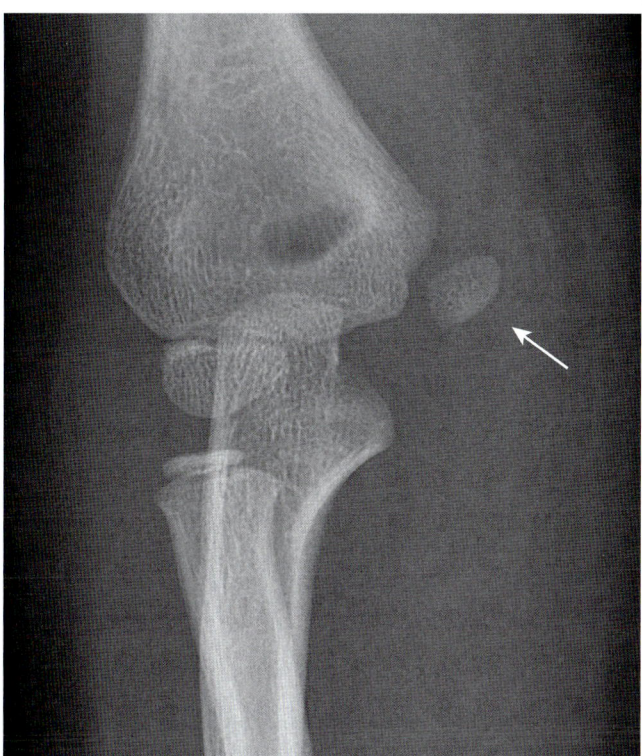

Figure 145-36 A 5-year-old girl with medial epicondylar avulsion fracture (*arrow*).

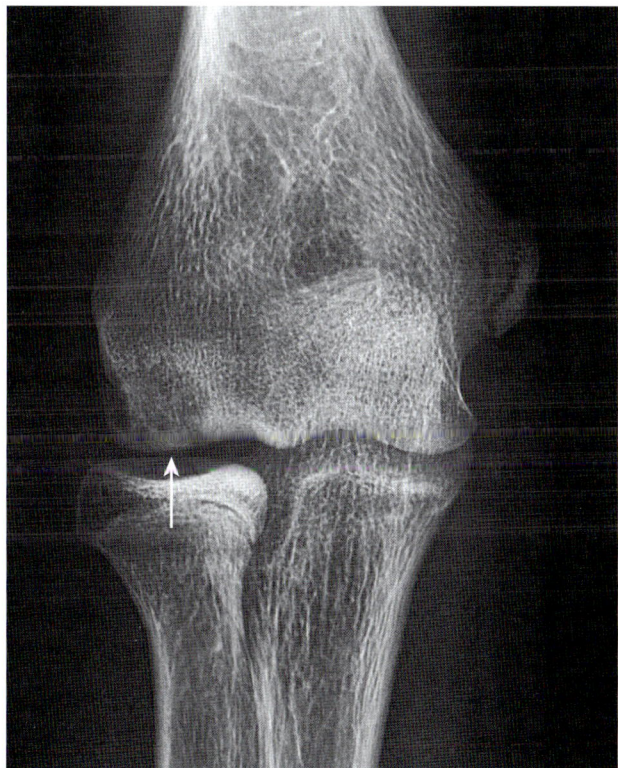

Figure 145-38 A 14-year-old boy with subchondral lucency and irregularity consistent with capitellar osteochondritis dissecans (*arrow*).

at its insertion on the sublime tubercle of the ulna which is best evaluated by magnetic resonance arthrography (e-Fig. 145-39).

Panner disease presents with diffuse sclerosis and fragmentation of the capitellum, with diffuse marrow edema seen on MRI. Osteochondral lesions of the capitellum are more likely to be seen in older children.

Treatment   Little league shoulder is treated nonsurgically with rest and activity modification. Surgical treatment is not indicated.[21]

For the elbow, medial epicondylitis and Panner disease are treated nonsurgically. Medial epicondylar avulsion fractures are surgically reduced if greater than 2 mm displacement exists. Anterior band ulnar collateral ligament tears are treated conservatively in most instances. In high-level athletes, reconstruction with tendon autograft may be performed.[22] Osteochondritis dissecans of the capitellum are surgically treated (debridement, microfracture technique) if MRI features of instability are present.

Internal Derangement of the Hip

Etiology   *Femoroacetabular impingement* describes a constellation of femoral head or acetabular anatomic deformities causing hip joint incongruity that may lead to early osteoarthritis and labral tears. Femoral-sided deformities are classified as *cam-type impingement*, and acetabular-sided deformities are classified as *pincer-type impingement*. Usually both cam-type and pincer-type impingements coexist.

The diagnosis of femoroacetabular impingement is controversial, since many patients may have the anatomic deformity present and yet be asymptomatic.[23,24] The diagnosis of femoroacetabular impingement may be suggested when positive clinical symptoms such as pain with hip flexion and hip internal rotation, as well as imaging findings of femoroacetabular impingement are present.

Common etiologies for cam-type femoroacetabular impingement in children include Perthes disease and slipped capital femoral epiphysis (SCFE).[25] Perthes disease is a primary cam-type femoroacetabular impingement because the femoral head becomes aspherical. A secondary pincer-type femoroacetabular impingement may occur because the acetabulum is relatively too large compared with the aspherical small femoral head. SCFE may lead to an abnormal femoral head–neck offset with a cam-type femoroacetabular bump, which may impinge on the labral acetabular rim, leading to labral tears and acetabular chondral injuries. In more severe cases, a "pistol grip" deformity (loss of the normal concavity of the lateral femoral neck) may occur.

Etiologies that may cause a pincer-type impingement include acetabular retroversion, sequelae of inflammatory arthritis, and acetabular protrusio deformity. *Acetabular version* describes the orientation of the acetabular cup, which is normally mildly anteverted. *Acetabular retroversion* describes a posteriorly oriented acetabular cup. Acetabular retroversion causes a pincer-type impingement due to anterosuperior overcoverage of the femoral head. Acetabular retroversion may be congenital or secondary as a developmental alteration caused by femoral head deformities (a congruent normal femoral head is necessary to develop a normal acetabulum,

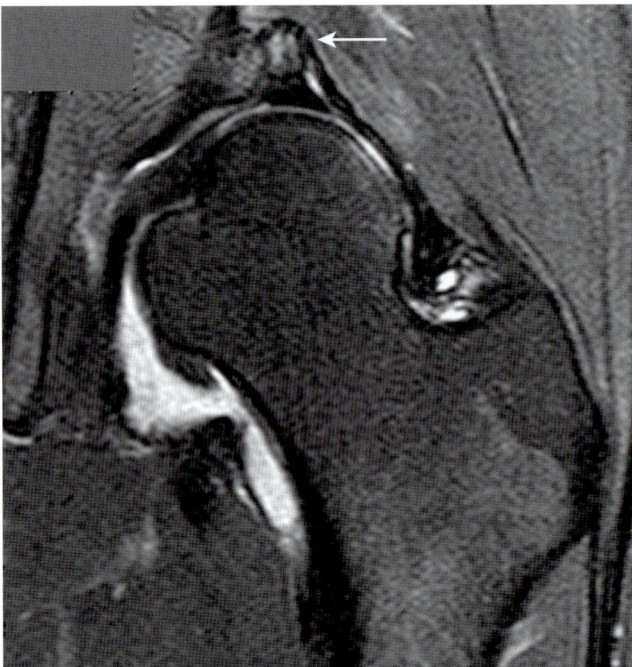

Figure 145-40 A 19-year-old girl with left-sided untreated developmental dysplasia of the hip. A T2-weighted fat suppression coronal sequence demonstrates size mismatch of relatively large femoral head and small acetabular fossa leading to cam-type impingement with resultant early labral degeneration with paralabral cysts (*arrow*).

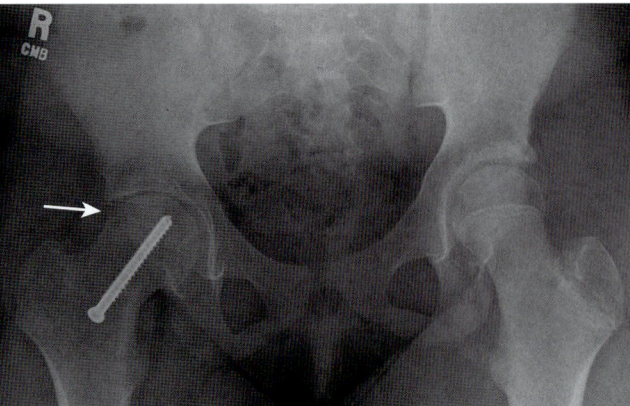

Figure 145-41 A 10-year-old girl with right-sided healed slipped capital femoral epiphysis with idiopathic chondrolysis and development of a junctional osteophyte (*arrow*), with resultant mixed cam-type and pincer-type femoroacetabular impingement.

and vice versa). Inflammatory arthritis may cause concentric narrowing of the joint, which leads to a pincer-type deformity from relative overcoverage of the femoral head. In the setting of inflammatory arthritis with uniform decreased joint space, less space is available for the femoral head to clear during hip motion. Acetabular protrusio deformity, which may also result from inflammatory arthritis, similarly leads to overcoverage of the femoral head, which causes a pincer-type deformity.

Developmental dysplasia of the hip (DDH) may cause a pincer-type impingement, cam-type impingement, or a combination of both. Cam-type femoroacetabular impingement results from a size mismatch between a small dysplastic acetabular cup and relatively large femoral head (Fig. 145-40). Subtrochanter varus osteotomy to relocate the hip may further exacerbate a cam-type impingement. Alternatively, periacetabular osteotomies such as a Salter osteotomy may increase the acetabular coverage, resulting in a pincer-type deformity.

Imaging Radiographic features of cam-type femoroacetabular impingement include junctional osteophytes at the level of the head–neck junction (Fig. 145-41). On MRI, anterosuperior labral tears are most frequently related to cam-type femoroacetabular deformities (Fig. 145-42). More obvious deformities leading to cam-type femoroacetabular impingement include Perthes disease (e-Fig. 145-43) and DDH (see Fig. 145-40). To assess labral tears, magnetic resonance arthrography with direct injection of diluted gadolinium is necessary.

On MRI or CT, an alpha-angle may be used to calculate the degree of femoral head deformity related to cam-type femoroacetabular impingement. The normal alpha-angle is less than 55 degrees. The alpha-angle is calculated by doing the following:

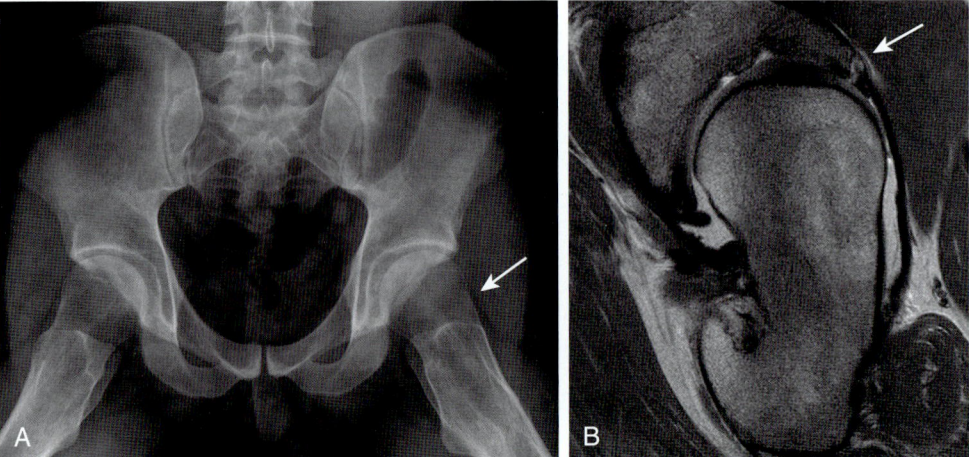

Figure 145-42 **A,** Cam-type femoroacetabular impingement with pistol-grip deformity and loss of normal femoral head–neck offset seen on frogleg lateral view (*arrow*). **B,** Proton density radial sequence again shows loss of femoral head-neck offset and anterosuperior labral tear (*arrow*).

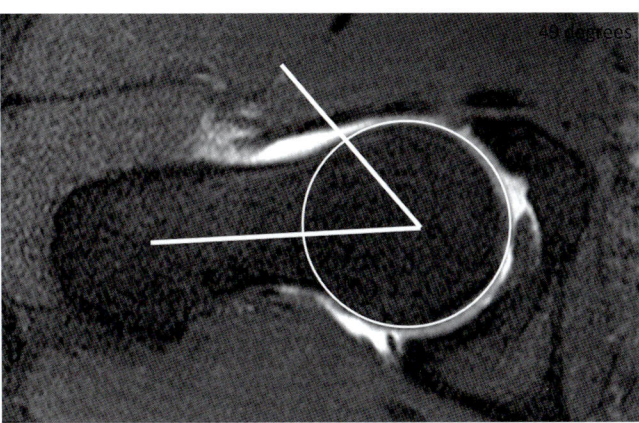

Figure 145-44 An oblique axial T1-weighted fat suppression with intraarticular contrast image demonstrating lines for calculating the alpha-angle.

1. Drawing a best-fit circle around the femoral head outlining the cortical margin
2. Drawing a parallel line with respect to the femoral neck terminating at the center of the circle
3. Drawing a line from the center of the circle and where the femoral head or neck protrudes from the circle
4. Calculating an angle between lines created from item 2 and 3 (Fig. 145-44)

Pincer femoroacetabular impingement changes identified on radiography include the cross-over sign (Fig. 145-45) and a center edge angle greater than 29 degrees (e-Fig. 145-46). On frontal radiographs of the pelvis, the anterior acetabular wall is normally more medial with respect to the posterior

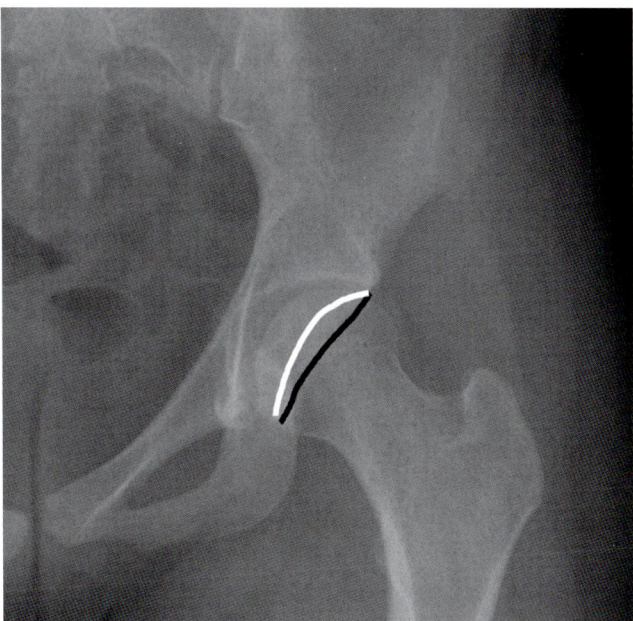

Figure 145-47 A normal anteroposterior radiograph of the hip showing no cross-over sign. The white line represents the anterior acetabular wall, the black line represents the posterior acetabular wall.

acetabular wall (Fig. 145-47). The cross-over sign occurs when the anterior and posterior acetabular wall lines intersect, indicative of acetabular retroversion (see Fig. 145-45). The normal acetabulum is usually in 19 degrees of anteversion in adult patients.[20] With acetabular retroversion, anterior overcoverage of the femoral head occurs. On CT or MRI, acetabular version should be calculated at the center of the hip joint.

Treatment Treatment is predicated on symptoms, not on the degree of imaging deformity. Surgical treatment may be indicated when the child has positive clinical findings for impingement with supportive imaging features. Treatment focuses on surgically removing the anatomic cause of the impingement deformity to improve acetabular and femoral head joint congruity so that the acetabulum and the femoral head–neck junction do not abnormally abut during normal range of hip motion.[27] This includes removing cam-type femoroacetabular osteophytes along the femoral head–neck junction as well as reshaping the femoral head to conform to a spherical shape and debridement of any labral tears or chondral injuries that may be present. This can be approached from an arthroscopic technique or an open technique. For pincer-type femoroacetabular deformity related to acetabular retroversion, a periacetabular rotational osteotomy may be performed to decrease the amount of anterior overcoverage.

Stress Injuries of Bone

Etiology A fatigue fracture occurs when supraphysiologic repetitive stress is applied to normal bone. Insufficiency fractures occur when normal stress is applied to abnormal osteopenic bone.[28] Stress injuries to bone can occur on either the compressive side or the tensile side of bone, leading to trabecular injury. A spectrum of bone changes may occur

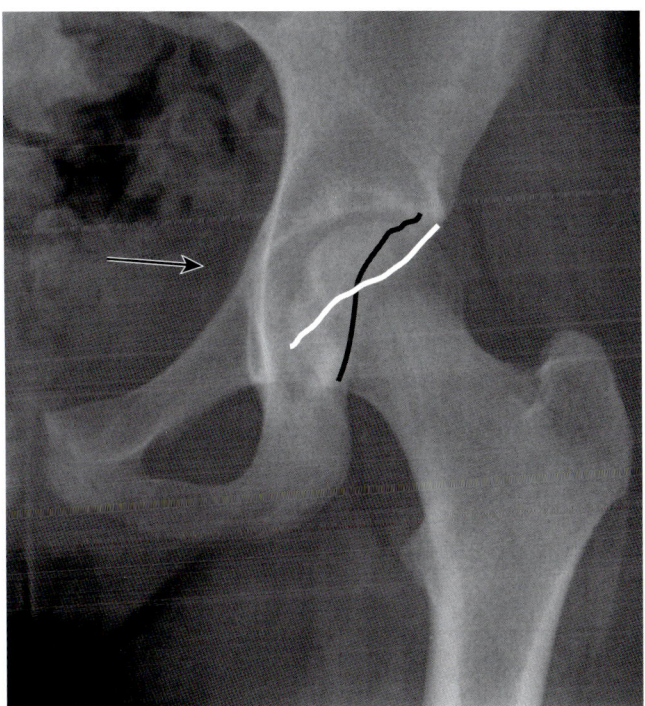

Figure 145-45 A radiograph of the cross-over sign indicative of acetabular retroversion. The white line represents the anterior acetabular wall, the black line represents the posterior acetabular wall. Note the ischial spine sign is present as well (arrow), an additional indicator of a pincer deformity.

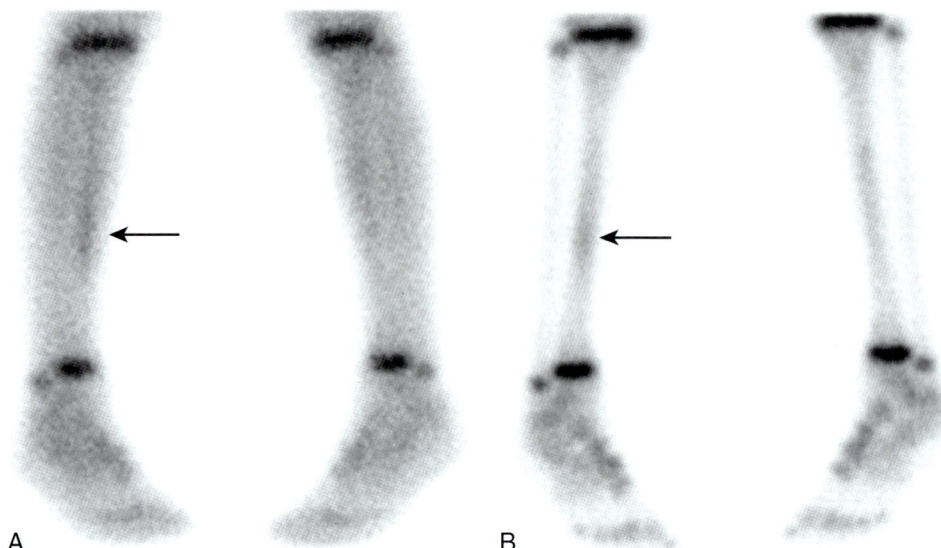

Figure 145-48 A triple phase bone scan demonstrating stress reaction (*arrow*) in the right midtibial diaphysis on blood-pool (**A**) and delayed-phase (**B**) images.

prior to the time a discrete fracture line may be seen on a radiograph or a cross-sectional image. These changes include periosteal edema, marrow edema, cortical edema, and micro-fractures (occult fractures not visible on imaging). With proper training, bone and muscle physiologic adaptation to repetitive stress is protective and may prevent stress reaction and stress fractures to bone.

Risk factors for stress injuries to bone include inadequate or improper athletic training, postpubertal females (female athlete triad: (1) menstrual irregularity, (2) disordered eating, (3) osteoporosis), and abnormal biophysical geometry of the child such as leg length discrepancies, varus alignment, abnormal femoral version, and pes cavus.[29]

Symptoms related to stress fractures are not present at rest but occur with physical activity.[29] *Shin splints*, or *medial tibial stress syndrome*, is a vague term to describe pain that occurs over the posteromedial aspect of the distal third of the tibia.[30] Proposed etiologies include muscle attachment inflammation, fascial edema, posterior compartment syndrome, and tibial stress fractures. Because of its nonspecific broad definition, shin splints should be reserved as a clinical diagnosis, not a radiologic diagnosis.

Imaging With radiography, the spectrum of stress reaction to bone includes normal (most common), periostitis, and discrete fracture. Radiographs are the first line of imaging when suspected fracture is present. Bone scintigraphy and MRI are complementary tools when radiographs are normal.

With technetium-99m scintigraphy, a three-phase bone scan should be performed. With acute fractures all three phases are abnormal due to hyperemia (Fig. 145-48). When stress fractures are subacute or chronic, only the delayed phases may be abnormal, with no abnormal uptake during the blood-flow and blood-pool phases. Bone scintigraphy alone is limited in the evaluation of stress fractures of bone because it only measures osteoblastic activity, which can be seen in nontraumatic entities such as osteomyelitis and primary bone neoplasms. Therefore, bone scintigraphy should always be interpreted in conjunction with radiography.

MRI is indicated when symptoms do not resolve with conservative management or failed physical rehabilitation in the setting of normal radiographs. When radiographs are abnormal, demonstrating a discrete nondisplaced stress fracture, MRI does not add additional value with regard to treatment in most cases. MRI will add value if the fracture has an intraarticular component, may involve the physis, or the fracture is pathologic because of an underlying primary neoplasm of bone.

MRI grading for bone stress injuries includes the spectrum from isolated periosteal edema (Fig. 145-49) to a true fracture (Fig. 145-50) (Table 145-3).[29] MRI may also suggest alternative soft tissue etiologies for symptoms such as muscle tears or DOMS.

Treatment Treatment will vary, depending on location of fractures and symptoms. For nondisplaced stress fractures, treatment includes local pain control, including physical therapy and nonsteroidal antiinflammatory drugs. Weight-bearing for normal activities is allowed. Eventually, return to athletic activity may begin if the child is pain-free for 10 to 14 days.[29]

Table 145-3

Grade	T2	T1
\multicolumn{3}{l}{**Magnetic Resonance Grading of Stress Injuries to Bone**}		
0	Normal	Normal
1	Periosteal edema, no marrow edema	Normal
2	Periosteal edema, marrow edema	Normal
3	Periosteal edema, marrow edema	Periosteal edema, marrow edema
4	Fracture line present	Fracture line present

Adapted from Fredericson M, Jennings F, Beaulieu C, et al. Stress fractures in athletes. *Top Magn Reson Imaging.* 2006;17(5):309-325.

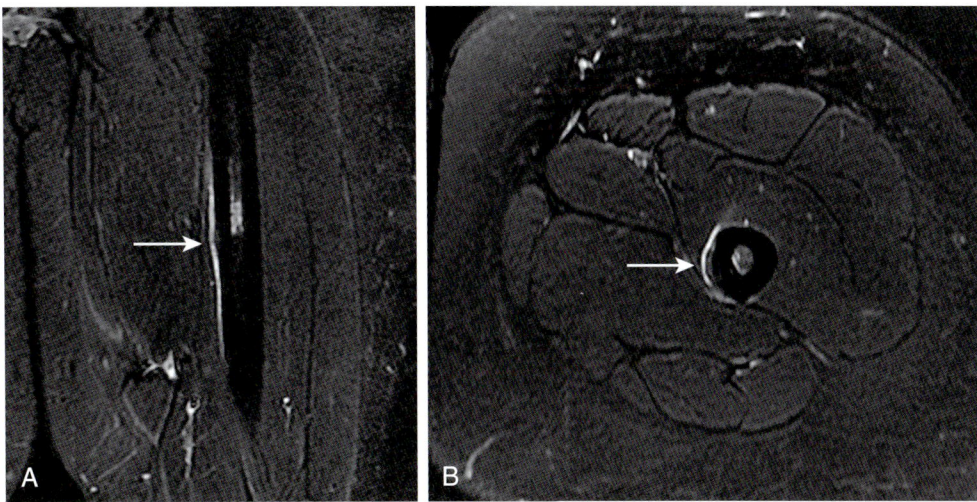

Figure 145-49 A 16-year-old boy with femoral stress reaction without discrete fracture seen on short tau inversion recovery axial (**A**) and coronal (**B**) sequences. Note the periosteal reaction and endosteal edema (*arrows*).

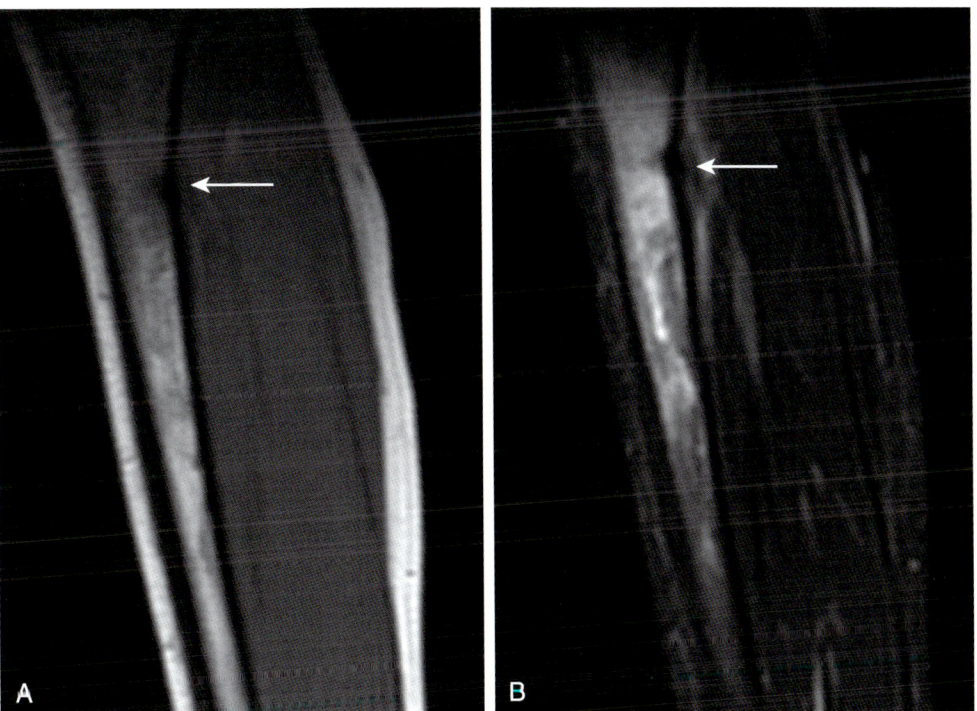

Figure 145-50 An 8-year-old boy with a nondisplaced proximal tibial stress fracture seen on T1-weighted sagittal (**A**) and short tau inversion recovery sagittal (**B**) sequences (*arrows*).

Key Points

Pelvic avulsion fractures are usually treated conservatively unless fracture displacement is greater than 2 cm.

In the setting of lateral patellar dislocation, the presence or absence of underlying patellofemoral dysplasia should always be noted.

Identification of loose bodies in acute patellar dislocation has more impact on surgical management than identifying bone contusions and medial retinacular injuries.

The Wrisberg variant of discoid lateral meniscus may occur in the setting of a meniscus of normal size and shape.

Among throwing athletes, skeletally immature children tend to develop medial epicondylitis and medial epicondylar avulsion fractures, whereas skeletally mature children tend to suffer flexor tendon and ulnar collateral ligament tears.

Femoroacetabular impingement treatment is predicated on both symptoms and imaging findings. Therefore, the imaging diagnosis without supportive clinical symptoms may generate unnecessary orthopedic referrals.

References

Full references for this chapter can be found on www.expertconsult.com.

Index

Page numbers followed by "f" indicate figures, "t" indicate tables, "b" indicate boxes, and "e" indicate online-only content.